Blood and
Bone Marrow
PATHOLOGY

Commissioning Editor: *Michael Houston*
Development Editors: *Ben Davie & Rachael Harrison*
Editorial Assistant: *Kirsten Lowson*
Project Manager: *Anita Somaroutu*
Design: *Kirsteen Wright*
Illustration Manager: *Bruce Hogarth*
Illustrator: *Robert Britton*
Marketing Managers (UK/USA): *Gaynor Jones & Cara Jespersen*

Blood and Bone Marrow PATHOLOGY

Anna Porwit MD, PhD
Professor
Department of Pathology
Karolinska University Hospital and Institute
Stockholm, Sweden;
Department of Laboratory Medicine and Pathobiology
University of Toronto
Toronto, ON, Canada

Jeffrey McCullough MD
Professor of Laboratory Medicine and Pathology
American Red Cross Professor of Transfusion Medicine
University of Minnesota
Minneapolis, MN, USA

Wendy N. Erber MD, DPhil, FRCPA, FRCPath
Consultant Hematologist
Addenbrooke's Hospital;
Hematology Department
University of Cambridge
Cambridge, UK

For additional online content visit expertconsult.com

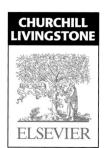

CHURCHILL LIVINGSTONE
ELSEVIER

Edinburgh   London   New York   Oxford   Philadelphia   St Louis   Sydney   Toronto   2011

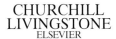

An Imprint of Elsevier Limited

© 2011, Elsevier Limited All rights reserved.
First edition 2002
Second edition 2011

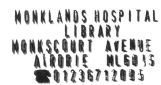

Notices

Knowledge and best practice in this field are constantly changing. As new research and experience broaden our understanding, changes in research methods, professional practices, or medical treatment may become necessary.

Practitioners and researchers must always rely on their own experience and knowledge in evaluating and using any information, methods, compounds, or experiments described herein. In using such information or methods they should be mindful of their own safety and the safety of others, including parties for whom they have a professional responsibility.

With respect to any drug or pharmaceutical products identified, readers are advised to check the most current information provided (i) on procedures featured or (ii) by the manufacturer of each product to be administered, to verify the recommended dose or formula, the method and duration of administration, and contraindications. It is the responsibility of practitioners, relying on their own experience and knowledge of their patients, to make diagnoses, to determine dosages and the best treatment for each individual patient, and to take all appropriate safety precautions.

To the fullest extent of the law, neither the Publisher nor the authors, contributors, or editors, assume any liability for any injury and/or damage to persons or property as a matter of products liability, negligence or otherwise, or from any use or operation of any methods, products, instructions, or ideas contained in the material herein.

Churchill Livingstone

British Library Cataloguing in Publication Data

Blood and bone marrow pathology.
  1. Blood – Diseases. 2. Bone marrow – Diseases. 3. Blood – Diseases – Histopathology. 4. Bone marrow – Diseases – Histopathology. I. Porwit, Anna. II. McCullough, Jeffrey J. III. Erber, Wendy N., 1957–
  616.1'5 – dc22

ISBN-13: 9780702031472

 your source for books, journals and multimedia in the health sciences
www.elsevierhealth.com

Working together to grow
libraries in developing countries
www.elsevier.com | www.bookaid.org | www.sabre.org

ELSEVIER   BOOK AID International   Sabre Foundation

The publisher's policy is to use paper manufactured from sustainable forests

Printed in China
Last digit is the print number: 9 8 7 6 5 4 3 2 1

Contents

Preface

In the time since the first edition of *Blood and Bone Marrow Pathology* was published in 2002, major advances have been made in all facets of the field of hematology. Much of this has resulted from progress in molecular genetics which has enhanced our understanding of the pathological basis of hematological disorders. The knowledge of the molecular basis of hematological diseases is now being used to both diagnose and classify non-malignant and malignant hematological disorders. This has had a major impact on the hemopoietic tumors where the World Health Organization classification is in large part based on this new biological information. This second edition of *Blood and Bone Marrow Pathology* has therefore been significantly updated and revised to incorporate these advances. Many chapters have been totally rewritten to encapsulate the advances in the understanding of the fundamentals of the pathology of blood and bone marrow in health and disease. This book truly focuses on the pathology of blood and bone marrow. Although clinical aspects of disease are alluded to along with treatment approaches, this is only given as a guide to the reader. The book is aimed at bridging pure cytology and histology with clinical hematology diagnostics.

The book was originally to be co-edited by Professor Sunitha Wickramasinghe, co-editor of the first edition and a major driving force behind *Blood and Bone Marrow Pathology*. It is with immense sadness we note the untimely death of Sunitha during the production of this second edition. His death has been a tremendous loss to hematology.

The book is divided into sections on normal blood and bone marrow, pathology of the bone marrow, disorders of erythroid cells and leukocytes, abnormalities of hemostasis and immunohematology. Within each section there are chapters devoted to specific aspects of each of these areas and which have been written by internationally recognized experts. We are most grateful to them for their outstanding contributions and the time they have devoted to this project.

We are also immensely grateful to the publishers and especially Michael Houston, Ben Davie and Rachael Harrison for their enormous help in bringing this project to fruition. We hope this second edition of *Blood and Bone Marrow Pathology* will be of benefit to clinical and laboratory hematologists, hematopathologists and those in training in gaining a better understanding of the pathology of blood and bone marrow.

Anna Porwit
Jeffrey McCullough
Wendy N. Erber
2011

Contributors

Kenneth C. Anderson MD, PhD
Director, Jerome Lipper Multiple Myeloma Center
Dana-Farber Cancer Institute
Kraft Family Professor of Medicine
Harvard Medical School
Boston, MA, USA

Daniel A. Arber MD
Professor and Associate Chair of Pathology
Department of Pathology
Stanford University
Stanford, CA, USA

Donald M. Arnold MDCM, MSc, FRCPC
Assistant Professor, Department of Medicine
Division of Hematology and Thromboembolism
Michael G. DeGroote School of Medicine
McMaster University
Canadian Blood Services
Hamilton, ON, Canada

Barbara J. Bain MB BS, FRACP, FRCPath
Professor in Diagnostic Hematology
Imperial College
Honorary Consultant Hematologist
Department of Hematology
St Mary's Hospital
London, UK

Marie Christine Béné Pharm Sci D, PhD
Professor of Immunology
Immunology Laboratory
Faculty of Medicine
Nancy University and University Hospital
Vandoeuvre-lès-Nancy, France

David H. Bevan FRCP FRCPath
Director and Consultant Hematologist
Centre for Hemostasis and Thrombosis
Guy's and St Thomas' NHS Foundation Trust
London, UK

Oliver Bock MD
Professor for Transplantation Pathology
Head Central Tissue and Specimen Bank
Institute of Pathology
Medizinische Hochschule Hannover
Hannover, Germany

Jeremiah C. Boles MD
Hematology/Oncology Fellow
Division of Hematology/Oncology
University of North Carolina at Chapel Hill
Chapel Hill, NC, USA

Gerben Bouma PhD
Research Associate
Molecular Immunology Unit
UCL Institute of Child Health
London, UK

Scott D. Boyd MD, PhD
Assistant Professor of Pathology
Department of Pathology
Stanford University
Stanford, CA, USA

Shannon M. Buckley PhD
Postdoctoral Research Fellow
Department of Pathology
New York University Medical Center
New York, NY USA

Guntram Büsche
Lecturer in Hematopathology
Institute of Pathology
Medizinische Hochschule Hannover
Hannover, Germany

Magdalena Czader MD, PhD
Director, Division of Hematopathology
Department of Pathology and Laboratory Medicine
Indiana University School of Medicine
Indianapolis, IN, USA

Geoff Daniels PhD, FRCPath
Head of Molecular Diagnostics and Senior Research Fellow
Bristol Institute for Transfusion Sciences and IBGRL
NHS Blood and Transplant
Bristol, UK

Faith E. Davies MBBCh, MD, MRCP, FRCPath
Hemato-oncology Unit
Royal Marsden Hospital
London, UK

Jean Delaunay MD, PhD
Professor of Genetics
INSERM
Faculté de Médecine Paris-Sud
Univ Paris-Sud
Le Kremlin-Bicêtre, France

Wendy N. Erber MD, DPhil, FRCPA, FRCPath
Consultant Hematologist
Addenbrooke's Hospital
Hematology Department
University of Cambridge
Cambridge, UK

Gines Escolar MD, PhD
Head of Department
Servicio de Hemoterapia y Hemostasia
Hospital Clinic, University of Barcelona, Medical School
Barcelona, Spain

David J. P. Ferguson BSc, PhD, DSc
Professor of Ultrastructural Morphology
Nuffield Department of Clinical Laboratory Science
University of Oxford
John Radcliffe Hospital
Oxford, UK

Edward C. Gordon-Smith MA, BSc, FRCP, FRCPath, FMedSci
Emeritus Professor of Hematology
St George's College, University of London
London, UK

Ralph Green MD, PhD, FRCPath
Professor and Chair Emeritus
Department of Pathology and Laboratory Medicine
University of California Davis School of Medicine
Sacramento, CA, USA

Carolyn S. Grove MBBS, FRACP, FRCPA
Clinical Research Training Fellow
Wellcome Trust Sanger Institute
Hinxton, UK

Georgina W. Hall MBBS, PhD, FRCP, FRCPath, FRCPCH
Consultant Paediatric Hematologist
Honorary Senior Lecturer
Paediatric Hematology/Oncology Unit
Children's Hospital
John Radcliffe Hospital
Oxford, UK

Nancy M. Heddle MSc., FCSMLS(D)
Professor
Michael G. DeGroote School of Medicine
Department of Medicine, Department of Pathology and
  Molecular Medicine
McMaster University
Hamilton, ON, Canada

Hans-Peter Horny MD
Professor of Pathology
Institute of Pathology
Ansbach, Germany

Carolyn Katovich Hurley PhD, D(ABHI)
Professor of Oncology and Microbiology and Immunology
Georgetown University Medical Center
Washington, DC, USA

John G. Kelton MD, FRCPC
Professor
Department of Medicine
Department of Pathology and Molecular Medicine
Michael G. DeGroote School of Medicine
McMaster University
Hamilton, ON, Canada

Nigel S. Key MB, ChB, FRCP
Harold R Roberts Distinguished Professor
Department of Medicine, Division of Hematology/Oncology
University of North Carolina at Chapel Hill
Chapel Hill, NC, USA

Hans H. Kreipe MD
Professor of Pathology, Director Institute of Pathology
Medizinische Hochschule Hannover
Hannover, Germany

Hans M. Kvasnicka MD
Professor of Pathology
Senkenberg Institute of Pathology
University of Frankfurt
Frankfurt, Germany

D. Mark Layton FRCP, FRCPCH
Consultant and Reader in Hematology
Department of Hematology
Imperial College
London, UK

Peter K. MacCallum MD, FRCP, FRCPath
Department of Hematology
Wolfson Institute of Preventive Medicine
Barts and The London School of Medicine and Dentistry
Queen Mary College, University of London
London, UK

Alison May PhD
Senior Research Fellow
Department of Hematology
Cardiff University School of Medicine
Cardiff, UK

Jeffrey McCullough MD
Professor of Laboratory Medicine and Pathology
American Red Cross Professor of Transfusion Medicine
University of Minnesota
Minneapolis, MN, USA

Mufaddal T. Moonim MD, FRCPath
Consultant Histopathologist
Department of Histopathology
Guy's and St Thomas' Hospitals
London, UK

Jane C. Moore BSc, ART
Assistant Professor
Michael G. DeGroote School of Medicine
Department of Medicine, Department of Pathology and
  Molecular Medicine
McMaster University
Hamilton, ON, Canada

Ishac Nazi PhD
Assistant Professor
Michael G. DeGroote School of Medicine
Department of Medicine, Department of Pathology and
  Molecular Medicine
Department of Biochemistry and Biomedical Sciences
McMaster University
Hamilton, ON, Canada

Adrian C. Newland CBE, MA, FRCP, FRCPath
Professor of Hematology
Department of Hematology
The Royal London Hospital
London, UK

Eva Norström MD, PhD
Medical Doctor
Department of Laboratory Medicine
Clinical Chemistry Malmö
Lund University
Lund, Sweden

Attilio Orazi MD, FRCPath
Professor of Pathology and Laboratory Medicine and Vice-
  Chair for Hematopathology
Director, Division of Hematopathology
Department of Pathology and Laboratory Medicine
Weill Medical College of Cornell University
New York, NY, USA

David J. Perry MD PhD, FRCPEdin, FRCPLond,FRCPath
Consultant Hematologist
Department of Hematology
Addenbrooke's Hospital
Cambridge, UK

Martin J. Pippard BSc, MB, ChB, FRCP, FRCPath
Emeritus Professor of Hematology
University of Dundee
Dundee, UK

Anna Porwit MD, PhD
Professor
Department of Pathology
Karolinska University Hospital and Institute
Stockholm, Sweden
Department of Laboratory Medicine and Pathobiology
University of Toronto
Toronto, ON, Canada

Phillip E. Posch PhD
Assistant Professor of Oncology
Georgetown University School of Medicine
Department of Oncology
Washington, DC, USA

Drew Provan MD, FRCP, FRCPath
Academic Hematology Unit – Pathology Group
Blizard Institute of Cell and Molecular Science
Barts and the London School of Medicine and Dentistry
London, UK

Raffaele Renella MD, PhD
MRC Molecular Hematology Unit
Weatherall Institute of Molecular Medicine
University of Oxford, UK
Children's Hospital Boston
Harvard Medical School
Boston, MA, USA

David R. Roper MSc, CSci, FIBMS
Principal Biomedical Scientist
Department of Hematology
Hammersmith Hospital
Imperial College Healthcare NHS Trust
London, UK

Richard Rosenquist MD, PhD
Professor of Molecular Hematology
Department of Genetics and Pathology
Rudbeck Laboratory
Uppsala University
Uppsala, Sweden

Benny Sørensen MD, PhD
Director of HRU
Honorary Lecturer
Associate Professor
Hemostasis Research Unit (HRU)
Centre for Hemostasis and Thrombosis
Guy's and St Thomas' NHS Foundation Trust
St Thomas' Hospital
London, UK

Swee Lay Thein MB, BS, FRCP, FRCPath, DSc, FMedSci
Professor of Molecular Hematology/Consultant Hematologist
King's College London/King's College Hospital NHS
    Foundation Trust
James Black Centre
London, UK

Adrian J. Thrasher PhD, FRCP, FRCPath, FMedSci
Professor of Paediatric Immunology
Molecular Immunology Unit
UCL Institute of Child Health
London, UK

Jon D. van der Walt MB, BCh, FRCPat
Consultant Histopathologist
Department of Histopathology
Guy's and St Thomas' Hospitals
London, UK

Catherine Verfaillie MD
Professor of Medicine
Director
Stamcelinstituut
Katholieke Universiteit Leuven
Leuven, Belgium

James G. White MD
Regents Professor
Departments of Laboratory Medicine and Pathology, and
    Pediatrics
University of Minnesota School of Medicine
Minneapolis, MN, USA

The late Sunitha N. Wickramasinghe
Formerly Emeritus Professor of Hematology, University of
    London
Visiting Professor of Hematology, University of Oxford
Formerly Head of the Department of Hematology
St Mary's Hospital Medical School
Imperial College of Science, Technology and Medicine
London, UK

Bridget S. Wilkins MB BCh, DM, PhD, FRCPath
Consultant Hematopathologist
Department of Cellular Pathology
Guy's and St Thomas' Hospitals NHS Foundation Trust
London, UK

William G. Wood PhD
Professor of Molecular Hematology
MRC Molecular Hematology Unit
Weatherall Institute of Molecular Medicine
University of Oxford
John Radcliffe Hospital
Oxford, UK

Gina Zini MD, PhD
Professor of Clinical Pathology
Institute of Hematology
Catholic University of Sacred Heart
Rome, Italy

Dedication
to Sunitha N. Wickramasinghe

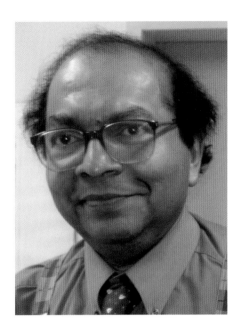

Sunitha N. Wickramasinghe, co-editor of the first edition of this book, died in June 2009, after a long and brave fight against a hematological neoplasm.

Sunitha was born in Sri Lanka (former Ceylon) in 1941, and received his medical training at the Royal College and Ceylon University. In 1964 he moved to England, and after postgraduate clinical and research training in Cambridge and Leeds was appointed as Professor of Hematology at St Mary's Hospital in London, soon to become the Imperial College Medical School. After retirement, he took a position in the Weatherall Institute of Molecular Medicine at the University of Oxford. He knew of his fatal disease in 2000, but continued to work on morphological and molecular aspects of hematopoesis until 2008.

Sunitha was an academic scholar in the genuine sense of the word. This is evident in the more than 200 internationally cited papers, mainly on abnormal red blood cell formation and the associated diseases. His monographs on human bone marrow, first published in 1973 and revised in 1975, are still widely utilized by scientists and clinical hematologists eager to understand the fundamentals of this work. Sunitha was also a superb methodologist. In the last 20 years, he became the leading authority on electron microscopy of the blood forming tissues. Driven by his scientific interest, he was always a hard worker. When he visited me in Ulm to analyze the specimens of my collection of bone marrow of patients with congenital dyserythropoietic anemia, he started work early each morning; all members of the electron microscopy department were highly impressed by his immense skill, knowledge and enthusiasm in this field.

I last met Sunitha in November 2008 at the second symposium on congenital dyserythropoietic anemia. Although already very ill and suffering from complications of recent chemotherapy he gave two lectures. On the night after his last presentation, he was admitted to the local hospital in a small town on Lake Como in Italy. He returned to England and with the support of his wife Priyanthi (to whom he had dedicated his monograph) survived another six months.

Sunitha was a talented teacher, keen to share his knowledge with students and younger colleagues. Not only were his postgraduate courses in the United Kingdom legendary, but he also found the time to return to Sri Lanka for lectures at the College of Hematologists. His intellectual curiosity and capacity for rigorous analysis, not only of the morphology of blood cells but also of other clinical and laboratory observations, made him a highly respected partner of clinicians and their patients.

Thanks to Sunitha's friendly, always helpful, modest and charming personality he had many friends all over the world. We all miss him, but we are all happy to have had the opportunity to work with him and to know him and his family.

Prof. Emerit. Dr. med.
Hermann Heimpel FRCPath
Medizinische Universitätsklinik
Ulm, Germany
2011

Section A

Normal blood and bone marrow cells

Normal blood cells

SN Wickramasinghe, WN Erber

Blood consists of plasma, a pale-yellow, coagulable fluid, in which various types of blood cells are suspended. The cells comprise erythrocytes, granulocytes, monocytes, lymphocytes and platelets. Blood also contains very small numbers of circulating hemopoietic stem cells and progenitor cells, mast cell progenitors, megakaryocytes and megakaryocyte bare nuclei.

Erythrocytes

Morphology

Erythrocytes are highly differentiated cells that have no nuclei or cytoplasmic organelles. Normal erythrocytes are circular biconcave discs with a mean diameter of 7.2 µm (range 6.7–7.7 µm) in dried fixed smears and about 7.5 µm in the living state. They are eosinophilic and consequently appear red with a central area of pallor in Romanowsky-stained smears (Fig. 1.1 A,B).

Red cell parameters

The three basic red blood cell parameters which can be measured are:[1]

1. the concentration of hemoglobin per unit volume of blood after lysis of the red cells (hemoglobin concentration) determined spectrophotometrically after conversion to cyanmethemoglobin.
2. the number of red blood cells per unit volume of blood (red cell count). The red cell count is determined using electrical impedance or light-scattering techniques.
3. the hematocrit. Prior to automation, blood was centrifuged in tubes of standard specification under a fixed centrifugal force for a fixed time to determine the packed cell volume (PCV). The hematocrit and PCV are not directly comparable as the value obtained for the PCV includes the volume of some plasma trapped between the red cells.

From the values obtained for the hemoglobin concentration, red cell count and hematocrit, it is possible to calculate the mean cell volume (MCV), mean cell hemoglobin (MCH) and mean cell hemoglobin concentration (MCHC) as shown in Table 1.1. Some automated blood-counting machines determine the MCV using electrical impedance or light-scattering techniques and calculate the hematocrit from the measured MCV and red cell count. Others determine the hematocrit directly by summing all the pulses in the red cell channel. The normal values for various red cell parameters at different ages are given in Tables 1.2 and 1.3; however, there are some differences based on the analyzer used and the method of measurement. Between the age of 2 years and the onset of puberty there is a gradual rise in the hemoglobin

©2011 Elsevier Ltd
DOI: 10.1016/B978-0-7020-3147-2.00001-8

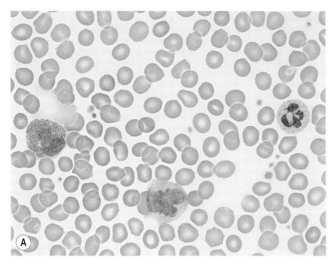

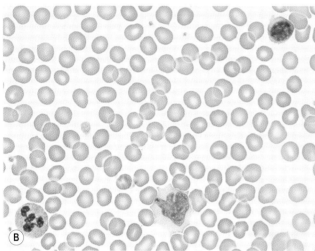

Fig. 1.1 (A, B) Cells from peripheral blood smears of normal individuals.
(A) Normochromic normocytic red cells, a normal neutrophil, eosinophil, monocyte and platelets. May–Grünwald–Giemsa stain. ×1000.
(B) Normochromic normocytic red cells, a normal neutrophil, lymphocyte, monocyte and platelets. May–Grünwald–Giemsa stain. ×1000.

Table 1.1 Calculation of red cell indices

MCV (fl)	= Hct[a] ÷ RBC per liter × 10^{15}
MCH (pg)	= Hb[b] ÷ RBC per liter × 10^{13}
MCHC (g/dl)	= Hb[b] ÷ Hct[a]

Hb, hemoglobin; Hct, hematocrit; MCH, mean corpuscular hemoglobin; MCHC, mean corpuscular hemoglobin concentration; MCV, mean corpuscular volume; RBC, red blood cells.

[a]Expressed as a fraction.

[b]In g/dl.

Table 1.2 95% reference limits for some hematologic parameters in healthy Caucasian adults (18–60 years) determined in the UK[48]

	Males (n = 100)	Females (n = 100)	Males and females (n = 200)
Hb (g/dl)	13.4–16.7	11.9–14.7	
Red cell count (10^{12}/l)	4.4–5.7	3.9–5.0	
PCV[a]	0.40–0.51	0.36–0.45	
MCV (fl)			82–99
MCH (pg)			27–32.8
MCHC (g/dl)			32–34
Platelet count (10^9/l)	168–411	188–445	

Hb, hemoglobin; MCV, mean corpuscular volume; MCH, mean corpuscular hemoglobin; MCHC, mean corpuscular hemoglobin concentration.

[a]3% correction for plasma trapping.

in unselected healthy adults is 82 fl, the corresponding figure for children between 1 and 7 years (who show no biochemical evidence of iron deficiency) is about 70 fl. The MCV increases progressively with age both in children and, to a much lesser extent, in adults.

Red cell life span

As red cells do not contain ribosomes, they cannot synthesize protein to replace molecules (e.g. enzymes, structural proteins) which become denatured. Red cells therefore have a limited life span of 110–120 days, at the end of which they are ingested and degraded by the macrophages of the marrow, spleen, liver and other organs. A variety of changes affect red cells as they age within the circulation. These include:

1. progressive decrease in MCV and surface area
2. progressive increase in density and osmotic fragility
3. decrease in deformability
4. decreased ability to reduce methemoglobin
5. decrease in the rate of glycolysis.

The critical change that causes a red cell to be destroyed at the end of its life span appears to be the formation of denatured/oxidized hemoglobin (hemichromes) which induces clustering of the integral membrane protein, band 3. This clustering generates an epitope on the red cell surface that binds naturally occurring IgG anti-band 3 antibodies and the antibody-coated aged erythrocytes are recognized and phagocytosed by macrophages.[2,3] A second mechanism that may be involved in the elimination of aged red cells by macrophages is the exposure of phosphatidylserine on the outer surface of their cell membrane; this is recognized by the macrophage scavenger receptor CD36 or, after combination with lactadherin, by macrophage integrin.[3,4] Aging red cells also extrude microvesicles containing denatured hemoglobin that have the same membrane changes and are phagocytosed by the same mechanisms as the residual red cell.[5]

concentration in both males and females. There is a subsequent further rise in males but not in females with the result that the mean hemoglobin is higher in adult males than in adult females. In healthy infants aged 4 months and over, and in healthy young children, the average MCV is lower than in healthy adults. Whereas the lower limit for the MCV

Table 1.3 Age-dependent changes in the mean values (and 95% reference limits) for red cell parameters in normal individuals

Age	n	Hb (g/dl)	RBC (× 10¹²/l)	MCV (fl)	Reference details
Cord blood	59	17.1 (13.5–20.7)	4.6 (3.6–5.6)	113 (101–125)	a
1 day	59	19.4 (15.1–23.7)	5.3 (4.2–6.4)	110 (99–121)	a
1 month*	240	13.9 (10.7–17.1)	4.3 (3.3–5.3)	101 (91–112)	b
2 months*	241	11.2 (9.4–13.0)	3.7 (3.1–4.3)	95 (84–106)	b
4 months*	52	12.2 (10.3–14.1)	4.3 (3.5–5.1)	87 (76–97)	b
6 months*	52	12.6 (11.1–14.1)	4.7 (3.9–5.5)	76 (68–85)	b
12 months	56*	12.7 (11.3–14.1)	4.7 (4.1–5.3)	78 (71–84)	b
	51	11.1 (7.7–14.5)	4.8 (3.8–5.8)	73 (58–88)	a
	163	10.1 (7.5–12.7)	4.7 (3.5–5.5)	72 (58–86)	c
10–17 months*	59			77 (70–84)	d
3 years	103	12.4 (10.1–14.7)	4.7 (3.9–5.5)	78 (68–88)	a
	128	11.0 (8.6–13.4)	4.5 (3.5–5.5)	78 (64–92)	c
18 months–4 years*	26			80 (74–86)	d
5 years	97	12.7 (10.7–14.7)	4.7 (3.7–5.6)	80 (72–88)	a
	24	11.8 (9.2–14.4)	4.4 (3.7–5.1)	83 (69–97)	
4–7 years*	42			81 (76–86)	d
7 years	103	12.9 (9.2–16.6)	4.8 (3.8–5.8)	79 (61–97)	a
7–8 years	151	12.5 (10.3–14.7)	4.6 (4.0–5.2)	81 (72–89)	e
10 years	111	13.2 (10.8–15.6)	4.8 (3.9–5.7)	81 (68–94)	a
14 years	45	13.6 (10.7–16.5)	4.9 (3.9–5.9)	81 (66–96)	a
20 years male	–	15.9 (13.7–18.3)	5.3 (4.6–6.2)	89 (78–99)	f
20 years female	–	13.8 (11.7–15.8)	4.6 (4.0–5.4)	89 (76–99)	f
60 years male	–	15.9 (13.8–18.4)	5.0 (4.3–5.9)	93 (82–103)	f
60 years female	–	13.9 (11.8–15.9)	4.6 (3.9–5.3)	90 (77–100)	f

*Data in which cases with iron deficiency were excluded.

a = Healthy and sick American whites; used microhematocrit and counting chambers.

b = Healthy full-term infants from Finland; continuous iron supplementation; normal transferrin saturation and serum ferritin level; used Coulter counter model S.

c = Healthy Jamaican blacks; cohort study; HbS and β-thalassemia excluded; used Coulter ZBI 6.

d = Healthy Caucasian, Asian and black children in America; Hb > 11.0 g/dl, transferrin saturation ≥20%, normal serum ferritin; hemoglobinopathy and β-thalassemia trait excluded; used Coulter counter model S.

e = Healthy individuals; mostly American blacks; used Coulter counter model S.

f = Reference intervals derived from 1744 healthy Americans (ethnic origin not stated) aged 16–89 years using Hemac 630 laser cell counter.

Functions of red cells

Normal function of the erythrocyte requires a normal red cell membrane and normal enzyme systems to provide energy and protect against oxidant damage. The erythrocyte membrane is composed of a lipid bilayer (containing integral proteins) and is bound to a submembranous cytoskeletal network of protein molecules including spectrin, actin and the proteins constituting bands 4.1a and 4.1b[6] (Chapter 7). This cytoskeletal network is responsible for maintaining the biconcave shape of a normal erythrocyte. The membrane also contains adenosine triphosphate (ATP)-dependent cation pumps that continuously pump Na^+ out and K^+ into the red cell, against concentration gradients, thereby counteracting a continuous passive diffusion of ions across the membrane in the opposite direction. Mature erythrocytes derive their energy from glycolysis by the Embden–Meyerhof pathway (Chapter 8). They can also metabolize glucose through the pentose phosphate pathway, which generates the reduction potential of the cell and protects the membrane, the hemoglobin and erythrocyte enzymes from oxidant damage (Chapter 8). Both a normal cell membrane and normal energy production are required to enable the biconcave red cells to repeatedly and reversibly deform during numerous transits through the microcirculation.

The prime function of the red cell is to combine with oxygen in the lungs and to transport and release this oxygen for utilization by tissues. The red cells also combine with CO_2 produced in tissues and release this in the lungs. The function of oxygen transport resides in the hemoglobin molecule which is ideally structured for this purpose. Most of the hemoglobin (Hb) of an adult is HbA which is a tetramer consisting of two α-globin chains and two β-globin chains. Each of these globin chains is associated with a heme molecule which is inserted deeply within a pocket which excludes water but allows O_2 to enter and interact with the iron atom at the center of the heme molecule. In the deoxygenated state, the iron atom is in the ferrous state (Fe^{++}) and has a 'spare' electron. In the oxygenated state there is a weak ionic link between the oxygen molecule and the iron atom as a result of the 'sharing' of the 'spare' electron, but the iron remains in the ferrous state. This reaction between the oxygen molecule and the iron atom of the heme ring is reversible and the oxygen is readily released at the low oxygen concentrations found in tissues. The importance of excluding water from the heme pocket is that the water could oxidize the iron atom to the ferric state by accepting the spare electron. Hemoglobin in which the iron atoms are in the ferric state is called methemoglobin and does not combine with oxygen.

The ability of red cells to combine with and release oxygen is illustrated in the oxygen dissociation curve (Fig. 1.2). The shape of the oxygen dissociation curve of HbA is sigmoid and this is a function of the interaction between the four monomers which make up its tetrameric structure (heme–heme interaction); the combination of one oxygen molecule with one heme group causes a slight shape change in the Hb molecule due to movement at the $α_1$–$β_2$ contact facilitating the binding of oxygen to the next heme group. The shape of the oxygen dissociation curve of the monomer, myoglobin, is hyperbolic. The advantage of the sigmoid curve over the hyperbolic curve is that much more oxygen is released from the hemoprotein at the low PO_2 values obtained in tissues (35–40 mmHg) with the former than with the latter. The percentage saturation of hemoglobin at this PO_2 is about 70%. The capacity of hemoglobin to combine with O_2 is referred to as its oxygen affinity and is expressed as the PO_2 required to cause 50% saturation (P_{50}). A decrease in pH leads to a shift of the oxygen dissociation curve to the right and a decrease in oxygen affinity. This effect, which is known as the Bohr effect, facilitates the release of oxygen at the low pH of tissues. A shift of the oxygen dissociation curve to the right also results from the combination of deoxyhemoglobin with 2,3-diphosphoglycerate (2,3-DPG) that is produced as a result of the metabolism of glucose via the Rapoport–Luebering shunt of the Embden–Meyerhof pathway (Chapter 8). In deoxyhemoglobin, the two β chains are separated slightly allowing one molecule of 2,3-DPG to enter and bind to the β chains; when hemoglobin combines with oxygen, the 2,3-DPG is ejected.

The CO_2 produced in the tissues enters the blood. Most of this CO_2 enters the red cells and is converted there to carbonic acid by the enzyme carbonic anhydrase. The hydrogen ions released from the dissociation of this weak acid combine with the hemoglobin, and are largely responsible for the Bohr effect referred to above. A small proportion of the CO_2 entering red cells combines with hemoglobin to form carbaminohemoglobin. When the blood circulates through the lungs, where the PCO_2 is lower than that in the blood, the CO_2 is released from the red cells into the alveolar air. The release of CO_2 from red cells results in a reversal of the Bohr effect (i.e. a shift of the oxygen dissociation curve to the left) and the uptake of considerable amounts of O_2. The oxygen saturation and PO_2 of arterial blood are, respectively, greater than 95% and 100 mmHg.

The biconcave shape of normal erythrocytes facilitates the diffusion of gases in and out of the cytoplasm and also imparts adequate flexibility and deformability to enable these cells repeatedly to traverse the microcirculation. The hemoglobin molecules within erythrocyes inactivate some of the endothelial cell-derived nitric oxide and consequently regulate the bioavailability of nitric oxide in the circulation. The inactivation results from the reaction of nitric oxide with oxyhemoglobin resulting in the formation of nitrite. Plasma nitrite may also be converted to nitric oxide by deoxyhemoglobin which has a nitrite reductase activity and by a nitric oxide synthase (NOS) located in the plasma membrane and cytoplasm of red cells. These three mechanisms affect nitric oxide-dependent vascular tone and nitric oxide generated by red cell NOS may affect red cell deformability.[6–8]

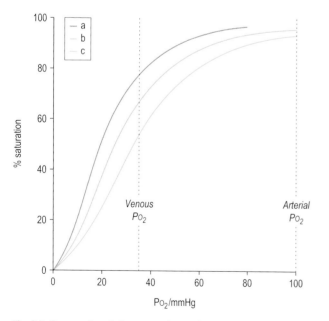

Fig. 1.2 Oxygen dissociation curve of normal adult blood and the effect of varying the pH. PO_2 and PCO_2 = partial pressure of O_2 and CO_2 respectively. a = pH 7.6 (PCO_2 25 mmHg); b = pH 7.4 (PCO_2 40 mmHg); c = pH 7.2 (PCO_2 61 mmHg).

Reticulocytes

These are the immediate precursors of mature erythrocytes. They are rounded anucleate cells that are about 20% larger in volume than mature red blood cells and appear faintly polychromatic when stained by a Romanowsky method. When stained with a supravital stain such as new methylene blue or brilliant cresyl blue, the diffuse basophilic material responsible for the polychromasia (i.e. ribosomal RNA) appears as a basophilic reticulum. Electron-microscope studies have shown that reticulocytes are rounded cells with a tortuous surface and that in addition to ribosomes they contain mitochondria and autophagic vacuoles. Circulating reticulocytes mature into red cells over a period of 1–2 days during which there is progressive degradation of ribosomes and mitochondria and the acquisition of a biconcave shape. Reticulocytes actively synthesize hemoglobin and non-hemoglobin proteins. They contain enzymes of the Embden–Meyerhof pathway and the pentose phosphate shunt and, unlike the mature red cells, can also derive energy aerobically via the Krebs cycle that operates in the mitochondria and oxidizes pyruvate to CO_2 and water. Supravitally stained preparations were traditionally used and are still frequently used to assess reticulocyte numbers by microscopy with an eyepiece micrometer disc to facilitate counting. In normal adults, the reference range for reticulocytes counted in this way is widely accepted to be 0.5–2.0% of the total circulating erythrocyte plus reticulocyte population. The usefulness of the reticulocyte percentage is increased by applying a correction for the hematocrit and the corrected reticulocyte percentage (usually corrected to a hematocrit of 0.45) is obtained by multiplying the observed percentage by [patient's hematocrit ÷ 0.45]. Although several laboratories still express reticulocyte counts as a percentage, the absolute reticulocyte count (i.e. the total number per liter of blood) is clinically more useful. The latter is directly proportional both to the rate of effective erythropoiesis and to the average maturation time of blood reticulocytes. In normal adults the absolute reticulocyte count determined by microscopy is $20–110 \times 10^9$/l. Reticulocytes can be counted using automated machines employing flow cytometry and laser light after staining their RNA with fluorescent reagents such as acridine orange, thioflavin T, thiazol orange or auramine O. There are also automated methods in which the RNA is stained with supravital basic dyes and the extent of staining quantified using light absorbance or scatter. Results obtained by these automated methods are more reproducible than when counted by the traditional manual method as much larger numbers of reticulocytes are counted. The accepted reference range for reticulocytes in adults when counted by automated fluorescent-based methods is $20–120 \times 10^9$/l.[9,10] The absolute reticulocyte count has also been shown to be higher in men than women. Reference values do depend on the method of measurement used and each laboratory should determine its own reference range. Semi-automated and fully automated discrete reticulocyte counters and some fully automated multiparameter hematology analyzers also provide various reticulocyte maturation parameters based primarily on the intensity of fluorescence (i.e. the amount of RNA), or, in the case of cells stained supravitally with a basic dye, on the extent of absorbance or scatter. These parameters include the immature reticulocyte fraction (immature reticulocytes have more RNA than mature ones), mean reticulocyte hemoglobin content and concentration and mean reticulocyte volume.[11–12] Although these parameters have been shown to be of value in the assessment of

certain clinical situations, they are not in regular use in clinical practice.

Granulocytes (polymorphonuclear leukocytes)

These cells contain characteristic cytoplasmic granules and a segmented nucleus. The latter consists of two or more nuclear masses (nuclear segments) joined together by fine strands of nuclear chromatin. The nuclear masses contain moderate quantities of condensed chromatin. The granulocytes are subdivided into neutrophil, eosinophil and basophil granulocytes according to the staining reactions of the granules.

Neutrophil granulocytes

Morphology and composition

Neutrophil granulocytes have a mean volume of 500 fl and, in dried fixed smears, a diameter of 9–15 μm. Their cytoplasm is slightly acidophilic and contains many very fine granules that stain with neutral dyes; the granules stain a faint purple color with Romanowsky stains (Figs 1.1 and 1.3). The nucleus usually contains two to five nuclear segments; the percentages of neutrophils with two, three, four and five or more segments are 32, 45, 20 and 3%, respectively, with a mean of 2.9 segments. In the female up to 17% of neutrophls contain a drumstick-like appendage attached by a fine chromatin strand to one of the nuclear segments. These appendages correspond to Barr bodies (inactivated X-chromosomes). Neutrophils possess a variety of surface receptors including those for C3 and IgG-Fc and the CXC chemokine receptors.

Neutrophils contain primary granules and specific (secondary) granules. Primary granules, first formed at the promyelocyte stage of differentiation, contain myeloperoxidase, lysozyme (muramidase), defensins, bacterial permeability inducer, acid phosphatase, β-glucuronidase, α-mannosidase, elastase, cathepsins B, D and G, and proteinase 3. On electron microscopy they are electron-dense, 0.5–1.0 μm in their

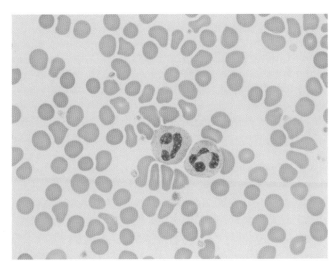

Fig. 1.3 Normal neutrophils. May–Grünwald–Giemsa stain. ×1000.

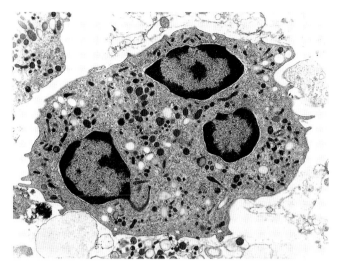

Fig. 1.4 Electron micrograph of a neutrophil granulocyte. The three nuclear segments contain a large quantity of condensed chromatin at their periphery. The cytoplasmic granules vary considerably in size, shape and electron-density. Uranyl acetate and lead citrate. ×5500.

Table 1.4 95% reference limits for the concentration of circulating leukocytes in peripheral venous blood of healthy adults[15,48]

Cell count × 10⁹/l	Caucasians		Blacks	
	Male (n = 100)	Female (n = 158)	Female (n = 226)	Male and female (n = 100)
Leukocytes	3.5–9.5	4.1–10.9	3.1–8.7	3.6–10.2
Neutrophils	1.6–6.0	2.0–7.3	1.1–6.1	1.3–7.4
Lymphocytes	1.2–3.5	1.4–3.2	1.0–3.6	1.45–3.75
Monocytes	0.2–0.8	0.3–0.8	0.14–0.77	0.21–1.05
Eosinophils	0.02–0.59	0.05–0.35	0.01–0.82	0.03–0.72
Basophils	0–0.15	0.01–0.06	0–0.08	0–0.16

long axis, and ellipsoidal in shape (Fig. 1.4). Specific granules are formed at the myelocyte (secondary granules) and metamyelocyte (tertiary granules) stages. They are less electron-dense and are very pleomorphic. Specific granules vary considerably in size, being frequently quite small (0.2–0.5 μm long), and the granule membrane contains NADPH oxidase (cytochrome b_{558}), vitronectin and laminin receptors, formylpeptide receptors and CR3. The granule proteins include lysozyme, transcobalamin I (vitamin B_{12} binding protein), collagenase, β2 microglobulin, lactoferrin or lactoferrin and gelatinase, SGP28 (specific granule protein of 28 kDa), hCAP-18 (human cationic antimicrobial protein) and NGAL (a matrix protein). A third type of granule contains gelatinase but little or no lactoferrin (gelatinase granules) and neutrophils also contain secretory vesicles with molecules such as β2-integrins, formylpeptide receptors and CD14. The secretory vesicles are involved in adhesion of neutrophils to the endothelium, the gelatinase granules in migration through basement membrane and the primary and specific granules mainly in phagocytosis, killing and digestion of microorganisms.[13–14] The alkaline phosphatase activity of neutrophils is present within membrane-bound intracytoplasmic vesicles called phosphosomes. In addition to the various organelles mentioned above, the cytoplasm contains a centrosome, a poorly developed Golgi apparatus, microtubules and microfilaments, a few small mitochondria, a few ribosomes, a little endoplasmic reticulum, occasional multivesicular bodies and numerous glycogen particles.

Number and life span

In the blood, the neutrophil granulocytes are distributed between a circulating granulocyte pool (CGP) and a marginated granulocyte pool (MGP). The latter, which is in a rapid equilibrium with the CGP, consists of cells that are loosely associated with the endothelial cells of small venules. The CGP accounts for 15–99% (mean 44%) of the total blood granulocyte pool in healthy subjects. Exercise and adrenaline both cause a rapid shift of cells from the MGP to the CGP; bacterial endotoxin causes a shift from the CGP to the MGP.

The number of neutrophil granulocytes in the peripheral venous blood of healthy Caucasians of different ages and genders are given in Tables 1.4 and 1.5. Healthy blacks have lower neutrophil counts than Caucasians (Table 1.4); Chinese and Indians have similar counts to those in Europeans.[15] A single nucleotide polymorphism in the Duffy antigen receptor/chemokine gene is strongly associated with the neutropenia in Afro-Caribbeans and Africans but the mechanism by which this mutation causes neutropenia is not yet clear.[16] Ethnic neutropenia has also been described in Yemenite Jews, Falashah Jews, black Bedouin and Jordanian Arabs.[17] Considerably lower total leukocyte and neutrophil counts have been reported from East Africa than those shown in Table 1.4 for black Americans, and black West Indians and Africans living in England. However, the former studies have not allowed for the skewed distribution of leukocyte numbers in calculating reference ranges, and thus have exaggerated the difference between the black and Caucasian populations. Despite this, total white cell and neutrophil counts are probably genuinely lower in Africans living in African countries, particularly if taking an African diet, than in Africans living in Western countries.

Once formed, the mature neutrophil is retained in the bone marrow through interaction of stromal cell-derived CXCL12 with its receptor CXCR4 on neutrophils.[18] After entering the blood by migration through the sinusoidal endothelium, neutrophil granulocytes leave the circulation in an exponential fashion with a $T_{1/2}$ of 2.6–11.8 h (mean 7.2 h) and appear in normal secretions (saliva, secretions of the respiratory and gastrointestinal tracts and urine) and in various tissues. They probably survive outside the blood for up to 30 h.

Functions

Neutrophils are highly motile cells. They move towards, phagocytose and degrade various types of particulate material such as bacteria and damaged tissue cells. Neutrophils are attracted to sites of infection or inflammation as a result of chemotactic gradients generated around such sites. The chemotactic factors include activated complement

Table 1.5 Age-related ranges for the concentration of circulating white blood cells ($\times 10^9$/l) in normal individuals.

Age	Leukocytes	Neutrophils[a]	Eosinophils	Basophils	Lymphocytes	Monocytes
Cord blood	5.0–23.0[b]	1.7–19.0	0.05–2.0	0–0.64	1.0–11.0	0.1–3.7
12 h	13.0–38.0	6.0–28.0	0.02–0.95	0–0.50	2.0–11.0	0.4–3.6
24 h	9.4–34.0	4.8–21.0	0.05–1.00	0–0.30	2.0–11.5	0.2–3.1
7–8 days	9.0–18.4	1.8–8.0	0.16–0.94	0–0.25	3.0–9.0	0.03–0.98
2 months	5.1–18.0	0.7–9.0	0.07–0.84	0.02–0.20	3.0–16.0	0.13–1.8
5–6 months	5.9–17.5	1.0–8.5	0.01–1.0	0.02–0.20	3.2–13.5	0.10–1.3
1 year	5.6–17.5	1.5–8.5	0.05–0.70	0.02–0.20	2.5–10.5	0.05–1.28
2 years	5.6–17.0	1.5–8.5	0.04–1.19	0.02–0.20	2.2–9.5	0.05–1.28
4 years	4.9–15.5	1.5–8.5	0.02–1.40	0.03–0.20	1.7–8.0	0.15–1.28
6 years	4.4–14.5	1.5–8.9	0.08–1.10	0.02–0.20	1.5–7.0	0.15–1.28
9–10 years	3.9–13.5	1.5–8.0	0.06–1.03	0.01–0.54	1.4–6.5	0.15–1.28
13–14 years	3.9–13.0	1.4–8.0	0.04–0.76	0.01–0.43	1.2–5.8	0.15–1.28
18 years	4.5–12.5	1.8–7.7	0–0.45	0–0.20	1.0–5.0	0–0.8

[a]Includes a small percentage of myelocytes during the first few days after birth.

[b]Includes 0.03–5.4 $\times 10^9$/l of erythroblasts.

components (C3a, C5a, C567), membrane phospholipids and other factors released from tissue cells, lymphokines released from activated lymphocytes, products of mononuclear phagocytes (e.g. tumor necrosis factor, IL-8), platelet-derived factors (platelet factor 4, the β-thromboglobulin neutrophil-activating peptide 2 (NAP-2), platelet-derived growth factor) and products of certain bacteria. IL-8, platelet factor 4 and NAP-2 bind to CXC chemokine receptors on the surface of neutrophils and activate these cells. Activated neutrophils adhere to endothelial cells via adhesion molecules on their cell membrane (Chapter 17). The arrival of neutrophils at sites of inflammation is probably facilitated by an increased permeability of adjoining blood vessels caused by activated complement components such as C3a and C5a.

The first stage in the phagocytosis of a particle such as a bacterium is the adherence of the neutrophil to the particle. The adherence is mediated through specific receptors on the neutrophil cell membrane: these include Fc (IgG_1, IgG_3) and C3 receptors. Both the adherence and the subsequent ingestion of such particles are enhanced by their interaction with opsonizing factors such as C3 generated via the classical or alternative complement activation pathway, antibody and mannose-binding lectin (Chapter 17). Following adhesion, pseudopodia form around the particle and progressively encircle it, probably via a zipper-like mechanism dependent on the interaction between receptors on the cell membrane and opsonizing factors present all over the particle. Both the movement of neutrophils towards a particle and the act of phagocytosis may be dependent on the activity of intracytoplasmic microfilaments composed of actin. The act of phagocytosis is associated with a burst of oxygen consumption (respiratory burst) and the production of hydrogen peroxide.

The ingestion of a particle is followed by the fusion of primary and specific granules with the membrane of the phagosome and the discharge of granule contents into the phagocytic vacuole. Neutrophils contain considerable quantities of glycogen that can be converted to glucose. They obtain much of their energy by breaking down glucose anaerobically via the Embden–Meyerhof pathway but can oxidize some glucose aerobically through the Krebs cycle. The killing of certain bacteria (e.g. *Staphylococcus aureus*, *Escherichia coli*, *Salmonella typhimurium*, *Klebsiella pneumoniae*, *Proteus vulgaris*) is oxygen dependent but for others (e.g. *Pseudomonas aeruginosa*, *Staphylococcus epidermidis*, 'viridans' streptococci, various anaerobes) is oxygen independent. The mechanisms responsible for the killing of bacteria are complex.

NADPH serves as the electron donor in the biochemical processes leading to the reduction of O_2 to O_2^- and oxygen-dependent killing; the bactericidal agents derived from O_2^- include hydrogen peroxide, hydroxyl radicals, hypochlorite ions (generated from halides by hydrogen peroxide in the presence of the enzyme myeloperoxidase) and chloramines. The generation of O_2^- requires the membrane-associated enzyme known as the respiratory burst oxidase, the components of which only assemble when the neutrophil is activated by various stimuli, including the phagocytosis of opsonized bacteria. These components are cytochrome b_{558} (the electron transferring oxidase), three phosphoproteins (p40-phox, p47-phox and p67-phox) and two GTP-binding proteins (Rac2 and Rap1a) (see also Chapter 17).

The substances mediating oxygen-independent killing include defensins (small peptides) that kill a variety of both Gram-negative and Gram-positive bacteria as well as yeasts by permeabilizing their membranes, and bactericidal/

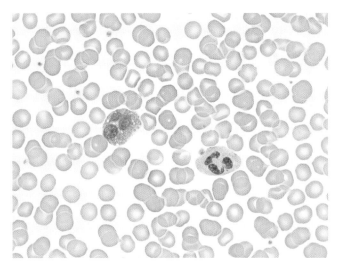

Fig. 1.5 Normal eosinophil with red-orange granules and a normal neutrophil. May–Grünwald–Giemsa stain. × 1000.

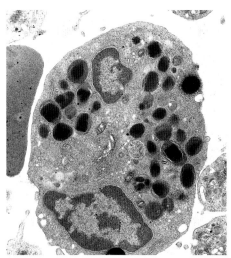

Fig. 1.6 Electron micrograph of a normal eosinophil. Uranyl acetate and lead citrate. The two nuclear segments contain a large quantity of condensed chromatin at their periphery. One homogeneous granule and several crystalloid-containing granules are present in the cytoplasm. There is a small Golgi apparatus at the center of the cell (this apparatus is usually somewhat better developed in eosinophils than in neutrophils). × 10 000.

permeability increasing protein. The latter binds to surface lipopolysaccharides of Gram-negative bacteria thereby damaging membranes and rendering them leaky. Defensins also have anti-viral effects against some enveloped viruses and prevent entry of some viruses into cells. Lysozyme and lactoferrin are also involved in oxygen-independent killing. At the acid pH of the phagocytic vacuole, lysozyme (muramidase) hydrolyses peptidoglycans in bacterial cell walls and consequently allows the osmotic swelling and lysis of certain bacteria. Lactoferrin is bacteriostatic as it binds iron at a low pH and thus deprives bacteria of this growth factor.

Eosinophil granulocytes

Morphology and composition

Eosinophil granulocytes (eosinophils) have a diameter of 12–17 μm in fixed smears. Their cytoplasm is packed with large rounded granules which stain red-orange with Romanowsky stains (see Figs 1.1A and 1.5). The percentage of cells with one, two, three and four nuclear segments are 6, 68, 22 and 4%, respectively (mean 2.2). Eosinophils possess surface receptors for IgG-Fc (FcγRII, FcγRIII), IgE, IgA, IgM, C4, C3b, C3d, cytokines (GM-CSF, IL-3 and IL-5) and the CC chemokine receptor 3.[19–20]

There are two types of eosinophil granules: a few rounded homogeneously electron-dense granules and many rounded, elongated or oval crystalloid-containing granules (Fig. 1.6) (see also Chapter 2).[21] Both homogeneous and crystalloid-containing granules contain an arginine- and zinc-rich basic protein, a peroxidase (distinct from neutrophil peroxidase) and acid phosphatase. Eosinophil granules also contain phospholipase B and D, histaminase, ribonuclease, β-glucuronidase, cathepsin and collagenase but not lysozyme. The eosinophil ribonucleases include eosinophil-derived neurotoxin (Rnase2) and eosinophil cationic protein (Rnase3). The Charcot–Leyden crystal protein, which has lysophospholipase activity and carbohydrate-binding properties, is found both in the cytosol and in some of the eosinophil granules.[22]

Number and life span

Table 1.4 gives the venous blood eosinophil counts for normal healthy adults. The eosinophil counts of healthy blacks and people from the Indian subcontinent do not differ from those of Caucasians.[15] Eosinophils leave the circulation in a random manner with a $T_{1/2}$ of about 4.5–8 h; they probably survive in the tissues for 8–12 days.

Functions

Eosinophils share several functions with neutrophils: both cell types are motile, respond to specific chemotactic agents and phagocytose and kill similar types of microorganisms.[23–24] Eosinophils tend to be slower at ingesting and killing bacteria than neutrophils but appear to be metabolically more active than these cells. Eosinophil granule contents are transported to and discharged at the surface via large vesicular-tubular structures (piecemeal degranulation).[24] Eosinophils also function as the effector cell (killer cell) in antibody-dependent damage to metazoal parasites. Eosinophils bind to IgG- and C3-coated helminths via their corresponding surface receptors and discharge their granule contents around the parasite. The killing of the parasite is caused by the eosinophilic cationic proteins which generate defects and pores in the cuticle and cell membrane and the major basic protein which is a potent toxin for helminths, as well as eosinophil peroxidase, which exerts its effect through the production of H_2O_2 and hypochlorous acid and superoxide. All three molecules are also toxic towards human tissues. The two eosinophil ribonucleases, Rnase2 and Rnase3, may be involved in defense against viruses.[25] Not only the stimulation of FcγRII and complement receptors but also binding of IgA to IgA receptors triggers degranulation and the respiratory burst. Eosinophils also have a role in regulating immediate-type hypersensitivity reactions. In these reactions chemical mediators of anaphylaxis such as histamine and leukotriene

C_4 (LTC$_4$) and LTB$_4$ (a component of a mixture of small peptides known as eosinophil chemotactic factor of anaphylaxis or ECF-A) are released from mast cells and basophils as a result of the interaction between specific antigen and IgE on the surface of these cells. Eosinophils are attracted to the site of the activated mast cells or basophils by mast cell- and basophil-derived ECF-A, platelet-activating factor (PAF) and leukotriene B$_4$ (LTB$_4$) and by several other chemoattractants (chemokines) produced at sites of allergic inflammation; some of the chemokines are also activators of eosinophils. The most potent eosinophil chemoattractants are eotaxin (produced by macrophages and some other tissue cells), RANTES (released from thrombin-activated platelets), the 5-lipoxygenase product 5-oxo-6,8,11,14-eicosatetraenoic acid and monocyte chemoattractant protein 3 (MCP3) (released from endothelial and other cells).[26] Eotaxin is a ligand of the CC chemokine receptor 3 (CCR3) that is expressed on eosinophils, basophils and T$_H$2 lymphocytes. C5a, monocyte-derived LTB$_4$ and PAF, and some lymphokines are also involved in attracting eosinophils. The attracted eosinophils then release prostaglandin E$_2$ (PGE$_2$) which inhibits further release of basophil- and mast-cell-derived mediators. Eosinophils also release specific enzymes that inactivate these mediators, including histaminase and phospholipase B and D which break down histamine and PAF, respectively. Eosinophil-derived arylsulphatase inactivates various chemotactic peptides and LTC$_4$. Eosinophils may enhance hypersensitivity reactions by their phospholipase-A$_2$-dependent synthesis and release of LTC$_4$ and PAF, and also via the release of eosinophil-derived major basic protein, peroxidase and cationic proteins that activate basophils and mast cells and cause histamine release. Recent studies have shown that eosinophils also function as antigen-presenting cells, constitutively express T$_H$1- and T$_H$2-associated cytokines including IL-4, IL-13, IL-6, IL-10, IL-12, IFN-γ and TNF-α, differentially release these cytokines, and modulate the function of T cells (promoting either a T$_H$1 or T$_H$2 response) as well as of dendritic cells, B cells, mast cells, neutrophils and basophils.[27,28]

Basophil granulocytes

Basophil granulocytes (basophils) represent the most infrequent type of leukocyte in the blood (see Tables 1.4 and 1.5). In Romanowsky-stained blood smears, basophil granulocytes have an average diameter of about 12 µm and display large round purple-black cytoplasmic granules (Fig. 1.7), some of which overlie the nucleus. The granules stain metachromatically (i.e. reddish-violet) with toluidine blue or methylene blue. The nucleus usually has two segments, although these can be difficult to see by light microscopy. Basophils stain strongly by the periodic acid-Schiff (PAS) reaction (due to the presence of glycogen aggregates) and do not stain for acid or alkaline phosphatase. Basophil granules undergo varying degrees of extraction during processing for electron microscopy and characteristically show a particulate substructure with each particle measuring about 20 nm in diameter (Fig. 1.8).[29] Basophils possess at their cell surface high-affinity receptors for IgE (FcεRI), low-affinity receptors for IgG (FcγRIIIB and FcγRII), receptors for C5a and histamine, and CC chemokine receptors (CCR3 and CCR2).[30]

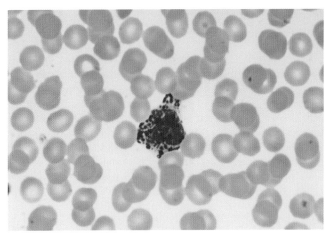

Fig. 1.7 A normal basophil showing the numerous large deeply violaceous granules. May–Grünwald–Giemsa stain. ×1000.

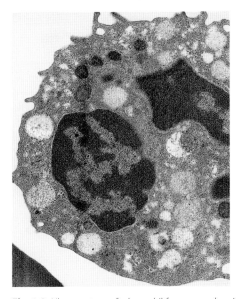

Fig. 1.8 Ultrastructure of a basophil from normal peripheral blood. Uranyl acetate and lead citrate. There are several large distinctive granules within the cytoplasm. Most of the granules have been partially or completely extracted during the processing for electron microscopy. ×18 300.

Basophil granules contain histamine (which is synthesized by the cell), sulphated mucopolysaccharides (predominantly chondroitin sulphate), peroxidase, low levels of chymase (a serine protease) and negligible amounts of tryptase. The mucopolysaccharides account for the metachromatic staining of the granules. Basophils also contain Charcot–Leyden crystal protein and possibly PAF (which causes platelets to aggregate and release their contents) and eosinophil chemotactic factor of anaphylaxis (ECF-A).[22]

Functions

Basophils play a key role in immediate-type hypersensitivity reactions and in the immune response to helminthic infections.[29–31] When IgE binds to FcεRI and the bound IgE reacts with specific antigen, basophils degranulate releasing histamine and chemotactic factors such as eosinophil chemotactic factor of anaphylaxis (ECF-A) and generate and release metabolites of arachidonic acid such as LTC₄ (that stimulate secretion of mucus and contraction of smooth muscle) as well as cytokines, especially TNF-α, IL-4, IL-5 and IL-6. Basophils and mast cells may also be activated to release histamine by the binding of monocyte chemoattractant protein-1 (MCP-1) (produced by endothelial and other cells) to CCR2 on their surface and to a lesser degree the binding of ligands to FcγRIIIB and C5a receptors. Basophils also have FcγRIIB on their surface and stimulation via this receptor generates inhibitory signals. The release of histamine and other substances from basophils (and mast cells) is mediated via the transport of vesicles between the secretory granules and plasma membrane (piecemeal degranulation).[32] The released histamine causes contraction of bronchial and gastrointestinal smooth muscle, inhibition of cytotoxic T-cell activity and lymphokine release, chemotactic attraction of other granulocytes, upregulation of C3b receptors on eosinophils and release of lysosomal enzymes from neutrophils. The accumulation of basophils at sites of hypersensitivity reactions is mediated by chemokines such as MCP-1 and eotaxins (produced by macrophages and some other cells such as fibroblasts, endothelial cells and epithelial cells). Eotaxin receptors (e.g. CCR3) are present not only on basophils but also on mast cells, eosinophils and T-helper type 2 cells (T_H2 cells) which have IL-4-induced CCR3, leading to the attraction of eosinophils and T_H2 cells to sites of allergic inflammation and parasitic infection. Basophils appear to be a major source of the immunomodulatory cytokine IL-4 in the body; mast cells do not produce this cytokine. Basophil-derived IL-4 may be important for the development of type 2 immunity via promotion of the development of T_H2 cells and consequently antibody synthesis, particularly IgE synthesis, by B-cells.

Monocytes

These are the largest leukocytes in peripheral blood. In stained smears, they vary considerably in diameter (15–30 μm) and in morphology (Figs 1.1 and 1.9). The nucleus is large and eccentric and may be rounded, kidney-shaped, horseshoe-shaped or lobulated. The nuclear chromatin has a skein-like or lacy appearance. The cytoplasm is plentiful, stains grayish-blue and contains few to many fine azurophilic granules. One or more intracytoplasmic vacuoles may be present. Cytochemical studies with the light microscope have shown the presence of many hydrolytic enzymes, including acid phosphatase, NaF-resistant esterase, galactosidases and lysozyme. Monocytes also contain defensins, myeloperoxidase, collagenase, elastase and coagulation system proteins (tissue factor, factors V, VII, IX, X and XIII, plasminogen activator) and have membrane receptors for IgG-Fc and C3. In addition, they have two CC chemokine receptors, CCR2 and CCR5, that bind various CC chemokines such as monocyte chemoattractant protein-1 (MCP-1), MCP-2, MCP-3, RANTES, macrophage inflammatory protein-1α (MIP-1α) and MIP-1β.

Under the electron microscope, monocyte granules vary considerably in size and shape and are relatively homogeneously electron-dense (Fig. 1.10). Some of the granules contain acid phosphatase and peroxidase. The

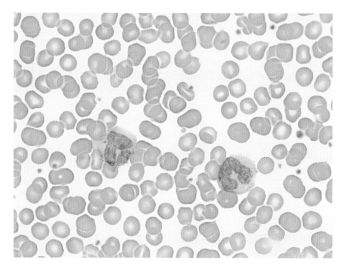

Fig. 1.9 Normal monocytes showing their large size, gray cytoplasm and horseshoe-shaped nuclei. May–Grünwald–Giemsa stain. ×1000.

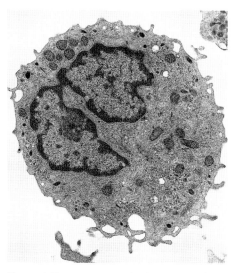

Fig. 1.10 Electron micrograph of a monocyte from normal peripheral blood. Uranyl acetate and lead citrate. The cytoplasm contains numerous mitochondria, several small pleomorphic electron-dense granules and short strands of rough endoplasmic reticulum. The nucleus has an irregular outline. It contains moderate quantities of condensed chromatin and a prominent nucleolus. ×11 300.

peroxidase-positive granules are characteristically smaller than those of neutrophils. In thin sections, monocytes display finger-like projections of their cell membrane. Their cytoplasm contains appreciable amounts of rough endoplasmic reticulum, moderate numbers of dispersed ribosomes, a well-developed Golgi apparatus, several mitochondria and bundles of microfibrils. The nucleus has moderate quantities of heterochromatin and nucleoli are commonly seen by electron microscopy.

Blood monocytes are, like neutrophils, distributed between a circulating and a marginated pool; there are, on average, 3.6 times more marginated than circulating cells. The number of circulating monocytes in the peripheral venous blood of healthy adults is given in Table 1.4. Monocytes leave the circulation in an exponential manner, with an average $T_{1/2}$ of 71 h. They then transform into macrophages in various tissues and may survive in this form for several months.

Monocytes are actively motile cells that respond to chemotactic stimuli (e.g. MCP-1, RANTES, MIP-1α and MIP-1β), phagocytose particulate material and kill microorganisms in a manner similar to that described for neutrophil granulocytes. Monocytes and monocyte-derived macrophages are conspicuous at sites of chronic inflammation. In addition to their role as a phagocytic cell, macrophages play important roles in various aspects of the immune response. These include the processing and presentation of antigen on class II major histocompatibility complex (MHC) molecules (Ia molecules) in a form recognizable by helper T-lymphocytes, and the degradation of excess antigen. They also secrete proinflammatory, immunoregulatory or anti-inflammatory cytokines such as IL-1β, IL-6, IL-8, IL-10, IL-12, IL-18, tumor necrosis factor alpha (TNF-α). The macrophages of the liver, spleen and bone marrow destroy senescent red cells and those in the marrow produce several cytokines regulating various aspects of hemopoiesis, including G-CSF, M-CSF, GM-CSF, erythropoietin and thymosin B_4. Macrophages also produce fibroblast growth factor and platelet-derived growth factor.

Lymphocytes

Lymphocytes have an average volume of approximately 180 fl and in stained smears have a diameter of 7–12 μm. Most of the lymphocytes in normal blood are small (Figs 1.1B and 1.11). In Romanowsky-stained smears, they have scanty bluish cytoplasm; the nucleus is round or slightly indented and there is considerable condensation of nuclear chromatin. The cytoplasm, which sometimes merely consists of a narrow rim around the nucleus, may contain a few azurophilic granules. Ultrastructural studies reveal that small lymphocytes contain a few scattered monoribosomes, an inactive Golgi apparatus, a few mitochondria, a few lysosomal granules and a small nucleolus (Fig. 1.12). About 10% of lymphocytes are large lymphocytes. These are about 12–16 μm in diameter and contain more cytoplasm and less condensed chromatin than small lymphocytes. In normal blood an occasional large lymphocyte has voluminous cytoplasm and several coarse azurophilic granules (large granular lymphocytes).

The concentration of lymphocytes in the blood is age-dependent: normal values are given in Tables 1.4 and 1.5. Lymphocytes leave the blood through endothelial cells of the postcapillary venules of lymphoid organs and eventually find their way back into lymphatic channels and re-enter the blood via the thoracic duct. The life span of lymphocytes varies considerably. The average life span in humans appears to be about 4 years but some cells survive for over 10 years.

Although most mature lymphocytes are morphologically similar to one another they can be divided into two major functionally distinct groups, B-lymphocytes (B-cells) and T-lymphocytes (T-cells).[33] Some characteristics of these two types of cell, including their various functions, are summarized in Table 1.6. On the basis of the nature of the two disulfide-linked chains of the T-cell receptor (TcR), T-cells are divided into αβ-T-cells (with αβ-TcR) and γδ-T-cells (with γδ-TcR); most T-cells are αβ-T-cells. Four functionally different groups of αβ-T-cells exist, termed helper cells or T_H cells, cytotoxic/suppressor T-cells or T_C cells, T-regulatory cells or Treg cells and T_H17 cells.[34] TH cells are CD4-positive, recognize antigen and release lymphokines involved in promoting the functions of B-cells and the maturation of other kinds of T-cells including T_C cells. T_H cells are subdivided into T_H1 cells and T_H2 cells. When the TcR of T_H1 cells reacts with antigen fragments on class II MHC molecules on dendritic cells, the antigen-presenting cells produce IL-12, IL-18 and

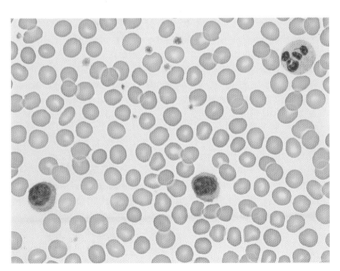

Fig. 1.11 Normal blood showing two lymphocytes and one neutrophil. Note one has a small number of azurophilic cytoplasmic granules. May–Grünwald–Giemsa stain. ×1000.

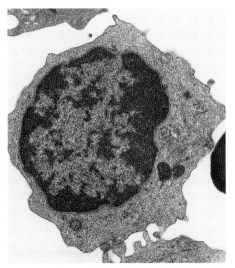

Fig. 1.12 Ultrastructural appearance of a normal lymphocyte from an adult. Uranyl acetate and lead citrate. The lymphocyte has a high nucleus:cytoplasm ratio, a rounded nuclear outline and large quantities of nuclear-membrane-associated condensed chromatin. The cytoplasm lacks granules but has a few mitochondria and a few moderately long strands of rough endoplasmic reticulum. ×14 200.

Table 1.6 Some characteristics of T- and B-lymphocytes[33]

		T-lymphocyte	B-lymphocyte
Characteristics		T-cell receptor associated with CD3	Surface membrane immunoglobulin (SmIg)
		Form rosettes with sheep red blood cells	Receptors for complement components C3b, C3d, C4
		Surface antigens CD2, CD5, CD6, CD4/CD8	Receptors for Fc end of immunoglobulin molecule in immune complex or in aggregated immunoglobulin (FcR) Surface antigens CD19, CD20, CD22 Receptors for Epstein–Barr virus
Origin		Derived from lymphoid stem cell initially detectable in fetal liver and subsequently in bone marrow; develop under the influence of thymic epithelium	Derived from a lymphoid stem cell initially detectable in fetal liver and subsequently in marrow
Relative distribution	Blood	70%	20–30%
	Bone marrow	70%	15%
	Lymph node	75% Paracortical distribution; medullary sinuses	25% Follicles; medullary cords
	Lymph	75%	25%
	Spleen	50% Periarteriolar lymph sheath	50% Follicles; marginal zone between T zone and red pulp
Function		Cellular immunity (e.g. against viruses, fungi, low-grade intracellular pathogens such as mycobacteria) Graft rejection Tumor rejection Delayed hypersensitivity Interaction with B-cells in production of antibodies against certain antigens Suppression of B-cell function Production of eosinophilia	Maturation into plasma cells for the production of antibodies (immunoglobulin)

IFN-γ which in turn stimulates T_H1 cells to secrete the inflammatory cytokines TNF-β and IFN-γ. These cytokines activate macrophages, thus promoting the killing of intracellular pathogens such as *Mycobacterium tuberculosis*, and also attract leukocytes. When activated by antigen fragments on dendritic cells, T_H2 cells produce cytokines such as IL-4 that affect growth and differentiation of B-cells (promoting the synthesis of antibody, including IgE), IL-13 that promotes IgE synthesis and recruits and activates basophils, and IL-5 that recruits and activates eosinophils. In this way they are involved in killing extracellular pathogens. After reaction with specific peptide antigens on class II MHC molecules, some CD4-positive T-cells may function directly as cytotoxic cells.[35] TC cells are CD8-positive, inhibit the functions of other lymphocytes and also have cytotoxic capability against malignant or virus-infected cells. They react with and are activated by peptides presented with class I MHC molecules on the abnormal cell. Activated TC cells acquire azurophilic cytoplasmic granules (lysosomes) containing perforin that forms pores in the target cell membrane and granzymes (serine proteases) that enter the cell via the pores and mediate target cell apoptosis. They also express more Fas ligand on their surface; this reacts with Fas on the target cell surface resulting in apoptosis. When activated by peptides presented on class II MHC molecules, another subset of T-cells, the T-regulatory cells (Treg cells), produce IL-10 that inhibits T_H1-mediated stimulatory effects on inflammation and T_H2-mediated stimulatory effects on antibody synthesis; these effects operate towards the end of an immune response.[36] A further subset of T-cells, T_H17 cells, is located near the skin and mucosal surfaces and when activated these produce TGF-β and IL-21 and eventually IL-17.[37] The antibacterial effects of T_H17 cells are mediated via the secretion of defensins and the attraction of neutrophils to the site of inflammation. Lymphocytes that are neither B-cells nor T-cells also exist. These were originally called null cells but are now called NK (natural killer) cells; they have the appearance of large granular lymphocytes.[38] NK cells lack antigen-specific receptors but have NK receptors that have an innate capacity to recognize virus-infected and tumor cells with low expression of class I MHC molecules, and kill such cells by exocytosis of perforin and granzymes. They also secrete the antiviral cytokine IFN-γ and the proinflammatory cytokine TNF-α.

T_H lymphocytes regulate normal hemopoiesis including eosinophil granulocytopoiesis and erythropoiesis.[39] Furthermore, abnormalities in T-cell subpopulations seem to play a role in the pathogenesis of the cytopenias in some cases of aplastic anemia, pure red cell aplasia associated with chronic lymphocytic leukemia and chronic idiopathic neutropenia (Chapters 17 and 28).

Platelets

Morphology and composition

Platelets are small fragments of megakaryocyte cytoplasm with an average volume of 7–8 fl.[40,41] When seen in Romanowsky-stained blood smears, most platelets have a diameter of 2–3 μm. They have an irregular outline, stain light blue and contain a number of small azurophilic granules that are usually concentrated at the center (Fig. 1.1). Newly formed platelets are larger than more mature ones and have a higher mean platelet volume (MPV).

Electron microscope studies have revealed that non-activated (resting) platelets are shaped like biconvex discs, have a convoluted surface and contain mitochondria, granules, two systems of cytoplasmic membranes (a surface-connected canalicular system and a dense tubular system), microfilaments, microtubules and many glycogen molecules (Fig. 1.13). The discoid shape is actively maintained by a cytoskeleton consisting of many short contractile microfilaments composed of actomyosin and an equatorial bundle of microtubules composed of tubulin. The microfilaments are situated between various organelles and may be attached to specific proteins at the inner surface of the cell membrane. In addition to maintaining cell shape, the microfilaments are probably involved in clot retraction. The equatorial bundle of microtubules is situated in an organelle-free sol-gel zone just beneath the cell membrane and appears to be connected to this membrane by filaments. When platelets change shape during activation, the microtubules break their connections with the cell membrane and contract inwards; the platelet granules also become concentrated at the center of the cell. The cell membrane of the resting platelet is extensively invaginated to form a surface-connected open canalicular system. This canalicular system provides a large surface area through which various substances, including the contents of platelet granules, can be released to the exterior via multiple openings in the cell membrane. It is thought that the contraction of the microfilaments during platelet activation brings the platelet granules close to special areas of this canalicular system which are capable of fusing with granules. The contraction of microtubules may also play a role in this process. The platelet also contains a specialized form of endoplasmic reticulum known as the dense tubular system, elements of which are found adjacent to the bundle of microtubules and in between the invaginations of the open canalicular system. This system is the main site of synthesis of thromboxane A_2 which plays an important role in the reactions leading to the release of the contents of platelet granules. In addition, the dense tubular system contains a high concentration of calcium ions when compared with that elsewhere in the cytoplasm and may regulate the activity of several calcium-dependent reversible cytoplasmic processes such as the activation of actomyosin, depolymerization of microtubules and glycogenolysis.

There are four types of platelet granules (Table 1.7):

1. Dense bodies (δ granules) are very electron-dense, usually show a bull's eye appearance because of the presence of an electron-lucent zone between the central electron-dense material and the limiting membrane and contain the storage pool of adenosine diphosphate (ADP) and ATP which is concerned with secondary platelet aggregation. They also contain calcium and adrenaline as well as 5HT (which causes both vasoconstriction and platelet aggregation).

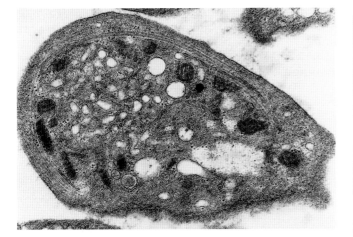

Fig. 1.13 Electron micrograph of a platelet sectioned in the equatorial plane showing the circumferential band of microtubules. Many electron-lucent vesicles belonging to the surface-connected canalicular system, a few mitochondria and some platelet granules (including one dense body) can be seen. The dense tubular system is present between the vesicles of the surface-connected canalicular system, but is only just visible at the present magnification. Uranyl acetate and lead citrate. ×20 000.

Table 1.7 Characteristics of the four types of platelet granules

Granule	Contents	Appearance
Dense bodies (δ granules)	Serotonin, calcium, storage pool of ATP and ADP, pyrophosphate	Very dense, may have 'bull's eye' appearance
α granules[a]	β-thromboglobulin, platelet factor 4, platelet-derived growth factor, fibrinogen, fibronectin, factor-VIII-related antigen (vWF), thrombospondin	Less electron-dense than dense bodies
Lysosomal granules[a] (λ granules)	Acid phosphatase, cathepsin, β-glucuronidase, β-galactosidase, arylsulphatase	Less electron-dense than dense bodies
Peroxisomes	Catalase	Smaller than α and λ granules

[a]Distinguished from each other by ultrastructural cytochemistry.

2. α granules: these are the most frequent type of platelet granule and contents include platelet factor 4 (which has heparin-neutralizing activity and may thus potentiate the action of thrombin), and platelet mitogenic factors that stimulate growth of endothelial and smooth muscle cells and of skin fibroblasts (Table 1.7).
3. Lysosomal (λ) granules: these are slightly larger than dense granules, and are moderately electron-dense. They contain acid phosphatase.
4. Peroxisomes: these are smaller than α and λ granules.

Disorders of platelet granules are discussed in more detail in Chapter 32.

Number and life span

The normal range for the platelet count in peripheral blood is about $150–450 \times 10^9/l$ (see Table 1.2); slightly lower values are seen during the first 3 months of life. Small cyclical variations in the platelet count may be seen in some individuals of both sexes, with a periodicity of 21–35 days; in premenopausal women the fall usually occurs during the 2 weeks preceding menstruation. The platelet counts of women are slightly higher than those of men.[42,43] There are also slight racial variations in the normal platelet count. For example, values lower than those quoted above have been reported in Australians of Mediterranean descent. In addition, Nigerians have lower platelet counts than Caucasians, as have Africans and West Indians living in the UK.[44] The life span of normal platelets is 8–10 days.

Functions

Large quantities of energy are used during various platelet functions. This energy is mainly derived from the metabolism of glucose by the glycolytic pathway and tricarboxylic acid cycle. The energy is held as ATP within a metabolic pool that is distinct from the storage pool of adenine nucleotides situated in the dense bodies.

Platelets play an essential role in the hemostatic mechanism. When endothelial cells of vessel walls are damaged and shed, platelets adhere to subendothelial connective tissue (basement membrane and non-collagen microfibrils) via von Willebrand factor (vWF) attached to a specific receptor on the platelet membrane, glycoprotein Ib-IX. This adhesion requires calcium ions. Platelets may also adhere to collagen via other specific membrane receptors. Adhesion is followed within seconds by the transformation of the platelet from its original discoid shape to a spiny sphere (a potentially reversible process) and within a few minutes by the release of the contents of some platelet granules (the release reaction). The release reaction may be mediated through thromboxane A_2 synthesized in the platelet from arachidonic acid released from membrane phospholipids (the conversion of arachidonic acid to thromboxane A_2 requires the enzymes cyclo-oxygenase and thromboxane synthase). Initially, the contents of the dense bodies are released; with stronger stimulation, some α granules are also discharged. The ADP released from the dense bodies, and possibly also traces of thrombin generated by the activation of the clotting cascade, cause an interaction of other platelets with the adherent platelets and with each other (secondary platelet aggregation) with further release of ADP from the aggregating platelets. Aggregation induced by ADP (and by adrenaline and collagen) is preceded by an alteration of the cell membrane leading to calcium-dependent binding of fibrinogen to specific platelet receptors on membrane glycoprotein IIb–IIIa; the fibrinogen molecules link adjacent platelets. To a lesser extent, aggregation may also be mediated by binding of vWF and vitronectin to glycoprotein IIb–IIIa. In addition, platelet- and endothelial-cell-derived thrombospondin stabilize aggregation after binding to receptors on glycoprotein IV. The process of secondary aggregation continues until a platelet plug occludes the damaged vessel. The formation of a fibrin clot around the platelet plug is initiated by tissue factor (TF)-VIIa complex; the TF is expressed and factor VII is activated at the site of injury (Chapter 31). The exposure of certain membrane phospholipids (platelet factor 3) in aggregated platelets plays a role in the formation of this fibrin clot. These platelet phospholipids participate in:

1. the formation of factor Xa through a reaction involving factors IXa, VIII, X and calcium
2. in the reaction between factors II, V, Xa and calcium.

In addition to their primary role in hemostasis, platelets have several other functions. They participate in the generation of the inflammatory response by releasing factors that increase vascular permeability and attract granulocytes. The α granules of the platelet contain mitogenic factors that may promote the regeneration of damaged/detached endothelial cells. These mitogenic factors also stimulate fibroblast proliferation and may therefore promote the healing of wounds. Furthermore, platelets remove the pharmacologically active substance 5HT from their microenvironment by taking it up and concentrating it in the dense granules; they thus serve as 'detoxifying' cells. Platelets also have a limited capacity for phagocytosis. Finally, platelets play a role in pathological processes such as thrombosis and the rejection of transplants and have also been implicated in the pathogenesis of atherosclerosis.

Platelet function may be tested *in vivo* or *in vitro*. Platelet functions that may be investigated *in vitro* include adhesion, aggregation, clot retraction and contribution to the intrinsic coagulation pathway (also see Chapter 31). Both adhesion and aggregation may be tested by passing blood through a glass bead column and determining the percentage of retained platelets; this test is difficult to standardize. Automated equipment has been developed to test these linked functions using whole blood. Aggregation is most readily tested by the use of an aggregometer which measures optical density of platelet-rich plasma; as aggregation is induced (e.g. by ADP, adrenaline [epinephrine], collagen or the antibiotic ristocetin) the optical density falls; if platelets disaggregate the optical density rises again. It is also possible to measure ATP release during platelet aggregation. Clot retraction is assessed by measuring the volume of serum expressed by whole blood that is allowed to clot in a glass tube at $37°C$ for 1 h; a high hematocrit may interfere with clot retraction. The contribution of the platelet to the intrinsic pathway of blood coagulation may be tested by the prothrombin consumption test (which shows defective conversion of prothrombin to thrombin when there is a deficiency of platelet number or function) or the platelet factor 3 availability test or the thromboplastin generation test (which test for the ability of the platelet to accelerate the intrinsic pathway of coagulation). A number of machines are available to test platelet function and coagulation at the bedside (see Chapter 31). For example, the platelet function analyzer (PFA100) measures the time taken for whole blood to occlude ADP- or epinephrine-impregnated membranes. Thromboelastography is a global test for hemostasis that measures viscoelastic changes induced by fibrin polymerization and evaluates platelet function as well as the rate of formation of a clot, its strength, stability, retraction and lysis.

Alterations in the blood in pregnancy

In most women, the hemoglobin level begins to fall at about the 6th to 8th week of a normal pregnancy, reaches its lowest level at about the 32nd week and increases slightly thereafter. The extent of fall varies markedly from woman to woman but hemoglobin levels less than 10 g/dl are probably abnormal.[45] The average fall is about 1.5–2 g/dl. This physiologic 'anemia' occurs despite an average increase in the red cell mass of about 300 ml and results from an increase in the plasma volume of about one liter. The reticulocyte count is initially unchanged but increases between week 25 and week 35. The mean corpuscular volume and MCH rise during pregnancy in the absence of any deficiency of vitamin B_{12} or folic acid. Serum iron falls. Transferrin synthesis increases due to a direct hormonal effect (similar changes are seen in subjects taking oral contraceptives); the transferrin concentration and total iron-binding capacity increase. The serum vitamin B_{12} level falls steadily throughout pregnancy reaching its lowest level at term; this is a physiological change and is not indicative of deficiency. About 10% of normal women have serum vitamin B_{12} levels below 100 ng/l during the last trimester. There is a return to non-pregnant levels by 6 weeks postpartum. Red cell and serum folate levels also fall and 20–30% of women have subnormal red cell folate levels at term. Physiologic needs for iron and folic acid are increased, and in subjects with reduced stores and/or poor intake (Chapters 11 and 12) deficiency may occur. The hemoglobin F level increases slightly. The percentage of F-cells is increased at mid-term but returns to non-pregnant levels by term. The erythrocyte sedimentation rate (ESR) rises early in pregnancy and is highest in the third trimester. The white cell count increases, due to an increase of neutrophils and monocytes. Total white blood cell counts (WBCs) of $10–15 \times 10^9$/l are common during pregnancy, and postpartum levels may reach $20–40 \times 10^9$/l. Metamyelocytes and myelocytes are seen in the blood in about a quarter of subjects and promyelocytes may also be present. 'Toxic' granulation and Döhle bodies (see Chapter 16) are common and are a physiologic change. The neutrophil alkaline phosphatase rises early in pregnancy and remains elevated; a further rise occurs during labor, with a return to non-pregnant levels by 6 weeks postpartum. The bactericidal capacity of neutrophils is increased and in 40–60% of subjects in the second and third trimester, an increased proportion of neutrophils are positive in the nitro-blue tetrazolium reduction test. Lymphocyte and eosinophil counts are decreased. The basophil count may rise. Some fall in the platelet count may occur in the third trimester and values in the range $80–150 \times 10^9$/l may be observed.[46]

A prothrombotic state develops during pregnancy. Throughout pregnancy, factors VII, VIIIC, VIIIR:Ag, X and fibrinogen increase progressively and markedly. Factors II and V are not significantly altered apart from a transient increase early in pregnancy and there is some increase in factor IX.[46,47] Pregnancy is also associated with a marked increase in α_1 antitrypsin, reduced protein S activity and with acquired activated protein C resistance. From 11–15 weeks onwards there is a marked decrease in fibrinolytic activity mainly due to large increases in endothelial cell-derived plasminogen activator inhibitor-1 (PAI-1) and placenta-derived plasminogen activator inhibitor-2 (PAI-2) in the plasma. Fibrin degradation products and D-dimer increase after 21–25 weeks in a proportion of subjects.

Fetal cells, for example fetal red cells and fetal lymphocytes, enter the maternal circulation during pregnancy as well as at delivery. This phenomenon is common enough to be regarded as physiologic, although it may have adverse effects when the mother becomes sensitized to fetal antigens (see Chapters 10 and 37).

References

1. Lewis S, Bain B, Bates I, editors. Dacie & Lewis Practical Haematology. 10th ed. Philadelphia: Elsevier; 2006.

2. Arese P, Turrini F, Schwarzer E. Band 3/complement-mediated recognition and removal of normally senescent and pathological human erythrocytes. Cell Physiol Biochem 2005;16(4–6):133–46.

3. Pantaleo A, Giribaldi G, Mannu F, et al. Naturally occurring anti-band 3 antibodies and red blood cell removal under physiological and pathological conditions. Autoimmun Rev 2008 Jun;7(6):457–62.

4. Boas FE, Forman L, Beutler E. Phosphatidylserine exposure and red cell viability in red cell aging and in hemolytic anemia. Proc Natl Acad Sci USA 1998 Mar 17;95(6):3077–81.

5. Bosman GJ, Willekens FL, Werre JM. Erythrocyte aging: a more than superficial resemblance to apoptosis? Cell Physiol Biochem 2005;16(1–3):1–8.

6. Marchesi VT. The red cell membrane skeleton: recent progress. Blood 1983 Jan;61(1):1–11.

7. Kleinbongard P, Schulz R, Rassaf T, et al. Red blood cells express a functional endothelial nitric oxide synthase. Blood 2006 Apr 1;107(7):2943–51.

8. Ozuyaman B, Grau M, Kelm M, et al. RBC NOS: regulatory mechanisms and therapeutic aspects. Trends Mol Med 2008 Jul;14(7):314–22.

9. Bowen D, Bentley N, Hoy T, Cavill I. Comparison of a modified thiazole orange technique with a fully automated analyser for reticulocyte counting. J Clin Pathol 1991 Feb;44(2):130–3.

10. Tarallo P, Humbert JC, Mahassen P, et al. Reticulocytes: biological variations and reference limits. Eur J Haematol 1994 Jul;53(1):11–5.

11. D'Onofrio G, Zini G, Rowan RM. Reticulocyte counting: methods and clinical applications. In: Rowan RM, van Assendelft OW, Preston FE, editors. Advanced Laboratory Methods in Haematology. London: Arnold; 2002.

12. Kim JM, Ihm CH, Kim HJ. Evaluation of reticulocyte haemoglobin content as

marker of iron deficiency and predictor of response to intravenous iron in haemodialysis patients. Int J Lab Hematol 2008 Feb;30(1):46–52.

13. Borregaard N. Development of neutrophil granule diversity. Ann N Y Acad Sci 1997 Dec 15;832:62–8.

14. Borregaard N, Lollike K, Kjeldsen L, et al. Human neutrophil granules and secretory vesicles. European Journal of Haematology 1993;51:187–98.

15. Bain B, Seed M, Godsland I. Normal values for peripheral blood white cell counts in women of four different ethnic origins. J Clin Pathol 1984 Feb;37(2):188–93.

16. Reich D, Nalls MA, Kao WH, et al. Reduced neutrophil count in people of African descent is due to a regulatory variant in the Duffy antigen receptor for chemokines gene. PLoS Genet 2009 Jan; 5(1):e1000360.

17. Shoenfeld Y, Alkan ML, Asaly A, et al. Benign familial leukopenia and neutropenia in different ethnic groups. Eur J Haematol 1988 Sep;41(3):273–7.

18. von Vietinghoff S, Ley K. Homeostatic regulation of blood neutrophil counts. J Immunol 2008 Oct 15;181(8):5183–8.

19. Tachimoto H, Bochner BS. The surface phenotype of human eosinophils. Chem Immunol 2000;76:45–62.

20. Anwar AR, Kay AB. Membrane receptors for IgG and complement (C4, C3b and C3d) on human eosinophils and neutrophils and their relation to eosinophilia. J Immunol 1977 Sep;119(3):976–82.

21. Dvorak AM, Weller PF. Ultrastructural analysis of human eosinophils. Chem Immunol 2000;76:1–28.

22. Calafat J, Janssen H, Knol EF, et al. Ultrastructural localization of Charcot–Leyden crystal protein in human eosinophils and basophils. Eur J Haematol 1997 Jan;58(1):56–66.

23. Butterworth AE, David JR. Eosinophil function. N Engl J Med 1981 Jan 15;304(3):154–6.

24. Rothenberg ME, Hogan SP. The eosinophil. Annu Rev Immunol 2006;24:147–74.

25. Rosenberg HF. Eosinophil-derived neurotoxin/RNase 2: connecting the past, the present and the future. Curr Pharm Biotechnol 2008 Jun;9(3): 135–40.

26. Powell WS, Ahmed S, Gravel S, Rokach J. Eotaxin and RANTES enhance 5-oxo-6,8,11,14-eicosatetraenoic acid-induced eosinophil chemotaxis. J Allergy Clin Immunol 2001 Feb;107(2):272–8.

27. Akuthota P, Wang HB, Spencer LA, Weller PF. Immunoregulatory roles of eosinophils: a new look at a familiar cell. Clin Exp Allergy 2008 Aug;38(8): 1254–63.

28. Spencer LA, Szela CT, Perez SA, Kirchhoffer CL, et al. Human eosinophils constitutively express multiple Th1, Th2, and immunoregulatory cytokines that are secreted rapidly and differentially. J Leukoc Biol 2009 Jan;85(1): 117–23.

29. Mitre E, Nutman TB. Basophils, basophilia and helminth infections. Chem Immunol Allergy 2006;90:141–56.

30. Sullivan BM, Locksley RM. Basophils: a nonredundant contributor to host immunity. Immunity 2009 Jan 16;30(1):12–20.

31. Ohnmacht C, Voehringer D. Basophil effector function and homeostasis during helminth infection. Blood 2009 Mar 19;113(12):2816–25.

32. Min B, Paul WE. Basophils and type 2 immunity. Curr Opin Hematol 2008 Jan;15(1):59–63.

33. Blom B, Spits H. Development of human lymphoid cells. 2006. Annu Rev Immunol 24:287–320.

34. Romagnani S. Regulation of the T cell response. Clin Exp Allergy 2006 Nov;36(11):1357–66.

35. van de Berg PJ, van Leeuwen EM, ten Berge IJ, van Lier R. Cytotoxic human CD4(+) T cells. Curr Opin Immunol 2008 Jun;20(3):339–43.

36. Askenasy N, Kaminitz A, Yarkoni S. Mechanisms of T regulatory cell function. Autoimmun Rev 2008 May;7(5):370–5.

37. Chen Z, O'Shea JJ. Th17 cells: a new fate for differentiating helper T cells. Immunol Res 2008;41(2):87–102.

38. Andoniou CE, Coudert JD, Degli-Esposti MA. Killers and beyond: NK-cell-mediated control of immune responses. Eur J Immunol 2008 Nov;38(11):2938–42.

39. Dent AL, Kaplan MH. T cell regulation of hematopoiesis. Front Biosci 2008;13:6229–36.

40. White JG. Platelet structural physiology: the ultrastructure of adhesion, secretion, and aggregation in arterial thrombosis. Cardiovasc Clin 1987;18(1):13–33.

41. Kaushansky K. Historical review: megakaryopoiesis and thrombopoiesis. Blood 2008 Feb 1;111(3):981–6.

42. Stevens RF, Alexander MK. A sex difference in the platelet count. Br J Haematol 1977 Oct;37(2):295–300.

43. Bain BJ. Platelet count and platelet size in males and females. Scand J Haematol 1985 Jul;35(1):77–9.

44. Bain BJ, Seed M. Platelet count and platelet size in healthy Africans and West Indians. Clin Lab Haematol 1986;8(1):43–8.

45. Perry D, Lowndes K. Blood disorders specific to pregnancy. 3rd ed. In: Warrell D, Cox T, Firth J, editors. Oxford Textbook of Medicine: Oxford University Press; 2010:2173–80.

46. Hellgren M. Hemostasis during normal pregnancy and puerperium. Semin Thromb Hemost 2003 Apr;29(2):125–30.

47. Brenner B. Haemostatic changes in pregnancy. Thromb Res 2004;114 (5–6):409–14.

48. Bain BJ, editor. Blood cells. A practical guide. 4th ed. Oxford: Blackwell Publishing; 2006.

CHAPTER 2

Normal bone marrow cells: development and cytology

SN Wickramasinghe, A Porwit, WN Erber

Chapter contents

The bone marrow (BM), the major site of hemopoiesis, is comprised of hemopoietic cells and stromal cells. This chapter will describe the morphological appearances, cytochemical characteristics and antigen expression profile of BM cells throughout their development. The emphasis will be to provide a broad understanding of normal BM development as a necessary baseline for further understanding of blood and BM pathology. Only brief mention will be made of cell ultrastructure. Although this method has provided significant insight into cell development, it now has little practical role in diagnostic hematology; for a detailed review of the ultrastructural appearances of BM cells the reader is referred to the previous edition of this book.

©2011 Elsevier Ltd
DOI: 10.1016/B978-0-7020-3147-2.00002-X

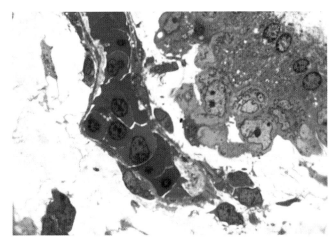

Fig. 2.1 Semithin section of a plastic-embedded chorionic villus biopsy taken at 7 weeks of gestation showing a blood vessel containing nucleated embryonic red cells. Toluidine blue stain.

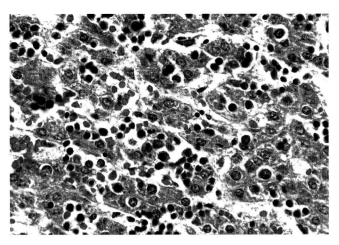

Fig. 2.2 Histologic appearances of normal fetal liver during the middle trimester of pregnancy. About 40% of the area of the section consists of erythropoietic cells which are present singly or in clusters between the plates of liver cells. Hematoxylin–eosin stain.

Hemopoietic cells

Hemopoiesis is the process by which mature blood elements of all lineages are derived from a common pluripotent stem cell. There are two types of hemopoietic systems:

1. 'primitive' hemopoiesis, derived from the yolk sac, which is transient and consists mainly of erythroid cells
2. 'definitive' hemopoiesis which is derived from pluripotent hemopoietic stem cells (HSC). All postnatal hemopoietic cells are derived from these pluripotent HSC which undergo differentiation via a number of intermediate cell types to generate mature blood cells of lymphoid and myeloid lineage.

Embryonic hemopoiesis

Hemopoiesis commences from a transient population of primitive HSC generated in the yolk sac. This commences on the 14th to 19th day of embryogenesis and persists there until the end of the 12th week of gestation. The yolk sac primarily produces nucleated erythroid cells that are megaloblastic and contain embryonic hemoglobins, Gower I ($\zeta_2\varepsilon_2$), Gower II ($\alpha_2\varepsilon_2$) and Portland I ($\zeta_2\gamma_2$) (Fig. 2.1). Yolk sac erythropoiesis is referred to as 'primitive'. In the 6th and 7th weeks of gestation, the blood islands within the yolk sac also contain a few megakaryocytes. Hemopoietic activity then occurs in a region of the para-aortic splanchopleural mesoderm. This region contains the dorsal aorta, gonadal ridge and mesonephros and is known as the aorta-gonad-mesonephros or AGM region.[1,2] Hemopoiesis in the AGM region develops from 'definitive' HSC that eventually populate the adult BM. Some adult-type HSC also develop in the yolk sac and the placenta.

HSC derived from the AGM migrate to the liver and erythropoietic foci are detectable in the 6th week of gestation. The liver remains the main site of erythropoiesis from the 3rd to the 6th month when erythroblasts account for about 50% of the nucleated cells of the liver. The erythroblasts are mainly extravascular (Fig. 2.2), located near and within Kupffer cells (emperipolesis) and continue their maturation

inside sinusoids.[3] Erythroblasts are initially megaloblastic but subsequently become macronormoblastic. Fetal hepatic erythropoiesis is associated with the synthesis of fetal hemoglobin (HbF; $\alpha_2\gamma_2$) and results in the production of nucleated, macrocytic red cells. The liver continues to produce red cells in decreasing numbers after the 6th month of gestation until the end of the 1st postnatal week.

Small foci of erythropoietic cells are present in the vascular connective tissue of some BM cavities from 2.5 to 4 months' gestation. From the 6th month the BM is the major site of hemopoiesis and the myeloid/erythroid (M/E) ratio is about 1:4. Erythropoiesis in fetal BM occurs extravascularly, is macronormoblastic and results in the production of macrocytic red cells containing HbF and HbA ($\alpha_2\beta_2$). The mean cell volume (MCV) in the cord blood of full-term newborns is 90–118 fl. Erythropoieisis in fetal BM appears to be regulated by erythropoietin produced extrarenally, probably in the liver. From the 6th month there is also proliferation of HSC in the fetal liver which generate erythroid, myeloid and some lymphoid cells. Small foci of erythroblasts, a few granulocytopoietic cells and occasional megakaryocytes also occur in many other embryonic and fetal tissues and organs (including lymph nodes, spleen and kidneys); however, their contribution to overall hemopoietic activity is small.

Postnatal changes in the distribution of hemopoietic marrow

At birth all BM cavities contain red marrow consisting mainly of hemopoietic cells. By 1 year virtually all the hemopoietic cells in the terminal phalanges are replaced by fat cells. After the first 4 years there is an increase in fat cells amongst the hemopoietic cells of other marrow cavities. Between 10 and 14 years, the hemopoietic cells in the middle of the shafts of the long bones become virtually completely replaced by fat cells. Subsequently, these zones of non-hemopoietic yellow marrow spread proximally and distally. Distal spread is the more rapid and by about the 25th year the only regions of the long bones that contain red, hemopoietic marrow are the proximal shafts of the femora and humeri. Other sites

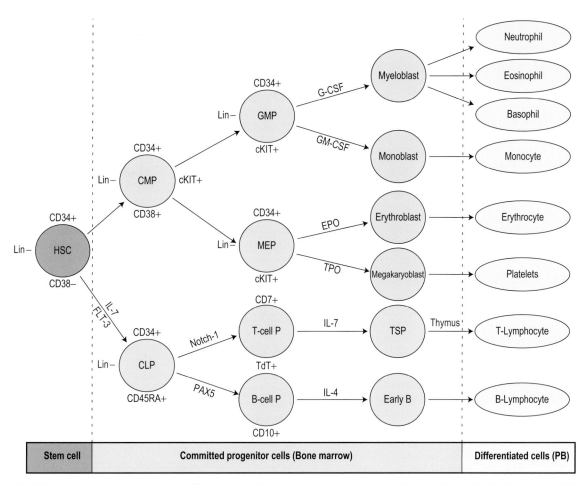

Fig. 2.3 Schematic diagram showing the differentiation of hemopoietic stem cells to mature blood cells. B-cell P, B-cell precursor; CLP, common lymphoid progenitor; CMP, common myeloid progenitor; GMP, granulocyte-macrophage progenitor; HSC, hemopoietic stem cell; MEP, megakaryocyte-erythroid progenitor; T-cell P, T-cell precursor; TSP, thymus-seeding progenitor.

of hemopoiesis in an adult are the skull, ribs, clavicles, scapulae, sternum, vertebrae and pelvis.

General characteristics of hemopoiesis

The formation of blood cells of all types involves two processes:

1. cell proliferation, which amplifies the number of mature cells produced from a cell that has become committed to any particular cell lineage
2. cell differentiation, or the progressive development of biochemical, functional and structural characteristics specific for a given cell type.

During intrauterine life and in the growing child, there is a progressive increase in the total number of hemopoietic and blood cells. In normal adults, the total number of hemopoietic and blood cells remains relatively constant. There is steady-state cell renewal with a relatively constant rate of loss of mature cells (erythrocytes, granulocytes, monocytes and platelets) balanced precisely by the production of new cells.

Hemopoietic stem cells and progenitor cells

The uncommitted HSC has the capacity for self-renewal and is pluripotent, that is, it has the ability to differentiate into

lineage-committed progenitors. It is not recognizable morphologically but can be identified by antigen expression profile. The differentiation of HSC generates multipotent myeloid progenitors and lymphoid progenitors (Fig. 2.3).[4] Evidence for the presence of pluripotent HSC has come from a number of pieces of evidence including:

1. Cytogenetic studies of chronic myeloid leukemia, which showed that the Philadelphia (Ph) chromosome is present in both myeloid (granulocytic, erythroid and megakaryocytic) and lymphoid cells.
2. The demonstration that in a case of sideroblastic anemia with glucose-6-phosphate-dehydrogenase (G6PD) mosaicism, a single G6PD isoenzyme was present in myeloid cells as well as T- and B-lymphocytes.
3. Studies of xenogeneic transplant models in immuno-incompetent animals.

All pluripotent HSC express CD34 antigen and are usually AC133[+], CD59[+]; Thy1[low]; CD38[−]; C-kit[−/low]; CD33[−]; lineage[−]. By flow cytometry (FCM) CD34[+] HSC constitute most cells of the CD45[dim]/SSC[low] (blast) region and are a heterogeneous cell population. A small fraction of pluripotent HSC with long-term repopulating cell activity have been associated with the CD34[+]/CD38[−] phenotype.[5,6] These cells are very rare in normal BM (usually <0.1%), but may increase in

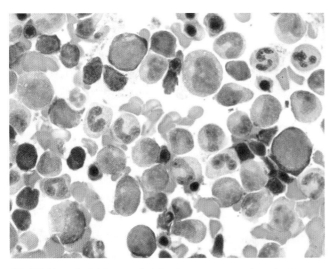

Fig. 2.4 Normal adult hemopoiesis in a bone marrow aspirate showing a range of normal erythroid and granulocytic progenitors at different stages of differentiation. May–Grünwald–Giemsa stain. ×400.

regenerating BM and in myelodysplastic syndromes.[7,8] CD34[+]/CD45[dim] cells include a major fraction of progenitor cells that are already committed to specific hematopoietic lineages (erythroid, neutrophil, monocytic, dendritic cell (DC), basophil, mast cell (MC), eosinophil and megakaryocytic) and variable numbers of CD34[+] B-cell precursors (BCP).[9]

The multipotent (or pluripotent) HSC undergo gradual restriction in their hemopoietic potential as they eventually give rise to unipotent progenitor cells[10,11] (Fig. 2.4). The progeny of HSC therefore become progressively restricted to one cell lineage and they lose the capacity to self-renew. The earliest branching between myeloid and lymphoid development is to committed progenitor cells of myeloid or lymphoid types, as follows:[11,12]

1. Common myeloid progenitor (CMP) which gives rise to cells of all myeloid lineages (i.e. granulocytic, erythroid, megakaryocytic). The CMP subsequently generates granulocyte-macrophage progenitors (GMP) and megakaryocyte-erythroid progenitors (MEP).
2. Common lymphoid progenitor (CLP), which gives rise to T- and B-lymphocytes and natural killer (NK) cells.

The complex mechanisms involved in the regulation of hemopoietic stem cells and progenitor cells are described in Chapter 4. Growth-promoting cytokines, such as granulocyte-macrophage colony stimulating factor (GM-CSF) and granulocyte colony stimulating factor (G-CSF), other cytokines and transcription factors are key regulators of hemopoiesis and may also enhance some functions of the mature cells.

Erythropoiesis

The CMP undergoes further differentiation to generate megakaryocyte-erythroid progenitors (MEP) or granulocyte-macrophage progenitors (GMP).[4,13] The bipotent MEP has potential to form erythroid or megakaryocytic cells, both of which require GATA-1 (globin transcription factor 1) for their terminal differentiation. The most immature

lineage-specific erythroid progenitor cells are the erythroid burst-forming units (BFU-E) and the most mature are the erythroid colony-forming units (CFU-E). The CFU-E develop into proerythroblasts, the earliest morphologically recognizable BM red cell precursors. Proerythroblasts progress through several morphologically defined cytologic classes. These are, in order of increasing maturity, the basophilic erythroblasts, early and late polychromatic erythroblasts and reticulocytes. Cell division occurs in the proerythroblasts, basophilic erythroblasts and early polychromatic erythroblasts but not in more mature cells. There are, on average, four cell divisions in the morphologically recognizable precursor pool so that one proerythroblast may give rise to 2^4 (16) red cells. In normal adults, the time taken for a proerythroblast to mature into BM reticulocytes and for reticulocytes to enter the circulation is about 7 days; of this, about 2.5 days is spent in the marrow reticulocyte pool. The time taken for blood reticulocytes to mature into erythrocytes is 1–2 days. In normal individuals erythrocytes circulate for approximately 120 days before they are removed and broken down by the mononuclear phagocyte system.

Within the BM, erythroblasts are present in erythroid islands composed of one or more central macrophages surrounded by one or two layers of erythroblasts (Fig. 2.5); fine processes of macrophage cytoplasm are found between the erythroid progenitors. Surface receptors on the macrophages are involved in macrophage–erythroblast interactions. One such receptor, erythroblast macrophage protein (Emp), mediates attachment of erythroid cells to macrophages in the erythroid island. Emp is required for normal erythroid differentiation and nuclear extrusion.[14] A receptor on erythroblasts, intercellular adhesion molecule-4, binds to alpha (V) integrins on macrophages and is important for the formation of erythroblastic islands.[15] Interactions between the macrophage and erythroblasts may modulate erythropoiesis by affecting gene expression and apoptosis and are required for iron delivery for the production of hemoglobin.[16,17]

Erythroid progenitor cells that do not develop successfully into erythrocytes undergo apoptosis and are phagocytosed by BM macrophages. The loss of potential erythrocytes, or 'ineffective' erythropoiesis, is small in normal BM but substantial in certain anemias.

Regulation of erythropoiesis

A key factor determining the rate of red cell production is the glycoprotein hormone erythropoietin (EPO) which, in the adult, is produced mainly by the peritubular cells of the kidney. EPO receptors are expressed on erythroid progenitor cells and the binding of EPO to its receptor results in the activation of JAK2 tyrosine kinase, which causes tyrosine phosphorylation in a number of proteins and triggers the activation of several signal transduction pathways involved in proliferation and in the prevention of apoptosis.[18] An important effect of EPO is, therefore, to maintain the viability and proliferation of erythroid progenitor cells, by preventing apoptosis. In synergy with stem cell factor (SCF), GM-CSF, interleukin (IL)-3 and insulin-like growth factor-1 (IGF-1), EPO stimulates the rate of differentiation of CFU-E to pronormoblasts. EPO also stimulates terminal differentiation and decreases the time taken for the maturation of a

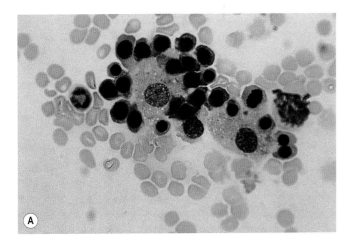

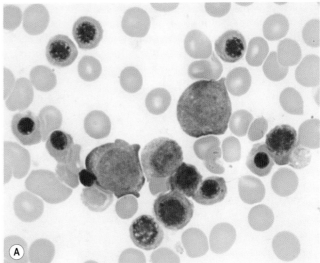

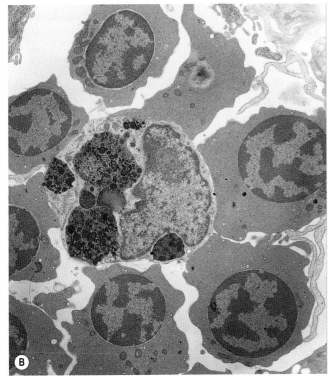

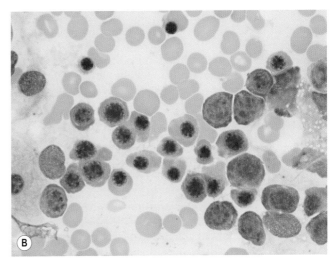

Fig. 2.6 (A, B) Erythroblasts in a normal bone marrow aspirate showing all stages of erythropoiesis from pronormoblast to late polychromatic normoblasts. May–Grünwald–Giemsa stain. ×400. (A) Two pronormoblasts and many late polychromatic normoblasts. (B) Early and late polychromatic normoblasts.

Fig. 2.5 (A, B) Erythroid islands in normal bone marrow. (A) Erythroid islands consisting of early and late polychromatic erythroblasts surrounding macrophages. May–Grünwald–Giemsa stain. ×400. (B) Electron micrograph of an erythroid island showing a macrophage (central) surrounded by a layer of erythroblasts. Uranyl acetate and lead citrate.

pronormoblast to a marrow reticulocyte and its release into the circulation. The plasma level of EPO is inversely related to the capacity of the blood to deliver oxygen to the kidneys and other tissues. Reduction of the oxygen supply to the kidney results in enhanced *EPO* gene expression via a hypoxia-regulated transcription factor, HIF (hypoxia-inducible factor).[19] Thus, in most anemic states there is an EPO increased level in the plasma, which in turn causes an enhancement of the rate of erythropoiesis.

Erythropoiesis is also influenced by the secretions of various endocrine glands. For example, hypofunction of the thyroid, testes, adrenal glands or anterior lobe of the pituitary gland result in mild to moderate anemia. Erythropoiesis is stimulated by thyroxine (stimulates terminal differentia-tion of erythroid progenitor cells), androgens (proliferation and expansion of erythroid progenitors) and growth hormone partly by an effect on the kidneys resulting in increased EPO production.[20] Corticosteriods enhance erythropoiesis by stimulating EPO production and by a direct effect on progenitor cells. There is some evidence that estrogens may inhibit erythropoiesis;[21] the sex difference in the hemoglobin levels of adults appears to be largely due to the higher androgen levels in males.

Light microscope cytology

The term erythroblast is used to define erythroid progenitors. When these appear normal the term normoblast is applied. In Romanowsky-stained normal BM smears morphologically identifiable erythroid cells have the following features (Figs 2.5 and 2.6):

- *Pronormoblasts:* large cells (diameter 12–20 μm) with a large rounded nucleus surrounded by a small amount of deeply basophilic cytoplasm; the intensity of cytoplasmic basophilia is greater than of myeloblasts. The cytoplasm may have a pale-staining area adjacent to the nucleus (corresponding to the Golgi apparatus). The nuclear chromatin has a finely granular or reticular appearance and there are prominent nucleoli. With maturation erythroid cells decrease in size and there is a progressive increase in cytoplasm relative to that of the nucleus.

- *Basophilic normoblast:* the cytoplasm is even more blue-staining than that of the pronormoblast. Its nuclear chromatin has a coarsely granular appearance and there are no nucleoli.
- *Early polychromatic normoblasts:* have polychromatic cytoplasm due to hemoglobinization and a nucleus containing clumps of condensed chromatin.
- *Late polychromatic normoblasts:* are smaller (diameter 8–10 μm), have faintly polychromatic cytoplasm and a small eccentric nucleus (diameter less than 6.5 μm) and contain large clumps of condensed chromatin. The nucleus becomes pyknotic, is extruded and rapidly phagocytosed by adjacent macrophages. The morphology of the resulting marrow reticulocytes is similar to that of circulating reticulocytes, as described in Chapter 1.

Cytochemistry

Perls' acid ferrocyanide stain identifies one small blue–black granule in up to 30% of polychromatic erythroblasts. These iron-containing siderotic granules are randomly distributed in the cytoplasm, and erythroblasts containing such granules are termed sideroblasts. Abnormalities of siderotic granulation include increased numbers of sideroblasts, increased granulation or abnormal granule localization. The term ring sideroblasts is used when there are five or more perinuclear siderotic granules. Erythroid cells at all stages of maturation frequently contain coarse acid phosphatase-positive paranuclear granules. Normal erythroblasts are periodic acid-Schiff (PAS)-, Sudan black- and myeloperoxidase (MPO)-negative. Occasional erythroblasts contain a few alpha-naphthol AS-D chloroacetate esterase-positive granules.

Antigen expression

Early erythroblasts have weak CD45 expression, are CD44 (strong), CD71, CD36, HLA-DR and CD117 positive. Glycophorin A (CD235a) is expressed at a low level at this stage. Maturation to the basophilic erythroblast is accompanied by a decrease in CD44, CD45 and acquisition of CD235a antigen. Transition to polychromatic erythroblast shows a further loss of CD45, HLA-DR and CD44, a mild decrease in CD36 expression and presence of hemoglobin.[22,23]

Ultrastructure

Electron microscope studies show that all erythroblasts contain characteristic surface invaginations which develop into small intracytoplasmic vesicles (rhopheocytotic vesicles) (Fig. 2.5B). Morphological changes can be seen with maturation from pronormoblasts to mature late polychromatic normoblasts. The major changes are an increase in the

amount of heterochromatin, decrease in the number of ribosomes, increase in the electron-density of the cytoplasm due to the accumulation of hemoglobin, a decrease in the number and size of mitochondria and aggregation of ferritin molecules into siderosomes. A Golgi apparatus persists in polychromatic normoblasts.

Megakaryopoiesis

Megakaryopoiesis is the process of development of megakaryocytes and platelets within the marrow. Humans generate 10^{11} platelets per day, and production can be increased 20-fold when in demand.[24] Megakaryocytes are derived following a cascade of differentiation from the megakaryocyte-erythroid progenitor (MEP). The bipotent MEP commits to megakaryopoiesis under the influence of thrombopoietin (TPO), the primary regulator of platelet production, IL-6 and IL-11 to generate megakaryocyte colony-forming units (CFU-MK). CFU-MK are a diploid cell population, in which DNA synthesis and nuclear division (karyokinesis) is followed by cell division (cytokinesis). CFU-MK undergo further maturation to megakaryoblasts, the earliest morphologically recognizable member of the megakaryocyte series.

Four types of megakaryocytic cells can be identified in Romanowsky-stained BM smears. These are, in increasing order of maturity (Fig. 2.7):

1. megakaryoblasts (group I megakaryocytes)
2. promegakaryocytes (group II megakaryocytes)
3. granular megakaryocytes (group III megakaryocytes), which produce platelets
4. 'bare' nuclei.

DNA synthesis occurs in 44% of megakaryoblasts, 18% of promegakaryocytes and in only 2% of granular megakaryocytes. DNA synthesis is not associated with cell division and therefore cycles of DNA synthesis result in the production of mononucleate polyploid cells. The DNA content of a megakaryoblast ranges from 4 n to 32 n (1 n = haploid DNA content) and that of the larger promegakaryocyte and granular megakaryocyte from 8 n to 64 n. These polyploid cells undergo massive cellular enlargement to enable large numbers of platelets to be formed; each megakaryocyte generates 1000–3000 platelets. The megakaryocyte cytoplasm contains a network of specialized membranes, the demarcation membrane system (DMS), dense bodies, secretory vesicles and other organelles. Long extensions from the DMS form branches and undergo evagination to form pro-platelet processes. Platelets, which form by the fragmentation of these cytoplasmic processes, have a diameter of 1–3 μm. During platelet release the granular megakaryocytes protrude cytoplasmic processes close to or directly into the marrow sinusoids, pieces of cytoplasm break away and fragment into platelets. The almost 'bare' nucleus that remains after the release of platelets is surrounded by a narrow rim of cytoplasm containing a few granules and other organelles. The time taken for a megakaryoblast to mature into a platelet-producing granular megakaryocyte is approximately 6 days. Although the majority of megakaryocytes are in the marrow, some enter the circulation via the sinusoids and become trapped in the lungs; some pulmonary megakaryocytes appear to produce platelets.

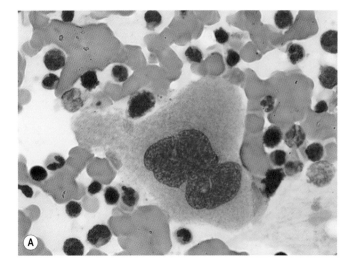

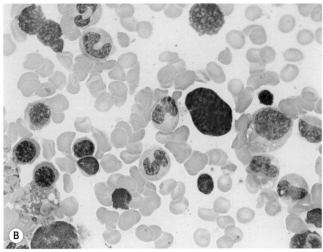

Fig. 2.7 (A, B) Megakaryocytes in normal bone marrow. May–Grünwald–Giemsa stain. ×400. (A) Granulated megakaryocyte. (B) The bare nucleus of a senescent megakaryocyte.

Light microscope cytology

Early megakaryoblasts are difficult to distinguish from BM myeloblasts (see later) but do have a distinct ultrastructural appearance and phenotype. Megakaryoblasts (20–30 µm diameter) have a single large oval, kidney-shaped or lobed nucleus with several nucleoli, a very high nucleus to cytoplasm ratio and deeply basophilic agranular cytoplasm. Promegakaryocytes are usually larger than megakaryoblasts and have a lower nucleus to cytoplasm ratio and less basophilic cytoplasm. They have overlapping nuclear lobes and the cytoplasm may contain azurophilic cytoplasmic granules. The granular megakaryocytes (Fig. 2.7) are up to 70 µm in diameter and possess abundant pale-staining cytoplasm and numerous azurophilic cytoplasmic granules. The nucleus has coarsely granular chromatin and multiple lobes which extend through much of the cell. Prior to the formation of platelets by the fragmentation of cytoplasmic processes, the nuclear lobes become fairly tightly packed together. Following completion of platelet formation, a 'bare' nucleus remains (Fig. 2.7B).

Antigen expression

Cells committed to the megakaryocyte lineage express platelet glycoproteins. The earliest is platelet glycoprotein IIIa (CD61; integrin αIIβ3) followed by glycoprotein IIb (CD41; integrin αIIb), glycoprotein Ib (CD42), glycoprotein V and factor VIII-related antigen. Thrombospondin receptor (CD36; glycoprotein IIIb) and platelet-endothelial cell adhesion moleculae (PECAM-1; CD31) are also expressed.

Ultrastructure

Extensive studies have been performed of megakaryocytes throughout differentiation; the reader is referred to the previous edition of this book and other references for details of the ultrastructural features.[25,26] Ultrastructural cytochemical studies have demonstrated platelet peroxidase (PPO), distinct from myeloperoxidase (MPO), in the endoplasmic reticulum and perinuclear space of promegakaryoblasts, megakaryoblasts and megakaryocytes. PPO is also present in the dense bodies and dense tubular system of platelets.

Emperipolesis

Emperipolesis describes the presence and movement of one cell within the cytoplasm of another; the 'engulfed' cell can subsequently leave the 'engulfing' cell and appears morphologically unaltered by the interaction.[27] Emperipolesis is most commonly seen within megakaryocytes and sometimes one megakaryocyte may contain several cells 'inside' it (Fig. 2.8). The engulfed cells may be neutrophils, eosinophils and their precursors, lymphocytes, erythroblasts or red cells. Megakaryocytic emperipolesis is of uncertain significance but may represent a transmegakaryocytic route for the entry of blood cells into the circulation; it has been suggested that some of the intramegakaryocytic cells may enter the circulation via the processes of megakaryocytic cytoplasm which protrude into adjacent marrow sinusoids. Emperipolesis has also been described in non-hemopoietic cells and malignant cells, including blast cells in the blast phase of chronic myelogenous leukemia.

Granulopoiesis and monocytopoiesis

Granulopoesis is the production of granulocytic cells (neutrophils, eosinophils and basophils, and cells of the monocyte–macrophage series) within the BM. Granulopoiesis commences with the differentiation of the HSC to the common myeloid progenitor (CMP). The CMP further develops into the bipotent granulocyte-macrophage progenitor (GMP). The GMP differentiates into cells that are irreversibly committed to mature into granulocytic cells (CFU-G) or macrophages (CFU-M). The granulocytic cells, including neutrophils, eosinophils and basophils, are all characterized by the presence of cytoplasmic granules (Table 2.1).

Neutrophil granulopoiesis

The formation of neutrophil granulocytes from the GMP is stimulated by G-CSF, GM-CSF and IL-3 and is also influenced M-CSF, SCF and IL-6. The transcription factor,

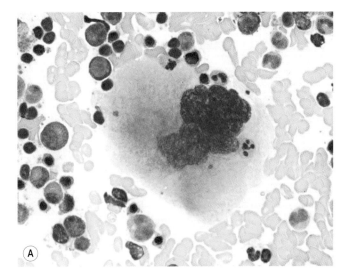

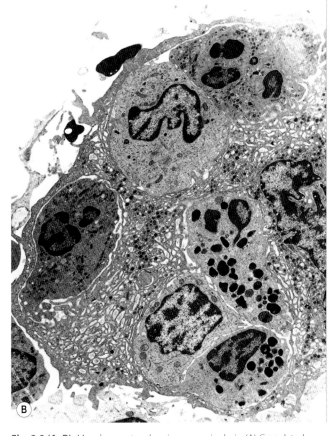

Table 2.1 The major granule proteins present in neutrophils, eosinophils, basophils and mast cells

Cell type	Primary granules	Specific granules

Neutrophil granulocytes	Myeloperoxidase
	Acid phosphatase
	Lysozyme
	Neutrophil elastase
	Defensins
	Bactericidal permeability-increasing protein
	Cathepsins
	α_1 antitrypsin
	Heparin-binding protein
	Sulphated mucosubstances
	Aryl sulphatase
	α-mannosidase
		Secondary:
		  Lysozyme
		  Lactoferrin
		  Transcobalamin I
		  Collagenase
		  Histaminase
		  Vitamin B_{12} binding protein
		Tertiary:
		  Gelatinase
		  Cathepsins
		  Arginase 1
		  Human cationic antimicrobial protein
		  α-mannosidase

Eosinophil granulocytes	Eosinophil peroxidase Eosinophil cationic protein Eosinophil major basic protein Aryl sulphatase	Eosinophil peroxidase Eosinophil cationic protein Eosinophil major basic protein Eosinophil-derived neurotoxin Histaminase Aryl sulphatase Gelatinase
Basophil granulocytes		Acid phosphatase Histamine Chondroitin sulphates Heparin Neutral proteases
Mast cells		Mast cell tryptase Chymase Cathepsin G Mast cell carboxypeptidase A Heparin Chondroitin sulphates Histamine 5-hydroxytryptamine (serotonin) Granzymes Neurolysin

Fig. 2.8 (A, B) Megakaryocytes showing emperipolesis. (A) Granulated megakaryocyte showing emperipolesis of a neutrophil granulocyte. May–Grünwald–Giemsa stain. ×400. (B) Electron micrograph of a megakaryocyte which is apparently showing an unusual degree of emperipolesis. Six cells (two eosinophil granulocytes, two neutrophil granulocytes and a monocyte) can be seen within the megakaryocyte profile. It is possible that at least some of these cells are not completely within the megakaryocyte but merely protruding into it. Uranyl acetate and lead citrate. ×6800.

lymphoid enhancer-binding factor 1 (LEF-1), also plays an important role in regulating proliferation, lineage commitment and differentiation during granulocytopoiesis.[28] In granulopoiesis the earliest morphologically recognizable cell is the myeloblast. The myeloblast undergoes sequential differentiation to the promyelocyte, myelocyte, metamyelocyte, 'band' form (also known as 'stab' form or juvenile neutrophil) and finally mature segmented neutrophil granulocytes. Cell division occurs up to and including the myelocyte stage whereas cell differentiation occurs in both the proliferating and non-proliferating cells. It takes 10–12 days for a myeloblast to differentiate into a mature neutrophil granulocyte, and for the latter to enter the circulation; about half of this time is spent in the proliferating cell pool. In healthy individuals the blood neutrophils leave the circulation with an average $T_{1/2}$ of 7.2 hours.

Light microscope cytology

In Romanowsky-stained BM smears, myeloblasts are round cells with a diameter of 10–20 μm, have a large rounded or

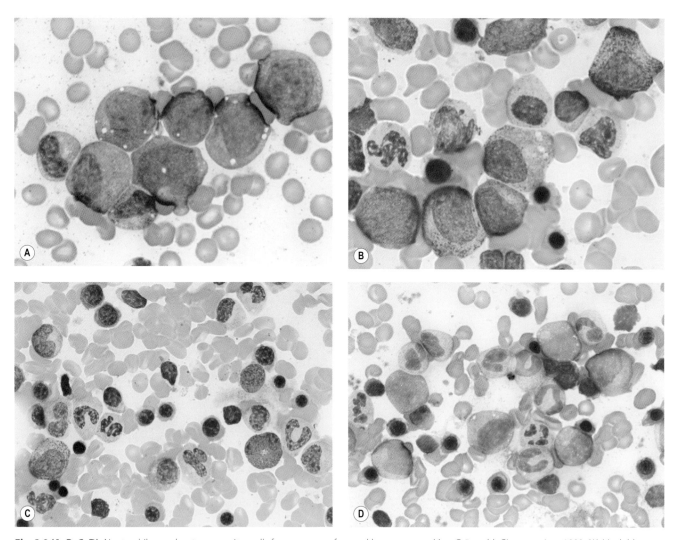

Fig. 2.9 (A, B, C, D) Neutrophil granulocyte progenitor cells from a smear of normal bone marrow. May–Grünwald–Giemsa stain. ×1000. (A) Myeloblasts and promyelocyte. (B) Neutrophil promyelocytes (center and top right). (C) Maturing granulocytic cells including neutrophil metamyelocytes, band forms and neutrophil myelocyte. (D) All stages of granulopoiesis.

oval nucleus with immature nuclear chromatin, two or more nucleoli and a relatively small quantity of agranular, moderately basophilic cytoplasm (Fig. 2.9A). The neutrophil promyelocyte is slightly larger and has an eccentrically located ovoid nucleus with coarser nuclear chromatin and prominent nucleoli. The cytoplasm retains some basophilia and contains a few to several azurophilic granules (primary granules) (Fig. 2.9B). The primary granules first formed at the promyelocyte stage remain in the more mature cells, including granulocytes, but lose their azurophilic property and are therefore not seen by light microscopy in metamyelocytes and more mature cells. The neutrophil myelocyte is smaller than the promyelocyte and has a greater volume of predominantly acidophilic cytoplasm. It contains many fine neutrophilic granules (specific granules) in addition to the primary azurophilic granules (see Table 2.1). The nucleus is rounded, oval, flattened on one side or slightly indented (Fig. 2.9C), has coarsely granular chromatin and usually lacks a nucleolus. Neutrophil metamyelocytes are smaller than myelocytes and have a C-shaped nucleus with greater nuclear chromatin condensation than the myelocyte nucleus. The cytoplasm is acidophilic and contains numerous

neutrophilic granules but few or no azurophilic granules. The 'band' form has a U-shaped or long, relatively narrow, band-like nucleus, which shows no further chromatin condensation. The nucleus may be twisted and may show one or more partial constrictions along its length (see Fig. 2.9C). The neutrophil granulocyte differs from the 'band' neutrophil in being slightly smaller and having a segmented nucleus in which there are 2–5 nuclear masses with condensed chromatin joined by fine stands of chromatin.

Cytochemistry

Myeloblasts stain diffuse pale red–purple in the PAS reaction and there may sometimes also be a fine granular positivity. They are Sudan black- and MPO-negative and, usually, alpha-naphthol AS-D chloroacetate esterase-negative. Neutrophil promyelocytes and more granulocytic cells show granular cytoplasmic staining with PAS, Sudan black, MPO and alpha-naphthol AS-D chloroacetate esterase reactions. The intensity of PAS staining and, to a lesser extent, Sudan black increases with cell maturity. Alpha-naphthyl acetate esterase activity is present in promyelocytes and myelocytes

Table 2.2 Surface marker expression during neutrophil development[6,48,51,80]

Antigen	Blasts	Promyelocytes	Myelocytes	Metamyelocytes	Band forms	Segmented neutrophils
CD10	–	–	–	–	–	++
CD11a	+	+	+	++	++	++
CD11b	–	–	+	++	++	++
CD11c	–	–	+	+	+	+
CD13	+	++	++/+	+	+	++
CD15	–/+	+/++	++	++	++	++
CD16	–	–	–	+	++	+++
CD18	++	++	+++	++	++	++
CD24	–	–	++	++	++	++
CD33	–/+/++	+++	++	+	+	+
CD34	++/+	–	–	–	–	–
CD35	–	–	–	–	+	+
CD44	+++	++	+	+	++	+++
CD45RA	+	–	–	–	–	–
CD45RO	–	+	+	+	++	+++
CD54	++	++	–/+	–/+	–/+	–/+
CD55	+++	+	+	+++	+++	+++
CD59	+++	+++	+++	+++	+++	+++
CD62L	++	++	++	++	++	++
CD64	+	+	++	++	–	–
CD65	–/+	+	++	++	+++	+++
CD66a	–	–	++	++	++	++
CD66b	–	+++	+++	++	++	++
CD66c	–	+++	+++	++	++	+
CD117	+	++	–	–	–	–
CD133	+	–	–	–	–	–

but not in mature neutrophil granulocytes. Promyelocytes and more mature cells are acid phosphatase-positive; the immature cells have stronger positivity than the mature ones. Segmented neutrophil granulocytes show weak to strong staining for alkaline phosphatase and a few metamyelocytes stain weakly.

Antigen expression

Multipotent myeloid stem cells are CD34[+], CD38[+] and CD33[+]. Several antigens change their expression intensity during granulopoiesis, especially CD13, CD11b, and CD16. The sequence of antigen expression during neutrophil differentiation is summarized in Table 2.2 and FCM findings illustrated in Fig. 2.10.[5,6,29,30] CD13 is expressed at high levels on CD34[+] stem cells and CD117[+] precursors (promyelocytes). CD13 is then down-regulated and is expressed more weakly on intermediate precursors (myelocytes); it is

gradually up-regulated as granulocytic cells differentiate into segmented neutrophils. CD11b and CD16 are initially expressed at low levels in granulocyte progenitors (myeloblasts), but expression increases during maturation.

The expression of CD33 is particularly useful if followed together with that of HLA-DR during granulocytic maturation. CD34[+] cells are HLA-DR positive and become weakly positive for CD33. With maturation there is loss of the CD34 antigen and CD33 expression is up-regulated; this is followed by down-regulation of HLA-DR and slight down-regulation of CD33 in most mature granulocytes.[31] CD15 and CD65 antigens are only expressed when cells are restricted to neutrophil differentiation. CD66, CD16 and CD10 are the markers of band forms and segmented neutrophil granulocytes.[30] MPO is present in myeloblasts through granulocytic differentiation to mature neutrophils and elastase from promyelocytes onwards. Lactoferrin is present in myelocytes, metamyelocytes and granulocytes.

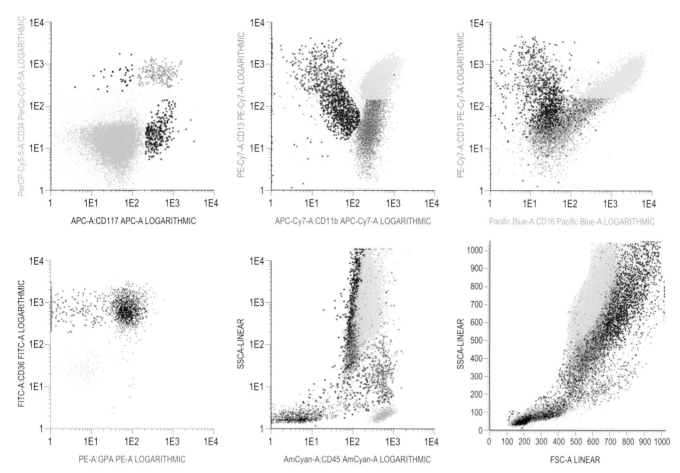

Fig. 2.10 Flow cytometry of normal bone marrow. Differentiation of normal granulopoietic precursors visualized by the antibody combination CD36-FITC / CD235a-PE / CD34-PerCP-Cy5.5 / CD117-APC / CD13-PE-Cy7 / CD11b-APC-Cy7 / CD16-PacBlue / CD45 AmCyan. Various cell populations are back-gated and visualized with different colors on the CD45/SSC plot (lower middle) and FSC/SSc plot (lower right). CD34 and/or CD117 positive precursors (brown, orange and dark purple, upper left plot) are localized in the CD45 dim blast area. Upper middle and right plots show various subpopulations of granulopoietic differentiation: CD13++/CD11b−/CD16− (light purple, promyelocytes), CD13dim/CD11dim/CD16− (blue, myelocytes), CD13dim/CD11b++/CD16-/dim (green, metamyelocytes/band) and CD13+/++/CD11c++/CD16+ (yellow, neutrophils). Erythropoietic precursors are CD36+/CD235a+/CD45− (lower left plot, red) and monocytes are CD36+/CD235a−/CD45++ (lower left plot, green).

Granule composition and ultrastructure

Neutrophil granulocytic cells contain primary and secondary granules, which appear at different stages of their differentiation. About 300 individual granule proteins are synthesized and stored in these granules at different times during granulocytopoiesis and these have important roles in neutrophil function.[32] There are three main types of granules (see Table 2.1):

1. Primary (azurophilic) granules, which develop at the promyelocyte stage, are large and electron-dense and are primarily involved in killing and degradation of microorganisms within the phagolysosome.
2. Specific granules which are first synthesized at the myelocyte stage of differentiation.[33] There are at least two types of specific granules:
   a. secondary granules which develop at the myelocyte stage
   b. tertiary granules (0.2–0.5 μm in their long axis) which develop at the metamyelocyte stage.

The granules contain antimicrobial and cytotoxic substances including MPO, defensins, lactoferrin and serine proteases. The neutrophil granules secrete these products for hydrolytic substrate degradation, microbial killing and to mediate a number of physiological processes, including inflammation.[34] Neutrophil granulocytes also contain small membrane-bound vesicles with alkaline phosphatase activity, called phosphosomes. The granule structure and other ultrastructural features of granulocytic progenitors have been well studied by electron microscopy (Fig. 2.11).

Eosinophil granulopoiesis

Eosinophils develop and mature in the BM from the common myeloid progenitor under the influence of IL-3, GM-CSF, IL-5 and IL-7. The eosinophil progenitor cell is the eosinophil colony-forming unit or CFU-Eo. The earliest morphologically recognizable eosinophil precursor is the eosinophil promyelocyte. This undergoes differentiation to generate the eosinophil myelocyte, eosinophil metamyelocyte, eosinophil band form and mature eosinophil. The CFU-Eo, eosinophil promyelocyte and eosinophil myelocyte undergo cell division, whereas the eosinophil metamyelocyte, band forms and eosinophils are non-dividing cells.

Light microscope cytology

In Romanowsky-stained smears, eosinophil promyelocytes resemble a neutrophil promyelocyte except that they contain

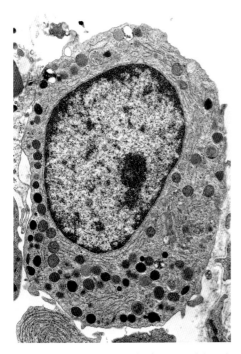

Fig. 2.11 Electron micrograph of a neutrophil myelocyte from normal bone marrow. The nucleus is rounded, contains a nucleolus and shows a small amount of nuclear-membrane-associated heterochromatin (condensed chromatin). The cytoplasm contains two morphologically distinct types of granules and many strands of rough endoplasmic reticulum. Uranyl acetate and lead citrate. × 11 100.

coarse granules, some of which are reddish-orange (eosinophilic) and others basophilic. Other maturing eosinophil progenitors (eosinophil myelocytes, metamyelocytes and band forms) resemble their neutrophil counterpart except that they have many typical eosinophil granules in the cytoplasm (Fig. 2.12A). The mature eosinophil granulocyte (described in Chapter 1) has a bisegmented nucleus and the cytoplasm is filled with eosinophil granules.

Cytochemistry

All cells of the eosinophil series have strong Sudan black positivity at the periphery of the granules whereas the core stains weakly or is negative. The granules are MPO- and acid phosphatase-positive, essentially alpha-naphthol AS-D chloroacetate esterase-negative, and contain lysozyme. Eosinophil granules do not stain by the PAS reaction, but PAS-positive material is found between the granules.

Antigen expression

Eosinophilic myelocytes express CD45 at a level slightly higher than that of neutrophilic myelocytes. By FCM they have low to intermediate intensity of CD11b, intermediate CD13, and low CD33 with bright CD66b without CD16. Mature eosinophils show increased levels of CD45 and CD11b with a decrease in CD33 and, in contrast to neutrophils, are negative for CD16 antigen.[23,35]

Eosinophil granules and ultrastructure

Eosinophils produce and store many granule proteins in primary and secondary granules. Primary granules are large, homogeneous and electron-dense on EM; secondary granules are derived from the maturation of primary granules, contain a crystalloid inclusion that is composed largely of polymerized major basic protein. Eosinophil promyelocytes contain several primary granules (larger and more rounded than those of neutrophil promyelocytes) and

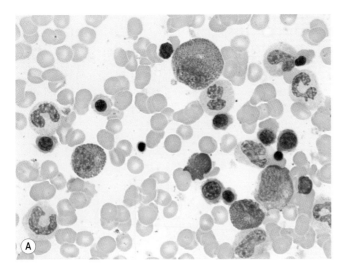

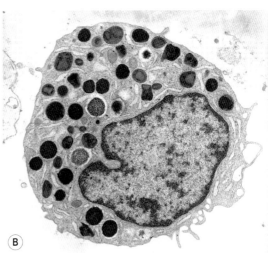

Fig. 2.12 (A, B) Eosinophil morphology. (A) Normal bone marrow showing an eosinophil promyelocyte, eosinophil metamyelocyte and eosinophil band form. May–Grünwald–Giemsa stain. × 400. (B) Electron micrograph of an early eosinophil myelocyte. The nucleus shows condensed chromatin. The majority of cytoplasmic granules are electron-dense primary granules with a few crystalloid-containing secondary granules. The cytoplasm contains many dilated sacs of rough endoplasmic reticulum. Uranyl acetate and lead citrate. × 8500.

an occasional secondary granule. Eosinophil myelocytes contain several granules of both types (Fig. 2.12B); secondary granules predominate in eosinophil metamyelocytes and mature eosinophils. Eosinophil granules contain a number of proteins including eosinophil cationic protein, eosinophil peroxidase, eosinophil-derived neurotoxin, an arginine- and zinc-rich major basic protein, histaminase and aryl sulphatase (Table 2.1). Eosinophil peroxidase is biochemically and immunochemically distinct from the MPO present in granules of the neutrophil granulocyte series.[36]

Basophil granulopoiesis

The basophil granulocyte is derived from the CMP via a committed progenitor cell, the basophil colony-forming unit (CFU-Baso), a progenitor cell that may be closely related to the mast cell progenitor.[37] IL-3, GM-CSF, IL-5 and nerve growth factor (NGF) all stimulate basophil differentiation.[38] The morphologically recognizable precursors of basophil granulocytes are basophil promyelocytes and myelocytes, which are round cells with a round or oval nucleus, and basophil metamyelocytes, which have C-shaped, unsegmented nuclei. Characteristically, in Romanowsky-stained smears these cell types all have large round deeply basophilic (blue–black) cytoplasmic granules that often overlie and obscure the nucleus. The mature basophil granulocyte is extensively granulated and the granules overlie and obscure the segmented nucleus (Table 2.1). Basophil granules are water-soluble and so their contents may be extracted during fixation and staining. Basophils are the least common granulocyte subset (0.5% of total blood leukocytes and about 0.3% of nucleated BM cells in healthy individuals).

With basic dyes such as toluidine blue or methylene blue, the more mature basophil granules stain metachromatically (i.e. reddish-violet). Basophil granules are PAS-negative (with PAS-positive deposits between the granules), Sudan black- and MPO-positive (most strongly in promyelocytes and myelocytes), acid-phosphatase-positive and essentially alpha-naphthol AS-D chloroacetate-esterase-negative (Table 2.2). By FCM, basophils express the following antigens: CD9, CD13, CD22 (weaker than B lymphocytes), CD25 (dim), CD33, CD36 (may be due to adherent platelets), CD38 (bright), CD45 (dimmer than lymphocytes; brighter than myeloblasts), and CD123 (bright). They are negative for CD3, CD4, CD19, CD34, CD64, CD117, and HLA-DR. In some individuals basophils are CD11b-positive.[39]

Monocytopoiesis: the mononuclear phagocyte system

Monocytopoiesis is the process by which peripheral blood monocytes and tissue macrophages are produced. The monocyte–macrophage lineage is derived from the GMP, the common progenitor for granulocytes and monocytes. Under the influence of GM-CSF, M-CSF and IL-3, and up-regulation of a basic leucine zipper (bZIP) transcription factor, MafB, the GMP commits to the monocyte maturation pathway.[40] The morphologically recognizable precursors of the monocyte series are, in order of increasing maturity, monoblasts, promonocytes and BM monocytes; only the first two of these

cell types undergoes division. The blood monocytes leave the circulation after 20–40 hours and transform into tissue macrophages. These are present in the BM, as well as other tissues, where they have a role in erythropoiesis and phagocytosis of cell debris (see below). In the normal steady state there is a constant loss of tissue macrophages (e.g. by shedding of alveolar macrophages), balanced by the formation of new macrophages from blood monocytes and to a small extent from the division of some existing macrophages. The system of cells concerned with macrophage production is called the mononuclear phagocyte system.

Light microscope cytology

Monoblasts are agranular cells of intermediate size with basophilic cytoplasm; they resemble myeloblasts except for the tendency of their nuclei to be slightly clefted or lobulated. Promonocytes are slightly larger, have a lower nucleus-to-cytoplasm ratio and have less cytoplasmic basophilia. They have a more ovoid or indented nucleus with one or more prominent nucleoli and a small number of azurophilic granules in the cytoplasm. Marrow and blood monocytes have a low nucleus-to-cytoplasm ratio, gray cytoplasm which sometimes contains vacuoles, and a greater number of azurophilic granules than promonocytes. The nucleus is eccentric, kidney-shaped, horse-shoe-shaped or lobulated with lacy chromatin.

Cytochemistry

Monocytes stain positively for alpha-naphthyl acetate esterase (nonspecific esterase) and alpha-naphthyl butyrate esterase but are alpha-naphthol AS-D chloroacetate-esterase-negative. The activity of both alpha-naphthyl acetate and butyrate esterase are inhibited by fluoride (in contrast to granulocytes). Monocytes have some granular PAS and Sudan black positivity, slight granular MPO positivity, strong staining for acid phosphatase and lack alkaline phosphatase activity. Monocytes contain lysozyme. Similar proportions of promonocytes, BM monocytes and blood monocytes have IgG-Fc, IgE-Fc and C3b receptors.

Antigen expression

CD14, CD36 and CD64 are considered as monocyte-associated markers, CD14, the lipopolysaccharide receptor, being the most specific. During maturation towards promonocytes, monoblasts down-regulate CD34 and CD117 and gain expression of CD64, CD33, HLA-DR, CD36 and CD15 antigens, with an initial mild decrease in CD13 and an increase in CD45 expression. Maturation toward mature monocytes leads to a progressive increase in CD14, CD11b, CD13, CD36 and CD45 expression, with a mild decrease in HLA-DR and CD15. Mature monocytes show expression of bright CD14, bright CD33, variably bright CD13, bright CD36, CD38 and CD64 and low CD15.[9,23]

Lymphopoiesis

The common lymphoid progenitor (CLP), the precursor of mature lymphocytes, arises from the differentiation of the

Table 2.3 Characteristics of human B-cell subsets in normal bone marrow[41]

	CLP	Early B	Pro-B	Pre-BI	Large pre-BII	Small pre-BII	Immature B	Mature B	Plasma cells
CD34	+	+	+	–	–	–	–	–	–
CD10	+	+	+	+	+	+	+/dim	–	–
IL7-Rα	+	+	+	–	–	–	–	–	–
CD19	–	–	+	+	+	+	+	+	+
CD79a	–	+	+	+	+	+	+	+	+
CD138	–	–	–	–	–	–	–	–	+
TdT	–	–	+	–	–	–	–	–	–
RAG	–	–	+	+	–	+	+	–	–
Vpre-B	–	+	+	+	+	–	–	–	–
μH	–	–	–/+	+	+	+	+	+	+
Pre-BCR	–	–	–	–	+	–	–	–	–
IgH	GL	DJ$_H$	V$_H$ DJ$_H$	V$_H$ DJ$_H$	V$_H$ DJ$_H$	V$_H$ DJ$_H$	V$_H$ DJ$_H$	V$_H$ DJ$_H$	V$_H$ DJ$_H$
κL	GL	GL	GL	GL	GL	V$_L$L$_L$	V$_L$L$_L$	V$_L$L$_L$	V$_L$L$_L$
Cycling	–	–	–	+	+	–	–	–	–
Pax 5	–	–	+	+	+	+	+	+	–
CD20	–	–	–	+	+	+	+	+	–
sIgM	–	–	–	–	–	–	+	+	–
sIgD	–	–	–	–	–	–	–	+	–

BCR, B-cell receptor; CLP, common lymphoid progenitor; GL, germline; H, heavy chain; L, light chain; PAX, paired box; RAG, recombination activating gene; s, surface; TdT, terminal deoxynucleotidyl transferase; VDJ, variable, diversity and joining genes; Vpre-B protein, product of the *Vpre-B* gene.

HSC under the influence of IL-7 and FLT3.[41-43] The common lymphoid progenitor cells exist in both fetal and postnatal hemopoietic tissues. These generate B-cell, T-cell and NK cell progenitors and give rise to all types of lymphocytes. Much of the lymphopoiesis that occurs in normal BM is independent of antigenic stimulation and serves to supply the body with mature B-lymphocytes or with T-lymphoid progenitors that mature into T-cells in the thymus. The newly-formed mature B- and T-cells enter the circulation and then migrate to peripheral lymphoid tissues (spleen, lymph nodes, Peyer's patches, Waldeyer's ring).

B-cell production commences in fetal life within the BM, fetal liver and omentum. Postnatally it is restricted to the BM where it is dependent on the interaction of the CLP and their progeny with marrow stromal cells. The main features of the development of a CLP cell into an antibody-secreting plasma cell are shown in Table 2.3; this development is characterized by the step-wise rearrangement of the V, D and J segments of the immunoglobulin (Ig) heavy and light chain gene loci and differential expression of the rearranged genes. The maturation of early B, pro-B, pre-B and immature B-cells is antigen-independent and occurs within the BM under the influence of PAX5 and IL-4. Mature B-cells that leave the marrow have both IgM and IgD on their surface. Newly formed B-cells that enter peripheral lymphoid tissues may undergo antigen-dependent proliferation within lymphoid tissue and further maturation into plasma cells. The activation of a mature B-cell results from the binding of surface antibody with unique antigen specificity (generated by immunoglobulin gene rearrangement) to the corresponding unprocessed antigen. B-cells may also be activated by processed antigen via a T-cell-dependent mechanism. Some B-cells undergo antigen-dependent development into plasma cells in the BM itself. Other antigen-activated B-cells develop into memory B-cells rather than plasma cells, allowing rapid antibody production in a secondary immune response.

T-cell production occurs predominantly in the thymus and this requires a supply of early progenitors (thymus-seeding progenitor cells) from the BM. The development of T-lymphocytes is dependent on an interaction of the precursor cells with the surface molecules and secretory products of the epithelial elements of the thymus. The stages in the development of CLP into mature peripheral blood T-cells in the thymus is shown in Table 2.4. During T-lymphopoiesis in the thymus, the thymus-seeding progenitor (TSP) matures sequentially from early thymic progenitors, through transitional stages to mature T-lymphocytes. During the early stages of T-cell ontogeny rearrangement of the T-cell receptor (TCR) genes occurs in the sequence δ, γ, β and then α. The TCR (the antigen receptor on the surface of a T-cell) is a heterodimer consisting of one α- and one β-chain in about

Table 2.4 Maturation of T-cells in normal bone marrow and thymus[9,41,55]

	CLP	TSP	ETP	Pre-T	Common thymocyte	Mature thymocyte	T-lymphocyte
	BM	Thymus					Blood
CD34	+	+	+	+	−	−	−
TdT	−	−	+	+	+	+	−
CD1a	−	−	−	+	+	−	−
iTCRβ	−	−	−	−	+	+	+
cCD3ε	−	−	+/−	+	+	+	+
CD2	−	−	+/−	+	+	+	+
sCD3	−	−	−	−	−	+	+
CD5	−	−	+/−	+	+	+	+
CD7	+	+	+	+	+	+	+
CD4	−	−	−	−	+	+/−	+/−
CD8	−	−	−	−	+	+/−	+/−
CD45RA	+	+	+	−	−	−	−
CD45RO	−	−	−	−	+/−	+	+
DJβ	−	−	+	+	+	+	+
V- DJβ	−	−	−	−	+	+	+
V-Jα	−	−	−	−	−	+	+

CLP, common lymphoid progenitor; ETP, early T-cell precursor; TSP, thymus-seeding progenitor.

95% of the mature thymocytes and mature T-cells and of one γ and one δ chain in the remainder. During thymic T-cell development the cell goes through a double-positive stage (common thymocyte) when both CD4 and CD8 antigens are expressed. The mature thymocytes and mature T-cells are either CD4+CD8− (T-helper cells) or CD4−CD8+ (cytotoxic T-cells).

The regulation of lymphopoiesis is complex, and involves cytokines, transcription factors and stromal cells; the same cytokine may affect development of different lineages. For B-cell lymphopoiesis stromal cell-derived IL-4 plays a key role as well as IL-5, IL-6, KL (kit ligand), FL (FLT3 ligand) and IL-11. Expression of the transcription factors EBF (early B-cell factor) and PAX5 commits the lymphoid progenitor cell to the B-lineage.[44] IL-7 has a critical role for the T-lineage and is indispensible for T-cell development. Other key cytokines are stem cell factor, FL, IL-2, IL-3, IL-4, IL-12 and IL-10. Binding of ligands in intrathymic niches to Notch-1 receptor and the glycosyl transferase lunatic fringe (Lfng) on the progenitor surface commits progenitors to the T-cell lineage.[45]

There is a high rate of cell death during antigen-independent lymphopoiesis in both the BM and the thymus that serves to delete clones of B- and T-cells recognizing self-antigens. For example, T-cells that fail to recognize MHC class I molecules plus self-peptides on thymic epithelium or that bind to this complex with high affinity undergo apoptosis. In fact, over 99% of T-cell-receptor-bearing cells generated in the thymus undergo apoptosis within this organ.

Light microscope cytology

Lymphoblasts are morphologically identifiable in marrow and are also known as hematogones, most of which are B-cell precursors. They are small to intermediate sized round mononuclear cells with a high nucleus-to-cytoplasm ratio, round or indented nuclei, homogeneous condensed chromatin, absent or inconspicuous nucleolus and minimal basophilic agranular cytoplasm (Fig. 2.13). They comprise up to 5% of cells in normal pediatric BM and up to 1% in adults. Mature marrow lymphocytes, in contrast, are smaller with a round nucleus, more coarsely clumped chromatin and no nucleolus. They have a moderately high nucleus-to-cytoplasm ratio and basophilic cytoplasm which is visible around the majority of the nucleus. Intermediate stages of lymphoid differentiation cannot be identified. The morphology of mature B- and T-lymphocytes do not differ. Large granular lymphocytes, which may be T-suppressor/cytotoxic or NK cells, are larger with an eccentrically located nucleus, more abundant cytoplasm and azurophilic granules. The distribution of lymphoid cells and plasma cells in the marrow is described in Chapter 3.

Antigen expression

The common lymphoid progenitor cell is CD34+, CD10+, CD45RA+, CD24− and does not express surface markers for T-, B- or NK cells. B- and T-cells then undergo an orderly

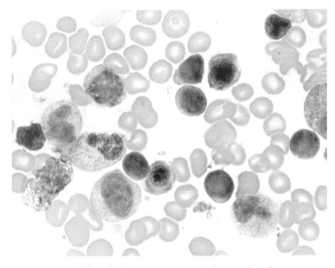

Fig. 2.13 Normal lymphoblasts (hematogones) in normal pediatric marrow. Lymphoblasts are larger than lymphocytes with finer, less condensed chromatin. May–Grünwald–Giemsa stain. × 1000.

sequence of antigen expression during differentiation (see Tables 2.3 and 2.4).

B-cells: there are characteristic patterns of antigen expression through B-cell differentiation in the normal human bone marrow (Table 2.3 and Fig. 2.14).[9,46–49] The current concept is that progenitor B-cells undergo differentiation as follows:[41]

1. B lineage-committed cells: CD34$^+$ CD10$^-$ TdT$^+$ cCD79a$^+$ CD19$^+$ common lymphoid progenitor or early B (E-B) stage.
2. Pro-B-cells: CD34$^+$ CD19$^+$ CD10$^+$ TdT$^+$ CD38^{++} CD20$^-$ cytIgM$^-$. MHC Class II molecules are expressed on pro-B-cells and more mature cells up to mature B-cells.
3. Pre-B-cells: down-regulation of CD34 and TdT to become CD34$^-$ CD19$^+$ CD10$^\pm$ CD38^{++} cytIgM$^+$ CD20$^\pm$. Pre-B-cells can be further subdivided in type I and II subsets (see Table 2.3).
4. Immature (IM) B-cells: CD34$^-$ CD19$^+$ CD20$^+$ CD38^{++}CD10$^{dim/-}$ sIgM$^{low/-}$ and TdT$^-$.
5. Mature B-cells: CD10$^-$ CD19$^+$ CD38$^{+/-}$ CD20$^+$ sIgM$^+$ sIgD and express light chains.

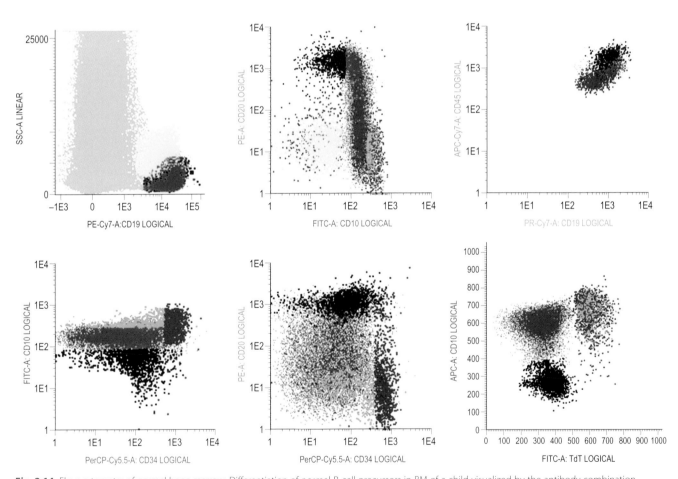

Fig. 2.14 Flow cytometry of normal bone marrow. Differentiation of normal B-cell precursors in BM of a child visualized by the antibody combination CD10-FITC / CD20-PE / CD34 PerCP-Cy5.5 / CD38-APC / CD19-Pe-Cy7 / CD45-APC-Cy7. CD19$^+$ lymphocytes were gated on CD19/SSC plot (upper left) and CD19/CD45 plot (upper right). CD19$^+$ plasma cells were painted yellow on a CD19/CD38 plot (not shown). CD34$^+$ most immature precursors (pro-B) are painted purple (lower left plot). The upper middle plot shows differential expression of CD10 and CD20 in three main subpopulations of B-cell precursors. CD34$^+$ cells show high CD10 expression. CD10$^+$ pre-B cells (orange) show variable CD20 expression and mature CD10- B-cells (blue) are CD20$^+$. The lower right plot illustrates the distribution of three main subsets or B-cell precursors in the CD19-gated B-cell population in CD10/TdT staining.

Rearrangements of the immunoglobulin (Ig) variable, diversity and joining (VDJ) heavy (H) chain loci are characteristic of pro-B-cells and require expression of the lymphocyte-specific recombination enzymes RAG1, RAG2 and TdT. Expression of the pre-B-cell receptor (BCR), composed of IgH chains and surrogate light (L) chains (VpreB and λ14.1), is a hallmark for the pre-B-cell population. Signaling through the pre-BCR promotes L chain (VJL) rearrangement and allelic exclusion at the IgH chain locus. Once VJ rearrangements are successful, L chains are expressed and combine with H chains as well as Igα/Igβ (CD79a, CD79b) to form a functional BCR expressed on IM-B cells.[41] Pre-B and IM B-cells constitute the majority of B-cells in children, while mature B-cells are most frequent in adult BM.[9,46] In children with BM regeneration after chemotherapy and transient hyperplasia of B-cell progenitors, subpopulations of IM and mature B-cells co-expressing CD5 have been identified.[50] CD5[+] B cells are the major population of B cells in fetal life, and their percentage decreases with age.[51]

T-cells: rare (<0.1%) T-cell restricted precursors, which express the pre-Tα protein on the cell surface and are CD34[+] CD7[+] CD45RA[+], can be identified in human BM.[41,52] Recently, it has been suggested that CD34[+] CD10[+] CD24[−] progenitors are present in both BM and thymus. These constitute a thymus-seeding population and may replace CD34[+] CD7[+] CD45RA[+] cells in the postnatal period. However, the frequency of these cells in normal BM is lower than 1×10^{-4}.[47] No TdT positive T-cells expressing cytoplasmic CD3 are found in normal BM. Most mature T-cells in the marrow co-express CD2, CD5, CD7 and membrane CD3 antigens, are either CD4 or CD8 positive and express CD45 brightly. However, minor subsets of CD7[+] cells lacking other 'pan-T' antigens, small subsets with co-expression of CD4 and CD8, and a subset lacking CD4 and CD8 have been reported.

Natural killer cells: there are two major subsets of NK cells: one expressing high levels of CD56 and low or no CD16 (CD56[hi] CD16[−]), and the second that is CD56[+] CD16[hi].[53] CD56[hi] CD16[±] cells have relatively lower cytolytic activity and produce more cytokines than the CD56[+] CD16[hi] cells, which are the cytotoxic effectors exerting their function through perforin and granzyme production. A putative committed NK cell precursor has been found within the CD34[lo] CD45RA[+] α4β7[hi]CD7[±]CD10[−] BM population and gives rise to CD56[hi]CD16[±] NK cells *in vitro*. The immature NK cells developing from committed NK cell precursors are defined by the expression of CD161 (NKR-P1).[54] These do not express CD56 or CD16 antigens. Immature NK cells can be induced to express these markers as well as the activating and inhibitory receptors, CD94- NKG2A and killer immunoglobulin receptors (KIR), upon culture with stromal cells and cytokines such as IL-15 or FLT3-L.[41]

Plasma cells

Plasma cells comprise less than 1% of cells in normal BM. The morphology of mature plasma cells in Romanowsky-stained smears varies markedly (Fig. 2.15). The majority are 14–20 μm in diameter and have deeply basophilic cytoplasm with a pale perinuclear zone corresponding to the site of the Golgi apparatus; the cytoplasm may have one or more vacuoles. The nucleus is eccentric and small relative to the

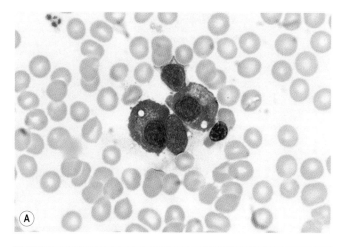

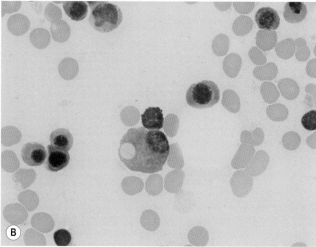

Fig. 2.15 (A, B) Plasma cell morphology. May–Grünwald–Giemsa stain. ×400. (A) Normal plasma cells. (B) Plasma cell showing a Russell body.

volume of the cytoplasm and contains moderate amounts of condensed chromatin. A small proportion of normal plasma cells may show various additional cytologic features, such as:

1. Russell bodies: very large, rounded, acidophilic, PAS-positive cytoplasmic inclusions; there is usually only one Russell body per cell (Fig. 2.15B). These result from the condensation of immunoglobulin within distended cisternae of the RER.
2. Mott cells (grape cells, or morular cells): plasma cells containing several smaller, slightly basophilic, rounded inclusions.
3. 'Flaming cells': peripheral cytoplasmic eosinophilia (occasionally the entire cytoplasm may take on an eosinophilic hue).
4. Azurophilic rods with a crystalline ultrastructure (rare) which resemble Auer rods. These are PAS-, Sudan black- and MPO-negative.

Normal plasma cells in the BM are CD19[dim]/ CD38[++]/ CD138[+/++]/ CD20[−]/ CD45[−]/ CD56[−]/ sIg[−] and express cytoplasmic immunoglobulin kappa or lambda.[55] They are negative for CD45, HLA-DR, CD117 and CD20.

Bone marrow stromal cells

The differentiation and proliferation of HSC requires interactions with the BM environment, the majority of which is cellular. BM stromal cells include osteoblasts, endothelial cells, macrophages, non-phagocytic reticular cells (including myofibroblasts and sinusoidal adventitial cells) and mesenchymal stem cells. The stromal cells are important in the regulation of hemopoiesis through direct contact and soluble mediators, that is, adhesive ligands, synthesis of extracellular matrix and production of signaling molecules and cytokines. Two niches exist in the bone marrow for pluripotent hemopoietic stem cells, one associated with the endosteum (in which osteoblasts play a key role) and the other with the sinusoids.[56]

Bone marrow sinusoids

Marrow sinusoids are thin-walled and composed of an inner complete layer of flattened endothelial cells, little or no associated basement membrane material, and an outer incomplete layer of adventitial cells. Thus some areas of the sinusoidal wall are only composed of thin endothelial cells. Endothelial cells overlap and may interdigitate extensively. They have numerous small pinocytotic vesicles along their luminal and abluminal surfaces. Marrow endothelial cells affect hemopoiesis by secreting stem cell factor, IL-6, IL-1α, IL-11, GM-CSF and G-CSF. They are also involved in controlling the entry and exit of hemopoietic stem cells and progenitor cells from the marrow and the exit of mature blood cells. The adventitial cells protrude long cytoplasmic processes; some of these lie on the external surface of the sinusoid and others are found between surrounding hemopoietic cells. Like the endothelial cells, the associated adventitial cells are likely to be involved in supporting hemopoiesis.

Bone marrow macrophages

Macrophages are derived from monocytes, as described above. Their role is to phagocytose cell debris and pathogens and to stimulate lymphocytes to respond to pathogens. They are located within erythroblastic islands (where they are involved in regulating erythropoiesis), plasma cell islands, lymphoid nodules, and adjacent to marrow sinusoids (forming part of the incomplete adventitial layer of the sinusoidal wall).

Macrophages contain the components of respiratory burst oxidase (NADPH oxidase) and phagocytosis is followed by a respiratory burst, the release of H_2O_2 and superoxide into phagosomes and, usually, killing of intracellular microorganisms. Oxygen-independent killing also occurs within phagosomes via defensins, lysozyme and hydrolytic enzymes. When activated, macrophages release reactive oxygen intermediates and nitric oxide extracellularly and can cause extracellular killing of parasites and microorganisms. Macrophages secrete a number of cytokines involved in inflammation and the immune response, including TNF-α, IL-1β, IL-6, IL-8 and IL-12. Bacterial endotoxin-stimulated macrophages secrete the chemokines macrophage inflammatory protein (MIP)-1α and MIP-1β that attract monocytes, neutrophils, NK cells and some T- and B-cells.

Light microscope cytology, cytochemistry and antigen expression

Macrophages are large (20–30 μm) irregularly shaped cells with a round or ovoid nucleus with lacy chromatin and may have a nucleolus (Fig. 2.16). They have abundant pale-staining cytoplasm with long cytoplasmic processes. The cytoplasm may be vacuolated and contain small azurophilic granules, vacuoles, lipid droplets and phagocytosed material, including extruded erythroblast nuclei and, occasionally, whole granulocytes. Phagocytosed degraded cells, extruded erythroid nuclei and other debris may be visible. Phagocytosed intact cells (hemophagocytosis) may also be seen. Macrophages are relatively fragile and their cytoplasm is frequently ruptured during the preparation of smears. The macrophages of iron-replete individuals contain blue granules when stained with Perls' acid ferrocyanide. Macrophages are PAS-positive, strongly alpha-naphthyl acetate esterase- and acid phosphatase-positive, NADH dehydrogenase- and succinate dehydrogenase-positive and alpha-naphthol AS-D chloroacetate esterase-negative. Most are Sudan black- and alkaline phosphatase-negative.

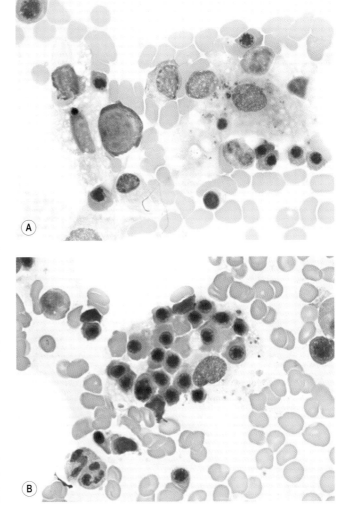

Fig. 2.16 (A, B) Macrophages. May–Grünwald–Giemsa stain. ×400. (A) Normal bone marrow macrophage. (B) Macrophage showing hemophagocytosis, predominantly of erythroblasts.

Macrophages express monocyte-associated cell surface antigens CD11b, CD14, CD64, CD68 and CD163 and are CD45 and HLA-DR-positive and their granules contain acid hydrolases and lysozyme.

Dendritic cells

Dendritic cells (DC) are derived from hemopoietic progenitor cells and process antigen which they then present to other immune cells. There are two main subpopulations: conventional DC (cDC) and interferon-producing plasmacytoid (pDC).

1. cDC are lineage (Lin)-negative (i.e. do not express myeloid or lymphoid lineage differentiation antigens), HLA-DR$^+$ cells that express high levels of CD11c and consist of a major blood dendritic cell antigen (BDCA)3$^-$ and a minor BDCA3$^+$ population. The major CD11c$^+$ HLA-DR$^+$ BDCA3$^-$ cDC population can be further subdivided into CD16$^+$ and CD16$^-$ subsets. cDC in lymphoid tissues arise from a population of committed cDC precursors (pre-cDC) that originate in the BM and migrate via peripheral blood. Spleen cDC arise from a population of Lin$^-$, CD11c$^+$ HLA-DR$^-$ immediate cDC precursors (pre-cDC). Pre-cDC originate from bone marrow Lin$^-$, CD117^{int}, Flt3$^+$, CD115$^+$ common DC progenitors.[57]
2. pDC are Lin$^-$ HLA-DR$^+$ and are defined by the absence of CD11c antigen and high levels of CD123 (the IL-3Rα chain) and BDCA2.[57] The direct progenitors of pDC (pro-pDC) are within the CD34^{lo} compartment of cord blood, fetal liver and BM. pro-pDC express CD45RA, CD4 and high levels of CD123.[41]

Mast cells

Mast cells differentiate from multipotent hemopoietic cells in the BM and have a close developmental relationship with basophils.[58,59] After initial differentiation in the BM the most mature mast cell progenitors enter the blood, circulate and migrate into tissues where they proliferate and mature into mast cells.[60] Mature mast cells are present in normal BM at a very low frequency (<0.03%). Stem cell factor (SCF), also known as Kit ligand, is crucial for the development, proliferation and maturation of mast cells from progenitors. SCF and Kit signaling are necessary for stimulating the proliferation of committed mast cell progenitors and homing and recruitment mast cells to tissues. Other factors that influence mast cell development are TPO, IL-3, a number of other cytokines and inflammatory mediators such as prostaglandin E, TNFα, IL-6 and IFNγ.[61-63]

Mast cells have an abundance of electron-dense secretory granules. These contain large amounts of mast cell mediators which include histamine, serotonin, cytokines (especially tumor necrosis factor), proteoglycans, lysosomal enzymes, heparin and chondroitin sulphates and mast-cell-specific proteases (Table 2.1).[64] Mast cells contain particularly large amounts of the serine proteases tryptase, chymase and carboxypeptidase A and these are stored in fully active form.[65,66] After activation by antigen and IgE, mast cell granule contents are released in massive amounts by a process termed piecemeal degranulation. Stimulated mast cells also release products of arachidonic acid oxidation such as leukotriene C4 (LTC4) and prostaglandin D2 (PGD2) as well as the cytokines such as tumor necrosis factor α (TNFα) and IL-4. Tissue mast cells have a principal role in immediate-type hypersensitivity and allergic reactions where they respond to antigen and release mast cell mediators. Mast cells (and basophils) also participate in IgE-dependent host defense against parasites and accumulate at sites of resolving inflammation. They may modulate inflammatory responses by releasing heparin (which prevents further fibrin deposition) and proteases (which may inhibit coagulation and promote fibrinolysis).

Light microscope cytology

Mast cells can be distinguished from basophils by their generally larger size and the coarse, purplish-black to red-purple granules (Romanowsky stain) that pack the cytoplasm but seldom overlie the nucleus (Fig. 2.17). The nucleus of the mast cell is small, round or oval and the chromatin is less condensed than that of a basophil. The nucleus is centrally or, occasionally, eccentrically placed. Mast cells stain metachromatically with toluidine blue and are less strongly PAS-positive than basophils. Unlike basophil granulocytes, mast cells may undergo mitosis.

Antigen expression

Bone marrow mast cells have characteristically strong CD117 expression and high light scatter by FCM. They express CD9, CD11c, CD29, CD33, CD43, CD44, CD45, CD49d, CD49e, CD51, CD54 and CD71 antigens and FcεRI. Other antigens such as CD11b, CD13, CD18, CD22, CD35, CD40 and CD61 display a variable expression in normal individuals. They are negative for CD34, CD38 and CD138 antigens.[67,68]

Osteoblasts

Osteoblasts are derived from pluripotent mesenchymal stem cells. They may be seen in BM smears as single cells or small groups. They are ovoid or elongated, have a single small eccentric nucleus with small quantities of condensed chromatin and one to three nucleoli (Fig. 2.18A). They have abundant lightly basophilic cytoplasm with indistinct margins. Although they superficially resemble plasma cells, they are larger and their Golgi zone is not immediately adjacent to the nucleus. Furthermore, the nucleus of an osteoblast does not show the heavily-stained coarse clumps of condensed chromatin that are characteristic of plasma cells. Osteoblasts are alkaline-phosphatase-positive and express CD56. Osteoblasts in the endosteum of trabecular bone interact with HSC via adhesion and signaling molecules and maintain them in a quiescent state (i.e. osteoblasts regulate the bone-associated HSC niche).[69,70] In addition, factors that regulate B-lymphopoiesis affect osteoblast and osteoclast formation and vice versa.[71]

Osteoclasts

Osteoclasts are derived from undifferentiated cells of the monocyte-macrophage lineage. Diffferentiation to

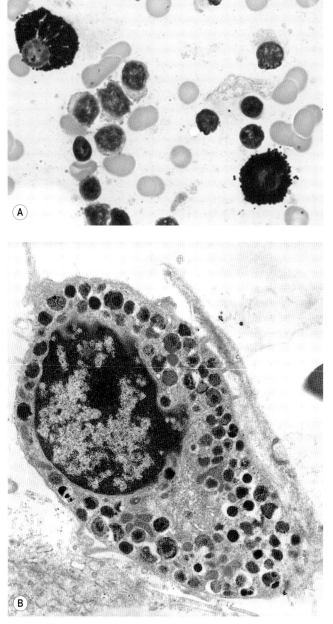

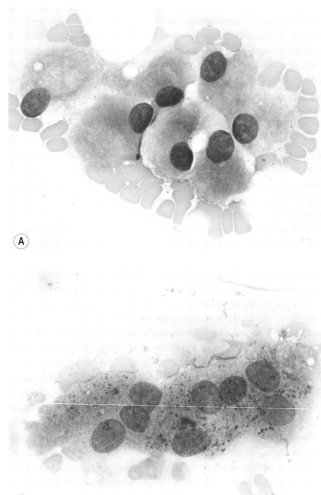

Fig. 2.18 (A, B) Osteoblasts and osteoclast in normal bone marrow. May–Grünwald–Giemsa stain. × 1000. (A) Osteoblasts in normal bone marrow. The cytoplasm of each cell contains a large pale-staining area (occupied by the Golgi apparatus). (B) A multinucleate osteoclast from a smear of normal bone marrow.

Fig. 2.17 (A, B) Mast cells. (A) Normal appearing mast cells in a case of Waldenström macroglobulinemia. The cytoplasm is packed with coarse granules only a few of which overlie the nucleus. May–Grünwald–Giemsa stain. × 1000. (B) Electron micrograph of a mast cell in normal bone marrow. The cytoplasmic granules vary considerably in their ultrastructure. There are long thin cytoplasmic projections at the cell surface. Uranyl acetate and lead citrate. × 8500.

terminally differentiated osteoclasts requires RANKL or osteoclast differentiation factor. Osteoclasts are giant multinucleate cells with abundant pale-staining cytoplasm containing many fine azurophilic granules (Fig. 2.18B). The individual nuclei within a single cell are small, round or oval, are uniform in size, and have a single prominent nucleolus. There is usually no overlap between adjacent nuclei within the same cell. Osteoclasts must be distinguished from megakaryocytes, the other polyploid giant cells in the marrow. Unlike multinucleated osteoclasts, normal megakaryocytes

have a single large lobulated nucleus. Osteoclasts are strongly acid-phosphatase-positive.

Mesenchymal stem cells

Mesenchymal stem cells (MSC) comprise a population of non-hemopoietic stromal cells and are found in the BM. They are rare cells in the BM (<0.01%) and possess multilineage potential with the capacity to differentiate and contribute to the regeneration of mesenchymal tissues but not blood cells. MSC also exist in the AGM region of the embryo and can differentiate *in vitro* into chondrocytes, adipocytes and osteocytes.[72] They express CD73, CD90 and CD105 antigens but not CD34, CD45 or HLA-DR. They are further characterized by their ability to adhere to tissue-culture plastic and capacity to generate osteoblasts, chondrocytes and adipocytes *in vitro*.[73]

Adipocytes

Adipocytes, the largest cell in the BM, share a common precursor with osteoblasts; it is unclear what influences their

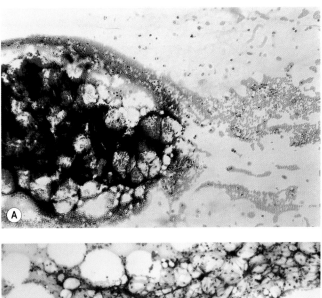
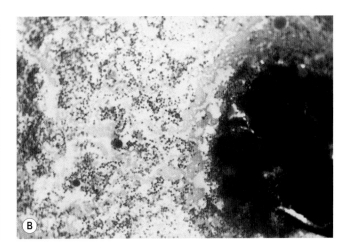
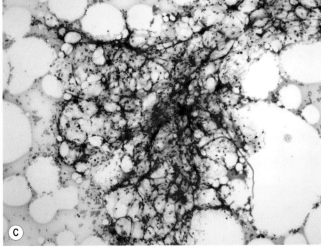

Fig. 2.19 (A, B, C) Bone marrow smears showing particles with different cellularity. May–Grünwald–Giemsa stain. × 100. (A) Normocellular fragments in which a little over half the volume of the fragment consists of hemopoietic cells (normal adult). (B) Hypercellular fragment showing virtually complete replacement of fat cells by hemopoietic cells (congenital dyserythropoietic anemia, type I). (C) Hypocellular fragment (cellularity <10% of the volume of the fragment) composed predominantly of stromal cells and few hemopoietic cells (aplastic anemia).

differentiation. The number of adipocytes is inversely related to the marrow cellularity (see below).

Assessment of marrow hemopoietic activity

Morphological assessment

BM activity can be assessed subjectively by morphological analysis of hemopoietic cells in aspirated material or on sections of a biopsy specimen by light microscopy; the latter is discussed in Chapter 3. The cellularity of the BM can be assessed in the aspirate by examining several marrow fragments in stained smears (Fig. 2.19). Cellularity varies according to age and the site from which the specimen was taken. Marrow cellularity is at its greatest at birth (>80% cellularity) and reduces with aging; by age 10 years the cellularity will have reduced to approximately 70%, by 30 years 50% and by 70 years to 30%. Although it is not established that the number of HSC declines with age, qualitative changes may affect their self-renewal potential and hence BM cellularity.

The overall BM cellularity is more accurately assessed in BM trephine biopsies or clot sections of aspirated marrow than smears, as discussed in Chapter 3.

Hemopoietic activity is determined by assessing the individual hemopoietic cell lineages, as described above. A bone marrow nucleated differential cell count (NDC) is used to assess the proportions of the different hemopoietic cell lineages against known reference ranges, and to quantify any abnormal cells that may be present.[74] The NDC should include the morphologically recognizable cells, that is, blast cells, promyelocytes, myelocytes, metamyelocytes, band forms, segmented neutrophil granulocytes, eosinophils, basophils, promonocytes and monocytes, lymphocytes, plasma cells and erythroblasts. It does not include megakaryocytes, macrophages, mast cells, osteoblasts, osteoclasts, stromal cells, smudged cells or non-hemopoietic cells such as metastatic tumor cells.

Changes occur in the cellular composition as well as the cellularity of the marrow during life (Tables 2.5–2.7). In the first 3 months of life there is a progressive fall in erythroid progenitors from 40% (range, 20–65%) on the first day to 10% (range, 0–20.5%) between days 8 and 10, and this

Table 2.5 Changes in the cellular composition of the marrow from birth to age 20 years (% cells)

	0–24 hours (n = 19)	2 months–1 year (n = 16)	2–20 years (n = 92)
Neutrophil series			
Mean	46.4	54.4	60.6
Range	20–73		45–77
Erythroblasts			
Mean	40	19.8	23.1
Range	18.5–65		12.7–19.3
Lymphocytes			
Mean	12.1	25.1	16.0
Range	2–22.5		12–28
Myeloid/ erythroid ratio			
Mean	1.16	3.5	2.9
Range		1.2–5.2	2.0–8.3

Table 2.6 Changes in the number of lymphocytes in the bone marrow from birth to age 29 years

			Percentage of lymphocytes	
Age	Number of cases	Mean	Range or ± 2 standard deviations
0–48 h	24	12.3	4.0–22.0
7–10 days	28	32.7	7.5–62.0
1 month	23	46.9	12.0–73.0
3 months	12	47.0	31.0–81.0
6 months	22	47.5	± 15.7
12 months	18	47.1	± 22.6
1–4 years	19	43.5	± 17.1
4–5 years	9	19.1	12.0–27.0
5–20 years	89	15.9	5.0–36.0
20–29 years	28	14.6	9.3–25.0

Table 2.7 Cellular composition of marrow in healthy adults: differential cell counts (% BM cells), mean and 95% confidence limits

Cell type	Age range and number of individuals			
	20–29 years n = 28 (Mean)	20–29 years (95% confidence limits)	20–29 years (Observed range)	20–93 years n = 63 (Observed range)
Myeloid cells				
Myeloblasts	1.21	0.75–1.67	0.75–1.80	0.75–1.90
Promyelocytes	2.49	0.99–3.99	1.00–3.75	
Myelocytes				
Neutrophil	17.36	11.54–23.18	12.25–22.65	12.00–24.35
Eosinophil	1.37	0–2.85	0.25–3.45	0.25–3.45
Basophil	0.08	0–0.21	0.00–0.25	0.00–0.25
Metamyelocytes				
Neutrophil	16.29	11.40–22.44	11.45–23.60	8.75–27.35
Eosinophil	0.63	0.07–1.19	0.25–1.30	0.15–1.70
Band forms	8.70	3.58–13.82	4.85–13.95	2.60–13.95
Polymorphs				
Neutrophil	13.42	4.32–22.52	8.70–28.95	6.40–28.95
Eosinophil	0.93	0.21–1.65	0.45–1.55	0.25–2.35
Basophil	0.20	0–0.48	0.05–0.50	0.05–0.65
Monocytes	1.04	0.36–1.72	0.65–2.10	0.50–2.95
Lymphocytes	14.60	6.66–22.54	9.35–25.05	6.85–25.05
Plasma cells	0.46	0–0.96	0.10–0.95	0.10–2.00
Erythroid cells				
Basophilic erythropoietic cells	0.92	0.40–1.44	0.50–1.60	0.50–1.60
Early polychromatic erythroblasts	6.76	2.56–10.96	3.30–12.20	1.80–12.20
Late polychromatic erythroblasts	11.58	6.16–1.70	7.85–19.55	6.15–19.90

remains low for about 3 weeks. It then gradually increases again to reach 15–20% in the 3-month-old infant. These changes appear to be secondary to an increase of arterial oxygen saturation to adult levels within 3 h of birth resulting in a suppression of erythropoietin production. Erythropoietin production increases again when the infant is 6–13 weeks old. The proportion of granulocytes and their precursors increases during the first 2 weeks after birth and decreases to stabilize at about 50% after the 2nd month (Table 2.5); a slight increase is seen after the age of 4 years. The proportion of lymphocytes is relatively low in the neonate, increases markedly during the first 7–10 days and remains high throughout the first year. Adult values are reached by the age of 4 years (Table 2.6). Plasma cells are rarely seen in the marrow at birth but increase progressively to reach adult values by the age of about 12 years.

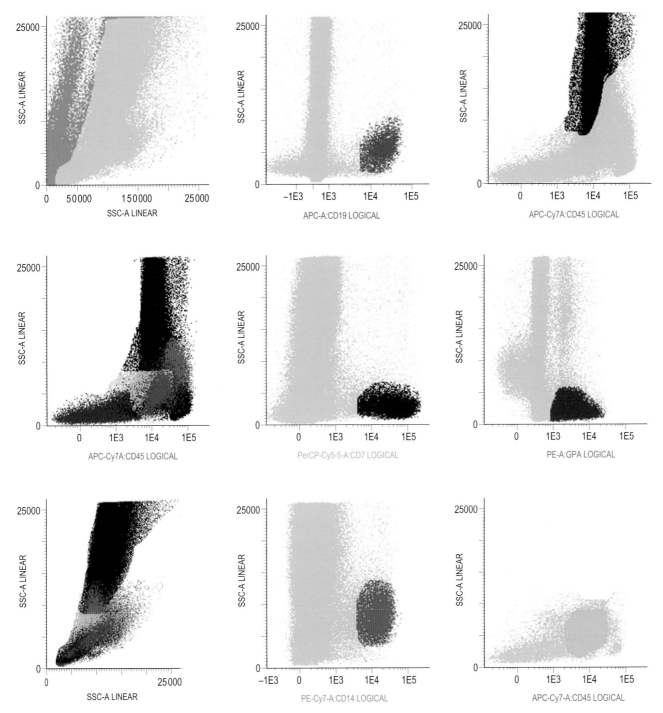

Fig. 2.20 Main subpopulations of hematopoietic cells in a bone marrow of a child are visualized on the forward scatter (FSC)/side scatter (SSC) plot (upper middle plot) by the back-gating of cells gated on the expression of characteristic markers and SSC. The antibody combination: CD61 FITC / CD235a PE / CD7 PerCP-Cy5.5 / CD19 APC / CD14 Pe-Cy7 / CD45 APC-Cy7 was applied. Dead cells were removed using FSC/SSC plot (upper left). Platelet aggregates were removed by gating CD61++ events (not shown). CD19+ B-cells (purple) are CD45dim/CD45+ due to the presence of a considerable B-cell precursor population. CD7+ T-cells (dark blue) are mainly located in the CD45++ area. Glycophorin-positive erythropoietic precursors (red) are mainly CD45-negative. CD14+ monocytes (green) are CD45++ and have higher SSC than lymphocytes. Granulopoietic precursors (brown) are gated on the basis of their high SSC and are CD45 dim. The blast area (cyan) is defined by gating CD45 dim cells that are left after removing cells stained by all used markers (lower right plot).

Phenotypic assessment

Multiparameter flow cytometry (FC) is a highly reproducible and objective way of assessing hemopoietic cells of all lineages and their stage of differentiation based on antigen expression. Knowledge of levels and expression patterns of various antigens in normal hemopoietic cells at different stages of development provides a frame of reference for recognition of abnormal differentiation patterns in the assessment of hematologic malignancies. Antigenic profiles of normal hemopoietic cells have been described in preceding sections of this chapter; these data have been based on reports by several groups that have rigorously assessed differentiation stages of various hematopoietic cell lineages.[9,31,46,47,75-77] Mapping of normal BM cell subpopulations can be achieved by gating cell populations on CD45 (leukocyte common antigen) expression and light side scatter (SSC) (Fig. 2.20).[78,79] This approach can be used to assess hemopoietic activity as cells of the following types can all be identified and analyzed:

- Early hematopoietic precursors of various lineages, including CD34[+] stem cells: low CD45 expression and low SSC
- Erythropoietic precursors: CD45-negative and low SSC
- Granulocytic precursors and mature granulocytes: weak CD45 expression (CD45[dim]) and variable SSC

- Monocytes: strong CD45 expression and higher SSC
- Mature lymphocytes: strong CD45 expression and low SSC.

The localization of these subpopulations on the CD45/SSC plot can be refined by multicolor labeling of lineage-associated antigens and visualization of cell populations positive for given antigen combinations (Fig. 2.20).[79] Further analysis of discrete cell subpopulations will depend on the clinical question and include antibodies to differentiation-associated antigens, as described above. Immunocytochemistry can also be used to detect normal hemopoietic cell types of all lineages; this will be described in Chapter 3.

References

1. Robin C, Ottersbach K, de Bruijn M, et al. Developmental origins of hematopoietic stem cells. Oncology Research 2003;13:315–21.
2. Dzierzak E, Speck NA. Of lineage and legacy: the development of mammalian hematopoietic stem cells. Nat Immunol 2008;9(2):129–36.
3. Lee W, Erm SK, Kim KY, Becker RP. Emperipolesis of erythroblasts within Kupffer cells during hepatic hemopoiesis in human fetus. Anatomical Record 1999;256:158–64.
4. Wickramasinghe S. Human bone marrow. Oxford: Blackwell Scientific Publications; 1975.
5. Yahata T, Muguruma Y, Yumino S, et al. Quiescent human hematopoietic stem cells in the bone marrow niches organize the hierarchical structure of hematopoiesis. Stem Cells 2008; 26(12):3228–36.
6. Huang S, Terstappen I.W. Lymphoid and myeloid differentiation of single human CD34[+], HLA-DR[+], CD38[-] hematopoietic stem cells. Blood 1994;83(6): 1515–26.
7. Bjorklund E, Gruber A, Mazur J, et al. CD34[+] cell subpopulations detected by 8-color flow cytometry in bone marrow and in peripheral blood stem cell collections: application for MRD detection in leukemia patients. Int J Hematol 2009;90(3):292–302.
8. Goardon N, Nikolousis E, Sternberg A, et al. Reduced CD38 expression on CD34[+] cells as a diagnostic test in myelodysplastic syndromes. Haematologica 2009;94(8):1160–3.
9. van Lochem EG, van der Velden VH, Wind HK, et al. Immunophenotypic differentiation patterns of normal hematopoiesis in human bone marrow: reference patterns for age-related changes and disease-induced shifts. Cytometry B Clin Cytom 2004;60(1):1–13.
10. Bellantuono I. Haemopoietic stem cells. Int J Biochem Cell Biol 2004;36(4): 607–20.

11. Buza-Vidas N, Luc S, Jacobsen SE. Delineation of the earliest lineage commitment steps of haematopoietic stem cells: new developments, controversies and major challenges. Current Opinion in Hematology 2007;14:315–21.
12. Giebel B, Punzel M. Lineage development of hematopoietic stem and progenitor cells. Biol Chem 2008;389(7):813–24.
13. Migliaccio AR, Papayannopoulou T. Erythropoiesis. In: Steinberg MH, Forget BG, Higgs DR, Nagel RL, editors. Cambridge: Cambridge University Press; 2001:52–71.
14. Hanspal M, Smockova Y, Uong Q. Molecular identification and functional characterisation of a novel protein that mediates the attachment of erythroblasts to macrophages. Blood Reviews 1998;92:2940–50.
15. Lee G, Lo Lee G, Lo A, et al. Targeted gene deletion demonstrates that the cell adhesion molecule ICAM-4 is critical for erythroblastic island formation. Blood Reviews 2006;(108):2064–71.
16. Chasis J. Erythroblastic islands: specialized microenvironmental niches for erythropoiesis. Current Opinion in Hematology 2006;13:137–41.
17. Manwani D, Bieker JJ. The erythroblastic island. Current Topics in Developmental Biology 2008;82:23–53.
18. Fisher J. Erythropoietin: physiology and pharmacology update. Experimental Biology and Medicine 2003;228:1–14.
19. Gleadle JM. Review article: How cells sense oxygen: lessons from and for the kidney. Nephrology (Carlton) 2009; 14(1):86–93.
20. Leberbauer C, Boulmé F, Unfried G, et al. Different steroids co-regulate long-term expansion versus terminal differentiation in primary human erythroid progenitors. Blood 2005;105:85–94.
21. Blobel G, Sieff CA, Orkin SH. Ligand-dependent repression of the erythroid transcription factor GATA-1 by the estrogen receptor. Molecular and Cellular Biology 1995;15:3147–53.

22. Chen K, Liu J, Heck S, et al. Resolving the distinct stages in erythroid differentiation based on dynamic changes in membrane protein expression during erythropoiesis. Proc Natl Acad Sci USA 2009;106(41): 17413–8.
23. Wood B. Multicolor immunophenotyping: human immune system hematopoiesis. Methods Cell Biol 2004;75:559–76.
24. Kaushansky K. Historical review: megakaryopoiesis and thrombopoiesis. Blood 2008;111(3):981–6.
25. Jean G, Lambertenghi-Deliliers G, Ranzim T, Poirier-Basseti M. The human bone marrow megakaryocyte. An ultrastructural study. Haematologia 1971;5:253–64.
26. Breton-Gorius J, Reyes F. Ultrastructure of human bone marrow cell maturation. International Review of Cytology 1976;46:251–321.
27. Larsen T. Emperipolesis of granular leukocytes within megakaryocytes in human hemopoietic bone marrow. American Journal of Clinical Pathology 1970;53:485–9.
28. Skokowa J, Welte K. LEF-1 is a decisive transcription factor in neutrophil granulopoiesis. Annals of the New York Academy of Sciences 2007;1106:143–51.
29. van Rhenen A, Feller N, Kelder A, et al. High stem cell frequency in acute myeloid leukemia at diagnosis predicts high minimal residual disease and poor survival. Clin Cancer Res 2005;11(18): 6520–7.
30. Elghetany MT, Ge Y, Patel J, et al. Flow cytometric study of neutrophilic granulopoiesis in normal bone marrow using an expanded panel of antibodies: correlation with morphologic assessments. J Clin Lab Anal 2004;18(1):36–41.
31. Kussick SJ, Wood BL. Using 4-color flow cytometry to identify abnormal myeloid populations. Arch Pathol Lab Med 2003;127(9):1140–7.
32. Cowland JB, Borregaard N. The individual regulation of granule protein mRNA levels during neutrophil maturation explains the heterogeneity of neutrophil granules.

Journal of Leukocyte Biology 1999;66:989–95.

33. Faurschou M, Kamp S, Cowland JB, et al. Prodefensins are matrix proteins of specific granules in human neutrophils. Journal of Leukocyte Biology 2005;78:785–93.

34. Jacobsen L, Theilgaard-Mönch K, Christensen EI, Borregaard N. Arginase 1 is expressed in myelocytes/metamyelocytes and localized in gelatinase granules of human neutrophils. Blood 2007;109:3084–7.

35. Bjornsson S, Wahlstrom S, Norstrom E, et al. Total nucleated cell differential for blood and bone marrow using a single tube in a five-color flow cytometer. Cytometry B Clin Cytom 2008;74(2): 91–103.

36. Egesten A, Calafat J, Weller PF, et al. Localization of granule proteins in human eosinophil bone marrow progenitors. International Archives of Allergy and Immunology 1997;114:130–8.

37. Zucker-Franklin D. Ultrastructural evidence for the common origin of human mast cells and basophils. Blood Reviews 1980;56(3):534–40.

38. Valent P. Cytokines involved in growth and differentiation of human basophils and mast cells. Experimental Dermatology 1995;4:255–9.

39. Han X, Jorgensen JL, Brahmandam A, et al. Immunophenotypic study of basophils by multiparameter flow cytometry. Arch Pathol Lab Med 2008;132(5):813–9.

40. Gemelli C, Montanari M, Tenedini E, et al. Virally mediated MafB transduction induces the monocyte commitment of human CD34+ hematopoietic stem/ progenitor cells. Cell Death and Differentiation 2006;13:1686–96.

41. Blom B, Spits H. Development of human lymphoid cells. 2006. Annu Rev Immunol 2006;24:287–320.

42. LeBien T, Tedder TF. B lymphocytes: how they develop and function. Blood 2008;112:1570–80.

43. Strominger J. Developmental biology of T cell receptors. Science 1989;244: 943–50.

44. Pongubala J, Northrup DL, Lanckim DW, et al. Transcription factor EBF restricts alternative lineage options and promotes B cell fate commitment independently of Pax5. Nature Immunology 2008;9: 203–15.

45. Visan I, Tan JB, Yuan JS, et al. Regulation of T lymphopoiesis by Notch1 and Lunatic fringe-mediated competition for intrathymic niches. Nature Immunology 2006;7:634–43.

46. Lucio P, Parreira A, van den Beemd MW, et al. Flow cytometric analysis of normal B cell differentiation: a frame of reference for the detection of minimal residual disease in precursor-B-ALL. Leukemia 1999;13(3):419–27.

47. Porwit-MacDonald A, Bjorklund E, Lucio P, et al. BIOMED-1 concerted action report: flow cytometric characterization of CD7+ cell subsets in normal bone marrow as a basis for the diagnosis and follow-up of T cell acute lymphoblastic leukemia (T-ALL). Leukemia 2000;14(5): 816–25.

48. McKenna RW, Washington LT, Aquino DB, et al. Immunophenotypic analysis of hematogones (B-lymphocyte precursors) in 662 consecutive bone marrow specimens by 4-color flow cytometry. Blood 2001;98(8):2498–507.

49. Campana D, Janossy G, Bofill M, et al. Human B cell development. I. Phenotypic differences of B lymphocytes in the bone marrow and peripheral lymphoid tissue. J Immunol 1985;134(3):1524–30.

50. Fuda FS, Karandikar NJ, Chen W. Significant CD5 expression on normal stage 3 hematogones and mature B lymphocytes in bone marrow. Am J Clin Pathol 2009;132(5):733–7.

51. Loken MR, Shah VO, Dattilio KL, Civin CI. Flow cytometric analysis of human bone marrow. II. Normal B lymphocyte development. Blood 1987;70(5): 1316–24.

52. Six EM, Bonhomme D, Monteiro M, et al. A human postnatal lymphoid progenitor capable of circulating and seeding the thymus. J Exp Med 2007;204(13): 3085–93.

53. Cooper MA, Fehniger TA, Caligiuri MA. The biology of human natural killer-cell subsets. Trends Immunol 2001 Nov;22(11):633–40.

54. Bennett IM, Zatsepina O, Zamai L, et al. Definition of a natural killer NKR-P1A+/ CD56-/CD16- functionally immature human NK cell subset that differentiates in vitro in the presence of interleukin 12. J Exp Med 1996;184(5):1845–56.

55. Jourdan M, Caraux A, De Vos J, et al. An in vitro model of differentiation of memory B cells into plasmablasts and plasma cells including detailed phenotypic and molecular characterization. Blood 2009;114(25): 5173–81.

56. Yin T, Li L. The stem cell niches in bone. Journal of Clinical Investigation 2006;116: 1195–201.

57. Dzionek A, Fuchs A, Schmidt P, et al. BDCA-2, BDCA-3, and BDCA-4: three markers for distinct subsets of dendritic cells in human peripheral blood. J Immunol 2000;165(11): 6037–46.

58. Okayama Y, Kawakami T. Development, migration, and survival of mast cells. Immunol Res 2006;34(2):97–115.

59. Denburg J, Richardson M, Telizyn S, Bienenstock J. Basophil/mast cell precursors in human peripheral blood. Blood Reviews 1983;61:775–80.

60. Kirshenbaum A, Kessler SW, Goff JP, Metcalfe DD. Demonstration of the origin of human mast cells from CD34+ bone marrow progenitor cells. Journal of Immunology 1991;146:1410–5.

61. Migliaccio A, Rana RA, Vannucchi AM, Manzoli FA. Role of thrombopoietin in mast cell differentiation. Annals of the New York Academy of Sciences 2007;1106:152–74.

62. Takemoto C, Lee YN, Jegga AG. Mast cell transcriptional networks. Blood Cells, Molecules and Diseases 2008;41:82–90.

63. Hu Z, Zhao WH, Shimamura T. Regulation of mast cell development by inflammatory factors. Current Medicinal Chemistry 2007;14:3044–50.

64. Pejler G, Ronnberg E, Waern I, Wernersson S. Mast cell proteases: multifaceted regulators of inflammatory disease. Blood 2010;115(24):4981–90.

65. dePaulis A, Minopoli G, Arbustini E, et al. Stem cell factor is localized in, released from, and cleaved by human mast cells. Journal of Immunology 1999;163: 2799–808.

66. Diao J, Zhao J, Winter E, Cattral MS. Recruitment and differentiation of conventional dendritic cell precursors in tumors. J Immunol 2010;184(3): 1261–7.

67. Orfao A, Escribano L, Villarrubia J, et al. Flow cytometric analysis of mast cells from normal and pathological human bone marrow samples: identification and enumeration. Am J Pathol 1996;149(5): 1493–9.

68. Escribano L, Navalon R, Nunez R, et al. Immunophenotypic analysis of human mast cells by flow cytometry. Curr Protoc Cytom 2001;Chapter 6:Unit 6.

69. Arai F, Suda T. Maintenance of quiescent hematopoietic stem cells in the osteoblastic niche. Annals of the New York Academy of Sciences 2007;1106: 41–53.

70. Porter R, Calvi LM. Communications between bone cells and hematopoietic stem cells. Archives of Biochemistry and Biophysics 2008;473:193–200.

71. Horowitz M, Bothwell AL, Hesslein DG, et al. B cells and osteoblast and osteoclast development. Immunological Reviews 2005;208:141–53.

72. Wang X, Lan Y, He WY. Identification of mesenchymal stem cells in aorta-gonad-mesonephros and yolk sac of human embryos. Blood Reviews 2008;111: 2436–43.

73. Dominici M, Le Blanc K, Mueller I, et al. Minimal criteria for defining multipotent mesenchymal stromal cells. The International Society for Cellular Therapy position statement. Cytotherapy 2006;8(4):315–7.

74. Lee SH, Erber WN, Porwit A, et al. ICSH guidelines for the standardization of bone marrow specimens and reports. Int J Lab Hematol 2008;30(5):349–64.

75. Terstappen LW, Huang S, Picker LJ. Flow cytometric assessment of human T-cell

differentiation in thymus and bone marrow. Blood 1992;79(3): 666–77.

76. Terstappen LW, Levin J. Bone marrow cell differential counts obtained by multidimensional flow cytometry. Blood Cells 1992;18(2):311–30; discussion 31–2.

77. Terstappen LW, Safford M, Loken MR. Flow cytometric analysis of human bone marrow. III. Neutrophil maturation. Leukemia 1990;4(9):657–63.

78. Stelzer GT, Shults KE, Loken MR. CD45 gating for routine flow cytometric analysis of human bone marrow specimens. Ann N Y Acad Sci 1993;677:265–80.

79. Arnoulet C, Bene MC, Durrieu F, et al. Four- and five-color flow cytometry analysis of leukocyte differentiation pathways in normal bone marrow: a reference document based on a systematic approach by the GTLLF and GEIL. Cytometry B Clin Cytom 2010;78(1): 4–10.

80. Campana D, Coustan-Smith E. Minimal residual disease studies by flow cytometry in acute leukemia. Acta Haematol 2004;112(1–2):8–15.

CHAPTER 3

Normal bone marrow histology

MT Moonim, A Porwit

Normal bone marrow – generalities and function

The term 'bone marrow' (BM) refers to the tissue occupying the cavities under the cortex within the honeycomb of trabecular bone. Normal marrow is either red, consisting of the hematopoietic tissue, or yellow, composed mainly of fat cells (adipose tissue). In children most bones contain hematopoietic marrow, almost to the exclusion of fat cells. In the adult, red marrow is found in the skull, sternum, scapulae, vertebrae, ribs, pelvic bones and the proximal ends of the long bones (e.g. femora and humeri). The hematopoietic marrow produces the mature blood cells, which have a finite life span and must be constantly replaced (see Chapter 2). The weight of the total BM is 1600–3700 g. The BM is composed of:

- the parenchyme: the hemopoietic cells including precursors and mature cells of the erythroid, myeloid and megakaryocytic lineages, i.e. various stages of red cells, white cells, megakaryocytes, lymphocytes, plasma cells and mast cells
- the stroma: fat cells, histiocytes/macrophages, fibroblasts, blood vessels and intercellular matrix.

The BM can be assessed in aspirated material and in biopsied tissue. This chapter will describe the histology of BM in the trephine biopsy.

Bone marrow structure

The constituents of the normal BM are closely packed within a hard bony 'container'. Hemopoiesis occurs in the intertrabecular space within marrow cavities. The bony trabeculae (cancellous bone) are lined by endosteum, osteoblasts and osteoclasts. The stromal elements form an extensive, closely woven network in which the hematopoietic precursors are embedded, attached in various ways and to different components by the adhesive proteins and by other cells, such as the central macrophages in the erythroid islands. Hematopoietic precursors receive their nutrients, vitamins, hormones, regulatory factors, cytokines and modulators through the extracellular matrix (ECM), which also contributes to the regulation of the cell cycle, cellular differentiation and apoptosis. The blood supply to the BM consists of two systems: periosteal arteries, which give off branches to the BM after they penetrate the bone, and nutrient arteries. Blood drains from the BM cavity through central veins. The BM receives approximately 2–4% of cardiac output. The

©2011 Elsevier Ltd
DOI: 10.1016/B978-0-7020-3147-2.00003-1

microvasculature of the BM comprises a network of sinusoids. Hemopoiesis only occurs in the interstital space between these sinusoids, thereby ensuring that hemopoietic progenitors are located close to the blood supply. Normal BM contains a network of fine branching reticulin fibers between parenchymal cells, which provide the extracellular matrix for the BM. There is a higher concentration of thicker fibers around arterioles and near the endosteum. The BM also has a nerve supply.

Bone marrow trephine biopsy

The process of obtaining a bone marrow trephine biopsy (BMTB) originates in the ancient procedure of trepanning.[1] Prior to the advent of BMTB needles, clot preparations of aspirated marrow were prepared for diagnostic purposes. BM biopsies were obtained only as a means of diagnosis if marrow was inaspirable, a 'dry tap'. The modification of needles by Jamshidi in the 1970s revolutionized the process of obtaining intact cores of bone and bone marrow for examination, primarily from the pelvis. The most common site biopsied is the posterior superior iliac crest. Other sites which can be biopsied include the anterior superior iliac crest, tibia, and vertebrae. Biopsy of the sternum is contraindicated due to the significant morbidity and mortality associated with this practice. The optimal length of a BMTB is 2–3 cm; shorter biopsies may not be representative and may not detect diseases that have a focal or patchy pattern of BM involvement.[2]

Processing and stains

A number of methods are available for fixation, decalcification and embedding of the BMTB[2] (Table 3.1). For optimal evaluation, sections are cut at a thickness of 1–3 μm. Conventional stains are hematoxylin and eosin (H&E) (Fig. 3.1A) and Giemsa (Fig. 3.1B) stains. Giemsa staining generally gives better discrimination of cell types based on cytoplasmic staining characteristics, that is:

1. myeloid/eosinophil granules: red
2. mast cell granules: purplish red
3. erythroid precursor cytoplasm: blue
4. plasma cell cytoplasm: purplish blue
5. perinuclear Golgi complex (hof) also seen as a pale area.

Other stains commonly used include the Perls stain for iron, silver stains for reticulin and Masson's trichrome stain or Martius scarlet blue stain for collagen. Immunohistochemistry (IHC) using monoclonal or polyclonal antibodies, and *in situ* hybridization using nucleic acid probes can be used to identify specific cell types and genetic aberrations; these are discussed in sections below.[3]

Marrow cellularity

The BMTB is particularly useful for the assessment of marrow cellularity. This is the relative amount of BM cells to adipocytes, which is assessed subjectively and should be interpreted in the context of the age of the patient. The terms normocellular (normal for age), hypercellular (increased

Table 3.1 The bone marrow trephine biopsy: processing techniques

Fixatives		Decalcification		Embedding
Neutral buffered formalin	18–24 h	**Chelators**		Paraffin
Bouin's solution	<24 h	EDTA	48 h	Routinely used in histopathology labs and so easily available Immunohistochemistry, FISH and PCR easily feasible
B5 (currently not widely used due to mercury content)	<24 h	Has the advantage of excellent preservation of morphology, antigens and nucleic acids. Only disadvantage is the time taken for decalcification. This can be shortened using heated oscillators, microwave / ultrasound technology		
Schaffer's solution	4–16 h	**Acids**		Plastic[25]
		Formic acid[26]	12–24 h	Not routinely used in most histopathology laboratories. Specialized reagents, equipment and skilled technical staff required. Semithin sections can be cut thus allowing excellent morphologic evaluation. Limited immunohistochemistry and PCR possible
		Nitric acid	6–18 h	
Buffered formalin or zinc formalin		Time for decalcification is dependent on the concentration of the acid. Preservation of antigens and DNA/RNA is directly proportional to the concentration of the acid		
		Quick decalcifiers as Rapid Decal or TBD1 Shandon decalcifier	15–60 min	
Combined fixatives and decalcification agents				
Acetic acid zinc formaldehyde[27]			18 h	
Rapid. Good morphology and antigen preservation. Poor nucleic acid preservation (authors' unpublished observations based on >40 cases run in parallel with EDTA)				
Commercial preparations			Various	
Microwave / ultrasound assisted fixation and decalcification			6–18 h	

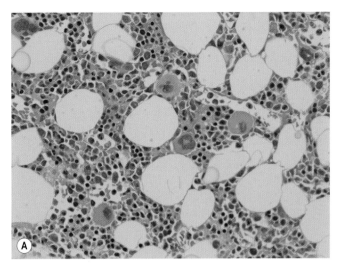
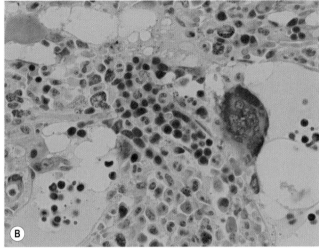

Fig. 3.1 (A, B) Normal bone marrow biopsy showing normal marrow cellularity and architecture. (A) Hematoxylin & Eosin stain. ×200. (B) Giemsa stain. ×400.

Table 3.2 Cellularity ranges for various age groups

Age	Cellularity
Newborn to 3 months	80–100%
Childhood	60–80%
20–40 years	60–70%
40–70 years	40–50%
>70 years	30–40%

cellularity for age) and hypocellular (reduced cellularity for age) are used. Cellularity reduces with increasing age (Table 3.2).[4,5] In practice, the formula (cellularity = 100 − patient age) can be applied for adults; however, it does not correlate with cellularity at the extremes of the age range. The intertrabecular spaces adjacent to the marrow cortex tend to be hypocellular and should not be assessed when determining overall BM cellularity.

Marrow architecture

The BMTB enables the assessment of bone marrow architecture, the distribution of cellular elements and the bone and stromal cells. The outermost elements of the biopsy are composed of collagenous periosteal connective tissue, followed by a zone of cartilage or cortical bone (depending on the age of the patient). After this the bone breaks up into a meshwork of trabeculae, between which are the intertrabecular spaces. Hemopoietic cells are present within these intertrabecular spaces and are supported by fat cells, stromal cells, histiocytes extracellular matrix and blood vessels (Fig. 3.2). The hemopoietic cells are located within the intertrabecular spaces. The intertrabecular areas can be divided into three zones which contain different hemopoietic cell types (Fig. 3.3):

1. *Endosteal or paratrabecular zone*: immediately adjacent to the trabecular bone and composed predominantly of myeloid precursor cells

2. *Intermediate zone*: contains erythroid colonies and maturing myeloid cells
3. *Central zone*: in the center of the intertrabecular space. In addition to erythroid cells and maturing myeloid cells, this contains sinusoids and megakaryocytes.

Small arteries and arterioles are often seen in the intermediate and central zones; these may be surrounded by cuffs of immature myeloid cells around them.

Hemopoiesis

The process of formation of blood elements from hemopoietic stem cells has been described in detail in Chapter 2. The BMTB enables the visualization of the spatial localization of the individual cell lineages during their development. Hemopoietic progenitors are present in cords, islands or clusters. Fully mature erythroid and granulocytic cells and platelets migrate through the sinusoidal endothelial cells to enter the bloodstream.

Erythropoiesis

Erythroid progenitors are found in small and large 'islands' called erythroid colonies within the intermediate and central zones of the marrow cavity. Erythroid islands are made up of concentric circles of immature erythroblasts (proerythroblasts) and a spectrum of maturing erythroid precursors leading to the late erythroblasts. Each erythroid island has a central iron-containing macrophage. The most primitive erythroid progenitor cells are present centrally around the macrophage and the maturing forms towards the periphery[6] (Fig. 3.4). The central macrophage possesses dendritic processes, which extend between the maturing erythroid precursors. Its function is to support and nurture the erythroblasts, act as a source of iron and remove debris from dying cells and extruded nuclei. The central macrophage is often difficult to identify in histologic sections. Erythroid precursors are easily identified by being in distinct islands with cells of varying maturity, their almost perfectly round nuclei and by a perinuclear halo, an artifact of fixation and processing.

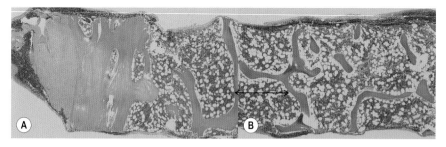

Fig. 3.2 (A, B) Low power view of a bone marrow biopsy. (A) Periosteal connective tissue is seen external to cortical bone. (B) Bone trabeculae with the intertrabecular spaces (one marked – arrow) containing hemopoietic cells and fat cells. ×40.

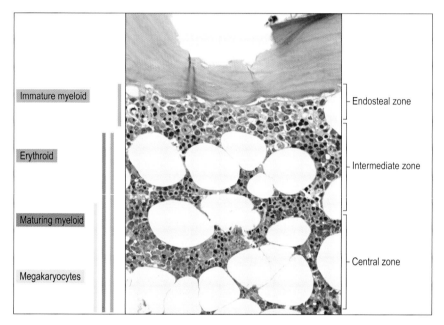

Fig. 3.3 Organization of the bone marrow: zones and distribution of various cell types. ×100.

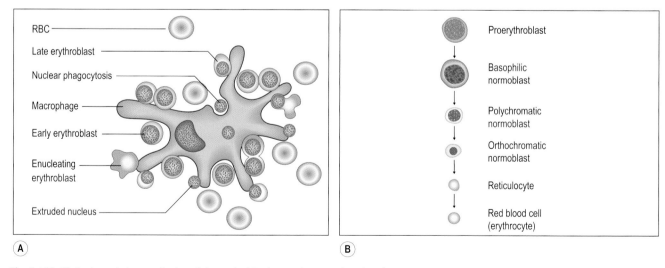

Fig. 3.4 (A, B) Erythropoiesis: organization of the erythroid colony and stages of erythroid maturation. *((A) Modified from Erythroblastic islands: niches for erythropoiesis. Blood 2008; 112: 470; (B) http://www.healthsystem.virginia.edu/internet/haematology/hessimages/erythropoiesis.jpg.)*

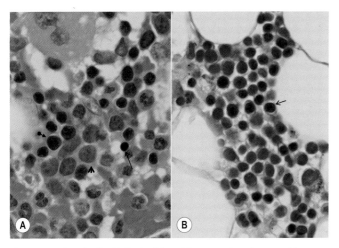

Fig. 3.5 Erythroid cells. (A) Erythroblasts (short arrow), early normoblasts (arrow with a dot) and an extruded erythroid nucleus (long arrow) are seen along with macrophage cytoplasm containing debris. ×400. (B) Erythroid cells showing the round, smooth, hyperchromatic nuclei along with the perinuclear halo artifact (arrow), ×400.

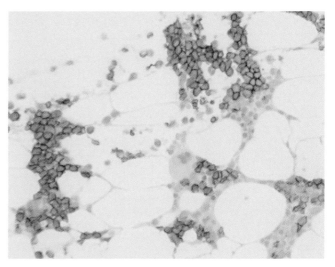

Fig. 3.6 Immunohistochemical staining for glycophorin A. Note nucleated erythroid precursors and RBCs have stained. ×200.

Proerythroblast. The earliest recognizable erythroid precursors (proerythroblasts) are medium to large round cells with minimal cytoplasm, large round nuclei with dispersed or open chromatin, many small nucleoli and a crisp nuclear membrane. A rim of weakly basophilic cytoplasm with a halo is also present (Fig. 3.5A).

Maturing erythroblast (also called normoblast). These are smaller than proerythroblasts, and differ in their nuclear and cytoplasmic characteristics. As a rule, with maturation, nuclear size reduces and the amount of cytoplasm increases. The nuclear chromatin becomes more condensed and acquires a uniform, condensed, hyperchromatic 'ink dot' appearance. It is this nuclear characteristic that enables late normoblasts to be distinguished from lymphocytes. As hemoglobin forms, the cells acquire rims of pale pink cytoplasm (orthochromatic erythroblast) which with further maturation acquires the crisp orangiophilia of mature RBCs (Fig. 3.5B).

Red blood cell. This is the terminally differentiated and most mature erythroid cell. Morphologically, it is an anucleate, orange biconcave disc, with an average size of about 8 μm.

Erythroid cells can be identified by IHC using antibodies to glycophorin A (CD235) or C and intracellular hemoglobin. Glycophorin A highlights both nucleated erythroid precursors and RBCs (Fig. 3.6) while hemoglobin A tends to be restricted to hemoglobinized nucleated erythroid precursors. *In situ* hybridization can also be performed using probes for hemoglobin A.

Granulopoiesis

The granulocytic series consists of neutrophils, eosinophils, basophils and mast cells. All the morphologic stages of myeloid maturation as seen in the BM aspirate can be identified on trephine sections. Most immature granulocytic cells (myeloblasts and promyelocytes) are arranged along the endosteal surface (paratrabecular zone) (Fig. 3.7A, B) or as periarteriolar cuffs (Fig. 3.7C, D); these constitute the granulocytic 'generation zones'; however, precursors are also scattered throughout the rest of the marrow as is often

seen on myeloperoxidase (MPO) staining (Fig. 3.7E, F). Maturing granulocytic cells occur in the intermediate and central intertrabecular zones.

Myeloblast. This is the earliest recognizable granulocytic cell in the BMTB. It is a medium sized cell with a centrally placed round-ovoid nucleus, with very open, pale-staining chromatin which contains one or more fine eosinophilic nucleoli. A small amount of cytoplasm is often present; granules are difficult to identify (Fig. 3.8A).

Promyelocyte. This is a slightly larger cell than the myeloblast with an ovoid nucleus and usually a single, prominent eosinophilic nucleolus. Promyelocytes have moderate amounts of heavily granulated cytoplasm. Promyelocytes often have a paranuclear pale-staining hof and are located in the endosteal zone (Fig. 3.8A).

Myelocyte. Myelocytes are seen in the intermediate zone of the intertrabecular space. They are smaller than promyelocytes with a smaller round to ovoid nucleus with coarser chromatin, and abundant granulated cytoplasm. Myelocytes do not have a nucleolus (Fig. 3.8B).

Metamyelocyte and band form. These are smaller than myelocytes and have an indented or horseshoe-shaped nucleus. Myelocytes and band forms are predominantly located in the central zone of the marrow (Fig. 3.8B).

Neutrophil. Neutrophils are also predominantly located in the central zone and can be identified by their small size and segmented nucleus. Histologically, one is usually able to identify about three segments per neutrophil (Fig. 3.8B). The granulation seen on Romanowsky-stained smears is not appreciable on H&E-stained biopsy sections.

Eosinophils and their precursors. These account for about 1–3% of all BM cells. Mature eosinophils are 10–12 μm sized cells with bi-segmented nuclei. They can be identified by their abundant, coarse eosinophilic cytoplasmic granules, which tend to be refractile. Eosinophil precursors follow the same morphologic maturation pathway as myeloid cells and eosinophil myelocytes and metamyelocytes are easily identified in sections (Fig. 3.9).

Basophils and their precursors. These account for <1% of all bone marrow cells and are difficult to identify on BMTB sections. Basophil granules are water-soluble and therefore do

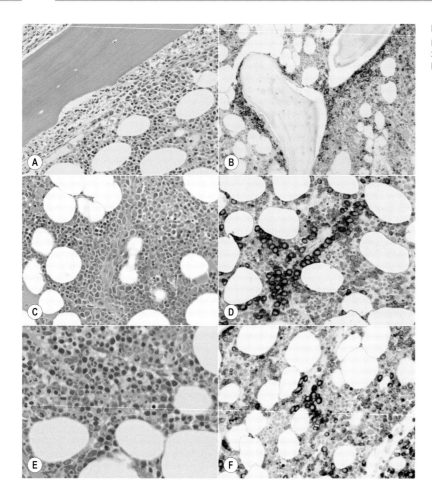

Fig. 3.7 Topography of early myelopoiesis: (A) paratrabecular, ×100; (C) periarteriolar, ×200; (E) interstitial, ×200; (B, D, F) represent the corresponding fields stained by immunohistochemistry for myeloperoxidase.

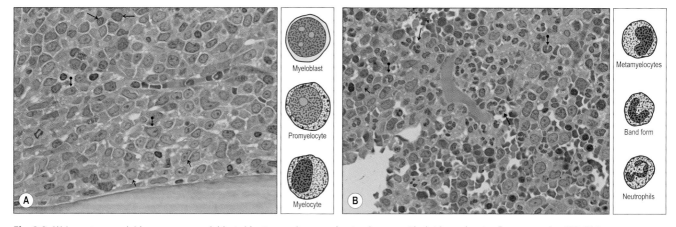

Fig. 3.8 (A) Immature myeloid precursors: myeloblasts (short arrows); promyelocytes (arrows with dots), myelocytes (long arrows). ×600. (B) Late myelopoiesis: metamyelocytes (short arrow); band forms (arrow with dot); neutrophils (long arrows). ×600.

not stain up as one would expect on H&E-stained slides. IHC for CD123 expression highlights basophils and specific antibodies for basophils (2D7, BB1) are available if these need to be visualized on sections.[7]

By immunohistochemistry, myeloid cells are positive for MPO, CD15, CD13, and CD33 (the latter two antibodies are available for use in paraffin sections but CD13 gives better results in flow cytometry). MPO is expressed weakly in myeloblasts, but is prominently expressed from the pro-myelocyte stage. Therefore, MPO preferentially highlights the immature myeloid precursors in the form of crisp, dense cytoplasmic staining, which allows easy visualization of their non-segmented nuclei. MPO staining is preferentially seen in the granulocytic cells that are distributed around the bony trabeculae and as cuffs around blood vessels (Fig. 3.7). Small groups of immature myeloid cells are also often seen in the interstitium away from both the trabeculae and vessels; these can present as cells of very large size with prominent nucleoli and should not be overinterpreted as atypical localization of immature precursors (ALIPs). Terminally differentiated myeloid cells express relatively lower amounts of MPO and thus the intermediate and central region of the intertrabecular space appears to stain weakly. CD15, in contrast, highlights the differentiated forms avidly and the intertrabecular area is therefore more intensely stained (Fig. 3.10A–D).

Myeloid : erythroid ratio

The myeloid : erythroid (M : E) ratio can be assessed in the BMTB on standard stains or with the aid of IHC. In the neonate, the M : E ratio is 1 : 3–4. During life there is an increase in granulocytic cells and reduction in erythroid precursors. In normal adults, the ratio is usually 2–5 : 1. Staining for CD15 is helpful in assessing this ratio as it rather uniformly stains all myeloid cells and if one mentally excludes the small number of megakaryocytes present, most of the remaining negative cells are erythroid cells (Fig. 3.10C).

Megakaryopoiesis

These are the largest cells normally present in the BM (Fig. 3.11). They range from 12 to 150 μm and show considerable variation in shape, size and nuclear configuration. The smaller ones are difficult to identify without IHC. As megakaryocytes develop, DNA synthesis proceeds as polyploidization goes through 8, 16, 32 or 64 n, while lobulation may continue after that; 95% of platelet-shedding megakaryocytes are 16–32 n.[8,9] Megakaryocytes and their precursors are

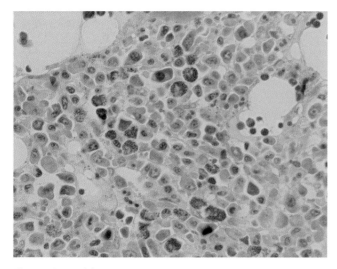

Fig. 3.9 Eosinophil precursors. Giemsa. ×400.

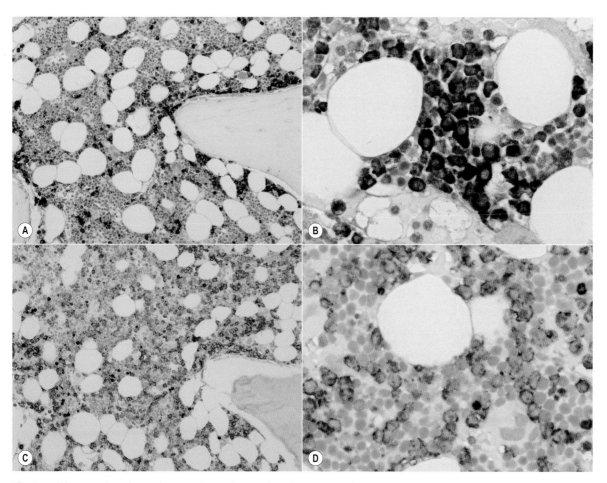

Fig. 3.10 (A) Immunohistochemical staining for myeloperoxidase shows increased staining paratrabecularly. ×100. (C) CD15 staining shows increased intertrabecular expression. ×100. The M : E ratio is also easily assessed on CD15 staining. Intracellular staining patterns of myeloid cells are different using MPO (B) and CD15 (D). ×400.

located centrally, within the BM intermediate and central zones. They are uniformly distributed as single cells and do not normally form clusters.

In sections of normal BM, the following differentiation stages can be recognized.

Megakaryoblast. Cells at this early stage of megakaryocyte development cannot be readily identified on H&E sections but are readily recognizable with immunohistochemical staining (e.g. CD41 and CD42). These cells are medium sized (up to 12–20 μm) and possess an ovoid or reniform nucleus with open, vesicular chromatin and inconspicuous cytoplasm.

Promegakaryocyte. Promegakaryocytes can be recognized in the BMTB. These cells are intermediate stage megakaryocytes (up to 80 μm) and the nucleus shows some lobation.

Mature megakaryocytes. These are large cells with abundant eosinophilic cytoplasm, a large nucleus with vesicular chromatin and small often inconspicuous nucleoli. The nucleus is multi-lobated in 3 dimensional studies and this can usually be appreciated in two dimensional histologic sections. However, depending on which part of the megakaryocyte is present in the plane of the section, the cells can appear spuriously small and the nuclei may appear mono- or hypolobated (Fig. 3.12). While this raises questions about the absolute definition of dysplastic megakaryocytes, the practical way to go about this is to see whether the change is uniform across megakaryocytes within the biopsy – if not then the changes are unlikely to represent dysmegakaryopoesis. Topographically, megakaryocytes are dispersed singly within the intermediate and central zones of the intertrabecular spaces and typically they abut or project into the sinusoids allowing direct platelet shedding. The presence of paratrabecular megakaryocytes indicates a marrow abnormality. Whole megakaryocytes or portions of their cytoplasm may also enter the sinuses and fragment in the vascular system.

Senescent megakaryocyte. After the megakaryocyte has finished shedding its cytoplasm as platelets, all that remains is a round hyperchromatic nucleus with inconspicuous cytoplasm around it. These senescent end-stage megakaryocytes

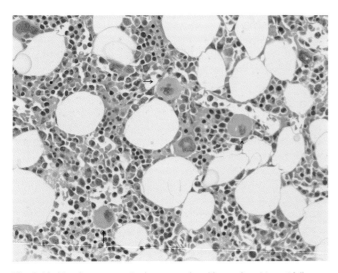

Fig. 3.11 Megakaryocytes, singly scattered and located perisinusoidally. Three cells are seen in close apposition to the sinusoidal wall, extending part of their cytoplasm into the lumen. ×100.

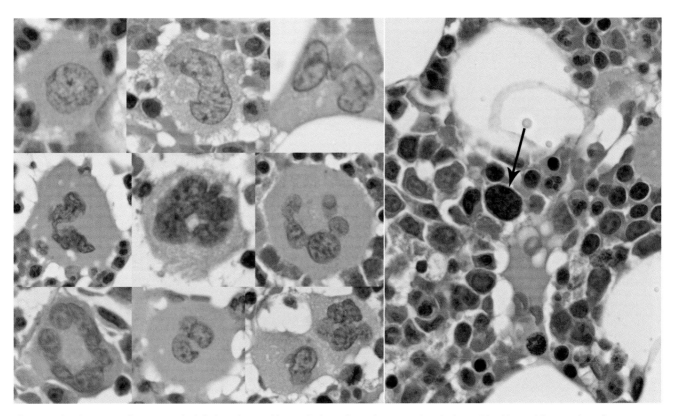

Fig. 3.12 The three rows of images on the left show the variable morphology of megakaryocytes in a single trephine biopsy. A bare nucleus of a senescent megakaryocyte is illustrated on the right (arrow).

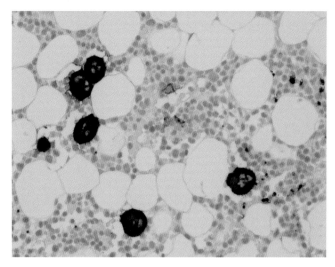

Fig. 3.13 CD61 immunohistochemistry showing normal megakaryocytes. ×200.

appear as 'naked' or 'bare' nuclei in the central zones (Fig. 3.12).

Micromegakaryocyte. This is a small mono- or binucleate megakaryocyte, approximately the size of a promyelocyte. These may be found in small numbers in biopsies from elderly patients and are characteristic in myelodysplasia (see Chapter 20).

There are also some morphologic changes which are uncommonly seen in normal BM. Emperipolesis, the presence of other intact cells (erythroblasts, granulocytes, lymphocytes) within megakaryocyte cytoplasm, may be found in megakaryocytes of any size. The 'engulfed' cells have not been phagocytosed but are passaging through the megakaryocyte cytoplasm (see Chapter 2). This is a benign reactive change with no specific association. Emperipolesis is increasingly common with age; it should not be interpreted as myelodysplasia unless florid or accompanied by other features of dysplasia.

Megakaryocytes have intense cytoplasmic positivity with CD61, CD41 and CD42 antibodies by immunohistochemistry (Fig. 3.13A). Platelets are also positive with these antibodies and these may be seen in the interstitium or vessels (Fig. 3.13B). Platelets can completely surround myeloid and erythroid precursors; these should not be interpreted as micromegakaryocytes or megakaryoblasts. The latter show either intense cytoplasmic staining with a small eccentric nucleus or a crisp membrane stain with negligible cytoplasm and all nucleus.

Macrophages, monocytes and dendritic cells

Macrophages (histiocytes) are present throughout the marrow, where they store and deliver iron to erythroid progenitors (Fig. 3.14) and remove cellular debris by phagocytosis. There are two main types of histiocytic cells in the marrow, the roving monocyte and the fixed, stroma-based dendritic histiocyte (Fig. 3.15A).

Monocyte. Although produced in the BM these are not easily recognized, as they are difficult to distinguish from granulocytic precursors. Monocytes are medium sized cells with oval to kidney-shaped vesicular nuclei and abundant

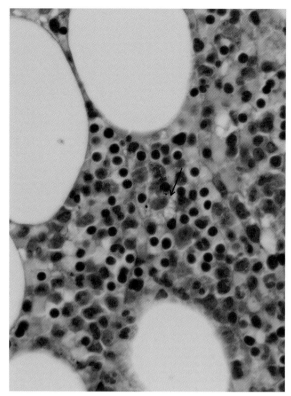

Fig. 3.14 An iron laden macrophage (arrow) in the center of an erythroid colony. ×400.

eosinophilic cytoplasm with no or variable granulation.[10] Monocytes can be identified using IHC for CD68 (PGM1 clone, Fig. 3.15B) and CD14.[11]

Dendritic macrophage. These are large, fixed, stroma based macrophages. CD68 or CD163 highlight their large size and extensively dendritic nature.[12] The dendritic processes of these cells insinuate between hemopoietic cells to form a meshwork which adds to the reticulin based support system (Fig. 3.15C). They have various functions, most revolving around phagocytosis of cellular debris (nuclei, cell membranes, granules, lipid) and iron storage. In cases where the macrophages are activated, CD68 highlights a more bubbly pattern of staining due to the increased number and size of cytoplasmic lysosomal vacuoles.

Iron-containing macrophage. These are responsible for iron storage and release to developing erythroblasts (Fig. 3.14). There are about 16 iron-containing macrophages per mm² of BM.[11] Iron is well demonstrated on H&E as golden brown hemosiderin pigment or on special stains as an olive green pigment (Giemsa) or blue colored reaction product (Perls stain). Iron within tissue reacts with decalcifying agents and biopsies which are decalcified using acids lose iron and are therefore unsuitable for exact quantitation of iron stores.[13] An increased number of iron-laden macrophages is a common finding in post-therapy biopsies and in cases of unsuspected hemachromatosis.

Plasmacytoid dendritic cell. These medium sized cells with vescicular nuclei are difficult to identify on conventional stains. They can be highlighted by CD123 which picks up a few cells in every intertrabecular space (Fig. 3.15D). CD123 is also co-expressed in a subset of granulopoietic precursors and basophils.

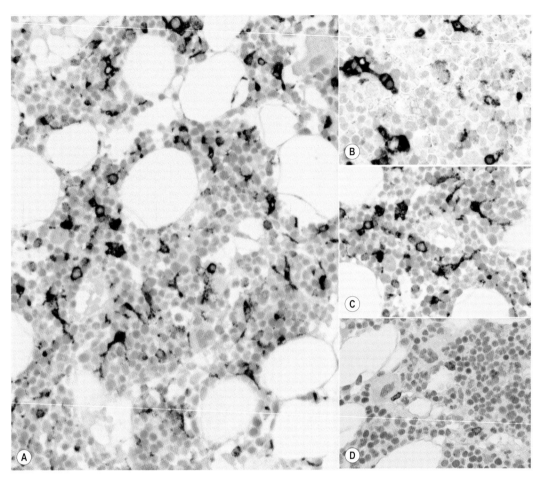

Fig. 3.15 CD68 immunohistochemistry. (A) Showing predominantly dendritic macrophages with fewer monocytes. (B) Monocytes showing peripheral cytoplasmic granular staining. (C) Detail of dendritic macrophages; the contents of the lysosomal vacuoles are unstained and appear as cytoplasmic bubbles. (D) CD123 highlighting a few immature precursors/plasmacytoid dendritic cells. ×200.

Mast cells

Mast cells are distributed throughout the BM; they lie adjacent to the endothelial cells of sinusoids, at the endosteal surface of the trabecular bone, in the periosteum, in the walls of small arteries, scattered in the BM, and frequently at the edges of and within lymphoid aggregates or nodules. Mast cells are round or oval cells characterized by medium sized oval to round hyperchromatic nuclei and moderate to abundant cytoplasm, which is densely packed with granules. The latter are eosinophilic on H&E staining, reddish – purple on Giemsa staining (Fig. 3.16A) and metachromatically purple on Toluidine blue staining. Mast cells can be identified using antibodies to mast cell tryptase and CD117 (Fig. 3.16B, C). Both of these stain normal mast cells in a granular cytoplasmic fashion. The granularity is better appreciated if the mast cell is partly degranulated. Within the periosteum or within zones of fibrosis, normal mast cells may be compressed into a spindle shape, thereby resembling neoplastic mast cells. The paucity of such cells and lack of CD25 and CD2 expression can be used to distinguish between benign and neoplastic cells (see Chapter 26).

Lymphocytes

Lymphoid cells are part of the normal BM population and may constitute 10–15% of the nucleated cells. This is slightly lower than what one sees in aspirates as there is contamination with peripheral blood in those samples. In newborns between 30% and 60% of the nucleated cells in the marrow may be lymphocytes; this figure reduces in adult life and increases again in the elderly, predominantly as a consequence of reduced hemopoiesis and appearance of reactive lymphoid nodules. In children, B-cells are numerous and most are CD10$^+$ precursors. In adults, most marrow lymphocytes are T-cells with few B-lymphocytes present. The B-cell : T-cell ratio is approximately 1 : 4.[14-16] Lymphocytes are rather inconspicuous on conventional stains and their number and distribution are only obvious on immunohistochemistry.

B-lymphocytes. These form a small proportion of adult BM cells. They are predominantly small in size with a few medium sized cells. They stain with B-cell markers PAX5, CD20, CD19 and CD79a and have the phenotype of naive B-cells, i.e. IgM$^+$, IgD$^+$.

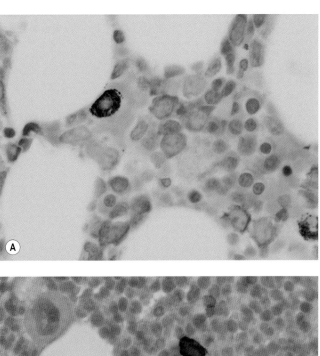

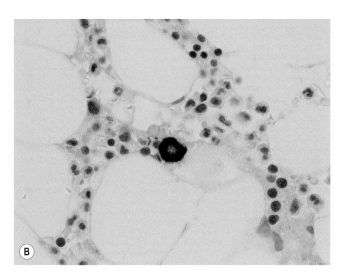

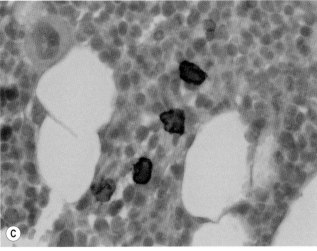

Fig. 3.16 Mast cells. (A) Giemsa. ×400. (B) Mast cells around a sinusoid stained with mast cell tryptase. ×400. (C) CD117. ×200.

T-lymphocytes. The majority of BM lymphocytes are of T-cell origin (CD3 positive) (Fig. 3.17F). The ratio between CD4 (T-helper) and CD8 (cytotoxic) is variable. Normally CD4+ cells are mostly found in lymphoid aggregates and CD8+ cells are diffusely distributed in the BM. It should be noted that weak CD4 staining can also be seen in monocytes/ macrophages and in some granulopoietic precursors. In reactive BM there is often a predominance of cytotoxic CD8+ T-cells and very few CD4+ T-cells. Other T-cell markers (i.e. CD2, CD5, CD7) are positive on most BM T-cells. The cytotoxic molecules TIA-1, granzyme B and perforin may be expressed in a significant number of BM lymphocytes; they are negative on some CD8+ cells. CD25 stains very occasional lymphocytes within the intertrabecular space.

Natural killer cells. These form a small population of BM lymphocytes. They are morphologically nondescript and can be highlighted by CD56, which shows them to have a lymphocyte-like or plasmacytoid appearance with an eccentric nucleus. CD56 staining highlights the wrinkled nature of the cytoplasmic membrane, which helps in differentiating

these from neoplastic plasma cells. One has to be aware that CD56 also stains osteoblasts and can be positive in tumors with neuroendocrine differentiation.

Lymphoid nodules. These are nodular aggregates of lymphocytes seen within the interstitium and are often termed as 'nodular interstitial lymphoid aggregates' (NILA). Their incidence increases with age, and it is estimated that biopsies from about 30–40% of elderly patients harbor these; especially females and those suffering from autoimmune conditions. All lymphoid nodules show an increased reticulin fiber content.[17] Three types are recognized:

1. *Nodular lymphoid aggregates*. These are round collections of lymphocytes with circumscribed but ill defined boundaries. They are composed predominantly of small lymphocytes with very few medium and large forms. Most of the cells within these are CD3+, CD4+ T-lymphocytes (Fig. 3.17A, B, C).
2. *Lymphoid nodules with germinal centers*. These display a germinal center often surrounded by a mantle zone

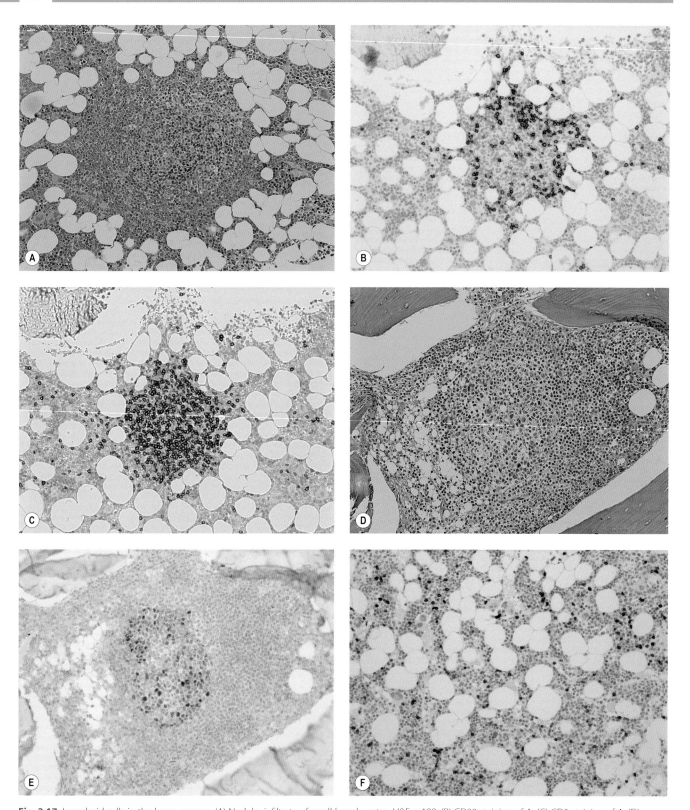

Fig. 3.17 Lymphoid cells in the bone marrow. (A) Nodular infiltrate of small lymphocytes. H&E. ×100. (B) CD20 staining of A. (C) CD3 staining of A. (D) Nodular infiltrate with germinal center. (E) Bcl-6 highlighting the germinal center cells in D. (F) CD3 positive T-cells present in the bone marrow.

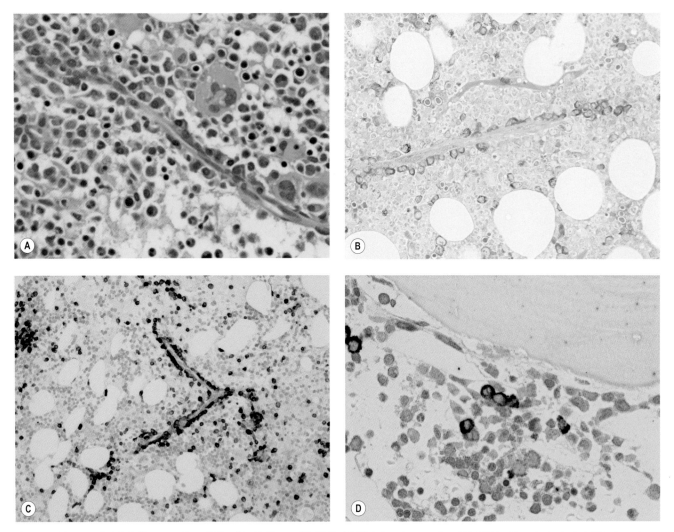

Fig. 3.18 Plasma cells. (A) Cuffing a capillary. H&E. ×400. (B) Giemsa. (C) CD138 highlighting plasma cells. ×200. (D) Double color *in situ* hybridization using kappa (brown) and lambda (red) probes. ×400.

(Fig. 3.17D, E). The germinal center cells are Bcl-6⁺, CD10⁺, Bcl-2-negative B-lymphocytes; the mantle cells express IgM and IgD. CD21⁺ follicular dendritic cell meshworks are present. Small numbers of T-cells are seen within and around these aggregates. BM involvement by marginal zone lymphoma often simulates this pattern and care must be taken to exclude this possibility. PCR to evaluate B-cell clonality is often needed for this discrimination.

3. *T-lymphocyte micronodules.* These are small collections of CD3⁺, CD8⁺ T-lymphocytes, and are often seen in marrows showing reactive changes. These are invariably accompanied by an increase in interstitial T-lymphocytes.

Plasma cells

Plasma cells account for about 2–4% of all BM nucleated cells and are found perivascularly, as single scattered cells, or as small groups of 2–3 cells within the interstitium (Fig. 3.18).[18] Plasma cells have an eccentric nucleus with a coarse cart-wheel chromatin pattern, a perinuclear hof and mildly basophilic or amphophilic cytoplasm. Immunohistochemically, normal plasma cells express CD19 (membrane), CD79a (intense cytoplasmic), CD138 (membrane) and MUM-1 (strong nuclear positivity with a lighter cytoplasmic blush); they are CD20 and CD45 negative. Plasma cells express cytoplasmic immunoglobulin heavy chains in the following proportion: IgG > IgA > IgM > IgD. Kappa and lambda light chains are expressed in a 2–3 : 1 ratio.

Hemopoietic stem cells and early precursor cells

These are pluripotent hemopoietic cells which are capable of self-replication or generating more differentiated hemopoietic cells (see Chapter 2 for details). These are difficult to identify on standard morphology as they make up only <1–4% of cells and do not have distinctive features. They are medium sized cells with a high nuclear : cytoplasmic ratio and inconspicuous or small nucleoli. Stem cell markers include CD34, CD117, HLA-DR and TdT. Evaluation of the normal BM with these antibodies highlights variable numbers and types of cells.

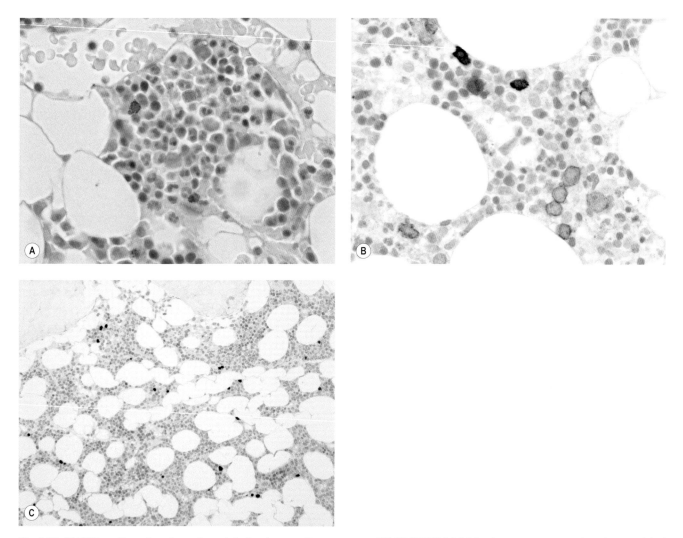

Fig. 3.19 (A) CD34 positive cells and vascular endothelium in normal bone marrow. ×100. (B) CD117 highlighting immature precursors (membrane staining) and mast cells (cytoplasmic staining). ×200. (C) TdT highlighting singly scattered hematogones. ×100.

CD34. This is the most useful marker for stem cells but also stains endothelial cells. Staining is granular and cytoplasmic and highlights medium sized, often ovoid cells scattered within the interstitium (Fig. 3.19A). Studies have shown that small numbers of these cells are found in normal and reactive marrows with an average of 1 cell for every 4–5 high power fields.[19,20] In normal BM, CD34+ cells account for <1% of all nucleated cells. In children, CD34+ cells are more numerous due to the presence of CD34-positive B-cell precursors. Interestingly, the positive cells are located interstitially and are not associated with either erythroid colonies or early myeloid progenitors on the endosteal surface.

CD117. Expression is seen in stem cells, promyelocytes and early erythroid precursors. Staining is membranous and usually highlights large cells which morphologically equate to erythroblasts and promyelocytes (Fig. 3.19B). These usually account for 1–3% of nucleated bone marrow cells. CD117 also stains some plasma cells (membrane or cytoplasmic staining, especially in myeloma) and mast cells (granulated forms: dense cytoplasmic positivity; degranulated forms: weak granular cytoplasmic positivity to rare membranous positivity).

Lymphoblasts or immature lymphoid cells. Lymphoblasts, or hematogones, are identified in large numbers in marrows from infants and children (324/mm²) but the numbers reduce markedly in adult life (6/mm²). Biopsies following therapy or transplantation characteristically show larger numbers of these cells. They can be identified by their expression of TdT (nuclear stain)[21] and in the adult marrow are seen as a few singly scattered interstitial cells without nodule formation. They also variably express CD34, CD38, CD79a, CD10 and PAX5 antigens but only small fractions are positive for CD20. Diagnostic difficulties arise while assessing post-therapy staging marrows from acute lymphoblastic leukemia patients. Nodule formation and an aberrant phenotype are useful indicators of relapsed disease.[22]

The bone marrow stroma

Stromal cells

The stroma provides the framework 'scaffolding' for hemopoiesis. The stroma consists of fat cells, histiocytic cells, fibroblasts and their fibrils, and blood vessels including the

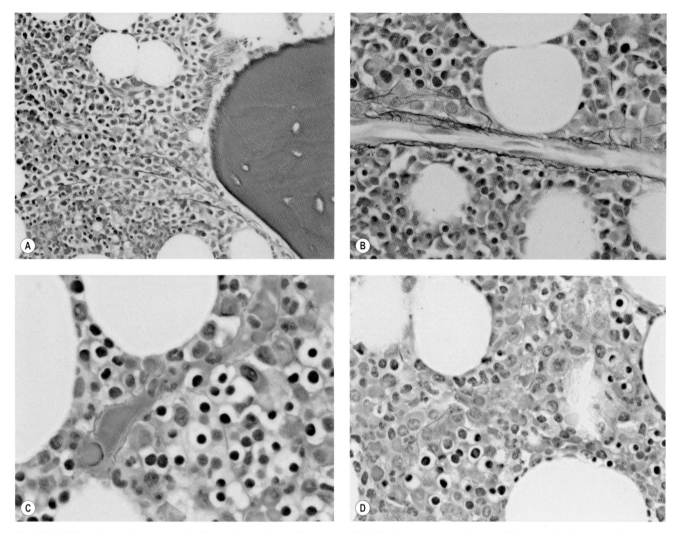

Fig. 3.20 (A) Reticulin attaching/originating from trabecular bone. Gomori stain. (B) Reticulin around a blood vessel. (C) Reticulin forming the wall of a sinusoid. ×400. (D) Typical distribution and density of reticulin in a normal adult marrow. ×200.

sinusoids. Fat cells occupy variable proportions of BM volume depending on the age of the patient. They serve a supporting, filling and metabolic function. Fibroblasts are spindle-shaped cells with elongated vesicular nuclei with small nucleoli and cytoplasmic processes. These are not readily identified on routine H&E sections, but are responsible for extracellular matrix and fiber production.

The extracellular matrix

The extracellular matrix (ECM) consists of a variety of components; these are mainly glycoproteins and proteoglycans, which are produced by the stromal cells. ECM components include cell adhesion molecules, collagen, fibronectin, vitronectin, as well as the growth and other factors involved in the highly complex regulatory mechanisms controlling the production of the formed elements of the blood. Histologically, ECM is seen only in reparative and pathologic conditions (e.g. post-chemotherapy, gelatinous transformation, etc.).

Reticulin

Hemopoietic cells are supported by a fine meshwork of reticulin fibers which act as scaffolding within the intertrabecular space. The fibers, which are produced by elongated fibroblasts, span the intertrabecular space and are tethered to the endosteal surface of the bone. They also form cuffs around blood vessels, provide the structural framework for sinusoids and frame adipocytes (Fig. 3.20). Reticulin fibers are best visualized by silver staining (Gömöri stain) and in sections of the normal marrow are seen as short, single, thin fibers which abruptly terminate without intersecting with other fibers (an artifact of section thickness) (Fig. 3.20). The amount of reticulin is graded semi-quantitatively; there is little reticulin in normal BM and the amount should be related to the total BM cellularity.

Collagen

In normal BM collagen is found around blood vessels and in the bone trabeculae. Masson's trichrome stain (Fig. 3.21)

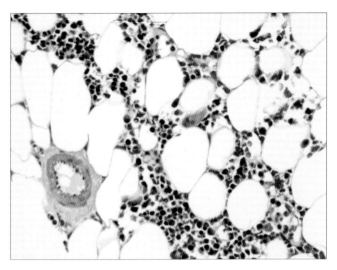

Fig. 3.21 Collagen fibers (green) seen around a blood vessel. Note the lack of collagen between the hemopoetic cells. Masson's trichrome stain. ×200.

Table 3.3 Grading systems for bone marrow fibrosis

Bauermeister/modified Bauermeister[23]		European consensus/WHO 2008[5]	
1	Occasional fine individual reticulin fibers and foci of a fine fiber network	0	Scattered linear reticulin with no intersections (crossovers) corresponding to normal bone marrow
2	Diffuse fine reticulin fiber network. No coarse fibers	1	Loose network of reticulin with many intersections, especially in perivascular areas
3	Scattered thick coarse reticulin fibers present. No collagen fibers	2	Diffuse and dense increase in reticulin with extensive intersections, occasionally with only focal bundles of collagen and/or focal osteosclerosis
4	Diffuse, often coarse reticulin fiber network. Collagen fibers present	3	Diffuse and dense increase in reticulin with extensive intersections, with coarse bundles of collagen often associated with significant osteosclerosis

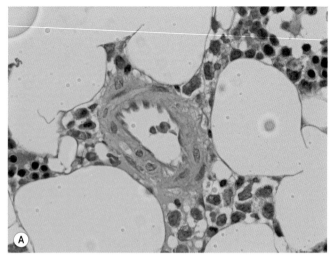

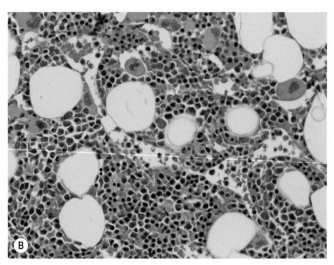

Fig. 3.22 Blood vessels in normal bone marrow. (A) Arteriole. ×400. (B) Sinusoid. ×100.

and Martius scarlet blue do not reveal any collagen fibers within the interstitium (i.e. in between hemopoetic cells).

Reticulin and collagen grading

The reticulin and collagen fiber content of BM is graded semi-quantitatively. The reticulin content may be increased or is the defining feature of various disease processes. Several scoring systems have been devised of which two are commonly used (Table 3.3).[5,23,24] There are several issues to be considered while evaluating reticulin fibers. Demonstration of cuffs of reticulin fibers around blood vessels and at the endosteal surface of bone where the fibers are easily visualized is evidence that the stain has worked appropriately. Only areas containing hemopoietic cells should be graded;

fibers around blood vessels, framing adipocytes, and those in or around lymphoid nodules should not be evaluated. Assesment of whether stains for collagen have worked is best done by looking for arterial blood vessels which always have a peripheral cuff of collagen.

Blood vessels

The medullary arteries enter via the cortical bone and branch within the BM and the trabeculae. The smaller branches divide into arterioles, then into capillaries and into the sinusoids. The sinusoidal wall is thin consisting of a single layer of endothelial cells, an incomplete outer covering of adventitia and, when large, a very loose network of reticulin fibers (Fig. 3.22). The sinusoids are present throughout the BM and drain into the periosteal veins. The endothelial cells of post-capillary, or post-sinusoidal venules may be plump, with vesicular nuclei and distinct nucleoli. The endothelium forms the interface between the intra- and the extravascular compartments through which the blood cells enter the circulation, and the sinus endothelial cells possibly contribute to regulation of entry of mature cells into the circulation. In histologic sections, megakaryocytes can often be seen close

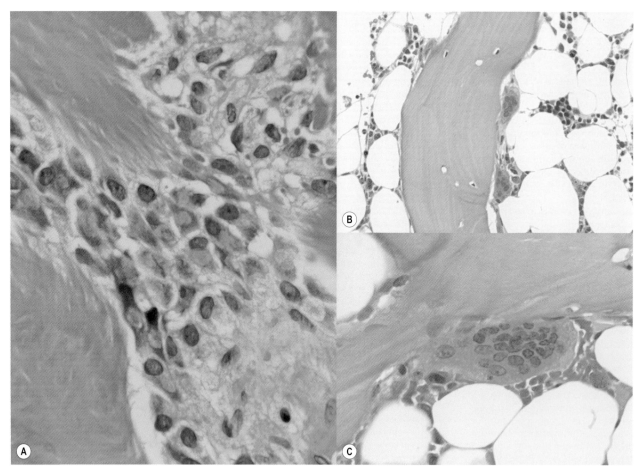

Fig. 3.23 (A) Osteoblasts. ×400. (B) Osteoclasts in Howship's lacunae. ×100. (C) Higher power view of an osteoclast. ×400.

to the sinusoids into which they discharge platelets. Sinusoids are often difficult to identify in histologic sections as they are collapsed. They are easily identified by the Gömöri stain which highlights the rim of reticulin fibers around the sinusoids. Immunohistochemically, endothelial cells express vascular markers, that is, CD34 and CD31. Blood vessels may supply additional information in diseases which affect them, especially amyloidosis.

Nerves

Nerves are rarely found in biopsy sections, but occasionally may be seen adjacent to blood vessels in the periosteum.

Bone

The bone is covered externally by a layer of dense collagenous tissue, the periosteum. This abuts a layer of cortical bone or cartilage (the latter is invariably seen in children and often in elderly patients). It is beyond the scope of this chapter to discuss the normal architecture of bone, but a few comments will be made about bone forming and resorbing cells. Trabeculae are composed of lamellar bone. Osteoblasts (Fig. 3.23A) produce new bone and are often seen lining the bone trabeculae when the latter are subject to stress. They are large cells with abundant eosinophilic cytoplasm, a prominent paranuclear hof and an eccentric vesicular nucleus and a prominent nucleolus. Osteoclasts (Fig. 3.23B, C) are very large multinucleated cells which resorb bone and are often seen in indentations of the trabeculae known as Howship lacunae. They have abundant cytoplasm and possess multiple small nuclei with nucleoli. The portion of the cytoplasm abutting bone is often ruffled and the bone surface is also ragged, thus illustrating the resorptive function of these cells. Osteocytes are present within bone and are seen within lacunae and have densely stained nuclei.

References

1. Parapia LA. Trepanning or trephines: a history of bone marrow biopsy. Br J Haematol 2007;139:14–9.
2. Lee SH, Erber WN, Porwit A, et al. ICSH guidelines for the standardization of bone marrow specimens and reports. Int J Lab Hematol 2008;30:349–64.
3. Torlakovic EE, Naresh K, Kremer M, et al. Call for a European programme in external quality assurance for bone marrow immunohistochemistry; report of a European Bone Marrow Working Group pilot study. J Clin Pathol 2009;62:547–51.
4. Foucar K. Bone Marrow Pathology 2nd ed. ASCP Press; Chicago, USA; 2001.

5. Thiele J, Kvasnicka HM, Facchetti F, et al. European consensus on grading bone marrow fibrosis and assessment of cellularity. Haematologica 2005;90: 1128–32.

6. Chasis JA, Mohandas N. Erythroblastic islands: niches for erythropoiesis. Blood 2008;112:470–8.

7. Agis H, Krauth MT, Mosberger I, et al. Enumeration and immunohistochemical characterisation of bone marrow basophils in myeloproliferative disorders using the basophil specific monoclonal antibody 2D7. J Clin Pathol 2006;59: 396–402.

8. Kaushansky K. Historical review: megakaryopoiesis and thrombopoiesis. Blood 2008;111:981–6.

9. Deutsch VR, Tomer A. Megakaryocyte development and platelet production. Br J Haematol 2006;134:453–66.

10. Dale DC, Boxer L, Liles WC. The phagocytes: neutrophils and monocytes. Blood 2008;112:935–45.

11. Naresh KN. Morphological evaluation of monocytes and monocyte precursors in bone marrow trephine biopsies – need for establishing diagnostic criteria. Haematologica 2009;94:1623–4.

12. Thiele J, Braeckel C, Wagner S, et al. Macrophages in normal human bone marrow and in chronic myeloproliferative disorders: an immunohistochemical and morphometric study by a new monoclonal antibody (PG-M1) on trephine biopsies. Virchows Arch A Pathol Anat Histopathol 1992;421:33–9.

13. Stuart-Smith SE, Hughes DA, Bain BJ. Are routine iron stains on bone marrow trephine biopsy specimens necessary? J Clin Pathol 2005;58:269–72.

14. Horny HP, Engst U, Walz RS, Kaiserling E. In situ immunophenotyping of lymphocytes in human bone marrow: an immunohistochemical study. Br J Haematol 1989;71:313–21.

15. Horny HP, Wehrmann M, Griesser H, et al. Investigation of bone marrow lymphocyte subsets in normal, reactive, and neoplastic states using paraffin-embedded biopsy specimens. Am J Clin Pathol 1993;99:142–9.

16. Thaler J, Greil R, Dietze O, Huber H. Immunohistology for quantification of normal bone marrow lymphocyte subsets. Br J Haematol 1989;73:576–7.

17. Thiele J, Zirbes TK, Kvasnicka HM, Fischer R. Focal lymphoid aggregates (nodules) in bone marrow biopsies: differentiation between benign hyperplasia and malignant lymphoma – a practical guideline. J Clin Pathol 1999;52:294–300.

18. Kass L, Kapadia IH. Perivascular plasmacytosis: a light-microscopic and immunohistochemical study of 93 bone marrow biopsies. Acta Haematol 2001;105:57–63.

19. Soligo D, Delia D, Oriani A, et al. Identification of CD34+ cells in normal and pathological bone marrow biopsies by QBEND10 monoclonal antibody. Leukemia 1991;5:1026–30.

20. Horny HP, Wehrmann M, Schlicker HU, et al. QBEND10 for the diagnosis of myelodysplastic syndromes in routinely processed bone marrow biopsy specimens. J Clin Pathol 1995;48:291–4.

21. Wolf E, Harms H, Winkler J, et al. Terminal deoxynucleotidyl transferase-positive cells in trephine biopsies following bone marrow or peripheral stem cell transplantation reflect vigorous B-cell generation. Histopathology 2005; 46:442–50.

22. Rimsza LM, Larson RS, Winter SS, et al. Benign hematogone-rich lymphoid proliferations can be distinguished from B-lineage acute lymphoblastic leukemia by integration of morphology, immunophenotype, adhesion molecule expression, and architectural features. Am J Clin Pathol 2000;114:66–75.

23. Bauermeister DE. Quantitation of bone marrow reticulin – a normal range. Am J Clin Pathol 1971;56:24–31.

24. Kuter DJ, Bain B, Mufti G, et al. Bone marrow fibrosis: pathophysiology and clinical significance of increased bone marrow stromal fibres. Br J Haematol 2007;139:351–62.

25. Krenacs T, Bagdi E, Stelkovics E, et al. How we process trephine biopsy specimens: epoxy resin embedded bone marrow biopsies. J Clin Pathol 2005; 58:897–903.

26. Wickham CL, Sarsfield P, Joyner MV, et al. Formic acid decalcification of bone marrow trephines degrades DNA: alternative use of EDTA allows the amplification and sequencing of relatively long PCR products. Mol Pathol 2000; 53:336.

27. Naresh KN, Lampert I, Hasserjian R, et al. Optimal processing of bone marrow trephine biopsy: the Hammersmith Protocol. J Clin Pathol 2006;59:903–11.

CHAPTER 4

Regulation of hematopoiesis

SM Buckley, C Verfaillie

Chapter contents

Introduction

Hematopoiesis, including both myelopoiesis and lymphopoiesis, is maintained throughout life by hematopoietic stem cells (HSC). Hematopoietic cells can first be detected in the yolk sac,[1] followed by the aorta-gonad-mesonephros (AGM) region of the embryo proper.[2,3] HSC then migrate from the AGM region to the fetal liver,[4] where they undergo extensive self-renewal to generate a sufficiently large pool of HSC to sustain hematopoiesis throughout adult life.[5] Prior to birth HSC seed the bone marrow (BM), and the BM becomes the primary site of hematopoiesis throughout adult life.[6] To ascertain that sufficient mature blood cells are generated, hematopoietic cell production is a highly regulated process in which the majority of HSC remain quiescent under steady-state conditions, but may be induced to proliferate under conditions of stress. By contrast, the first descendants from HSC, hematopoietic progenitor cells (HPC), proliferate extensively prior to maturing to terminally differentiated cells. Although significant insights have been gained in the processes that regulate self-renewal and differentiation of HSC, which will be reviewed here, these processes remain incompletely understood. This chapter will highlight a number of the processes that are responsible for

coordinating self-renewal and differentiation of HSC and HPC to ensure the controlled generation of mature blood elements under steady-state conditions and conditions of stress. Although we do address mechanisms underlying leukemogenesis or syndromes of hematopoietic failure, it follows that if any of the delicately controlled processes that will be discussed fail, insufficient or excess cells can be produced leading to these disease states.

Characteristics of hematopoietic stem and progenitor cells

The minimal definition of an HSC is a cell capable of extensive self-renewal as well as generation of both myeloid and lymphoid progeny. The concept of the hematopoietic stem cell was first proposed in the 1950s after researchers discovered that lethally irradiated mice could be rescued from BM aplasia by transplanting cells from healthy mouse BM or spleen.[7] Subsequent studies demonstrated that HSC possess the unique property to self-renew and maintain the hematopoietic system throughout life. The HSC is capable of generating all blood cell lineages. During postnatal life, HSC reside in the BM where they constitute less than 0.01%

©2011 Elsevier Ltd
DOI: 10.1016/B978-0-7020-3147-2.00004-3

of the total cell population.[8] Many studies over the last two to three decades have developed tools to characterize HSC and their descendants. This has led to the development of a hematopoietic cell hierarchy wherein HSC are at the top of the hierarchy generating progressively more lineage committed cells which coincides with decreased self-renewal and proliferative potential.

HSC are the only cells that reconstitute hematopoiesis long term, and proliferate rarely *in vivo*. Studies using BrdU labeling in mouse HSC estimate the frequency of HSC division to be somewhere around once every month;[9] however, studies using biotin label or histon 2B-GFP transgenic mice have suggested that multiple populations of HSC exist with different division kinetics and that slow dividing HSC only very rarely exist. The division rate of these different populations of HSC ranges between 0.5% per day and once every 145 days.[10–12] In larger mammals, felines and non-human primates, both retroviral marking and telomere length have been used to evaluate frequency of HSC division.[13,14] HSC divide in felines about once every 8 weeks,[13] in non-human primates once every 25–35 weeks,[14] and in humans once every year.[15] Hematopoietic progenitor cells (HPC), by contrast, cannot reconstitute the hematopoietic system for the life of the recipient. However, in contrast to HSC, HPC proliferate actively to generate the millions of hematopoietic cells generated daily. At the bottom of the hierarchy are the terminally differentiated hematopoietic cells.

Phenotypic characterization

Although HSC in the mouse have been enriched to 100% purity,[16] the exact phenotype of human HSC is not known, because of lack of accurate functional assays that allow enumeration of human HSC. The CD34+ population of hematopoietic cells has been shown to possess the majority of hematopoietic repopulating activity in humans, and is known to enrich for hematopoietic progenitors.[17–19] Primitive human progenitors that can initiate long-term cultures or can repopulate immunodeficient animals are lineage−, CD34+, CD133+, CD38−, HLA-DR^{low}, c-Kit+ and Thy1^{low}, and Lin−CD34+CD38− cells contain approximately 0.1% primitive progenitors that can repopulate the hematopoietic system of severe combined immunodeficient (SCID) mice (SCID-repopulating cells (SRC)).[17,20–23] Although HPC are also CD34+, they co-express CD38, as well as cell surface proteins associated to specific lineages, such as CD33 (myeloid lineage),[24] CD19 and CD10 (B-lymphoid) or CD7 (NK and T-lymphoid).[25–27] Recent studies have indicated that some of the cell surface antigens previously thought to be expressed only on more differentiated cells may be present on HSC, making the characterization of human HSC even more difficult. For instance, CD33 which had been thought only to be on myeloid cells is also expressed on cord blood HSC.[28]

As stem cells are quiescent, they are spared from cell cycle-specific cytotoxic agents such as 5-fluorouracil, a method used frequently to enrich murine BM for HSC.[29,30] In addition, stem cells express functional multidrug resistance proteins, such as p-glycoprotein (MDR1),[31] and breast cancer related protein (BCRP),[32] which extrude toxins from the cell. This allows selection of stem cells based on their ability to, for instance, extrude the dyes Rhodamine or

Hoechst 33342.[31,33] Combining these functional characteristics of HSC to cell-surface markers further enriches for human HSC, and 1/30 Rho^{lo}Lin−CD34+CD38− cells are SRC.[34]

Functional characterization

Even if we now can enrich for HSC using fluorescent activated cell sorting procedures, identification of HSC continues to depend on assays that measure stem cell function. Committed HPC can be assessed using colony-forming assays, where colony forming unit (CFU)- granulocyte-macrophage (GM), burst-forming-unit (BFU)-E, CFU-Mix can be enumerated. An additional primitive HPC subset is the high proliferative potential colony-forming cells (HPP-CFC).[35] Even though HPP-CFC generate visible myeloid cell colonies and can be replated to generate new HPP-CFC, demonstrating their extensive self-renewal ability, they do not correspond to HSC.

Dexter and colleagues demonstrated in the late 1970s that long-term hematopoiesis could be established *in vitro*, by plating BM cells in the presence of fetal calf and horse serum. They demonstrated that this leads to the establishment of an adherent feeder of stromal cells, where hematopoietic progenitors proliferate for several weeks while generating more mature progeny.[36] Subsequent adaptations of this culture system, wherein hematopoietic supportive stromal feeders are first established, whereupon hematopoietic cells can be seeded, has allowed investigators to quantify primitive hematopoietic progenitors, also termed long-term culture initiating cells (LTC-IC). LTC-IC can generate more committed CFC in a sustained manner (5 to more than 20 weeks).[37,38] Although there is evidence in mice that the number of LTC-IC may correlate with repopulating HSC as progeny are only of the myeloid lineage, this assay cannot assess the frequency of true HSC.[39] *In vitro* assays have also been developed to assess the lymphoid potential of human primitive progenitor cells, all of which also require specific microenvironments (BM stroma or stromal cell lines for B-lymphocytes, NK and dendritic cell differentiation, and either thymus derived feeders or other feeders engineered to express Notch ligands for T-cell differentiation).[40–44] As is true for the LTC-IC assays described above, only lymphoid differentiation can be assessed in the latter assays, and thus again not true HSC activity. To assess the ability of cells to generate both myeloid and lymphoid progeny, 'switch' cultures have been developed in which the ability of single cells to give rise to both myeloid and lymphoid long-term culture initiating cells can be tested.[43,45,46] Enumeration of the frequency of single cells that have the ability to generate both myeloid and lymphoid progeny comes close to assessment of HSC; however, it cannot address homing and engraftment, nor the true long-term expansion ability of cells.

In mice, HSC can be assessed by transplantation into irradiated animals. When this is done in competition with a known source of repopulating cells, the ability of putative HSC to compete with other HSC can be assessed, and when this is combined with limiting dilution analyses, the absolute frequency of repopulating cells can be measured.[47–50] In general engraftment is evaluated at 4 months following transplantation; it is, however, clear that the cells generating progeny for only 4 months *in vivo* may not represent long-term repopulating (LTR-)HSC. Therefore, some groups evaluate engraftment at 8–10 months after transplantation to demonstrate presence of LTR-HSC,[51] whereas others perform secondary transplantations to allow assessment of self-renewal ability of HSC.[52,53] The development of xenogeneic transplant models in immuno-incompetent animals (immunodeficient mice such as severe combined immunodeficient (SCID) mice,[54] non-obese diabetic (NOD)-SCID mice[22] or NOD-SCID mice also lacking the gamma-c receptor ($\gamma c^{-/-}$),[55] beige-nude-SCID (BNX) mice[56] and Rag2$^{-/-}$ $\gamma c^{-/-}$,[57] or preimmune fetal lambs[58]) has provided in vivo models that allow not only demonstration of multilineage differentiation but also self-renewal and repopulating ability of human cells. As human HSC have to repopulate a xenogeneic microenvironment, which may support homing, growth and differentiation of human HSC with decreased efficiency compared with a syngeneic human microenvironment, it remains to be proven that these assays enumerate all human HSC. Researchers are therefore trying to further improve mouse models for human HSC transplantation by for instance humanizing certain growth factors that poorly cross-react with human cells and/or HLA antigens to increase the efficiency of human cells to repopulate xenogeneic animal models and develop into a fully competent hematopoietic system.[59] Finally, testing of the effect of certain manipulations on stem cells can also be done in large animals including non-human primate or canine models.[60–63]

Hematopoietic stem cell fate decisions: symmetrical vs. asymmetrical

To continually replenish mature hematopoietic cells (many millions a day), HSC must divide to generate progenitors, while at the same time mechanisms need to be in place to ascertain that HSC pool is maintained. As already discussed above, HSC rarely divide in postnatal life, and proliferation is mainly seen in the more committed progenitor pool. Nevertheless, under steady-state conditions HSC divide intermittently and this is increased under stress conditions. To ascertain that the HSC pool is maintained, HSC need to undergo, at a minimum, asymmetrical cell divisions whereby one of the daughter cells is a new HSC or under conditions of stress, such as after transplantation of a small number of HSC, symmetrical cell divisions such that both daughter cells retain HSC characteristics and the small HSC pool is expanded. Exactly how self-renewal of HSC is regulated is not yet fully understood and much less yet is known regarding mechanisms underlying asymmetric and symmetric self-renewing cell divisions. It is thought that both extrinsic cues that regulate stem cell division, provided by the microenvironment wherein they reside (also termed niche), as well as events intrinsic to the HSC are responsible in combination to regulate HSC fate.

That asymmetrical vs. symmetrical divisions occur in stem cell compartments has most elegantly been demonstrated in the model organisms such as Caenorhabditis elegans and Drosophila. One example is the fate of Drosophila germ stem cells (GSC). In the Drosophila testes, approximately 12 non-dividing somatic hub cells, located at the apical tip, make up the niche to which 5–9 GSC are attached in a characteristic rosette pattern.[64] When GSC divide, one spindle pole associates with the GSC-niche interface.[65] The daughter cell that remains attached to the hub cell continues to have stem cell properties, whereas the second cell, no longer attached to the hub, differentiates. The location of the GSC in Drosophila directs the fate of the cells, which has been shown to depend in part on Notch, TGFβ, and Jak/Stat signaling.

It has been shown in both C. Elegans and Drosophila that the plane of the mitotic spindle also appears to predict which daughter cell remains a progenitor/stem cell and which daughter cell differentiates. As the exact niche for HSC is not known, in vivo studies related to symmetrical and asymmetrical divisions of HSC depend on in vitro studies. These studies have shown that when primitive hematopoietic progenitor cells are cultured in vitro, they divide asymmetrically yielding one daughter cell with characteristics of the original cell and the other daughter cell having more differentiated characteristics.[66] There is also preliminary evidence that a number of molecules, such as CD53, CD62L/L-selectin, CD63/lamp-3, and CD71/transferrin receptor, distribute asymmetrically which may govern the fate decisions.[67]

Early during development, HSC undergo symmetrical self-renewing cell divisions to generate the pool of stem cells required throughout adult life. This occurs between e14 and e18 of fetal liver development in mice. It is believed that characteristics intrinsic to the HSC as well as factors provided by the fetal liver (FL) niche must be responsible for the symmetrical divisions of HSC, and hence the net increase in HSC during this period of development. Bowie et al. demonstrated that HSC in the fetal liver are indeed significantly less quiescent than those found early postnatally.[68–70] They also demonstrated that this can be explained by a number of cell intrinsic differences between FL HSC and BM HSC, including expression of some but not all of the known transcription factors and cell cycle proteins known to be involved in self-renewal of HSC, as well as differences in response to exogenous cytokines, including SCF and CXCL12. Whether the nature of the cell extrinsic signals in fetal liver stem cell niches differ from those in postnatal BM niches, to favor expansion of HSC, is not yet known but deserves further study as this may aid in developing strategies that allow HSC expansion, even postnatally or in vitro. During postnatal life HSC self-renewal occurs rarely and in an asymmetric fashion, yielding one new HSC and a cell that partakes in extensive proliferation in the transient amplifying pool to generate all mature cells. It is believed that only under stress conditions, HSC may divide symmetrically either yielding two new HSC to recreate the pool of HSC or giving rise to two differentiating cells.[71]

The hematopoietic stem cell niche

The notion that HSC reside in microenvironments or niches that regulate their behavior (cell quiescence vs. symmetric divisions vs. asymmetric divisions vs. differentiation) was put forward first by Schofield in 1978,[72,73] even though it was not until recently that the nature of these niches has become elucidated. The bone marrow microenvironment in which HSC reside in postnatal life consists of both hematopoietic and 'stromal' cells.[74,75] These stromal cells include

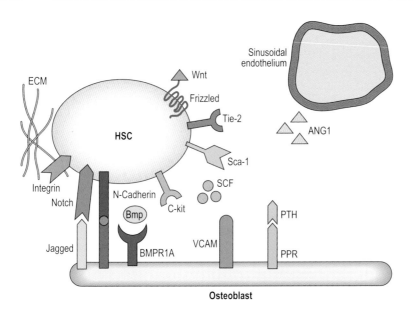

Fig. 4.1 The hematopoietic stem cell niche. The HSC niche consists of the extracellular matrix, the neighboring cells and secreted factors that regulate the stem cell fate. Some of the important regulators in the HSC microenvironment are illustrated. ANG1, angiopoietin-1; BMP, bone morphogenetic protein; BMPRIA, BMP receptor IA; ECM, extracellular matrix; HSC, hematopoietic stem cells; PPR, PTH/PTH related protein receptor; PTH, parathyroid hormone; SCF, stem cell factor; TIE2, tyrosine kinase receptor 2.

endothelial cells, fibroblasts, myocytes, adipocytes and osteoblasts. Stromal cells produce and deposit a complex extracellular matrix (ECM) and produce hematopoietic cytokines that induce or inhibit progenitor proliferation and differentiation.[76,77] Hematopoietic cells interact through cell-surface receptors with either immobilized or secreted cytokines, with adhesive ligands present on stromal cells or ECM components, and other hematopoietic cells. The combined effect of cell–cytokine, cell–cell and cell–ECM interactions governs the normal hematopoietic process.

The fact that one can now identify murine HSC based on cell surface antigens to near homogeneity has allowed investigators to determine that HSC can be found either in close proximity with endosteal osteoblasts (the osteoblastic niche)[78,79] or near small blood vessels (the vascular niche)[16] (Figure 4.1). The osteoblastic niche may be providing a favorable environment to maintain the HSC in a quiescent state, whereas the vascular niche may be providing signals for differentiation and mobilization to the peripheral blood.

Osteoblastic niche

The development of bone has long been linked to the formation and function of the bone marrow.[80] A direct role *in vivo* has more recently been established by a number of studies. In the adult mouse, HSC reside near the endosteum lining the BM cavity.[78,79] The finding that osteoblasts play a role in HSC homeostasis comes from studies in which the osteoblast compartment of the bone was expanded by overexpression of parathyroid hormone (Pth) and its receptors,[81] and a second series of studies in which the BMP-receptor-1a was knocked out, both leading to an increase in HSC.[82] In both studies an increase in osteoblasts correlated with an increase in HSC.[81] Osteoblasts and HSC were found to interact through N-cadherin interactions, although the role of this interaction is unclear.[81] As these genetic manipulations increase HSC numbers,[83] it is believed that the osteoblastic niche regulates HSC maintenance and self-renewal, perhaps by direct cell–cell interactions via the Notch[84] and N-

cadherin pathways.[85] There is evidence that multiple receptor ligand interactions may affect HSC localized in the osteoblastic niche; many of these will be discussed later in this chapter. They include the morphogens BMP4 and Wnt3a,[86,87] interactions between Notch on HSC and Jagged-1 in the niche,[88] Tie2 expressed on HSC and angiopoietin-1;[83] c-Kit and c-Kit-L;[89] or β1 integrins that interact with both VCAM-1[90] and osteopontin.[91,92] Osteoblasts also appear to affect adjacent cells including osteoclasts[93] that then affect HSC fate decisions. Likewise, there is evidence that RANK-L produced by osteoclast mediated breakdown of the bone also influences HSC behavior.[94] However, other studies demonstrated that ablation of osteoblasts using a Collagen-1a1 conditional knockout mouse leads first to the depletion of more committed progenitors and later to depletion of the HSC compartment, which contradicts the notion that osteoblasts would preserve the HSC pool.[95] Like murine HSC, human primitive progenitors can be found in close proximity with the endosteal lining of the marrow cavity,[6] although the molecular mechanisms underlying these interactions and the role of endosteal cells in human HSC regulation are unknown.

Vascular niche

In vivo, endothelial cells line the sinusoids of the BM cavity. As in other tissues, entry and exit from the marrow requires that HSC/HPC and mature blood cells pass through the endothelial barrier of the sinusoids. Unlike most sinusoids, BM sinusoids only have a single layer of endothelial cells, which allows for increased permeability.[96] Aside from serving as a gatekeeper for cell entry and exit from the BM, it is believed that BM endothelial cells also play a role in regulating hematopoiesis. Aside from endothelial cells, additional cells in the vicinity which may regulate HSC *in vivo* include pericytes (thought to be the *in vivo* mesenchymal progenitor cell), megakaryocytes and perivascular reticular cells. Although identification of murine HSC via the SLAM receptors has shown that HSC reside near endothelial cells,[16] the exact contribution of the different cell types in the vascular niche to HSC proliferation and differentiation control are, however, less well understood.

Intrinsic regulation of hematopoiesis

HSC behavior is controlled in part by factors exogenous to the HSC, but also in part by cell intrinsic mechanisms. The latter is the result of a complement of transcription factors (TFs) expressed specifically in HSC but not HPC, which can bind to the promoter regions of specific target genes to allow their transcription and ultimate production of the proteins typical for HSC and not HPC. TFs also recruit co-factors that can modify the chromatin surrounding target genes, to allow easier or more difficult transcription of certain regions of the genome, which is part of the epigenetic regulation of gene expression. The latter consist of methylation and acetylation of histones, proteins to which the DNA is bound, as well as of methylation of CpG islands in the promoter regions of target genes, which prevent binding of TFs to allow transcription. The role of these basic processes, important in all steps of development to allow orderly process of lineage commitment and specification, in hematopoiesis has recently been extensively reviewed by Rice et al., and we refer readers to that exhaustive review for more detailed information.[97]

This section will focus specifically on four classes of cell intrinsic genes that play a role in the correct regulation of hematopoiesis:

1. hematopoietic stem and progenitor-specific genes
2. homeobox (HOX) genes
3. Polycomb genes
4. cell cycle regulator genes.

For many of these genes, aberrant expression is associated with abnormal hematopoiesis, in many instances leukemia development. For instance, recurrent chromosomal translocations in human leukemias that deregulate expression and/or function of genes such as TAL1, LMO2, NOTCH1, and HOX genes[98–102] result in aberrant proliferation of HSC/HPC without maturation, findings that have led to the identification of these genes as key regulators of hematopoiesis.

Hematopoietic stem and progenitor cell specific genes

A number of genes have been identified that are indispensable for the creation of HSC and their lineage specific progeny during development. These include, among others, LMO2, TAL1, GATA2, GATA1 and PU.1.[103–107] LMO2, TAL1 and GATA2 are expressed already in the hemangioblast, or the mesodermal cell that can generate both endothelium and hematopoietic cells.[104–110] Loss of any of these three genes inhibits the emergence of HSC during development. Subsequent commitment to lineage specific hematopoietic cells such as erythroid vs. myeloid and B-cells is then governed by the lineage specific expression of GATA1 and PU.1, respectively.[111]

Homeobox genes

This is a family of highly preserved genes containing a DNA-binding domain, termed homeodomain, that play important roles in many aspects of development, including normal as well as malignant hematopoiesis.[112–117] Aside from the typical HOX genes, there is a second family of homeodomain-containing genes, the three amino acid loop extension (TALE) family of transcription factors, which include PBX1 and MEIS1.[118,119] HOX proteins interact with PBX1 to form a complex with MEIS1, and regulate gene expression.[120–122] Mice deficient in either PBX1 or MEIS1 are embryonic lethal.[123,124] MEIS1 may play a role in expansion of fetal liver HSC as MEIS1$^{-/-}$ fetal liver cells have impaired competitive repopulation abilities.[124,125]

The HOX family consists of four clusters (A–D) which are located on different chromosomes. Within each cluster, HOX genes are further subclassified from the 3′ to 5′ end in 13 paralog groups, based on sequence homology. Different HOX genes are expressed in HSC and HPC, with HSC being characterized by presence of HOXB3, HOXB4 and HOXA4,[125,126] whereas HOXA9 is more highly expressed in HPC that will give rise to granulopoiesis and T- and B-cell lymphopoiesis.[113] Although these genes are very important regulators of hematopoiesis, loss of a single homeobox gene does not always lead to hematopoietic defects due to redundancy between different HOX genes. For instance loss of HOXB4 or HOXB3 alone does not lead to defective hematopoiesis, and even combined loss of HOXB4 and HOXB3 only results in a moderate decrease in hematopoietic cell output. By contrast, aberrant expression of HOX genes has been associated with different types of leukemia, including HOXA9 and HOXC13, pointing to their role in HSC and HPC self-renewal and differentiation. When the HSC specific HOXB4 gene is force expressed in murine and human HSC, significant increased proliferation of cells with HSC characteristics in vitro is observed. When grafted in competitive repopulation assays in vivo, HOXB4 transduced cells outcompete normal HSC, without significant skewing of hematopoiesis or frank leukemia development.[112,117,127] As increased self-renewal of HSC may also be possible by simple HOXB4 protein transfection, this strategy is being contemplated to induce HSC expansion clinically.[128] Kyba et al. also demonstrated that forced expression of HOXB4 in murine embryonic stem cell (ESC) aids in the generation and engraftment of competent HSC from ESC, possibly by inducing the expression of the chemokine receptor CXCR4.[129,130] Although HOXB4 does not seem to promote leukemia, deregulation of other HOX family members is linked to hematopoietic malignancies such as leukemia. A number of HOX genes are found fused with NUP98 in human leukemia,[131,132] and expression of HOXA9 is associated with a poor prognosis in patients with acute myelogenous leukemia.

Polycomb genes

Upstream regulators of HOX genes are among others the mixed-lineage leukemia (MLL), a common target of chromosomal translocations in human acute leukemias, which induces gene expression during development and the Polycomb gene (PcG) family, responsible for suppression of gene expression. Both of these are believed to regulate gene expression by complex epigenetic mechanisms. The Polycomb group (PcG) represents a gene family of transcriptional repressors first identified in Drosophila. They play a key role in many developmental processes by regulating self-renewal and proliferation, senescence and cell death,[133–137] and this via interactions with the initiation transcription machinery[138,139] as well as chromatin-condensation proteins and histones.[140,141] The PcG proteins are organized in Polycomb regulatory complexes (PRC). Two PRC complexes have been identified, consisting of *EZH, EED* and *SUZ12* (PRC2) whereas *BMI1* and *RAE28* are part of the PRC1 complex.[142] A number of PcG genes are expressed in differentiating hematopoietic cells, whereas *BMI1* and *RAE28* are found highly expressed in HSC.[136,143–145] The role of *BMI1* in HSC has been elucidated using both knock-out studies and by forced expression in HSC. HSC from *BMI1*[−/−] mice fail to long-term repopulate lethally irradiated recipients suggesting that *BMI1* plays a role in HSC self-renewal. In addition, the HSC compartment in *BMI1*[−/−] senesces significantly faster than in WT mice. Similar defects are also seen in other stem cell compartments of *BMI1*[−/−] mice.[146–148] By contrast, forced expression of *BMI1* enhances self-renewal *in vivo*.[136,149,150] Similar findings were seen in *RAE28*[−/−] fetal liver HSC, which have impaired engraftment potential.[144] *MEL18*, another PcG gene, which is expressed in a reciprocal fashion with *BMI1*, by contrast inhibits HSC self-renewal.[151,152] There is also evidence for a role of PcG proteins part of the PRC2 complex in HSC proliferation, including *EED, EZH2* and *SUZ12*.[153–156] Aside from being upstream regulators of HOX genes, several of the PcG genes may act by modifying the expression of cell cycle regulators *p16*INK4a/*p19*ARF.[151]

Cell cycle regulators

In postnatal life, the majority of HSC are in a quiescent state which is associated with the finding that many inhibitors of the cell cycle are highly expressed in HSC. Cell proliferation is driven by cyclin-dependent kinases (CDKs) and their corresponding cyclins. CDK activity is blocked by a number of cyclin-dependent kinase inhibitors (CDKIs). CDKIs are separated into two groups, the CIP/KIP (*p21*CIP1, *p27*KIP1, *p57*KIP2) and INK4 (*p14*ARF, *p15*INK4b, *p16*INK4a, *p18*INK4c, *p19*ARF) families, based on the specific CDKs they inhibit. Loss of *p21*CIP1 results in an increased pool of HSC. However, when *p21*CIP1[−/−] HSC are stressed, such as after multiple serial transplantations, HSC exhaustion occurs.[157] siRNA mediated knockdown of *p21*CIP1 in human CD34[+]CD38[−] cells also leads to a modest increase in SRC.[158] Whereas loss of *p21*CIP1 leads to expansion of the HSC compartment (albeit with eventual exhaustion), loss of *p27*KIP1 leads to minimal increases in HSC but a significant expansion of the HPC pool.[159] Members of the INK4/ARF family also play a role in HSC control. As discussed above, *p16*INK4a/*p19*ARF expression is regulated by the PcG gene *BMI1*: loss of *BMI1* leads to increased expression of *p16*INK4a/*p19*ARF,[160] and the associated senescence of HSC seen in *BMI1*[−/−] mice can be ascribed to the higher levels of *p16*INK4a/*p19*ARF.[161] As is seen in *p21*CIP1[−/−] mice, the HSC compartment in mice wherein *p18*INK4c has been knocked out is increased, but unlike *p21*CIP1[−/−] HSC, *p18*INK4c[−/−] HSC are not exhausted over the lifetime of the animal, but demonstrate a competitive advantage compared with WT HSC.[162,163] Moreover, loss of *p18*INK4c can compensate for the early exhaustion and senescence seen in the HSC compartment of *p21*CIP1[−/−] mice.[157,162] The mechanism underlying these differences remains to be elucidated. Finally, loss of Rb, which

plays a central role in the regulation of the G(1)-S phase of the cell cycle, has minimal or no effects on HSC function.[164] Concluding, although loss or gain of cell cycle regulators have some effect on HSC behavior, these effects are relatively mild.

Extrinsic regulation of hematopoiesis

A large number of cytokines have been identified that regulate hematopoietic cells. However, as can be seen from the many studies attempting to expand HSC *ex vivo*, most cytokines cannot sustain self-renewal of HSC and lead to their differentiation. As discussed above in the section on the osteogenic niche, a number of factors provided by the niche affect HSC renewal and differentiation. These will be discussed in the sections below.

Classical cytokines

Over the last three decades, a large number of hematopoietic cytokines and growth factors and their receptors have been identified. Stem and progenitor cells are thought to express most cytokine receptors, a phenomenon also known as stem cell priming.[165] Tyrosine kinase receptors include c-Kit, the receptor for steel factor or stem cell factor (SCF),[166] and the fetal liver tyrosine kinase receptor-3 (FLT3) which binds to FLT3-L.[167] All HSC express c-Kit and SCF, its ligand, is expressed on osteoblasts *in vivo*. Although SCF plays a role in self-renewing cell divisions, loss of either SCF or its receptor does not cause complete aplasia,[168,169] and c-Kit can also not support long-term self-renewal of HSC *in vitro*.[170,171] Likewise, loss of FLT3 or its ligand FLT3-L does not lead to aplasia,[172,173] and although FLT3-L may improve self-renewal cell divisions of HSC *in vitro*, it can again not prevent differentiation of HSC.[170,174,175] Combined loss of SCF and FLT3-L or the two receptors causes near aplasia,[172] suggesting that the combination of the two cytokines plays a role in HSC self-renewal *in vivo*. The second family is the cytokine receptor family, which lacks endogenous tyrosine kinase activity but recruits and activates non-receptor tyrosine kinases such as Jak/Stat and Ras/MAPK.[176,177] Ligands for these receptors include interleukin (IL)-3[176] and thrombopoietin (TPO), both of which are active on primitive progenitors. However, IL-3 functions chiefly to induce differentiation, as addition of high concentrations to *ex vivo* cultured HSC/HPC induces terminal differentiation and loss of primitive HPC.[178,179] TPO, initially discovered as a cytokine important for thrombopoiesis, also pays an important role in HSC biology.[180,181] Like SCF, TPO is expressed by osteoblasts.[181] In TPO[−/−] mice, postnatal HSC frequency and function are normal, but significantly more HSC proliferation is seen, which leads eventually to HSC exhaustion, as is also seen in *p16*INK4a/*p19*ARF[−/−] mice.[180] The third family consists of the gp130 family, which includes receptors for IL-6,[182] IL-11,[183] oncostatin-M[184] and leukemia inhibitory factor (LIF).[185]

Morphogens

Hedgehog signaling

The hedgehog (Hh) family consists of three ligands, Sonic Hh (Shh), Indian Hh (Ihh), and desert Hh (Dhh), which bind to patched (Ptch). This leads to the activation of the intracellular signaling molecule, smoothened (Smo), which is normally inhibited by Ptch when not bound to Hh. As in many developmental processes, Shh and Ihh are involved in hematopoietic emergence and specification from zebrafish to mouse.[186-188] *In vitro* studies with human HSC found that Ihh expanded HSC,[189] and *in vivo* murine studies have shown that Hh may play a role in HSC expansion.[190] However, the latter studies also demonstrate that sustained activation of the Hh signaling pathway, causing extensive HSC cycling, leads to exhaustion of the HSC pool. A recent study has also shown that complete loss of Hh signaling, via conditional knockout of Smo in HSC, does not affect hematopoiesis, suggesting that although Hhs may affect HSC behavior, it is not required for maintenance of adult hematopoiesis.[191,192]

Wnt signaling

The Wnt family consists of 19 different secreted glycoproteins that signal through a number of receptors including 10 transmembrane receptors of the frizzled (Fzd) family, retinoid orphan receptor 2 (Ror2), and two co-receptors, LRP5/6. Wnt proteins are commonly grouped according to the downstream signaling cascade that they activate, most commonly but not limited to 'canonical' or β-catenin dependent and 'non-canonical' or β-catenin independent proteins. Canonical Wnts bind to cell-surface-expressed frizzled receptors. This causes complex formation between cytoplasmic β-catenin[193] and the lymphoid enhancing binding/T-cell transcription factor (LEF/TCF) family of transcription factors. As a result of this complex formation, β-catenin–LEF/TCF translocates to the nucleus,[194] where LEF/TCF induces transcription of a number of genes, among which are HOX genes as well as cell cycle regulatory genes.

There is a significant body of evidence that canonical Wnt signaling plays a role in postnatal hematopoiesis. Forced expression of Dickkopf1 (Dkk1), an inhibitor of canonical Wnt signaling, in osteoblasts *in vivo* significantly reduces the number and repopulation ability of HSC harvested from these mice.[87] Addition of Wnt3a to *ex vivo* cultures of murine HSC leads to improved maintenance and expansion of HSC, which can be mimicked by forced expression of an active form of β-catenin and can be inhibited by forced expression of axin, an inhibitor of β-catenin.[86,195] Consistent with this, e12.5 FL cells from Wnt3a⁻/⁻ mice contain significantly fewer HSC, which leads to severely reduced reconstitution capacity as measured in secondary transplantation assays.[196] However, other studies question the role of β-catenin in hematopoiesis *in vivo*. β-catenin⁻/⁻ mice have no aberrations in hematopoiesis, nor do mice in which, aside from β-catenin, γ-catenin has also been knocked out,[197,198] whereas mice expressing a constitutively active form of β-catenin have a decreased number of HSC.[199,200] To confuse matters further, loss of adenomatous polyposis coli (APC), which together with axin and GSK3-β phosphorylates and ubiquitinates β-catenin leading to proteasomal degradation of β-catenin, causes a severe hematopoietic phenotype, with a severe reduction in the HSC and HPC pool, due to increased apoptosis, as well as increased proliferation.[201] It should be noted that APC may also have effects on HSC via mechanisms independent of the canonical Wnt signaling pathway. However, the role of canonical Wnt signaling in adult hematopoiesis remains not fully understood.

There is also evidence that the non-canonical Wnts may play a role in hematopoiesis. Austin *et al.* and Van Den Berg *et al.* demonstrated that Wnt5a increases proliferation *in vitro* of primitive murine and human hematopoietic progenitors, respectively.[202,203] Wnt5a appears to also affect HSC. Although exposure of human CD34⁺ cells to Wnt5a *in vitro* did not significantly affect their proliferation or differentiation, administration of Wnt5a containing conditioned medium to mice transplanted with human umbilical cord blood CD34⁺CD38⁻Lin⁻ cells increased the repopulation ability of these cells. Although suggestive that Wnt5a affects HSC, this study did not address whether the effect of Wnt5a was directly on HSC.[204] More recently, evidence was provided for a direct effect of Wnt5a on HSC, as culture of highly enriched murine HSC with Wnt5a alone under serum free conditions increased in short term repopulating HSC, possibly by increasing the maintenance of a quiescent state of the *ex vivo* cultured HSC.[204] As no clear-cut increase in β-catenin was observed, the authors concluded that this occurred via non-canonical signaling.

TGFβ superfamily

The TGFβ family consists of 35 ligands, including TGFβs, activins, nodal and BMP, which regulate cell proliferation, apoptosis and differentiation.[205] The TGFβ family, and members of the BMP family in particular, are important during development for the specification of mesoderm. The TGFβ and BMP signaling pathways activate the Smad signaling cascade and the complex is translocated to the nucleus where they function as transcriptional regulators by binding directly to DNA or to other transcription factors.[206]

Tgfβ1⁻/⁻ mice are embryonic lethal with defects in yolk sac formation, including erythroid cell development, with a similar phenotype also seen in *TgfβrII⁻/⁻* mice suggesting an important role of TGFβ in hematopoietic development.[207-209] By contrast, *Tgfβr⁻/⁻* mice have increases in early erythroid cells suggesting that TGFβ is not important in early hematopoietic development.[207-209] The addition of TGFβ to *in vitro* HSC cultures inhibits proliferation of HSC and primitive progenitors but not more mature progenitor populations.[209] Neutralization of TGFβ by blocking antibodies in BM cultures leads to increased repopulation of murine HSC.[210,211] How TGFβ influences hematopoietic cells is not fully understood, even though there is evidence that it regulates cell cycle progression and apoptosis.[212]

As *Bmp4⁻/⁻* mice are embryonically lethal, its role in mammalian development as well as postnatal hematopoiesis is unclear.[213] BMP4 is thought to play a role in initiation of mammalian HSC as it is highly expressed in the AGM region where the first HSC are found[214] as well as in the ICM region of zebrafish, where HSC are born. Studies in which BMP4 was added to *ex vivo* expansion cultures of human HSC demonstrated that BMP4 acts in a dosage dependent manner to increase human SRC *ex vivo*.[215] On the other hand, BMP4 was found to have no effect on mouse HSC cultured *ex vivo*.[216] Forced expression of the inhibitory Smad, Smad-7, in BM cells resulted in reduced proliferation of KLS *in vitro*; however *in vivo*, Smad7-overexpressing HSC demonstrated increased self-renewal and engraftment ability.[217] *Smad5⁻/⁻*

mice, activated by BMP, die early in development with defects in yolk sac development, but they have increased numbers of HPP-CFC in the yolk sac.[218] As most mice in which BMPs or Smads, activated by BMPs, are embryonic lethal the role of BMP signaling in adult hematopoiesis remains incomplete.[219]

Notch pathway

Differentiation into multiple cell types from a population of initially equivalent cells is a fundamental process in the development of all multicellular organisms.[220–223] Studies initially in *Drosophila* and later in mammalian cells have shown that intercellular signaling through the Notch/LIN-12 transmembrane receptors is imperative for normal growth and differentiation during the development of all species. The Notch family is made up of five ligands, Jagged-1/2 and Delta-1/3/4. Binding of the Notch receptor to its ligand causes proteolysis of the Notch receptor.

Both Notch and Notch ligands are expressed in primitive hematopoietic cells as well as in the hematopoietic micro-environment.[88,224,225] Overexpression of the activated form of Notch in murine HSC causes lymphoid leukemia.[226] The human homolog of one of the Notch ligands, Jagged-1, is expressed in human-marrow-derived stromal cells that support growth of primitive human hematopoietic progenitors *in vitro*.[227] Another Notch family member, Delta-1, when engineered in immobilized form, expanded human HPC in *ex vivo* cultures.[84,228] Also, an increase of HSC is found *in vivo* when the parathyroid-hormone-related receptor is activated on osteoblasts, which results in increased expression of Jagged-1 by the osteoblast. This increase in Jagged-1 correlates with an increase in Notch-1 activation on HSC.[88] Although in a transgenic Notch reporter mouse, BM c-Kit$^+$ cells express the active Notch reporter,[229] Notch-1 deficient HSC engraft Jagged-1 deficient mice and reconstitute the hematopoietic system normally.[224] Studies have also shown that other ligands for Notch, Delta-4 and delta like (Dlk) act as regulators of primitive hematopoietic progenitors.[230,231]

Angiopoietin-like proteins

The interaction between Tie2, a receptor tyrosine kinase, and its ligand angiopoietin-1 has been found to play a role in HSC maintenance in the osteoblastic niche. Tie2 is expressed on HSC that are in the quiescent state, and angiopoietin is expressed by osteoblasts lining the bone marrow cavity.[83] Arai *et al.* found that angopoietin-1 enhanced HSC binding

to the osteoblast and promoted HSC quiescence enabling maintenance of HSC by its niche.[83] They also found that injection of recombinant angiopoietin-1 protein in mice resulted in protection from myeloablation after irradiation,[83] suggesting an important role of Tie2/angiopoietin in maintaining the HSC pool within the BM.

Insulin-like growth factors

Insulin-like growth factor (IGF)-1 and -2 hormones are produced by osteoblasts in the bone and are regulated by PTH signaling.[232] HSC cultured with cells expressing IGF-1 and -2 leads to expansion of HSC.[233] Although IGFs are produced by osteoblast in the BM and are important in maintaining bone, it is unclear whether they directly interact with HSC *in vivo*.

Conclusions

Regulation of hematopoiesis takes place in the BM, where it is believed that HSC reside in 'niches' that control the fate of stem cells by presenting factors that control self-renewal vs. differentiation. It is noteworthy that factors that appear to play a role in the extrinsic control of HSC are not solely the classical cytokines and hematopoietic growth factors; they also include such molecules as angiopoietin-like proteins,[83,234] IGFs,[233] members of the TGFβ family and Wnts,[195,204] as well as cell–cell interactions via Notch and N-cadherin. Although many signals from the microenvironment have been identified that affect HSC, it remains clear that intrinsic regulation also plays a key role in cell fate decisions. There is also mounting evidence that HSC and their microenvironment may differ at different stages of development. For instance, the proliferative behavior of HSC found in fetal liver differs from that of adult HSC. Further elucidation of the differences in both intrinsic and extrinsic control of FL vs. BM HSC may aid in developing methods for HSC expansion.[69,70,180,181]

Recent insights have provided a clearer understanding of how the intrinsic program and extrinsic cues regulate molecular mechanisms of hematopoietic cell fate decisions. These not only provide a more detailed understanding of normal hematopoiesis, but also give insight into the development of hematopoietic malignancies and potential novel targets for anti-leukemic therapy. Many questions still remain and a future challenge lies in understanding the intrinisic targets of extrinisic cues, and how the two types of molecular mechanisms collaborate to regulate cell fate decisions.

References

1. Yoder MC, Hiatt K, Mukherjee P. In vivo repopulating hematopoietic stem cells are present in the murine yolk sac at day 9.0 postcoitus. Proceedings of the National Academy of Sciences of the United States of America 1997;94(13):6776–80.

2. Medvinsky A, Dzierzak E. Definitive hematopoiesis is autonomously initiated by the AGM region. Cell 1996;86(6):897–906.

3. de Bruijn MF, Speck NA, Peeters MC, Dzierzak E. Definitive hematopoietic stem cells first develop within the major arterial regions of the mouse embryo. EMBO J 2000;19(11):2465–74.

4. Dzierzak E, Medvinsky A. Mouse embryonic hematopoiesis. Trends Genet 1995;11(9):359–66.

5. Morrison SJ, Hemmati HD, Wandycz AM, Weissman IL. The purification and characterization of fetal liver

hematopoietic stem cells. Proceedings of the National Academy of Sciences of the United States of America 1995;92(22):10302–6.

6. Charbord P, Tavian M, Humeau L, Peault B. Early ontogeny of the human marrow from long bones: an immunohistochemical study of hematopoiesis and its microenvironment. Blood 1996;87(10):4109–19.

7. Jacobson LO, Simmons EL, Marks EK, Eldredge JH. Recovery from radiation injury. Science (New York, NY) 1951;113(2940):510–11.

8. Morrison SJ, Uchida N, Weissman IL. The biology of hematopoietic stem cells. Annual Review of Cell and Developmental Biology 1995;11: 35–71.

9. Cheshier SH, Morrison SJ, Liao X, Weissman IL. In vivo proliferation and cell cycle kinetics of long-term self-renewing hematopoietic stem cells. Proceedings of the National Academy of Sciences of the United States of America 1999;96(6):3120–5.

10. Wilson A, Laurenti E, Oser G, et al. Hematopoietic stem cells reversibly switch from dormancy to self-renewal during homeostasis and repair. Cell 2008;135(6):1118–29.

11. Nygren JM, Bryder D. A novel assay to trace proliferation history in vivo reveals that enhanced divisional kinetics accompany loss of hematopoietic stem cell self-renewal. PloS one 2008;3(11): e3710.

12. Foudi A, Hochedlinger K, Van Buren D, et al. Analysis of histone 2B-GFP retention reveals slowly cycling hematopoietic stem cells. Nature Biotechnology 2009;27(1):84–90.

13. Abkowitz JL, Catlin SN, McCallie MT, Guttorp P. Evidence that the number of hematopoietic stem cells per animal is conserved in mammals. Blood 2002; 100(7):2665–7.

14. Shepherd BE, Kiem HP, Lansdorp PM, et al. Hematopoietic stem-cell behavior in nonhuman primates. Blood 2007;110(6):1806–13.

15. Shepherd BE, Guttorp P, Lansdorp PM, Abkowitz JL. Estimating human hematopoietic stem cell kinetics using granulocyte telomere lengths. Experimental Hematology 2004; 32(11):1040–50.

16. Kiel MJ, Yilmaz OH, Iwashita T, et al. SLAM family receptors distinguish hematopoietic stem and progenitor cells and reveal endothelial niches for stem cells. Cell 2005;121(7):1109–21.

17. Huang S, Terstappen LW. Lymphoid and myeloid differentiation of single human CD34+, HLA–DR+, CD38– hematopoietic stem cells. Blood 1994;83(6):1515–26.

18. Osawa M, Hanada K, Hamada H, Nakauchi H. Long-term lymphohematopoietic reconstitution by a single CD34-low/negative hematopoietic stem cell. Science (New York, NY) 1996;273(5272):242–5.

19. Tavian M, Coulombel L, Luton D, et al. Aorta-associated CD34+ hematopoietic cells in the early human embryo. Blood 1996;87(1):67–72.

20. Sharma Y, Astle CM, Harrison DE. Heterozygous Kit mutants with little or no apparent anemia exhibit large defects in overall hematopoietic stem cell function. Experimental Hematology 2007;35(2):214–20.

21. Baum CM, Weissman IL, Tsukamoto AS, et al. Isolation of a candidate human hematopoietic stem-cell population. Proceedings of the National Academy of Sciences of the United States of America 1992;89(7):2804–8.

22. Larochelle A, Vormoor J, Hanenberg H, et al. Identification of primitive human hematopoietic cells capable of repopulating NOD/SCID mouse bone marrow: implications for gene therapy. Nature Medicine 1996;2(12): 1329–37.

23. Sutherland HJ, Eaves CJ, Eaves AC, et al. Characterization and partial purification of human marrow cells capable of initiating long-term hematopoiesis in vitro. Blood 1989;74(5):1563–70.

24. Terstappen LW, Huang S, Safford M, et al. Sequential generations of hematopoietic colonies derived from single nonlineage-committed CD34+CD38– progenitor cells. Blood 1991;77(6):1218–27.

25. Galy A, Travis M, Cen D, Chen B. Human T, B, natural killer, and dendritic cells arise from a common bone marrow progenitor cell subset. Immunity 1995;3(4):459–73.

26. Miller JS, Alley KA, McGlave P. Differentiation of natural killer (NK) cells from human primitive marrow progenitors in a stroma-based long-term culture system: identification of a CD34+7+ NK progenitor. Blood 1994;83(9):2594–601.

27. LeBien TW. B-cell lymphopoiesis in mouse and man. Current Opinion in Immunology 1998;10(2):188–95.

28. Pearce DJ, Taussig DC, Bonnet D. Implications of the expression of myeloid markers on normal and leukemic stem cells. Cell Cycle (Georgetown, Tex) 2006;5(3):271–3.

29. Randall TD, Weissman IL. Phenotypic and functional changes induced at the clonal level in hematopoietic stem cells after 5-fluorouracil treatment. Blood 1997;89(10):3596–606.

30. Hodgson GS, Bradley TR. Properties of haematopoietic stem cells surviving 5-fluorouracil treatment: evidence for a pre-CFU-S cell? Nature 1979;281(5730): 381–2.

31. Chaudhary PM, Roninson IB. Expression and activity of P-glycoprotein, a multidrug efflux pump, in human hematopoietic stem cells. Cell 1991;66(1):85–94.

32. Morita Y, Ema H, Yamazaki S, Nakauchi H. Non-side-population hematopoietic stem cells in mouse bone marrow. Blood 2006;108(8):2850–6.

33. Goodell MA, Brose K, Paradis G, et al. Isolation and functional properties of murine hematopoietic stem cells that are replicating in vivo. Journal of Experimental Medicine 1996;183(4): 1797–806.

34. McKenzie JL, Takenaka K, Gan OI, et al. Low rhodamine 123 retention identifies long-term human hematopoietic stem cells within the Lin-CD34+CD38– population. Blood 2007;109(2):543–5.

35. McNiece IK, Robinson BE, Quesenberry PJ. Stimulation of murine colony-forming cells with high proliferative potential by the combination of GM-CSF and CSF-1. Blood 1988;72(1): 191–5.

36. Dexter TM, Allen TD, Lajtha LG. Conditions controlling the proliferation of haemopoietic stem cells in vitro. Journal of cellular physiology 1977; 91(3):335–44.

37. Fraser CC, Szilvassy SJ, Eaves CJ, Humphries RK. Proliferation of totipotent hematopoietic stem cells in vitro with retention of long-term competitive in vivo reconstituting ability. Proceedings of the National Academy of Sciences of the United States of America 1992;89(5):1968–72.

38. Hao QL, Thiemann FT, Petersen D, et al. Extended long-term culture reveals a highly quiescent and primitive human hematopoietic progenitor population. Blood 1996;88(9):3306–13.

39. Ploemacher RE, van der Sluijs JP, van Beurden CA, et al. Use of limiting-dilution type long-term marrow cultures in frequency analysis of marrow-repopulating and spleen colony-forming hematopoietic stem cells in the mouse. Blood 1991;78(10): 2527–33.

40. Miller JS, McCullar V, Verfaillie CM. Ex vivo culture of CD34+/Lin-/DR-cells in stroma-derived soluble factors, interleukin-3, and macrophage inflammatory protein-1alpha maintains not only myeloid but also lymphoid progenitors in a novel switch culture assay. Blood 1998;91(12):4516–22.

41. Schmitt TM, Zuniga-Pflucker JC. Induction of T cell development from hematopoietic progenitor cells by delta-like-1 in vitro. Immunity 2002;17(6):749–56.

42. Berardi AC, Meffre E, Pflumio F, et al. Individual CD34+CD38lowCD19-CD10-progenitor cells from human cord blood generate B lymphocytes and granulocytes. Blood 1997;89(10): 3554–64.

43. Punzel M, Wissink SD, Miller JS, et al. The myeloid-lymphoid initiating cell (ML-IC) assay assesses the fate of multipotent human progenitors in vitro. Blood 1999;93(11):3750–6.

44. Whitlock CA, Robertson D, Witte ON. Murine B cell lymphopoiesis in long term culture. J Immunol Methods 1984;67(2):353–69.

45. Whitlock CA, Witte ON. Long-term culture of B lymphocytes and their precursors from murine bone marrow. Proceedings of the National Academy of Sciences of the United States of America 1982;79(11):3608–12.

46. Hao QL, Smogorzewska EM, Barsky LW, Crooks GM. In vitro identification of single CD34+CD38– cells with both lymphoid and myeloid potential. Blood 1998;91(11):4145–51.

47. Spangrude GJ, Heimfeld S, Weissman IL. Purification and characterization of mouse hematopoietic stem cells. Science (New York, NY) 1988;241(4861):58–62.

48. Lemischka IR, Raulet DH, Mulligan RC. Developmental potential and dynamic behavior of hematopoietic stem cells. Cell 1986;45(6):917–27.

49. Jordan CT, McKearn JP, Lemischka IR. Cellular and developmental properties of fetal hematopoietic stem cells. Cell 1990;61(6):953–63.

50. Szilvassy SJ, Fraser CC, Eaves CJ, et al. Retrovirus-mediated gene transfer to purified hemopoietic stem cells with long-term lympho-myelopoietic repopulating ability. Proceedings of the National Academy of Sciences of the United States of America 1989;86(22):8798–802.

51. Zhong RK, Astle CM, Harrison DE. Distinct developmental patterns of short-term and long-term functioning lymphoid and myeloid precursors defined by competitive limiting dilution analysis in vivo. J Immunol 1996;157(1):138–45.

52. Iscove NN, Nawa K. Hematopoietic stem cells expand during serial transplantation in vivo without apparent exhaustion. Curr Biol 1997;7(10):805–8.

53. Jordan CT, Lemischka IR. Clonal and systemic analysis of long-term hematopoiesis in the mouse. Genes and Development 1990;4(2):220–32.

54. McCune JM, Namikawa R, Kaneshima H, et al. The SCID-hu mouse: murine model for the analysis of human hematolymphoid differentiation and function. Science (New York, NY) 1988;241(4873):1632–9.

55. Ishikawa F, Yasukawa M, Lyons B, et al. Development of functional human blood and immune systems in NOD/SCID/IL2 receptor γ chain(null) mice. Blood 2005;106(5):1565–73.

56. Nolta JA, Hanley MB, Kohn DB. Sustained human hematopoiesis in immunodeficient mice by cotransplantation of marrow stroma expressing human interleukin-3: analysis of gene transduction of long-lived progenitors. Blood 1994;83(10):3041–51.

57. Hiramatsu H, Nishikomori R, Heike T, et al. Complete reconstitution of human lymphocytes from cord blood CD34+ cells using the NOD/SCID/gammacnull

mice model. Blood 2003;102(3):873–80.

58. Srour EF, Zanjani ED, Cornetta K, et al. Persistence of human multilineage, self-renewing lymphohematopoietic stem cells in chimeric sheep. Blood 1993;82(11):3333–42.

59. Pearson T, Greiner DL, Shultz LD. Creation of 'humanized' mice to study human immunity. Current Protocols in Immunology, edited by John E Coligan 2008; Chapter 15:Unit 15 21.

60. Norol F, Drouet M, Pflumio F, et al. Ex vivo expansion marginally amplifies repopulating cells from baboon peripheral blood mobilized CD34+ cells. British Journal of Haematology 2002;117(4):924–34.

61. Andrews RG, Bryant EM, Bartelmez SH, et al. CD34+ marrow cells, devoid of T and B lymphocytes, reconstitute stable lymphopoiesis and myelopoiesis in lethally irradiated allogeneic baboons. Blood 1992;80(7):1693–701.

62. Tisdale JF, Hanazono Y, Sellers SE, et al. Ex vivo expansion of genetically marked rhesus peripheral blood progenitor cells results in diminished long-term repopulating ability. Blood 1998;92(4):1131–41.

63. Horn PA, Thomasson BM, Wood BL, et al. Distinct hematopoietic stem/progenitor cell populations are responsible for repopulating NOD/SCID mice compared with nonhuman primates. Blood 2003;102(13):4329–35.

64. Kiger AA, Jones DL, Schulz C, et al. Stem cell self-renewal specified by JAK-STAT activation in response to a support cell cue. Science (New York, NY) 2001;294(5551):2542–5.

65. Tulina N, Matunis E. Control of stem cell self-renewal in *Drosophila* spermatogenesis by JAK-STAT signaling. Science (New York, NY) 2001;294(5551):2546–9.

66. Giebel B, Zhang T, Beckmann J, et al. Primitive human hematopoietic cells give rise to differentially specified daughter cells upon their initial cell division. Blood 2006;107(5):2146–52.

67. Giebel B, Beckmann J. Asymmetric cell divisions of human hematopoietic stem and progenitor cells meet endosomes. Cell Cycle (Georgetown, Tex) 2007;6(18):2201–4.

68. Bowie MB, Kent DG, Copley MR, Eaves CJ. Steel factor responsiveness regulates the high self-renewal phenotype of fetal hematopoietic stem cells. Blood 2007;109(11):5043–8.

69. Bowie MB, McKnight KD, Kent DG, et al. Hematopoietic stem cells proliferate until after birth and show a reversible phase-specific engraftment defect. Journal of Clinical Investigation 2006;116(10):2808–16.

70. Bowie MB, Kent DG, Dykstra B, et al. Identification of a new intrinsically

timed developmental checkpoint that reprograms key hematopoietic stem cell properties. Proceedings of the National Academy of Sciences of the United States of America 2007;104(14):5878–82.

71. Attar EC, Scadden DT. Regulation of hematopoietic stem cell growth. Leukemia 2004;18(11):1760–8.

72. Schofield R. The relationship between the spleen colony-forming cell and the haemopoietic stem cell. Blood Cells 1978;4(1–2):7–25.

73. Quesenberry PJ, Crittenden RB, Lowry P, et al. In vitro and in vivo studies of stromal niches. Blood Cells 1994;20(1):97–104; discussion 104–6.

74. Lemischka IR. Microenvironmental regulation of hematopoietic stem cells. Stem Cells (Dayton, Ohio) 1997;15(Suppl. 1):63–8.

75. Clark BR, Keating A. Biology of bone marrow stroma. Annals of the New York Academy of Sciences 1995;29;770:70–8.

76. Yoder MC, Williams DA. Matrix molecule interactions with hematopoietic stem cells. Experimental Hematology 1995;23(9):961–7.

77. Verfaillie C, Hurley R, Bhatia R, McCarthy JB. Role of bone marrow matrix in normal and abnormal hematopoiesis. Critical Reviews in Oncology/Hematology 1994;16(3):201–24.

78. Gong JK. Endosteal marrow: a rich source of hematopoietic stem cells. Science (New York, NY) 1978;199(4336):1443–5.

79. Nilsson SK, Johnston HM, Coverdale JA. Spatial localization of transplanted hemopoietic stem cells: inferences for the localization of stem cell niches. Blood 2001;97(8):2293–9.

80. Patt HM, Maloney MA. Bone formation and resorption as a requirement for marrow development. Proc Soc Exp Biol Med 1972;140(1):205–7.

81. Zhang J, Niu C, Ye L, et al. Identification of the haematopoietic stem cell niche and control of the niche size. Nature 2003;425(6960):836–41.

82. Park C, Afrikanova I, Chung YS, et al. A hierarchical order of factors in the generation of FLK1- and SCL-expressing hematopoietic and endothelial progenitors from embryonic stem cells. Development (Cambridge, England) 2004;131(11):2749–62.

83. Arai F, Hirao A, Ohmura M, et al. Tie2/angiopoietin-1 signaling regulates hematopoietic stem cell quiescence in the bone marrow niche. Cell 2004;118(2):149–61.

84. Varnum-Finney B, Brashem-Stein C, Bernstein ID. Combined effects of Notch signaling and cytokines induce a multiple log increase in precursors with lymphoid and myeloid reconstituting ability. Blood 2003;101(5):1784–9.

85. Haug JS, He XC, Grindley JC, et al. N-cadherin expression level distinguishes reserved versus primed states of hematopoietic stem cells. Cell Stem Cell 2008;2(4):367–79.

86. Willert K, Brown JD, Danenberg E, et al. Wnt proteins are lipid-modified and can act as stem cell growth factors. Nature 2003;423(6938):448–52.

87. Fleming HE, Janzen V, Lo Celso C, et al. Wnt signaling in the niche enforces hematopoietic stem cell quiescence and is necessary to preserve self-renewal in vivo. Cell Stem Cell 2008;2(3):274–83.

88. Calvi LM, Adams GB, Weibrecht KW, et al. Osteoblastic cells regulate the haematopoietic stem cell niche. Nature 2003;425(6960):841–6.

89. Kent D, Copley M, Benz C, et al. Regulation of hematopoietic stem cells by the steel factor/KIT signaling pathway. Clin Cancer Res 2008;14(7):1926–30.

90. Hidalgo A, Sanz-Rodriguez F, Rodriguez-Fernandez JL, et al. Chemokine stromal cell-derived factor-1alpha modulates VLA-4 integrin-dependent adhesion to fibronectin and VCAM-1 on bone marrow hematopoietic progenitor cells. Experimental Hematology 2001;29(3):345–55.

91. Nilsson SK, Johnston HM, Whitty GA, et al. Osteopontin, a key component of the hematopoietic stem cell niche and regulator of primitive hematopoietic progenitor cells. Blood 2005;106(4):1232–9.

92. Stier S, Ko Y, Forkert R, et al. Osteopontin is a hematopoietic stem cell niche component that negatively regulates stem cell pool size. Journal of Experimental Medicine 2005;201(11):1781–91.

93. Porter RL, Calvi LM. Communications between bone cells and hematopoietic stem cells. Arch Biochem Biophys 2008;473(2):193–200.

94. Adams GB, Chabner KT, Alley IR, et al. Stem cell engraftment at the endosteal niche is specified by the calcium-sensing receptor. Nature 2006;439(7076):599–603.

95. Visnjic D, Kalajzic Z, Rowe DW, et al. Hematopoiesis is severely altered in mice with an induced osteoblast deficiency. Blood 2004;103(9):3258–64.

96. Tavassoli M. Structure and function of sinusoidal endothelium of bone marrow. Progress in Clinical and Biological Research 1981;59B:249–56.

97. Rice KL, Hormaeche I, Licht JD. Epigenetic regulation of normal and malignant hematopoiesis. Oncogene 2007;26(47):6697–714.

98. Goldfarb AN, Greenberg JM. T-cell acute lymphoblastic leukemia and the associated basic helix-loop-helix gene SCL/tal. Leukemia and Lymphoma 1994;12(3–4):157–66.

99. Rabbitts TH, Bucher K, Chung G, et al. The effect of chromosomal translocations in acute leukemias: the LMO2 paradigm in transcription and development. Cancer Research 1999;59(Suppl. 7):1794s–8s.

100. Abramovich C, Humphries RK. Hox regulation of normal and leukemic hematopoietic stem cells. Current Opinion in Hematology 2005;12(3):210–6.

101. Jundt F, Schwarzer R, Dorken B. Notch signaling in leukemias and lymphomas. Current Molecular Medicine 2008;8(1):51–9.

102. McGonigle GJ, Lappin TR, Thompson A. Grappling with the HOX network in hematopoiesis and leukemia. Front Biosci 2008;13:4297–308.

103. Scott EW, Simon MC, Anastasi J, Singh H. Requirement of transcription factor PU.1 in the development of multiple hematopoietic lineages. Science (New York, NY) 1994;265(5178):1573–7.

104. Tsai FY, Keller G, Kuo FC, et al. An early haematopoietic defect in mice lacking the transcription factor GATA-2. Nature 1994;371(6494):221–6.

105. Warren AJ, Colledge WH, Carlton MB, et al. The oncogenic cysteine-rich LIM domain protein rbtn2 is essential for erythroid development. Cell 1994;78(1):45–57.

106. Robb L, Lyons I, Li R, et al. Absence of yolk sac hematopoiesis from mice with a targeted disruption of the SCL gene. Proceedings of the National Academy of Sciences of the United States of America 1995;92(15):7075–9.

107. Shivdasani RA, Mayer EL, Orkin SH. Absence of blood formation in mice lacking the T-cell leukaemia oncoprotein tal-1/SCL. Nature 1995;373(6513):432–4.

108. Patterson LJ, Gering M, Eckfeldt CE, et al. The transcription factors Scl and Lmo2 act together during development of the hemangioblast in zebrafish. Blood 2007;109(6):2389–98.

109. Gering M, Rodaway AR, Gottgens B, et al. The SCL gene specifies haemangioblast development from early mesoderm. Embo J 1998;17(14):4029–45.

110. Gering M, Yamada Y, Rabbitts TH, Patient RK. Lmo2 and Scl/Tal1 convert non-axial mesoderm into haemangioblasts which differentiate into endothelial cells in the absence of Gata1. Development (Cambridge, England) 2003;130(25):6187–99.

111. Maeno M, Mead PE, Kelley C, et al. The role of BMP-4 and GATA-2 in the induction and differentiation of hematopoietic mesoderm in Xenopus laevis. Blood 1996;88(6):1965–72.

112. Sauvageau G, Thorsteinsdottir U, Eaves CJ, et al. Overexpression of HOXB4 in hematopoietic cells causes the selective expansion of more primitive populations in vitro and in vivo. Genes and Development 1995;9(14):1753–65.

113. Lawrence HJ, Helgason CD, Sauvageau G, et al. Mice bearing a targeted interruption of the homeobox gene HOXA9 have defects in myeloid, erythroid, and lymphoid hematopoiesis. Blood 1997;89(6):1922–30.

114. Sauvageau G, Thorsteinsdottir U, Hough MR, et al. Overexpression of HOXB3 in hematopoietic cells causes defective lymphoid development and progressive myeloproliferation. Immunity 1997;6(1):13–22.

115. Thorsteinsdottir U, Sauvageau G, Humphries RK. Hox homeobox genes as regulators of normal and leukemic hematopoiesis. Hematology/oncology clinics of North America 1997;11(6):1221–37.

116. Thorsteinsdottir U, Sauvageau G, Hough MR, Dragowska W, Lansdorp PM, Lawrence HJ, et al. Overexpression of HOXA10 in murine hematopoietic cells perturbs both myeloid and lymphoid differentiation and leads to acute myeloid leukemia. Molecular and cellular biology 1997;17(1):495–505.

117. Antonchuk J, Sauvageau G, Humphries RK. HOXB4-induced expansion of adult hematopoietic stem cells ex vivo. Cell 2002;109(1):39–45.

118. Shen WF, Montgomery JC, Rozenfeld S, et al. AbdB-like Hox proteins stabilize DNA binding by the Meis1 homeodomain proteins. Molecular and Cellular Biology 1997;17(11):6448–58.

119. Shen WF, Rozenfeld S, Lawrence HJ, Largman C. The Abd-B-like Hox homeodomain proteins can be subdivided by the ability to form complexes with Pbx1a on a novel DNA target. Journal of Biological Chemistry 1997;272(13):8198–206.

120. Swift GH, Liu Y, Rose SD, et al. An endocrine-exocrine switch in the activity of the pancreatic homeodomain protein PDX1 through formation of a trimeric complex with PBX1b and MRG1 (MEIS2). Molecular and Cellular Biology 1998;18(9):5109–20.

121. Shen WF, Rozenfeld S, Kwong A, et al. HOXA9 forms triple complexes with PBX2 and MEIS1 in myeloid cells. Molecular and Cellular Biology 1999;19(4):3051–61.

122. Jacobs Y, Schnabel CA, Cleary ML. Trimeric association of Hox and TALE homeodomain proteins mediates Hoxb2 hindbrain enhancer activity. Molecular and Cellular Biology 1999;19(7):5134–42.

123. DiMartino JF, Selleri L, Traver D, et al. The Hox cofactor and proto-oncogene Pbx1 is required for maintenance of definitive hematopoiesis in the fetal liver. Blood 2001;98(3):618–26.

124. Hisa T, Spence SE, Rachel RA, et al. Hematopoietic, angiogenic and eye

defects in Meis1 mutant animals. Embo J 2004;23(2):450–9.

125. Pineault N, Helgason CD, Lawrence HJ, Humphries RK. Differential expression of Hox, Meis1, and Pbx1 genes in primitive cells throughout murine hematopoietic ontogeny. Experimental Hematology 2002;30(1):49–57.

126. Argiropoulos B, Humphries RK. Hox genes in hematopoiesis and leukemogenesis. Oncogene 2007; 26(47):6766–76.

127. Thorsteinsdottir U, Sauvageau G, Humphries RK. Enhanced in vivo regenerative potential of HOXB4-transduced hematopoietic stem cells with regulation of their pool size. Blood 1999;94(8):2605–12.

128. Amsellem S, Pflumio F, Bardinet D, et al. Ex vivo expansion of human hematopoietic stem cells by direct delivery of the HOXB4 homeoprotein. Nature Medicine 2003;9(11):1423–7.

129. Kyba M, Perlingeiro RC, Daley GQ. HoxB4 confers definitive lymphoid-myeloid engraftment potential on embryonic stem cell and yolk sac hematopoietic progenitors. Cell 2002;109(1):29–37.

130. Kyba M, Perlingeiro RC, Daley GQ. Development of hematopoietic repopulating cells from embryonic stem cells. Methods in Enzymology 2003; 365:114–29.

131. Nakamura T. NUP98 fusion in human leukemia: dysregulation of the nuclear pore and homeodomain proteins. International Journal of Hematology 2005;82(1):21–7.

132. Slape C, Aplan PD. The role of NUP98 gene fusions in hematologic malignancy. Leukemia and Lymphoma 2004;45(7): 1341–50.

133. Sparmann A, van Lohuizen M. Polycomb silencers control cell fate, development and cancer. Nat Rev Cancer 2006;6(11): 846–56.

134. Dietrich N, Bracken AP, Trinh E, et al. Bypass of senescence by the polycomb group protein CBX8 through direct binding to the INK4A-ARF locus. Embo J 2007;26(6):1637–48.

135. Guo WJ, Datta S, Band V, Dimri GP. Mel-18, a polycomb group protein, regulates cell proliferation and senescence via transcriptional repression of Bmi-1 and c-Myc oncoproteins. Molecular Biology of the Cell 2007; 18(2):536–46.

136. Lessard J, Sauvageau G. Bmi-1 determines the proliferative capacity of normal and leukaemic stem cells. Nature 2003;423(6937):255–60.

137. Loring JF, Porter JG, Seilhammer J, et al. A gene expression profile of embryonic stem cells and embryonic stem cell-derived neurons. Restorative Neurology and Neuroscience 2001;18(2–3): 81–8.

138. Dellino GI, Schwartz YB, Farkas G, et al. Polycomb silencing blocks transcription initiation. Molecular Cell 2004;13(6): 887–93.

139. Wang L, Brown JL, Cao R, et al. Hierarchical recruitment of polycomb group silencing complexes. Molecular Cell 2004;14(5):637–46.

140. Breiling A, Bonte E, Ferrari S, et al. The *Drosophila* polycomb protein interacts with nucleosomal core particles in vitro via its repression domain. Molecular and Cellular Biology 1999;19(12): 8451–60.

141. Ogawa H, Ishiguro K, Gaubatz S, et al. A complex with chromatin modifiers that occupies E2F- and Myc-responsive genes in G0 cells. Science (New York, NY) 2002;296(5570):1132–6.

142. Lund AH, van Lohuizen M. Polycomb complexes and silencing mechanisms. Current Opinion in Cell Biology 2004;16(3):239–46.

143. Raaphorst FM, Otte AP, Meijer CJ. Polycomb-group genes as regulators of mammalian lymphopoiesis. Trends in Immunology 2001;22(12):682–90.

144. Ohta H, Sawada A, Kim JY, et al. Polycomb group gene rae28 is required for sustaining activity of hematopoietic stem cells. Journal of Experimental Medicine 2002;195(6):759–70.

145. Lessard J, Sauvageau G. Polycomb group genes as epigenetic regulators of normal and leukemic hemopoiesis. Experimental Hematology 2003;31(7):567–85.

146. Molofsky AV, Pardal R, Iwashita T, et al. Bmi-1 dependence distinguishes neural stem cell self-renewal from progenitor proliferation. Nature 2003;425(6961): 962–7.

147. Molofsky AV, He S, Bydon M, et al. Bmi-1 promotes neural stem cell self-renewal and neural development but not mouse growth and survival by repressing the p16Ink4a and p19Arf senescence pathways. Genes and Development 2005;19(12):1432–7.

148. Zhang HW, Ding J, Jin JL, et al. Defects in mesenchymal stem cell self-renewal and cell fate determination lead to an osteopenic phenotype in Bmi-1 null mice. J Bone Miner Res 2010;25(3): 640–52.

149. Park IK, Qian D, Kiel M, et al. Bmi-1 is required for maintenance of adult self-renewing haematopoietic stem cells. Nature 2003;423(6937):302–5.

150. Iwama A, Oguro H, Negishi M, et al. Enhanced self-renewal of hematopoietic stem cells mediated by the polycomb gene product Bmi-1. Immunity 2004; 21(6):843–51.

151. Kajiume T, Ninomiya Y, Ishihara H, et al. Polycomb group gene mel-18 modulates the self-renewal activity and cell cycle status of hematopoietic stem cells. Experimental Hematology 2004;32(6): 571–8.

152. Kajiume T, Ohno N, Sera Y, Kawahara Y, Yuge L, Kobayashi M. Reciprocal expression of Bmi1 and Mel-18 is associated with functioning of primitive hematopoietic cells. Experimental hematology 2009;37(7):857–66, e2.

153. Kamminga LM, Bystrykh LV, de Boer A, et al. The Polycomb group gene Ezh2 prevents hematopoietic stem cell exhaustion. Blood 2006;107(5):2170–9.

154. De Haan G, Gerrits A. Epigenetic control of hematopoietic stem cell aging: the case of Ezh2. Annals of the New York Academy of Sciences 2007;1106:233–9.

155. Majewski IJ, Blewitt ME, de Graaf CA, et al. Polycomb repressive complex 2 (PRC2) restricts hematopoietic stem cell activity. PLoS Biology 2008;6(4):e93.

156. Lessard J, Schumacher A, Thorsteinsdottir U, et al. Functional antagonism of the Polycomb-Group genes eed and Bmi1 in hemopoietic cell proliferation. Genes and Development 1999;13(20): 2691–703.

157. Cheng T, Rodrigues N, Shen H, et al. Hematopoietic stem cell quiescence maintained by p21cip1/waf1. Science 2000;287(5459):1804–8.

158. Stier S, Cheng T, Forkert R, et al. Ex vivo targeting of p21Cip1/Waf1 permits relative expansion of human hematopoietic stem cells. Blood 2003;102(4):1260–6.

159. Cheng T, Rodrigues N, Dombkowski D, et al. Stem cell repopulation efficiency but not pool size is governed by p27(kip1). Nature Medicine 2000; 6(11):1235–40.

160. Oguro H, Iwama A, Morita Y, et al. Differential impact of Ink4a and Arf on hematopoietic stem cells and their bone marrow microenvironment in Bmi1-deficient mice. Journal of Experimental Medicine 2006;203(10):2247–53.

161. Janzen V, Forkert R, Fleming HE, et al. Stem-cell ageing modified by the cyclin-dependent kinase inhibitor p16INK4a. Nature 2006;443(7110): 421–6.

162. Yu H, Yuan Y, Shen H, Cheng T. Hematopoietic stem cell exhaustion impacted by p18 INK4C and p21 Cip1/Waf1 in opposite manners. Blood 2006; 107(3):1200–6.

163. Yuan Y, Shen H, Franklin DS, et al. In vivo self-renewing divisions of haematopoietic stem cells are increased in the absence of the early G1-phase inhibitor, p18INK4C. Nature Cell Biology 2004;6(5):436–42.

164. Walkley CR, Orkin SH. Rb is dispensable for self-renewal and multilineage differentiation of adult hematopoietic stem cells. Proceedings of the National Academy of Sciences of the United States of America 2006;103(24): 9057–62.

165. Billia F, Barbara M, McEwen J, et al. Resolution of pluripotential

intermediates in murine hematopoietic differentiation by global complementary DNA amplification from single cells: confirmation of assignments by expression profiling of cytokine receptor transcripts. Blood 2001;97(8): 2257–68.

166. Hamel W, Westphal M. The road less travelled: c-kit and stem cell factor. Journal of Neuro-oncology 1997; 35(3):327–33.

167. Lyman SD, Williams DE. Biology and potential clinical applications of flt3 ligand. Current Opinion in Hematology 1995;2(3):177–81.

168. McCulloch EA, Siminovitch L, Till JE, et al. The cellular basis of the genetically determined hemopoietic defect in anemic mice of genotype Sl-Sld. Blood 1965;26(4):399–410.

169. McCulloch EA, Siminovitch L, Till JE. Spleen-Colony Formation in Anemic Mice of Genotype Ww. Science (New York, NY) 1964;144:844–6.

170. Zandstra PW, Conneally E, Petzer AL, et al. Cytokine manipulation of primitive human hematopoietic cell self-renewal. Proceedings of the National Academy of Sciences of the United States of America 1997;94(9):4698–703.

171. Audet J, Miller CL, Eaves CJ, Piret JM. Common and distinct features of cytokine effects on hematopoietic stem and progenitor cells revealed by dose-response surface analysis. Biotechnology and Bioengineering 2002;80(4):393–404.

172. Mackarehtschian K, Hardin JD, Moore KA, et al. Targeted disruption of the flk2/flt3 gene leads to deficiencies in primitive hematopoietic progenitors. Immunity 1995;3(1):147–61.

173. McKenna HJ, Stocking KL, Miller RE, et al. Mice lacking flt3 ligand have deficient hematopoiesis affecting hematopoietic progenitor cells, dendritic cells, and natural killer cells. Blood 2000;95(11):3489–97.

174. Miller CL, Eaves CJ. Expansion in vitro of adult murine hematopoietic stem cells with transplantable lympho-myeloid reconstituting ability. Proceedings of the National Academy of Sciences of the United States of America 1997;94(25): 13648–53.

175. Ueda T, Tsuji K, Yoshino H, et al. Expansion of human NOD/SCID-repopulating cells by stem cell factor, Flk2/Flt3 ligand, thrombopoietin, IL-6, and soluble IL-6 receptor. Journal of Clinical Investigation 2000;105(7): 1013–21.

176. Bagley CJ, Woodcock JM, Stomski FC, Lopez AF. The structural and functional basis of cytokine receptor activation: lessons from the common beta subunit of the granulocyte-macrophage colony-stimulating factor, interleukin-3 (IL-3), and IL-5 receptors. Blood 1997; 89(5):1471–82.

177. Liu KD, Gaffen SL, Goldsmith MA. JAK/STAT signaling by cytokine receptors. Current Opinion in Immunology 1998;10(3):271–8.

178. Petzer AL, Zandstra PW, Piret JM, Eaves CJ. Differential cytokine effects on primitive (CD34+CD38-) human hematopoietic cells: novel responses to Flt3-ligand and thrombopoietin. Journal of Experimental Medicine 1996;183(6): 2551–8.

179. Petzer AL, Hogge DE, Landsdorp PM, et al. Self-renewal of primitive human hematopoietic cells (long-term-culture-initiating cells) in vitro and their expansion in defined medium. Proceedings of the National Academy of Sciences of the United States of America 1996;93(4):1470–4.

180. Qian H, Buza-Vidas N, Hyland CD, et al. Critical role of thrombopoietin in maintaining adult quiescent hematopoietic stem cells. Cell Stem Cell 2007;1(6):671–84.

181. Yoshihara H, Arai F, Hosokawa K, et al. Thrombopoietin/MPL signaling regulates hematopoietic stem cell quiescence and interaction with the osteoblastic niche. Cell Stem Cell 2007;1(6):685–97.

182. Peters M, Muller AM, Rose-John S. Interleukin-6 and soluble interleukin-6 receptor: direct stimulation of gp130 and hematopoiesis. Blood 1998;92(10): 3495–504.

183. Nandurkar HH, Robb L, Begley CG. The role of IL-II in hematopoiesis as revealed by a targeted mutation of its receptor. Stem Cells (Dayton, Ohio) 1998; 16(Suppl. 2):53–65.

184. Miyajima A, Kinoshita T, Tanaka M, et al. Role of oncostatin M in hematopoiesis and liver development. Cytokine and Growth Factor Reviews 2000;11(3): 177–83.

185. Taupin JL, Pitard V, Dechanet J, et al. Leukemia inhibitory factor: part of a large ingathering family. International Reviews of Immunology 1998;16(3–4): 397–426.

186. Peeters M, Ottersbach K, Bollerot K, et al. Ventral embryonic tissues and hedgehog proteins induce early AGM hematopoietic stem cell development. Development (Cambridge, England) 2009;136(15):2613–21.

187. Dyer MA, Farrington SM, Mohn D, et al. Indian hedgehog activates hematopoiesis and vasculogenesis and can respecify prospective neurectodermal cell fate in the mouse embryo. Development (Cambridge, England) 2001;128(10): 1717–30.

188. Baron M. Induction of embryonic hematopoietic and endothelial stem/progenitor cells by hedgehog-mediated signals. Differentiation 2001;68(4–5): 175–85.

189. Kobune M, Ito Y, Kawano Y, et al. Indian hedgehog gene transfer augments

hematopoietic support of human stromal cells including NOD/SCID-beta2m$^{-/-}$ repopulating cells. Blood 2004;104(4): 1002–9.

190. Trowbridge JJ, Scott MP, Bhatia M. Hedgehog modulates cell cycle regulators in stem cells to control hematopoietic regeneration. Proceedings of the National Academy of Sciences of the United States of America 2006;103(38): 14134–9.

191. Gao J, Graves S, Koch U, et al. Hedgehog signaling is dispensable for adult hematopoietic stem cell function. Cell Stem Cell 2009;4(6):548–58.

192. Hofmann I, Stover EH, Cullen DE, et al. Hedgehog signaling is dispensable for adult murine hematopoietic stem cell function and hematopoiesis. Cell Stem Cell 2009;4(6):559–67.

193. Willert K, Nusse R. Beta-catenin: a key mediator of Wnt signaling. Current opinion in genetics and Development 1998;8(1):95–102.

194. Hsu SC, Galceran J, Grosschedl R. Modulation of transcriptional regulation by LEF-1 in response to Wnt-1 signaling and association with beta-catenin. Molecular and Cellular Biology 1998;18(8):4807–18.

195. Reya T, Duncan AW, Ailles L, et al. A role for Wnt signalling in self-renewal of haematopoietic stem cells. Nature 2003;423(6938):409–14.

196. Luis TC, Weerkamp F, Naber BA, et al. Wnt3a deficiency irreversibly impairs hematopoietic stem cell self-renewal and leads to defects in progenitor cell differentiation. Blood 2009;113(3): 546–54.

197. Koch U, Wilson A, Cobas M, et al. Simultaneous loss of beta- and gamma-catenin does not perturb hematopoiesis or lymphopoiesis. Blood 2008;111(1): 160–4.

198. Cobas M, Wilson A, Ernst B, et al. Beta-catenin is dispensable for hematopoiesis and lymphopoiesis. Journal of Experimental Medicine 2004;199(2):221–9.

199. Kirstetter P, Anderson K, Porse BT, et al. Activation of the canonical Wnt pathway leads to loss of hematopoietic stem cell repopulation and multilineage differentiation block. Nature Immunology 2006;7(10):1048–56.

200. Scheller M, Huelsken J, Rosenbauer F, et al. Hematopoietic stem cell and multilineage defects generated by constitutive beta-catenin activation. Nature Immunology 2006;7(10): 1037–47.

201. Qian Z, Chen L, Fernald AA, et al. A critical role for Apc in hematopoietic stem and progenitor cell survival. Journal of Experimental Medicine 2008;205(9): 2163–75.

202. Van Den Berg DJ, Sharma AK, Bruno E, Hoffman R. Role of members of the Wnt

gene family in human hematopoiesis. Blood 1998;92(9):3189–202.

203. Austin TW, Solar GP, Ziegler FC, et al. A role for the Wnt gene family in hematopoiesis: expansion of multilineage progenitor cells. Blood 1997;89(10):3624–35.

204. Nemeth MJ, Topol L, Anderson SM, et al. Wnt5a inhibits canonical Wnt signaling in hematopoietic stem cells and enhances repopulation. Proceedings of the National Academy of Sciences of the United States of America 2007; 104(39):15436–41.

205. Mishra L, Derynck R, Mishra B. Transforming growth factor-beta signaling in stem cells and cancer. Science (New York, NY) 2005;310(5745): 68–71.

206. Piek E, Heldin CH, Ten Dijke P. Specificity, diversity, and regulation in TGF-beta superfamily signaling. FASEB J 1999;13(15):2105–24.

207. Dickson MC, Martin JS, Cousins FM, et al. Defective haematopoiesis and vasculogenesis in transforming growth factor-beta 1 knock out mice. Development (Cambridge, England) 1995;121(6):1845–54.

208. Martin JS, Dickson MC, Cousins FM, et al. Analysis of homozygous TGF beta 1 null mouse embryos demonstrates defects in yolk sac vasculogenesis and hematopoiesis. Annals of the New York Academy of Sciences 1995;752:300–8.

209. Larsson J, Goumans MJ, Sjostrand LJ, et al. Abnormal angiogenesis but intact hematopoietic potential in TGF-beta type I receptor-deficient mice. EMBO J 2001;20(7):1663–73.

210. Soma T, Yu JM, Dunbar CE. Maintenance of murine long-term repopulating stem cells in ex vivo culture is affected by modulation of transforming growth factor-beta but not macrophage inflammatory protein-1 alpha activities. Blood 1996;87(11):4561–7.

211. Fortunel NO, Hatzfeld A, Hatzfeld JA. Transforming growth factor-beta: pleiotropic role in the regulation of hematopoiesis. Blood 2000;96(6): 2022–36.

212. Jacobsen FW, Stokke T, Jacobsen SE. Transforming growth factor-beta potently inhibits the viability-promoting activity of stem cell factor and other cytokines and induces apoptosis of primitive murine hematopoietic progenitor cells. Blood 1995;86(8):2957–66.

213. Zhao GQ. Consequences of knocking out BMP signaling in the mouse. Genesis 2003;35(1):43–56.

214. Marshall CJ, Kinnon C, Thrasher AJ. Polarized expression of bone morphogenetic protein-4 in the human aorta-gonad-mesonephros region. Blood 2000;96(4):1591–3.

215. Bhatia M, Bonnet D, Wu D, et al. Bone morphogenetic proteins regulate the developmental program of human hematopoietic stem cells. Journal of Experimental Medicine 1999; 189(7):1139–48.

216. Utsugisawa T, Moody JL, Aspling M, et al. A road map toward defining the role of Smad signaling in hematopoietic stem cells. Stem Cells (Dayton, Ohio) 2006;24(4):1128–36.

217. Blank U, Karlsson G, Moody JL, et al. Smad7 promotes self-renewal of hematopoietic stem cells. Blood 2006;108(13):4246–54.

218. Liu B, Sun Y, Jiang F, et al. Disruption of Smad5 gene leads to enhanced proliferation of high-proliferative potential precursors during embryonic hematopoiesis. Blood 2003;101(1): 124–33.

219. Canalis E, Economides AN, Gazzerro E. Bone morphogenetic proteins, their antagonists, and the skeleton. Endocr Rev 2003;24(2):218–35.

220. Weinmaster G. The ins and outs of notch signaling. Molecular and Cellular Neurosciences 1997;9(2):91–102.

221. Simpson P. Notch signalling in development: on equivalence groups and asymmetric developmental potential. Current Opinion in Genetics and Development 1997;7(4):537–42.

222. Muskavitch MA. Delta-notch signaling and *Drosophila* cell fate choice. Developmental Biology 1994;166(2): 415–30.

223. Dale TC. Signal transduction by the Wnt family of ligands. Biochemical Journal 1998;329(Pt 2):209–23.

224. Mancini SJ, Mantei N, Dumortier A, et al. Jagged1-dependent Notch signaling is dispensable for hematopoietic stem cell self-renewal and differentiation. Blood 2005;105(6):2340–2.

225. Milner LA, Kopan R, Martin DI, Bernstein ID. A human homologue of the *Drosophila* developmental gene, Notch, is expressed in CD34+ hematopoietic precursors. Blood 1994;83(8):2057–62.

226. Pear WS, Aster JC, Scott ML, et al. Exclusive development of T cell neoplasms in mice transplanted with bone marrow expressing activated Notch alleles. Journal of Experimental Medicine 1996;183(5):2283–91.

227. Varnum-Finney B, Purton LE, Yu M, et al. The Notch ligand, Jagged-1, influences the development of primitive hematopoietic precursor cells. Blood 1998;91(11):4084–91.

228. Ohishi K, Varnum-Finney B, Bernstein ID. Delta-1 enhances marrow and thymus repopulating ability of human CD34(+)CD38(-) cord blood cells. Journal of Clinical Investigation 2002;110(8):1165–74.

229. Duncan AW, Rattis FM, DiMascio LN, et al. Integration of Notch and Wnt signaling in hematopoietic stem cell maintenance. Nature Immunology 2005;6(3):314–22.

230. Moore KA, Pytowski B, Witte L, et al. Hematopoietic activity of a stromal cell transmembrane protein containing epidermal growth factor-like repeat motifs. Proceedings of the National Academy of Sciences of the United States of America 1997;94(8):4011–6.

231. Karanu FN, Murdoch B, Miyabayashi T, et al. Human homologues of Delta-1 and Delta-4 function as mitogenic regulators of primitive human hematopoietic cells. Blood 2001; 97(7):1960–7.

232. LeRoith D, Werner H, Burguera B, et al. The insulin-like growth factor family of peptides, binding proteins and receptors: their potential role in tissue regeneration. Advances in Experimental Medicine and Biology 1992;321:21–8; discussion 9–30.

233. Zhang CC, Lodish HF. Insulin-like growth factor 2 expressed in a novel fetal liver cell population is a growth factor for hematopoietic stem cells. Blood 2004;103(7):2513–21.

234. Zhang CC, Kaba M, Iizuka S, et al. Angiopoietin-like 5 and IGFBP2 stimulate ex vivo expansion of human cord blood hematopoietic stem cells as assayed by NOD/SCID transplantation. Blood 2008;111(7):3415–23.

Section B

Pathology of the marrow

Pathology of the marrow: general considerations and infections/reactive conditions

BJ Bain

Chapter contents

Bone marrow (BM) function is altered in a large number of pathologic states. However, there is a relatively limited range of cytologic and histologic changes that can be detected in the marrow in disease. This chapter provides a summary of the various types of physiologic or pathologic alterations that may be seen. Details of abnormalities encountered in particular diseases are given in subsequent chapters.

Principles of bone marrow examination

The bone marrow may be examined after aspiration through a special wide-bore needle. The aspirate and trephine biopsy specimens are complementary and when both are obtained, they permit a comprehensive evaluation of the bone marrow. Guidelines based on preferred best practices have been published by the International Council for Standardization in Hematology.[1] The usual sites of aspiration are the posterior or anterior iliac crest or manubrium sterni in adults, the posterior superior iliac spine in infants and children and the medial aspect of the upper end of the tibia in neonates. The aspirate, which consists of fragments of marrow tissue, individual nucleated marrow cells and a variable quantity of blood, is spread on glass slides and examined after fixation and staining. Examination of marrow smears allows a detailed analysis of the morphology and cytochemistry of cells and the percentages of various cell types (see Chapter 2 for details). However, differential counts performed on marrow smears do not give accurate data on the prevalence of some cell types, such as megakaryocytes and macrophages, which are relatively resistant to aspiration or have a tendency to remain attached to the aspirated marrow fragments during the preparation of the smears. This drawback may be overcome, to a large extent, by examining preparations obtained by crushing marrow fragments between two glass slides and pulling the slides apart. Apart from its use for cytologic studies with the light microscope, aspirated BM can be used for immunophenotypic, cytogenetic, molecular genetic, biochemical and electron microscope studies.

The histology of the BM is investigated by examining sections of aspirated marrow particles (either in clotted aspirates or after concentration of the particles in various ways) or by examining sections of a core of bone obtained using a specially-constructed trephine needle. The usual site of trephine biopsy is the posterior superior iliac spine. Unlike marrow smears, histologic sections of trephine biopsies permit an appreciation of intercellular relationships and particularly of the relationship between hemopoietic cells, non-hemopoietic cells, the blood vessels and bone (see Chapter 3). Such sections are therefore useful for the detection of granulomas and focal accumulations of malignant cells. They also allow a study of the quantity and distribution of reticulin and collagen in marrow and make possible the diagnosis of myelofibrosis. Histologic sections are usefully stained with hematoxylin and eosin (H&E), Giemsa stain and a reticulin stain. Some laboratories also stain for hemosiderin routinely but an alternative is to apply this stain selectively, only when an aspirate for a Perls stain with an adequate number of fragments is not available.

Alterations of the marrow in disease

The BM alterations include changes in cellularity, alterations in the proportions or morphology of various types of BM cells, hemophagocytosis, changes in iron stores and intraerythroblastic iron, the presence of specific microorganisms and the formation of granulomas, infiltration by malignant cells, fibrosis, presence of storage cells, necrosis, gelatinous transformation, deposition of amyloid, and vascular and embolic lesions. BM cells may also show various cytogenetic or molecular genetic abnormalities in some diseases and these are discussed in sections dealing with specific disorders; such abnormalities are usually acquired but sometimes they are inherited or constitutional abnormalities, such as trisomy 21, that are relevant to the subsequent development of a hematologic disorder.

Alterations in cellularity

The method of assessing the proportion of the marrow tissue that is composed of hemopoietic cells as opposed to fat cells (percentage cellularity) and the normal values for this parameter are discussed in Chapters 2 and 3. Hypocellularity (i.e. cellularity <25%) is seen in the acquired aplastic or hypoplastic anemias, Fanconi anemia, paroxysmal nocturnal hemoglobinuria, rare cases of acute leukemia, and in normal adults over the age of 70 years. Hypercellularity (cellularity >75%) may be seen in a variety of conditions, including hemolytic anemia, hemorrhage, megaloblastic and sideroblastic anemias, the congenital dyserythropoietic anemias, polycythemia vera and other chronic myeloproliferative neoplasms (MPN), infections, malignant disease, myelodysplastic syndromes (MDS), the leukemias and in normal infants and young children.

Alterations in the frequency and morphology of various types of bone marrow cells

Erythroblasts and neutrophil precursors

Myeloid:erythroid ratio

The myeloid:erythroid ratio (M:E ratio) is often defined as the ratio between the number of cells of the neutrophil granulocyte series (including mature granulocytes) and the number of erythroblasts. The normal range for this ratio in adults has been reported as 2.0–8.3 and 1.1–5.2 in BM smears and 1.5–3.0 in histologic sections.[1,2] Some hematologists include eosinophils, basophils and monocytes, and their precursors in the 'myeloid' figure but this has only a slight effect on the values for the M:E ratio in normal subjects. The M:E ratio can be used as an index of total erythropoietic activity in patients in whom there is reason to assume that the total number of marrow granulocytes and their precursors is normal (e.g. in patients with normal counts of circulating granulocytes). Conversely, the M:E ratio may be used as an index of total granulocytopoietic activity, provided that the total number of erythroblasts in the body can be assumed to be normal. Some causes of a reduced or increased M:E ratio are listed in Box 5.1.

Morphologic changes in erythroblasts

Most of the erythroblasts in normal BM are uninucleate, show synchrony between nuclear and cytoplasmic maturity and do not display any peculiar cytologic features. In a study of normal BM, only 0.31% of erythroblasts were binucleate (range 0–0.57%), 0.24% (range 0–0.91%) of normal erythroblasts showed basophilic stippling of the cytoplasm, up to 0.7% had vacuolated cytoplasm, 2.38% (range 0.72–4.77%) had intererythroblastic cytoplasmic bridges and 0.22% (range 0–0.55%) possessed markedly irregular or karyorrhectic nuclei.[3] Howell–Jolly bodies were found in 0.18% (range 0–0.39%) and asynchrony between nuclear and cytoplasmic maturation was found very infrequently. In various diseases accompanied by a disturbance of erythropoiesis, the frequency of such cytologic features ('dysplastic' changes) is increased; hence these cytologic 'aberrations' are described as dyserythropoietic changes. Morphologic abnormalities that are not encountered in normal BM, such as internuclear chromatin bridges and giant erythroblasts, may also be found in a few diseases (Table 5.1). Dyserythropoiesis occurs in a number of congenital and acquired disorders. The congenital disorders include some thalassemia syndromes, homozygosity for hemoglobin C or E, some unstable hemoglobins, hereditary sideroblastic anemias, thiamine-responsive anemia, homozygosity for pyruvate kinase deficiency, and the congenital dyserythropoietic anemias. The acquired disorders include vitamin B_{12} and folate deficiency, iron deficiency anemia, alcohol abuse, MDS, acute myeloid leukemia (AML), aplastic anemia, paroxysmal nocturnal hemoglobinuria, acquired immunodeficiency syndrome (AIDS), *Plasmodium falciparum* and *P. vivax* malaria, kala azar and liver disease. Dyserythropoietic changes have also been reported after excess ingestion of kelp tablets (containing arsenic) and after BM transplantation.

Increased vacuolation of the cytoplasm of erythropoietic cells has been observed during treatment with chloramphenicol and as an effect of taking excess ethanol. It has also been

Reduced M:E ratio due to increased erythropoiesis:

Hemorrhagic and hemolytic states

Thalassemia major and intermedia

Megaloblastic anemias

Sideroblastic anemias

Congenital dyserythropoietic anemias

Erythropoietin administration

Polycythemia vera

Secondary polycythemia

Myelodysplastic syndromes

Erythroleukemia

Reduced M:E ratio due to decreased total granulocytopoiesis:

Certain drugs

Radiotherapy

Some cases of aplastic anemia

Some severe congenital neutropenia

Increased M:E ratio due to erythroid hypoplasia:

Pure red cell aplasia including that due to parvovirus infection

Some cases of anemia of chronic disorders

Increased M:E ratio due to increased total granulocytopoiesis:

Infections

Tissue necrosis

Non-infective inflammatory disease

Chronic myelogenous leukemia

Acute myeloid leukemia

Non-hematologic malignant disease

Hypersplenism

During recovery from marrow suppression

Administration of cytokines such as G-CSF

reported in aplastic anemia associated with glue sniffing, in protein-energy malnutrition, riboflavin and phenylalanine deficiency, AML and hyperosmolar diabetic coma.[4] Increased vacuolation of both erythroid cells and granulocyte precursors is observed in Pearson syndrome (a mitochondrial cytopathy) and in copper deficiency.

When there is asynchrony between nuclear and cytoplasmic maturation in a substantial proportion of erythroblasts, erythropoiesis is described as being megaloblastic. A detailed description and the causes of megaloblastic erythropoiesis are given in Chapter 12.

Morphologic changes in the neutrophil series

Morphological abnormalities in the neutrophil series may be of cell size, or shape of nucleus or cytoplasm. There may be abnormalities in the differentiation pathway with left shift or maturation arrest. These changes may be inherited or acquired; the latter may be the result of hematinic deficiencies, infections, drugs, cytokine administration or malignancy. Cytoplasmic abnormalities include the absence of specific granules in the myelocytes and metamyelocytes in acute leukemia and MDS, the reduction of nuclear segmentation in the marrow granulocytes in cases of the inherited and acquired Pelger–Huët anomaly and the formation of giant

Table 5.1 Morphologic abnormalities in erythroblasts that may be detected in pathologic states using the light microscope

Feature	Abnormality	Examples of causative disorder
Cell size	Large	Megaloblastic anemia Parvovirus B19 infection Congenital dyserythropoietic anemia
	Small (micronormoblast)	Iron deficiency anemia Thalassaemia Anemia of chronic disease (when severe) Congenital sideroblastic anemia
Nuclei	N:C asynchrony	Megaloblastic anemia Myelodysplastic syndrome and erythroleukemia
	Irregular shape	Myelodysplastic syndrome Non-neoplastic dysplasia Congenital dyserythropoietic anemia
	Nuclear bridges	Myelodysplastic syndrome Congenital dyserythropoietic anemia
	Multinuclearity	Myelodysplastic syndrome and erythroleukaemia Congenital dyserythropoietic anemia
	Karyorrhexis	Myelodysplastic syndrome Non-neoplastic dysplasia
Cytoplasm	Vacuolation	Alcohol Sideroblastic anemia Chloramphenicol Copper deficiency
	Cytoplasmic bridging	Myelodysplastic syndrome Congenital dyserythropoietic anemia
	Basophilic stippling	Myelodysplastic syndrome Thalassaemia
Sideroblasts	Reduced	Iron deficiency Anemia of chronic disease
	Increased	Iron overload Megaloblastic anemia Myelodysplastic syndrome
	Ring sideroblasts	Congenital sideroblastic anemia Mitochondrial cytopathy (Pearson syndrome) Myelodysplastic syndrome Lead poisoning Drug-induced sideroblastic anaemia

metamyelocytes and macropolycytes in vitamin B_{12} or folate deficiency. Giant metamyelocytes may also be found, usually in small numbers, in the absence of evidence of vitamin B_{12} or folate deficiency, in iron deficiency, infections, malignant disease, falciparum malaria (especially chronic falciparum malaria) and protein-energy malnutrition. They are seen quite often in the BM of patients with AIDS.[5] Macropolycytes are also not specific for vitamin B_{12} or folate deficiency, being found in infections, myeloproliferative neoplasms, drug-induced marrow damage and protein-energy malnutrition. Increased numbers of binucleate cells of the neutrophil series occur in protein-energy malnutrition and to a lesser extent in vitamin B_{12} or folate deficiency. Macropolycytes and binucleate cells are sometimes seen in MDS. An increased proportion of neutrophils with ring- or doughnut-shaped nuclei may be seen in chronic myelogenous leukemia (CML), AML, MDS, AIDS and falciparum malaria.

Vacuolation of the neutrophil precursors, usually from the promyelocyte/myelocyte stage onwards, may be seen in patients with acute alcoholic intoxication, severe infections, drug-induced marrow damage (e.g. chloramphenicol toxicity), protein-energy malnutrition and certain rare conditions such as the Chédiak–Higashi syndrome, severe congenital neutropenia, hereditary transcobalamin II deficiency,[6] neutral lipid storage disease with and without ichthyosis and carnitine deficiency. The term Jordan's anomaly is sometimes used to designate familial vacuolation of leukocytes; Jordan's original patient may have had carnitine deficiency.[7] Giant metamyelocytes, whatever the condition with which they are associated, may also be vacuolated.

Detached nuclear fragments in neutrophils, resembling Howell–Jolly bodies in erythrocytes, are occasionally seen as a reversible drug-induced anomaly but more often they are indicative of human immunodeficiency virus (HIV) infection (see below).

Eosinophil series

An increase of eosinophils and their precursors, sometimes without an associated eosinophilia in the peripheral blood (PB), may be seen in parasitic infections, allergic disorders, certain skin diseases, Hodgkin lymphoma, non-Hodgkin lymphoma, acute lymphoblastic leukemia (ALL), carcinoma, sarcoma and collagen vascular diseases. A BM and PB eosinophilia is also seen in CML, eosinophilic leukemias including those associated with rearrangement of *PDGFRA*, *PDGFRB* and *FGFR1* (see Chapter 25), other chronic myeloproliferative neoplasms, occasional cases of AML and the idiopathic hypereosinophilic syndrome.

Basophils

An increase of BM basophils may be seen in CML, primary myelofibrosis and other myeloproliferative neoplasms. Basophils are not detected in H&E-stained sections of paraffin-embedded tissues, since basophil granules are water soluble, but they can be identified by immunohistochemistry.

Mast cells

Mast cells may be increased in the marrow in infection and inflammation, renal failure, aplastic anemia, paroxysmal nocturnal hemoglobinuria, lymphoplasmacytic lymphoma including Waldenström macroglobulinemia, chronic lymphocytic leukemia, non-Hodgkin lymphoma, MDS, scleroderma, systemic mastocytosis (in which the mast cells are neoplastic; see Chapter 26), some chronic eosinophilic leukemias (see Chapter 25) and less often in a variety of other conditions. Mast cells are difficult to recognize in sections stained with H&E but are detectable when sections are stained with a Giemsa stain, which stains the granules

purple. The granules also stain by the periodic acid-Schiff (PAS) reaction, are α-naphthyl AS-D chloroacetate esterase-positive (positive Leder stain) and stain metachromatically with toluidine blue. They are readily identified with an immunohistochemical stain for mast cell tryptase and may also express mast cell chymotryptase, CD68 and CD117.

Megakaryocytes

Conditions associated with an increased number of megakaryocytes include CML, polycythemia vera, essential thrombocythemia, primary myelofibrosis, infections, chronic alcoholism, reactive changes due to generalized malignant disease, Hodgkin lymphoma, non-Hodgkin lymphoma and hemorrhage. Megakaryocytes are also increased in diseases such as 'idiopathic' (autoimmune) thrombocytopenic purpura and thrombotic thrombocytopenic purpura in which thrombocytopenia is primarily caused by a reduced platelet life span (see Chapter 33).

A decreased number of megakaryocytes is seen in acute leukemia, Fanconi anemia and other constitutional aplastic anemias, the syndrome of thrombocytopenia with absent radii, and acquired aplastic anemia. The morphological abnormalities that may affect megakaryocytes in HIV infection are described later in this chapter. Those found in inherited disorders are reviewed in Chapter 32 and those in the myeloproliferative neoplasms in Chapters 22–27.

Lymphocytes

Lymphocytes are more numerous in the BM in children than in adults (Chapters 2 and 3). An artifactual increase in the percentage of lymphocytes occurs if a BM aspirate is much diluted with PB. BM lymphocytes are increased in many reactive and malignant conditions in which there is a PB lymphocytosis (e.g. infectious mononucleosis, chronic lymphocytic leukemia). In addition, BM lymphocytes may be increased in the absence of a PB lymphocytosis in non-Hodgkin lymphoma. The majority of lymphocytes in normal BM are T cells, but BM infiltration is more likely to be seen in B-lymphoproliferative disorders.

A trephine biopsy will show whether a lymphocytic infiltrate is diffuse or focal and whether any focal infiltration is paratrabecular or nodular (with or without follicle formation) (see Chapter 3). In normal BM, lymphocytes are spread diffusely through the marrow but small aggregates or nodules also develop, and rarely they may have germinal centers.[8] The incidence of such lymphoid aggregates rises with age, and an increased incidence is seen in pernicious anemia, chronic myeloproliferative neoplasms, hemolytic states, inflammatory reactions and autoimmune conditions such as rheumatoid arthritis and secondary to immunotherapy (e.g. rituximab treatment of lymphoma patients). BM biopsy specimens showing lymphoid aggregates are more likely than other BM specimens to show lipid granulomas and plasmacytosis. A malignant lymphocytic infiltrate may be diffuse or focal and occasionally a nodular pattern is seen (detailed description in Chapters 28 and 29).

Plasma cells

There are less than 1–2% of plasma cells in normal BM. An increased percentage of BM plasma cells may be found in a wide range of pathologic conditions (Box 5.2). In various non-neoplastic conditions, up to 50% of nucleated BM cells may be plasma cells (reactive plasmacytosis). It is sometimes difficult to distinguish between reactive plasmacytosis and multiple myeloma on the basis of the morphologic characteristics of the plasma cells and definitive diagnosis requires immunohistochemistry.[9] Some features useful in differential diagnosis are listed in Table 5.2. Russell bodies, Mott cells (plasma cells containing multiple Russell bodies) and apparently intranuclear inclusions resembling Russell bodies (Dutcher–Fahey bodies) may be seen in both reactive conditions and multiple myeloma but apparently intranuclear inclusions (which represent invagination of a cytoplasmic inclusion into the nucleus) are more often seen in myeloma (see Chapter 30). Cells with flaming cytoplasm may be found in both reactive plasmacytosis and myeloma but a substantial proportion of such cells is more likely in myeloma. Examination of the distribution of plasma cells in histologic sections of BM is of considerable value in elucidating the cause of plasmacytosis since homogeneous nodules of these cells, with little supporting stroma, are found in myeloma but not in reactive plasmacytosis (Table 5.2). Myeloma cells may show hemophagocytosis. Hemosiderin-containing granules are sometimes found in the cytoplasm of plasma cells in alcoholics and in copper deficiency, porphyria cutanea tarda, megaloblastic anemia, refractory normoblastic anemia and iron overload.

Box 5.2 Causes of plasmacytosis in the bone marrow

Reactive polyclonal plasmacytosis

Infection and inflammation

Viral infection including AIDS
Bacterial infection
Leishmaniasis
Pyrexia of unknown origin
Chronic inflammatory disorders

Malignant disease

Carcinoma
Hodgkin lymphoma
Non-Hodgkin lymphoma
Chronic myelogenous leukemia
Acute myeloid leukemia

Immunologic disorders

Hypersensitivity states
Autoimmune disorders including AITP

Miscellaneous

Iron deficiency anemia
Megaloblastic anemia
Marrow hypoplasia
Cirrhosis

Monoclonal plasmacytosis

Monoclonal gammopathy of undetermined significance
Light-chain-derived amyloidosis
Systemic light chain disease
Multiple myeloma

AITP, autoimmune thrombocytopenic purpura.

Macrophages (histiocytes)

An increase of BM macrophages is common in a wide variety of hematologic and non-hematologic conditions. These include various infective and inflammatory disorders, conditions associated with increased blood cell destruction or increased ineffective hemopoiesis and post-granulocyte-macrophage colony-stimulating factor (GM-CSF) therapy. The macrophages range from immature cells showing little phagocytic activity to mature cells containing phagocytosed material or having foamy cytoplasm. In most instances the increase in macrophages is reactive. However, in the rare neoplastic condition designated malignant histiocytosis the increase results from the proliferation of cells of a neoplastic clone.[10] The histiocytic disorders are defined by their constitutive cell type[11] (Box 5.3). The two morphological features that distinguish malignant histiocytosis from reactive macrophage hyperplasia are: 1) pleomorphism of macrophages, with immature and atypical features such as a prominent nucleolus, distinct and thick nuclear membrane, irregular

Table 5.2 Characteristics of bone marrow plasma cells in reactive plasmacytosis and multiple myeloma

	Reactive plasmacytosis	Multiple myeloma
Number	Up to 10–20%, rarely up to 50%	Usually 30–90%
Cytology	Most cells are mature and look like normal plasma cells Majority of cells are mononucleate; four nuclei per cell rare Nucleoli only in occasional cells Nucleocytoplasmic asynchrony usually not a prominent feature	More cells show features of immaturity; cells are either pleomorphic or monomorphic; occasionally lymphoid Multinuclearity common Nucleoli common Nucleocytoplasmic asynchrony common
Distribution	Interstitial infiltrate, especially perivascular; some cells may be aggregated around macrophages Small clusters of plasma cells may be present but large homogeneous nodules are absent Broad band-like infiltrates very rare	Commonly near endosteal surface as well as perivascular Large homogeneous nodules of plasma cells with little intervening hemopoietic tissue common Broad band-like infiltrates common
Immunocytochemistry	κ:λ ratio about 2:1 CD19 positive CD56 negative	Monotypic κ- or λ-chains CD19 negative CD56 positive (90% cases)

Benign disorders of varying biologic behavior

a. *Dendritic cell related*
   Solitary form of Langerhans cell histiocytosis*
   Juvenile xanthogranuloma and related disorders including:
   – Erdheim-Chester disease
   – Solitary histiocytomas with juvenile xanthogranuloma
     phenotype
   – Secondary dendritic cell disorders

b. *Monocyte/macrophage related (see Box 5.4)*
   Hemophagocytic lymphohistiocytosis
   – Familial
   – Sporadic
   Secondary hemophagocytic syndromes

Sinus histiocytosis with massive lymphadenopathy (Rosai–Dorfman disease)

Solitary histiocytoma of macrophage phenotype

*Solitary form of Langerhans cell histiocytosis is a clonal neoplastic proliferation of Langerhans cells' but clinically behaves in a benign manner.

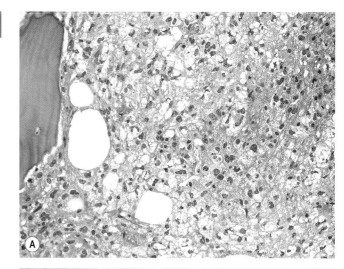

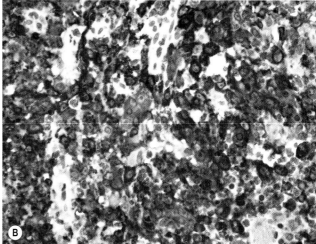

Fig. 5.2 (A, B) Trephine biopsy section of the bone marrow of a patient with histiocytic sarcoma *(courtesy of Professor Stefano A. Pileri, Haematopathology Unit, Bologna University School of Medicine, Bologna, Italy)*. (A) Giemsa stain. (B) CD163 immunohistochemistry. *Courtesy of Dr N Francis.*

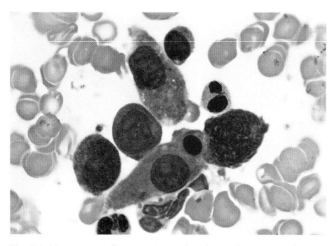

Fig. 5.1 Marrow smear from a patient with malignant histiocytosis showing a monoblast, a promonocyte and two macrophages. May–Grünwald–Giemsa (MGG) stain. Objective ×100.

nuclear chromatin and multinuclearity; and 2) the presence among the macrophages and large multinucleate cells of many monoblasts and promonocytes[12] (Fig. 5.1). The number of malignant cells in the BM varies from 5 to 90%[12] and the infiltration of the marrow may be focal or diffuse (Fig. 5.2). The demonstration of positivity for CD163 (to differentiate from other mesenchymal tumors that may express CD68 shared by monocytes/macrophages) and a clonal cytogenetic abnormality in BM cells provides strong supporting evidence. Cytochemical reactions of the malignant cells are similar to those of monocytes and macrophages; they are positive for nonspecific esterase, acid phosphatase and lysozyme. Immunohistochemical analysis distinguishes tumors derived from Langerhans cells (Langerhans cell histiocytosis and sarcoma), follicular dendritic cell sarcoma and interdigitating cell sarcoma from true histiocytic sarcoma and malignant histiocytosis.[13] Primary bone marrow involvement in these tumors is relatively rare. The blood count may show

anemia, leukopenia, thrombocytopenia and eosinophilia and the PB film may contain macrophages and small numbers of monoblasts. A minor degree of hemophagocytosis is common. It is now apparent that the majority of patients initially described as having malignant histiocytosis actually had a reactive hemophagocytic syndrome, which could have been associated with malignant lymphoma and/or Epstein–Barr virus (EBV) infection.[14–16]

Hemophagocytic syndromes

The hemophagocytic syndrome, also called hemophagocytic lymphohistiocytosis (HLH), is a collection of non-malignant but frequently life-threatening disorders, associated with an ever growing list of genetic and acquired causes[17,18] (Box 5.4). In HLH, there is a deregulation of T-lymphocytes and excessive production of cytokines leading to macrophage hyperplasia, enhanced macrophage activity and increased phagocytosis by macrophages of red cells, granulocytes, platelets and hemopoietic cells. The clinico-pathologic features of the syndrome include fever, hepatosplenomegaly, lymphadenopathy, skin rash, neurologic abnormalities, cytopenias, hypertriglyceridemia, high serum ferritin level

Box 5.4 Classification of hemophagocytic syndromes

Primary or genetic hemophagocytic syndrome

Familial hemophagocytic lymphohistiocytosis

- Perforin gene (*PRF1*) mutations
- *SH2D1A* (*SAP*) mutations
- *UNC13D* mutation (encoding MUNC13-4)
- *STX11* mutations

Immune deficiency syndromes

- Chédiak–Higashi syndrome
- Griscelli syndrome
- X-linked lymphoproliferative syndrome
- Wiskott–Aldrich syndrome
- Severe combined immunodeficiency
- Lysinuric protein intolerance
- Hermansky–Pudlak syndrome

Secondary or reactive hemophagocytic syndrome

Infection-associated hemophagocytic syndromes

Viral infections

Human immunodeficiency virus (HIV)
Epstein–Barr virus (EBV)
Cytomegalovirus (CMV)
Human herpesvirus-6 (HHV-6)
Human herpesvirus-7 (HHV-7)
Human herpesvirus-8 (HHV-8)
Other herpesviruses, e.g. herpes simplex, varicella zoster
Parvovirus B19
Hepatitis viruses B, C or A
Hantavirus
Adenovirus
Parainfluenza type III
Rubella
Measles
Dengue
Coxsackie virus
Influenza A

Bacterial infection

Pyogenic bacteria
Mycobacterium tuberculosis
Atypical mycobacteria

Brucellosis
Salmonella typhi
Mycoplasma pneumoniae
Legionella pneumophila
Ehrlichiosis
Chlamydia

Rickettsial infection

Rocky Mountain spotted fever
Q fever
Rickettsia tsutsugamushi

Fungal infection

Histoplasmosis
Candidiasis
Trichosporonosis
Cryptococcosis

Parasitic infection

Leishmania donovani
Toxoplasma gondii
Pneumocystis jiroveci
Malaria

Drug associated

Phenytoin

Malignancy-associated hemophagocytic lymphohistiocytosis

Lymphomas
Breast cancer
Gastric cancer
Lung cancer
Medulloblastoma
Acute myeloid leukemias
Acute lymphoblastic leukemia
Prolymphocytic leukemia
Myeloma

Macrophage activation syndrome (associated with autoimmune diseases)

Systemic lupus erythematosus
Juvenile idiopathic arthritis, systemic form (SoJIA)

Other

Weber–Christian disease

and coagulopathy. In the 'primary' hemophagocytic syndrome (familial hemophagocytic lymphohistiocytosis), there is an inherited immune defect. Many cases of acquired hemophagocytic syndrome have an underlying predisposing condition leading to immunosuppression such as HIV infection, renal transplantation, malignant disease and autoimmune disease. The most frequent cause of a virus-associated hemophagocytic syndrome is EBV. The many other causes of infection-associated hemophagocytic syndrome include tuberculosis and *P. falciparum* malaria (Fig. 5.3). Reactive macrophages containing phagocytosed blood or BM cells can be distinguished on the basis of cytologic and cytochemical characteristics from other malignant cells showing hemophagocytic activity (Box 5.4).

Increased phagocytosis only of granulocyte lineage cells may be seen in drug-induced agranulocytosis and increased erythrophagocytosis may be observed in hemolytic states such as autoimmune hemolytic anemia, paroxysmal cold hemoglobinuria, malaria and sickle cell anemia.

An increase of BM macrophages that do not show excessive hemophagocytic activity is commonly seen in reactive conditions such as viral infections, bacterial endocarditis, mycobacterial infections and histoplasmosis.

In lysosomal storage diseases, BM macrophages are laden with lipid or mucopolysaccharide.

Osteoblasts and osteoclasts

BM smears contain increased numbers of osteoblasts and osteoclasts when there is enhanced bone remodeling. Osteoblasts and osteoclasts are more frequent in aspirates from children than in those from adults. An increase is often seen

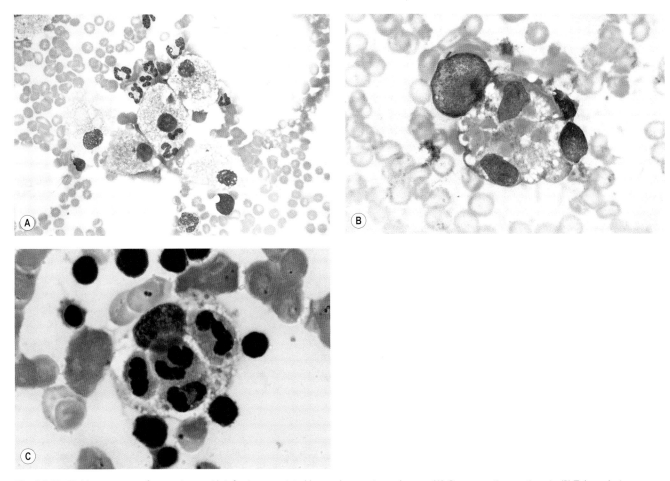

Fig. 5.3 (A–C) Marrow smears from patients with infection-associated hemophagocytic syndromes. (A) Gram-negative septicemia. (B) Tuberculosis. (C) Acute *Plasmodium falciparum* malaria. The central foamy macrophage in (A) contains two ingested neutrophils and an ingested red cell. The macrophage in (B) contains several red cells and that in (C) contains four granulocytes. May–Grünwald–Giemsa stain.

in BM aspirates containing metastatic malignant cells. Strongly PAS-positive, vacuolated osteoblasts have been reported in Pompe's disease (type II glycogen storage disease).

Changes in iron stores and intraerythroblastic iron

Iron stores

In the BM, storage iron is normally present in the form of ferritin and hemosiderin and is mainly within the macrophages but also in endothelial cells. The stores of hemosiderin can be assessed by examining BM smears or histologic sections of either trephine biopsy sections or aspirated marrow fragments. In unstained smears and sections and in H&E-stained sections, hemosiderin granules appear as golden-yellow or brown refractile particles. In preparations stained by Perls acid ferrocyanide method (Prussian blue method), the hemosiderin appears as blue or bluish-black granules that may vary considerably in size. Various methods of grading hemosiderin stores semiquantitatively have been employed by different authors but in practice, it is adequate to grade hemosiderin iron as absent (or greatly reduced), present or increased.[1] In examining BM smears it is necessary to examine a minimum of seven particles before

concluding that hemosiderin is absent.[19] BM hemosiderin stores are either absent or virtually absent in iron deficiency anemia from any cause. Rarely, patients recently treated with large doses of iron dextran develop iron deficiency anemia in the presence of stainable BM iron; in this situation the stainable iron is in a form that is unavailable for rapid mobilization.

Increased marrow hemosiderin may be found in hereditary hemochromatosis, transfusion-induced hemosiderosis, anemia of chronic disease, hemolytic anemias with predominantly extravascular hemolysis (e.g. sickle cell anemia, pyruvate kinase deficiency, glucose-6-phosphate dehydrogenase (G6PD) deficiency), aplastic anemia and anemias associated with increased ineffective erythropoiesis. The latter include megaloblastic and sideroblastic anemias, certain thalassemia syndromes even in the absence of repeated transfusions, congenital dyserythropoietic anemia and MDS. A number of mechanisms operate to increase marrow hemosiderin stores in various types of anemia. As two-thirds of the total body iron is normally present as hemoglobin within circulating erythrocytes, an anemia that is not primarily due to iron deficiency and is unassociated with hemorrhage will result in a redistribution of body iron with some increase of storage iron. In addition, because iron absorption via the gut is proportional to total erythropoiesis, patients with anemia associated with increased effective or ineffective erythropoiesis have an absolute increase in their total body iron due to increased iron absorption. The increase in iron absorption may, even in untransfused patients, eventually lead to hemosiderosis. Repeated transfusion for chronic anemia also causes a progressive increase of iron stores as the body has no effective mechanism for getting rid of excess iron. Signs and symptoms of hepatic, cardiac and endocrine dysfunction due to hemosiderosis are usually only seen after the transfusion of about 50 l of blood (equivalent to a total of about 25 g of iron).

There is a reasonable correlation between the cytochemical assessment of iron stores in stained preparations of marrow and biochemical determinations such as the iron content of the marrow or liver or, with certain exceptions, the serum ferritin level. The causes of alterations in the serum ferritin level are given elsewhere (Chapter 11).

Alterations in stainable non-hemoglobin iron within erythroblasts

When normal BM smears are stained by Perls acid ferrocyanide method and examined at high magnification (e.g. as high as ×950) using an oil immersion lens, 20–90% of the polychromatic erythroblasts are sideroblasts containing one or a few (up to five) very small (usually barely visible) blue-staining siderotic granules randomly distributed in the cytoplasm.[20] Ultrastructural studies indicate that the siderotic granules present in normal erythroblasts correspond to intracytoplasmic aggregates of altered ferritin molecules (siderosomes or ferritin bodies) that may be membrane-bound (Fig. 5.4). In iron deficiency anemia and the anemia of chronic diseases, the percentage of sideroblasts is decreased. By contrast, in a wide variety of diseases associated with an increase in the percentage saturation of transferrin (e.g. hemolytic anemia, megaloblastic anemia, thalassemia, hereditary and secondary hemochromatosis), the number (per erythroblast) and size of siderotic granules are increased, but the granules remain randomly distributed. Erythroblasts showing this phenomenon are described as abnormal sideroblasts. Most of the siderotic granules of such erythroblasts also consist of siderosomes (albeit abnormally large ones) but a few consist of iron-laden mitochondria. In the sideroblastic anemias there is an increase in both the coarseness and number (per erythroblast) of siderotic granules but additionally the majority of the granules tend to be distributed in either a partial or complete perinuclear ring; cells showing such perinuclear rings are termed ring sideroblasts; ring sideroblasts have been defined as erythroblasts containing at least five perinuclear granules.[21] Ultrastructural studies indicate that most of the siderotic granules within a ring sideroblast consist of iron-laden mitochondria. The sideroblastic anemias are discussed in Chapter 14.

Infections and the bone marrow

In acute bacterial infections the BM shows increased cellularity and an increased M:E ratio due to increased neutrophil granulocytopoiesis. Even when the cellularity of the marrow is greatly increased, some fat cells persist. The neutrophil series may show toxic granulation and the formation of Döhle bodies. The marrow may also contain occasional

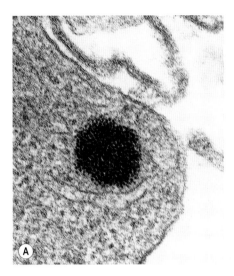

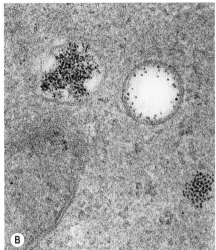

Fig. 5.4 (A, B) Different ultrastructural appearances of siderosomes in two erythroblasts from normal bone marrow. (A) Siderosome consisting of a densely packed aggregate of hemosiderin molecules. The aggregate does not appear to be enclosed within a membrane. (B) Siderosome consisting of a membrane-bound collection of hemosiderin granules (top left). The electron micrograph also shows a smaller aggregate of ferritin molecules (bottom right) and a rhopheocytotic vesicle lined by ferritin molecules. Uranyl acetate and lead citrate. (A) ×11300; (B) ×120400.

giant metamyelocytes. In severe infections there may be a marked reduction of the proportion of neutrophil granulocytes. In histologic sections of marrow, the spatial distribution of the granulocyte precursors is normal, with myeloblasts and promyelocytes located near the bone trabeculae. Some degree of erythroid hypoplasia is frequent in many infections and there are reduced numbers of siderotic granules within erythroblasts.

In microbial infections associated with monocytosis, the marrow may show an increased proportion of cells of the mononuclear phagocyte system. In occasional patients with some types of infection the macrophages show prominent hemophagocytosis (see Box 5.4 and Fig. 5.3). Certain infections are characterized by granulomatous lesions in the BM (see below).

Microscopic examination of BM smears and sections after staining with specific stains may be useful in diagnosing

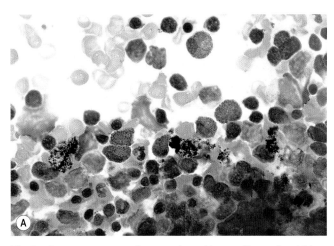
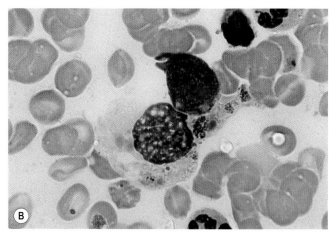

Fig. 5.5 Bone marrow smear from a patient with acute *Plasmodium falciparum* malaria. (A) Edge of a marrow fragment showing three macrophages laden with malarial pigment. (B) Higher power view of a macrophage with pigment. May–Grünwald–Giemsa stain.

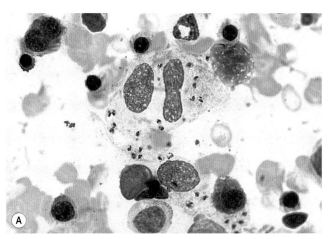
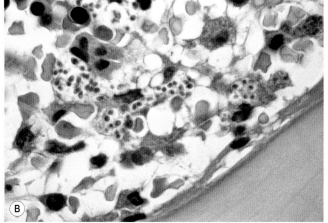

Fig. 5.6 (A, B) (A) Macrophages containing several Leishman–Donovan bodies, from a marrow smear of a patient with kala azar. Each parasite has a large ovoid or rounded nucleus and a rod-like kinetoplast situated more or less at right-angles to the nucleus. Both the nucleus and the kinetoplast stain reddish-violet. May–Grünwald–Giemsa stain. (B) Trephine biopsy section of the bone marrow of a patient with AIDS, showing Leishman–Donovan bodies within macrophage cytoplasm. H&E.

certain mycobacterial and fungal infections, especially but not exclusively in patients with granulomas. Fungi are usually seen in the marrow in immunocompromised patients and may be found extracellularly and within macrophages. In Whipple's disease, *Tropheryma whipplei* (previously *Tropheryma whippelii*), which stain violet with Romanowsky stains and black with methenamine silver, may be seen within BM macrophages.[22]

In certain bacterial and fungal infections, the organisms can be cultured from marrow. In histoplasmosis, cryptococcosis, candidiasis, blastomycosis and coccidioidomycosis organisms may be demonstrated both by microscopy of smears or histologic sections and by culture.[23]

Chronic *Plasmodium falciparum* malaria in young children is associated with a marked increase of dyserythropoiesis and ineffective erythropoiesis.[24] Dyserythropoiesis is also seen in severe acute falciparum malaria, especially cerebral malaria. BM aspiration is not usually performed for the diagnosis of malaria and there is limited information on its value. A BM aspirate is helpful in making a retrospective diagnosis of *Plasmodium falciparum* malaria in an undiag-

nosed but treated patient; in this situation, malarial pigment will be present in BM macrophages (Fig. 5.5). In post-mortem examinations of patients who have had recurrent attacks of falciparum malaria, malarial pigment is found in the marrow, spleen and liver.

Leishmaniasis may be diagnosed by studies of BM smears or sections although culture of the BM aspirate is more sensitive (Fig. 5.6); occasionally, the organisms may also be seen in PB monocytes. As in the case of chronic falciparum malaria, the erythroblasts of patients with leishmaniasis show nonspecific morphologic abnormalities indicative of dyserythropoiesis[25] (Fig. 5.7).

In viral infections, the BM contains an increased number of normal or atypical lymphocytes. Especially in herpesvirus infections, macrophages may show hemophagocytosis. In cytomegalovirus (CMV) infection the marrow may contain the typical giant cells with eosinophilic intranuclear inclusions.[26] Infection by parvovirus B19 causes transient red cell aplasia and, consequently, severe anemia occurs in patients with an underlying hemolytic state (e.g. sickle cell anemia, thalassemia intermedia, hereditary spherocytosis and pyru-

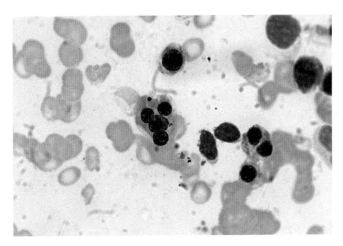

Fig. 5.7 Erythroblast with four nuclei and a micronucleus in a marrow smear from a patient with kala azar. May–Grünwald–Giemsa stain.

vate kinase deficiency).[27] Chronic pure red cell aplasia with resultant anemia can occur in parvovirus B19-infected patients with congenital or acquired immune deficiency, who are unable to mount an immune response that is adequate to clear the virus. In some cases of the congenital rubella syndrome, thrombocytopenia is at least partly due to reduced numbers of megakaryocytes in the marrow. In other cases the thrombocytopenia is mainly caused by a decreased platelet life span and is associated with normal or increased numbers of BM megakaryocytes.

HIV infection

A variety of hematologic abnormalities may be found in HIV infection,[28] especially at the later stages of infection. These include cytopenias, dysplastic changes affecting all hemopoietic cell lineages and changes in the BM resulting from opportunistic infections.

Changes in the peripheral blood

During the primary infection with HIV, which is associated with fever, sore throat and cervical lymphadenopathy, there is an initial lymphopenia followed by lymphocytosis. Atypical lymphocytes are present in the blood film and false positive results may be obtained in tests for glandular fever. Other changes may include a mild normocytic normochromic anemia, with or without neutropenia or thrombocyto-

penia, and pancytopenia. The PB picture returns to normal after seroconversion.

During the phase of clinically latent infection that follows the primary infection there is a slowly progressive CD4$^+$ lymphopenia. The total lymphocyte count may be initially normal because of a CD8$^+$ lymphocytosis. The prevalence of various cytopenias increases with progression of infection (i.e. increasing viral load). In a study of over 32 000 HIV-infected patients in the USA, an Hb <10 g/dl was found in 37% of patients with AIDS and 12% of patients without AIDS but with a CD4$^+$ lymphocyte count <0.2×10^9/l.[29] When isolated thrombocytopenia occurs during the clinically latent phase, platelet-associated immune-complexes are frequently present and the antibody in some such complexes may have specificity against HIV antigens. Rarely, an immune thrombocytopenia and autoimmune hemolysis may develop as may a microangiopathic hemolytic anemia and thrombocytopenia resembling that seen in the hemolytic uremic syndrome or thrombotic thrombocytopenic purpura.[30]

The blood film in AIDS may show various changes. The red cells are normocytic and normochromic or macrocytic; macrocytosis may occur even in the absence of zidovudine therapy. There may be reticulocytopenia, monocytopenia and atypical lymphocytes with lobulated nuclei. Some neutrophils may show various dysplastic changes including Howell–Jolly-body-like nuclear fragments, hypogranularity, the acquired Pelger–Huët anomaly, a high nucleocytoplasmic ratio, bizarre nuclear shapes and binuclearity.[5,31] There may also occasionally be circulating giant metamyelocytes and giant neutrophils. Neutrophils may also show changes related to infection, such as toxic granulation, vacuolation, Döhle bodies and a 'left-shift'.

Changes in the bone marrow

The various abnormalities found in trephine biopsy sections from patients with AIDS and their prevalence are shown in Table 5.3. The BM is hypercellular at the early stages and hypocellular in advanced AIDS. Polymorphous lymphoid aggregates are seen in the absence of lymphoma or opportunistic infections and appear to be at least partly a manifestation of the HIV infection itself; they are aggravated by opportunistic infections. The reticulin fibrosis is usually mild or moderate and leads to the marrow sinusoids being held open in paraffin-embedded trephine biopsy sections.

Gelatinous transformation occurs late in the disease and affects patients with considerable weight loss. The gelatinous

Table 5.3 Various abnormalities[a] found in trephine biopsy sections from patients with AIDS *(From Wickramsinghe SN 1994 Bone marrow damage in AIDS. In: Bhatt HR, James VHT, Besser GM et al. (eds) Advances in Thomas Addison's diseases, vol 1. Journal of Endocrinology, Bristol, 339–355)*

Abnormality	% Cases affected	Abnormality	% Cases affected
Hypercellular	35–55	Gelatinous transformation	9–20
Hypocellular	13–33	Granulomas	11–16
Plasmacytosis	25–98	Burkitt lymphoma	1–5
Lymphoid aggregates	16–32	Hodgkin lymphoma	<1–3
Reticulin fibrosis	20–55	Acid-fast bacilli	1–7

[a]Other malignant diseases encountered include other non-Hodgkin lymphomas and Kaposi sarcoma.

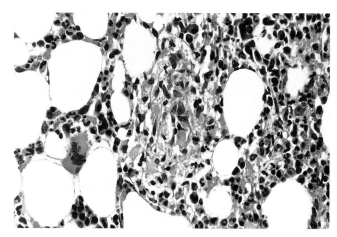

Fig. 5.8 Granuloma in a trephine biopsy section of bone marrow from a patient with AIDS and disseminated atypical mycobacterial infection. H&E.

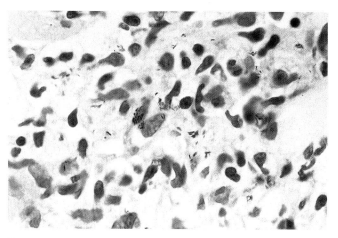

Fig. 5.9 Bone marrow granuloma from a patient with AIDS and disseminated *Mycobacterium avium intracellulare* infection. The macrophages contain many acid-fast bacillli. Ziehl–Neelsen stain.

material, which is composed of hyaluronic acid and sulfated glycosaminoglycan, first appears around the fat cells as these decrease in size but eventually appears between hemopoietic cells, presumably because of the replacement of the fat cells by this extracellular material. Trilineage myelodysplasia occurs in AIDS (38–86% of cases) and AIDS-related complex (18%). Many dysplastic changes may be observed. These changes may be seen in patients without current opportunistic infections.

Opportunistic infections in AIDS[32–35] may be due to:

1. Bacteria: *Mycobacterium tuberculosis* (common in Africa), *Mycobacterium avium intracellulare* and other atypical mycobacterial infections (common in UK), rarely Bartonella species (causing focal epithelioid angiomatosis).
2. Viruses: CMV, EBV, parvovirus B19.
3. Fungi: *Cryptococcus neoformans*, *Histoplasma capsulatum* (reported especially from USA, Central and South America), Candida species, *Penicillium marneffei* (reported from the Far East).
4. Parasites: leishmaniasis, toxoplasmosis, histoplasmosis, American trypanosomiasis.

In keeping with the virulence *of Mycobacterium tuberculosis*, this organism becomes disseminated in patients whose CD4+ lymphocyte count is not severely reduced and, consequently, well-formed granulomas may be found in the marrow. However, less-virulent opportunistic organisms (e.g. atypical mycobacteria and fungi) generally provoke poorly formed granulomas (Fig. 5.8). BM trephine biopsies are more useful than aspirates in detecting such infections. Sections should be stained by the Ziehl–Neelsen stain to look for mycobacteria (Fig. 5.9), by the PAS stain or Grocott's methenamine silver stain to look for fungi such as *Cryptococcus neoformans* (Fig. 5.10), *Histoplasma capsulatum* and *Candida albicans* and the Giemsa stain, to look for protozoa such as *Toxoplasma gondii* and *Leishmania donovani*. These organisms may be found within poorly formed granulomas or diffusely in the marrow, within macrophages.

A number of different mechanisms interact to cause the hematologic abnormalities in HIV infection[5,36–38] and the relative importance of the different mechanisms may vary from patient to patient. The possible mechanisms are:

1. HIV infection of stem cells.
2. Disordered regulation of hemopoiesis due to stromal cell damage.
3. Anemia of chronic disease secondary to opportunistic infections.
4. Drug-related hematological disturbances. BM suppression may result from antiretroviral drugs (e.g. zidovudine), drugs against opportunistic viral infections (e.g. ganciclovir for CMV infection) and drugs against HIV-associated neoplasms.
5. BM infiltration by neoplastic cells, including Hodgkin lymphoma and non-Hodgkin lymphoma such as Burkitt's lymphoma and diffuse large B-cell lymphoma. Rarely Kaposi's sarcoma infiltrates the marrow. Both monoclonal gammopathy of undetermined significance and multiple myeloma may occur.
6. Other mechanisms. Reduced serum levels of vitamin B12 and other hematinics and abnormal Schilling test results may be found in AIDS secondary to an HIV-induced gastropathy and enteropathy; however, treatment with vitamin B12 does not usually result in substantial clinical improvement.

Bone marrow granulomas

A granuloma is a compact collection of mature cells of the mononuclear phagocyte system. The types of monocyte-derived cells that may be found in granulomas include epithelioid cells, macrophages, Langhans-type giant cells (containing numerous small nuclei situated around the periphery of the cell) and foreign body-type giant cells (containing a smaller number of nuclei scattered throughout the cell). Granulomas may also contain lymphocytes, plasma cells, neutrophils, eosinophils, fibroblasts and necrotic or caseating areas. BM granulomas are seen in many conditions characterized by the formation of granulomas in other tissues[39] (Box 5.5). Immunodeficient patients may fail to generate granulomas in response to organisms that evoke granuloma formation in immunocompetent subjects. This is because the development of granulomas requires normal lymphocyte functions; in experimental animals granuloma

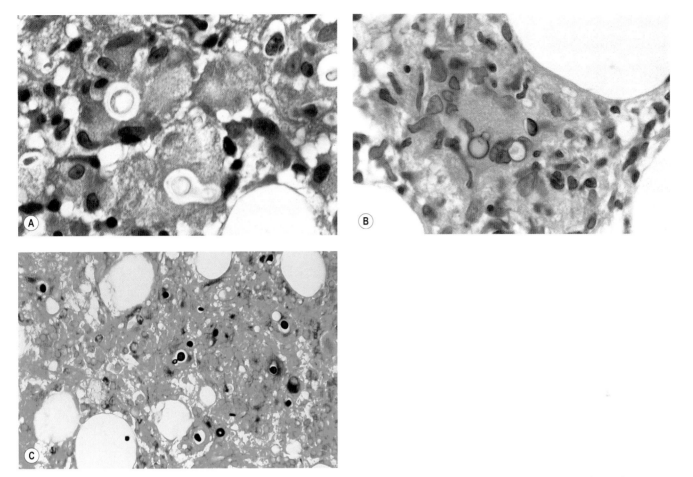

Fig. 5.10 (A–C) Poorly formed granuloma in trephine biopsy sections of bone marrow from patients with AIDS, showing budding yeast forms of *Cryptococcus neoformans*. (A) H&E; (B) PAS stain; (C) Grocott's methenamine silver stain.

formation is suppressed by neonatal thymectomy and anti-lymphocyte serum.

Epithelioid cells may rarely be seen in Romanowsky-stained BM smears suggesting the possibility of granuloma formation. In BM smears, epithelioid cells tend to occur in groups and have abundant blue-gray to dark blue cytoplasm and round, oval or reniform nuclei. However, BM granulomas are best detected in histologic sections of trephine biopsy specimens or clot sections of aspirated marrow (Fig. 5.11).

Patients being investigated for infections that generate granulomas, for example those with pyrexia of unknown origin, should not only have a trephine biopsy for histologic studies but also a BM aspiration for culture of mycobacteria and fungi and, if they have visited or lived in an endemic area, leishmaniasis. If granulomas are found, sections should be stained by the Ziehl–Neelsen stain for mycobacteria and the PAS and silver stains for fungi.

BM granulomas are found in 15–40% of patients with miliary tuberculosis, including some patients with normal chest radiology. In tuberculous granulomas, Langhans-type giant cells are usually found, caseation is present in about 50% of patients and acid-fast bacilli are usually absent or, when present, found in small numbers. In disseminated *Mycobacterium avium intracellulare* infection, granulomas of variable size and appearance are seen in about half the cases.

Giant cells and necrosis are uncommon and macrophages are packed with organisms and may appear foamy. The organisms are best demonstrated using the Ziehl–Neelsen stain; they are acid-fast but longer, more curved and more coarsely beaded than *Mycobacterium tuberculosis* and unlike the latter are PAS-positive. *Mycobacterium tuberculosis* and atypical mycobacteria may be cultured from the BM sometimes even in patients in whom the Ziehl–Neelsen stain has not revealed organisms. Patients with hairy cell leukemia and those with AIDS may have absent or impaired granuloma formation with mycobacterial infection of the BM.[40]

Granulomas with large foamy macrophages may be found in typhoid fever and the bacilli may be seen within macrophages; the organisms can usually be cultured from the BM. In leprosy, the *Mycobacterium leprae* may appear as bacilliform 'ghosts' within macrophages in Romanowsky-stained marrow smears, and the acid-fast organisms can be demonstrated by the Fite stain. The ghosts of mycobacteria have also been observed free and within macrophages in atypical mycobacterial infection in AIDS.[41] BM granulomas are frequently found in brucellosis and these are smaller and less distinct than those in tuberculosis and sarcoidosis. Large granulomas, often with Langhans-type giant cells and scanty organisms and sometimes with caseation, may occur in patients with histoplasmosis and reasonably normal immunity. By contrast, patients with immune suppression usually

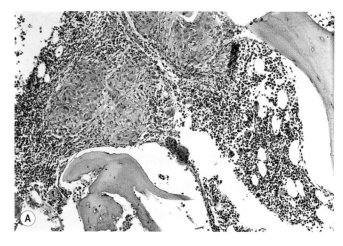

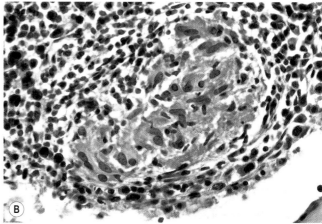

Fig. 5.11 (A, B) Trephine biopsy sections of bone marrow showing sarcoid granulomas. H&E. (A) ×94; (B) ×375.

have a marked and diffuse increase in macrophages and BM necrosis. In both types of patient, the yeast form of the organism is found within macrophages. The yeast forms appear blue in Romanowsky-stained films and are 2–5 μm in diameter. In histologic sections, they may be seen after staining with H&E but are best demonstrated when stained by the PAS reaction and by Gömöri's methenamine silver stain. The fungi can be cultured from BM aspirates in 60–75% of patients with disseminated infection. Granulomas may also be seen in the marrow in disseminated *Cryptococcus neoformans* infection. The organisms (yeasts) are 5–10 μm in diameter, have a thick capsule that appears as a clear halo in sections stained with H&E and they show unequal budding (see Fig. 5.10). The capsule is PAS-positive and also stains with mucicarmine (red) and Alcian blue.

Small BM granulomas are fairly frequently seen in infectious mononucleosis. Giant cells are uncommon and caseation does not occur but there may be focal necrosis. Similar granulomas are less commonly found in varicella zoster infection, CMV infection and some other viral infections.

BM granulomas may also be seen in infections with the protozoa, *Leishmania donovani* and *Toxoplasma gondii*.

BM granulomas are found in some cases of sarcoidosis (Fig. 5.11) and in one-third of cases the granulomas contain Langhans-type giant cells.[42] It is not always possible to distinguish between granulomas in sarcoidosis and tuberculosis or other microbial infections on histologic features alone. Caseation is characteristic of tuberculosis but is neither invariably present nor restricted to it. Furthermore, non-caseating granulomas with no detectable acid-fast bacilli may sometimes be due to tuberculosis rather than sarcoidosis. Both tuberculous and sarcoid granulomas may have associated eosinophils and lymphocytes and these features are not helpful in making a distinction between them. Although sarcoid granulomas do not caseate they may show eosinophilic coagulative necrosis and, in the healing stage, hyaline fibrosis. They may also show asteroid bodies.[43]

In Hodgkin and non-Hodgkin lymphomas, malignant infiltration of the marrow may be accompanied by granuloma formation. In these conditions, BM granulomas (or liver or spleen granulomas) may also be found in the absence of malignant infiltration of the tissue either as a reaction to an infection or as a non-infiltrative manifestation of the disease.

Poorly circumscribed BM granulomas may occur as part of a hypersensitivity reaction to drugs such as phenytoin, procainamide, oxyphenbutazone, chlorpropamide, sulphasalazine, ibuprofen, indometacin, allopurinol and amiodarone. The granulomas may coexist with other adverse reactions such as neutropenia, eosinophilia, rash and fever.

Lipid granulomas in which fat globules are present both within macrophages and extracellularly do not have any diagnostic significance. They may contain plasma cells, lymphocytes and eosinophils and frequently occur near sinusoids or lymphoid nodules.

Lesions seen in the BM in systemic mastocytosis and in angioimmunoblastic T-cell lymphoma need to be distinguished from granulomas. In systemic mastocytosis the lesions are composed of mast cells, eosinophils, lymphocytes and collagen fibers (see Chapter 26) and in angioimmunoblastic T-cell lymphoma of immunoblasts, plasma cells, lymphocytes, histiocytes, eosinophils, arborizing capillaries and reticulin fibers.

Metastatic tumors in bone marrow

Patients with metastatic tumor cells in the BM usually have a normochromic normocytic anemia and, less commonly, a hypochromic microcytic anemia, thrombocytopenia or neutropenia. In less than half the patients with BM metastases, the blood film contains some erythroblasts and neutrophil precursors (leukoerythroblastic anemia)[44] and the presence of such cells reflects the extent of myelofibrosis. Circulating malignant cells may occasionally be seen, especially in children with small cell tumors and, more rarely, in adults with carcinoma. The PB may also show abnormalities not directly related to the BM infiltration such as the anemia of chronic disease, iron deficiency anemia, red cell fragmentation, neutrophilia, thrombocytosis, eosinophilia and features of hyposplenism (as a result of splenic infiltration).

A BM trephine biopsy is generally more useful in detecting metastatic tumor cells in the marrow than a section of aspirated BM and the latter is more useful than a smear.[44,45] However, the three procedures should be regarded as complementary. Another advantage of histologic sections (either particle sections or of trephine biopsy specimens) over smears is that they can better reveal intercellular organization such as the formation of rosettes in neuroblastoma or acini in adenocarcinoma (Fig. 5.12A) and can demonstrate fibrosis and osteoblastic reactions that may be associated with tumor metastases (Fig. 5.12B). BM fibrosis in response to tumor metastases is particularly marked in carcinomas of the breast, stomach and prostate and correlates with the occurrence of a leukoerythroblastic anemia. BM fibrosis can make aspiration impossible or lead to only peripheral blood from BM sinusoids being aspirated. In this circumstance, detection of metastases is dependent on the trephine biopsy.

In adults, the tumors that most commonly metastasize to the marrow are carcinomas of the prostate, breast, gastroin-

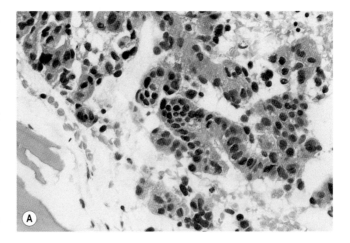

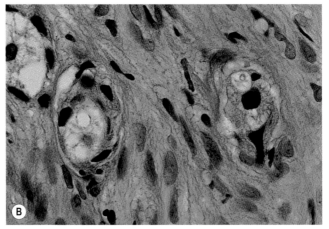

Fig. 5.12 (A, B) (A) Trephine biopsy section of bone marrow showing metastases from an adenocarcinoma. The carcinoma cells are arranged in a well-defined tubular pattern. H&E. ×94. (B) Trephine biopsy section of bone marrow showing myelofibrosis and osteosclerosis secondary to the presence in the marrow of scattered metastatic tumor cells from an unidentified primary tumor. H&E. ×940.

testinal tract, lung, thyroid and kidney[44] and in children they are neuroblastoma, rhabdomyosarcoma, Ewing tumor and retinoblastoma.[46]

Metastatic carcinoma cells can usually be readily recognized in BM smears because they are larger than all hemopoietic cells other than megakaryocytes and tend to occur in clumps (Fig. 5.13A). Generally, carcinoma cells are markedly pleomorphic and have a moderate quantity of slightly or moderately basophilic cytoplasm, sometimes with vacuoles. Some cells are multinucleate and there may be a high mitotic index. Usually, it is not possible to identify the primary tumor on the basis of the morphologic features of the metastatic cells in BM smears. However, some melanomas can be identified by the presence of intracytoplasmic melanin pigment (which stains positively with the Masson–Fontana or Schmorl stains for melanin) and renal carcinoma may be suspected if the cells have abundant foamy cytoplasm and small nuclei ('clear cell' morphology). Mucin-secreting adenocarcinoma cells possess foamy or vacuolated cytoplasm. The mucin may push the nucleus to the periphery, thus giving the cell a 'signet-ring' appearance. Stains for mucin (combined diastase-treated PAS/Alcian blue stain) can be used to identify mucin-secreting carcinoma cells.

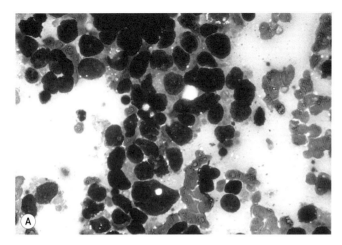

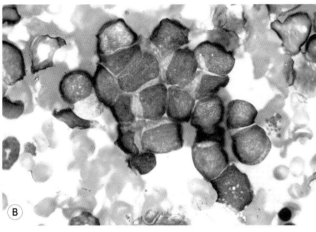

Fig. 5.13 (A, B) Clumps of metastatic tumor cells in bone marrow smears. (A) Carcinoma of the bronchus. (B) Neuroblastoma. May–Grünwald–Giemsa stain.

Patients with metastatic carcinoma frequently have increased numbers of macrophages and plasma cells in their BM. When there is associated osteosclerosis, the BM smears may also contain increased numbers of osteoblasts and osteoclasts. Sometimes, there is necrosis of the infiltrated BM and necrotic material may be seen in both smears and histologic sections.

Information on the nature of malignant cells may be obtained by immunocytochemistry and immunohistochemistry. Monoclonal antibodies against antigens such as human milk fat globulin, epithelial membrane antigen (an antigen found in carcinoma of the breast but also in other adenocarcinomas) or cytokeratin have proved most useful in detecting carcinoma cells either in histologic sections of biopsy specimens or in BM smears.[47,48] Antibody against S100 protein reacts with most malignant melanomas, including amelanotic melanomas. The detection of metastatic prostatic carcinoma cells requires the use of antibodies against both prostate-specific antigen and prostatic acid phosphatase.

Metastatic tumor cells of neuroblastoma (Fig. 5.13B), medulloblastoma, retinoblastoma, rhabdomyosarcoma and Ewing sarcoma are small and round with relatively little cytoplasm and may be difficult to distinguish from the blast cells of ALL and lymphoblastic lymphoma. In some cases of neu-

roblastoma, medulloblastoma and rhabdomyosarcoma, the small tumor cells are present in the circulation.[49] Metastatic small round cell tumors can sometimes be distinguished from acute leukemia on morphologic criteria alone. However, in other cases this distinction requires cytochemical, ultrastructural and immunochemical studies. In neuroblastoma, both BM smears and sections may show characteristic rosettes of tumor cells near fibrillar extracellular material that stains blue-gray by Romanowsky methods and eosinophilic by H&E.[50] However, these features are often absent and the diagnosis may then be made by immunohistochemistry, flow cytometry and/or PCR.[51] Rhabdomyosarcoma cells are usually heavily vacuolated, reflecting glycogen in the cytoplasm, and can be identified by electron microscopy on the basis of the presence of cross-striated myofibrils and by the immunohistochemical demonstration of myosin, desmin or myoglobin. In Ewing sarcoma histologic sections may show small numbers of 'pseudorosettes' around blood vessels. In medulloblastoma, tumor cells may display hemophagocytosis and autophagocytosis. The malignant cells of ALL give positive reactions with monoclonal antibodies against lymphoid-associated antigens (see Chapter 19) whereas the malignant cells from neuroblastoma, rhabdomyosarcoma and Ewing sarcoma give negative reactions. The blasts of ALL also usually show terminal deoxynucleotidyl transferase (TdT) expression while neuroblastoma and retinoblastoma cells do not.

Bone marrow fibrosis

An increase in the reticulin or reticulin and collagen in the BM is referred to as bone marrow fibrosis.[52,53] Reticulin fibers are collagen precursors and are produced by fibroblasts. A scheme for grading bone marrow fibrosis is discussed in Chapter 3. Patients with advanced myelofibrosis may also have osteosclerosis.

Increased reticulin deposition (reticulin fibrosis) (detected by silver stains) is a common abnormality which does not help to make a specific diagnosis. It is seen in a variety of conditions, including CML, AML (particularly acute megakaryoblastic leukemia and acute panmyelosis, which often present with the clinical picture of 'acute myelofibrosis'), multiple myeloma, chronic lymphocytic leukemia, ALL, malignant mastocytosis, hairy cell leukemia, lymphoplasmacytic lymphoma (including Waldenström macroglobulinemia) and in infections such as kala azar. Although reticulin fibrosis does not help to make a specific diagnosis it may serve to attract attention to an area of abnormal bone marrow, for example the site of a granuloma or a malignant infiltrate, so the corresponding area in an H&E-stained section should be re-examined.

Myelofibrosis may be generalized or focal. Generalized myelofibrosis occurs as in so-called 'primary' myelofibrosis and also in association with a number of diseases with widely differing etiology (Box 5.6).

The development of myelofibrosis in patients with myeloproliferative neoplasms may be related to secretion of platelet-derived growth factor, transforming growth factor β and platelet factor 4 (which inhibits collagenase) by megakaryocytes. Similarly, myelofibrosis is commonly found in acute megakaryoblastic leukemia and in acute panmyelosis (in which dysplastic megakaryocytes are part of the neoplas-

Box 5.6 Conditions associated with myelofibrosis

Generalized:

Chronic myeloproliferative
   neoplasms
   Primary myelofibrosis[a]
   Polycythemia vera
   Essential thrombocythemia[b]
   Chronic myelogenous leukemia
Acute leukemias
   Acute myeloid leukemia
      (particularly acute
      megakaryoblastic leukemia
      and acute panmyelosis)
   Acute lymphoblastic leukemia
Other malignant diseases
   Secondary carcinoma
   Hodgkin lymphoma
   Non-Hodgkin lymphoma
   Multiple myeloma[a]
   Systemic mastocytosis[a]
   Waldenström macroglobulinemia
Bone diseases
   Nutritional and renal rickets
   Primary hyperparathyroidism
   Marble bone disease –
      osteopetrosis
   Osteomalacia
   Primary hypertrophic
      osteoarthropathy
Miscellaneous
   Tuberculosis
   Other granulomatous disorders
   Myelodysplastic syndrome
      (especially therapy-related)
   Paroxysmal nocturnal
      hemoglobinuria
   Gaucher disease
   Gray platelet syndrome
   Systemic lupus erythematosus
   Systemic sclerosis
   Administration of thrombopoietin
      analogs or mimetic agents

Focal or localized:

Osteomyelitis
Paget disease
Following bone marrow
   necrosis
Following irradiation of bone
   marrow
Adult T-cell leukemia/
   lymphoma
Healing fracture site
Old trephine biopsy site

[a]There may also be osteosclerosis.

[b]As this condition is defined in the 2008 WHO Classification of Tumours of
Hematopoietic and Lymphoid Tissues, reticulin is no more than minimally
increased at diagnosis and fibrosis develops rarely.

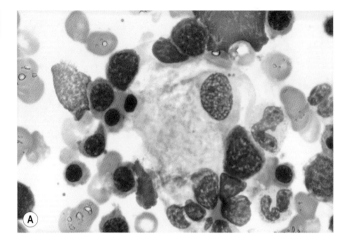

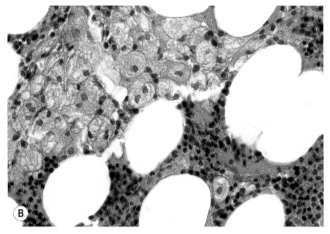

Fig. 5.14 (A, B) (A) Gaucher cell from the marrow smear of a patient with
Gaucher disease. May–Grünwald–Giemsa stain. ×940. (B) Trephine biopsy
section from a case of Gaucher disease. H&E.

tic population) and it is likely that cytokines secreted by
megakaryocytes are again relevant. In primary myelofibrosis,
necrotic megakaryocytes have been noted in fibrotic areas.
In CML and polycythemia vera the degree of fibrosis has
been related to the total number of megakaryocytes and the
number of atypical megakaryocytes respectively. In the congenital defect gray platelet syndrome it has been hypothesized that associated myelofibrosis may be consequent on
the release of granule contents (which could include platelet-
derived growth factor) from abnormal megakaryocytes.
When myelofibrosis is secondary to non-hemopoietic malignancy it is likely that the tumor cells themselves promote
fibrosis, since they may do so in sites other than the bone
marrow. When myelofibrosis is secondary to a non-
hemopoietic disorder, reversal of the fibrosis may occur
when the primary condition is effectively treated. This is also

true if effective treatment can be given for a hematological
malignancy with associated fibrosis.

Whenever extensive dense fibrosis occurs, for example
in patients with metastatic carcinoma, the hematological
findings may mimic those of primary myelofibrosis.
Extramedullary hemopoiesis may occur in secondary as well
as in 'primary' myelofibrosis.

Storage cells in lysosomal storage diseases

Lysosomes catabolize lipids, carbohydrates, proteins and
nucleotides. In a group of inherited diseases, mutations
in one of the genes encoding a lysosomal hydrolytic
enzyme lead to the intracellular accumulation of abnormal
amounts of various substances and consequent clinical
manifestations.

Sphingolipidoses

Gaucher disease

In Gaucher disease, which is usually inherited as an autosomal recessive character, there is defective production of the
lysosomal enzyme glucocerebroside β-glucosidase leading
to the intracellular accumulation of abnormal quantities
of glucocerebrosides.[54] Typical storage cells are seen in the
BM (Fig. 5.14A) as well as in other tissues; these cells are

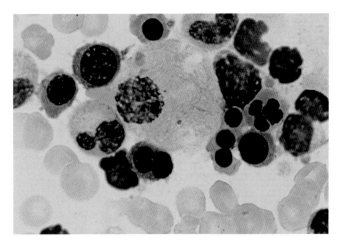

Fig. 5.15 Pseudo-Gaucher cell from the marrow smear of a patient with congenital dyserythropoietic anemia, type II. May–Grünwald–Giemsa stain. ×940.

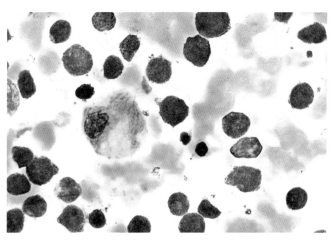

Fig. 5.16 Sea-blue histiocyte in a marrow film from a patient with chronic lymphocytic leukemia. May–Grünwald–Giemsa stain.

macrophages distended by glucocerebrosides. Gaucher's cells are large, round or oval, and have pale blue cytoplasm with a wrinkled appearance due to the presence of many fibrillar structures (Romanowsky stain). The cytoplasm is Sudan Black B- and PAS-positive. Gaucher cells also stain positively for nonspecific esterase and tartrate-resistant acid phosphatase. Stains for iron give weak positive reactions. In histologic sections, Gaucher cells are often found in clumps or sheets and their abundant cytoplasm has a crumpled appearance (Fig. 5.14B). The affected marrow may show an increase in reticulin and collagen. Electron microscopy reveals that the cytoplasm is packed with large elongated sacs containing characteristic tubes, 30–40 nm wide, each of which is made up of spirally arranged fibrils. Occasionally, particularly after splenectomy, Gaucher cells are seen in the PB. Cells resembling Gaucher cells under the light microscope are seen in the marrow in a variety of hematologic disorders including CML, acute leukemia, thalassemia major, the congenital dyserythropoietic anemias (Fig. 5.15), sickle cell anemia, Hodgkin lymphoma, non-Hodgkin lymphoma, multiple myeloma and after many platelet transfusions. However, such cells (pseudo-Gaucher cells) are ultrastructurally and by immunohistochemistry different from Gaucher cells.[55] Pseudo-Gaucher cells result from an increased phagocytic load (e.g. of abnormal red cells or erythroblasts or leukemic cells) on the macrophages resulting in the production of lipid in excess of that which can be metabolized, with consequent intracellular accumulation. Morphologically somewhat similar cells can be seen in *Mycobacterium avium intracellulare* infection but in this instance the abnormal staining characteristics of the macrophages ('pseudo-pseudo-Gaucher's cells') result from the presence of very large numbers of mycobacteria within the macrophages.

Sea-blue histiocyte syndrome

Sea-blue histiocytosis is an inherited group of disorders in which large macrophages containing coarse granules that stain sea-blue or blue-green (Romanowsky stain) are seen in the spleen, liver, BM and other organs.[56] The characteristic color of these granules after Romanowsky staining is attrib-

uted to the presence of ceroid; when unstained the granules are yellow or brown. The granules stain with oil red O and Sudan Black B; as the pigment ages it develops autofluorescence and, subsequently, PAS-positivity followed by acid-fast positivity. Ceroid is histochemically similar to lipofuscin. Ultrastructural studies have revealed that the granules are pleomorphic and that some of them contain concentric arrangements of membrane (myelin figures). Sea-blue histiocytes have also been observed in the BM in conditions other than the inherited sea-blue histiocyte syndrome (Fig. 5.16). These include acquired disorders such as CML, polycythemia vera, multiple myeloma, lymphoproliferative disorders (including Hodgkin lymphoma), autoimmune thrombocytopenic purpura and rheumatoid arthritis as well as various inherited disorders such as sickle cell anemia, thalassemia, chronic granulomatous disease, Niemann–Pick disease, Tay–Sachs disease, Fabry disease, Hurler disease, Wolman disease, lecithin-cholesterol acyltransferase deficiency, type V hyperlipidemia, and Hermansky–Pudlak syndrome.

Niemann–Pick disease

Niemann–Pick disease is usually inherited as an autosomal recessive condition and is often due to a deficiency of sphingomyelinase.[57] This leads to the accumulation of excess sphingomyelin within the macrophages of the BM and other organs. The cytoplasm of affected macrophages appears foamy, being filled with rounded lipid-containing inclusions (Fig. 5.17). The inclusions stain faint blue with Romanowsky stains and variably with the PAS reaction and lipid stains. Some sea-blue histiocytes are present. The cytoplasm of the foamy cells appears pale-yellow to yellow-brown in sections stained with H&E. The inclusions within these cells vary in their ultrastructure but often show myelin figures towards their periphery. Blood monocytes and lymphocytes in cases of Niemann–Pick disease have lipid-containing inclusions similar to those in macrophages. Foamy macrophages are not specific for Niemann–Pick disease. They are also seen in some other storage diseases and in hyperlipidemias. They may also be found in certain infections, fat necrosis, BM infarction and in Langerhans cell histiocytoses (eosinophilic

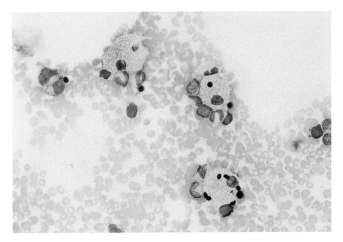

Fig. 5.17 Three foamy macrophages from the marrow smear of a patient with Niemann–Pick disease. May–Grünwald–Giemsa stain.

granuloma, Letterer–Siwe disease and Hand–Schüller–Christian disease).

Fabry disease

Fabry disease is an X-linked recessive disorder due to deficiency of α-galactosidase.[58] This leads to the accumulation of globotriaosylceramide and other neutral glycolipids in BM macrophages. The cytoplasm of the abnormal macrophages appears foamy, being crowded with small globular structures staining pale blue with Romanowsky stains and strongly with PAS, Sudan Black B, Luxol fast blue, oil red O, and stains for acid phosphatase. In sections stained with H&E, the cytoplasmic globules appear pink.

Mucopolysaccharidoses

In Hurler syndrome and other mucopolysaccharidoses, there is a deficiency of enzymes involved in the metabolism of the carbohydrate component of glycoproteins leading to an accumulation within lysosomes of mucopolysaccharides and glycolipids.[59] The abnormal lysosomes inside BM macrophages, plasma cells and lymphocytes may appear as metachromatic granules; the granules stain lilac or purple with Romanowsky stains (Alder–Reilly bodies). The cytoplasm of macrophages may be packed with basophilic inclusions of varying size which are surrounded by a clear halo. In histologic sections, the macrophage cytoplasm appears foamy due to extraction of the mucopolysaccharides.

Other storage diseases and hyperlipidemias

Foamy histiocytes resembling those seen in Niemann–Pick disease and Fabry disease may also be seen in the BM in Wolman disease, neuronal ceroid lipofuscinosis, hypercholesterolemia, hyperchylomicronemia, late-onset cholesterol ester storage disease and in Tangier disease (familial high-density lipoprotein deficiency).

Bone marrow necrosis

In some pathologic conditions, there is necrosis of both the hemopoietic and the non-hemopoietic cells of the red

Box 5.7 Conditions associated with bone marrow necrosis

Relatively common:

    Sickle cell anemia[a]

    Hemoglobin SC disease,[a] hemoglobin S/β[+]-thalassemia[b]

Acute myeloid leukemia

Acute lymphoblastic leukemia

Metastatic carcinoma

Caisson disease

Uncommon:

    Essential thrombocythemia

    Chronic myelogenous leukemia

    Primary myelofibrosis

    Lymphoma, both non-Hodgkin and Hodgkin lymphoma

    Chronic lymphocytic leukemia

    Multiple myeloma

    Malignant histiocytosis

    Other hemoglobinopathies (Hb SD, hemoglobin SE,[b] sickle cell trait)

    Disseminated intravascular coagulation

    Antiphospholipid syndrome

    Tumor embolism of the marrow

    Embolism from vegetations on cardiac valves

    Systemic lupus erythematosus

    Hyperparathyroidism

    Megaloblastic anemia

Infections:

    Cytomegalovirus infection

    Parvovirus B19 infection

    HIV infection (AIDS)

    Miliary tuberculosis

    Gram-positive infections (e.g. infection by streptococcus, staphylococcus)

    Gram-negative infections (e.g. *Escherichia coli* infection)

    Typhoid fever

    Fusobacterium necrophorum infection

    Diphtheria

    Q fever

    Histoplasmosis

    Mucormycosis

[a]Particularly during pregnancy.
[b]With parvovirus infection.

marrow and there may also be necrosis of adjacent bone.[60] BM necrosis is a common finding at autopsy but is less often diagnosed during life. It may be widespread and can recur. The necrosis may be caused by interference with the blood supply or a failure to meet increased metabolic demands from a hypercellular marrow, or both, and may sometimes be related to high concentrations of tumor necrosis factor in the blood.[61]

The conditions associated with BM necrosis are given in Box 5.7. In sickle cell anemia, Hb SC disease (heterozygous state for both hemoglobin S and hemoglobin C), hemoglobin S/β[+]-thalassemia and, rarely, heterozygosity for both hemoglobins S and E (plus parvovirus infection), necrosis may occur due to occlusion of the BM microvasculature by

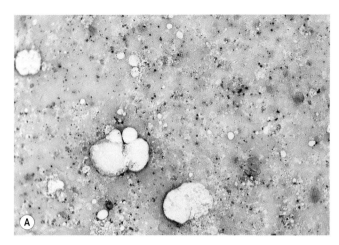

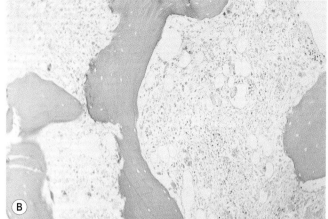

Fig. 5.18 (A, B) (A) Bone marrow smear showing necrosis of the marrow cells. May–Grünwald–Giemsa stain. ×940. (B) Trephine biopsy section of bone marrow showing necrosis of both the bone and the marrow. The lacunae within the bone do not contain osteocytes and appear empty. H&E. ×375.

sickled cells. In sickle cell disease pregnancy increases the degree of BM hyperplasia and, thereby, further increases the likelihood of BM infarction and also of death from the embolism of necrotic BM to the lungs.

In mucormycosis, the mucorales invade vessel walls and cause thrombosis and infarction.[62] In caisson disease (acute decompression illness) and disseminated intravascular coagulation (DIC) the microvasculature is occluded by bubbles of nitrogen and thrombi, respectively. In acute leukemia, carcinomatous infiltration of the BM and megaloblastic anemia plus infection, the increased metabolic needs of a hyperplastic BM may play a role in the pathogenesis of the BM necrosis. In addition, in leukemia and carcinomatosis, the malignant cells may compress vessels, invade vessel walls and occlude their lumina or cause thrombosis.

BM necrosis is accompanied by bone pain and fever. Extensive necrosis causes a leukoerythroblastic blood picture and pancytopenia. The macroscopic appearance of the aspirated BM fragments may be abnormal with the fragments appearing opaque and white/pale yellow, or plum-colored. In a Romanowsky-stained smear of necrotic BM, little cellular detail is discernible (Fig. 5.18A); the blurred outlines of cells are seen in a background of amorphous pink material. In some patients with BM necrosis secondary to metastatic carcinoma, an aspirate may show a mixture of intact tumor cells and necrotic tumor and hemopoietic cells. If BM aspirated from one site shows only necrosis and leukemia or metastatic carcinoma is suspected, a second aspiration from another site may be useful in demonstrating infiltration by malignant cells. The appearance of the trephine biopsy depends on the time after infarction as well as the underlying disorder. Initially, the cells have indistinct margins, granular cytoplasm and pyknotic nuclei. Later, cell outlines are unrecognizable and there is karyorrhexis. Necrosis of the adjacent bone is common, with loss of osteoclasts, osteoblasts and osteocytes (Fig. 5.18B). Recovery is accompanied by repopulation with hemopoietic tissue but small fibrotic scars or, rarely, large areas of fibrous tissue may develop (Fig. 5.19); new bone is laid down on the spicules of dead bone. Radiologic examination shows no abnormality initially and may show sclerotic changes after some time.

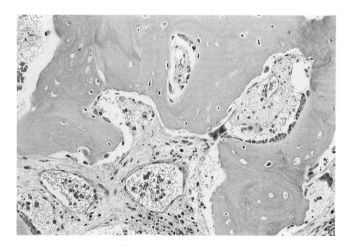

Fig. 5.19 Bone marrow fibrosis and osteosclerosis following bone marrow necrosis in a case of Ph-positive chronic myelogenous leukemia. H&E.

However, in the acute phase, bone scanning with ^{99m}Tc-sulfur-colloid shows lack of reticuloendothelial function in the infarcted area. The scan gradually returns to normal. Extramedullary hemopoiesis may develop in patients with extensive BM necrosis.

Gelatinous transformation

The BM of most patients with severe malnutrition contains a gelatinous material which consists of acid mucopolysaccharide. This may be seen in severe anorexia nervosa, some patients with cachexia secondary to AIDS and chronic disorders (e.g. tuberculosis, carcinoma) and occasional cases of leukemia post-chemotherapy and of systemic lupus erythematosus (SLE). Gelatinous transformation has also been reported in other conditions including severe hypothyroidism, intestinal lymphangiectasia (Waldman disease) and leishmaniasis.[63] The gelatinous material is amorphous, granular or fibrillar, stains pink-purple with Romanowsky stains or H&E (Fig. 5.20A,B) and stains positively with Alcian blue (particularly at a high pH) and the PAS stain.

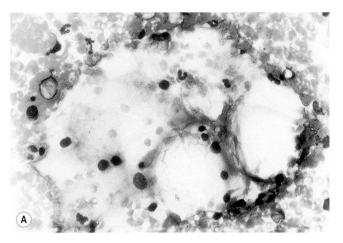
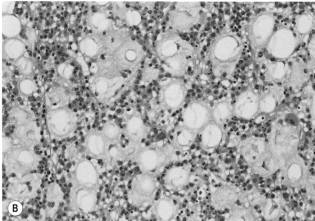

Fig. 5.20 (A, B) (A) Very small marrow fragment from a bone marrow smear of a patient with AIDS showing gelatinous transformation. In this photomicrograph, the pink-purple gelatinous material is mainly found between the fat cells. May–Grünwald–Giemsa stain. ×94. (B) Trephine biopsy section of bone marrow from a patient with AIDS showing gelatinous transformation. H&E. ×375.

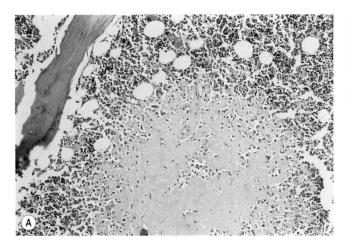
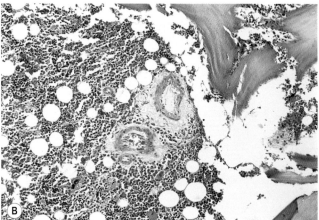

Fig. 5.21 (A, B) Amyloid deposition in the bone marrow. (A) Much of the normal hemopoietic tissue is replaced by a nodule of amyloid that appears faintly eosinophilic and homogenous. (B) Two arterioles showing advanced amyloid deposition in their walls and occlusion of their lumina with amyloid. In arterioles and small arteries, amyloid deposition commences in subendothelial tissues and gradually spreads outwards. H&E. (A) ×90; (B) ×90.

The hemopoietic cells are reduced in number and embedded within the gelatinous material and there is an absence or marked reduction of fat cells. BM fragments showing gelatinous transformation do not smear properly. A deficiency of carbohydrates and calories may underlie the gelatinous transformation and the excessive accumulation of acid mucopolysaccharide may serve to fill the BM space normally occupied by fat cells. Interestingly, young children with protein-energy malnutrition do not show gelatinous transformation.

Amyloidosis

Amyloid deposits may be seen in the BM both in smears of aspirated material, infrequently, and in histologic sections. In Romanowsky-stained smears amyloid appears pink to purple, waxy to transparent, and has been described as resembling a cumulus cloud.[64] In histologic BM sections, amyloid has the same appearance and staining characteristics as in other tissues (Fig. 5.21). It is seen most often in

vessel walls but sometimes in the interstitium. BM amyloid is observed most frequently in light-chain-associated amyloidosis (sometimes referred to as primary amyloidosis) but is also observed in secondary amyloidosis, for example in familial Mediterranean fever and secondary to chronic inflammatory conditions such as rheumatoid arthritis. In light-chain-associated amyloidosis the BM may show, in addition, a slight to moderate increase in monotypic plasma cells or overt multiple myeloma.

Vascular and embolic lesions

The BM may show arteritis and arteriolitis in any form of generalized arteritis, including giant cell arteritis.[65] Hypersensitivity reactions to drugs may cause granulomatous vasculitis and in polyarteritis nodosa there may be vasculitic lesions with fibrinoid necrosis.

Trephine biopsy specimens may reveal arteriosclerotic and thromboembolic lesions. Emboli that are acellular or composed of hyaline material or cholesterol crystals may be

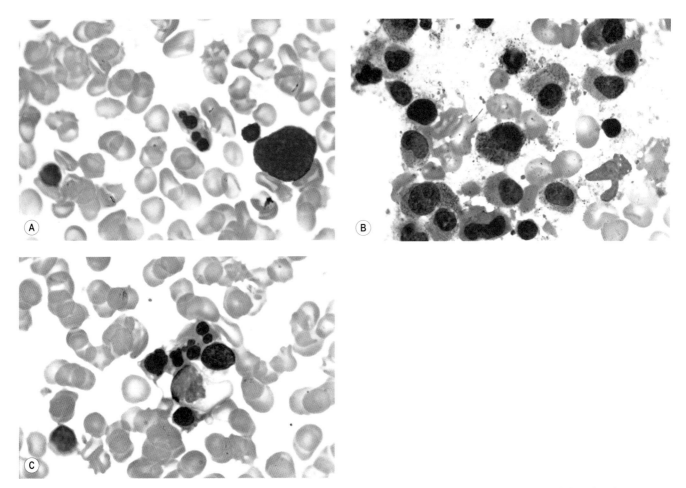

Fig. 5.22 (A–C) Marrow smear prepared from aspirates taken 30 and 82 h post mortem. (A) Two erythroblasts showing dumb-bell-shaped nuclei. (B) Normal-looking and degenerating cells of the neutrophil series. The latter have many coarse cytoplasmic granules and round nuclei. (C) Five erythroblasts. Two of these show nuclear budding, one has a dumb-bell-shaped nucleus and another shows lobulation of the nucleus. May–Grünwald–Giemsa stain.
(Courtesy of Dr N Francis).

derived from atheromatous plaques and cause a multisystem disease characterized by anemia, leukocytosis, eosinophilia and elevated erythrocyte sedimentation rate.[66] BM emboli are found in 20% of these cases at autopsy and may also be seen in biopsy material. Vessels are partly or completely occluded by acellular material with cholesterol clefts and there may be intimal hyperplasia and infiltration of vessel walls initially with granulocytes and subsequently with mononuclear cells and giant cells.

Tumor emboli may be seen in patients with carcinoma and may be accompanied by microangiopathic hemolytic anemia. In thrombotic thrombocytopenic purpura, intravascular and subendothelial hyaline deposits and platelet thrombi may be seen in BM vessels.

Aluminum deposition

In patients on hemodialysis and other patients with chronic renal failure aluminum may be deposited both in bone (at the osteoid/mineralized tissue junction) and in BM cells as coarse granules. The aluminum is derived from oral intake and dialysis fluids and may cause dementia.[67] Aluminum may be demonstrated by a specific stain (Irwin stain on an undecalcified trephine biopsy). The BM cell that contains the aluminum may be the macrophage.

Post-mortem bone marrow changes

A variety of morphologic changes occur fairly rapidly in marrow cells post mortem[68] (Fig. 5.22). This applies particularly to the neutrophil metamyelocytes and granulocytes which are rich in hydrolytic enzymes. Post-mortem BM aspirations and tissue sampling with a trephine needle should therefore be performed as soon after death as possible and preferably not more than 3 h after death. Vacuolation of the cytoplasm of granulocytes may be first seen in BM smears aspirated 1.5–7 h after death and the vacuolation increases progressively thereafter. Swelling of the nuclei of neutrophil metamyelocytes and granulocytes may be detected as early as 2 h after death; the swelling causes the affected metamyelocytes to look like myelocytes. By 8–12 h post mortem, most of the nuclei of the neutrophil metamyelocytes and granulocytes appear rounded, with a loosening of the nuclear chromatin and the appearance of structures resembling small nucleoli. The nuclear membrane is ruptured and many of the cells have indistinct cell membranes. The neutrophil myelocytes begin to lyse after 7–12 h. Karyorrhexis and budding, lobulation or segmentation of erythroblast nuclei may begin as an agonal event or during the first 2 h after death; in occasional cases, over 20% of erythroblasts show nuclear abnormalities 25 min following death, but in others marked changes do not develop in less than 3 h. Macrophages are greatly increased in number in aspirates taken within hours of death, probably mainly because they are released into the aspirate more readily than from living marrow. The post-mortem appearances of marrow aspirated 10–20 h after death differ markedly from those obtained during life and are sufficiently confusing to have led to the incorrect diagnosis of leukemia or malignant infiltration.

References

1. Lee SH, Erber WN, Porwit A, et al. ICSH guidelines for the standardization of bone marrow specimens and reports. Int J Lab Hematol 2008;30:349–64.

2. Bain BJ. The bone marrow aspirate of healthy subjects. Br J Haematol 1996; 94:206–9.

3. Wickramasinghe SN, Lee MJ, Furukawa T, et al. Composition of the intra-erythroblastic precipitates in thalassaemia and congenital dyserythropoietic anaemia (CDA): identification of a new type of CDA with intra-erythroblastic precipitates not reacting with monoclonal antibodies to alpha- and beta-globin chains. Br J Haematol 1996;93:576–85.

4. Lehane DE. Vacuolated erythroblasts in hyperosmolar coma. Arch Intern Med 1974;134:763–5.

5. Bain BJ. The haematological features of HIV infection. Br J Haematol 1997;99: 1–8.

6. Niebrugge DJ, Benjamin DR, Christie D, Scott CR. Hereditary transcobalamin II deficiency presenting as red cell hypoplasia. J Pediatr 1982;101:732–5.

7. Oshima Y, Hirota H, Nagai H, et al. Images in cardiovascular medicine. Specific cardiomyopathy caused by multisystemic lipid storage in Jordan's anomaly. Circulation 2002;106:280–1.

8. Thiele J, Zirbes TK, Kvasnicka HM, Fischer R. Focal lymphoid aggregates (nodules) in bone marrow biopsies: differentiation between benign hyperplasia and malignant lymphoma – a practical guideline. J Clin Pathol 1999;52:294–300.

9. Ioannou MG, Stathakis E, Lazaris AC, et al. Immunohistochemical evaluation of 95 bone marrow reactive plasmacytoses. Pathol Oncol Res 2009;15:25–9.

10. Sohn BS, Kim T, Kim JE, et al. A case of histiocytic sarcoma presenting with primary bone marrow involvement. J Korean Med Sci 2010;25:313–6.

11. Filipovich A, McClain K, Grom A. Histiocytic disorders: recent insights into pathophysiology and practical guidelines. Biol Blood Marrow Transplant 2010;16: S82–9.

12. Lampert IA, Catovsky D, Bergier N. Malignant histiocytosis: a clinico-pathological study of 12 cases. Br J Haematol 1978;40:65–77.

13. Pileri SA, Grogan TM, Harris NL, et al. Tumours of histiocytes and accessory dendritic cells: an immunohistochemical approach to classification from the International Lymphoma Study Group based on 61 cases. Histopathology 2002;41:1–29.

14. Shimada A, Kato M, Tamura K, et al. Hemophagocytic lymphohistiocytosis associated with uncontrolled inflammatory cytokinemia and chemokinemia was caused by systemic anaplastic large cell lymphoma: a case report and review of the literature. J Pediatr Hematol Oncol 2008;30:785–7.

15. Chuang HC, Lay JD, Hsieh WC, Su IJ. Pathogenesis and mechanism of disease progression from hemophagocytic lymphohistiocytosis to Epstein–Barr virus-associated T-cell lymphoma: nuclear factor-kappa B pathway as a potential therapeutic target. Cancer Sci 2007;98: 1281–7.

16. Koh MJ, Sadarangani SP, Chan YC, et al. Aggressive subcutaneous panniculitis-like T-cell lymphoma with hemophagocytosis in two children (subcutaneous panniculitis-like T-cell lymphoma). J Am Acad Dermatol 2009;61:875–81.

17. Rouphael NG, Talati NJ, Vaughan C, et al. Infections associated with haemophagocytic syndrome. Lancet Infect Dis 2007;7:814–22.

18. Tiab M, Mechinaud F, Harousseau JL. Haemophagocytic syndrome associated with infections. Baillière's Best Pract Res Clin Haematol 2000;13:163–78.

19. Hughes DA, Stuart-Smith SE, Bain BJ. How should stainable iron in bone marrow films be assessed? J Clin Pathol 2004;57:1038–40.

20. Kaplan E, Zuelzer WW, Mouriquand C. Sideroblasts: a study of stainable nonhemoglobin iron in marrow normoblasts. Blood 1954;9:203–13.

21. Mufti GJ, Bennett JM, Goasguen J, et al. Diagnosis and classification of myelodysplastic syndrome: International Working Group on Morphology of myelodysplastic syndrome (IWGM-MDS) consensus proposals for the definition and enumeration of myeloblasts and ring sideroblasts. Haematologica 2008;93: 1712–7.

22. Krober SM, Kaiserling E, Horny HP, Weber A. Primary diagnosis of Whipple's disease in bone marrow. Hum Pathol 2004;35: 522–5.

23. Pasternak J, Bolivar R. Histoplasmosis in acquired immunodeficiency syndrome (AIDS): diagnosis by bone marrow examination. Arch Intern Med 1983; 143:2024.

24. Wickramasinghe SN, Abdalla SH. Blood and bone marrow changes in malaria. Baillière's Best Pract Res Clin Haematol 2000;13:277–99.

25. Dhingra KK, Gupta P, Saroha V, et al. Morphological findings in bone marrow biopsy and aspirate smears of visceral kala azar: a review. Indian J Pathol Microbiol 2010;53:96–100.

26. Penchansky L, Krause JR. Identification of cytomegalovirus in bone marrow biopsy. South Med J 1979;72:500–1.

27. Brown KE. Haematological consequences of parvovirus B19 infection. Baillière's Best Pract Res Clin Haematol 2000; 13:245–59.

28. Evans RH, Scadden DT. Haematological aspects of HIV infection. Baillière's Best Pract Res Clin Haematol 2000;13:215–30.

29. Sullivan PS, Hanson DL, Chu SY, et al. Epidemiology of anemia in human immunodeficiency virus (HIV)-infected persons: results from the multistate adult and adolescent spectrum of HIV disease surveillance project. Blood 1998;91:301–8.

30. Nair JM, Bellevue R, Bertoni M, Dosik H. Thrombotic thrombocytopenic purpura in patients with the acquired immunodeficiency syndrome (AIDS)-related complex. A report of two cases. Ann Intern Med 1988;109:209–12.

31. Candido A, Rossi P, Menichella G, et al. Indicative morphological myelodysplastic alterations of bone marrow in overt AIDS. Haematologica 1990;75:327–33.

32. Huang L, Crothers K. HIV-associated opportunistic pneumonias. Respirology 2009;14:474–85.

33. Lawn SD, Churchyard G. Epidemiology of HIV-associated tuberculosis. Curr Opin HIV AIDS 2009;4:325–33.

34. Cello JP, Day LW. Idiopathic AIDS enteropathy and treatment of gastrointestinal opportunistic pathogens. Gastroenterology 2009;136:1952–65.

35. Currier JS, Havlir DV. Complications of HIV disease and antiretroviral therapy. Top HIV Med 2009;17:57–67.

36. Moses A, Nelson J, Bagby GC Jr. The influence of human immunodeficiency virus-1 on hematopoiesis. Blood 1998; 91:1479–95.

37. Bain BJ. Pathogenesis and pathophysiology of anemia in HIV infection. Curr Opin Hematol 1999;6: 89–93.

38. Bain BJ. Lymphomas and reactive lymphoid lesions in HIV infection. Blood Rev 1998;12:154–62.

39. Eid A, Carion W, Nystrom JS. Differential diagnoses of bone marrow granuloma. West J Med 1996;164:510–5.

40. Cohen RJ, Samoszuk MK, Busch D, Lagios M. Occult infections with M. intracellulare in bone-marrow biopsy specimens from patients with AIDS. N Engl J Med 1983;308:1475–6.

41. Bain BJ. The importance of a negative image. Am J Hematol 2008;83:410.

42. Browne PM, Sharma OP, Salkin D. Bone marrow sarcoidosis. JAMA 1978;240: 2654–5.

43. Bain BJ, Clark DM, Wilkins B. Bone marrow pathology. Oxford: Blackwell Wiley; 2010.

44. Singh G, Krause JR, Breitfeld V. Bone marrow examination: for metastatic tumor: aspirate and biopsy. Cancer 1977; 40:2317–21.

45. Savage RA, Hoffman GC, Shaker K. Diagnostic problems involved in detection of metastatic neoplasms by bone-marrow aspirate compared with needle biopsy. Am J Clin Pathol 1978;70:623–7.

46. Anner RM, Drewinko B. Frequency and significance of bone marrow involvement by metastatic solid tumors. Cancer 1977; 39:1337–44.

47. Bain BJ, Clark DM, Wilkins B. Bone marrow pathology. Oxford: Blackwell Wiley; 2010.

48. Cotta CV, Konoplev S, Medeiros LJ, Bueso-Ramos CE. Metastatic tumors in bone marrow: histopathology and advances in the biology of the tumor cells and bone marrow environment. Ann Diagn Pathol 2006;10:169–92.

49. Morandi S, Manna A, Sabattini E, Porcellini A. Rhabdomyosarcoma presenting as acute leukemia. J Pediatr Hematol Oncol 1996;18:305–7.

50. Smith SR, Reid MM. Neuroblastoma rosettes in aspirated bone marrow. Br J Haematol 1994;88:445–7.

51. Beiske K, Burchill SA, Cheung IY, et al. Consensus criteria for sensitive detection of minimal neuroblastoma cells in bone marrow, blood and stem cell preparations by immunocytology and QRT-PCR: recommendations by the International Neuroblastoma Risk Group Task Force. Br J Cancer 2009;100:1627–37.

52. McCarthy DM. Annotation. Fibrosis of the bone marrow: content and causes. Br J Haematol 1985;59:1–7.

53. Kuter DJ, Bain B, Mufti G, et al. Bone marrow fibrosis: pathophysiology and clinical significance of increased bone marrow stromal fibres. Br J Haematol 2007;139:351–62.

54. Pastores GM. Gaucher's Disease. Pathological features. Baillière's Clin Haematol 1997;10:739–49.

55. Florena AM, Franco V, Campesi G. Immunophenotypical comparison of Gaucher's and pseudo-Gaucher cells. Pathol Int 1996;46:155–60.

56. Varela-Duran J, Roholt PC, Ratliff NB Jr. Sea-blue histiocyte syndrome. A secondary degenerative process of macrophages? Arch Pathol Lab Med 1980;104:30–4.

57. Kolodny EH. Niemann–Pick disease. Curr Opin Hematol 2000;7:48–52.

58. Mehta AB. Anderson–Fabry disease: developments in diagnosis and treatment. Int J Clin Pharmacol Ther 2009; 47(Suppl 1):S66–74.

59. Clarke LA. The mucopolysaccharidoses: a success of molecular medicine. Expert Rev Mol Med 2008;10:e1.

60. Janssens AM, Offner FC, Van Hove WZ. Bone marrow necrosis. Cancer 2000;88:1769–80.

61. Knupp C, Pekala PH, Cornelius P. Extensive bone marrow necrosis in patients with cancer and tumor necrosis factor activity in plasma. Am J Hematol 1988;29:215–21.

62. Caraveo J, Trowbridge AA, Amaral BW, et al. Bone marrow necrosis associated with a Mucor infection. Am J Med 1977;62:404–8.

63. Bohm J. Gelatinous transformation of the bone marrow: the spectrum of underlying diseases. Am J Surg Pathol 2000;24:56–65.

64. Stavem P, Larsen IF, Ly B, Rorvik TO. Amyloid deposits in bone marrow aspirates in primary amyloidosis. Acta Med Scand 1980;208:111–3.

65. Enos WF, Pierre RV, Rosenblatt JE. Giant cell arteritis detected by bone marrow biopsy. Mayo Clin Proc 1981;56:381–3.

66. Muretto P, Carnevali A, Ansini AL. Cholesterol embolism of bone marrow clinically masquerading as systemic or metastatic tumor. Haematologica 1991;76:248–50.

67. McClure J, Fazzalari NL, Fassett RG, Pugsley DJ. Bone histoquantitative findings and histochemical staining reactions for aluminium in chronic renal failure patients treated with haemodialysis fluids containing high and low concentrations of aluminium. J Clin Pathol 1983;36:1281–7.

68. Findlay AB. Bone marrow changes in the post mortem interval. J Forensic Sci Soc 1976;16:213–8.

Recommended reading

Bain BJ, Clark DM, Wilkins BS. Bone Marrow Pathology. 4th ed. Oxford: Wiley-Blackwell; 2010.

Torlakovic EE, Naresh KN, Brunning RD. Bone Marrow Immunohistochemistry. Chicago: American Society for Clinical Pathology Press; 2009.

Foucar K, Viswanatha DS, Wilson CS. Non-Neoplastic Disorders of Bone Marrow (Atlas of Nontumor Pathology). Washington: AFIP; 2008.

Section C

Disorders affecting erythroid cells

CHAPTER 6

Investigation and classification of anemia

WN Erber

Definition and causes of anemia

Anemia is defined as a reduction in the concentration of hemoglobin in the peripheral blood below the reference range for the age and gender of an individual (see Table 1.3 for reference ranges). It may be inherited or acquired and results from an imbalance between red cell production and red cell loss (Table 6.1). In general terms the causes of anemia are:

1. reduced red cell production: a reduction in, or failure of, erythropoiesis within the marrow, or
2. increased red cell destruction or cell loss: accelerated loss of red cells in the periphery may be due to intrinsic red cell defects or extrinsic effects. Anemia develops when the bone marrow erythropoietic activity cannot adequately compensate for the degree of reduction in red cell life span
3. relative or dilutional anemia.

This chapter outlines the clinical features of anemia and the process for investigation and classification of anemia. It will set the scene for the following chapters which detail the specific mechanisms of anemia.

Clinical features of anemia

A detailed clinical history is critical in determining the cause of anemia. Table 6.2 lists some of the important personal, dietary, drug and family history issues to be explored. The symptoms and signs of anemia result from decreased tissue oxygenation leading to organ dysfunction as well as from adaptive changes, particularly in the cardiovascular system.[1,2] The nature and severity of symptoms is influenced by:

1. speed of onset of the anemia
2. status of the cardiovascular and respiratory systems, e.g. significant coronary artery or chronic obstructive airways disease may result in the development of symptoms with only mild anemia
3. patient age. Neonates, young children and the elderly have a reduced ability to compensate for changes in hemoglobin.

Symptoms of anemia include lassitude, easy fatigability, dyspnea on exertion, palpitations, angina and intermittent claudication, headache, vertigo, light-headedness, visual disturbances, drowsiness, anorexia, nausea, bowel disturbances, menstrual disturbances and loss of libido. Physical signs include pallor, signs of a hyperkinetic circulation (tachycardia, wide pulse pressure with capillary pulsation, cardiac murmurs), signs of congestive cardiac failure, and hemorrhages and exudates in the retina. Severe anemia may also cause slight proteinuria, mild impairment of renal function and low-grade fever.

A moderate degree of chronic anemia is usually associated with only mild symptoms accompanied by slight increases in cardiac output at rest and slight decreases in mixed venous PO_2. This is because there is a substantial shift of the oxygen dissociation curve to the right (see Chapter 1), mainly due to an adaptive increase in the levels of red cell 2,3-diphosphoglycerate. When the hemoglobin falls below

©2011 Elsevier Ltd
DOI: 10.1016/B978-0-7020-3147-2.00006-7

Table 6.1 Mechanisms of anemia

Mechanism	Pathogenesis
Reduced or ineffective erythropoiesis	Decreased marrow erythropoiesis Inadequately increased total erythropoiesis Increased ineffective erythropoiesis
Increased red cell loss or reduced red cell life span	Acute or chronic blood loss Increased red cell destruction Splenic pooling and sequestration
Dilutional anemia	Plasma volume expansion

Table 6.2 Clinical history in the investigation of anemia

History	Mechanism	Examples
Current illness	Acute hemorrhage	Epistaxis, menorrhagia, hematemesis, melaena
	Chronic blood loss	Menorrhagia, melaena
	Infection	Parvovirus
	Hemolysis	Jaundice
Past medical history	Anemia of chronic disease	Chronic infection Liver disease Renal impairment Hypothyroidism Malignancy
	Malabsorption	Gastrectomy Gastric bypass Celiac disease Ileal surgery
Travel history	Intra-erythrocytic parasites	Malaria
Dietary history	Vegetarian or veganism Iron intake Excess alcohol	Vitamin B_{12} deficiency Iron deficiency Liver disease
Drugs	Antiplatelet agents Anticoagulants Oxidant drugs Myelosuppressive agents	Aspirin, clopidogrel Warfarin Salazopyrin, dapsone Methotrexate Cytotoxic chemotherapy
Exposure to toxins	Toxins or chemicals that interfere with erythropoiesis	Lead, aluminum
Family history	Inherited red cell abnormality	Hereditary spherocytosis G6PD deficiency Thalassemia Other hemoglobinopathy
	Autoimmune disorders	Pernicious anemia Rheumatoid arthritis
	Bleeding disorders	Hemophilia von Willebrand disease

Table 6.3 Practical classification of anemia based on mean cell volume

Types	Mean cell volume	Conditions
Microcytic	<80 fl	Iron deficiency Anemia of chronic disease Hemoglobinopathies Hereditary sideroblastic anemia
Normocytic	Within reference range (80–100 fl)	Blood loss Hemolysis Failure of erythropoiesis
Macrocytic	>80 fl	Deficiency of folate or vitamin B_{12} Myelodysplasia Liver disease Hypothyroidism

2. redistribution of blood flow: vasoconstriction in the skin and kidneys and increased perfusion of the heart, brain and muscle

3. reduction of the mixed venous PO_2 which increases the arterial–venous oxygen difference.

The blood count and red cell indices in anemia

The mean cell volume (MCV) is the most useful red cell parameter for the assessment of the underlying cause of anemia. By using the MCV, anemias can be categorized by red cell size as microcytic (MCV <80 fl), normocytic (normal MCV) or macrocytic (MCV >100 fl). This provides a practical and rapid way of assessing possible causes and guiding further investigations (see below and Table 6.3). The mean cell hemoglobin (MCH) and mean cell hemoglobin concentration (MCHC) are generally of less value than the MCV in the assessment of anemia. The red cell distribution width (RDW), a quantitative measure of the degree of variation in red cell size, can be useful in the assessment of some types of anemia. Usually erythrocytes are of a standard size (6–8 μm) and the RDW is 12–14%. A high RDW indicates that there is variation in erythrocyte size and gives a quantitative measure of anisocytosis. For example, in microcytic anemias, a normal RDW is generally seen in thalassemias whereas in iron deficiency it is mildly elevated. The graphical depiction of red cell features on blood count histograms, such as red cell number versus MCV, may also give an indication of anisocytosis, or the presence of dimorphic populations of erythrocytes.

The reticulocyte count can be used as a guide to distinguish between reduced bone marrow erythropoiesis and accelerated red cell loss as the primary cause of the anemia. An inappropriately low reticulocyte count for the degree of anemia indicates that there is impaired marrow erythroid response to the anemia, i.e., the underlying cause is interfering with marrow erythropoiesis. This may be due to a chronic infective or inflammatory process, bone marrow failure or

7–8 g/dl symptoms usually become more marked. The intra-erythrocytic adaptation cannot by itself maintain adequate oxygen delivery to the tissues and other compensatory mechanisms come into effect. These include:

1. an increase in stroke volume, heart rate and cardiac output at rest

infiltration, reduced hematinics, ineffective erythropoiesis (dyserythropoiesis) or inadequate erythropoietin as occurs in renal failure. In contrast an appropriate reticulocytosis is evidence that the marrow is responding to the anemia and the cause is likely to be peripheral (i.e. hemolysis or blood loss). Other red blood cell measurements, such as the nucleated red cell count and immature reticulocyte fraction, do not generally add significant value to the investigation of anemia.

The leukocyte and platelet counts will distinguish isolated anemia from pancytopenia. Neutrophilia and/or thrombocytosis can be seen in response to acute blood loss and hemolysis. The presence of abnormal leukocytes in the presence of anemia (e.g. blast cells) may indicate underlying bone marrow failure as a result of a neoplastic infiltrate.

Red cell morphology in anemia

Blood film examination to review red cell morphology has a critical role in the investigation and diagnosis of anemia. The identification of red cell morphological abnormalities may lead to a definitive or differential diagnosis and guide further investigations (Fig. 6.1A–F). The film should be prepared from a freshly collected blood sample, well-stained and coverslipped. Blood stored for >6 hours in anticoagulant prior to the preparation of the film can result in artifacts (e.g. red cell crenation) that can interfere with interpretation of the true red cell morphology. Morphological artifacts can also result from the blood being stored at incorrect temperatures (hot or cold) prior to preparation of the blood film. The film should be examined in an area where only occasional red cells overlap. In such an area normal red cells are primarily round and show a central area of pallor which occupies less than a third of the diameter of the cell. The film should be assessed systematically for:

1. *Red cell size.* An erythrocyte is normocytic, microcytic or macrocytic when its diameter appears to be normal, smaller than normal or larger than normal, respectively. Macrocytes may be round or ovoid (Fig. 6.1A). Anisocytosis refers to increased degree of variation in cell diameter compared with normal.
2. *Red cell shape.* Assess for specific morphological features associated with different causes of anemia. Poikilocytosis is variation in cell shape: poikilocytes may be oval, teardrop-shaped, sickle-shaped or irregularly contracted.
3. *Red cell color* (chromasia). The terms normochromic and hypochromic are applied to red cells in which the area of central pallor is, normal in size and greater than normal, respectively. Severely hypochromic red cells have a very large central area of pallor surrounded by a narrow rim of hemoglobinized cytoplasm (Fig. 6.1B). Spherocytes lack central pallor and appear hyperchromic (Fig. 6.1C). Polychromasia is a morphological indicator of the reticulocyte response.
4. *Red cell inclusions.* Red cells should be assessed for the presence of basophilic stippling (Fig. 6.1A, C) and intra-erythrocytic parasites.
5. *Red cell distribution.* Rouleaux formation and agglutination may indicate the presence of a proteinemia.

6. *Leukocytes and platelet number and morphology.* These may show numerical or morphological abnormalities associated with specific types of anemia, for example, hypersegmented neutrophils in megaloblastic anemia or spherocytosis of autoimmune hemolytic anemia secondary to chronic lymphocytic leukemia. A leukoerythroblastic blood film may indicate the presence of marrow infiltration or fibrosis.

Some of the important diagnostic red cell morphological features are described together with their disease associations below and in Table 6.4:[3,4]

Target cells. These are abnormally thin red cells with a well-stained hemoglobinized zone in the middle of the usual central area of pallor (Fig. 6.1D). This morphology is due to a disproportionate increase in red cell membrane due to abnormal lipid content. They are seen in liver disease (especially cholestatic), hyposplenism and hemoglobinopathies such as hemoglobin C and E disease.

Spherocytes. Spherocytes, small, round, deeply-staining (hyperchromic) red cells without central pallor, have lost their biconcave shape and therefore have a spherical form. They occur due to loss of cell membrane and are a feature of hereditary spherocytosis, warm autoimmune hemolytic anemia and clostridial septicemia (Fig. 6.1C).

Schistocytes. These are fragmented red cells with sharp points and occur in fragmentation hemolysis as a result of their interaction with fibrin strands, diseased vessel walls or foreign surfaces (e.g. cardiac valve prostheses). Conditions in which they are seen include disseminated intravascular coagulation, thrombotic thrombocytopenic purpura, hemolytic uremic syndrome and graft-versus-host disease (Fig. 6.1D).

Bite cells. Bite cells are characterized by a cup-shaped defect in the red cell membrane. They form as a result of the removal of oxidized hemoglobin (Heinz bodies) as they pass through the spleen, as seen in oxidative hemolytic anemia, e.g. glucose 6-phosphate dehydrogenase (G6PD) deficiency.

Stomatocytes. These are red cells with a slit-like area of pallor across the center instead of the circular area of pallor. They are associated with hereditary stomatocytosis and Southeast Asian ovalocytosis (see Chapter 7).[5,6] They can also be seen in alcoholic liver disease or as artifact on a poorly spread blood film.

Sickle cells. Sickle-shaped or crescentic red cells occur as a result of deoxygenation of hemoglobin S (Fig. 6.1E). Deoxygenated hemoglobin S is about 50 times less soluble than deoxygenated hemoglobin A and, under appropriate conditions, forms long fibers (tactoids) which deform the red cell. Sickle cells are found in hemoglobin S homozygotes and in double heterozygotes for hemoglobin S and β-thalassemia or other abnormal hemoglobins, such as hemoglobin C, E, O-Arab, D-Punjab or Lepore.

Echinocytes ('burr' cells). Echinocytes are spiculated red cells with 10–30 short projections of similar length that are evenly distributed over the cell surface. They are seen in renal imapirment.[7,8]

Acanthocytes ('spur' cells). These are spiculated red cells with 5–10 projections of varying length and thickness that are irregularly spaced over the cell surface. These commonly lack central pallor (Fig. 6.1F). Acanthocytes are seen in

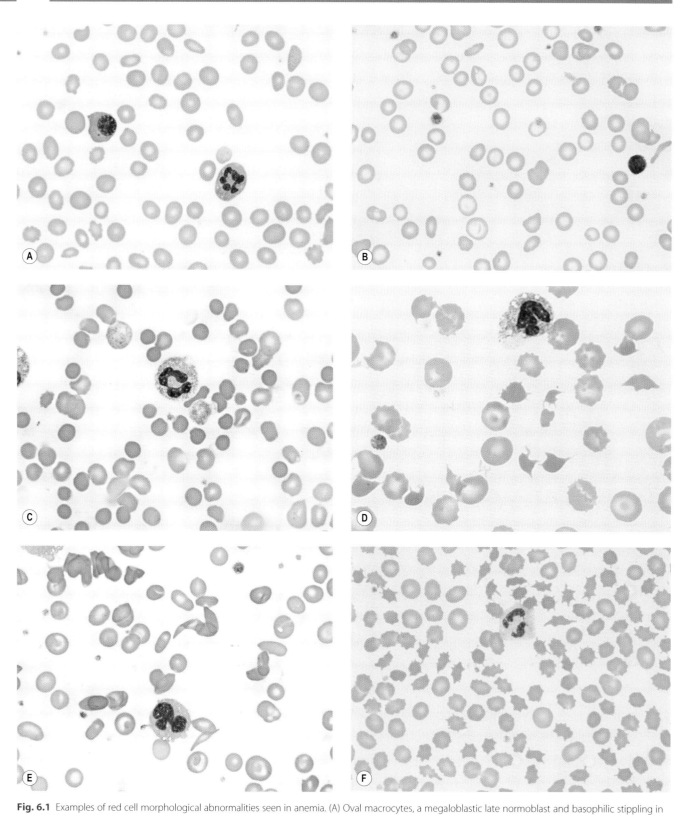

Fig. 6.1 Examples of red cell morphological abnormalities seen in anemia. (A) Oval macrocytes, a megaloblastic late normoblast and basophilic stippling in megaloblastic anemia due to folate deficiency. (B) Hypochromic red cells and mild poikilocytosis in severe iron deficiency anemia. (C) Spherocytes and basophilic stippling in hemolytic anemia secondary to clostridial septicemia. (D) Schistocytes, target cells, echinocytes, acanthocytes and polychromasia in sepsis with disseminated intravascular coagulation, renal and hepatic impairment. (E) Sickle-shaped red cells in sickle cell disease. Target cells are also present. (F) Acanthocytes in end-stage liver disease ('spur' cell anemia). May–Grünwald–Giemsa stain. ×1000.

Table 6.4 Morphological abnormalities of red cells in anemia (see also Fig. 6.1)

Morphological feature	Pathogenesis	Disorders (examples)
Microcytosis	Impaired synthesis of heme or globin	Iron deficiency, thalassemias, congenital sideroblastic anemia, congenital atransferrinemia, aluminum-induced anemia (dialysis patients)
Macrocytosis	Dyserythropoiesis or accelerated release of reticulocytes	Megaloblastic erythropoiesis e.g. vitamin B_{12} or folate deficiency, congenital dyserythropoietic anemia types I, III, non-megaloblastic (e.g. liver disease, alcohol, hypothyroidism)
Hypochromasia	Impaired synthesis of heme	Iron deficiency, anemia of chronic disease
Anisocytosis	Nonspecific evidence of a perturbation of erythropoiesis	Various
Target cells	Increased surface area relative to volume	Thalassemias, hemoglobinopathies, (HbAC, HbCC, HbEE), liver disease, obstructive jaundice, hyposplenism
Stomatocytes	Cation leak	Hereditary stomatocytosis, Rh null phenotype, alcohol, drugs
Spherocytosis	Abnormality of cell membrane	Hereditary spherocytosis, immune-hemolytic anemia
Elliptocytosis	Abnormality of cell membrane	Hereditary elliptocytosis
Acanthocytes	Membrane lipid imbalance	Liver disease, anorexia nervosa, hyposplenism, abetalipoproteinemia, McLeod phenotype
Echinocytes	Extrinsic effects	Uremia
Sickle cells	Abnormal globin chain	Sickle cell disease, HbS/β-thalassemia, HbSC disease, HbS/O-Arab, HbS/D-Punjab, HbS/Lepore
Schistocytes	Red cell fragmentation	Microangiopathic hemolytic anemias, hemolytic uremic syndrome, thrombotic thrombocytopenic purpura, disseminated intravascular coagulation, malignant hypertension, cardiac valve prostheses
Bite cells	Removal of oxidized hemoglobin	Oxidant stress, glucose-6-phosphate dehydrogenase deficiency, drugs (e.g. dapsone, salazopyrin, antimalarials)
Teardrop poikilocytes	Marrow fibrosis	Primary or secondary marrow fibrosis
Basophilic stippling	Ribosomes or RNA	Accelerated erythropoiesis, dyserythropoiesis, lead poisoning, thalassemias, pyrimidine 5′-nucleotidase deficiency
Pappenheimer bodies	Iron	Lead poisoning, sideroblastic anemias, hemolytic anemias, hyposplenism
Howell–Jolly bodies	Nuclear remnants	Hyposplenism, megaloblastic hemopoiesis
Polychromasia and nucleated red cells	Increased erythropoiesis and red cell release	Marrow erythroid response to anemia, especially hemolytic anemia and blood loss

hepatic failure, Zieve's syndrome ('spur' cell anemia), malnutrition, abetalipoproteinemia and McLeod syndrome (inherited Kell blood group abnormality associated with hemolysis). Spiculated cells are also seen in pyruvate kinase deficiency.

Teardrop poikilocytes (dacrocyte). Teardrop poikilocytes have a single elongated point giving the appearance of a teardrop. They are associated with primary or secondary causes of marrow fibrosis.

Basophilic stippling. Fine or coarse basophilic stippling indicates the presence of ribosomes, generally within reticulocytes or young mature red cells, or RNA. Stippling indicates increased erythropoietic response to anemia or dyserythropoiesis (Fig. 6.1A).

Pappenheimer bodies. These are single or multiple coarse unevenly distributed basophilic red cell inclusions. They stain positively for iron with the Prussian blue reaction. Red cells containing iron-positive granules are called siderocytes.

Howell–Jolly bodies. Howell–Jolly bodies are single round, dark magenta-colored red cell inclusions associated with hyposplensim. They consist of nuclear material and are formed within erythroblasts either by karyorrhexis or from chromosome fragments which become isolated outside the nucleus when the nuclear membrane is reformed during telophase.

Intra-erythrocytic parasites. Malaria, babesiosis and bartonellosis may be evident on the blood film.

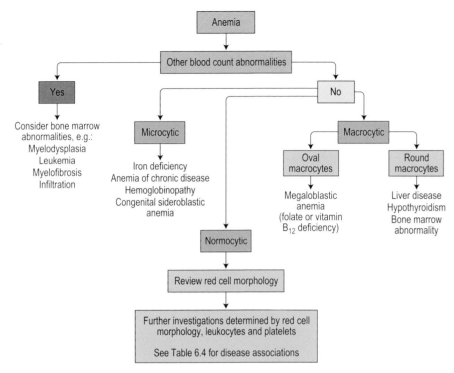

Fig. 6.2 Pathway for the investigation of anemia based on the mean cell volume and blood film morphology.

Investigation of the cause of anemia

The further laboratory investigation of the cause of anemia should be guided by the MCV, red cell morphology and the reticulocyte count (Fig. 6.2).

Microcytic anemias

Microcytic anemias are due to deficient synthesis of hemoglobin (Fig. 6.1B). This may be due to inadequate heme production (e.g. iron deficiency, anemia of chronic disease and hereditary sideroblastic anemia) or abnormalities of globin chain synthesis (i.e. hemoglobinopathies).[9,10] The laboratory investigation should therefore include assessment of body iron status, i.e. ferritin, serum iron, transferrin and transferrin saturation (see Chapters 11 and 14). Evaluation of hemoglobin (e.g. high-performance liquid chromatography (HPLC); hemoglobin electrophoresis) may be required if a hemoglobinopathy is suspected (see Chapter 9). Bone marrow examination may be indicated especially to assess iron stores and its incorporation into sideroblasts.

Macrocytic anemias

Macrocytic anemias may be megaloblastic or non-megaloblastic, a distinction which can often be made on the blood film (see below and Chapter 12). The megaloblastic anemias are due to deficiencies of folate or vitamin B_{12} and cause a failure of DNA synthesis and resultant impaired cell division. Macrocytes in megaloblastic anemia tend to be oval with associated hypersegmented neutrophils and megaloblastic erythroid progenitors (Fig. 6.1A).[11] In non-megaloblastic macrocytic anemias the macrocytes are round. There are many possible etiologies, which may be intrinsic to the marrow (e.g. myelodysplasia) or due to extrinsic causes (e.g. liver disease, hypothyroidism, drug therapy, reticulocytosis, myelodysplasia).[12] Accompanying cytopenias, neutrophil morphological abnormalities and the presence of blast cells may suggest myelodysplasia. Serum and red cell folate and serum vitamin B_{12} levels should be measured in all cases. The requirement for analysis of hepatic and thyroid function and other biochemical analyses should be based on the clinical scenario. Bone marrow examination may be required if myelodysplasia is a consideration or the etiology cannot be determined following the above-mentioned investigations.

Normocytic anemias

Normocytic anemias may be secondary to hemorrhage, hemolysis, dilution (plasma volume expansion) or failure of erythropoiesis (prior to the reticulocyte response). There are many possible causes of a normocytic anemia and therefore the laboratory investigation can be complex. The clinical history and red cell morphology may lead to a differential diagnosis and enable a structured approach to further investigations. Iron, folate and vitamin B_{12} measurements may be appropriate if there are relevant clinical or early morphological features on the blood film. Investigations for features of hemolysis, including direct antiglobulin test, bilirubin, lactate dehydrogenase and haptoglobins, may be appropriate if there are suggestive features from the history and blood film.

If spherocytes are present investigation should be performed for a possible inherited (i.e. hereditary spherocytosis) or acquired (e.g. immune mediated hemolytic anemia) cause of spherocytic hemolytic anemia (see Chapter 10). Schistocytes (Fig. 6.1D) should prompt investigation for causes of possible microangiopathic hemolytic anemia (e.g. D-dimer, ADAMTS13). The presence of teardrop poikilocytes may require bone marrow examination to exclude underlying fibrosis. Inherited red cell enzyme defects, for example G6PD deficiency and pyruvate kinase deficiency, can also present with a normocytic anemia. The blood film may, however, show distinctive red cell abnormalities such as bite cells and spiculated cells, respectively. See Chapter 8 for the approach to the diagnosis of these conditions.

Normocytic anemia in the absence of any specific morphological abnormality or reticulocytosis may be due to acute or chronic infective or inflammatory conditions, hepatic, renal or endocrine conditions, red cell aplasia, dilution, or paroxysmal nocturnal hemoglobinuria (PNH). The clinical history, biochemical studies demonstrating the underlying abnormality and iron studies (changes associated with the anemia of chronic disease) may assist in establishing the cause. A bone marrow examination may be required in unresolved cases. PNH may require flow cytometry to demonstrate deficient expression of CD55 and CD59 antigens (see Chapter 10).

A normocytic anemia occurs following acute hemorrhage.[13,14] The hemoglobin is initially normal but normocytic normochromic anemia occurs with plasma volume expansion; the hemoglobin is at its lowest 36–72 hours following blood loss. The reticulocyte count increases slightly after 1–2 days, reaches a peak with a few circulating normoblasts at 7–10 days and returns to normal by 2 weeks. Chronic blood loss eventually results in iron deficiency and a hypochromic microcytic anemia (see Chapter 11).

Assessment of the erythropoietic response to anemia

Overall erythropoietic activity is the total of 'effective' and 'ineffective' erythropoiesis (Table 6.5). Effective erythropoiesis is the rate of release of newly-formed red cells from the marrow. Ineffective erythropoiesis is the rate of loss of potential erythrocytes (as a result of apoptosis of progenitor cells) and phagocytosis of defective erythropoietic cells by bone marrow macrophages. In practice, the most readily measured parameters of the erythropoietic response are the peripheral blood reticulocyte count, and, in the bone marrow, the myeloid:erythroid ratio, morphology of erythropoiesis (for evidence of dyserythropoiesis) and phagocytosis of erythroblasts by macrophages. Serum transferrin receptor, a truncated soluble form of the surface receptor mainly produced by erythroblasts, can also be used. Serum transferrin receptor is increased in erythroid hyperplasia as well as in iron deficiency; in the absence of iron deficiency, it is a measure of total erythropoietic activity.[15,16]

Table 6.5 Indices of erythropoietic activity

Erythropoietic activty	Measurement
Total erythropoiesis	Myeloid:erythroid (M:E) ratio in the bone marrow Marrow erythropoiesis Serum transferrin receptor Plasma iron turnover Total marrow iron turnover Fecal urobilinogen excretion
Effective erythropoiesis	Absolute reticulocyte count Red cell turnover Red cell ^{59}Fe utilization Red cell iron turnover
Ineffective erythropoiesis	Difference between indices of total and effective erythropoiesis Morphologic evidence of increased dyserythropoiesis Erythroblast phagocytosis by macrophages

The classification of anemia

The pathophysiologic or mechanistic classification is based on the etiology of the anemia: whether it is 'true' (absolute) or 'relative' (dilutional), the underlying defect and whether the anemia is inherited or acquired (Table 6.1). These are listed as follows and detailed in Table 6.6:

1. Reduced erythropoiesis: e.g. iron deficiency, red cell aplasia, bone marrow failure, bone marrow infiltration.
2. Ineffective erythropoiesis: e.g. megaloblastic anemia, myelodysplasia, congenital sideroblastic and dyserythropoietic anemias.
3. Reduced red cell lifespan secondary to:
   a. blood loss, which may be acute hemorrhage or chronic blood loss
   b. hemolysis: a hemolytic state occurs when the red cell survival in the circulation is reduced below normal (i.e. less than 120 days) due to intravascular (within the circulation) or extravascular (premature destruction by cells of the mononuclear phagocyte system) hemolysis, or both. Table 6.5 provides a detailed sub-classification of inherited and acquired causes of hemolysis[17-21]
   c. red cell pooling: e.g. splenic sequestration.
4. Relative or dilutional anemia: due to plasma volume expansion, e.g. as occurs in the third trimester of pregnancy, secondary to proteinemia or within hours following acute hemorrhage.

Detailed descriptions of each of these causes of anemia are in the following chapters.

Table 6.6 Pathophysiologic classification of anemia

Anemia	Mechanism	Inherited or acquired	Defect	Disorders (examples)
Absolute	Reduced or ineffective red cell production	Inherited	Progenitor cell defect	Congenital dyserythropoietic anemia Congenital sideroblastic anemia Hemoglobinopathies
		Acquired	Bone marrow failure Failure of or inadequate erythropoiesis	Aplastic anemia Bone marrow infiltration, e.g. leukemia; myelodysplasia Pure red cell aplasia Renal failure Anemia of chronic disease Iron deficiency Megaloblastic anemia
	Increased red cell destruction/ reduced red cell lifespan (Hemolysis and blood loss)	Inherited	Cell membrane defect Cell enzyme defect Globin defect	Herditary spherocytosis Hereditary stomatocytosis Hereditary pyropoikilocytosis G6PD deficiency Pyruvate kinase deficiency Pyrimidine 5′-nucleotidase deficiency Hemoglobinopathies and thalassemias
		Acquired	Immune (antibody-mediated) Non-immune	Autoimmune hemolytic anemia Allo-immune hemolytic anemia Drug-induced hemolytic anemia Blood loss Hypersplenism Microangiopathic hemolytic anemia Liver disease Renal failure Intra-erythrocytic parasites Drug-mediated
Relative	Dilutional anemia	Acquired	Plasma volume expansion	Pregnancy Proteinemias Within hours of acute hemorrhage

References

1. Wickramasinghe SN, Weatherall DJ. The pathophysiology of erythropoiesis. In: Hardisty RM, Weatherall DJ, editors. Blood and its Disorders. 2nd ed. Oxford: Blackwell Scientific Publications; 1982. p. 101.

2. Means RT, Glader B. Anaemia: general considerations. In: Greer JP, Foerster J, Rodgers GM, et al. editors. Wintrobe's Clinical Hematology. 12th ed. Philadelphia: Wolters Kluwer/Lippincott, Williams & Wilkins; 2009.

3. Pierre RV. Red cell morphology and the peripheral blood film. Clin Lab Haem 2002;22(1):25–61.

4. Bain BJ. Morphology in the diagnosis of red cell disorders. Hematology 2005;10(Suppl. 1):178–81.

5. Bruce LJ. Hereditary stomatocytosis and cation leaky red cells – recent developments. Blood Cells, Molecules and Diseases 2009;42(3):216–22.

6. Wong P. A hypothesis of the stomatocytosis in individuals with the phenotype Rh(null). Medical Hypotheses 2001;57:770–1.

7. Bessis M. Living blood cells and their ultrastructure. Berlin: Springer; 1973. p. 197.

8. Brecher G, Bessis M. Present status of spiculed red cells and their relationship to the discocyte–echinocyte transformation: a critical review. Blood 1972;40:333–44.

9. Camaschella C. Recent advances in the understanding of inherited sideroblastic anaemia. British Journal of Haematology 2008;143(1):27–38.

10. Camaschella C. Hereditary sideroblastic anaemia: pathophysiology, diagnosis and treatment. Seminars in Hematology 2009;46(4):371–7.

11. Wickramasinghe SN. Diagnosis of megaloblastic anaemias. Blood Reviews 2006;20(6):299–318.

12. Morse EE. Mechanisms of hemolysis in liver disease. Annals of Clinical and Laboratory Science 1990;20: 169–74.

13. Adamson J, Hillman RS. Blood volume and plasma protein replacement following acute blood loss in normal man. Journal of the American Medical Association 1968;205:609–12.

14. Wallace J, Sharpey-Shafer EP. Blood changes following controlled haemorrhage in man. Lancet 1941;ii:393.

15. Beguin Y, Clemons GK, Pootrakul P, Fillet G. Quantitative assessment of

erythropoiesis and functional classification of anaemia based on measurements of serum transferrin receptor and erythropoietin. Blood 1993;81: 1067–76.

16. Beguin Y. Soluble transferrin receptor for the evaluation of erythropoiesis and iron status. Clinica Chimica Acta 2003;329: 9–22.

17. Dacie JV. The Haemolytic Anaemias, vol 1: The Hereditary Haemolytic Anaemias, part

1. 3rd ed. Edinburgh: Churchill Livingstone; 1985.

18. Dacie JV. The Haemolytic Anaemias, vol 2: The Hereditary Haemolytic Anaemias, part 2. 3rd ed. Edinburgh: Churchill Livingstone; 1988.

19. Dacie JV. The Haemolytic Anaemias, vol 3: The Auto-Immune Haemolytic Anaemias. 3rd ed. Edinburgh: Churchill Livingstone; 1992.

20. Dacie JV. The Haemolytic Anaemias, vol 4: Secondary or Symptomatic Haemolytic Anaemias. 3rd ed. New York: Churchill Livingstone; 1995.

21. Dacie JV. The Haemolytic Anaemias, vol 5: Drug- and Chemical-Induced Haemolytic Anaemias; Paroxysmal Nocturnal Haemoglobinuria; Haemolytic Disease of the Newborn. 3rd ed. New York: Churchill Livingstone; 1999.

CHAPTER 7

Abnormalities of the red cell membrane

J Delaunay

Chapter contents

A number of hereditary hemolytic anemias result from mutations affecting the quality and/or amount of proteins that belong to the red cell membrane, its skeleton, or the attachment systems (nexuses) of the latter to the former. Most proteins participate in complexes (Fig. 7.1). They play a role in erythrocyte resilience and elastic deformability, either mechanically, through the skeleton and its attaching systems, or osmotically, through a variety of transporters and pumps. Major proteins and their genes are listed in Table 7.1. The ever increasing number of mutations, too numerous to detail here, have given insight into the function of such protein domains and the regulatory regions of some genes. A selection of abnormally-shaped red cells is shown in Fig. 7.2.

It should be pointed out that although the genes involved are expressed in a wide range of cell types as isoforms (spliceoforms in particular), genetic disorders are usually confined to the erythroid line. Naturally affected animals and animals with experimentally invalidated genes are helpful, although they do not necessarily mirror the human diseases.

Hereditary spherocytosis

Hereditary spherocytosis (HS) is the most common genetic disorder of the red cell membrane in Western countries. Its incidence has been estimated as 1 in 2000 live births and there is a wide spectrum of clinical severity. In typical cases the hemolytic anemia is moderate, with an increased reticulocyte count a reticulocytosis, intermittent jaundice, gallstones and splenomegaly. Severe cases are rare and may cause death *in utero* or shortly after birth. In contrast, patients with mild HS may be over 60 years of age when diagnosed. Parvovirus B19 infection commonly occurs. Blood films show a variable percentage of spherocytes. The diagnosis relies on an increased percentage of hyperdense cells and a reduction in osmotic resistance, and on a number of tests, including polyacrylamide gel electrophoresis of the red cell membrane proteins in the presence of sodium dodecylsulfate (SDS-PAGE). The main treatment is splenectomy, though the need for this should be carefully weighed owing to its complications, namely severe infections and a statistically significant increase in thromboembolic accidents.[1] Transfusions may be necessary.

Most cases of HS result from reduced or absent proteins. Consequently, the lining of the inner surface of the lipid bilayer by the skeletal meshwork is less dense. Microvesicles bud out of naked bilayer patches. The surface area shrinks and the normal discoid cells gradually turn into spherocytes. The six genes most commonly involved in HS are discussed below.

©2011 Elsevier Ltd
DOI: 10.1016/B978-0-7020-3147-2.00007-9

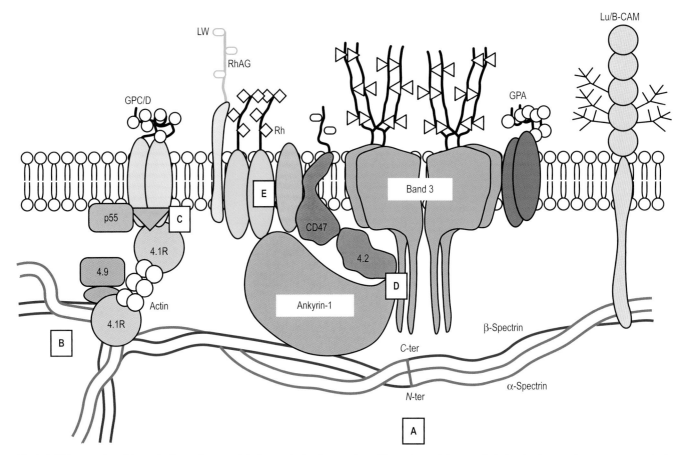

Fig. 7.1 Major proteins of the red cell membrane and their organization in complexes. The major proteins, usually belonging to complexes, are represented. Not all proteins mentioned are shown. *Box A: the spectrin self-association site.* Spectrin $\alpha_2\beta_2$ tetramers form a network lining the inner surface of the lipid bilayer. The α- and β-chains are antiparallel and contain 22 and 17 repeats, respectively. Two dimers associate side-by-side, a process set off at the nucleation sites on both chains, near the *C*- and *N*-terminal regions of the α- and β-chains, respectively. Dimers associate head-to-head, α-chain *N*-terminal region vs. β-chain *C*-terminal region, at the self-association site, in order to generate tetramers, or higher order oligomers. Spectrin, through its α4 repeat (away from *Box A*), interacts with the Lu-BCAM protein. *Box B: the 4.1R-based multiprotein complex: (i) the junctional complex.* Several converging spectrin tetramers interact with oligomeric β-actin, whose length is limited by tropomodulin. 4.1R strengthens this interaction through its 10 kDa domain, which binds to a site located in the spectrin β-chain *N*-terminal region. Many additional proteins participate in the junctional complex: dematin (protein 4.9), tropomyosin, α- and β-adducin, and several others. *Box C: the 4.1R-based multiprotein complex: (ii) the 4.1R-glycophorin C/D-p55 complex.* 4.1R interacts through its 30 kDa domain with transmembrane glycophorin C/D and p55 in a triangular fashion. *Box D: the band 3-based multiprotein complex: (i) the band 3 complex, stricto sensu.* Band 3 appears as a tetramer. The bulky part of each band 3 monomer represents 12 transmembrane segments of band 3. The stalky part accounts for its cytoplasmic domain which serves as an anchor to ankyrin-1, protein 4.2 and many cytoplasmic proteins. Ankyrin-1, in turn, binds to spectrin β-chain (*C*-terminal region). Recently, band 3 has also been demonstrated to be present in the 4.1R multiprotein complex, making the interactions much more complicated (not shown). *Box E: the band 3-based multiprotein complex: (ii) the Rh complex.* It includes the Rh polypeptides (RhD/RhCE) and the RhAG protein (Rh-associated glycoprotein), being arranged as a trimer; the latter is associated with CD47, the Landsteiner–Wiener glycoprotein (LW, also called ICAM-4) and glycophorin B.

ANK1 gene mutations

Ankyrin-1 is encoded by *ANK1*.[2] It connects the skeleton to band 3, i.e. the anion exchanger-1. Approximately 60% of HS are due to *ANK1* gene mutations and have reduced ankyrin-1. HS due to *ANK1* mutations is relatively severe and has a dominant inheritance pattern, although *de novo* mutations may occur. Homozygosity is bound to be lethal. (One case has been recently described, however.) This may not be evident due to the elevated reticulocyte count, as young cells have a higher ankyrin-1 content. Spectrin α- and β-chains, and protein 4.2, interacting with ankyrin-1, are secondarily decreased.

SLC4A1 gene mutations

Band 3, encoded by *SLC4A1*, is the pillar of the band 3 complex *stricto sensu*, which is itself attached to the Rh complex. Both complexes are linked through protein 4.2-

CD47[3] and Rh/RhAG-ankyrin-1 contacts.[4] In the heterozygous state, mutations in *SLC4A1* produce a mild, dominantly inherited HS (approximately 20% of HS cases). Band 3 is uniformly reduced, along with a proportional decrease in protein 4.2. Scores of mutations have been reported since the first report.[5] More severe cases are seen in compound heterozygotes. Two homozygous cases, leading to missing or strongly reduced band 3, have been reported. They were associated with a dramatic picture. Spherocytes were replaced in part by poikilocytes (see below).[6,7] The absence of band 3 is likely to be lethal unless intensive care is provided prior to and following birth. An early subtotal splenectomy, to be completed later, is indicated. These cases are accompanied by distal renal tubular acidosis, due to the fact that α-intercalated cells of the distal tubule basolateral membrane contain an isoform of band 3, lacking the 65 first amino acids of the erythroid isoform. The prognosis is

Table 7.1 Major membrane proteins, their genes and related diseases

There may be slight differences between websites (http://genome.ucsc.edu and http://www.ensembl.org). The total number of exons is provided, though the number of exons actually used in the red cells may be different. The length of the proteins is given for the erythrocyte. Associated diseases are shown (non-bold and bold fonts are used for recessive and dominant mode of inheritance, respectively).

Components	Genes (strand)	Location	Size[a] (kbp)/ exons	Amino acids (TM domains)	N-glycans	Copies[a] ×10³/RBC	Related diseases
Spectrin self-association site (*Box A* in Fig. 7.1)							
Spectrin α-chain	*SPTA1* (−)	1q23.1	76/52	2419 (none)	None	242	**HE**, **HP**, HS
Spectrin β-chain	*SPTB* (−)	14q23.3	113/32	2137 (none)	None	242	**HE**, **HP**, **HS**
The 4.1R-based multiprotein complex: (i) the junctional complex (*Box B* in Fig. 7.1)							
4.1R	*EPB41* (+)	1p35.3	>233/21	641 (none)	None	200	**HE**, **HP**
Spectrin β-chain (cf. *Box A*)							
β-Actin[b]	*ACTB* (−)	7p22.1	2.5/5	375 (none)	None	500	
Protein 4.9[c]	*EPB49* (+)	8p21.3	16/15	405 (none)	None	140	
The 4.1R-based multiprotein complex: (ii) the 4.1R-glycophorin C/D-p55 complex (*Box C* in Fig. 7.1)							
4.1R (cf. *Box B*)							
GPC/D[d]	*GYPC* (+)	2q14.3	41/4	128 (1)/107 (1)	Present	200	HE
p55[e,f]	*MPP1* (−)	Xq28	27/12	466 (none)	None	/	
The band 3-based multiprotein complex: (i) band 3 complex, *stricto sensu* (*Box D* in Fig. 7.1)							
Band 3	*SLC4A1* (−)	17q21.31	20/20	911 (12)	Present	1000	**HS**, **SAO**, **CHC1**
Ankyrin-1	*ANK1* (−)	8p11.21	224/43	1897 (none)	None	120	**HS**
Protein 4.2[e]	*EPB42* (−)	15q15.2	24/13	721 (none)	None	200	HS
GPA	*GYPA* (−)	4q31.22	31/7	137 (1)	Present	1000	
The band 3-based multiprotein complex: (ii) Rh complex (*Box E* in Fig. 7.1)							
RhD	*RHD* (+)	1p36.11	58/10	417 (12)	None	200	
RhCE	*RHCE* (−)	1p36.11	68/12	401/(12)	None	200	
RhAG	*RHAG* (−)	6p12.3	32/10	409 (12)	Present	200	HS,**OHSt**
CD47	*CD47* (−)	3q13.12	48/11	323	None	/	
LW	*ICAM4* (+)	19p13.2	1.5/3	271 (1)	Present	3–5	
GPB	*GYPB* (−)	4q31.22	22/5	100 (1)	Present	200	
Other proteins of interest (not shown in Fig. 7.1)							
Stomatin	*EPB72*(−)	9q33.2	31/7	288 (1)	None	/	
α-Adducin[g]	*ADD1*(+)	4p16.3	86/15	737 (none)	None	30	
β-Adducin[g]	*ADD2*(−)	2p13.3	106/16	727 (none)	None	30	

[a]Approximate values.

[b]β-Actin is organized as oligomers of *c.* 14–16 monomers.

[c]aka dematin.

[d]GPD starts at Met 22 (exon 2) of GPC.

[e]Heavily fatty-acylated protein.

[f]Member of the MAGUK family (membrane-associated guanylate kinase homologs).

[g]α- and β-adducin are organized as a heterodimer.

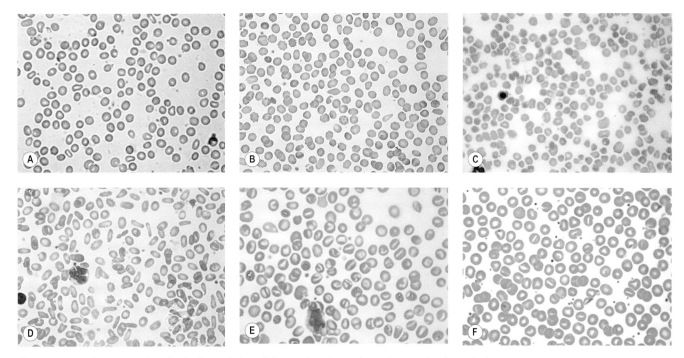

Fig. 7.2 (A–F) Selected examples of red cell morphological abnormalities. (A) Moderate dominantly inherited spherocytosis (mutation unknown). (B) Mild, recessively inherited spherocytosis due to the total absence of protein 4.2. (C) Severe, recessively inherited hereditary spherocytosis, with a strong touch of poikilocytosis (mutations in the *SPTA1* gene). (D) Asymptomatic, dominantly inherited elliptocytosis due to the partial absence of 4.1R. (E) Dehydrated hereditary stomatocytosis (gene unknown). (F) Overhydrated hereditary stomatocytosis (mutation in the *RHAG* gene). May–Grünwald–Giemsa. × 1000. *(Courtesy of Dr Thérèse Cynober.)*

obscured by nephrocalcinosis. A third case of homozygosity was described free of renal disorders because the mutation lay in the missing region of the renal isoform of band 3.

SPTB gene mutations

SPTB encodes spectrin β-chain. Mutations generate a dominantly inherited, relatively severe form of HS (20% of HS in Europe).[8] There is an isolated reduction in spectrin (α- and β-chains) on SDS-PAGE. *De novo* mutations may occur. Homozygous cases have never been reported.

EPB42 gene mutations

Mutations in *EPB42*, encoding protein 4.2, engender a relatively rare recessively inherited form of HS which is not absolutely typical. Spherocytes are bulky. A mutation has shown some frequency in Japan (Ala142Thr).[9]

SPTA1 gene mutations

SPTA1 encodes spectrin α-chain. Mutations in *SPTA1* are rare and show a recessive inheritance pattern. Homozygosity, or compound heterozygosity (involving peremptory mutations: stop codon or frameshift), has never been reported. In contrast, compound heterozygosity for a peremptory HS mutation and a rather common weak allele of the *SPTA1* gene, allele α^LEPRA, has been observed, causing a severe picture with poikilocytosis.[10]

RHAG gene mutations

RHAG encodes the Rh-associated glycoprotein (RhAG). The exceptional absence of RhAG (Rh-deficiency of the regulator type) results in a severe hemolytic anemia which has been classified as HS, although this issue has never been assessed thoroughly.

Hereditary elliptocytosis and poikilocytosis

Hereditary elliptocytosis (HE) has a much lower incidence in Caucasians than HS but occurs with the same frequency as HS in black Africans. The clinical phenotype is usually mild with peripheral blood elliptocytes but it can be moderately severe. In severe forms that achieve hereditary poikilocyotosis (HP), large red cell fragments are torn off, appearing as schistocytes and leaving erythrocytes with marked poikilocytosis.

SPTA1 gene mutations

SPTA1 mutations account for approximately 60% of HE and HP. Their mode of inheritance is dominant. Mutations are located from the *N*-terminal region of the spectrin α-chain down to repeat α9.[11] As a consequence, the self-association process is impaired, loosening the meshwork at a critical junction. Homozygosity or compound heterozygosity has a moderate to severe presentation depending on the mutation(s). Severe forms display an HP phenotype. The same situation happens when an HE mutation lies in *trans* to a frequent, worldwide, low-expression allele of the *SPTA1* gene, allele α^LELY.[12] Splenectomy should only be considered in the most severe cases.

SPTB gene mutations

SPTB mutations are rarer than *SPTA1* mutations and are associated with HE or HP. They are sporadic and dominantly transmitted. Mutations are situated in the C-terminal region (repeat β17) of the spectrin β-chain, in the self-association site, and with the same consequences as the facing mutations in the α-chain.[11] Homozygosity may be life-threatening.

EPB41 gene mutations

The *EPB41* gene encodes protein 4.1R. Mutations in *EPB41* account for 20–30% of HE in Caucasians. In the heterozygous state, 20–30% of 4.1R is missing. The 4.1R (–) trait, which is dominantly transmitted, is symptomless. In the homozygous state,[13] in which 4.1R is absent, HP is severe in the newborn but tends to improve later on. Early subtotal splenectomy may accelerate the improvement.

Genetic disorders of the monovalent cation leak across the membrane

Disorders of monovalent cation leak across the membrane, or cation leak, encompass conditions that remain poorly understood. Most include hemolytic anemia, jaundice and splenomegaly, erythrocyte shape abnormalities and macrocytosis. They have a major tendency to iron overload, an alteration of intra-erythrocytic cation concentrations, and an increase in the cation leak. The leak is defined as the fluxes that remain when the Na^+, K^+ ATPase and the Na^+, K^+, $2Cl^-$ co-transporter are inhibited by ouabain and bumetanide, respectively. The leak assumes various curves as a function of temperature. In a subset of cases, the leak diminishes with a fall in temperature from 37°C to 20°C, and then resumes, sometimes dramatically, at lower temperatures, warranting the prefix 'cryo-'. The inheritance pattern is dominant. Splenectomy is contraindicated in most of these conditions due to the risk of thromboembolic accidents, which may be lethal.[14]

A pleiotropic syndrome revolving around dehydrated hereditary stomatocytosis

Dehydrated hereditary stomatocytosis (DHSt) may occur alone, as first reported by Oski *et al.*[15] The presentation is mild and sometimes revealed only at a late stage by its major complication, an iron overload (hemochromatosis). Anemia is well compensated, and the reticulocyte count is elevated. Stomatocytes are scarce and incompletely formed. There is a borderline macrocytosis. The osmotic resistance is increased. *De novo* mutations may occur. In the homozygous state it is lethal. The curve: cation leak as a function of temperature is monophasic and has a 'shallow' slope. One responsible gene has been mapped to 16q23-ter in a large Irish kindred.[16] The region of interest was recently narrowed down to 16q24.1-ter in an extended French kindred.[17] However, there must be another or other gene(s) involved. DHSt is associated with pseudohyperkalemia and/or perinatal fluid effusions, resulting in a pleiotropic syndrome.[18]

Pseudohyperkalemia designates an increase in potassium when collected blood is left at room temperature for a few hours. DHSt-related pseudohyperkalemia is similar to familial pseudohyperkalemia (FP), a dominantly inherited trait.[19] Although extremely rare, it has been mapped to 16q23-ter[20] and to 2q35-36[21] in distinct (Scottish and Flemish) extended families. The first location coincides with that of some cases of DHSt, strengthening the idea that FP is a truncated form of the pleiotropic syndrome.

Perinatal fluid effusion is characterized by mild (sonography discovery) to dramatic edema (hydrops fetalis). When severe, the edema must be treated in order to ease mechanical constraints on the fetus. These effusions, which are sometimes chylous, recede prior to birth or in the following months, never to reappear. Whether DHSt-related fluid effusions can occur alone has not been systematically investigated.

Overhydrated hereditary stomatocytosis

Overhydrated hereditary stomatocytosis (OHSt) is an exceedingly rare form of stomatocytosis. The first case of stomatocytosis ever described was an OHSt.[22] The presentation is quite pronounced with anemia (sometimes requiring transfusions), marked macrocytosis, a strong tendency to iron overload and a reduced osmotic resistance. Stomatocytes are numerous and fully fledged. *De novo* mutations are frequent. A salient feature is the sharp decrease in, or the absence of, stomatin (not shown in Fig. 7.1). The responsible gene is *RHAG*.[23]

Hereditary cryohydrocytosis

Hereditary cryohydrocytosis with normal stomatin (CHC1) is also an exceedingly rare disorder, first described by Miller *et al.*[24] CHC 1 presents like a stomatocytosis (though of the dehydrated type, with elevated mean corpuscular hemoglobin concentration (MCHC)). Pseudohyperkalemia may be present. The salient feature is the resumption of the leak at low temperature. Mutations have been found in the *SLC4A1* gene.[25] Rare, atypical forms of HS (on the basis of the curve: leak as a function of temperature) displayed mutations in the involved region of band 3 (but with no reduction, as seen above); they were eventually related to CHC1.[25]

Hereditary cryohydrocytosis with low or missing stomatin (CHC2) presents as OHSt. Only two cases have been reported worldwide.[26] Various neurological signs were found to be associated with the condition. There was a soaring resumption of the leak at low temperatures. No mutations were found in the *RHAG* gene.

Southeast Asian ovalo-stomatocytosis

Southeast Asian ovalo-stomatocytosis is a dominantly inherited condition. It is a symptomless trait. The red cells are oval and show a longitudinal slit or two transverse ridges. This condition is classified with disorders of cation leak because an increased leak is present at low temperatures. The red cell membrane is very rigid and it is this feature which accounts for the associated resistance to malaria. The genetic alteration is a deletion of 27 nucleotides in *SLC4A1*, generating a deletion of 9 amino acid at the junction of the cytoplasmic and membrane domains of band 3.[27] Homozygosity is bound to be lethal, in keeping with the other disorders of cation leak.

Paroxysmal exertion-induced dyskinesia

Paroxysmal exertion-induced dyskinesia is characterized by disorders induced by prolonged exercise. They include epilepsy, mild developmental delay and reduced cerebrospinal fluid glucose level. Some forms are associated with a hemolytic anemia and echinocytosis, altered intra-erythrocytic cation concentrations and an increased cation leak. In one family, a deletion of four highly conserved amino acids was found GLUT1 encoded by *SLC2A1*.[28]

Conclusion

Defining the genetic abnormalities of red cell membrane disorders is critical for their classification, leading both to more accurate diagnosis and to more appropriate treatment.

References

1. Schilling RF, Gangnon RE, Traver MI. Delayed adverse vascular events after splenectomy in hereditary spherocytosis. J Thromb Haemost 2008;6:1289–95.

2. Eber SW, Gonzalez JM, Lux ML, et al. Ankyrin-1 mutations are a major cause of dominant and recessive hereditary spherocytosis. Nature Genetics 1996; 13:214–8.

3. Bruce LJ, Beckmann R, Ribeiro ML, et al. Evidence for a band 3-based membrane macrocomplex: a potential gas exchange metabolon. Blood 2003;101: 4180–8.

4. Nicolas V, Le Van Kim C, Gane P, et al. Rh-RhAG/ankyrin-R, a new interaction site between the membrane bilayer and the red cell skeleton, is impaired by Rh(null)-associated mutation. Journal of Biological Chemistry 2003;278:25526–33.

5. Jarolim P, Rubin HL, Liu SC, et al. Duplication of 10 nucleotides in the erythroid band 3 (AE1) gene in a kindred with hereditary spherocytosis and band 3 protein deficiency (band 3 PRAGUE). Journal of Clinical Investigation 1994; 93:121–30.

6. Ribeiro L, Alloisio N, Almeida H, et al. Near lethal hereditary spherocytosis and distal tubular acidosis associated with the total absence of band 3. Blood 2000; 96:1602–4.

7. Toye AM, Williamson RC, Khanfar M, et al. Band 3 Courcouronnes (Ser667Phe): a trafficking mutant differentially rescued by wild type band 3 and glycophorin A. Blood 2008;111:5380–9.

8. Hassoun H, Vassiliadis JN, Murray J, et al. Molecular basis of spectrin deficiency in β spectrin Durham. A deletion within β spectrin adjacent to the ankyrin-binding site precludes spectrin attachment to the membrane in hereditary spherocytosis. Journal of Clinical Investigation 1995; 96:2623–9.

9. Bouhassira EE, Schwartz RS, Yawata Y, et al. An alanine-to-threonine substitution in protein 4.2 cDNA is associated with a Japanese form of hereditary hemolytic anemia (protein 4.2^{NIPPON}). Blood 1992;79:1846–54.

10. Wichterle H, Hanspal M, Palek J, et al. Combination of two mutant alpha spectrin alleles underlies a severe spherocytic hemolytic anemia. Journal of Clinical Investigation 1996;98:2300–7.

11. Maillet P, Alloisio N, Morlé L, Delaunay J. Spectrin mutations in hereditary elliptocytosis and hereditary spherocytosis. Human Mutation 1996;8:97–107.

12. Wilmotte R, Maréchal J, Morlé L, et al. Low expression allele α^{LELY} of red cell spectrin is associated with mutations in exon 40 ($\alpha^{V/41}$ polymorphism) and intron 45 and with partial skipping of exon 46. Journal of Clinical Investigation 1993;91:2091–6.

13. Dalla Venezia N, Gilsanz F, Alloisio N, et al. Homozygous 4.1(−) hereditary elliptocytosis associated with a point mutation in the downstream initiation codon of protein 4.1 gene. Journal of Clinical Investigation 1992;90:1713–7.

14. Stewart GW, Amess JAL, Eber SW, et al. Thrombo-embolic disease after splenectomy for hereditary stomatocytosis. British Journal of Haematology 1996;93:303–10.

15. Oski FA, Naiman JL, Blum SF, et al. Congenital hemolytic anemia with high-sodium, low-potassium red cells. Studies of three generations of a family with a new variant. New England Journal of Medicine 1969;280:909–16.

16. Carella M, Stewart G, Ajetunmobi JF, et al. Genomewide search for dehydrated hereditary stomatocytosis (hereditary xerocytosis): mapping of locus to chromosome 16 (16q23-qter). American Journal of Human Genetics 1998;63: 810–6.

17. Beaurain G, Mathieu F, Grootenboer S, et al. Dehydrated hereditary stomatocytosis mimicking familial hyperkalaemic hypertension: clinical and genetic investigation. European Journal of Haematology 2007;78:253–9.

18. Grootenboer S, Schischmanoff PO, Laurendeau I, et al. Pleiotropic syndrome of dehydrated hereditary stomatocytosis, pseudohyperkalemia and perinatal edema maps to 16q23-q24. Blood 2000;96: 2599–605.

19. Stewart GW, Corral RJ, Fyffe JA, et al. Familial pseudohyperkalemia. A new syndrome. Lancet 1979;2(8135):175–7.

20. Iolascon A, Stewart G, Ajetunmobi JF, et al. Familial pseudohyperkalemia maps to the same locus as dehydrated hereditary stomatocytosis (hereditary xerocytosis). Blood 1999;93:3120–3.

21. Carella M., Pio d'Adamo A, Grootenboer-Mignot S, et al. A second locus mapping to 2q35-36 for familial pseudohyperkalaemia. European Journal of Human Genetics 2004;12:1073–6.

22. Lock SP, Sephton Smith R, Hardisty RM. Stomatocytosis: a hereditary red cell anomaly associated with haemolytic anaemia. British Journal of Haematology 1961;7:303–14.

23. Bruce LJ, Guizouarn H, Burton NM, et al. The monovalent cation leak in over-hydrated stomatocytic red blood cells results from amino acid substitutions in the Rh associated glycoprotein (RhAG). Blood 2009;113:1350–7.

24. Miller G, Townes PL, MacWhinney JB. A new congenital hemolytic anemia with deformed erythrocytes (? 'stomatocytes') and remarkable susceptibility of erythrocytes to cold hemolysis in vitro. I. Clinical and hematologic studies. Pediatrics 1965;35:906–15.

25. Bruce LJ, C Robinson H, Guizouarn H, et al. Monovalent cation leaks in human red cells caused by single amino-acid substitutions in the transport domain of the band 3 chloride-bicarbonate exchanger, AE1. Nature Genetics 2005; 37:1258–63.

26. Fricke B, Jarvis HG, Reid CDL, et al. Four new cases of stomatin-deficient hereditary stomatocytosis syndrome. Association of the stomatin-deficient cryohydrocytosis variant with neurological dysfunction. British Journal of Haematology 2004; 125:796–803.

27. Jarolim P, Palek J, Amato D, et al. Deletion of erythrocyte band 3 gene in malaria-resistant Southeast Asian ovalocytosis. Proceedings of the National Academy of Sciences USA 1991;88: 11022–6.

28. Weber YG, Storch A, Wuttke TV, et al. GLUT1 mutations are a cause of paroxysmal exertion-induced dyskinesias and induce hemolytic anemia by a cation leak. Journal of Clinical Investigation 2008;118:2157–68.

CHAPTER 8

Erythroenzyme disorders

DM Layton, DR Roper

Chapter contents

Introduction

To achieve optimal performance as an oxygen transporter the mature red cell has sacrificed metabolic versatility.[1] Red cell structural and functional integrity depend on catabolism of glucose via the anerobic Embden–Meyerhof pathway to replenish adenosine triphosphate (ATP) required for cation homeostasis and other energy-dependent processes in conjunction with the oxidative pentose phosphate pathway (hexose monophosphate shunt) to maintain redox capacity. In the resting state 90% of glucose is catabolized anerobically through the Embden–Meyerhof pathway, which also serves to generate nicotinamide adenine dinucleotide in its reduced form (NADH) required as a cofactor for cytochrome b5 reductase for the conversion of methemoglobin to hemoglobin (Fig. 8.1). The pentose phosphate pathway serves mainly to supply the reduced form of nicotinamide adenine dinucleotide phosphate (NADPH) necessary to regenerate reduced glutathione (GSH), which acts as a sacrificial reductant to protect the membrane and contents of the red cell against oxidative damage (Fig. 8.2). Glucose-6-phosphate dehydrogenase (G6PD) catalyzes the first and rate limiting step, the conversion of glucose-6-phosphate (G6P) to 6-phosphogluconate (6PG), in this pathway. Synthesis of the tripeptide glutathione from its constituent amino acids and nucleotide salvage complete the essential metabolic repertoire active in the red cell cytosol. Conservation of adenine nucleotides to maintain intracellular ATP and elimination of pyrimidine nucleotides is facilitated through the action of pyrimidine 5′-nucleotidase (P5N) which specifically dephosphorylates pyrimidine nucleoside-5′-monophosphates formed by RNA breakdown. This permits removal of toxic pyrimidines by passive diffusion and prevents their accumulation within the red cell. Defects in each of these key pathways produces hemolytic anemia.

With the exception of polymorphic G6PD variants (Fig. 8.3) estimated to affect up to 400 million people worldwide, most inherited disorders of red cell metabolism are uncommon. Pyruvate kinase (PK) deficiency is the most commonly encountered defect of the Embden–Meyerhof pathway with around 500 cases reported to date. Heterozygote frequencies based on biochemical population studies vary from 0.14% in the US[2] to 6% in Saudi Arabia.[3] There is some evidence that reduced red cell PK activity affords protection against malaria.[4] Mice deficient in PK are protected from malaria and the growth of *Plasmodium falciparum* is impaired in PK-deficient red cells. The impact of this on populations in areas of malarial endemicity is, however, likely to be small compared with the selective advantage conferred by the more common genetic red cell variants, G6PD deficiency and the hemoglobinopathies.

After PK the most common enzyme deficiencies implicated in hemolytic anemia are in approximate order of frequency: glucosephosphate isomerase (GPI); class I G6PD variants (associated with chronic hemolytic anemia); phosphofructokinase (PFK), triosephosphate isomerase (TPI), phosphoglycerate kinase (PGK) and hexokinase (HK). Deficiencies of P5N,[5] which has been described in populations of diverse geographic origin, and glutathione synthetase[6] occur at a comparable frequency. Other erythroenzyme disorders are rare.

Clinical features

In the patient with suspected congenital hemolytic anemia several clinical features may assist in the diagnosis of an underlying enzyme disorder. The pattern of hemolysis, whether episodic or chronic, and likely mode of inheritance discerned from the family history are often informative. In

©2011 Elsevier Ltd
DOI: 10.1016/B978-0-7020-3147-2.00008-0

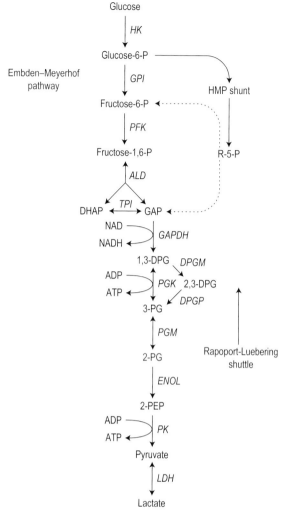

Fig. 8.1 Glycolytic pathways in the human red cell. ALD, aldolase; 2,3-DPG, 2,3-diphosphoglycerate; DPGM, diphosphoglycerate mutase; DPGP, diphosphoglycerate phosphatase; ENOL, enolase; GAPDH, glyceraldehyde-3-phosphate dehydrogenase; GPI, glucosephosphate kinase; HK, hexokinase; HMP, hexose monophosphate pathway; LDH, lactate dehydrogenase; PFK, phosphofructokinase; PGK, phosphoglycerate kinase; PGM, phosphoglycerate mutase; PK, pyruvate kinase; TPI, triosephosphate isomerase.

general, defects of the Embden–Meyerhof glycolytic pathway, essential for energy (ATP) generation in the steady state, result in chronic hemolytic anemia, whereas those of the pentose phosphate and glutathione pathways typically are associated with acute hemolysis after oxidative challenge. Overlap in the pattern of hemolysis renders this a useful though not infallible distinction.

The presence of neurological, myopathic or other non-hematologic manifestations is of considerable diagnostic value. Neurodevelopmental abnormalities must be interpreted with caution since severe neonatal hyperbilirubinemia sufficient to cause kernicterus has been described in deficiency of several red cell enzymes including G6PD and PK. Distinctive features of erythroenzymopathies are summarized in Table 8.1.

The pattern of somatic abnormalities manifest in individual enzyme disorders is determined by several factors. Deficiency of an isoenzyme, expression of which is restricted (e.g. pyruvate kinase-L/R), generally causes isolated hemolysis. Conversely, defects of ubiquitously expressed enzymes (e.g. triosephosphate isomerase) often result in a more generalized phenotype. The physiochemical properties of a mutant enzyme also influence clinical expression. Enzyme variants associated with impaired catalytic efficiency generally produce greater metabolic perturbance than those resulting in structural instability, the consequences of which are offset in tissues which retain the capacity for protein synthesis. This is reflected in a correspondingly more severe clinical phenotype. Examples include stable GPI mutants associated with multisystem[7] disease and high Km class I G6PD variants which in addition to hemolysis manifest impaired leukocyte function or cataract due to reduction of enzyme activity in non-erythroid tissues.[8]

Blood cell morphology

Red cell enzyme defects have traditionally been grouped under the heading congenital non-spherocytic hemolytic anemia. While morphological atypia in the red cells are usually apparent, these overlap with other causes of hemolysis and are seldom exclusive to a specific enzyme defect. A notable exception is the striking basophilic stippling associated with P5N deficiency which may be seen in up to 5% of red cells on a freshly stained blood film prepared from an ethylenediaminetetraacetic acid (EDTA) sample (Fig. 8.4). Stippling may disappear if the stain is delayed by more than a few hours, presumably because EDTA chelates metal ions required for ribonucleoprotein aggregation. This problem may be circumvented by examination of blood taken into lithium heparin. Conspicuous punctate basophilia akin to that in P5N deficiency accompanies unstable hemoglobin variants and CDP-choline phosphotransferase deficiency,[9] a putative defect of nucleotide metabolism described in only a few families. Lead is a potent inhibitor of P5N activity. This explains the finding of punctate basophilia in plumbism. The presence of other clinical and morphologic stigmata, the latter including red cell hypochromia and microcytosis, reticulocytosis or sideroblastic erythropoiesis, usually render distinction from primary P5N deficiency straightforward. Basophilic stippling may also be found in a wide range of congenital and acquired dyserythropoietic states including

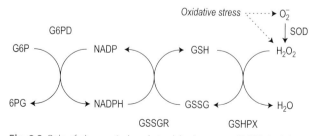

Fig. 8.2 Role of glucose-6-phosphate dehydrogenase (G6PD) in defense against oxidative damage. GSH, glutathione; GSHPX, glutathione peroxidase; GSSG, oxidized glutathione; GSSGR, glutathione reductase; H_2O_2, hydrogen peroxide; SOD, superoxide dismutase.

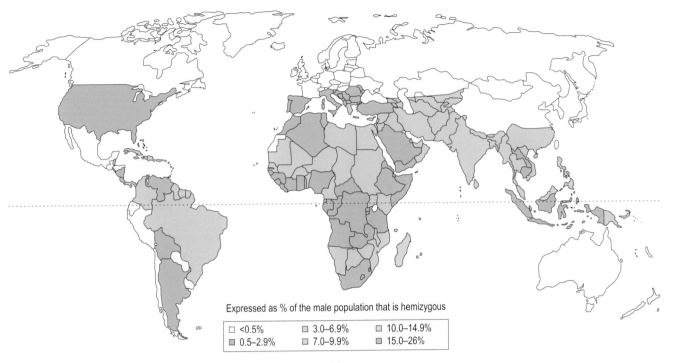

Expressed as % of the male population that is hemizygous

☐ <0.5%   ☐ 3.0–6.9%   ☐ 10.0–14.9%
☐ 0.5–2.9%   ☐ 7.0–9.9%   ☐ 15.0–26%

Fig. 8.3 World distribution of glucose-6-phosphate dehydrogenase (G6PD) deficiency.

Table 8.1 Distinctive clinical features associated with erythroenzymopathies

Enzyme	Inheritance	Neurological	Myopathy	Other
Glycolytic pathway				
Hexokinase	AR			Poor effort tolerance, erythrocytosis
Glucosephosphate isomerase	AR	+ rare	+ rare	Fetal hydrops, recurrent infection, priapism
Phosphofructokinase	AR		+/−	Myoglobinuria, hyperuricemia, erythrocytosis
Aldolase	AR	(+)	+/−	
Triosephosphate isomerase	AR	+	+	Recurrent infection, sudden cardiac death
Phosphoglycerate kinase	XL	+/−	+/−	Myoglobinuria
Diphosphoglycerate mutase	AR			Erythrocytosis
Enolase	AD?			Spherocytosis
Pyruvate kinase L/R	AR, rarely AD			Fetal hydrops, iron overload
Lactate dehydrogenase M (B)	AR		+	
Glutathione biosynthesis or regeneration				
γ-Glutamylcysteine synthetase	AR	+/−		
Glutathione synthetase	AR	+/−		Acidosis, 5-oxoprolinuria, recurrent infection
Glutathione reductase	AR			Favism, cataract
Nucleotide metabolism				
Pyrimidine 5'-nucleotidase	AR	(+)		Basophilic stippling
				Acquired deficiency in plumbism, transient erythroblastopenia of childhood and thalassemia
CDP-choline phosphotransferase	AR			Basophilic stippling
Adenosine deaminase	AD			
Adenylate kinase	AR	+/−		

AD, autosomal dominant; AR, autosomal recessive; XL, X-linked.

Parentheses denote link is unproven.

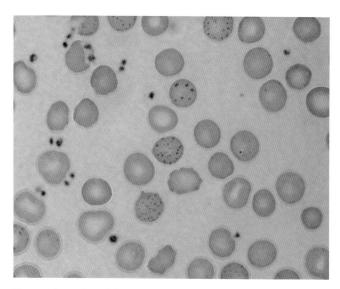

Fig. 8.4 Coarse basophilic stippling in pyrimidine 5'-nucleotidase deficiency. May–Grünwald–Giemsa. ×1000.

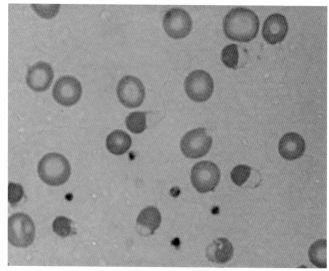

Fig. 8.5 Blood film during acute hemolytic episode in G6PD deficiency. May–Grünwald–Giemsa. ×1000.

Table 8.2 Drugs and chemicals associated with hemolysis in glucose-6-phosphate dehydrogenase (G6PD) deficiency

Class of drug	Examples
Antimalarials	Primaquine, pentaquine, pamaquine, chloroquine*
Sulfonamides and sulfones	Sulfanilamide, sulfacetamide, sulfapyridine, sulfamethoxazole (including co-trimoxazole), dapsone
Other antibacterial agents	Nitrofurantoin, nalidixic acid, chloramphenicol, ciprofloxacin*
Analgesic/antipyretic	Acetanilid, acetylsalicylic acid (aspirin)[†], paracetamol (acetaminophen)[†]
Miscellaneous	Probenecid
	Dimercaprol
	Vitamin K analogs
	Naphthalene (moth balls)
	Methylene blue
	Ascorbic acid
	Trinitrotoluene

*Possible association.

[†]Only after high doses or overdose.

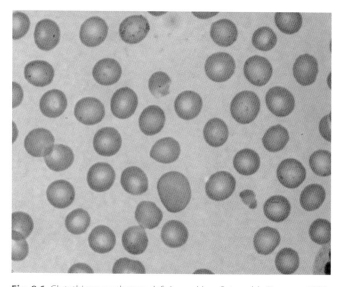

Fig. 8.6 Glutathione synthetase deficiency. May–Grünwald–Giemsa. ×1000.

thalassemia and occasionally in some glycolytic defects (e.g. pyruvate kinase or phosphofructokinase deficiency).

Features of oxidative damage to red cells are most commonly associated with, though not confined to, G6PD deficiency. These are most remarkable during hemolytic crises following exposure to oxidant drugs (Table 8.2) or fava bean (broad bean) consumption and include irregularly contracted hyperchromic erythrocytes, some of which display a characteristic 'bite' or 'hemighost' appearance (Fig. 8.5). 'Bite' cells in which the surface of the erythrocyte is breached producing an irregular gap are thought to be generated by removal of Heinz bodies during transit through the spleen. Erythrocyte 'hemighosts' are forms in which the hemoglobin appears condensed and is retracted to one side leaving an empty space in the cell. In the common polymorphic G6PD variants (e.g. G6PD A⁻ or Med) these morphologic abnormalities are visible only during hemolytic episodes. Following acute hemolysis in G6PD deficiency rapid clearance of damaged cells by the spleen ensues and during the recovery phase polychromasia and macrocytosis predominate. Similar though usually less marked features of oxidative damage may be seen in defects which impair glutathione biosynthesis (Fig. 8.6) or regeneration due to deficiency of γ-glutamylcysteine synthetase,[10] glutathione synthetase[6,11] or glutathione reductase[12] as well as neonatal hemolysis due to deficiency of glutathione peroxidase (Fig. 8.7).[13] The latter condition which does not conform to the laws of Mendelian inheritance may reflect a transient reduction in enzyme

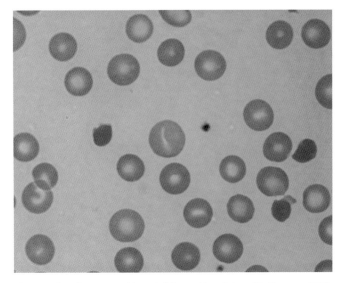

Fig. 8.7 Glutathione peroxidase deficiency. May–Grünwald–Giemsa. ×1000.

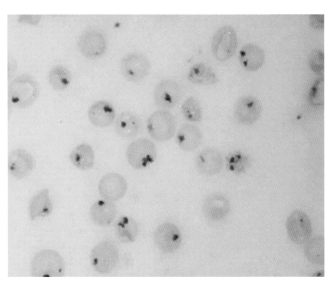

Fig. 8.8 Methyl violet stain showing numerous Heinz bodies. ×1000.

activity due to impaired selenium homeostasis in the mother or neonate. Selenium is an essential co-factor for glutathione peroxidase which serves to detoxify harmful peroxides in the red cell. Glutathione peroxidase deficiency produces an acute and usually self-limiting hemolytic anemia in the newborn period. The diagnosis may be confirmed by assay of neonatal and maternal selenium levels and red cell glutathione peroxidase. Defects of other enzymes in the pentose phosphate pathway, 6-phosphogluconolactonase[14] and phosphogluconate dehydrogenase[15] have been described, albeit rarely, and should be considered if changes suggestive of oxidative damage are evident and more common causes excluded.

Examination of a blood film for Heinz bodies should be performed in cases of suspected oxidative hemolysis. These intraerythrocytic inclusions, first characterized in experimental studies of acetylphenylhydrazine toxicity, are visualized after staining supravitally with the basic dyes methyl violet or brilliant cresyl blue (Fig. 8.8). Heinz bodies, formed from denatured globin which attaches to the inner surface of the erythrocyte membrane, develop either spontaneously in the case of unstable hemoglobin variants or after oxidative challenge in susceptible (e.g. G6PD-deficient) red cells. The number of Heinz bodies increases dramatically after splenectomy. Similar inclusions due to precipitation of surplus α-globin chains may be visible in some thalassemia syndromes. It should be noted that unstable hemoglobin variants which produce a Heinz-body hemolytic anemia often escape detection by conventional separation techniques either because they result from structural alteration within the interior of the hemoglobin molecule and therefore do not alter surface charge or are so unstable as to undergo rapid degradation *ex vivo*. Stability tests in combination with mass spectrometry[16] provide a reliable approach to the detection of unstable hemoglobins which should be undertaken in cases where oxidative changes or Heinz bodies are present before detailed studies of red cell metabolism are embarked upon. Similarly, if drug or toxin ingestion is suspected, screening for sulphemoglobin and methemoglobin by absorbance at 620 and 630 nm respectively is indicated to

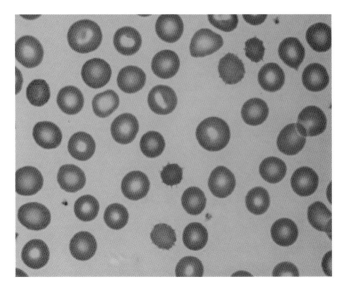

Fig. 8.9 Triosephosphate isomerase deficiency. May–Grünwald–Giemsa. ×1000.

exclude drug- or chemical-induced hemolysis which may follow severe oxidant stress in the absence of any intrinsic red cell defect.

True spherocytes, such as seen in hereditary spherocytosis in which both the normal discoid shape of the erythrocyte is lost and cell volume reduced, are generally not seen in erythroenzymopathies. A possible exception is enolase 1 deficiency, a disorder hitherto described in only a single kindred with a dominant mode of inheritance and spherocytosis but normal acidified glycerol lysis test. Morphologic variants, particularly spheroechinocytes, derived from the Greek for sea urchin (*Echinus*), are frequently present in variable numbers in glycolytic disorders (Fig. 8.9). These crenated cells have multiple short spicules of uniform appearance and represent effete red cells in which ATP depletion has led to failure of cation homeostasis and cellular dehydration. They are most striking in, though not specific to, PK deficiency where the number of such cells often

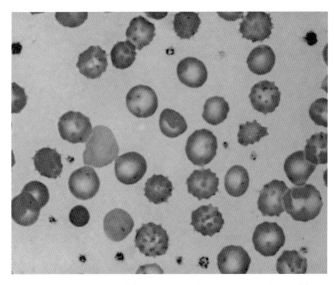

Fig. 8.10 Pyruvate kinase deficiency post-splenectomy. May–Grünwald–Giemsa. ×1000.

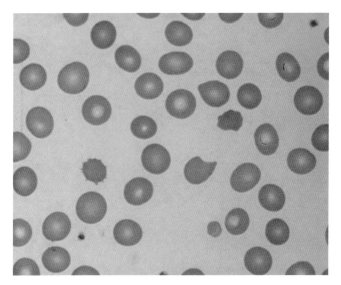

Fig. 8.11 Dyserythropoietic features in pyruvate kinase deficiency. May–Grünwald–Giemsa. ×1000.

increases dramatically (up to 30% of red cells) after splenectomy (Fig. 8.10). Poikilocytosis with elliptocytic, ovalocytic and dacrocytic (tear-drop) forms may also be seen in PK deficiency (Fig. 8.11). These findings are nonspecific and may be ascribable to dyserythropoiesis. Evidence of ineffective erythropoiesis with defective utilization of ^{59}Fe has been observed in some cases and experimental models indicate PK deficiency is associated with increased apoptosis of erythroid progenitors.[17]

Biochemical investigation of erythroenzyme disorders

Initial investigation of a patient in whom enzymopathy is suspected often necessitates the exclusion of other mechanisms of shortened red cell survival, specifically immune

hemolysis, a membrane cytoskeleton defect, unstable or thalassemic hemoglobinopathies and paroxysmal nocturnal hemoglobinuria. An increased rate of autohemolysis not corrected by exogenous glucose (type 2), first recognized by Dacie, is a characteristic though not consistent feature of glycolytic disorders. Autohemolysis pattern and osmotic fragility, though both abnormal in some enzyme disorders, have been largely superseded by direct estimation of enzyme activity or intermediate metabolites and their utility lies mainly in the exclusion of membrane defects as a cause of unexplained hemolytic anemia.

While useful screening methods[18] exist for detection of some more common enzyme defects (e.g. G6PD and PK deficiency) definitive diagnosis relies on quantitation of enzyme activity in red cells in conjunction with physiochemical properties of the mutant enzyme.[19] Rigorous removal of leukocytes in which residual enzyme activity is substantially higher or reflects expression of a different isoenzyme from that in red cells potentially masking deficiency and correction for the higher activity of some enzymes (HK, PK, aldolase, G6PD and P5N) in younger red cells by comparison with a control matched for a reticulocyte count or another red cell age-dependent enzyme is essential. In most clinical erythroenzymopathies residual enzyme activity in red cells is 5–40% of normal. Higher levels do not exclude an erythroenzyme disorder and particular care must be taken in interpretation of studies performed in patients who have received transfusion due to interference from donor red cells and neonates. Significant differences in erythrocyte metabolism have been observed between neonatal and adult red cells. These include a higher activity for some enzymes (PK, GPI, G6PD) and lower activity for others (PFK, glutathione peroxidase, adenylate kinase) in erythrocytes from cord blood. Under the saturating substrate conditions employed for quantitation of enzyme activity *in vitro* relatively stable mutants with impaired catalytic efficiency *in vivo* may elude detection. If a strong suspicion of enzymopathy remains, measurement of enzyme activity at low substrate concentration or studies of enzyme kinetics and response to physiologic modulators may be necessary (Fig. 8.12A, B).

Quantitation of the major red cell metabolites 2,3-diphosphoglycerate (2,3-DPG) and GSH by spectrophotometry is of value in the diagnosis of glycolytic disorders and hemolytic anemias due to impaired defense against oxidative damage to the red cell. The ratio of 2,3-DPG to ATP specifically may localize a defect in glycolysis to the proximal or distal part of the Embden–Meyerhof pathway (Table 8.3). A reduced GSH concentration is found in G6PD deficiency, other pentose phosphate pathway defects and enzyme disorders directly affecting glutathione biosynthesis or regeneration. A low red cell GSH level is, however, a relatively nonspecific finding which may be seen in other causes of hemolytic anemia particularly unstable hemoglobins as well as some glycolytic (e.g. GPI deficiency) and membrane defects. Marked reduction in GSH implies a defect in glutathione biosynthesis due to γ-glutamylcysteine synthetase or glutathione synthetase deficiency.

To overcome the limitation of *in vitro* measurement of enzyme activity under conditions which may not accurately reflect enzyme function *in vivo*, defects in the Embden–Meyerhof pathway may be identified by measurement of the

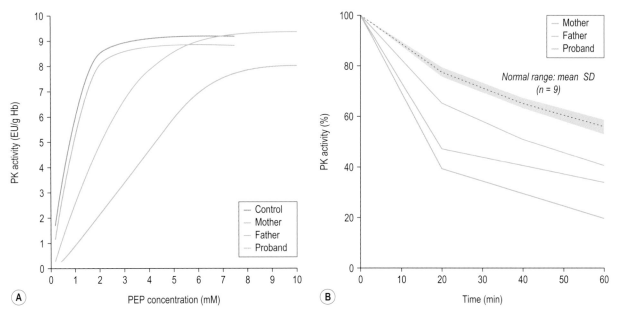

Fig. 8.12 (A, B) Pyruvate kinase (PK) kinetics. (A) Although the maximum PK activity is normal, enzyme activity at 50% phosphoenolpyruvate (PEP) saturation is reduced in the proband and father. (B) Residual PK activity after incubation at 55°C. The results indicate both the parents and proband have an unstable enzyme variant.

Table 8.3 2,3-diphosphoglycerate (2,3-DPG) and ATP patterns in some hereditary hemolytic anemias

Defect	2,3-DPG	ATP	Comments
Proximal glycolytic HK, GPI, PFK	N or ↓	N or ↓	Variable ↓2,3-DPG also seen in DPGM deficiency. Stomatocytosis ADA, overexpression and some cases of HS before splenectomy
Distal glycolytic PGK, PK	↑↑	N or ↓	↑2,3-DPG:ATP useful in PK deficiency. Also seen in Zieve's syndrome

ADA, adeonsine deaminase; ATP, adenosine triphosphate;
DPGM, diphosphoglycerate mutase; GPI, glucosephosphate isomerase;
HK, hexokinase; HS, hereditary spherocytosis; N, normal; PFK, phosphofructokinase;
PGK, phosphoglycerate kinase; PK, pyruvate kinase.

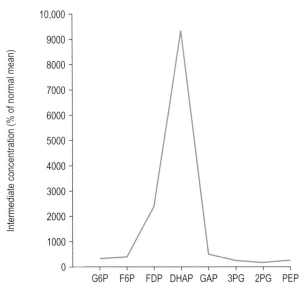

Fig. 8.13 Pattern of glycolytic intermediates in a patient with triosephosphate isomerase (TPI) deficiency demonstrating markedly elevated dihydroxyacetone phosphate (DHAP) concentration. Values are expressed as a percentage of the normal mean. F6P, fructose-6-phosphate; FDP, fructose-1,6-diphosphate; G6P, glucose-6-phosphate; GAP, glyceraldehyde-3-phosphate; PEP, phosphoenolpyruvate; 2PG, 2-phosphoglycerate; 3PG, 3-phosphoglycerate.

concentration of intermediate metabolites in a deproteinized red cell extract. Typically, metabolic block is indicated by accumulation of intermediates proximal and depletion distal to the step catalyzed by the deficient enzyme. In some instances substrate accumulation may be dramatic and the resulting intermediate profile pathognomonic of a specific disorder (Fig. 8.13). Unfortunately, in many countries, the reagents required for quantitation of glycolytic intermediates are no longer readily available. Prenatal diagnosis by biochemical or molecular analysis has been undertaken for several severe erythroenzymopathies including deficiencies of TPI, GPI, PK and G6PD.[20–23]

Molecular basis of erythroenzyme disorders

Over the past decade the molecular defects that underlie hematologically important erythroenzyme disorders have been elucidated. This has revealed a striking bias towards missense mutations mainly affecting conserved residues in the encoded protein (Fig. 8.14).[24–26] The paucity of null

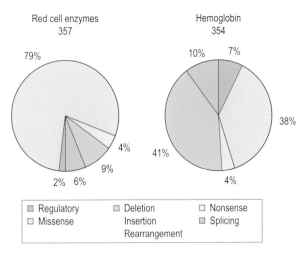

Red cell enzymes
357

Hemoglobin
354

79%

10% 7%

38%

4%

41%

9%

2% 6%

4%

☐ Regulatory   ☐ Deletion   ☐ Nonsense
☐ Missense   Insertion   ☐ Splicing
               Rearrangement

Fig. 8.14 Distribution of gene mutations in human erythroenzyme (n = 357) and hemoglobin (n = 354) disorders.

mutations found among patients with clinical enzyme deficiencies is consistent with evidence from murine models that complete disruption of the Embden–Meyerhof, pentose phosphate or glutathione biosynthetic pathways is lethal during embryogenesis. Exceptions to this are severe forms of PK deficiency due to mutations that abolish PK-L/R expression, for example the PK Gypsy mutation, a 1149bp deletion which results in the loss of exon 11. Surviving homozygotes may be rescued from what would otherwise be a lethal phenotype by persistence of the muscle isoenzyme PK-M2, normally expressed during early erythroid differentiation, which is encoded by a separate genetic locus.[27] Relatively few examples of regulatory mutations have been implicated in erythroenzyme disorders, exceptions being the −72G and −83C mutations which disrupt conserved elements in the promoter of the PK-L/R gene. Sequence variation within the TATA box and other essential promoter elements of the TPI

gene is widely distributed in human populations and has been linked to a reduction of enzyme activity *in vivo*.[26]

In certain populations individual mutations account for a high proportion of deficient alleles. This applies not only to G6PD deficiency where the prevalence of individual variants reflects evolutionary selection due to protection against malaria but is also evident in PK deficiency in which 1529A(Arg510Gln) and 1456T(Arg466Trp) substitutions together account for approximately 40% and 30% of mutations in patients of northern and southern European descent respectively. Among reported Japanese PK deficient patients the most frequently found mutation is1468T(Arg490Trp).[17] Even greater homogeneity is evident in TPI deficiency where a single missense mutation Glu104Asp accounts for the majority of reported cases. Haplotype studies support a single origin for these mutations. Genotype–phenotype correlations are beginning to emerge for the erythroenzyme disorders informed by the study of patients homozygous for individual mutations. Homozygotes for the 994A(Gly332Ser) mutation of the PK-L/R gene manifest a severe clinical course with transfusion-dependent anemia. At the other end of the spectrum it has been proposed, based on disparity in observed and predicted allele frequencies, that some genotypes such as homozygosity for the 1456T mutation may escape clinical detection due to their mild phenotype. Distant genetic factors may also exert an influence on the clinical course of erythroenzyme disorders. The level of unconjugated bilirubin in G6PD[28] and PK[27] deficiency correlates with inheritance of the (TA)₇ allele of the uridinine diphosphate glucuronosyltransferase gene (UGT1A1) promoter associated with Gilbert syndrome which has been shown to potentiate gallstone formation in other hemolytic states. Coinheritance of hereditary hemochromatosis may accelerate iron loading, though the high prevalence of this complication in pyruvate kinase deficiency suggests the contribution of other mechanisms, for example ineffective erythropoiesis, may be more important.

References

1. Beutler E. The red cell. In: editors. Haemolytic Anemia in Disorders of Red Cell Metabolism. New York: Plenum; 1978. p. 1–21.

2. Mohrenweiser HW. Frequency of enzyme deficiency variants in erythrocytes of newborn infants. Proceedings of the National Academy of Sciences USA 1981;78:5046–50.

3. El-Hazmi MAF, Al-Swailem AR, Al-Faleh FZ, Warsy AS. Frequency of glucose-6-phosphate dehydrogenase, pyruvate kinase and hexokinase deficiency in the Saudi population. Human Hereditory 1986;36:45–9.

4. Allison AC. Genetic control of resistance to human malaria. Current Opinion in Immunology 2009;21:499–505.

5. Vives Corrons JL. Chronic non-spherocytic haemolytic anaemia due to congenital pyrimidine 5′ nucleotidase deficiency: 25

years later. Baillière's Best Practice and Research in Clinical Haematology 2000;13:103–18.

6. Ristoff E, Mayatepek E, Larsson A. Long-term clinical outcome in patients with glutathione synthetase deficiency. Journal of Pediatrics 2001;139: 79–84.

7. Schroter W, Eber SW, Bardosi A, et al. Generalized glucosephosphate isomerase (GPI) deficiency causing hemolytic anemia, neuromuscular symptoms and impairment of granulocytic function: a new syndrome due to a new stable GPI variant and diminished specific activity (GPI Homburg). European Journal of Pediatrics 1985;144:301–5.

8. Luzzatto L, Mehta A, Vulliamy T. Glucose-6-phosphate dehydrogenase deficiency. In: Scriver CR, Beaudet AL, Sly WS, Valle D, editors. The metabolic

and molecular basis of inherited disease. McGraw-Hill; 2001. p. 4517–53.

9. Paglia DE, Valentine WN, Nakatani M, et al. Selective accumulation of cytosol CDP-choline as an isolated erythrocyte defect in chronic haemolysis. Proceedings of the National Academy of Sciences USA 1983;80:3081–5.

10. Konrad PN, Richards F II, Valentine WN, Paglia DE. Gammaglutamyl-cysteine synthetase deficiency. New England Journal of Medicine 1972;286:557–61.

11. Hirono A, Iyori H, Skine I, et al. Three cases of hereditary non-spherocytic haemolytic anemia associated with red blood cell glutathione deficiency. Blood 1996;87:2071–4.

12. Loos H, Roos D, Weening R, Houwerzijl J. Familial deficiency of glutathione reductase in human blood cells. Blood 1976;48:53–62.

13. Necheles TF, Steinberg MH, Cameron D. Erythrocyte glutathione-peroxidase deficiency. British Journal of Haematology 1970;19:605–12.

14. Beutler E, Kuhl W, Gelbert T: 6-Phosphogluconolactonase deficiency, a hereditary erythrocyte enzyme deficiency: possible interaction with glucose-6-phosphate dehydrogenase deficiency. Proceedings of the National Academy of Sciences USA 1985;82:3876–8.

15. Vives Corrons JL, Colomer D, Pujades A, et al. Congenital 6-phosphogluconate dehydrogenase (6PGD) deficiency associated with chronic hemolytic anemia in a Spanish family. American Journal of Hematology 1996;53:221–7.

16. Wild BJ, Green BN, Cooper EK, et al. Rapid identification of hemoglobin variants by electrospray ionization mass spectrometry. Blood Cells, Molecules and Diseases 2001;27:691–704.

17. Zanella A, Fermo E, Bianchi P, et al. Pyruvate kinase deficiency: the genotype-phenotype association. Blood Reviews 2007;21:217–31.

18. Beutler E, Blume KG, Kaplan JC, et al. International Committee for Standardization in Haematology: recommended screening test for glucose-6-phosphate dehydrogenase (G-6-PD) deficiency. British Journal of Haematology 1979;43:469–77.

19. Beutler E. Red Cell Metabolism. A Manual of Biochemical Methods. 2nd ed. Orlando, FL. Grune and Stratton; 1984.

20. Ayra R, Lalloz MRA, Nicolaides KH, et al. Prenatal diagnosis of triosephosphate isomerase deficiency. Blood 1996;87:4507–9.

21. Whitelaw AGL, Rogers PA, Hopkinson DA, et al. Congenital haemolytic anaemia resulting from glucose phosphate isomerase deficiency: genetics, clinical picture and prenatal diagnosis. Journal of Medical Genetics 1979;16:189–96.

22. Baronciani L, Beutler E. Prenatal diagnosis of pyruvate kinase deficiency. Blood 1994;84:2354–6.

23. Beutler E, Kuhl W, Fox M, et al. Prenatal diagnosis of glucose-6-phosphate dehydrogenase deficiency. Acta Haematologica 1992;87:103–10.

24. Stenson PD, Ball E, Howells K, et al. Human Gene Mutation Database: towards a comprehensive central mutation database. Journal of Medical Genetics 2008;45:124–6.

25. Mehta A, Mason PJ, Vulliamy TJ. Glucose-6-phosphate dehydrogenase deficiency. Baillière's Best Practice and Research in Clinical Haematology 2000;13:21–38.

26. Marinaki AM, Escuredo E, Duley JA, et al. Genetic basis of hemolytic anemia caused by pyrimidine 5'-nucleotidase deficiency. Blood 2001;97:3327–32.

27. Zanella A, Bianchi P. Red cell pyruvate kinase deficiency: from genetics to clinical manifestations. Baillière's Best Practice and Research in Clinical Haematology 2000;13:57–81.

28. Samipietro M, Lupica L, Perrero L, et al. The expression of uridine diphosphate glucuronsyltransferase gene is a major determinant of bilirubin level in heterozygous thalassaemia and in glucose-6-phosphate dehydrogenase deficiency. British Journal of Haematology 1997;99:437–9.

CHAPTER 9

Abnormalities of the structure and synthesis of hemoglobin

SL Thein

Chapter contents

Introduction

Hemoglobin (Hb) is the protein in red blood cells that is responsible for the delivery of oxygen from the lungs to the tissues and the transport of carbon dioxide from the tissues back to the lungs. All human hemoglobins have a tetrameric structure consisting of two identical α-like (α and ζ) and two β-like (ε, γ, δ or β) globin chains, each linked to a heme group, the moeity that is responsible for the reversible binding and transfer of oxygen. Different types of hemoglobin are expressed at different stages of development. In the human embryo, the main hemoglobins include Hb Portland ($\zeta_2 \gamma_2$), Hb Gower I ($\zeta_2\varepsilon_2$), and Hb Gower II ($\alpha_2\varepsilon_2$); in the fetus, fetal hemoglobin (HbF $\alpha_2\gamma_2$) predominates and in adults, HbA ($\alpha_2\beta_2$) comprises over 95% of the total hemoglobin with a minor component of HbA$_2$ ($\alpha_2\delta_2$) in the red blood cells. Erythrocytes containing embryonic and fetal hemoglobins have a higher affinity for oxygen than those containing adult hemoglobin, an adaptation facilitating the efficient transfer of oxygen across the placenta from the maternal to the fetal circulation during development.

Normal human hemoglobin: structure and synthesis

The switch from embryonic to fetal hemoglobin production begins as early as week 5 of gestation and is completed by week 10 (Fig. 9.1). β-globin expression starts as early as week 8 but the synthesis remains low, increases to approximately 10% at weeks 30–35 of gestation with a dramatic up-regulation

DOI: 10.1016/B978-0-7020-3147-2.00009-2

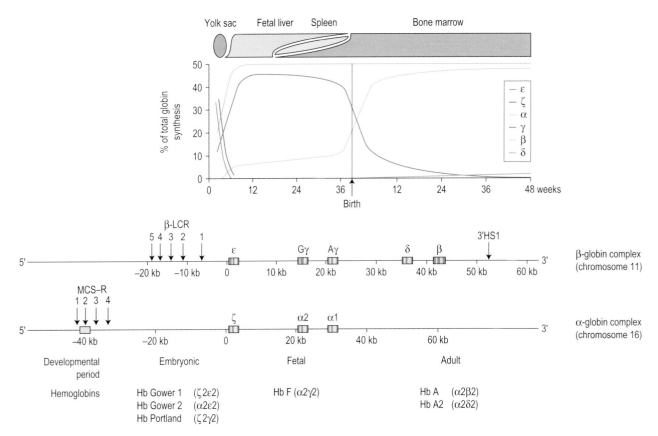

Fig. 9.1 Sequence of human hemoglobin synthesis (above) and the organization of the globin gene clusters on chromosome 11p and 16p (below) with the types of hemoglobin synthesized during the different developmental periods. Solid arrows represent the deoxyribonuclease I hypersensitive sites (HSs) in the β cluster. HSs 1 to 5 upstream of the β cluster form the β-LCR; the 3'HS1 site is a downstream enhancer.

of β-globin synthesis just before birth, coinciding with a precipitous decline in γ-globin expression. At birth, HbF ($\alpha_2\gamma_2$) comprises 60–80% of the total hemoglobin, falling to ~5% at 6 months of age and eventually reaching the adult level of about 1% at 2 years, by which stage mutations affecting the adult β-globin gene should become apparent. The switch from fetal to adult hemoglobin production is not total; γ-globin production persists at a low level throughout adult life, with the residual amounts of HbF restricted to a small subset (0.2–7%) of erythrocytes termed F cells.[1]

Each of the α-like and β-like globin chains are encoded by genetically distinct gene clusters, the α-like cluster on the tip of chromosome 16p (5'-ζ-α_2-α_1-3'), and the β-like cluster on chromosome 11p15.5 (5'-ε-$^G\gamma$-$^A\gamma$-δ-β-3') (Fig. 9.1). In both clusters, the genes are arranged along the chromosome in the order in which they are expressed during development, suggesting that gene order may be important in the program of their expression. The coding region of each globin gene is interrupted by two intervening sequences (IVSs) or introns. In the β-like globin genes, IVS-1 (122–130 bp) interrupts the sequence between codons 30 and 31, and IVS-2 (850–900 bp), between codons 104 and 105. In the α-like globin genes, IVS-1 interrupts the coding region between codons 30 and 31, and IVS-2, between codons 99 and 100. In addition to the primary *cis*-determinants of individual globin gene expression which are found in the promoter region immediately upstream of each gene, there are other local regulatory elements known as enhancers which are located at variable distances from the individual genes.[1]

Throughout development, the appropriate genes of the two globin gene clusters are coordinately expressed, maintaining a tight balance in the production of α- and β-like globins needed for the synthesis of normal hemoglobin; imbalance between the different proteins may lead to anemia. Expression of the individual genes within each cluster is controlled by complex interactions between the local regulatory sequences within each gene and regulatory elements upstream of the cluster, mediated by a series of transcription factors. In the β cluster, the upstream element is referred to as the β locus control region (β-LCR), which consists of five DNase I hypersensitive sites (designated HSs1–5) distributed between 5 and 25 kb upstream of the ε-globin gene (Fig. 9.1). The region was originally implicated in patients with anemia due to β-globin chain deficiency despite carrying normal β-globin genes. These patients were subsequently shown to be carrying mutations that deleted sequences upstream of the ε-globin gene. These natural mutants prompted experiments that demonstrated the absolute importance of the β-LCR for high levels of globin gene expression and led to a general definition of LCRs: elements that confer high levels of tissue-specific expression to a *cis*-linked gene dependent on copy-number but independent of position of integration site. The corresponding region in the α globin cluster consists of the four multispecies conserved sequence regions (MCS-Rs), lying 30–70 kb upstream of the α-globin genes termed MCS-R1 to R4.[2] Of these elements, only MCS-R2, which consists of a single DNase hypersensitive site, has been shown to be essential for α-globin expression. MCS-R2, which lies 40 kb upstream of the cluster, is also known as HS-40. The β-LCR establishes a transcriptionally active chromatin domain that encompasses the whole β-globin cluster and acts as a unique enhancer while the α-globin HS-40 is most similar to HS2 of the β-LCR and acts as an enhancer. In both clusters, full expression of the downstream genes is critically dependent on the presence of the upstream regulatory elements.

The precise molecular mechanisms by which the globin genes are expressed in a tissue- and developmental-stage-specific manner are still poorly understood. Each cluster contains various binding sites for both erythroid-specific and more ubiquitous DNA-binding proteins in the upstream regulatory elements as well as in the local promoters of the genes. Tissue-specific expression may be explained by the presence of the binding sites for the erythroid-specific transcription factors. These motifs include (A/T) GATA (A/G) binding the tissue-restricted zinc finger proteins (GATA-1 and GATA-2), and their cofactors (FOG1 and FOG2); 'CACCC' binding the erythroid Krüppel-like factors (EKLF and FLKL) and, 'TGA(C/G)TCA' (NF-E2/AP-1 like) elements, binding the b-Zip family of proteins (NF-E2, Nrf1, Nrf2, Nrf3, Bach1 and Bach2).[1,3] These transcription factors can both activate and repress gene expression. They are modular proteins and their dual functions are mediated via the distinct domains either through direct DNA binding or interaction with other proteins. Recent work has also shown that part of the function of these transcription factors involves modification of chromatin states. It seems likely that these erythroid-specific transcription factors form part of a network of factors that commit hemopoietic cells to erythroid differentiation. Elucidation of the complexity of transcription factor function has been facilitated in recent years by a series of technological advancements that included 'chromosome conformation capture' (3C, 4C and 3C-sequencing), RNA TRAP (tagging and recovery of associated proteins), chromatin immunoprecipitation (ChIP), and microarray analysis to identify gene targets of the transcription factors.[4] The 3C technique can be used to demonstrate interactions among chromosomal fragments and indeed, showed that the β-LCR and actively transcribed globin genes are in close spatial proximity in a cluster referred to as an active chromatin hub (ACH).[5]

The mechanisms by which developmental regulation is controlled are less clear and rely on two mechanisms, autonomous gene silencing and gene competition.[6] It appears that the ε and ζ genes are switched on in embryonic cells and autonomously switched off in definitive cells (liver and bone marrow) in which they cannot be substantially reactivated. The regulatory sequences mediating silencing of the ε-globin gene have been mapped to its distal and proximal promoters. The second switch from γ to β gene expression is more complex and involves both autonomous silencing of the γ genes and competition between the γ and β genes for the β-LCR. The LCR up-regulates only one gene at a time, and the genes compete with each other for activation by the LCR.[7] The main determinant for activation of a gene is the relative distance from the LCR. In human adult tissues, the switch leading to expression of the further downstream located β and δ genes is achieved by autonomous silencing of the fetal γ genes. The balance between the γ- and β-gene expression is thought to be mediated by changes in the rep-

ertoire and/or abundance of various nuclear factors favoring particular promoter–LCR interactions. A variety of nuclear factors involved in the transcriptional regulation and hemoglobin switching have been suggested, including BCL11A, SOX6, GATA-1, KLF1, NF-E4, COUP-TF, DRED /TR2 /TR4, Ikaros-PYR and BRG1 (SW1/SNF).[8] KLF1 (Krüppel-like factor 1), also known as erythroid Krüppel-like factor (EKLF) is restricted mainly to erythroid cells; it is also a highly promoter-specific activator, binding with high affinity to the β-globin CACCC box.[9] Mutations found in β-globin gene CACCC box abrogate EKLF binding result in reduced β-globin expression and β thalassemia.[10]

BCL11A (B cell lymphoma/leukemia 11A), also known as *Evi9*, CTIP1, is a zinc finger transcriptional factor, essential for normal lymphoid development.[11] Its role in hemoglobin switching was originally implicated in genetic association studies on HbF levels in humans.[12,13] Subsequent collective clinical and functional studies suggest that BCL11A acts as a stage-specific repressor of γ-globin expression.[14,15]

Hemoglobin switching has been the subject of intensive investigation for two main reasons: 1) the globin system provides an excellent model for understanding developmental gene regulation, and 2) understanding how switching is controlled is expected to lead to the development of strategies for the treatment of hemoglobinopathies. Thus, *BCL11A* appears as an attractive target for reactivation of HbF in patients with β thalassemia or sickle cell disease.

Inherited disorders of hemoglobin

The vast majority of disorders affecting hemoglobin are inherited; it is estimated that ~7% of the world's population are carriers for different inherited disorders of hemoglobin, making them the commonest monogenic diseases.[16] The disorders can be divided into two main groups, those in which there is a structural change in a globin chain (hemoglobin variants) and the thalassemias, which result from a quantitative deficiency in one or more of the globin chains of hemoglobin. Hemoglobin variants cause a wide range of clinical problems including sickle cell disease, unstable hemoglobin, decreased oxygen affinity and increased oxygen affinity, but the majority of hemoglobin variants cause no significant change in hemoglobin properties or clinical problems. Some hemoglobin variants are synthesized at a reduced rate, resulting in a phenotype of thalassemia. The most common example is HbE, β26 (Glu→Lys), in which the substitution at β-codon 26 (GAG→AAG) that causes HbE also causes alternative splicing of the β-globin mRNA, leading to a reduction of the normally spliced β message that encodes the variant. Other hemoglobin variants result in a thalassemic phenotype due to its extreme instability leading to a functional deficiency of the globin chain variants; for example, Hb Geneva, a dominantly inherited β thalassemia,[17] and Hb Constant Spring (an α thalassemia variant).[1] Some hemoglobin disorders are acquired; these can also be classified into those characterized by a reduced synthesis of the globin chain (e.g. acquired HbH disease) and those which alter the structure and function of hemoglobin so that oxygen transport is affected (e.g. carboxyhemoglobinemia, methemoglobinemia).[1]

There is another group of β-thalassemia-like disorders referred to as δβ thalassemias and hereditary persistence of fetal hemoglobin (HPFH). These are caused by mutations that alter the switch from fetal to adult hemoglobin, and are distinguishable from β thalassemias by the substantial increases in HbF levels.[1]

Thalassemias

Background

Thalassemia was first recognized by Cooley and Lee in 1925[18] as a form of severe anemia associated with splenomegaly and bone changes in children. The term thalassemia is derived from the Greek φαλασσα (the sea) since many of the early cases came from the Mediterranean region. However, it is now clear that the disorder is not limited to the countries around the Mediterranean but occurs throughout the world, being also prevalent in the tropical and subtropical regions including the Middle East, parts of Africa, the Indian subcontinent and Southeast Asia. It appears that heterozygotes for thalassemia are protected from the severe effects of falciparum malaria and natural selection has increased and maintained their gene frequencies in these malarious regions.

The thalassemias are classified into α, β, δβ, γδβ, δ, γ and εγδβ thalassemias according to the type of globin chain(s) that is reduced. The two major categories are the α and β thalassemias while the rare forms include the δβ, γδβ and εγδβ thalassemias. Hereditary persistence of fetal hemoglobin (HPFH) refers to the group of disorders in which the switch from fetal to adult hemoglobin production is altered and high levels of fetal hemoglobin are synthesized in individuals. Because of their concomitant increase in HbF levels, the δβ and γδβ thalassemias are often considered with the HPFH syndromes. In many populations the α and β thalassemias coexist with a variety of different structural hemoglobin variants. In these populations it is quite common to inherit a combination of α and/or β thalassemia and/or structural hemoglobin variant genes; these complex interactions give rise to an extremely wide spectrum of clinical phenotypes which together constitute the thalassemia syndromes.[10]

Most thalassemias are inherited in a Mendelian recessive fashion. Heterozygotes are normally symptomless, although they can often be recognized by simple hematological analysis. Severely affected individuals have inherited two copies of mutant hemoglobin gene, homozygotes for α or β thalassemia, or compound heterozygotes for different molecular forms of α or β thalassemia and a hemoglobin variant. It has been estimated that about 300 000 individuals severely affected with thalassemia are born each year, posing a heavy burden on the health services.[10] Due to recent population movements, these hemoglobin disorders have become an important part of clinical practice in all countries, including the UK.[19]

β Thalassemias

The β thalassemias pose by far the most important public health problems because they are common and usually produce severe anemia in individuals who have inherited two copies of the β thalassemia gene.

Genetic basis of disease

Molecular analysis of the β thalassemia genes has demonstrated a striking heterogeneity. Although almost 300 β thalassemia alleles (including deletions) have been characterized, population studies indicate that probably only 20 β thalassemia alleles account for >80% of the β thalassemia mutations in the whole world.[1,10] This is because in each of the high-frequency areas, only a few (4–6) mutations are common, reflecting the local selection from malaria, with a varying number of rare ones. Each of these populations has its own unique group of mutations.

Unlike α thalassemia, in which deletions in the α-globin gene cluster account for most of the mutations, the molecular defects causing β thalassemia are usually point mutations involving one (or a limited number of nucleotides) within the β gene or its immediate flanking regions.[1,10,20]

These point mutations involve the critical sequences that interfere with gene function at either the transcriptional or the post-transcriptional level, including translation (Fig. 9.2). Approximately half of these mutations completely inactivate the β gene with no β-globin production causing β° thalassemia. Other mutations allow the production of some β-globin, and are classified as β+ or β++ thalassemia, depending on the degree of quantitative reduction in the output of the β chains. The β-globin chains that are synthesized are usually structurally normal. Mutations affecting the conserved sequences in the 5′ promoter, i.e. TATA box, proximal CACCC and distal CACCC box, typically cause a 70–80% reduction in promoter activity and are often very mild. Mutations affecting the polyadenylation signal (AATAAA) at the 3′ end, also generally result in a mild β+ thalassemia phenotype.

A few β thalassemia mutations are 'silent'; carriers do not have any evident hematological phenotypes with near normal red cell indices and HbA$_2$ levels, the only abnormality being an imbalanced globin chain synthesis. These β thalassemia mutations have usually been ascertained by finding individuals with intermediate forms of β thalassemia resulting from compound heterozygosity for one typical β thalassemia mutation in combination with a very mild β+ thalassemia allele. In this case, one parent has typical β° thalassemia trait and the other, apparently normal. Overall, the 'silent' β° thalassemia alleles are uncommon except for the −101 C→T mutation which has been observed fairly frequently in the Mediterranean region where it interacts with a variety of more severe β thalassemia mutations to produce milder forms of β thalassemia.[21]

The β° thalassemia alleles are mostly caused by premature termination of translation, either by single base substitution to a nonsense codon, or through a frameshift mutation. Studies show that the different in-phase termination mutants exhibit a 'positional' effect and are subjected to a surveillance mechanism (nonsense mediated RNA decay or NMD) to prevent the accumulation of mutant mRNAs coding for truncated peptides.[22,23] Frameshifts and nonsense mutations that result in premature termination early in the sequence (in exon 1 and 2) are associated with minimal amounts of mutant β-mRNA.[24] In such cases, no β chain is produced from the mutant allele, resulting in a phenotype of typical heterozygous β thalassemia in the carrier. However, some mutations that produce in-phase terminations later in the β

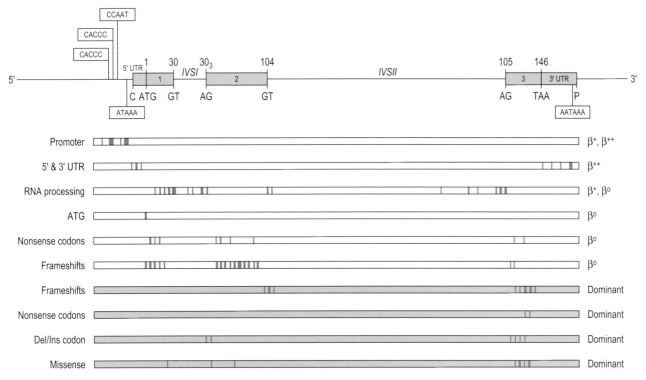

Fig. 9.2 Point mutations causing β thalassemia. The β globin gene is represented by 3 exons (gray) interrupted by 2 introns with the 5′ and 3′ untranslated regions (UTRs, striped boxes). The vertical lines within the open rectangular boxes represent the sites of the different mutations which can be found in the UTRs, exons and introns, and causing typical recessively inherited β thalassemia. Mutations in the hatched rectangular boxes are dominantly inherited. They include mutations that lead to premature termination due to frameshifts or nonsense codons, insertions or deletions of intact codons and amino acid substitutions.

sequence, in exon 3 and the 3′ half of exon 2[25] escape NMD, and are associated with substantial amounts of abnormal β-mRNA from the mutant allele. The mutant β-mRNA leads to a synthesis of abnormal β chain variants that are often highly unstable and non-functional, and are not able to form viable tetramers, thus effectively causing a functional deficiency of β-globin chain.[1] Not only are these abnormal β-globin chain variants non-functional, but they prove to be an additional nuisance as they precipitate in the erythroid precursors, overloading the proteolytic mechanism and accentuating the ineffective erythropoiesis. Carriers for such β thalassemia alleles have fairly severe anemias, hence the term 'dominantly inherited β thalassemia'. For a detailed review of the dominantly inherited β thalassemias, see Thein & Wood 2009[1] and Thein 1999.[26]

β thalassemia is rarely caused by deletions. Of these, only the 619 bp deletion at the 3′ end of the β gene is common, but even that is restricted to the Sind populations of India and Pakistan where it constitutes ~30% of the β thalassemia alleles.[1,27] The other deletions, although extremely rare, are of particular clinical interest because they are associated with an unusually high level of HbA$_2$ in heterozygotes. The mechanism underlying the markedly elevated levels of HbA$_2$ and the variable increases in HbF in heterozygotes for these deletions is postulated to be related to the removal of the 5′ promoter region of the β-globin gene which removes competition for the upstream β-LCR and limiting transcription factors, resulting in an increased interaction of the LCR with the γ and δ genes in *cis*, thus enhancing their expression (Fig. 9.3). This mechanism may also explain the unusually high

HbA$_2$ levels associated with the promoter mutations at positions –88 and –29.

Unusual causes of β thalassemia, although rare, illustrate the numerous molecular mechanisms of down-regulating the β-globin gene.[1] They include transposable elements which may disrupt and inactivate human genes. The insertion of such an element, a retrotransposon of the LI family into intron 2 of the β-globin gene, has been reported to cause β$^+$ thalassemia.[28] Mutations in other genes distinct from the β-globin complex (*trans*-acting mutations) can down-regulate β-globin expression. Such *trans*-acting mutations have been described affecting the XPD protein that is part of the general transcription factor TF11H,[29] and the erythroid-specific GATA-1 protein.[30] Somatic deletions of the β-globin gene have been reported as the contributory cause for the unusually severe anemia in three unrelated families of French and Italian origin[31,32] (see intermediate forms of β thalassemia). Unipaternal isodisomy of chromosome 11p15.5 that encompassed the β-globin gene cluster contributed to thalassemia major in a Chinese patient.[33]

Pathophysiology

The molecular defects in β thalassemias result in absent or reduced β chain production while α chain synthesis proceeds at a normal rate. This imbalance in globin synthesis in β thalassemia gives rise to excess α chains which are extremely unstable and precipitate in the red cell precursors forming inclusion bodies (Fig. 9.4). These inclusions interfere with the red cell maturation and are responsible for the

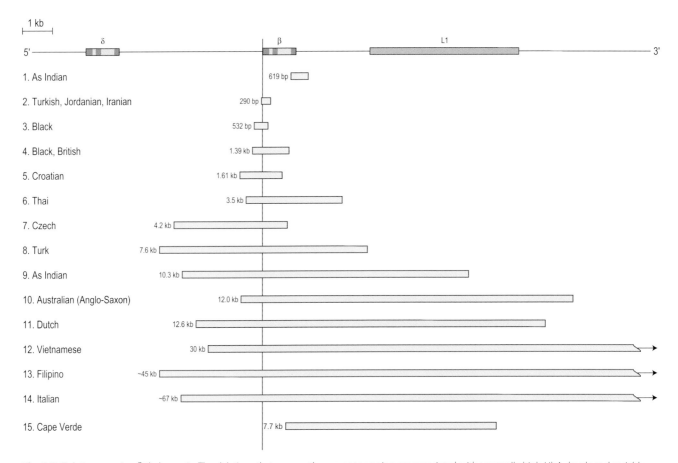

Fig. 9.3 Deletions causing β thalassemia. The deletions that remove the promoter region are associated with unusually high HbA₂ levels and variably increased HbF levels in the heterozygous state.

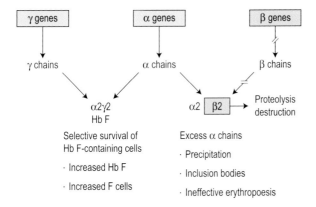

Fig. 9.4 Diagrammatic representation of the pathophysiology of β thalassemia.

intramedullary destruction of the erythroid precursors and hence the ineffective erythropoiesis that characterizes all β thalassemias. The anemia of β thalassemia results from a combination of underproduction of hemoglobin and ineffective erythropoiesis and, ultimately, correlates well with the degree of α- to non α-globin chain imbalance and the amount of free α chains. The complications of splenomegaly, bone disease, endocrine and cardiac damage are related to the severity of anemia and the hypercatabolic state, and the subsequent degree of iron loading resulting from the increased gastrointestinal iron absorption and from repeated blood transfusion.

Genotype-phenotype correlation

Typically, β thalassemia is inherited as haploinsufficient Mendelian recessives. The most severe end of the clinical spectrum, β° thalassemia, is characterized by the complete absence of HbA ($\alpha_2\beta_2$) and results from the inheritance of two β° thalassemia alleles (homozygous or compound heterozygous states). This normally results in the transfusion-dependent state of β thalassemia major and, at worst, the patients present within 6 months of life with profound anemia and, if not treated with regular blood transfusions, die within their first 2 years. Individuals who have inherited a single β thalassemia allele, whether β° or β⁺, have thalassemia trait. They are clinically asymptomatic but may have a mild anemia with characteristic hypochromic microcytic red blood cells, elevated levels of HbA₂ ($\alpha_2\delta_2$) and variable increases of HbF ($\alpha_2\gamma_2$). Inheritance of two β thalassemia alleles, however, does not always lead to thalassemia major; many patients with two β thalassemia alleles have a milder disease, ranging from a condition that is slightly less severe than transfusion-dependence to one that is asymptomatic and often mistaken for thalassemia trait. The diverse collection of phenotypes between the two extremes of thalassemia major and trait constitute the clinical syndrome of thalassemia intermedia.

The heterozygous states for β thalassemia also show a tremendous phenotypic diversity, comparable to that for the inheritance of two β thalassemia alleles. In some cases, the β thalassemia allele is so mild that it is phenotypically

Table 9.1 Thalassemia intermedia: the common genetic interactions that underlie the phenotype of thalassemia intermedia

I	**Homozygous or compound heterozygous state for β thalassemia**
	(a) Inheritance of mild β thalassemia alleles, β 'silent' and β⁺⁺, in homozygous or compound heterozygous states Phenotype depends on the sum total of β-globin output
	(b) Co-inheritance of α thalassemia Phenotype depends on severity of imbalance between α/non-α globin reflecting severity of α and β-globin deficit
	(c) Increased HbF response – β-globin gene promoter mutations (deletional or non-deletional) – Co-inheritance of HbF quantitative trait loci (QTLs) for HbF on 6q (HBS1L-MYB intergenic polymorphisms, BCL11A on 2p, Xmn1-ᴳγ on HBB cluster)
II	**Heterozygous state for β thalassemia**
	(a) Co-inheritance of extra α globin genes (ααα/αα,ααα/ααα,αααα/αα,αααα/αααα, and segmental duplication of whole α-globin gene cluster)
	(b) Dominantly inherited β thalassemia (Hyperunstable β-globin chain variants)
	(c) Somatic deletion of the other β-globin locus – mosaicism
III	**Compound heterozygotes for β thalassemia and β chain variants** e.g. HbE/β thalassemia
IV	**Compound heterozygotes for β thalassemia and HPFH or δβ thalassemia** A considerable variation in clinical phenotype of these genetic interactions has been observed

'silent,' with no anemia or hematological abnormalities. In others, the heterozygous state causes a phenotype almost as severe as the major forms, that is, the β thalassemia allele is dominantly inherited.

Unraveling the molecular basis of the clinical diversity in the intermediate state has provided tremendous insights on genotype-phenotype correlation and clues for the development of molecular therapy for the β thalassemias.

The main genetic interactions that result in a phenotype of thalassemia intermedia are summarized in Table 9.1. Thalassemia intermedia can result from the inheritance of one or two β thalassemia alleles. In 60–90% of the cases[34–36] the patients have inherited two β thalassemia alleles and the reduced disease severity can be explained by the inheritance of the milder forms (β⁺⁺ and 'silent' β thalassemia alleles) that allow the production of a significant proportion of β-globin chains. Co-inheritance of a single α-globin gene deletion (αα/α–) has very little effect on β° thalassemia, but individuals with two α-globin gene deletions (α–/α– or αα/––) and β⁺ thalassemia have a mild disease requiring intermittent transfusions. The role of increased HbF response as an ameliorating factor becomes evident in the group

of thalassemia intermedia patients who are mildly affected despite having minimal amounts or no HbA (α2β2), and without α thalassemia. Three major QTLs – Xmn1-Gγ, HBS1L-MYB on chromosome 6q, and BCL11A on chromosome 2p – recently identified in genome-wide association studies (GWAS) have been shown to impact HbF levels, not only in healthy individuals, but also patients with β thalassemia and sickle cell disease (SCD).[13,37,38] In Sardinia, BCL11A and HBS1L-MYB with α thalassemia accounts for 75% of variable phenotypic severity of β thalassemia,[39] and in Thailand, the three HbF QTLs are associated with both disease severity and HbF levels in HbE/β thalassemia.[40]

Other HbF determinants within the cluster are related to the mutation itself. Small deletions or mutations that involve the promoter sequence of the β-globin gene are associated with variable increases in HbF and unusually high HbA₂ levels, and reflect the competition between the γ and β globin gene promoters for interaction with the upstream β-LCR. Hence, although such deletions cause a complete absence of β-globin product, the severity of the phenotype is offset by the concomitant increase in hemoglobin F.

Inheritance of single copies of β thalassemia gene can also lead to thalassemia intermedia. In the majority of cases this is caused by the co-inheritance of extra α-globin genes, the severity of outcome depends on the total number of α-globin genes inherited (from one or two copies of triplicated (/ααα), or quadruplicated (/αααα) α-globin complexes), and the type of β thalassemia mutation (β° or β⁺).[41,42] More recently, another mechanism of inheriting extra α-globin genes has been described which involved segmental duplication of the whole α-globin gene cluster.[43,44] The additional α-globin genes have no phenotype in normal people but the small excess of α chains in heterozygous β thalassemia appears to tip the balance, crossing the critical threshold of α-globin excess with phenotypic consequences.

In a number of cases, the unusually severe heterozygous state is associated with a normal α-globin genotype. In such cases, the β thalassemia mutation itself leads to the synthesis of highly unstable, structurally abnormal β-globin chain variants.[17] The hyperunstable β chain variants are rapidly destroyed in the erythroid precursors, giving rise to a functional deficiency of β chains and simulating a phenotype of β thalassemia. The non-functional β chain variants together with the unmatched α-globin chains aggravate the ineffective erythropoiesis causing a disease phenotype even when present in a single copy. Hence, the term 'dominantly inherited β thalassemia'.

Finally, although rare, somatic mosaicisms of the β-globin gene in β thalassemia heterozygotes have been reported causing thalassemia intermedia. The individuals from three different families had moderately severe anemia despite being constitutionally heterozygous for a common β thalassemia mutation; they also had a normal α (αα/αα) genotype.[31,32] Subsequent investigations revealed that these individuals had a somatic deletion including the β-globin complex, on the other chromosome 11p15, in a subpopulation (~80%) of erythroid cells giving rise to a somatic mosaic: about 20% of the erythroid cells were heterozygous with one normal copy of β-globin gene and the rest hemizygous (i.e. without any normal β-globin gene). The sum total of the β-globin product is thus about 80% less than the asymptomatic β thalassemia trait. These unusual cases once again illustrate that the severity of anemia in β thalassemia reflects the quantitative deficiency of β-globin production.

Given the differences in the spectrum of β thalassemia mutations and differences in the frequency of the different α thalassemia variants, the relative importance of these genetic factors would vary accordingly in different population groups. It is also important to note that the genotypic factors are not mutually exclusive.

Tertiary modifiers affect complications of the disease; the severity of osteopenia and osteoporosis, iron loading and jaundice may be affected by polymorphisms of genes involved in the metabolic pathways concerned with these complications.[45] Bone mass is a quantitative trait under strong genetic control involving multiple quantitative trait loci (QTLs) and the QTLs implicated include estrogen receptor gene, vitamin D receptor (*VDR*), collagen type a1 genes and transforming growth factor β1 (*TGFβ1*).[46] The elevations of bilirubin and incidence of gallstones in thalassemia, as in other hemolytic anemias, are influenced by a polymorphic variant (seven (TA) repeats) in the promoter of the uridine diphosphate-glucuronosyltransferase 1A (*UGT1A1*) gene, also referred to as Gilbert's syndrome.[47,48] Iron loading in β thalassemia is also variable and results not just from blood transfusion but also from increased iron absorption. Variants in the *HFE* gene have a modulating effect on iron absorption,[49] and as other genes in iron homeostasis become uncovered, it is likely that there will be genetic variants in these loci that influence the different degrees of iron loading in β thalassemia.[50] For instance, recent genome wide association studies have identified variants in *HFE*, and the *TMPRSS6* (transmembrane protease serine 6 gene that regulates hepcidin expression) associated with iron status, erythrocyte volume and concentration.[51–53]

Diagnosis

In β thalassemia major, untransfused hemoglobin levels are usually less than 5 g/dl but can be as low as 2–3 g/dl. Mean corpuscular volume (MCV) and mean corpuscular hemoglobin (MCH) are low, with a very wide red cell distribution width (RDW), marked anisopoikilocytosis, target cell formation, and basophilic stippling. Poorly hemoglobinized nucleated red cells are frequently found in the peripheral blood, and may reach very high levels after splenectomy. The reticulocyte count is elevated but less than expected for the degree of anemia in keeping with the ineffective erythropoiesis. A bone marrow aspirate is not essential to make the diagnosis, but if performed shows marked erythroid hyperplasia characterized by poorly hemoglobinized normoblasts and dyserythropoiesis. Supravital staining (e.g. methyl violet) shows ragged inclusions in many of the erythroid precursor cells; similar inclusions are found in the peripheral red blood cells after splenectomy. Immunoelectron microscopy confirms that these inclusions consist of precipitated α-globin chains (Figs 9.5 and 9.6). Increased iron deposition is also seen in the bone marrow; the majority of the iron granules are randomly distributed. Biochemical evidence of hemolysis such as elevated bilirubin, aspartate transaminase (AST) and lactate dehydrogenase (LDH) with a normal alanine transaminase (ALT) and progressive iron loading is observed. Other biochemical changes may include evidence

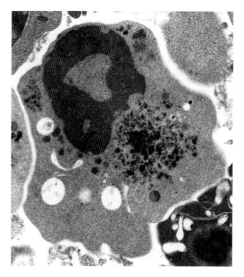

Fig. 9.5 Electron micrograph of a late erythroblast from a homozygote for β thalassemia. The cytoplasm contains multiple small rounded masses of electron-dense material, some of which have fused together to form larger masses. The masses probably consist of precipitated α chains. Uranyl acetate and lead citrate. ×11 625. *(Courtesy of Professor SN Wickramasinghe).*

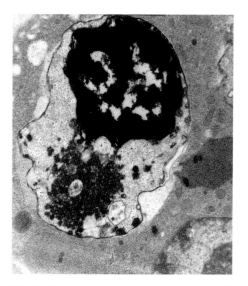

Fig. 9.6 Bone marrow macrophage from a case of homozygous β thalassemia. The macrophage contains a phagocytosed late erythroblast within which intracytoplasmic α chain precipitates can be recognized. Uranyl acetate and lead citrate. ×11 150. *(Courtesy of Professor SN Wickramasinghe).*

of diabetes and endocrine dysfunction such as parathyroid or thyroid insufficiency.

Hemoglobin analysis is needed to confirm the diagnosis, typically using electrophoretic or chromatographic techniques. The findings on Hb electrophoresis vary with the β thalassemia genotype and are informative only in the previously untransfused patient. Absence of HbA in pretransfused samples confirms a diagnosis of β° thalassemia, and the hemoglobin consists of F and A₂ only. In β⁺ thalassemia (homozygous or compound heterozygotes), a variable amount of HbA is present. The HbF is usually elevated and varies from 10 to almost 100% of the total hemoglobin in the case of β° thalassemia. The HbA₂ level is of no diagnostic value. *In vitro* globin chain biosynthesis of peripheral blood reticulocytes or bone marrow shows globin chain imbalance with a marked excess of α over β and γ chain production. Obviously, in β° thalassemia there is a complete absence of β-globin chain synthesis.

The heterozygous state for β thalassemia (β° or β+) is remarkably uniform hematologically. Anemia, if present, is mild and the diagnosis is based on a low mean corpuscular volume (MCV) and mean cell hemoglobin (MCH) accompanied by an increased proportion of HbA_2, from 3.5 to 5.5%, with the exception of a subgroup that has a normal level of HbA_2. Globin chain biosynthesis shows α chains in excess of about twofold. The hematological and hemoglobin electrophoresis profiles are usually sufficient to make a diagnosis of β thalassemia, although DNA analysis, where available, is often used to confirm the diagnosis.

Normal HbA_2 heterozygous β thalassemia may be difficult to distinguish hematologically from heterozygous α thalassemia since both cases have low MCVs and low MCHs, and normal HbA_2 levels. The distinction is made by globin chain biosynthesis (where available) and DNA analysis; family studies are useful. Type 1 normal HbA_2 β thalassemia, otherwise known as 'silent' β thalassemia, has almost normal red cell indices; it results from very mild mutations which cause only a minimal deficit in β chain production. The other group of normal HbA_2 β thalassemia (type 2) results from the co-inheritance of δ thalassemia in *cis* or in *trans* to the β thalassemia gene; in the latter, family studies show independent segregation of the thalassemia indices and normal HbA_2 levels.

Clinical features and management

The clinical phenotypes of β thalassemia range from very severe (major) to a completely silent carrier state, with a huge range of intermediate phenotypes (thalassemia intermedia) between the two ends of the spectrum.[10]

Thalassemia major. In many developed countries, infants affected with severe forms of β thalassemia will be first identified by neonatal screening programs, before the development of any symptoms; antenatal screening of the parents and possibly prenatal diagnosis may have identified the infant to be at risk of severe β thalassemia before birth. The severely affected child is likely to require regular red blood cell transfusions. To meet the aims of correcting the anemia and suppressing the abnormal endogenous erythroid hyperplasia, the trough hemoglobin levels need to be above 9.5 g/dl. In practice, this means maintaining pretransfusion hemoglobin of 9–10 g/dl.

Inadequately transfused children develop the typical features of Cooley's anemia. They show marked retardation of growth and development with progressive hepatosplenomegaly. A typical 'thalassemic' facies develops with frontal bossing, prominent cheek bones and protruding upper jaw due to erythroid hyperplasia in the skull and facial bones. Radiography of the skull shows the typical 'hair-on-end' appearance. The long bones and phalanges become rarefied from marrow expansion and show a lacy, trabecular pattern on radiography. These changes may be associated with repeated pathological fractures. Occasionally the expanding marrow extends from the rib or vertebrae and forms large paraspinal extramedullary masses. The massive marrow expansion causes a hypermetabolic state accompanied by intermittent fevers and weight loss. Gallstones and leg ulcers are common complications. Without any transfusion, death occurs within the first 2 years. 'Palliative' transfusion allows the child to live somewhat longer but the bony deformities remain unchanged and the child ultimately succumbs to an overwhelming infection. If these children survive to puberty, they develop complications of iron overload. Iron accumulation results from an increased rate of gastrointestinal absorption as well as that derived from the blood transfusions.

Adequately transfused children grow and develop normally until early puberty. Iron overload inevitably complicates regular blood transfusions, and progress of their disease then depends on whether they have received regular iron chelation. If not, they begin to show signs of progressive hepatic, cardiac and endocrine disturbances including diabetes, hypoparathyroidism and delayed or absent secondary sexual development. The endocrinopathies and cardiac disease are ascribed to the labile, more toxic forms of iron that appear in cells and plasma, referred to as non-transferrin bound iron (NTBI). Throughout their teenage life these children suffer from a variety of complications due to different endocrine deficiencies. Unless iron overload is controlled by regular chelation therapy, death results in the second or third decade, from acute or intractable congestive cardiac failure. Children who are adequately transfused and fully compliant with iron chelation therapy grow and develop normally, with few or no skeletal abnormalities, and achieve sexual maturity. Even within this group there is a high frequency of growth retardation and retarded sexual maturity, with variable complications relating to iron metabolism, bone disease, endocrine abnormalities and liver disease.[54]

Iron chelation is usually started after 1 year of monthly blood transfusions.[55,56] Currently, three iron chelating agents are available for use: desferrioxamine (DFO), deferiprone and deferasirox. DFO has been in use since the 1970s and is known to be safe and effective; side-effects seem to occur when the drug is used in high doses or when iron stores are low. The main problem with DFO is that it has to be given parenterally, and due to its short half-life, the regimen involves continuous subcutaneous infusions given over 8 hours using a syringe driver or balloon pump. Deferiprone was the first oral iron chelator to be used; it was licensed in Europe in 1999. Arthropathy and agranulocytosis (which can be fatal) are potential serious side-effects, and patients taking deferiprone are recommended to have weekly blood counts. Deferiprone seems to be particularly effective in removing cardiac iron, a therapeutic effect ascribed to its low molecular weight. Deferiprone is increasingly used in combination with DFO.[57] Deferasirox is a once-daily oral iron chelator, approved in the USA and Europe since the mid-2000s.[58] Large clinical trials have demonstrated its efficacy in removing liver iron in thalassemia, with increasing evidence that it also removes cardiac iron. All patients on regular blood transfusion and iron chelation therapy should be monitored regularly with a yearly review for assessment of growth, including tests for endocrine and cardiac function, iron loading (serum ferritin, MRI for liver iron concentration) and adverse effects related to therapy.[56]

Bone marrow transplantation (BMT) is considered the treatment of choice if there is a HLA-identical sibling. BMT should be considered only if it is clear that the child is transfusion-dependent and should be considered early as the success of BMT is reduced as the child gets older, with increasing iron overload and iron-related organ damage.[59]

Thalassemia intermedia. Thalassemia intermedia (TI) includes patients with a wide range of clinical phenotypes. To a large extent, whether a patient is classified as thalassemia intermedia or major depends on a doctor deciding if the patients would benefit from regular blood transfusions; this decision is based not only on clinical factors (such as failure to grow and frequent infections) but also on non-clinical factors such as experience of the doctor, availability of blood and wishes of the patient.

The clinical sequelae of TI results from the ineffective erythropoiesis, chronic anemia and iron overload. The severity may change with increasing age due to iron loading from increased intestinal absorption and decreased tolerance of anemia due to reducing cardiovascular fitness. A wide range of other problems is particularly associated with TI, including pulmonary hypertension, hypercoagulability, pseudoxanthoma elasticum and other connective tissue disorders, hypersplenism, leg ulceration, folate deficiency, extramedullary hemopoietic tumor masses in the chest and skull, gallstones and a marked proneness to infection. There are currently no clear guidelines for managing patients with TI. Because of the extreme variability of these disorders, management is highly dependent on the course that is likely to evolve in an individual patient; all patients should be followed from early childhood and carefully monitored in terms of growth and iron loading.

Intermittent blood transfusions in TI are often necessary due to falls in hemoglobin caused by fever, infection and specifically human parvovirus B19 infection. It can be difficult to decide who would benefit from a short period of regular blood transfusions and when to start them. In countries with a ready supply of safe blood there is an increasing tendency to start regular transfusions, even in children maintaining hemoglobins greater than 8 g/dl, to avoid the emerging complications of skeletal deformities, pulmonary hypertension and osteopenia. There is also some evidence that this improves the quality of life, particularly with emerging options for oral iron chelation. This is not possible in much of the world and management consists of reserving transfusion for severe symptomatic anemia. The initiation of iron chelation depends on the degree of iron overload (as indicated by liver iron concentration), but as with other aspects of the management of TI, there are no clear guidelines.[60]

Pharmacological treatment to increase HbF and total hemoglobin levels is potentially applicable to TI, in that relatively small increases in hemoglobin levels with a corresponding reduction in ineffective erythropoiesis could help a patient thrive who would otherwise require regular transfusions.[1] Hydroxyurea is the most widely used drug in this context, with encouraging results in some patients. Butyrate and other short-chain fatty acid derivatives also promote HbF synthesis, and have been used with limited clinical success in TI. A number of newer drugs are being developed which may boost HbF to a greater extent, most notably the new generation of short-chain fatty acid derivatives (SCFADs) and immunomodulatory drugs such as pomalidomide and lenalidomide.

Thalassemia minor. Individuals with β thalassemia minor (i.e. carriers) are typically asymptomatic. Splenomegaly is rare.

Disease Prevention. The thalassemias are a major health problem in many populations. Apart from bone marrow transplantation, there is no definitive treatment; hence major efforts are concentrated on prevention of the disease.

Preventive programs in most countries now combine education, pre-conceptual, antenatal and neonatal screening, heterozygote detection and genetic counseling for a comprehensive approach in the public health management of the disease.[61] Many screening programs are centered at antenatal clinics and concentrate on identifying women who are thalassemia carriers in the first trimester of pregnancy. This is done by varying combinations of blood tests and identifying women at high risk of carrying thalassemia based on their ethnic origin; this latter approach is particularly effective in areas with a low prevalence of thalassemia in the native population, such as northern Europe. If a woman is found to be a carrier, screening is then offered to her partner, and if both are carriers, they are counseled about the risk of the fetus inheriting a severe form of thalassemia and offered prenatal diagnosis, usually from 11–12 weeks' gestation by chorionic villus sampling or amniocentesis. Parents can then make an informed choice to terminate the pregnancy if the fetus is affected. However, chorionic villus sampling and amniocentesis are invasive with an increased risk of miscarriage of about 1%. This has led to research to develop non-invasive methods of prenatal diagnosis based on maternal blood sampling. Maternal blood contains small numbers of fetal cells and also cell-free fetal DNA, both of which could potentially be used to diagnose fetal thalassemia.

Some couples at risk of having an affected child find prenatal diagnosis and selective termination unacceptable. Pre-implantation genetic diagnosis (PGD) involves the use of *in vitro* fertilization techniques to generate 5–15 embryos; at the eight-cell stage, one embryonic cell can be removed and tested for thalassemia alleles; it is then possible to implant only embryos without thalassemia.[62] PGD, however, is currently a difficult, stressful and expensive procedure, with only 10–20% of couples taking home a baby.

Newborn screening detects the majority of babies with severe thalassemia, either using cord blood or, more commonly, from the neonatal blood spot; this is taken onto a piece of blotting paper and also screened for other conditions such as phenylketonuria. If hemoglobin analysis shows only HbF, with no HbA or other hemoglobin variants, it is likely that the baby has inherited a severe form of β thalassemia and may be transfusion-dependent; less severe possibilities include thalassemia intermedia and homozygosity for hereditary persistence of fetal hemoglobin. Babies identified in this way can then be followed up closely rather than waiting until they present following a period of prolonged illness. Parents can also be tested and given advice concerning the risk to future pregnancies.

β Thalassemia in association with other hemoglobin variants

In many populations, due to the high incidence of both β thalassemia and various hemoglobin variants, it is not uncommon for an individual to inherit a β thalassemia allele from one parent and a gene for a hemoglobin variant from the other. Three common interactions of this type include HbE/β thalassemia, HbS/β thalassemia and HbC/β thalassemia.

HbE/β thalassemia

This is the commonest severe form of thalassemia in Southeast Asia and parts of the Indian subcontinent. Recent demographic changes, however, have resulted in HbE/β thalassemia becoming a health problem in other parts of the world, such as North America.[63]

The β^E allele is mildly thalassemic as the mutation at β codon 26 (GAC→AAG, Glu→Lys) that gives rise to HbE, also activates a cryptic splice site, and when inherited together with β° thalassemia, results in a marked deficiency of β chain production. The clinical and hematological changes of HbE /β thalassemia are variable, ranging from severe anemia and transfusion dependency to thalassemia intermedia.[10,63] There is nearly always anemia (hemoglobin values range from 4–9 g/dl) and splenomegaly.

While a large part of this phenotypic variability can be explained by the severity of the β thalassemia alleles, this cannot be the only answer since an equally broad range of clinical phenotypes has been encountered in HbE/β° thalassemic individuals who all carry null β thalassemia mutations.[1,64] It can be difficult to differentiate homozygous HbE (HbE/E) from HbE/β° thalassemia on Hb electrophoresis alone since only HbE and F are observed in both cases. Genetic studies would be definitive since both parents would be HbE carriers in HbE/E, but HbE trait in one parent and β thalassemia trait in the other, in HbE/β thalassemia. Clinically, homozygotes for HbE have mild anemia and are asymptomatic, while HbE/β° thalassemia can result in transfusion-dependent thalassemia major. Variable quantities of HbA are found in HbE/β+ thalassemia cases, and the condition is milder than HbE/β° thalassemia.

HbS/β thalassemia

(See other sickling disorders.)

HbC/β thalassemia

This is restricted to West Africans, some North Africans and southern Mediterranean populations.[1] HbC/β thalassemia is largely asymptomatic and characterized by a mild hemolytic anemia and splenomegaly. A blood smear shows numerous target cells and polychromasia due to the mildly elevated reticulocyte count. Hemoglobin electrophoresis shows a preponderance of HbC and variable quantities of HbA depending on whether it is a β+ or β° thalassemia allele. The diagnosis is confirmed by demonstrating HbC trait in one parent and β thalassemia in the other.

The δβ-, γδβ-thalassemias and HPFH syndromes

This group of β-like thalassemia disorders is characterized by a reduced or absent synthesis of β- and δ-globin chains and a variable compensatory increase in γ chain production.[65] They are much less common than β thalassemia. The distinction between δβ thalassemias and the HPFH syndromes is subtle and originally made on what appeared to be clear-cut

clinical and hematological grounds. However, with the elucidation of the molecular basis of these conditions, it became increasingly clear that this broad classification is rather arbitrary, and that there is considerable overlap in many of the parameters that were initially used to differentiate them. It also became clear that the subtle difference between the two subgroups relates to the relatively higher compensatory increase in HbF levels in HPFH compared to the δβ thalassemias.

Heterozygotes for δβ thalassemia have a red cell picture similar to β thalassemia, with hypochromic microcytic red cells, but normal levels of HbA_2 (<3.0%). In addition, however, there is an increased level of HbF (5–15%) that was unevenly distributed (heterocellular) among the erythrocytes. Homozygotes for δβ thalassemia or compound heterozygotes with β thalassemias are not common but have been reported to have clinical phenotypes ranging from mild anemia to thalassemia major.[66] In contrast, HPFH heterozygotes have essentially normal red cell indices, normal levels of HbA_2 and higher levels of HbF (15–30%) with a homogeneous pancellular distribution of the HbF. HPFH homozygotes are clinically normal, their hemoglobin levels may be increased with mildly hyochromic microcytic red cells. Individuals with HPFH/β thalassemia may have a mild anemia but are clinically asymptomatic.

These conditions are remarkably heterogeneous genotypically; at the molecular level they can be classified into two groups:

1. Those due to varying deletions of the β-globin cluster removing the β and δ, or the β, δ and $^A\gamma$ genes producing an increase of both $^G\gamma$ and $^A\gamma$ chains [$^G\gamma^A\gamma$ (δβ)° thalassemia or HPFH] or only $^G\gamma$ chain [$^G\gamma$ ($^A\gamma$ δβ)° thalassemia], respectively.
2. Non-deletional type in which there is an increase of only the $^G\gamma$- or $^A\gamma$-globin chains and usually due to point mutations (single base substitutions or minor deletions) in the respective γ-globin promoters.

The non-deletion mutations are clustered in regions of the promoters that contain binding sites for ubiquitous and erythroid-specific transcription factors. Altered binding of the transcription factors due to the point mutations is thought to be the cause of the elevated HbF levels that range from 5–35% in heterozygotes.

A non-deletion form of δβ thalassemia due to a point mutation inactivating the β gene in *cis* with a point mutation in the γ gene promoter up-regulating HbF production has also been described.[67] δβ Thalassemia and HPFH are clearly defined by a significant increase in HbF levels in carriers; the molecular defects are inherited in a Mendelian fashion as alleles of the β-globin complex.

About 10–15% of the healthy adult population have modest increases of HbF (1–5%) in which the inheritance patterns are less clear-cut and traditionally referred to as heterocellular HPFH because the HbF is unevenly distributed among the erythrocytes. Heterocellular HPFH was previously known as Swiss-type HPFH, after the original report in which some members of a group of Swiss soldiers were found to have slight increases in HbF levels.[68,69] It is now clear that heterocellular HPFH represents the high values of HbF and F cells at the upper tail of the common HbF trait distribution.

Although of no consequence to healthy adults, when co-inherited with β thalassemia or sickle cell disease (SCD), heterocellular HPFH leads to increases in HbF that have a major ameliorating effect on the severity of disease.[34,70] Heterocellular HPFH is inherited as a complex trait; multiple genes contribute to the increase in HbF levels. Recent genome wide association studies (GWAS) have mapped three major quantitative trait loci (QTLs) – *Xmn1-HBG2*, *HBS1L-MYB* intergenic region (*HMIP*) on chromosome 6q and *BCL11A* on chromosome 2p – that account for 50% of the F cell variance in healthy Europeans.[12,13,71] These loci have been shown to impact HbF levels and disease severity in patients from diverse ethnic groups with SCD and β thalassemia.[37–40,72,73]

εγδβ Thalassemia

These are rare conditions.[10] Affected newborns may present with severe hemolysis and anemia, which is self-limited. In some cases, blood transfusions are necessary during the neonatal period. It is recognized in adults by the hematological phenotypes of β thalassemia trait with normal levels of HbA$_2$ and HbF. Only heterozygotes have been identified; presumably the homozygous state would not survive early gestation. The molecular defects result from large deletions of the β-globin gene cluster which involve the β-LCR.[65,74–76] The deletions fall into two categories: group I removes all, or a greater part of the complex including the β-globin gene and the β-LCR; group II removes extensive remote upstream regions including the β-LCR but leaving the β-globin gene itself intact, despite which, its expression is silenced because of the absence of the upstream β-LCR. There is no output from the globin genes of the affected cluster. The associated phenotypes of the two groups of deletions are similar.

α Thalassemias

α thalassemia can be regarded as α$^+$ or α$^\circ$, reflecting either a reduction or complete absence of α-globin synthesis from the affected chromosome.[1,77] The geographical distribution of α thalassemia is very similar to that of β thalassemia; in some parts of the tropical and subtropical regions where it is prevalent, carrier frequency for the mild form (α$^+$) reaches 90%. The more severe defect, α$^\circ$ thalassemia, is prevalent in the Mediterranean region and southeast Asia where carrier frequency can reach 10%. Although the α thalassemias are more common than β thalassemias, they pose less of a public health problem since the severe homozygous states cause death *in utero* and the milder forms that survive into adulthood do not cause a major disability.

Genetic basis of disease

Normal individuals have four α-globin genes arranged as linked pairs, α$_2$ and α$_1$, at the tip of each chromosome 16, the normal α genotype being written as αα/αα.[1] α Thalassemia most commonly results from deletion of one (−α/) or both (−−/) α genes of the linked pair from chromosome 16, causing a reduction (α$^+$) or absence (α$^\circ$) of α-globin from the affected chromosome, respectively. The homozygous and heterozygous states for α$^\circ$ thalassemia are represented as −−/−− and αα/−−, respectively; while those for α$^+$ thalassemia are −α/−α and αα/−α, respectively. As for the β-like

genes, full expression of the α-like globin genes is critically dependent on the presence of the major upstream regulatory element (MCS-R2 or HS-40) which lies 40 kb upstream of the cluster. Although more than 50 deletions removing one (−α/) or both (−−/) genes have been characterized, the majority of α thalassemia is caused by six deletions (/−α$^{3.7}$, /−α$^{4.2}$, /−−^{SEA}, /−−^{MED},/ − (α)$^{20.5}$, and /−−^{FIL}).[1]

The common α$^\circ$ thalassemias are caused by complete or partial deletion of both the structural α-globin genes. These deletions vary in size and are geographically isolated, with two particularly common ones, one in southeast Asia (/−−^{SEA}) and the other in the Mediterranean region (/−−^{MED}). Rarely, α$^\circ$ thalassemias arise from deletions of the upstream α-globin regulatory elements (MCS-R) with the downstream α-globin genes intact but completely inactivated. These deletions are highly variable in size (up to 150 kb have been reported); the smallest of these remove MCS-R1 (HS-48) and MCS-R2 (HS-40), demonstrating the importance of these elements in expression of the α-globin genes.[78]

The molecular basis of α$^+$ thalassemia is more complicated; the commonest forms result from deletion of one of the linked pairs of globin genes (/−α$^{3.7}$or /−α$^{4.2}$).[1] Less commonly, both the α-globin genes are intact, and α$^+$ thalassemia results from point mutations (T) that inactivate one of the pair. These point mutations involve the critical sequences that control the various stages of gene expression as encountered in the β thalassemias. To date, 69 causes of non-deletion α thalassemia have been described; 46 of these occur in the dominant α$_2$ gene (/α^{T}α), 17 in the α$_1$ gene (/αα^T), and the others on a /−α chromosome (/−α^T). In general, the non-deletional α thalassemia determinants have a more severe effect on α-globin output and hematological phenotype than simple deletions that remove one or the other α-globin gene. This may be explained by the majority of mutations affecting the dominant α$_2$ gene, where expression predominates over the α$_1$ gene. Another explanation is that, unlike deletional α thalassemia, there appears to be no compensatory increase in expression of the linked functional α gene when the other is inactivated by a point mutation.

A common non-deletion α thalassemia variant in Southeast Asia is Hb Constant Spring (HbCS, /α^{CS}α) which is due to a single base substitution (TAA→CAA) in the α$_2$ globin termination codon. This results in readthrough of the 3′ untranslated sequence until another in-phase termination codon is encountered 31 codons later producing an elongated α chain variant of 172 residues, 31 amino acids from the natural Arginine at codon 141. Three other variants (Hb Icaria, HbSeal Rock and Hb Koya Dora) involving different base substitutions in the α$_2$ termination codon have been identified. Non-deletional α thalassemia can also arise from single base substitutions causing structural α-globin variants that are highly unstable, for example, Hb Quong Sze α125 Leu→Pro (/α^{QS}α).

Pathophysiology

There is a fundamental difference in the pathophysiology of the α and β thalassemias (Fig. 9.7). Because γ$_4$ and β$_4$ tetramers are soluble, they do not precipitate to a significant degree in the bone marrow, i.e. erythropoiesis is more effective than in β thalassemia. However, these β$_4$ tetramers do precipitate

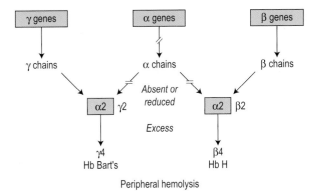

Fig. 9.7 Diagrammatic representation of the pathophysiology of α thalassemia

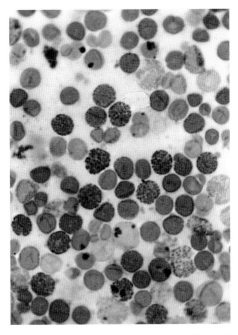

Fig. 9.8 Golfball-like appearance of many of the red cells of a case of HbH disease after supravital staining with brilliant cresyl blue. ×1000. *(Courtesy of Professor SN Wickramasinghe).*

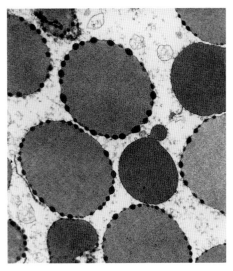

Fig. 9.9 Ultrastructure of red cells from a case of HbH disease after incubation with brilliant cresyl blue for 1 h. The HbH-containing cells show membrane-bound, redox-dye-induced masses of denatured HbH. Uranyl acetate and lead citrate. ×6650. *(Courtesy of Professor SN Wickramasinghe).*

as the red cells age, forming inclusion bodies in the mature erythrocytes, resulting in peripheral hemolysis due to the red cell membrane damage and obstruction in the spleen (Figs 9.7 and 9.8). The degree of anemia and the amount of the tetramers (HbH and Bart's) produced reflects the severity of the reduction in the output of the α-globin chain.

Genotype-phenotype correlation

Loss of one functioning α gene (αα/–α) is almost completely silent with normal or only slightly hypochromic red cells. Loss of two α genes (−−/αα or −α/−α) produces a mild hypochromic microcytic anemia, the α thalassemia trait. Homozygotes for α° thalassemia (−−/−−) have a lethal condition with intrauterine hemolytic anemia called the Hb Bart's hydrops fetalis syndrome. Deficiency of α chains gives rise to an excess of γ chains (in fetal life) or β chains (in adult life) which form γ_4-tetramers (Hb Bart's) and β_4-tetramers

(HbH), respectively. The presence of Hb Bart's or HbH is thus diagnostic of α thalassemia.

HbH disease lies between the two ends of the clinical spectrum, the asymptomatic α thalassemia trait and Hb Bart's hydrops fetalis. As in β thalassemia intermedia, HbH disease spans a wide range of clinical and hematological phenotypes,[79,80] the diagnostic feature being the presence of HbH inclusions in the peripheral red blood cells (Figs 9.8 and 9.9). The most severe forms can be lethal late in gestation or in the perinatal period (HbH hydrops fetalis).[1] The molecular basis of this order is equally heterogeneous, varying with the geographic distribution of the different α thalassemia variants.[79,80] HbH disease most commonly results from the interaction of α° and deletional α+ thalassemia (−−/−α). Less often it can result from the interaction of α° thalassemia with non-deletional forms of α thalassemia (−−/αᵀα) or from homozygous non-deletional α thalassemia (αᵀα/αᵀα). A less severe form of HbH disease in southeast Asia commonly arises from homozygosity or compound heterozygosity for Hb Constant Spring (αᶜˢα/αᶜˢα) or (αᶜˢα/−−). Very low levels of this elongated α-globin chain (5–8% of the total hemoglobin in homozygotes) are found; the defective αᶜˢ chain production is a consequence of the instability of the αᶜˢ mRNA.[81]

Diagnosis

Diagnosis is based on the hemoglobin level, red cell indices, examination of the peripheral blood smear and hemoglobin analysis.

Bart's hydrops fetalis

Infants with Hb Bart's hydrops are severely anemic with hemoglobin levels of 6–8 g/dl. The blood film shows severe thalassemic changes with numerous hypochromic nucleated red cells. There is no HbA or F, the hemoglobin consists mainly of Hb Bart's (γ_4 tetramers) with small amounts of embryonic hemoglobin and HbH (β_4 tetramers). Biosynthetic studies confirm the complete absence of α chains.

HbH disease

Patients with HbH disease run an hemoglobin level of 7–10 g/dl with moderate reticulocytosis. Again, typical thalassemic changes are seen in the blood film. On incubation of the red cells with brilliant cresyl blue, numerous inclusion bodies are generated by precipitation of the HbH which are tetramers of β chain (β_4), forming typical 'golf balls' (Fig. 9.8). Hemoglobin analysis shows 5–40% HbH, with the major component being HbA and a normal or reduced level of HbA$_2$. Sometimes, there is also a small amount of Hb Bart's.

Carriers

Carriers for α thalassemia may be slightly anemic with hypochromic microcytic red cells or 'silent' with minimal hematologic changes. The Hb electrophoretic pattern is normal and globin biosynthetic studies show a deficit of α chain production.

Diagnosis of α thalassemia is confirmed by DNA analysis which commonly reveals deletions of the α gene cluster, removing one or both α genes. Less commonly, the genes are present and α thalassemia is caused by point changes within the α_2 gene or its immediate flanking regions.

Clinical features

The clinical disorders resulting from α thalassemia range from death in utero (Hb Bart's hydrops syndrome) to a completely silent carrier state.[1] Hemoglobin Bart's hydrops, caused by homozygosity for $\alpha°$ thalassemia, occurs only in populations where $\alpha°$ thalassemia is common, notably in the Mediterranean and in Southeast Asia. Affected infants are usually stillborn with gross pallor, generalized edema and massive hepatosplenomegaly. The placenta is enlarged and friable and frequently causes obstetric difficulties. All these findings are caused by severe intrauterine anemia. There is no production of α chain, and hence neither fetal nor adult hemoglobin. The hemoglobin consists of approximately 80% Hb Bart's (γ_4 tetramers) and 20% Hb Portland ($\zeta_2\gamma_2$). Presumably affected infants survive to term because they continue to produce embryonic hemoglobin. Apart from fetal death, there is a high incidence of toxemia of pregnancy and obstetric complications due to the large placenta.

The intermediate form of α thalassemia is HbH disease, commonly seen in the Mediterranean, Middle East and Southeast Asia. As in β thalassemia intermedia, HbH disease spans a broad spectrum of hematological and clinical severity. Generally, these individuals have a moderately severe anemia and splenomegaly but are usually transfusion independent except during episodes of hemolysis associated with infection, or worsening of the anemia due to progressive hypersplenism. The skeletal deformities and growth retardation characteristic of β thalassemia are not unusually seen. Hemoglobin values range from 7–10 g/dl and the peripheral blood film shows typical thalassemia changes with hypochromia, polychromasia and anisopoikilocytosis; reticulocyte count is normally increased (3–6%). Rarely, the very severe forms of HbH disease can present with hydrops fetalis.

α Thalassemia trait is clinically asymptomatic; the hematological phenotype depends on the number of existing functional α-globin genes. Carriers for $\alpha°$ thalassemia may have very mild hypochromic anemia with red cell indices similar to those of the β thalassemia trait; the MCH is less than 25 pg and the HbA$_2$ level is normal. Occasional HbH bodies (β_4 tetramers) may be present in the red cell on supravital staining. Deletional α^+ thalassemia carriers have near-normal hematological findings. The heterozygous states for the non-deletion forms of α^+ thalassemia are sometimes associated with very mild hypochromic anemia; Hb Constant Spring can be identified by the presence of trace amounts of the variant on hemoglobin electrophoresis at an alkaline pH.

$\alpha°$ Thalassemia carriers can be identified with more certainty in the neonatal period, when they have 5–10% Hb Bart's (γ_4 tetramers), which disappears over the first few months of life and is replaced by HbH (β_4 tetramers). Some newborn carriers of α^+ thalassemia have slightly increased levels of Hb Bart's, in the 1–3% range, but its absence does not exclude the diagnosis.

α Thalassemia with mental retardation (ATR) syndromes

These are rare forms of α thalassemias found in association with a variety of developmental abnormalities, in particular with mental retardation, and hence they are often referred to as α thalassemia with mental retardation (ATR) syndromes.[1] One group, ATR-16, results from extensive deletions and rearrangements of 1–2 Mb removing many genes including the α globin genes, from the tip of chromosome 16.[1,82] The other group, ATR-X, describes a syndrome that includes α thalassemia and multiple developmental abnormalities, such as urogenital anomalies and mental retardation due to mutations in the *ATRX* gene, located on the X chromosome (Xq13.1–q21.1).

ATR-16 shows a remarkable variation in severity of α thalassemia, mental retardation and associated developmental abnormalities. The sub-telomeric deletion/rearrangement is *de novo* in all cases, and in many cases, neither parent is a carrier for α thalassemia, and the patient has a phenotype of severe α thalassemia trait ($\alpha\alpha$/——). However, less commonly, one parent may be a carrier for mild α thalassemia ($\alpha\alpha$/-α) that has been transmitted to the child resulting in HbH disease (——/-α) with mental retardation. Analysis of the length and characteristics of the rearrangements suggest that sub-telomeric deletions of up to ~900 kb appear to be associated with a normal phenotype. The region between 900 and 1700 kb from the 16p telomere contains 16 genes and is deleted in all families with the characteristic features of ATR-16. Deletions beyond 2000 kb result in a contiguous gene syndrome characterized by α thalassemia with tuberous sclerosis and polycystic kidney disease.[1] However, the critical genes responsible for the mental retardation and other developmental abnormalities associated with ATR-16 have yet to be identified.

ATR-X, because of its mode of inheritance, affects boys; the mental retardation is much more severe when compared to ATR-16, and although the dysmorphic features are widespread, they have a remarkably characteristic facial appearance. More than 150 families have now been characterized with considerable variation in the hematological phenotypes. In these cases, the α-globin cluster is intact and the underlying mutations reside in the *trans*-acting *ATR-X* gene on the X-chromosome. The *ATR-X* gene is a member of the SNF2 family of chromatin-remodeling proteins involved in a variety of cellular functions including transcription, cell cycle control, and DNA repair. ATR-X is likely to perturb the expression of multiple genes during early development including the α-globin genes. Although detailed genotype/phenotype correlations have elucidated the critical functional domains of the protein, the relationship with α thalassemia is less clear. There is no consistent relationship between the severity of α thalassemia and the predicted severity of the *ATR-X* mutations. Patients with identical *ATR-X* mutations may have very different degrees of α thalassemia suggesting that the effect of ATR-X protein on α globin expression may be modified by other genetic factors.

Acquired α thalassemia

Very rarely, α thalassemia can be acquired in patients with a variety of hematological disorders within the myelodysplastic syndromes (MDS).[1] These individuals are predominantly elderly males of northern European origin. They have a normal complement of α globin genes (αα/αα) and in all cases where data is available, there is no evidence of pre-existing α thalassemia and thus the α thalassemia and abnormal erythropoeisis is presumably acquired as a clonal genetic abnormality of the MDS. The blood films of such patients show dimorphic features with populations of red blood cells containing HbH inclusions. The marked hypochromic microcytic anemia is associated with an almost absent α-globin chain synthesis. Acquired mutations in the *ATR-X* have been found[83] and thought to have been acquired as passenger mutations as part of the pre-leukemic disorder.

Structural hemoglobin variants

More than 1000 structurally different hemoglobin variants have been described (http://globin.cse.psu.edu/globin/hbvar/), but only three, sickle hemoglobin (HbS), HbC and HbE, occur at a high frequency in different populations.[1] Many of the hemoglobin variants are harmless and have been discovered in population surveys using electrophoretic analyses of human hemoglobin. Since only variants which alter the charge of the hemoglobin molecule are detectable in routine electrophoresis, this number is probably an underestimate. Diseases resulting from structural abnormalities of hemoglobin are shown in Table 9.2. In this section only those abnormal hemoglobins of clinical importance are described.

Sickle cell disease

Background

Sickle cell disease (SCD) was first described by James Herrick from Chicago in 1910 in a student from Grenada.[84] Presence of peculiar elongated and sickle-shaped red blood cells in the peripheral blood films suggested the term sickle cell anemia. In 1949 Pauling *et al* demonstrated that this sickling phenomenon was related to an abnormal hemoglobin

Table 9.2 Clinical disorders due to structural hemoglobin variants

1.	Sickle syndromes causing hemolysis and vaso-occlusion: HbSS HbS and interaction of HbS with other Hb variants (Hbs S/C, S/O-Arab and S/D-Punjab) Compound heterozygosity of HbS with β thalassemia HbS/β thalassemia)
2.	Chronic hemolysis – unstable hemoglobin variants (congenital Heinz body anemia, CHBA), e.g. Hb Köln, Hb Bristol
3.	Congenital polycythemia – high oxygen affinity Hb variants
4.	Congenital cyanosis – low oxygen affinity Hb variants M hemoglobins
5.	Hypochromic microcytic anemia (thalassemic hemoglobinopathy), e.g. HbE – β structural variant Hb Constant Spring – α structural variant δβ fusion variants – e.g. Hb Lepore
6.	Drug induced hemolysis, e.g. Hb Zurich

present in all patients with sickle cell anemia.[85] Subsequently, in 1956 Ingram showed that the sickle hemoglobin differed from normal adult hemoglobin (HbA, $\alpha_2\beta_2$) by the single substitution of glutamic acid to valine at position 6 in the β subunit.[86]

The sickling disorders occur predominantly in black African populations but they are also prevalent throughout the Mediterranean, Middle East and parts of India. Carriers for the β^S gene are protected from *Plasmodium falciparum*, thus explaining the high gene frequencies in those malarious regions, although the mechanisms underlying such protection are still not clear. The β^S gene in these diverse population groups is caused by the same molecular defect (β codon 6 GAG to GTG), found on four different β haplotypes in Africa, known as the Senegal, Benin, Central African Republic (or Bantu) and the Cameroon types. In addition, it is associated with a different β haplotype (Arab-India) in Saudi Arabian and Asian Indian sickle patients.[1] The evidence suggests multiple independent origins of the β^S mutation although gene conversion on regionally specific β haplotypes cannot be excluded.

Genetic basis and pathophysiology

Apart from the homozygous state for the β^S gene, the syndrome of sickle cell disease (SCD), can also arise from the compound heterozygous state for HbS and β thalassemias (HbS/β thalassemia) and other structural variants such as HbS C (HbSC disease) and D (HbSD) (Table 9.3).

Fundamental to the pathophysiology of sickle cell disease is the polymerization of the sickle hemoglobin (HbS) which is dependent on several factors – concentration of the HbS itself, oxygen saturation, pH, temperature and other factors such as the 2,3-diphosphoglycerate concentration (2,3-DPG) (Fig. 9.10). Fully oxygenated HbS cannot enter the polymer phase whereas partially oxygenated or deoxygenated HbS can.[87] Mixed hybrids of HbS with non-S hemoglobins, e.g. HbA ($\alpha_2\beta\beta^S$) and HbC ($\alpha_2\beta^C\beta^S$), have a 0.5 probability of entering the polymer phase while those with HbF, i.e. ($\alpha_2\gamma\beta^S$) and HbA$_2$ ($\alpha_2\delta\beta^S$), cannot enter the polymer phase.

Table 9.3 The major sickling disorders

	β Genotype	α Genotype	Hb Electrophoresis
Sickle cell trait	β^A/β^S	αα/αα	HbS ~45%; HbA₂ normal; rest HbA
Sickle cell trait[a]	β^A/β^S	−α/αα −α/−α	HbS ~25–30%; HbA₂ increased (3.2–3.7%)
Sickle cell anemia	β^S/β^S	αα/αα	HbS 80–100%; HbF 0–20%, No HbA
SC disease	β^S/β^C	αα/αα	HbS 50%; HbC 50%
SO-Arab disease[b]	$\beta^S/\beta^{D\text{-}Punjab}$	αα/αα	HbS, HbO Arab
SD-Punjab disease[c]	β^S/β^C		HbS 50%; HbD Punjab 50%
Sβ⁺ thal	β^S/β^{Th}	αα/αα	HbS 50–80%; HbF 0–20%; HbA 1–30%; HbA₂ 3–6%
Sβ thal	β^S/β^{Th}		HbS 75–100%; HbF 0–20%; HbA₂ 3–6%; no HbA
S HPFH	β^S/β^*	αα/αα	HbS 70–80%; HbF 20–30%; HbA₂ decreased; no HbA

[a]Co-inheritance of α thalassemia (−α/−α or αα/−α) with sickle cell trait can be difficult to differentiate from HbS/mild β⁺ thalassemia; both demonstrate hypochromic microcytic red cells and raised A₂ levels.

[b]HbC, HbO-Arab and HbE are not separated on routine alkaline electrophoresis.

[c]Quantitation based on agar gel electrophoresis.

β* Deletion of β-globin cluster.

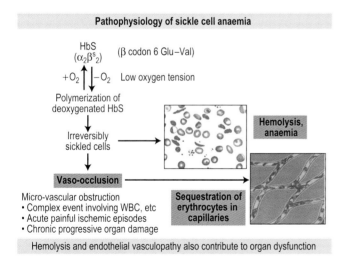

Pathophysiology of sickle cell anaemia

HbS
($\alpha_2\beta^S_2$)   (β codon 6 Glu–Val)

+O₂ ↕ −O₂   Low oxygen tension

Polymerization of deoxygenated HbS

↓

Irreversibly sickled cells → Hemolysis, anaemia

↓

Vaso-occlusion →

Micro-vascular obstruction
• Complex event involving WBC, etc
• Acute painful ischemic episodes
• Chronic progressive organ damage

Sequestration of erythrocytes in capillaries

Hemolysis and endothelial vasculopathy also contribute to organ dysfunction

Fig. 9.10 Pathophysiology of sickle cell anemia.

When a polymer-free solution is deoxygenated, there is a time delay before any polymer is detected. The delay time is exquisitely dependent on the concentration of the deoxy HbS, and also pH and temperature. Delay time shortens as deoxy HbS increases, pH falls and temperature rises. This explains the harmful effects of over-exercise, fever and dehydration. These red blood cells continue to sickle and unsickle, eventually reaching a threshold when sickling becomes irreversible. Although polymerization of HbS is critical, the irreversibly sickled red cells alone are not sufficient for initiating or maintaining the vaso-occlusion that triggers the complications of SCD. Vaso-occlusion is also dependent on factors extrinsic to the cell, such as the state of the vascular endothe-lium, vascular tone (balance of vasoconstrictors and vasodilators) and activation of platelets and white cells involving cytokines and adhesion molecules. The anemia in SCD is primarily hemolytic, a consequence of the shortened survival of the irreversibly sickled red cells which have a half-life of 20 days compared to a normal RBC life span of 120 days. Survival of the red cells is indirectly related to the level of HbF since red cells containing HbF are less likely to sickle.

Despite the identical sickle mutation, SCD has long been appreciated to exhibit extraordinary phenotypic variability which reflects the genetic background of the individual and the co-inheritance of different modifying genes interacting with the different environmental backgrounds.[88] Two case reports and a pilot twin study[89] suggest that environmental factors may be of greater importance in determining clinical expression and complications of SCD. These reports showed that, despite identical β- and α-globin genotypes with similarities in growth, hematological and biochemical parameters, the identical twins had quite different acute pain rate and sickle-related complications.

Nonetheless, genetic factors that influence the primary event of HbS polymerization, such as the causative genotype (HbSS vs. HbSC, HbSβ thalassemia), co-inheritance of α thalassemia and genetic determinants for producing HbF are major predictors of SCD severity. HbF levels are a major predictor of survival and complications in SCD; the risk of early death is inversely associated with HbF levels.[70] The beneficial effect of HbF is twofold: i) HbF inhibits HbS polymerization, and ii) its presence in the red blood cells reduces the concentration of intracellular HbS. The three recently identified HbF loci have also been shown to impact sickle phenotype.[13,37,73] α Thalassemia which is present in about 30% of SCD patients is associated with less hemolysis, higher hematocrit and hemoglobin levels, lower mean corpuscular volume (MCV) of the red blood cells, and lower reticulocyte counts. The resulting increased hematocrit and blood viscosity may increase certain vaso-occlusive complications such as acute painful episodes, acute chest syndrome and avascular necrosis.

At the secondary level, it is likely that genetic variants controlling differences in vascular hemodynamics, endothelial adhesion, red cell membrane proteins and red cell hydration account for much of the individual variability in vaso-occlusive complications and hemolysis. Genetic studies based on candidate genes have associated several genes with some complications of SCD including stroke, leg ulcers, priapism and avascular necrosis.[90] However, candidate genes were selected based on our understanding of the sickle pathophysiology. Genome wide association studies (GWAS) that permit a hypothesis-free and unbiased assessment of all genes should enlighten us on the key pathways and molecular mechanisms underlying the sickle pathophysiology. For such a complex disease, GWAS will require large numbers (thousands) of well characterized patients.

Diagnosis

Diagnosis is established by a combination of several tests for the detection and quantification of HbS plus the other Hbs for the elucidation of the different genetic interactions: hemoglobin electrophoresis on cellulose acetate (pH 8.6) and agar (pH 6.2) and positive sickling or solubility tests.[91] In sickle cell anemia (HbSS), it is usual to see sickled cells, Howell–Jolly bodies and changes typical of hyposplenism. In HbSC disease target cells are prominent and HbC crystals may be present and in HbSβ thalassemia (or HbS with α thalassemia) hypochromic microcytic target cells are present.

Because the gene for HbS (and the structural hemoglobin variants, HbC and HbE) and the thalassemias (both α and β) occur together at high frequency in many populations, it is not uncommon for an individual to inherit genes for both types of condition, posing difficulties in diagnosis. Although these diagnostic difficulties can normally be resolved by family studies, often family members may not be accessible and one has to rely on a careful assessment of the hemoglobin electrophoresis and the red cell indices. In sickle cell trait (Table 9.3) uncomplicated by α or β thalassemia the level of HbS varies between 40% and 45% and is always less than 50%. This is because the β^S chain is positively charged and is less able to compete with the negatively charged β^A chains for the positively charged α-globin subunits.[92,93] Carriers for α thalassemia and HbS have lower HbS levels, varying from ~25% (in −α/−α) to ~35% (in αα/−α). Electrophoretically there may be little difference between HbSS with high levels of HbF and HbS/β° thalassemia but the latter is accompanied by hypochromic microcytic red cells and an elevated HbA_2 level. These features are also present in HbS/β^+ thalassemia, but in this case, there is some HbA and the HbS is, of course, more than 50%. However, increased levels of HbA_2 do not always reflect the co-existence of β thalassemia. In terms of electrostatic attraction for the α globin subunit, the δ globin subunit lies between that of β^A and β^S. Since the δ globin chain has a greater affinity for the

α subunit compared to β^S, co-inheritance of α thalassemia with HbS can mimic HbS/β thalassemia. In both scenarios, the HbS level is lower than expected, the red cells hypochromic microcytic and the level of HbA_2 increased.

Clinical features

Sickle cell trait (carrier status) is a benign condition and generally does not cause any clinical disability. However, under certain extreme conditions, such as severe pneumonia, flying in unpressurized aircraft or rigorous physical exercise with ensuing dehydration, vaso-occlusive episodes can occur.[94,95]

SCD causes a chronic debilitating illness characterized by hemolytic anemia interrupted by episodic acute pain and acute clinical events resulting in end-organ damage and a reduced life span. A main determinant of disease severity is the causal genotype. Individuals homozygous for the β^S gene (HbSS, sometimes referred to as sickle cell anemia) and individuals with HbSβ° thalassemia, whose hemoglobin composition is almost all HbS, tend to have the most severe disease, followed by HbSC and HbS β^+ thalassemia. Compared to HbSS, HbSC patients have less hemolysis and thus are less anemic. All complications that occur in HbSS patients have also occurred in HbSC patients although at a lower frequency and they appear at a later age. Complications related to blood viscosity and microvascular occlusions such as avascular necrosis and proliferative retinopathy are just as frequent in HbSC patients. However, even within identical genotypic groups, the clinical course is remarkably variable; at one extreme are the completely asymptomatic patients with SCD discovered by chance on routine hematological examination such as during antenatal screening and at the other are patients who present with dactylitis in early childhood, followed by recurrent hospital admissions due to frequent acute pain. Most patients fall between the two extremes and are able to lead a relatively normal life. All SCD patients have a shortened life span; the life span of HbSC patients is shortened when compared to control populations but is longer than that of HbSS patients.

Sickle cell anemia (HbSS) normally presents in infancy after 6 months of life with attacks of dactylitis, manifested as painful swelling of the fingers and feet, the so-called 'hand-foot syndrome'. At this stage, the infant is usually anemic with mild jaundice and the spleen palpable. Splenomegaly usually resolves due to repeated infarctions of the spleen, the 'autosplenectomy' manifested by typical postsplenectomy changes in the peripheral blood film, visible as early as 10–12 months of age. Typically, these children have a chronic hemolytic anemia with a hemoglobin level that varies between 6 and 8 g/dl and a reticulocyte count of 10–20%. Serum bilirubin levels are elevated and peripheral blood smear shows polychromasia and poikilocytosis with a variable number of sickled erythrocytes.

The chronic hemolysis of sickle cell anemia is punctuated by acute clinical events termed sickling crises traditionally classified as vaso-occlusive, sequestration, aplastic or hemolytic, but in reality each acute clinical event has varying components of the different crises. The most common are the acute painful episodes due predominantly to vaso-occlusion in localized areas of bone marrow leading to infarction. Commonly affected areas are long bones, ribs, sternum and lumbosacral spine; often multiple sites are affected. The patient experiences a rapid onset of deep, throbbing bone pain in the affected areas, usually without physical findings but sometimes accompanied by local tenderness, warmth and swelling. Marrow aspirated from areas of bone tenderness have revealed infarction of the marrow tissue. Occasionally, abdominal pain is the major symptom and can pose a difficult problem in differential diagnosis. The abdominal crisis is accompanied by distension and rigidity with loss of bowel sounds, findings typical of an acute surgical abdomen. Acute cholecystitis and gallstones should also be considered.

Acute chest syndrome is characterized by acute dyspnea, pleuritic pain and fever, accompanied by a new pulmonary infiltrate on chest X-ray. It is often accompanied by a significant fall in the hemocrit which may reflect sequestration of the sickled cells in the pulmonary vessels. The distinction from pulmonary infection is often very difficult, particularly as infection and infarction usually co-exist. Acute chest syndrome is a frequent cause of admission but can be triggered by acute pain; it is the commonest cause of death in young patients.[70] The brain is the major site of morbidity in children; acute vaso-occlusion in the CNS usually presents in childhood, either as fits, transient neurological symptoms resembling ischemia attacks, or with a fully developed stroke.[96] Overt stroke affects about 6% of 10-year-olds with a peak between the ages of 2 and 5 years (incidence of 1.02 per 100 patient years), being rare in infants less than 1 year of age. Recurrent attacks are common; 70% of patients experience a recurrence within 3 years and many are left with permanent motor and intellectual disabilities. Long-term/lifetime blood transfusion is recommended for secondary prevention of stroke. Children with HbSS are at highest risk followed by HbS/β° thalassemia and HbSC disease. Priapism, defined as a sustained, painful and unwanted erection, is a well recognized complication in young men with SCD. It results from vaso-occlusion of the outflow vessels from the corpora cavernosa by sickled erythrocytes. This complication may present as multiple short-lived episodes ('stuttering' priapism) which may progress to 'severe prolonged' priapism lasting several days and leading to permanent penile dysfunction.

Transient marrow aplasia can have a profound effect with reticulocytopenia and a very sudden drop in hematocrit. These aplastic crises appear to result from intercurrent infections, particularly due to human parvovirus B19, and often occur in epidemics, frequently involving more than one sibling in the same family.

Sequestration crises commonly involve the spleen in the first two years of life. Definition of splenic sequestration includes a sudden, massive enlargement of the spleen concomitant with a drop in hemoglobin concentration (≥20 g/l) with substantial reticulocytosis. As the crisis progresses, a large proportion of the circulating red cell mass may be trapped in the spleen leading to profound anemia and death. Splenic sequestration shows a tendency to recur in the same individual and splenectomy is often recommended after a recurrence. A similar type of sequestration may occur in the liver in adult life, causing a dramatic fall in the hematocrit.

Patients with sickle cell disease are particularly susceptible to infection, due to *Streptococcus pneumoniae*, Salmonella, *Escherichia. coli* and *Hemophilus influenzae*. Osteomyelitis is common and results from infection of bone infarcts. Pneumococcal pneumonia and overwhelming septicemia are particularly important causes of death in infancy and childhood because of hyposplenism.

Repeated vaso-occlusive events and vasculopathy related to the chronic hemolysis ultimately result in end-organ damage and almost any organ can be affected. An observational study noted that by the fifth decade, ∼50% of patients would have one or more of sickle-related end-organ damage.[97] Avascular necrosis of the femoral head may lead to total disability, frequently requiring a total hip replacement. Virtually every patient with sickle cell anemia has some form of renal impairment. Sickling of the erythrocytes is enhanced in the hypertonic, hypoxic and acidotic environment of the renal medulla leading to progressive infarction of the medullary papillae. There is progressive inability to concentrate urine, polyuria, nocturia and enuresis, which is common in children. Eventually the glomerular damage causes end-stage renal failure, particularly in patients over 40 years of age. Due to the chronic hemolysis, pigment gallstones are very common and are seen in one third of SS patients by the age of 10 years. However, it is difficult to assess its clinical significance as not all patients develop clear-cut cholecystitis. Gilbert's disease, which is present in about 30% of Africans, is a predisposing factor. Recurrent chronic leg ulceration is common and can be a major handicap (Fig. 9.11). The lesions normally occur just above the medial or lateral malleoli and seem to be more common in those patients with severe anemia. Proliferative retinopathy leading to progressive visual loss is an important ocular complication although this is more common in HbSC disease.

Patients with SCD have a shortened life expectancy. Among HbSS patients in Jamaica, a life expectancy of 58 years for men and 66 years for women has been estimated, while in the United States a median age of death of 42 years for men and 48 years for women was reported in 1994.

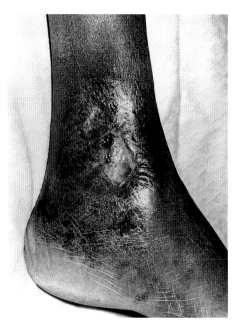

Fig. 9.11 Chronic leg ulcer in an adult with sickle cell anemia. Note the increased pigmentation of the skin around the ulcer.
(Courtesy of Professor SN Wickramasinghe).

Management

Bone marrow transplantation offers the only hope of cure for SCD, available and appropriate for a minority of patients. For the majority of SCD patients, care remains primarily reactive and preventive. Two non-transplant options have a major impact on management of SCD – blood transfusion and hydroxyurea therapy.

In general, management requires a multidisciplinary team effort and consists of continuous general medical care, attention to good nutrition, immunization, avoidance of extremes of temperature and dehydration, and treatment of complications as they arise.[98] In untreated patients, mortality is highest in the first year of life. In high risk populations, neonatal screening programs should be established to identify affected babies which should be referred to a specialist center and a comprehensive care plan initiated as soon as possible. These babies should be started on prophylactic penicillin at 3–4 months of age followed by polyvalent pneumococcal vaccine at the age of 6–12 months. There should be a systematic approach to education of parents (and later on, the child) on recognition of the different acute clinical events and signs of illness that play a critical role in successful management of children with SCD.

Most patients with SCD generally tolerate the relatively low Hb levels and blood transfusion is usually not required. Over the last decade, however, blood transfusion therapy is increasingly used in SCD with an ever expanding list of indications. Transfusion of normal blood provides benefit by correcting the low oxygen-carrying capacity as well as improving microvascular circulation by decreasing the population of sickled red cells. Regular blood transfusion also suppresses endogenous erythropoiesis and production of HbS. The choice of transfusion therapy – simple top-up, automated exchange (erythrocytapheresis), and partial exchange transfusion – depends on the needs of the patient. Except for severe anemia, exchange transfusion offers many advantages, and is increasingly used. Top-up transfusion is indicated when there is a sharp fall in the hemoglobin level due to bone marrow failure (aplastic crisis) or increased hemolysis (see Table 9.4 for indications for transfusion therapy in SCD).

Episodes of infection should be treated early and sudden exposure to cold and high altitudes avoided. All but the mildest crises should be managed in hospital. The patient should be examined for any underlying infection, kept warm and adequately hydrated, orally or intravenously, and given appropriate antibiotics. Prompt and adequate relief of pain is of prime importance. In selected patients, exchange transfusion may be effective in preventing recurrent painful crises.

Proliferative retinopathy may require photocoagulation or diathermy to reduce the risk of vitreous hemorrhage. Between 10% and 20% of HbSS patients develop leg ulcers which may become chronic and painful; they may respond to conservative treatment such as rest and elevation of the affected limb and zinc sulphate dressings. Occasionally, a regimen of regular blood transfusion for a limited period is helpful. Priapism is common in HbSS male patients (varies from 50% to 70% depending on study). Etilefrine may be effective in preventing a major episode in patients with so-called 'stuttering' priapism. Initial management should be conservative and include sedation, adequate hydration and

Table 9.4 Indications for blood transfusion in sickle cell disease

Acute/episodic	Long-term management

• Anemia   – severe
             – hemolytic
             – aplastic
• Splenic sequestration
• Stroke
• Acute chest syndrome
• Multiple organ failure syndrome
• Preoperative (selected cases)
• Malaria-associated severe hemolytic anemia
	• Heart failure
	• Prophylaxis against recurrent stroke
	• Prevention of first episode of stroke in high-risk pediatric patients
	• Chronic pulmonary hypertension
	• Refractory congestive heart failure
	• Hydroxyurea non-responders
	• Previous splenic sequestration in children aged ≤2–3 years
	• Chronic pain
	• Leg ulcers, avascular necrosis, etc.

analgesia. Failure to respond after 4 hours requires immediate hospital attention and may require surgical drainage.

There is no special treatment during pregnancy except for close supervision and folate supplementation. Blood transfusions are not normally indicated except when there is a significant drop in hemoglobin level or recurrent crises. In such cases a regular transfusion regimen may be considered throughout pregnancy until delivery. Although there is no evidence that oral contraceptives increase the risk of veno-occlusive episodes, it may be prudent to use a low estrogen preparation. Any surgical procedure should be undertaken with caution and scrupulous care taken to avoid factors known to precipitate crisis, including hypoxia, dehydration, cold, acidosis and circulatory stasis. Major surgical procedures may be best carried out after exchange transfusions.

Ischemic stroke is one of the most devastating complications in young children with SCD. Early cerebrovascular disease can be detected by transcranial Doppler (TCD) scanning demonstrating increased blood flow velocity in the middle cerebral artery, and studies have shown that starting blood transfusions at this stage can prevent progressive vasculopathy and overt stroke (STOP 1 study).[99] It is therefore recommended that children over 2 years of age should undergo TCD screening annually and those children at risk (abnormal blood flow velocities) started on prophylactic blood transfusion. A follow-up study (STOPI 2)[100] provided evidence that discontinuing blood transfusion after reversion to normal TCD velocity led to new CNS complications. Thus, it is recommended that prophylactic blood transfusion for primary prevention of stroke is indefinite. Adolescents and adults should be screened for pulmonary hypertension by transthoracic echocardiogram. Regular screening for proteinuria and institution of ACE inhibitors in those with significant proteinuria (>1 g in 24 hours) may slow the progress of sickle nephropathy.

Anti-sickling therapy. Therapeutic approaches to reducing vaso-occlusion and hemolysis in SCD are constantly evolving. The major therapies to date have been designed to inhibit the primary event of HbS polymerization, including anti-sickling agents and induction of HbF synthesis, and rehydration of the red blood cell.[1]

Numerous chemical anti-sickling agents, including cyanate, have been promoted but none can be regarded as safe and effective. The rationale of inhibiting erythrocyte dehydration by inducing hyponatremia, thereby causing an osmotic swelling of red cells, is sound but too cumbersome and risky. Agents that inhibit potassium and water loss from sickle cell erythrocytes by inhibiting the Gardos channel include clotrimazole which showed promise in sickle mouse models. However, a recent Phase III trial of the red cell membrane Gardos-potassiuim channel inhibitor (ICA-17403) in SCD patients was terminated due to negative results.

Other therapies – anti-adhesive, antithrombotic and anti-inflammatory – target the downstream pathways following HbS polymerization. These include anti-P-selectin antibodies, heparin, nitric oxide, statin, oral glutamine, aspirin, dipyridamole and others but none is in current routine use.

Induction of HbF as a form of therapy was initially based on clinical and epidemiological observations which showed that even slight elevations of fetal Hb have an ameliorating effect on the clinical severity.[70,101] An increase in intracellular HbF effectively reduces the concentration of HbS and mixed hybrids of HbS and HbF ($\alpha_2\gamma\beta^S$) do not form polymers. Pharmacological agents used include 5-azacytidine, a potent inhibitor of DNA methylation, arabinosylcytosine (Ara-C), hydroxyurea, erythropoietin and the butyrate analogues.[102] Hydroxyurea (HU) is the agent of choice and the only agent currently approved for treatment of SCD by the US Food and Drug Administration (FDA) and the European Medicines Agency (EMeA). Hydroxyurea has now been in use for patients with SCD for 25 years and has proven efficacy for reducing acute pain and acute chest syndrome.[103] An observational follow-up study also suggested that HU therapy was associated with reduced mortality in SCD patients.[104] However, only 60–80% of SCD patients respond to hydroxyurea.[105] The clinical benefits of hydroxyurea are not solely dependent on HbF increases but likely to be associated with the increased nitric oxide (promoting vasodilation), the accompanying reduction in the levels of neutrophils, monocytes and reticulocytes, and improved red cellular hydration, all of which are mitigating factors of vaso-occlusion. Genetic factors may also play a role in the individual response to HU.[106] Clinical indications for initiating HU include frequent acute pain and acute chest syndrome. However, potential expanding indications may include prevention of renal damage (indication significant proteinuria) and CNS damage (indication elevated TCD velocity). HU is relatively nontoxic, its myelosuppressive effects are reversible and limited evidence suggests that HU treatment in adults does not increase secondary malignancy. Despite the large body of evidence for its efficacy, HU remains under-prescribed in patients with SCD. Three reviews of the use of HU in SCD have recently been published.[107-109]

Bone marrow transplantation offers potential cure for sickle cell disease and may have a role in certain cases of sickle cell disease.[110] Allogeneic, cord blood and chimeric marrow transplantation are theoretically attractive ways to cure SCD but until more is known about the natural history of the disease and the ability to predict the disease severity, bone marrow transplant as a form of curative treatment for all cases is not recommended.

Hemosiderosis in SCD is a growing problem, and inevitable with simple top-up blood transfusions. The pathophysiology of transfusional loading in SCD appears to be different to that in thalassemia major but a major factor may be related to the total duration of transfusion.[1,111] Nonetheless, current recommendations are that patients should receive chelation therapy after twenty top-up transfusions or if liver iron concentration is more than 7 mg/g DW. (NIH publication, http://www.nhlbi.nih.gov/health/prof/blood/sickle/sc_mngt.pdf; Sickle Cell Society, UK, 2008, at http://www.sicklecellsociety.org/pdf/SCSPackageCareProp.pdf.)

Other sickling disorders

These include mainly the compound heterozygous states for HbS together with Hbs C, O-Arab, and D-Punjab as well as the inheritance of the β^S gene with the different forms of thalassemia (see Table 9.3).[91]

HbS/β thalassemia is the most common sickling disorder in individuals of Mediterranean origin. The severity of disease ranges from a completely asymptomatic state to one similar to that seen in sickle cell anemia. Much of this heterogeneity depends on the type of β thalassemia mutation and the amount of HbA produced. Because the majority of the β thalassemia alleles in Africans causes a minimal deficit in β chain production, HbS/β thalassemia in Africans is generally milder than in the Mediterranean populations. The presence of β thalassemia is indicated by the presence of hypochromic microcytic red cells, a HbS level of more than 50% on electrophoresis and an elevated level of HbA$_2$. Family studies are often crucial in distinguishing between the two disorders. Globin chain biosynthetic studies are also useful; in HbS/β thalassemia the β^S/α ratio is 0.5 while in SS disease, it is close to one.

Other hemoglobin variants

The other hemoglobin variants that are encountered commonly are Hbs C and E (see Table 9.5 and section on β thalassemias and sickle cell disease). HbC is the second most common variant among individuals of African ancestry. HbC is less soluble than HbA and tends to crystallize within the red cells leading to their reduced deformability. The

Table 9.5 Molecular abnormalities observed in thalassemic hemoglobinopathies

Abnormality	Example
Unstable variants	Hb Suan Dok ($\alpha2^{109\,Leu\rightarrow Arg}$)
Hyperunstable variants	Hb Quong Sze ($\alpha2^{125\,Leu\rightarrow Pro}$) Hb Showa Yakushiji ($\beta^{110\,Leu\rightarrow Pro}$)
Variants that cause abnormal splicing	HbE ($\beta^{26\,Leu\rightarrow Lys}$) Hb Knossos ($\beta^{27\,Ala\rightarrow Ser}$)
Variants with mutations in the termination codon	Hb Constant Spring ($\alpha2^{142\,Term\rightarrow Gln}$)*
Variants linked to thalassemic mutation	HbG-Philadelphia (/–α^{G-Phil})
δ/β fusion globin subunits	Hb Lepore

*Hb Constant Spring is a particularly common form of non-deletion α thalassemia in Thailand.

important interactions of HbC are with HbS (to produce HbSC disease)[1] and β thalassemia.

HbE (β26 Glu→Lys) is probably the most common hemoglobin variant in the world, occurring in a region extending from Bangladesh through to China, including Southeast Asia (see also section on HbE/β thalassemia). Gene frequencies of 50–70% have been recorded in parts of Thailand, Laos and Kampuchea.

After HbE/β thalassemia, other symptomatic forms of HbE-associated conditions include its interaction with the different genotypic forms of HbH disease.[1,64] However, inclusions and HbH (β_4) are present only in HbAE but not HbE/E or HbE/β° thalassemia; presumably the abnormal β^E-subunits do not form tetramers. Interaction of HbE with HbS produces sickle cell disease (HbSE).

The diagnosis of HbE is based on detection or quantitation of the variant by electrophoretic or chromatographic separation of the hemoglobin in peripheral blood. Separation of hemoglobins using routine techniques, including HPLC columns, cannot differentiate HbE from HbA_2. In uncomplicated heterozygous HbE, the variant forms ~35% of the total hemoglobin. As with β^S, the β^E globin variant is positively charged and is less able to compete with the negatively charged β-globin for the positively charged α subunits.[93] Hence, in the presence of limiting amounts of α-globin when α thalassemia is co-inherited with heterozygous HbE, the proportion of HbE is reduced: ~10% (in —/—α), 20–22% (in —/αα or −α/−α) and 27–30% (in αα/−α).

Unstable hemoglobin disorders

Structural changes in the globin subunits can lead to instability of the hemoglobin molecule causing it to precipitate intracellularly, detectable by supravital staining as globular aggregates known as Heinz bodies. These inclusions reduce the life span of the erythrocytes and cause variable hemolysis, an integral part of the syndrome of congenital Heinz body hemolytic anemia (CHBA).[91] The true incidence of CHBA is not known; according to the Globin Gene Server (http://globin.cse.psu.edu), more than 25% of the 1000 hemoglobin variants were designated 'unstable' and associated with varying degrees of reticulocytosis and hemolytic anemia. Many of the unstable variants are also associated with a thalassemic phenotype.[17,26] A basis for the phenotypic variation of these disorders lies in the variable instability of the abnormal globin subunits. Those at the severe end of the spectrum are not able to form functional tetramers and precipitate in the red cell precursors causing a functional deficiency and a thalassemic phenotype, while the less unstable globin variants are able to form a hemoglobin tetramer that survives the different stages of red cell maturation only to precipitate in the mature red cell causing hemolysis in the peripheral circulation. Hemolysis is highly variable in intensity and often precipitated by infections and exposure to chemical oxidants.

The majority of CHBA follows an autosomal dominant pattern of inheritance; affected individuals are almost exclusively heterozygotes.[91] Unstable hemoglobins are not common, generally limited to single families, and only the proband is affected, suggesting that the mutation has arisen by a *de novo* mutation. There are two exceptions: Hb Köln

(β98 Val→Met) has been reported in various ethnic groups and often observed as a *de novo* mutation.[20] Hb Hasharon (α47 Asp→His) is found in Italian families and Ashkenazi Jews, and causes hemolytic anemia in newborns.[20]

Blood films are not specific, and show typical features of hemolysis including prominent reticulocytosis and polychromia, but the red cell morphology may be normal. Heinz bodies are present in the peripheral blood after splenectomy and can be detected by incubating the erythrocytes with a supravital stain such as new methyline blue or crystal violet. The most characteristic feature of the unstable hemoglobins is their heat instability which can be demonstrated by the presence of flocculent precipitates on heating a dilute hemoglobin solution at 50°C for 15 minutes. A similar effect can be induced by the addition of isopropanol at lower temperature. Some of these variants can be seen on hemoglobin electrophoresis and often appears as a diffuse band, but others, because they result from a neutral amino acid substitution, produce no electrophoretic changes. DNA sequencing of the α- and β-globin genes provides a definitive diagnosis.

Most patients with CHBA do not require treatment. General supportive measures include folic acid supplements, prompt treatment of infection and reduction of fever. Oxidant drugs should be avoided. Intermittent transfusions may be needed, such as during an aplastic crisis or if hemolysis is very severe. In cases with very severe hemolysis, splenectomy may be beneficial although experience is limited. Bone marrow transplantation should be considered.

Hemoglobin variants with abnormal oxygen binding

The molecular basis underlying the abnormal oxygen binding of these structural hemoglobin variants lies in the perturbance of the transitional state between hemoglobin conformations – R or 'relaxed' in which it has a high affinity for oxygen, and low affinity for effectors such as 2,3-DPG, and T or 'tense' when it has a relatively low affinity for oxygen and high affinity for the allosteric affectors.[112]

The transition between these two conformations requires 'heme–heme interaction' which involves a series of structural changes. Thus mutations that result in a structural alteration which affects the equilibrium between the R and T states would have a marked effect on hemoglobin binding of oxygen. Both high and low oxygen affinity variants have been described.

Mutations for high oxygen affinity variants have been described only in the heterozygous form with the exception of one α chain variant, Hb Tarrent (α126 Asp→Asn) in which, on the basis of the Hb electrophoresis quantitation, two of the four α-globin genes were affected.[113] Since most of the affected individuals are likely to have four α-globin genes (αα/αα), α-globin variants cause a less clinically significant condition compared to those of the β subunit.

The increased oxygen affinity causes a functional anemia and tissue hypoxia, which in turn leads to increased output of erythropoietin and an elevated red cell mass. High affinity hemoglobin variants follow an autosomal dominant inheritance pattern; all affected individuals are heterozygotes.[91] A positive family history is useful but occasionally the variants arise from *de novo* mutations. Most affected individuals are completely healthy and identified through a routine blood count which shows increased hemoglobin or hematocrit. The individual may also have a ruddy complexion. There is no splenomegaly and, apart from an increased hemoglobin concentration and hematocrit, the white cell and platelet counts are within normal limits. Diagnosis is made by excluding other causes for erythrocytosis, and by demonstrating a left-shifted oxygen dissociation curve with a reduced P50 value, and a normal 2,3-diphosphoglycerate (2,3-DPG) value. Diagnosis is confirmed by hemoglobin analysis, using either mass spectrometry or DNA sequence analysis. A normal hemoglobin electrophoresis or HPLC does not exclude a diagnosis of high affinity hemoglobin.

In asymptomatic persons, no treatment is necessary. The difficulty arises if there is associated vascular disease, particularly coronary or cerebral artery insufficiency. As these patients require a high hemoglobin level for oxygen transport, venesection should be carried out with great caution. Venesection is undertaken because of increased risk of vascular complications, and typically the aim is to keep the hematocrit below 0.55, although there is little evidence to support this.

Far fewer hemoglobin variants with low oxygen affinity have been described but should always be considered in any patient with unexplained congenital cyanosis, the differential diagnosis being methemoglobinemia. Cyanosis is present from birth in some carriers of α-globin variants, while cyanosis associated with the β-globin variants presents in the second half of the first year of life when β-globin gene expression predominates.

Diagnosis of a low oxygen affinity hemoglobin is made by excluding other causes of cyanosis, especially cardiopulmonary, and differentiation of the cyanosis from that of methemoglobinemia.[1] A simple test is to expose the individual's blood to pure oxygen when it will turn bright red in cases of low oxygen affinity hemoglobin and cardiopulmonary disease. In contrast, in the blood of patients with methemoglobinemia, M hemoglobins and sulfhemoglobinemia retain their abnormal color despite exposure to pure oxygen. Most of the low oxygen affinity hemoglobin variants are unstable, and determination of the whole blood P50 is not always reliable. Hemoglobin electrophoresis, mass spectrometry of hemoglobin and DNA sequence analysis are useful tools for diagnosis.

Hemoglobins M

A striking clinical feature of the M hemoglobins is the dusky blue appearance of the skin and mucous membranes.[91] In the vast majority of cases, the cyanosis is due to an excess of deoxyhemoglobin in the blood from a congenital cardiopulmonary defect. Rarely, it can be caused by a low oxygen affinity hemoglobin variant. Next in the differential diagnosis are the methemoglobinemias or sulfhemoglobinemias, usually caused by a deficiency of the enzyme cytochrome b5 reductase.[114] The enzyme enables red cell hemoglobin to be maintained in a reduced form and deficiency of the enzyme results in oxidized hemoglobin and a cyanotic appearance. A much rarer cause of methemoglobinemia is the presence of one of the M hemoglobins. The M hemoglobins are inherited in an autosomal dominant pattern. Affected individuals present with cyanosis that varies from brownish to slate grey but are otherwise asymptomatic. If cyanosis is present from birth, it is normally due to an α chain variant, whereas β chain HbM produces cyanosis after the first few months of life when adult hemoglobin ($\alpha_2\beta_2$) synthesis becomes established.

Seven M hemoglobins have been described, of which two affect the α-, three the β-, and two, the γ-globin subunit. Six of the seven subunits have substitutions of tyrosine for the proximal (F8) or distal (E7) histidine, creating an abnormal microenvironment for stabilization of the heme iron in the ferric form. As a result of these substitutions, these Hbs M are resistant to reduction by methemoglobin reductase. The M hemoglobins are also functionally abnormal with a decreased oxygen affinity and they are mildly unstable.

The most reliable diagnostic test is based on examination of the hemolysate by recording spectrophotometry which shows an abnormal pattern that is similar to, but not identical with, that of methemoglobin.

Hb electrophoresis is of limited value unless the entire hemolysate is converted to methemoglobin prior to electrophoresis. Diagnosis is confirmed by hemoglobin analysis using mass spectrometry or DNA sequence analysis of the globin genes.

Thalassemic hemoglobinopathies

This group of hemoglobin disorders includes structural hemoglobin mutants associated with a thalassemia phenotype, that is, hypochromia and microcytosis with or without anemia.[10] The phenotype ranges from the mild forms of heterozygous thalassemia to that resembling thalassemia intermedia. In some cases, chronic severe hemolytic anemia with splenomegaly is a feature. The molecular abnormalities are remarkably heterogeneous and includes single amino acid mutations causing hemoglobin variants such as Hbs E and Knossos with abnormal splicing, amino acid deletions, elongated or truncated globin chains and fusion globins such as Hb Lepore (Table 9.5).

Some of the α-globin mutants are invariably linked to a tandem α-globin gene deletion and hence the concomitant deficiency, for example HbG-Philadelphia (/-α^G-Phil). Thalassemic hemoglobinopathies also include an increasing number of α and β structural variants in which the amino acid substitutions confer such instability that they are readily degraded in the bone marrow erythroid precursors resulting in an ineffective erythropoiesis and a thalassemic phenotype.[17]

Acknowledgment

I thank Claire Steward for preparation of the manuscript.

References

1. Steinberg MH, Forget BG, Higgs DR, Weatherall DJ, editors. Disorders of Hemoglobin: Genetics, Pathophysiology, and Clinical Management. 2nd ed. Cambridge, UK: Cambridge University Press; 2009. p. 826.

2. Higgs DR, Wood WG. Long-range regulation of alpha globin gene expression during erythropoiesis. Curr Opin Hematol 2008;15(3):176–83.

3. Cantor AB, Orkin SH. Hematopoietic development: a balancing act. Curr Opin Genet Dev 2001;11(5):513–9.

4. Blobel GA, Weiss MJ. Nuclear factors that regulate erythropoiesis. In: Steinberg MH, Forget BG, Higgs DR, Weatherall DJ, editors. Disorders of Hemoglobin: Genetics, Pathophysiology, and Clinical Management. Cambridge, UK: Cambridge University Press; 2009. p. 62–85.

5. Tolhuis B, Palstra RJ, Splinter E, et al. Looping and interaction between hypersensitive sites in the active beta-globin locus. Mol Cell 2002;10(6): 1453–65.

6. Stamatoyannopoulos G. Control of globin gene expression during development and erythroid differentiation. Exp Hematol 2005; 33(3):259–71.

7. Wijgerde M, Grosveld F, Fraser P. Transcription complex stability and chromatin dynamics in vivo. Nature 1995;377:209–13.

8. Sankaran VG, Xu J, Orkin SH. Advances in the understanding of haemoglobin switching. Br J Haematol 2010;149(2): 181–94.

9. Feng WC, Southwood CM, Bieker JJ. Analyses of β-thalassemia mutant DNA interactions with erythroid Krüppel-like factor (EKLF), an erythroid cell-specific transcription factor. Journal of Biological Chemistry 1994;269:1493–500.

10. Weatherall DJ, Clegg JB. The Thalassaemia Syndromes. 4th ed. Oxford: Blackwell Science; 2001.

11. Liu P, Keller JR, Ortiz M, et al. Bcl11a is essential for normal lymphoid development. Nat Immunol 2003;4(6): 525–32.

12. Menzel S, Garner C, Gut I, et al. A QTL influencing F cell production maps to a gene encoding a zinc-finger protein on chromosome 2p15. Nat Genet 2007; 39(10):1197–9.

13. Uda M, Galanello R, Sanna S, et al. Genome-wide association study shows BCL11A associated with persistent fetal hemoglobin and amelioration of the phenotype of beta-thalassemia. Proc Natl Acad Sci USA 2008;105(5): 1620–5.

14. Sankaran VG, Menne TF, Xu J, et al. Human fetal hemoglobin expression is regulated by the developmental stage-specific repressor BCL11A. Science 2008;322(5909):1839–42.

15. Sankaran VG, Xu J, Ragoczy T, et al. Developmental and species-divergent globin switching are driven by BCL11A. Nature 2009;460(7259):1093–7.

16. Weatherall DJ, Clegg JB. Thalassemia – a global public health problem. Nature Medicine 1996;2(8):847–9.

17. Thein SL. Structural variants with a beta-thalassemia phenotype, In: Steinberg MH, Forget BG, Higgs DR, Weatherall DJ, editors. Disorders of Hemoglobin: Genetics, Pathophysiology, and Clinical Management. Cambridge, UK: Cambridge University Press; 2001. p. 342–55.

18. Cooley TB, Lee P. A series of cases of splenomegaly in children with anemia and peculiar bone changes. Trans Am Pediatr Soc 1925;37:29.

19. Modell B, Darlison M, Birgens H, et al. Epidemiology of haemoglobin disorders in Europe: an overview. Scand J Clin Lab Invest 2007;67(1):39–69.

20. A Database of Human Hemoglobin Variants and Thalassemias. Online. Available from: http://globin.cse.psu.edu/globin/hbvar/.

21. Maragoudaki E, Kanavakis E, Traeger-Synodinos J, et al. Molecular, haematological and clinical studies of the −101 C→T substitution in the β-globin gene promoter in 25 β-thalassaemia intermedia patients and 45 heterozygotes. British Journal of Haematology 1999;107(4):699–706.

22. Frischmeyer PA, Dietz HC. Nonsense-mediated mRNA decay in health and disease. Human Molecular Genetics 1999;8:1893–900.

23. Hentze MW, Kulozik AE. A perfect message: RNA surveillance and nonsense-mediated decay. Cell 1999; 96:307–10.

24. Huang S-C, Benz EJJ. Posttranscriptional factors influencing the hemoglobin content of the red cells. In: Steinberg MH, Forget BG, Higgs DR, Weatherall DJ, editors Disorders of Hemoglobin: Genetics, Pathophysiology, and Clinical Management. Cambridge, UK: Cambridge University Press; 2001. p. 252–76.

25. Isken O, Maquat LE. Quality control of eukaryotic mRNA: safeguarding cells from abnormal mRNA function. Genes Dev 2007;21(15):1833–56.

26. Thein SL. Is it dominantly inherited beta thalassaemia or just a beta-chain variant that is highly unstable? Br J Haematol 1999;107(1):12–21.

27. Thein SL, Old JM, Wainscoat JS, et al. Population and genetic studies suggest a single origin for the Indian deletion beta zero thalassaemia. British Journal of Haematology 1984;57:271–8.

28. Kimberland ML, Divoky V, Prchal J, et al. Full-length human L1 insertions retain the capacity for high frequency retrotransposition in cultured cells. Hum Mol Genet 1999;8(8):1557–60.

29. Viprakasit V, Gibbons RJ, Broughton BC, et al. Mutations in the general transcription factor TFIIH result in beta-thalassaemia in individuals with trichothiodystrophy. Hum Mol Genet 2001;10(24):2797–802.

30. Yu C, Niakan KK, Matsushita M, et al. X-linked thrombocytopenia with thalassemia due to a mutation affecting DNA-binding contribution of the N-finger of transcription factor GATA-1 [abstract]. Blood 2000;96(11):495a.

31. Badens C, Mattei MG, Imbert AM, et al. A novel mechanism for thalassaemia intermedia. The Lancet 2002;359(9301): 132–3.

32. Galanello R, Perseu L, Perra C, et al. Somatic deletion of the normal beta-globin gene leading to thalassaemia intermedia in heterozygous beta-thalassaemic patients. Br J Haematol 2004;127(5):604–6.

33. Chang JG, Tsai WC, Chong IW, et al. Beta-thalassemia major evolution from beta-thalassemia minor is associated with paternal uniparental isodisomy of chromosome 11p15. Haematologica 2008;93(6):913–6.

34. Ho PJ, Hall GW, Luo LY, et al. Beta thalassemia intermedia: is it possible to consistently predict phenotype from genotype? British Journal of Haematology 1998;100(1):70–8.

35. Camaschella C, Mazza U, Roetto A, et al. Genetic interactions in thalassemia intermedia: analysis of beta-mutations, alpha-genotype, gamma-promoters, and beta-LCR hypersensitive sites 2 and 4 in Italian patients. American Journal of Hematology 1995;48:82–7.

36. Rund D, Oron-Karni V, Filon D, et al. Genetic analysis of β-thalassemia intermedia in Israel: diversity of mechanisms and unpredictability of phenotype. Am J Hematol 1997;54(1): 16–22.

37. Lettre G, Sankaran VG, Bezerra MA, et al. DNA polymorphisms at the BCL11A, HBS1L-MYB, and beta-globin loci associate with fetal hemoglobin levels and pain crises in sickle cell disease. Proc Natl Acad Sci USA 2008;105(33): 11869–74.

38. Sedgewick AE, Timofeev N, Sebastiani P, et al. BCL11A is a major HbF quantitative trait locus in three different populations with beta-hemoglobinopathies. Blood Cells Mol Dis 2008;41(3):255–8.

39. Galanello R, Sanna S, Perseu L, et al. Amelioration of Sardinian beta-zero thalassaemia by genetic modifiers. Blood 2009;114(18):3935–7.

40. Nuinoon M, Makarasara W, Mushiroda T, et al. A genome-wide association identified the common genetic variants influence disease severity in beta(0)-thalassemia/hemoglobin E. Hum Genet 2010;127(3):303–14.

41. Traeger-Synodinos J, Kanavakis E, Vrettou C, et al. The triplicated alpha-globin gene locus in beta-thalassaemia heterozygotes: clinical, haematological, biosynthetic and molecular studies. Br J Haematol 1996;95(3):467–71.

42. Camaschella C, Kattamis AC, Petroni D, et al. Different hematological phenotypes caused by the interaction of triplicated alpha-globin genes and heterozygous beta-thalassemia. American Journal of Hematology 1997;55(2):83–8.

43. Harteveld CL, Refaldi C, Cassinerio E, et al. Segmental duplications involving the alpha-globin gene cluster are causing beta-thalassemia intermedia phenotypes in beta-thalassemia heterozygous patients. Blood Cells Mol Dis 2008;40(3):312–6.

44. Sollaino MC, Paglietti ME, Perseu L, et al. Association of alpha globin gene quadruplication and heterozygous beta thalassemia in patients with thalassemia intermedia. Haematologica 2009;94(10):1445–8.

45. Thein SL. Genetic modifiers of beta-thalassemia. Haematologica 2005;90(5):649–60.

46. Wonke B. Bone disease in beta-thalassaemia major. British Journal of Haematology 1998;103:897–901.

47. Galanello R, Perseu L, Melis MA, et al. Hyperbilirubinaemia in heterozygous beta-thalassaemia is related to co-inherited Gilbert's syndrome. British Journal of Haematology 1997;99(2):433–6.

48. Galanello R, Cipollina MD, Dessì C, et al. Co-inherited Gilbert's syndrome: a factor determining hyperbilirubinemia in homozygous beta-thalassemia. Haematologica 1999;84(2):103–5.

49. Piperno A, Mariani R, Arosio C, et al. Haemochromatosis in patients with beta-thalassaemia trait. Br J Haematol 2000;111(3):908–14.

50. Andrews NC. Molecular control of iron metabolism. Best Pract Res Clin Haematol 2005;18(2):159–69.

51. Andrews NC. Genes determining blood cell traits. Nat Genet 2009;41(11):1161–2.

52. Ganesh SK, Zakai NA, van Rooij FJ, et al. Multiple loci influence erythrocyte phenotypes in the CHARGE Consortium. Nat Genet 2009;41(11):1191–8.

53. Soranzo N, Spector TD, Mangino M, et al. A genome-wide meta-analysis identifies 22 loci associated with eight hematological parameters in the HaemGen consortium. Nat Genet 2009;41(11):1182–90.

54. Borgna-Pignatti C, Rugolotto S, De Stefano P, et al. Survival and complications in patients with thalassemia major treated with transfusion and deferoxamine. Haematologica 2004;89(10):1187–93.

55. Angelucci E, Barosi G, Camaschella C, et al. Italian Society of Hematology practice guidelines for the management of iron overload in thalassemia major and related disorders. Haematologica 2008;93(5):741–52.

56. Cappellini M-D, Cohen A, Eleftheriuo A, et al. Guidelines for the Clinical Management of Thalassaemia. 2nd ed. Nicosia, Cyprus: Thalassaemia International Federation; 2008. p. 199.

57. Borgna-Pignatti C, Cappellini MD, De Stefano P, et al. Cardiac morbidity and mortality in deferoxamine- or deferiprone-treated patients with thalassemia major. Blood 2006;107(9):3733–7.

58. Vichinsky E. Clinical application of deferasirox: practical patient management. Am J Hematol 2008;83(5):398–402.

59. Gaziev J, Sodani P, Polchi P, et al. Bone marrow transplantation in adults with thalassemia: treatment and long-term follow-up. Ann N Y Acad Sci 2005;1054:196–205.

60. Taher A, Isma'eel H, Cappellini MD. Thalassemia intermedia: revisited. Blood Cells Mol Dis 2006;37(1):12–20.

61. Cao A, Galanello R, Rosatelli MC. Prenatal diagnosis and screening of the haemoglobinopathies. In: Rodgers GP, editor. Baillière's Clinical Haematology. London: Baillière Tindall; 1998. p. 215–38.

62. Braude P, Pickering S, Flinter F, et al. Preimplantation genetic diagnosis. Nat Rev Genet 2002;3(12):941–53.

63. Vichinsky E. Hemoglobin E syndromes. Hematology Am Soc Hematol Educ Program 2007;79–83.

64. Fucharoen S. Hemoglobin E disorders. In: Steinberg MH, Forget BG, Higgs DR, Weatherall DJ, editors. Disorders of Hemoglobin: Genetics, Pathophysiology, and Clinical Management. Cambridge, UK: Cambridge University Press; 2001. p. 1139–54.

65. Thein SL, Wood WG. The molecular basis of β thalassemia, δβ thalassemia, and hereditary persistence of fetal hemoglobin. In: Steinberg MH, Forget BG, Higgs DR, Weatherall DJ, editors. Disorders of Hemoglobin: Genetics, Pathophysiology, and Clinical Management. Cambridge, UK: Cambridge University Press; 2009. p. 323–56.

66. Rochette J, Craig JE, Thein SL. Fetal hemoglobin levels in adults. Blood Reviews 1994;8:213–24.

67. Ottolenghi S, Giglioni B, Pulazzini A, et al. Sardinian δβ-thalassemia: A further example of a C to T substitution at position -196 of the $^A\gamma$ globin gene promoter. Blood 1987;69(4):1058–61.

68. Marti HR. Normale und anormale menschliche Haemoglobine. Berlin: Springer Verlag; 1963.

69. Marti HR, Butler R. Hämoglobin F- und Hämoglobin A2-Vermehrung bei der Schweizer Bevölkerung. Acta Haematologia (Basel) 1961;26:65–74.

70. Platt OS, Brambilla DJ, Rosse WF, et al. Mortality in sickle cell disease: life expectancy and risk factors for early death. New England Journal of Medicine 1994;330(23):1639–44.

71. Thein SL, Menzel S, Peng X, et al. Intergenic variants of HBS1L-MYB are responsible for a major quantitative trait locus on chromosome 6q23 influencing fetal hemoglobin levels in adults. Proc Natl Acad Sci USA 2007;104(27):11346–51.

72. So CC, Song YQ, Tsang ST, et al. The HBS1L-MYB intergenic region on chromosome 6q23 is a quantitative trait locus controlling fetal haemoglobin level in carriers of beta-thalassaemia. J Med Genet 2008;45(11):745–51.

73. Creary LE, Ulug P, Menzel S, et al. Genetic variation on chromosome 6 influences F cell levels in healthy individuals of African descent and HbF levels in sickle cell patients. PLoS ONE 2009;4(1):e4218.

74. Game L, Bergounioux J, Close JP, et al. A novel deletion causing $(\varepsilon\gamma\delta\beta)$ thalassemia in a Chilean family. Br J Haematol 2003;123(1):154–9.

75. Rooks H, Bergounioux J, Game L, et al. Heterogeneity of the epsilon gamma delta beta-thalassaemias: characterisation of three novel English deletions. Br J Haematol 2005;128(5):722–9.

76. Harteveld CL, Voskamp A, Phylipsen M, et al. Nine unknown rearrangements in 16p13.3 and 11p15.4 causing α- and β-thalassaemia characterised by high resolution multiplex ligation-dependent probe amplification. J Med Genet. 2005 Dec;42(12):922-31.

77. Higgs DR, Weatherall DJ. The alpha thalassaemias. Cell Mol Life Sci 2009;66(7):1154–62.

78. Viprakasit V, Harteveld CL, Ayyub H, et al. A novel deletion causing alpha thalassemia clarifies the importance of the major human alpha globin regulatory element. Blood 2006;107(9):3811–2.

79. Kanavakis E, Papassotiriou I, Karagiorga M, et al. Phenotypic and molecular diversity of haemoglobin H disease: a Greek experience. Br J Haematol 2000;111(3):915–23.

80. Fucharoen S, Viprakasit V. Hb H disease: clinical course and disease modifiers. Hematology Am Soc Hematol Educ Program, 2009:26–34.

81. Liebhaber SA, Schrier SL. Pathophysiology of α thalassaemia. In: Steinberg MH, Forget BG, Higgs DR, Weatherall DJ, editors. Disorders of Hemoglobin: Genetics, Pathophysiology, and Clinical Management. Cambridge, UK: Cambridge University Press; 2001. p. 391–404.

82. Wilkie AO, Buckle VJ, Harris PC, et al. Clinical features and molecular analysis of the alpha-thalassemia/mental retardation syndromes. I. Cases due to deletions involving chromosome band 16p13.3. American Journal of Human Genetics 1990;46:1112–26.

83. Gibbons RJ, Pellagatti A, Garrick D, et al. Identification of acquired somatic mutations in the gene encoding chromatin-remodeling factor ATRX in the alpha-thalassemia myelodysplasia syndrome (ATMDS). Nat Genet 2003; 34(4):446–9.

84. Herrick JB, Peculiar elongated and sickle-shaped red blood corpuscles in a case of severe anemia. Arch Intern Med 1910;6:517–21.

85. Pauling L, Itano HA, Singer SJ, et al. Sickle cell anemia: a molecular disease. Science 1949;110:543–8.

86. Ingram VM, A specific chemical difference between the globins of normal human and sickle-cell anaemia haemoglobin. Nature 1956;178:792–4.

87. Noguchi C, Schechter AN, Rodgers GP. Sickle cell disease pathophysiology. In: Higgs DR, Weatherall DJ, editors. Baillière's Clinical Haematology: The Haemoglobinopathies. London: Baillière Tindall; 1993. p. 57–91.

88. Steinberg MH, Thein SL. Genetic modulation of sickle cell disease, in Renaissance of sickle cell disease research in the genome era, B. Pace, Editor. London, UK: Imperial College Press; 2007. p. 193–206.

89. Weatherall MW, Higgs DR, Weiss H, et al. Phenotype/genotype relationships in sickle cell disease: a pilot twin study. Clin Lab Haematol 2005;27(6):384–90.

90. Thein SL. Genetic modifiers of the beta-haemoglobinopathies. Br J Haematol 2008;141(3):357–66.

91. Bunn HF, Forget BG. Hemoglobin: molecular, genetic and clinical aspects. Philadelphia, PA: W.B. Saunders Company; 1986.

92. Bunn HF, McDonald MJ. Electrostatic interactions in the assembly of human hemoglobin. Nature 1983;306:498–500.

93. Bunn HF, Subunit assembly of hemoglobin: an important determinant of hematologic phenotype. Blood 1987;69:1–6.

94. Embury SH, Hebbel RP, Mohandas N, et al. Sickle Cell Disease: Basic Principles and Clinical Practice. New York, NY: Raven Press; 1994.

95. Kark JA, Ward FT. Exercise and hemoglobin S. Semin Hematol 1994; 31(3):181–225.

96. Ohene-Frempong K. Stroke in sickle cell disease: demographic, clinical, and therapeutic considerations. Seminars in Hematology 1991;28(3):213–9.

97. Powars DR, Chan LS, Hiti A, et al. Outcome of sickle cell anemia: a 4-decade observational study of 1056 patients. Medicine (Baltimore) 2005;84(6):363–76.

98. Steinberg MH. Management of sickle cell disease. New England Journal of Medicine 1999;340(13):1021–30.

99. Adams RJ, McKie VC, Hsu L, et al. Prevention of a first stroke by transfusions in children with sickle cell anemia and abnormal results on transcranial doppler ultrasonography. New England Journal of Medicine 1998;339(1):5–11.

100. Adams RJ, Brambilla D. Discontinuing prophylactic transfusions used to prevent stroke in sickle cell disease. N Engl J Med 2005;353(26):2769–78.

101. Platt OS, Thorington BD, Brambilla DJ, et al. Pain in sickle cell disease: Rates and risk factor. New England Journal of Medicine 1991;325(1):11–6.

102. Bunn HF. Induction of fetal hemoglobin in sickle cell disease. Blood 1999;93: 1787–9.

103. Charache S, Terrin ML, Moore RD, et al. Effect of hydroxyurea on the frequency of painful crises in sickle cell anemia. Investigators of the Multicenter Study of Hydroxyurea in Sickle Cell Anemia. New England Journal of Medicine 1995; 332(20):1317–22.

104. Steinberg MH, Barton F, Castro O, et al. Effect of hydroxyurea on mortality and morbidity in adult sickle cell anemia: risks and benefits up to 9 years of treatment. Jama 2003;289(13):1645–51.

105. Steinberg MH, Lu ZH, Barton FB, et al. Fetal hemoglobin in sickle cell anemia: determinants of response to hydroxyurea. Multicenter Study of Hydroxyurea. Blood 1997;89(3):1078–88.

106. Ma Q, Wyszynski DF, Farrell JJ, et al. Fetal hemoglobin in sickle cell anemia: genetic determinants of response to hydroxyurea. Pharmacogenomics J 2007;7(6):386–94.

107. Brawley OW, Cornelius LJ, Edwards LR, et al. National Institutes of Health Consensus Development Conference statement: hydroxyurea treatment for sickle cell disease. Ann Intern Med 2008;148(12):932–8.

108. Lanzkron S, Strouse JJ, Wilson R, et al. Systematic review: hydroxyurea for the treatment of adults with sickle cell disease. Ann Intern Med 2008;148(12): 939–55.

109. Strouse JJ, Lanzkron S, Beach MC, et al. Hydroxyurea for sickle cell disease: a systematic review for efficacy and toxicity in children. Pediatrics 2008;122(6): 1332–42.

110. Vermylen C. Bone marrow transplantation in sickle cell anemia. In: Steinberg MH, Forget BG, Higgs DR, Weatherall DJ, editors. Disorders of Hemoglobin: Genetics, Pathophysiology, and Clinical Management. Cambridge, UK: Cambridge University Press; 2001. p. 1073–83.

111. Vichinsky E, Butensky E, Fung E, et al. Comparison of organ dysfunction in transfused patients with SCD or beta thalassemia. Am J Hematol 2005;80(1): 70–4.

112. Perutz MF. Molecular anatomy and physiology of hemoglobin. In: Steinberg MH, Forget BG, Higgs DR, Weatherall DJ, editors. Disorders of Hemoglobin: Genetics, Pathophysiology, and Clinical Management. Cambridge, UK: Cambridge University Press; 2001. p. 174–96.

113. Ibarra B, Vaca G, Cantú JM, et al. Heterozygosity and homozygosity for the high oxygen affinity hemoglobin Tarrant or alpha 126 (H9) Asp replaced by Asn in two Mexican families. Hemoglobin 1981;5(4):337–48.

114. Percy MJ, Lappin TR. Recessive congenital methaemoglobinaemia: cytochrome b(5) reductase deficiency. Br J Haematol 2008;141(3):298–308.

CHAPTER 10

Acquired hemolytic anemia

DM Arnold, I Nazi, JC Moore, NM Heddle, JG Kelton

Chapter contents

Introduction

Accelerated red blood cell (RBC) destruction is called hemolysis. When bone marrow compensation is adequate, hemoglobin levels remain unchanged; however, if RBC destruction surpasses production, anemia will result. Hemolytic anemia is traditionally categorized as either congenital or acquired. The term 'acquired hemolytic anemia' was first coined in the early 1900s[1] and it is now commonly used to describe hemolytic anemia caused by antibodies (with or without complement), drugs or mechanical trauma to RBCs. Acquired hemolytic anemia can be classified as immune (autoimmune, alloimmune or drug-induced) and non-immune (infection-induced, mechanical trauma and paroxysmal nocturnal hemoglobinuria) and different causes of hemolytic anemia can overlap; for example, drug-induced hemolysis may be caused by immune mechanisms or by direct damage to the RBC membrane. In this chapter, the pathogenesis, clinical presentation and treatment of acquired hemolytic anemia will be reviewed.

Clinical and laboratory features of hemolytic anemia

The symptoms of acquired hemolytic anemia relate to the severity of the anemia and the rate of RBC destruction. Anemia may lead to cardiovascular symptoms such as dyspnea, angina and tachycardia; or nonspecific complaints of generalized malaise and dizziness. Rapid destruction of RBCs can be associated with fever, abdominal pain, back pain or limb pain, whereas patients with hemolytic anemia that develops gradually are often asymptomatic. Signs of anemia include dyspnea, pallor, jaundice and brown-discolored urine and in massive acute hemolysis, shock and renal failure can occur.

The laboratory tests useful for the diagnosis of acquired hemolytic anemia include peripheral blood film examination, reticulocyte count, direct antiglobulin test (Coombs' test), lactate dehydrogenase (LDH), bilirubin, aspartate aminotransferase (AST), haptoglobin, hemoglobinemia, methemalbumin and hemopexin, hemoglobinuria and

DOI: 10.1016/B978-0-7020-3147-2.00010-9

Table 10.1 Laboratory features of intravascular and extravascular hemolysis

	Intravascular	**Extravascular**
Serum bilirubin	Elevated	Elevated
Serum lactate dehydrogenase	Elevated	Elevated
Serum haptoglobin	Reduced or absent	Reduced or absent
Hemoglobinemia	Present	Absent (may be present with severe extravascular hemolysis)
Hemoglobinuria	Present	Absent
Urine hemosiderin	Present	Absent
Hemopexin-heme	Present	Absent (may be present with severe extravascular hemolysis)
Methemalbumin	Present	Absent
Morphology	Schistocytes, spherocytes, agglutination	Spherocytes, bite cells, blister cells, dense fragments, elliptocytes, ovalocytes, normal

hemosiderinuria. Bone marrow examination may be useful to uncover an underlying cause. The determination of RBC life span with radioactive isotope-labeled RBCs is rarely indicated. Laboratory tests can help determine whether the hemolytic anemia is occurring predominantly in the intravascular or extravascular space (Table 10.1). IgG-mediated autoimmune hemolysis is generally *extravascular* because the RBCs are destroyed by tissue macrophages in the spleen and liver. Hemolysis caused by malaria, major ABO blood group incompatibility, mechanical trauma to RBCs, thrombotic thrombocytopenic purpura (TTP) and paroxysmal nocturnal hemoglobinuria (PNH) is *intravascular* because RBC destruction occurs within the blood vessel.

Mechanisms of hemolysis

The principal mechanisms of hemolysis include:

1. Fc receptor (FcR)-mediated RBC clearance by phagocytic cells. This is the major mechanism in autoimmune and alloimmune hemolytic anemia syndromes which are primarily caused by IgG antibodies.
2. Complement-induced destruction of RBCs. This is the principal mechanism of RBC destruction caused by IgM antibodies, including some cases of drug-induced hemolysis.
3. Mechanical damage to the RBC membrane due to excess sheer forces, oxidative injury or temperature extremes.

FcR-mediated red cell clearance

Immunoglobulins and C3b on the RBC surface target these cells for destruction by macrophages in the spleen and less

frequently by Kupffer cells in the liver. These phagocytic cells express Fcγ receptors (FcγR) on their surface which bind to the Fc portion of IgG antibodies causing IgG-coated RBCs to be internalized and destroyed. Fcγ receptors are divided into three types depending on their structure, binding affinity and signalling ability: FcγRI (CD64), FcγRII (CD32) and FcγRIII (CD16). There are two extracellular immunoglobulin-like domains for FcγRII and FcγRIII, while FcγRI has three immunoglobulin-like domains. FcγRI mediates cytotoxic activity in vitro.[2] It is a 72 kDa high affinity receptor ($Ka = 10^8 - 10^9$ M^{-1}) capable of binding monomeric and multimeric IgG, preferentially IgG1 and IgG3; IgG3 is the most efficient IgG subclass in causing extravascular hemolysis in vivo.[3,4] FcγRI is expressed on monocytes, macrophages, neutrophils and dendritic cells and is required for antibody-dependent cell-mediated cytotoxicity (ADCC), endocytosis and phagocytosis,[5–8] the latter being an important mechanism of RBC destruction in IgG-mediated hemolytic anemia. Expression of FcγRI can be induced by interferon (IFN)-γ, tumor necrosis factor (TNF)-α or granulocyte colony-stimulating factor G-CSF.[9–12] The family of FcγRI receptors is further divided into FcγRIA, B and C each with different affinities for binding Fc (FcγRIA with the highest and FcγRIC with the lowest) and encoded by unique genes.

FcγRII is an inhibitory receptor and acts as a negative regulator of B-cell and mast cell activation.[13,14] FcγRII are low affinity receptors (Ka $<10^7$ M^{-1}) with molecular weights of 40–43 kDa and specificity for IgG1 and IgG3. Similar to FcγRI, FcγRII is divided into FcγRIIA, B and C. FcγRIIA is more widely distributed on platelets and immune cells such as monocytes, macrophages and neutrophils and delivers signals required for phagocytosis, ADCC and cellular activation.[15–17]

FcγRIIB is expressed on B-cells, basophils, mast cells, monocytes, macrophages and dendritic cells and functions as an inhibitory FcR by down-regulating downstream activation signals.[12,18,19] FcγRIIC is abundant on neutrophils.

FcγRIII receptors are highly glycosylated with molecular weights of 50–80 kDa. They bind multimeric IgG with an intermediate affinity (Ka $= 2 - 3 \times 10^7$ M^{-1}) and have the highest specificity for IgG1 and IgG3. The transmembrane form, FcγRIIIA, is found on monocytes, macrophages and eosinophils, and the GPI-linked FcγRIIIB is present on neutrophils and NK cells.[12,20,21]

A typical splenic macrophage has 30 000–40 000 FcR per cell.[22] As a result of infection or immunization the number and affinity of FcR are upregulated through cytokines such as IFN-γ,[23] which can worsen hemolysis if present. The density of FcR is also increased once IgG-coated RBCs become trapped in the spleen (and liver) and bind the FcR on the surface of phagocytes leading to receptor clustering. This effectively brings the cytoplasmic domains of multiple FcRs in close proximity, each of which share a common tyrosine-containing sequence motif called the immunoreceptor tyrosine-based activation motif (ITAM).[24] The tyrosine residues are phosphorylated by Src tyrosine kinase which creates Src homology 2 (SH2)-binding sites required for signal transduction involving other members of the tyrosine kinase family. A series of downstream signals leads to the internalization of the target cell and release of cytokines.[25–27]

The amount and type of antibodies bound to the RBC surface is a major determinant of hemolysis.[28] IgM may synergistically enhance IgG-mediated hemolysis, which is more severe when both IgG and IgM are present.[29] In addition, IgG3 subclass is a more efficient mediator of phagocytosis than IgG1. IgA autoantibodies are rarely associated with autoimmune hemolysis.

Complement-mediated red cell destruction

The complement system is made up of a number of plasma proteins most of which are zymogens proteases that are activated only after they have been cleaved by another enzyme (or convertase).[30,31] Many of the proteins in the complement system require calcium and activation of the complement system triggers a cascade that results in amplification of activating and inhibitory pathways[32] (Fig. 10.1).

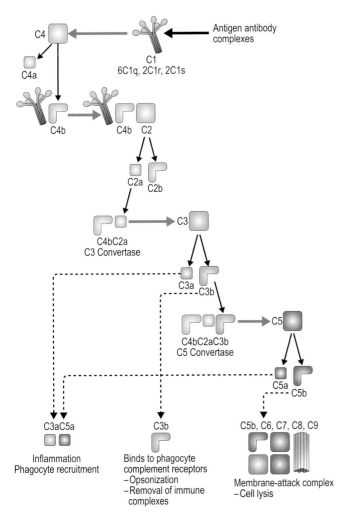

Fig. 10.1 The classical complement cascade. The complement cascade is composed of a number of proteases (zymogens) that are activated (red arrows) after they are bound to other specific proteins or have been cleaved by other enzymes (convertases). Activation of the complement cascade begins once C1q binds to the Fc portion of immunoglobulin on the target cell. Sequential progression (black arrows) and amplification of the remaining complement components results in the formation of the membrane attack complex (C5b6789) causing cell lysis. The released complement components, C3a and C5a, mediate inflammation and phagocyte recruitment. C3b down-regulates the complement cascade.

Once complement binds to RBCs, downstream events lead to the formation of the membrane attack complex and intravascular hemolysis. Complement binding is typically induced by IgM, and less frequently IgG antibodies on the surface of RBCs. Of the IgG antibodies IgG3 is most efficient at activating complement, followed by IgG1 and IgG2 (IgG4 does not). Only one bound IgM molecule is required to initiate complement activation, whereas multiple molecules of bound IgG are required. IgG dimers must be tethered within 30–40 nm (300 ångströms) of each other. The early breakdown products of complement, C3b and iC3b, are recognized by receptors on macrophages which act to contain complement activation; however, once the complement cascade proceeds to C3dg formation, the capacity for down-regulation is exceeded.[30]

The classical pathway of complement activation begins with binding of C1q to the Fc portion of immunoglobulin on the surface of the targeted cell, and ends with the formation of the membrane attack complex. C1q is a component of the calcium-dependent C1 complex along with two molecules of C1r and two molecules of C1s. C1q has six identical subunits with globular heads and long collagen-like tails, and upon binding to Fc induces a conformational change in the C1r:C1s complex.[31,33] This conformational change leads to activation of enzymatic C1r which then cleaves C1s generating an active serine protease. Activated C1s cleaves C4 producing C4b which can bind C2, anchoring it for cleavage by C1s and resulting in the production of C2a. The combined C4b2a remains covalently linked to antibody and is known as C3 convertase, the initiating factor of the classical complement pathway. C3 convertase cleaves C3; this generates C3b which covalently binds to the cell surface, and C3a which initiates a local inflammatory response. C3 is one of the most abundant proteins in plasma (1.2 mg/ml), thus providing a rich source of complement available for binding. C5 convertase (C4b2a3b) is formed by the binding of C3b to C4b2a complexes. C5 is bound to C3b and cleaved by the protease activity of C2a generating C5a and C5b.[32]

Once C5b is generated, a complex of C5b67 is formed. C7 undergoes conformational change and a hydrophobic site is exposed which inserts into the lipid bi-layer of the cell. Similarly once C8 and C9 are bound to this complex, they too bind through hydrophilic sites. C8β binds to C5b resulting in the hydrophilic domain of C8α-γ inserting into the bi-layer. C8α-γ also induces polymerization of 10–16 molecules of C9, ultimately forming the membrane-attack complex (C5b-9). The membrane-attack complex contains a hydrophobic external face allowing association with the lipid bi-layer and a hydrophobic internal channel allowing the free transport of solutes and water across the lipid bi-layer, effectively punching a hole in the target cell membrane and ultimately resulting in cell destruction.

There are two other pathways of complement activation: the lectin pathway and the alternative pathway. The lectin pathway occurs when proteins similar to C1q, such as mannose-binding lectin, activate the complement cascade. The alternative pathway results from spontaneous hydrolysis of C3 by a distinct C3 convertase, C3bBb, and does not need a pathogen-binding protein. The classical pathway is the major pathway of complement activation in hemolytic anemia.[32,34]

Complement regulation

Localization of complement activation to the cell surface ensures regulation of the complement cascade.[31,35] Complement activation is also controlled by inhibitor proteins including C1 inhibitor, a plasma serine protease (serpin). C1 inhibitor binds to C1r:C1s, dissociating these components from C1q, thus limiting the ability of C1s to cleave C4 and C2. Similar protective mechanisms are in place to prevent excess binding of C3 and C4. Specifically, factor I rapidly cleaves unbound C3b to iC3b (and then to C3bg), and C4b to the inactive proteins C4c and C4d. Membrane co-factor protein (MCP; CD46) acts as a co-factor for factor I by cleaving C3b and C4b, and decay-accelerating factor (DAF; CD55) also binds C3b to limit the extent of complement activation.[36] DAF also promotes dissociation of the C3 convertase. Complement receptor 1 (CR1) is another membrane-bound protein that regulates complement activation by binding complement-coated particles.[37] Other plasma co-factors which control C3 and C5 convertase include C4b-binding protein (C4bp) that cleaves C4b, and factor H and factor H-like protein 1 (FHL-1) that cleave C3b in the fluid phase.[38] Protective mechanisms including vitronectin (S-protein) and membrane inhibitor of reactive lysis (MILR; CD59) also control the insertion of the membrane-attack complex.[37,39,40]

Examples of complement-mediated hemolytic anemia

IgM anti-RBC antoantibodies: Cold reactive antibodies tend to be IgM and fix C3. They often show specificity for the Ii blood group system, expressed on the ABO precursor polysaccharides.[41] Binding of cold reactive autoantibodies to RBCs occurs in the peripheral circulation where temperatures are lower than the body core and may result in peripheral necrosis. Once the cells re-enter the warmer body core, the antibody dissociates but complement remains cell-bound leading to intravascular and/or extravascular hemolysis.[42]

Drug-induced hemolytic anemia: While most cases of drug-induced hemolysis are due to drug-dependent IgG antibodies (see later), IgM antoantibodies may also co-exist and cause intravascular hemolysis by fixing complement.[42]

Paroxysmal nocturnal hemoglobinuria (PNH): DAF (CD55) and MIRL (CD59) are linked to the cell surface by a phosphatidyl-inositol-glycerol (PIG) linkage. PNH is a syndrome caused by a somatic mutation in the PIG gene resulting in the functional failure of both DAF and MIRL,[43] thus rendering the cells susceptible to complement attack (discussed later).

Immune hemolytic anemia

Immune hemolytic anemia is the most common form of acquired hemolytic anemia and may be autoimmune, alloimmune or drug-induced. Autoimmune hemolytic anemia (AIHA) involves the premature destruction of RBCs by autoantibodies and may be secondary to underlying disorders such as malignancy, drugs, infection and connective tissue diseases.[44] RBC autoantibodies are *warm* or *cold*, based on the thermal range of activity.

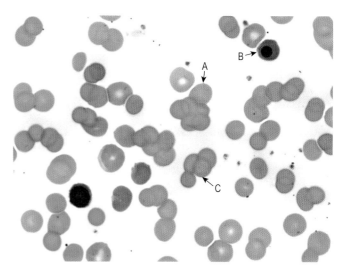

Fig. 10.2 Peripheral blood smear showing microspherocytosis (A), nucleated red cell (B) and red cell clumps (C) in a patient with immune-mediated hemolysis. The spherocytes lack a central halo of normal red cells and they are smaller than the nucleus of a normal lymphocyte. Wright stain. ×1000.

Warm autoimmune hemolytic anemia (AIHA)

Warm AIHA accounts for more than 70% of AIHAs[4] and is caused by IgG (particularly IgG1 and IgG3) directed against RBCs.[28] Warm AIHA generally results in extravascular hemolysis by FcR-mediated immune clearance and is characterized by spherocytes on the blood film (Fig. 10.2); however, some degree of intravascular hemolysis may occur simultaneously because of the properties of certain IgG autoantibodies or the co-existence of IgM autoantibodies.[29]

Specificity of IgG autoantibodies in AIHA

In initial serologic testing, most warm autoantibodies are panagglutinins, meaning that they react with all common RBCs. These panagglutinins can be classified into different categories based on Rh specificity: (1) antibodies that react with Rh-positive cells, but not Rh-null or partially deleted RhD cells; (2) antibodies that react with a specific part of the Rh antigen system and thus show reactivity with normal RhD antigens or partially deleted RhD antigens, but not Rh-null cells; and (3) antibodies that react to all cells including Rh-null cells.[45] Most warm autoantibodies (50–70%) show specificity for several antigens within the Rh antigen system;[46] in one series of 150 persons with warm autoantibodies, only four were specific to a single Rh antigen (i.e. anti-e or anti-c).[47] Because Rh antigens have a relatively low density on the RBC surface, autoantibodies against Rh do not cluster sufficiently to activate complement.

Up to 50% of warm autoantibodies with specificity for antigens other than Rh react with band 3 and glycophorin A.[48,49] Band 3, an anion transport protein, requires a portion of glycophorin A to form the Wright(b) [Wr(b)] antigen. Di(b), an antigen of Diego system, is also carried on protein band 3 but is an uncommon target for autoantibodies.[47] Decreased expression of certain blood group antigen, including Kell, Rh, MNS, Duffy, and the Kidd system[50,51] may occur with the development of autoantibodies. The mechanism of this phenomenon is unknown; however, it may imply that some RBC antigens protect against hemolysis.

Some warm autoantibodies appear to have specificity against RBC antigens, yet the antibodies can still be absorbed by RBC lacking the corresponding antigen. Even the eluates made from the RBCs used for this absorption procedure demonstrate specificity for that particular antigen. The cause of this 'pseudo-specificity' is unclear, but has been described for the Kell, Duffy, Kidd and MNS blood group systems.[50] Clinically, pseudo-specificity of the autoantibody is not directly associated with the severity of hemolysis, but it can cause confusion in the interpretation of serologic testing, especially when autoantibodies with real and pseudo-specificity co-exist.[50,52] This is of practical importance when selecting compatible blood for patients with warm autoimmune hemolytic anemia.

Diagnostic evaluation of a patient with suspected AIHA

The most useful test to detect warm antibodies is the direct antiglobulin test (DAT), or Coombs' test, using anti-IgG or anti-C3d polyclonal or monoclonal antibodies. However, the presence of antibodies and/or complement on the RBC surface does not necessarily indicate hemolysis and the strength of reactivity of the DAT is not related to clinical severity. A positive DAT without evidence of hemolysis occurs in about one per 10 000 healthy blood donors (usually IgG1). Both IgG and C3 are detected in 50% of such patients; IgG alone in 23% and C3 alone in 27%. Conversely, DAT-negative AIHA occurs in about 2% of patients with hemolysis, which may be explained by: (1) a low level of antibody sensitization; (2) hemolysis due to IgA or other immunoglobulins;[53,54] or (3) variable expression of RBC antigens during the course of disease.[55]

The lower limit of immunoglobulin detection using the DAT is estimated to be about 100–300 antibody molecules per cell.[56] Tests such as ^{125}I-radioimmune direct antiglobulin test,[57] enzyme-linked direct antiglobulin test,[58,59] two-stage immunoradiometric assay with ^{125}I-staphylococcal protein A,[60] or eluate concentration may increase the sensitivity of antibody detection;[4] however, the significance of these findings is uncertain.[61] Before the diagnosis of Coombs' negative autoimmune hemolytic anemia is made, other non-immune causes of hemolysis must be excluded.

In addition to detectable antibodies on the RBC surface, most patients with AIHA will have antibodies detectable in plasma (a positive *indirect* antiglobulin test); 57.4% of patients will have detectable antibodies on routine antibody screen, and up to 88.9% will have detectable antibody using enzyme-treated RBCs.[62] If the patient requires transfusion, the challenge is to uncover co-existing *allo*antibodies, which may be associated with transfusion reactions, using techniques such as autoabsorption or antibody titration.

Management of patients with warm AIHA

The goal of treatment for AIHA is to suppress autoantibody production; however, the effect of immunosuppressive therapy may be delayed. Transfusion of RBCs is often required until definitive therapy is achieved. Compatible RBC units for patients with severe hemolysis and RBC

antibodies may be difficult to obtain; thus, if clinically indicated, incompatible (or more precisely, the least *incompatible*) blood can be transfused with special care to avoid ABO and Rh incompatibility. The additional exposure to blood transfusion may further aggravate alloantibody formation;[50] however, transfusion therapy is still an important supportive measure in patients whose anemia has put them at risk of serious complications.

Corticosteroids are first line therapy for AIHA,[4] typically prednisone 1–1.5 mg/kg/day. The median time to response is 7–10 days. Mechanisms of steroid therapy include suppression of RBC clearance by the reticuloendothelial system,[63] down-regulation of FcR,[64] inhibition of release of lysosomal enzymes by macrophages and suppression of autoantibody production.[65] Corticosteroids can reduce the concentration of autoantibody, but have no effect on alloantibody production.[50] When hematologic improvement is seen, doses should be gradually reduced over several months to minimize complications of long-term corticosteroid use. In 60–70% of patients, complete remission can be achieved, but often maintenance therapy is required and up to 50% may relapse. If no response to corticosteroids is observed by the end of the first 3 weeks, continued therapy as sole treatment is usually ineffective. Up to 40% of patients with AIHA become dependent or resistant to corticosteroids.[66,67]

High-dose intravenous gamma-globulin (IVIg) results in improvement in hemolytic anemia in approximately 30–40% of patients.[68–76] It is less effective than for immune thrombocytopenia (ITP) and higher doses of IVIg may be required.[77] The therapeutic effect of IVIgG is usually short-lived, and further immunosuppressive therapy is often required to maintain clinical remission. The mechanism of action of IVIg therapy is likely FcR blockade,[78–81] although other mechanisms such as anti-idiotype antibodies,[78,82–84] interference with T-cell signaling and activation of T-suppressor cells,[85–88] inhibition of B-cell maturation[89–91] and dendritic-cell regulatory activity[92] have been described.

Splenectomy is effective in about half of patients with AIHA,[93] and like IVIg, is considerably less effective than in patients with ITP. Splenectomy removes the major site of antigen presentation and, in turn, reduces antibody production.[50,94] With the advance of laparoscopic splenectomy, the incidence of severe surgical complications has been significantly reduced;[95,96] however, infection, particularly with encapsulated organisms, occurs in up to 3% of patients;[97] therefore, vaccination against *Streptococcus pneumoniae*, *Neisseria meningitidis* and *Hemophilus influenzae type b* is recommended for all patients at least 2 weeks prior to splenectomy.

Immunosuppressive therapies, including vinca alkaloids, azathioprine and cyclophosphamide, are beneficial for up to 50% of patients with AIHA,[66] although the therapeutic effect may be delayed for 3–6 months and maintenance is often required. Danazol can induce long-lasting remissions in some patients;[98,99] possible mechanisms include reduction in RBC-bound C3d, immunomodulation by alteration of T-cell subsets and downregulation of FcR in the reticuloendothelial (RE) system.[100] Side-effects of danazol include virilization and dose-dependent hepatic toxicity.

Rituximab, a CD20 monoclonal antibody indicated for the treatment of lymphoma and rheumatoid arthritis, has been assessed in a variety of autoimmune disorders. In one report,

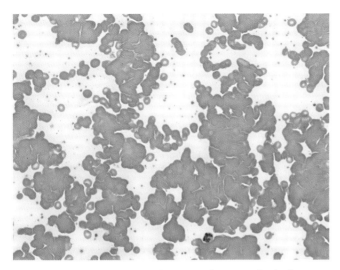

Fig. 10.3 Peripheral blood smear showing agglutination of red cells in a patient with Waldenström's macroglobulinemia and cold AIHA. The background of the smear is bluish because of high protein content, which contains IgM hemagglutinin. Wright stain. ×400.

25 of 27 (93%) patients with primary or secondary AIHA responded to a course of rituximab after a mean of 6 weeks (range 2–16 weeks).[101] Response was maintained in 18 (72%) patients after a mean of 21 months. Rituximab has been known to cause reactivation of hepatitis B[102] and has been linked to the development of progressive multifocal leukoencephalopathy (PML), a rare life-threatening demyelinating disease caused by reactivation of JC polyomavirus in the brain.[103]

Cold autoimmune hemolytic anemia

Cold AIHA (IgM-mediated), also known as cold agglutinin disease, is much less common than warm AIHA. The antibodies react best at cold temperatures (below 30°C). In a large prospective cohort study,[4] 391/2390 patients (16.4%) undergoing investigations for RBC autoantibodies had cold autoantibodies while another 10 patients (0.4%) had both warm and cold autoantibodies. In another series of patients with AIHA,[104] the co-existence of warm and cold autoantibodies was reported in 8% of patients. At room temperature, peripheral blood examination of patients with cold AIHA typically shows agglutination of RBCs (Fig. 10.3). Cold autoantibodies are mainly IgM (85%);[4] however, the IgG biphasic Donath–Landsteiner antibody accounts for approximately 15% of such autoantibodies, especially in children.[4,105]

Red cell sensitization by cold IgM usually occurs in the body extremities (e.g. fingers, ears, nose) where temperatures may fall below 30°C, allowing antibody binding to occur. The complement cascade is then activated, which may result in intravascular hemolysis, giving rise to the characteristic clinical features of Raynaud's phenomenon, acrocyanosis or gangrene; however, most patients with cold AIHA have mild symptoms or are asymptomatic. If the inhibitors of complement stop the cascade, RBCs (now coated with C3b) can be removed through extravascular phagocytosis. However, eventually C3b is degraded to C3d which does not induce clearance by reticuloendothelial tissues, but is detectable with the anti-C3d reagent used in the DAT. The most common antibody specificity is the I ('big I') blood group antigen, typical following *Mycoplasma pneumoniae* infection; anti-i ('little i') is often associated with infectious mononucleosis. Other less frequent specificities include P, Pr, A1, D, Vo, Gd (glycolipid dependent gangliosides),[106] Lud,[107] F1,[108] Ju and IA.[4,109] Specificity will be apparent at temperatures between 15 and 20°C. Clinically, the specificity of the antibody is less important than its thermal amplitude.

Thermal range and titer of cold agglutinins is readily demonstrated in the laboratory. Addition of albumin to tests of thermal range improves clinical correlation. The presence of a cold agglutinin often causes problems with ABO and Rh phenotype cross-matching, which can be overcome by washing the RBCs with warm saline. The cross-match and antibody screen should be done using a prewarmed sample and monospecific anti-IgG to avoid false positive reactions. The DAT, using monoclonal reagents, is usually negative for IgG and positive for C3d from an ethylene diamine tetra-acetic acid (EDTA) sample.

Cold avoidance is the cornerstone of management of patients with cold agglutinin disease. Corticosteroids and alkylating agents are usually ineffective, and the likelihood of remission with splenectomy is low. Plasmapheresis can be used to treat acute hemolytic episodes since it effectively removes the IgM autoantibody; this is best performed in a warm environment with prewarmed tubing and equipment. Blood transfusion, when needed, is infused at room temperature; it remains controversial whether a blood warmer offers additional benefit. If cold AIHA is secondary to an underlying neoplastic disease, chemotherapy including alkylating agents may reduce the production of cold autoantibody. Preliminary observations with rituximab are encouraging, resulting in an increase in hemoglobin concentration by 4 g/dl and a decrease in IgM levels in 54% of patients.[110,111]

Paroxysmal cold hemoglobinuria

Paroxysmal cold hemoglobinuria (PCH) was one of the first recognized anemias described in the mid-1800s.[109] For years, PCH was believed to be a rare form of acquired AIHA associated with congenital syphilis. It then became recognized that PCH caused up to 40% of acute transient hemolytic anemia in young children[112] during viral infections such as measles, mumps, chickenpox and influenza. Due to the transient nature of the disease, establishing the diagnosis is often difficult. The biphasic IgG antibody (Donath–Landsteiner antibody) is directed against globoside glycosphingolipid (P antigen) and causes hemolysis by a unique mechanism: the antibody binds to RBCs in the cooler temperatures of the peripheral circulation and activates complement causing intravascular hemolysis when RBCs return to the warmer body core. Donath–Landsteiner antibodies are more potent than IgM cold agglutinins in initiating intravascular hemolysis because they retain their binding affinity even when the RBCs return to warmer temperatures.[44,113] IgG3 is the major immunoglobulin subclass for Donath–Landsteiner antibodies.[114]

Direct and indirect Donath–Landsteiner tests establish the diagnosis of PCH.[115] The direct test is done by incubating a whole blood sample at 0°C for 1 h, and then at 37°C for an additional 30 min. If the Donath–Landsteiner antibody is present, it will bind to RBC during the cold incubation phase and lyse the cells during the warm phase. As a control, a whole blood sample maintained at 37°C should show no evidence of hemolysis. The indirect test is done by mixing the patient's serum with ABO compatible P-positive RBCs in the presence of fresh serum as a source of complement. The indirect test has a much higher sensitivity than the direct test because of: (1) the addition of a complement source; (2) the ability to adjust the serum to cell ratio; and (3) the increased susceptibility of donor RBCs to lyse (compared with patient cells, which are coated with C3d). The sensitivity of the test can be increased further by using enzyme-treated RBCs. False positive results occur with IgM hemolytic antibodies with a high thermal range. False negative results may be seen with low antibody titers or if soluble globoside (P antigen) is present in the added fresh normal serum.[105]

The management of PCH may require urgent blood transfusion depending on the level of anemia and clinical symptoms. Theoretically, P antigen-negative RBCs may minimize *in vivo* hemolysis; however, P-negative blood is usually not available and the transfusion of P-positive RBCs can be beneficial. Transfusions should be administered slowly while the patient is kept warm.[116] Neither washing RBCs[117] (to remove complement proteins in donor plasma) nor corticosteroid therapy have been shown to be effective in PCH.[105]

Alloimmune hemolytic anemia

Alloimmune hemolytic anemia occurs when antibodies form in response to foreign RBC alloantigens. Typically, this occurs following a blood transfusion, pregnancy or hematopoietic stem cell transplantation. Exposure to environmental antigens (unrelated to erythrocytes) can also lead to sensitization but these antibodies are typically IgM with low thermal activity (i.e. anti-M, anti-N, anti-S, or anti-P_1) and are unlikely to cause hemolysis.

Transfusion reactions due to immune-mediated hemolysis

The incidence of clinically relevant immune-mediated hemolytic reactions due to ABO incompatibility is estimated to occur approximately once per 40 000 RBC transfusions.[118] Subclinical hemolysis is more common and the severity of the reaction depends on the amount of antibody on the RBC surface, the degree of complement activation and the affinity for FcR binding in reticuloendothelial tissues.

Immune-mediated hemolysis following blood transfusion may be acute or delayed. More than 80% of acute hemolytic transfusion reactions are caused by ABO incompatible RBC transfusions.[119] Although fewer than 10% of ABO incompatible transfusions result in a fatal outcome, mortality increases with larger volumes of incompatible blood and prolonged delays in recognition of the clinical syndrome. Transfusion reactions characterized by intravascular hemolysis are generally more severe than extravascular hemolytic reactions. IgM antibodies to ABO antigens are the classic example, but some IgG alloantibodies, including anti-Kell, anti-Kidd and anti-Duffy antibodies, can also fix complement and cause intravascular hemolysis.[119–121] Patients may experience fever, chills, joint pain, shock, renal failure and/or disseminated intravascular coagulation (DIC).

Delayed hemolytic transfusion reactions are typically caused by an increase in pre-formed IgG antibodies following re-exposure to a RBC antigen (anamnestic response). The increase in IgG titer generally occurs 7–14 days after the transfusion which coincides with the timing of hemolysis. Although most patients have been previously alloimmunized through a transfusion in the past, over time antibody levels fall below detection limits prior to the next transfusion; consequently, it is difficult to prevent this type of transfusion reaction.[50] The severity of delayed hemolytic transfusion reactions ranges from asymptomatic DAT-positivity only, to severe intravascular hemolysis as seen with anti-Kidd antibodies.

Differentiating immune hemolytic transfusion reactions from other types of transfusion reactions can be difficult. Similar clinical syndromes can occur with pseudo (or non-immune) hemolytic transfusion reactions whereby transfused RBCs are subject to excessive thermal, osmotic, mechanical or chemical injury.[120] Febrile non-hemolytic transfusion reactions and bacterial contamination of blood products may also mimic hemolytic reactions. Hypotension and shock may also occur in transfusion-related acute lung injury or severe allergic symptoms.

Hemolytic disease of the newborn

Hemolytic disease of the newborn (HDN) is characterized by hemolysis in the fetus caused by transplacental transfer of maternal IgG directed against fetal RBC antigens. Maternal sensitization typically occurs at delivery or after minor trauma during pregnancy, including amniocentesis, resulting in subclinical alloimmunization. In subsequent pregnancies, the secondary immune response may trigger the production of high titer IgG antibodies detectable in the fetal circulation as early as 12 weeks' gestation.[50] Hence, HDN caused by RhD incompatibility seldom affects the first pregnancy but typically becomes progressively more severe with subsequent pregnancies. Conversely, HDN caused by ABO incompatibility may affect the firstborn infant since ABO antibodies are pre-formed, and a previously affected child is not predictive of recurrence.[50] The transplacental transfer of maternal IgG is mediated by specific FcRs on placental cells and the rate of IgG transfer increases progressively with gestational age.[50,122,123]

Erythroblastosis fetalis is the most severe outcome in HDN characterized by edema, gross hepatosplenomegaly, portal hypertension and hepatic failure due to fetal anemia and extramedullary erythropoiesis,. More commonly, the affected fetus may present only with hyperbilirubinemia and anemia within the first 24 h of life which may progress to kernicterus unless proper treatment is instituted. Laboratory evidence of HDN without clinical findings are often described as maternal–fetal blood group incompatibility.[50]

Antibodies against Rh antigens used to be the most important cause of HDN; however, routine screening and prevention has decreased the frequency of anti-RhD HDN by 95%[124] such that currently anti-ABO and anti-Kell antibodies are more frequent causes.[125] Universal screening of pregnant women allows the identification of Rh-negative women in their first trimester who are at risk of forming antibodies.

Those women receive passive immunization with Rh immune globulin (RhIg) at approximately 28 weeks' gestation and again within 72 h of delivery. RhIg should also be given after invasive procedures therapeutic abortions or any fetal-maternal hemorrhage. Approximately 10 μg of RhIg is required to neutralize a 1 ml fetal-maternal hemorrage. The Kleihauer–Betke test or flow cytometry can be used to assess the volume of fetal cells in the maternal circulation. The efficacy of RhIg in preventing HDN is estimated to be approximately 95%. In addition to RhIg prophylaxis, Rh-negative women of childbearing potential should receive Rh-negative blood transfusions to avoid Rh sensitization.

The prenatal management of women at risk of HDN varies. For Rh-negative women without known anti-RBC antibodies, an antibody screening should be performed at the first prenatal visit and again at week 28 weeks when RhIg is given.[126] If a RBC alloantibody is detected early in the pregnancy, antibody testing should be repeated at regular intervals to detect a rising antibody titer.[127] If the antibody titer increases significantly (usually 1 : 16 or higher), other measurements are required to estimate the degree of fetal anemia including: (1) ultrasonography to detect the evidence of extramedullary hematopoiesis;[128,129] (2) amniocentesis to measure total bile pigment in the amniotic fluid;[130] and/or (3) percutaneous umbilical blood sampling to measure fetal hemoglobin concentration.[131] A recent advance in noninvasive testing is the measurement of the peak systolic velocity in the middle cerebral artery by fetal ultrasonography[132] which has been shown to be as predictive of fetal anemia as amniocentesis.[133]

Antenatal treatment of mothers aimed at preventing fetal morbidity and mortality from severe HDN include IVIg, starting at week 10–12, given at a dose of 1 g/kg every 1–3 weeks until delivery. For women with affected infants discovered early in pregnancy, maternal plasmapheresis may be useful until the 24th week of gestation at which time intrauterine transfusion can be performed; however, this procedure requires personnel with specialized training because of the risk of fetal hemorrhage and adverse pregnancy outcomes. Donor blood should be blood group O (or ABO specific), fresh, irradiated, cytomegalovirus (CMV)-negative and antigen-negative.[50] Preterm induction of delivery is usually done around week 35. After delivery, phototherapy and/or exchange transfusion may be used to reduce hyperbilirubinemia and the risk of kernicterus. IVIg has been shown to reduce the need for exchange transfusion in affected newborns.[134] If the infant is severely anemic, small volume transfusion may be required during the first few months of life.

Drug-induced immune hemolytic anemia

Drug-induced hemolytic anemia occurs in 1 in 1 million individuals.[135] Although rare, many drugs have been implicated (Table 10.2). In 1980 the most common cause of drug-induced immune hemolytic anemia was α-methyldopa followed by penicillin; currently, second and third generation cephalosporins, in particular cefotetan and ceftriaxone, are the most commonly implicated drugs. Drug-induced antibodies can be *drug-independent*, indistinguishable from autoantibodies, or *drug-dependent* if the addition of the drug is required for antibody detection *in vitro*.[135] Some drugs cause both drug-independent and drug-dependent

antibodies; examples are phenacetin, streptomycin, and non-steroidal anti-inflammatories.[136–139] Table 10.3 describes the principle mechanisms by which drugs can cause hemolysis. A detailed drug history is essential for any patients with hemolytic anemia, and demonstration of drug-dependent antibodies in vitro is confirmatory (although not widely available).

Drug-independent antibodies

Drug-independent antibodies have the same chacteristics of idiopathic AIHA, and while the precise pathogenesis is unknown, presumably the drug induces an autoimmune response possibly through the inhibition of suppressor T-cell function.[140] Such drug-induced autoantibodies have been associated with cladribine, fludarabine, procainamide, mefenamic acid, levodopa and α-methyldopa.

True autoantibody induction by α-methyldopa provides a human model for studying the mechanism underlying autoimmune disorders. Even though it is one of the most extensively studied drug reactions, the exact mechanism of α-methyldopa-induced autoantibody formation is still unclear. Up to 20% of patients on α-methyldopa develop a positive DAT; however, only 0.3–0.8% are associated with hemolysis.[141] Kelton et al.[142] showed that patients with a positive DAT, but without hemolysis, have significant impaired retriculoendothelial cell function. The development of a positive DAT in patients on α-methyldopa depends on the dose and duration of therapy; typically patients have been exposed to the drug continuously for 3 years or more.[143] Hemolysis resolves once the drug is stopped, although the serologic abnormalities resolve more gradually. The autoantibody induced by α-methyldopa is IgG and, in many patients, shows specificity for Rh antigens.[138,144,145] Other autoantibodies may co-exist including antinuclear antibody, rheumatoid factor and factor VIII inhibitor.[146]

Drug-dependent antibody

Drug-dependent antibodies can be classified according to their binding characteristics in the presence of the drug. Hapten type antibodies react with drug-treated RBCs and are inhibited by the addition of soluble drug; and 'immune complex type' or 'neoantigen type' antibodies are those that only react with RBCs in the presence of the drug.[135] Drugs associated with the *hapten-type* of reaction, including penicillins and cephalosporins, bind covalently to the RBC membrane and are not easily washed off *in vitro*. Only rarely will these antibodies cause overt hemolysis, which is usually extravascular.[147] Penicillin-induced hemolytic anemia typically occurs in patients treated with high-dose penicillin for 7–14 days intravenously, or in patients with renal failure and reduced drug clearance.[50,148] Drugs associated with the *immune complex* type of reaction, including ceftriaxone and quinine/quinidine, do not bind covalently to the RBC membrane but induce antibodies that bind to RBCs, activate complement and cause severe intravascular hemolysis. These antibodies are either adsorbed onto the RBC surface or bind a neoantigen which may be independent of the drug, or may include a portion of the drug and the RBC membrane. In addition, immunoglobulins (and other proteins) can be adsobed nonspecifically onto the surface of drug-treated

Table 10.2 Drugs associated with hemolytic anemia and/or positive direct antiglobulin test *(from Arndt and Garraty, Seminars in Hematology 2005;42:137–144, reproduced with permission)*

Aceclofenac	Diphenylhydantoin	p-Aminosalicylic acid
Acetaminophen	Dipyrone	Penicillin G
Aminopyrine/pyramidon	Erythromycin	Phenacetin
Amoxicillin	Etodolac	Piperacillin
Amphotericin B	Fenoprofen	Probenacid
Ampicillin	Fludarabine	Procainamide
Antazoline	Fluorescein	Propyhenazone
Butizide	Fluoroquinolones (e.g. temafloxacin)	Quinidine
Carbenicillin	Fluorouracil	Quinine
Carbimazole	Glafenine	Ranitidine
Carboplatin	Hydrochlorothiazide	Rifampicin
Carbromal	9-hydroxy-methyl-ellipticinium	Sodium Pentothal/thiopental
Catergen/cyanidanol	Ibuprofen	Stibophen
Cefamandole	Indene derivatives (e.g. sulindac)	Streptokinase
Cefazolin	Insulin	Streptomycin
Cefixime	Interferon	Sulbactam sodium
Cefotaxime	Interleukin-2	Sulindac
Cefotetan	Isoniazid	Sulfonamides
Cefoxitin	Latamoxef	Sulfasalazide
Ceftazidime	Levodopa	Sulfonylurea derivatives (e.g. chlorpropamide and tolbutamide)
Ceftizoxime	Mefenamic acid	Suprofen
Ceftriaxone	Mefloquine	Tazobactam sodium
Cephalexin	Melphalan	Teicoplanin
Cephaloridine	6-Mercaptopurine	Temafloxacin
Cephalothin	Methicillin	Teniposide
Chlordiazepoxide	Methotrexate	Tetracycline
Chlorinated hydrocarbons	Methyldopa	Ticarcillin
Chlorpromazine	Metrizoate-based radiographic contrast media	Tolbutamide
Chlorpropamide	Naficillin	Tolmetin
Cianidanol	Nomifensine	Triamterene
Cisplatin	Norfloxacin	Trimetallic anhydride
Cladribine	Oxaliplatin	Zomepiric
Clavulanate potassium		
Diclofenac		
Diethylstilbestrol		

Table 10.3 Principal mechanisms, laboratory features and clinical manifestations of drug-induced hemolytic anemia

Mechanism of hemolysis (drug examples)	Direct antiglobulin test	Details of reaction and *in vitro* testing	Clinical manifestations
Drug adsorption (e.g. penicillin)	Positive for IgG, C3d*	Antibody reacts with drug-coated RBCs. Eluates react only with drug-coated RBCs.	Moderate degree of hemolysis; usually extravascular.
Drug-dependent antibody (e.g. cefotetan)	Positive for C3d	Antibody reacts with RBCs only when drug is present. Antibody is IgG or IgM. Eluates react with RBCs only when drug is present	Abrupt onset of severe intravascular hemolysis. Renal failure.
Autoimmune induction (e.g. α-methyldopa)	Positive for IgG	Auto-antibodies against RBCs. Eluate reacts with RBCs.	Mild-to-moderate degree of extravascular hemolysis.
Direct damage to membrane (e.g. copper, sulpha drugs in G6PD deficiency)	Negative	Oxidative damage to RBC membrane.	Intravascular hemolysis which may be acute.

*Present in approximately 40% of penicillin-induced immune hemolytic anemia. C3d, cleavage product of complement component 3; DAT, direct antiglobulin test; IgG, immunoglobulin G; IgM, immunoglobulin M; RBC, red blood cell.

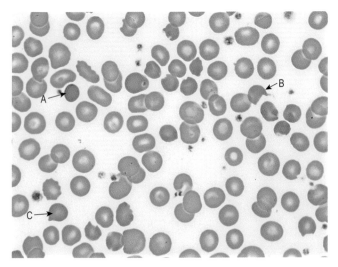

Fig. 10.4 Peripheral blood smear showing spherocytosis (A), bite cells (B) and blister cells (ghost cells) (C) in a patient with drug-induced oxidative hemolysis. Wright stain. × 1000.

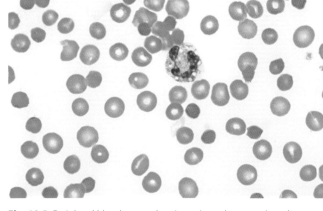

Fig. 10.5 Peripheral blood smear showing microspherocytosis and cytoplasmic vacuolation in neutrophils in a patient with clostridial infection. Wright stain. × 1000.

RBCs which not only causes a positive direct antiglobulin test *in vivo*,[149] but may be associated with hemolysis.[150]

Oxidative injury to red cells

Some drugs and industrial toxins (e.g. copper and arsine) directly damage the RBC membrane or induce oxidative changes in the cells by non-immune mechanisms. RBCs are also prone to oxidation and denaturation because of the rich oxygen content of hemoglobin, if the anti-oxidative protective mechanisms of the RBC are overwhelmed. The amount of oxidative hemolysis is determined by the strength and concentration of the oxidant, and the integrity of the glucose-6-phosphate dehydrogenase (G6PD) and glutathione-dependent pathways. The characteristic features of oxidative hemolysis include the formation of methemoglobin, sulfhemoglobin and Heinz bodies. Clinically, methemoglobin and sulfhemoglobin may present as bluish discoloration indistinguishable from cyanosis. Heinz bodies are the microscopic appearance of denatured hemoglobin. Moreover, examination of a peripheral blood smear may also reveal 'bite cells',[151] blister cells[120] and eccentrocytes[151] (Fig. 10.4). Bite cells are semicircular remnants of RBCs that remain after being partially phagocytosed or after extrusion of the Heinz body.[152] If the denatured hemoglobin shifts to one side of the RBC, the cell is called a blister cell, which is usually an indicator of brisk hemolysis. Drugs that can cause oxidative hemolysis include nitrofurantoin, amniosalicylic acid, dapsone and pyridium (phenazopyridine). Rarely, high-dose oxygen therapy can result in oxidative injury to RBCs, particularly in patients with vitamin E deficiency.[119,121,153]

Non-immune hemolytic anemia

Infection-induced hemolytic anemia

Microorganisms may cause injury to RBCs by various mechanisms including: (1) physical invasion of RBCs (e.g. malaria); (2) hemolysin secretions leading to direct RBC damage (e.g.

Clostridium perfringens) (Fig. 10.5); (3) infection that triggers formation of antibody (anti-I) against RBCs (e.g. *Mycoplasma*); (4) microangiopathic hemolysis caused by DIC; or (5) hemolytic complications of antibiotic drugs. In some cases, multiple mechanisms co-exist, which often poses a diagnostic challenge.

Mechanical injury to red cells

Mechanical injury to RBCs can occur with excessive shear forces due to a high-pressure gradient in the circulation, direct external impact and microangiopathic hemolysis.[154] On examination of a peripheral blood smear, burr cells and schistocytes of variable shapes, such as crescents, helmets, microspherocytes and fragments, are apparent; this is commonly called schistocytic hemolytic anemia (Fig. 10.6). Other non-specific features include aniso-poikilocytosis, polychromatic macrocytosis, thrombocytopenia and/or procoagulant activation.

Schistocytic hemolytic anemia can be classified according to the size of the blood vessels where hemolysis occurs. Schistocytic hemolytic anemia may occur in large vessels as a result of malignant hypertension or prosthetic heart valves. Small-vessel schistocytic hemolytic anemia, also called microangiopathic hemolytic anemia, occurs in march hemoglobinuria, autoimmune vasculitis, DIC, and thrombotic thrombocytopenic purpura–hemolytic uremic syndrome (TTP-HUS).

Thrombotic thrombocytopenic purpura–hemolytic uremic syndrome

In 1924, Moschowitz identified what is now called thrombotic thrombocytopenic purpura (TTP) in a 16-year-old girl; hemolytic uremic syndrome (HUS) was first described by Gasser in 1955. Only about half of patients present with the full pentad of symptoms (thrombocytopenia, anemia, renal impairment, fever and neurological dysfunction) and the diagnosis should be suspected in any patient with thrombocytopenia and schistocytic anemia. Renal failure is more

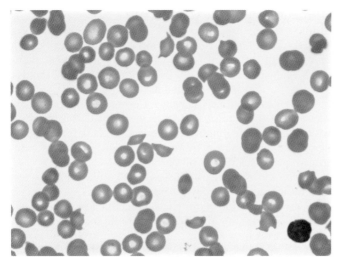

Fig. 10.6 Peripheral blood smear showing fragments of red cells and thrombocytopenia in a patient with thrombotic thrombocytopenic purpura. The size of red cells is approximately equal to the size of the nucleus in a non-reactive lymphocyte. Similar features may be present in patients with hemolytic uremic syndrome or microangiopathic hemolysis. Wright stain. ×1000.

common in classic HUS, while neurological symptoms including hemiparesis, aphasia, seizure, fluctuating mental function and coma are typically associated with TTP. Because of the overlap in the clinical and pathologic features, TTP and HUS may actually represent a spectrum of the same disorder. TTP usually occurs sporadically in adults while HUS typically occurs in children following a diarrheal illness caused by enterotoxin-producing *Escherichia coli* (OH157). TTP may occur in association with: vaccinations; drugs (e.g. quinine, quinidine, ticlopidine and mithramycin); pregnancy; collagen vascular disease; human immunodeficiency virus (HIV); malignancy such as adenocarcinoma; and bone marrow transplantation. Secondary TTP is often resistant to treatment.

The pathogenesis of TTP involves a deficiency of the enzyme ADAMTS13 (*A Disintegrin And Metalloprotease with ThromboSpondin-1-like repeats*). ADAMTS13 is the enzyme responsible for cleaving large multimers of von Willebrand factor (VWF) as they exit the Weibel–Palade bodies in endothelial cells. When ADAMTS13 is deficient (usually defined as <5% of normal), abnormally large multimers of VWF are formed and cause disseminated platelet-rich thrombi,[155] which lead to microvascular ischemia. Mutations in ADAMTS13 have been uncovered in patients with familial TTP[156] and decreased levels, either as a result of congenital deficiency or anti-ADAMTS13 antibodies have been implicated in the familial and the acquired forms. Not all patients with TTP have low levels of ADAMTS13 or functional anti-ADAMTS13 antibodies, and ADAMTS13 deficiency has been observed in other disorders.[157]

Without definitive treatment, mortality of patients with TTP exceeds 90%; however, if treated promptly, mortality is reduced to approximately 20%. The primary treatment is plasma exchange with fresh frozen or VWF-poor (cryosupernatant) plasma[158] using 1–1.5 times the plasma volume for the exchange. Plasma infusion is less effective than plasma exchange[159] likely because less plasma volume is being replaced.[160] Periodic plasma infusion has been used in familial TTP patients. Neurological symptoms may recover within hours after plasmapheresis and LDH and thrombocytopenia usually normalize within days. If possible, platelet transfusions should be avoided in patients with TTP or HUS, although evidence for harm from platelet transfusions in patients with TTP has recently been questioned.[161] Antiplatelet therapy such as aspirin, ticlopidine or dipyridamole may be considered when the platelet count is above $50 \times 10^9/l$; however, evidence is lacking in support of this practice. Evidence for corticosteroids derives from anecdotal reports and one retrospective study;[162] and IVIG, splenectomy and vincristine should be reserved for refractory or resistant TTP patients.

In non-randomized studies, rituximab has been used to treat patients with refractory and or relapsing TTP with remarkable success. In a review of 73 TTP patients treated with rituximab, 95% achieved a complete remission within weeks of the first dose.[163] Relapse-free survival was 10 months, reflecting the short duration of follow-up. Propsective studies of the use of rituximab for TTP are ongoing.

Over 90% of all childhood HUS is caused by Shiga toxin-producing enterohemorrhagic *E. coli* or invasive pneumococcal infection. The remainder are mostly associated with disorders of complement regulation, usually due to mutations in complement factor H, factor I or membrane co-factor protein; or precipitated by other conditions such as pregnancy, HIV or malignancy. Most patients with acute HUS survive; however, long-term complications include hypertension and chronic renal failure.[164]

Cardiac valve hemolysis

Almost any intracardiac lesion that alters the hemodynamics and generates excessive shear force can cause intravascular hemolysis. Traumatic hemolysis may occur after cardiac surgery such as heart valve replacement or repair. Synthetic material, small valvular area, and complications such as thrombotic valve and perivalvular leaks increase the risk of significant hemolysis. Hemolysis also occurs in patients with native valvular lesions including severe aortic stenosis, coarctation of aorta and ruptured aneurysm of the sinus of Valsalva. In addition, aortofemoral bypass has been associated with traumatic hemolysis.[154]

External impact on red cells

March hemoglobinuria, a well-described but uncommon condition of intravascular hemolysis, typically occurs after strenuous marching or running on a hard surface in susceptible individuals who wear thin-soled shoes. There is usually no underlying intrinsic erythrocyte abnormality. In patients with extensive burn injuries, RBC denaturation and fragmentation occur because of thermal damage. Hemolysis due to osmotic damage of RBCs may occur in fresh water or salt water drowning because of abrupt osmotic changes in the pulmonary circulation.

Other causes of hemolytic anemia

Paroxysmal nocturnal hemoglobinuria (PNH). PNH is a rare clonal hematopoietic stem cell disease characterized by bone marrow failure, hemolytic anemia, smooth muscle dystonias and thrombosis.[165] The disease arises from an acquired mutation the *PIG-A* gene located on the X chromosome (Xp22.1), which encodes for glycosyl phosphatidylinositol (GPI), a glycoplipid moiety that anchors a number of proteins to the plasma membranes of cells.[166] Without this anchor, many surface proteins are missing,[167] including CD55 and CD59, key complement regulatory proteins, thus rendering PNH erythrocytes susceptible to complement-mediated hemolysis. CD55 inhibits C3 convertase and CD59 blocks the formation of the membrane attack complex. The diagnosis of PNH uses flow cytometry to demontrate a combined deficiency of CD55 and CD59 on granulocytes, monocytes or erythrocytes. Characteristically, patients with PNH have a hypoplastic bone marrow in spite of significant hemolysis. PNH can arise de novo or in the setting of aplastic anemia.[168]

Treatment of PNH should generally be reserved for symptomatic patients with transfusion dependence, thrombosis or other symptoms such as disabling fatigue or pain paroxysms. The only curative therapy is hematopoietic stem cell transplantation;[169] however, recently, the complement inhibitor eculizumab, a humanized monoclonal antibody against complement protein C5, has been approved for PNH based on results of two phase 3 clinical trials.[170,171] Eculizumab resulted in stabilization of hemoglobin and transfusion independence in approximately 50% of patients, reduction in intravascular hemolysis and improvements of anemia and quality of life. The treatment is given intravenously at a dose of 600 mg weekly for the first 4 weeks, then 900 mg every second week indefinitely. Inhibition of C5 increases the risk of neisserial infections; thus all patients should be vaccinated against *N. meningitidis*. Even with vaccination, the risk of neisserial sepsis is estimated at 0.5% per year.[165]

Venom-induced hemolytic anemia. Cobras, pit vipers, spiders such as *Loxosceles* (also known as violin spider), and black widow spiders (belonging to *Latrodectus* genus), produce a hemolytic venom that activates coagulation and causes widespread intravascular hemolysis.[172]

Wilson's disease. Wilson's disease is a condition characterized by the accumulation of copper in body organs and is associated with acute hemolytic anemia due to excess copper in the blood stream. The diagnosis should be considered in a patient with liver dysfunction and neuropsychiatric symptoms. Occular Kayser–Fleischer rings are pathognomonic of Wilson's disease. Treatment with penicillamine can halt the hemolysis.

Acknowledgments

We thank Andrew McFarlane for his expert input on laboratory test for hemolysis, James Smith for his help with the tables and figures, Aurelio Santos for his help with the illustrations and Genie Leblanc for administrative support.

References

1. Mack P, Freedman J. Autoimmune hemolytic anemia: a history. Transfus Med Rev 2000;14(3):223–33.

2. Davis W, Harrison PT, Hutchinson MJ, Allen JM. Two distinct regions of FC gamma RI initiate separate signalling pathways involved in endocytosis and phagocytosis. EMBO J 1995;14(3):432–41.

3. Von dem Borne AE, Beckers D, van der Meulen FW, Engelfriet CP. IgG4 autoantibodies against erythrocytes, without increased haemolysis: a case report. Br J Haematol 1977;37(1):137–44.

4. Engelfriet CP, Overbeeke MA, Von dem Borne AE. Autoimmune hemolytic anemia. Semin Hematol 1992;29(1):3–12.

5. Allen JM, Seed B. Isolation and expression of functional high-affinity Fc receptor complementary DNAs. Science 1989;243(4889):378–81.

6. Ernst LK, Van de Winkel JG, Chiu IM, Anderson CL. Three genes for the human high affinity Fc receptor for IgG (Fc gamma RI) encode four distinct transcription products. J Biol Chem 1992;267(22):15692–700.

7. Peltz G, Frederick K, Anderson CL, Peterlin BM. Characterization of the human monocyte high affinity Fc receptor (hu FcRI). Mol Immunol 1988;25(3):243–50.

8. Van de Winkel JG, Ernst LK, Anderson CL, Chiu IM. Gene organization of the human high affinity receptor for IgG, Fc gamma RI (CD64). Characterization and evidence for a second gene. J Biol Chem 1991;266(20):13449–55.

9. Fischer G, Schneider EM, L Moldawer LL, et al. CD64 surface expression on neutrophils is transiently upregulated in patients with septic shock. Intensive Care Med 2001;27(12):1848–52.

10. Kerst JM, Van de Winkel JG, Evans AH, et al. Granulocyte colony-stimulating factor induces hFc gamma RI (CD64 antigen)-positive neutrophils via an effect on myeloid precursor cells. Blood 1993;81(6):1457–64.

11. Uciechowski P, Schwarz M, Gessner JE, et al. IFN-gamma induces the high-affinity Fc receptor I for IgG (CD64) on human glomerular mesangial cells. Eur J Immunol 1998;28(9):2928–35.

12. Van de Winkel JG, Capel PJ. Human IgG Fc receptor heterogeneity: molecular aspects and clinical implications. Immunol Today 1993;14(5):215–21.

13. Daeron M, Latour S, Malbec O, et al. The same tyrosine-based inhibition motif, in the intracytoplasmic domain of Fc gamma RIIB, regulates negatively BCR-, TCR-, and FcR-dependent cell activation. Immunity 1995;3(5):635–46.

14. Muta T, Kurosaki T, Misulovin Z, et al. A 13-amino-acid motif in the cytoplasmic domain of Fc gamma RIIB modulates B-cell receptor signalling. Nature 1994;369(6478):340.

15. Kiener PA, Rankin BM, Burkhardt AL, et al. Cross-linking of Fc gamma receptor I (Fc gamma RI) and receptor II (Fc gamma RII) on monocytic cells activates a signal transduction pathway common to both Fc receptors that involves the stimulation of p72 Syk protein tyrosine kinase. J Biol Chem 1993;268(32):24442–8.

16. Edberg JC, Lin CT, Lau D, et al. The Ca2+ dependence of human Fc gamma receptor-initiated phagocytosis. J Biol Chem 1995;270(38):22301–7.

17. Indik ZK, Park JG, Hunter S, Schreiber AD. The molecular dissection of Fc gamma receptor mediated phagocytosis. Blood 1995;86(12):4389–99.

18. Cassel DL, Keller MA, Surrey S, et al. Differential expression of Fc gamma RIIA, Fc gamma RIIB and Fc gamma RIIC in hematopoietic cells: analysis of transcripts. Mol Immunol 1993;30(5):451–60.

19. de HM, Vossebeld PJ, von dem Borne AE, Roos D. Fc gamma receptors of phagocytes. J Lab Clin Med 1995; 126(4):330–41.

20. Radeke HH, Gessner JE, Uciechowski P, et al. Intrinsic human glomerular mesangial cells can express receptors for IgG complexes (hFc gamma RIII-A) and the associated Fc epsilon RI gamma-chain. J Immunol 1994;153(3): 1281–92.

21. Hartnell A, Kay AB, Wardlaw AJ. IFN-gamma induces expression of Fc gamma RIII (CD16) on human eosinophils. J Immunol 1992;148(5): 1471–8.

22. Hunt JS, Beck ML, Tegtmeier GE, Bayer WL. Factors influencing monocyte recognition of human erythrocyte autoantibodies in vitro. Transfusion 1982;22(5):355–8.

23. Unanue ER. Antigen-presenting function of the macrophage. Annu Rev Immunol 1984;2:395–428.

24. Cambier JC. Antigen and Fc receptor signaling. The awesome power of the immunoreceptor tyrosine-based activation motif (ITAM). J Immunol 1995;155(7):3281–5.

25. Johnson SA, Pleiman CM, Pao L, et al. Phosphorylated immunoreceptor signaling motifs (ITAMs) exhibit unique abilities to bind and activate Lyn and Syk tyrosine kinases. J Immunol 1995;155(10):4596–603.

26. Keegan AD, Paul WE. Multichain immune recognition receptors: similarities in structure and signaling pathways. Immunol Today 1992; 13(2):63–8.

27. Oksanen K, Ebeling F, Kekomaki R, et al. Adverse reactions to platelet transfusions are reduced by use of platelet concentrates derived from buffy coat. Vox Sang 1994;67(4):356–61.

28. Sokol RJ, Hewitt S, Booker DJ, Bailey A. Erythrocyte autoantibodies, subclasses of IgG and autoimmune haemolysis. Autoimmunity 1990;6(1–2):99–104.

29. Sokol RJ, Hewitt S, Booker DJ, Bailey A. Red cell autoantibodies, multiple immunoglobulin classes, and autoimmune hemolysis. Transfusion 1990;30(8):714–7.

30. Garratty G. The James Blundell Award Lecture 2007: do we really understand immune red cell destruction? Transfus Med 2008;18(6):321–34.

31. Sim RB, Tsiftsoglou SA. Proteases of the complement system. Biochem Soc Trans 2004;32(Pt 1):21–7.

32. Kinoshita T. Biology of complement: the overture. Immunol Today 1991;12(9): 291–5.

33. Sim RB, Reid KB. C1: molecular interactions with activating systems. Immunol Today 1991;12(9):307–11.

34. Dodds AW. Which came first, the lectin/classical pathway or the alternative pathway of complement? Immunobiology 2002;205(4–5): 340–54.

35. Tomlinson S. Complement defense mechanisms. Curr Opin Immunol 1993;5(1):83–9.

36. Lambris JD, Lao Z, Oglesby TJ, et al. Dissection of CR1, factor H, membrane co-factor protein, and factor B binding and functional sites in the third complement component. J Immunol 1996;156(12):4821–32.

37. Gotze O, Muller-Eberhard HJ. Lysis of erythrocytes by complement in the absence of antibody. J Exp Med 1970;132(5):898–915.

38. Zipfel PF, Skerka C, Hellwage J, et al. Factor H family proteins: on complement, microbes and human diseases. Biochem Soc Trans 2002; 30(Pt 6):971–8.

39. Thompson RA, Lachmann PJ. Reactive lysis: the complement-mediated lysis of unsensitized cells. I. The characterization of the indicator factor and its identification as C7. J Exp Med 1970;131(4):629–41.

40. Meri S, Morgan BP, Davies A, et al. Human protectin (CD59), an 18,000–20,000 MW complement lysis restricting factor, inhibits C5b-8 catalysed insertion of C9 into lipid bilayers. Immunology 1990;71(1):1–9.

41. Gertz MA. Cold hemolytic syndrome. Hematology Am Soc Hematol Educ Program 2006;19–23.

42. Dhaliwal G, Cornett PA, Tierney Jr LM. Hemolytic anemia. Am Fam Physician 2004;69(11):2599–606.

43. Trivedi DH, Bussel JB. 21. Immunohematologic disorders. J Allergy Clin Immunol 2003;111(Suppl. 2): S669–76.

44. Sokol RJ, Booker DJ, Stamps R. The pathology of autoimmune haemolytic anaemia. J Clin Pathol 1992;45(12): 1047–52.

45. Weiner W, Vos GH, Serology of acquired hemolytic anemias. 1. Blood 1963; 22:606–13.

46. Vos GH, Petz LD, Fudenberg HH. Specificity and immunoglobulin characteristics of autoantibodies in acquired hemolytic anemia. J Immunol 1971;106(5):1172–6.

47. Issitt PD, Pavone BG, Goldfinger D, et al. Anti-Wrb, and other autoantibodies responsible for positive direct antiglobulin tests in 150 individuals. Br J Haematol 1976;34(1):5–18.

48. Leddy JP, Falany JL, Kissel GE, et al. Erythrocyte membrane proteins reactive with human (warm-reacting) anti- red cell autoantibodies. J Clin Invest 1993;91(4):1672–80.

49. Leddy JP, Wilkinson SL, Kissel GE, et al. Erythrocyte membrane proteins reactive with IgG (warm-reacting) anti- red blood cell autoantibodies: II. Antibodies coprecipitating band 3 and glycophorin A. Blood 1994;84(2):650–6.

50. Issitt PD, Anstee DJ. Applied Blood Group Serology. 4th ed. Durham, North Carolina, U.S.A.: Montgomery Scientific Publications; 1998.

51. Seyfried H, Gorska B, Maj S, et al. Apparent depression of antigens of the Kell blood group system associated with autoimmune acquired haemolytic anaemia. Vox Sang 1972;23(6): 528–36.

52. Issitt PD, Pavone BG. Critical re-examination of the specificity of auto-anti-Rh antibodies in patients with a positive direct antiglobulin test. Br J Haematol 1978;38(1):63–74.

53. Clark DA, Dessypris EN, Jenkins Jr DE, Krantz SB. Acquired immune hemolytic anemia associated with IgA erythrocyte coating: investigation of hemolytic mechanisms. Blood 1984;64(5): 1000–5.

54. Wolf CF, Wolf DJ, Peterson P, et al. Autoimmune hemolytic anemia with predominance of IgA autoantibody. Transfusion 1982;22(3):238–40.

55. Issitt PD, Wilkinson SL, Gruppo RA. Depression of Rh antigen expression in antibody-induced haemolytic anaemia [letter]. Br J Haematol 1983;53(4): 688.

56. Merry AH, Thomson EE, Rawlinson VI, Stratton F. Quantitation of IgG on Erythrocytes: correlation of number of IgG molecules per cell with the strength of the direct and indirect antiglobulin tests. Vox Sang 1984;47(1):73–81.

57. Schmitz N, Djibey I, Kretschmer V, et al. Assessment of red cell autoantibodies in autoimmune hemolytic anemia of warm type by a radioactive anti-IgG test. Vox Sang 1981;41(4):224–30.

58. Sokol RJ, Hewitt S, Booker DJ, Stamps R. Small quantities of erythrocyte bound immunoglobulins and autoimmune haemolysis. J Clin Pathol 1987;40(3): 254–7.

59. Sokol RJ, Hewitt S, Booker DJ, Stamps R. Enzyme linked direct antiglobulin tests in patients with autoimmune haemolysis. J Clin Pathol 1985;38(8): 912–4.

60. Salama A, Mueller-Eckhardt C, Bhakdi S. A two-stage immunoradiometric assay with 125I-staphylococcal protein A for the detection of antibodies and complement on human blood cells. Vox Sang 1985;48(4):239–45.

61. Stratton F, Rawlinson VI, Merry AH, Thomson EE. Positive direct antiglobulin test in normal individuals. II. Clin Lab Haematol 1983;5(1):17–21.

62. Petz LD, Garratty G. Acquired Immune Hemolytic Anemias. 1st ed. New York, N.Y., USA: Churchill Livingstone Inc.; 1980.

63. Atkinson JP, Schreiber AD, Frank MM. Effects of corticosteroids and

splenectomy on the immune clearance and destruction of erythrocytes. J Clin Invest 1973;52(6):1509–17.

64. Fries LF, Brickman CM, Frank MM. Monocyte receptors for the Fc portion of IgG increase in number in autoimmune hemolytic anemia and other hemolytic states and are decreased by glucocorticoid therapy. J Immunol 1983;131(3):1240–5.

65. Gibson J. Autoimmune hemolytic anemia: current concepts. Aust N Z J Med 1988;18(4):625–37.

66. Murphy S, LoBuglio AF. Drug therapy of autoimmune hemolytic anemia. Semin Hematol 1976;13(4):323–34.

67. Rosse WF. Autoimmune hemolytic anemia. Hosp Pract (Off Ed) 1985; 20(8):105–9.

68. Argiolu F, Diana G, Arnone M, et al. High-dose intravenous immunoglobulin in the management of autoimmune hemolytic anemia complicating thalassemia major. Acta Haematol 1990;83(2):65–8.

69. Besa EC. Rapid transient reversal of anemia and long-term effects of maintenance intravenous immunoglobulin for autoimmune hemolytic anemia in patients with lymphoproliferative disorders. Am J Med 1988;84(4):691–8.

70. Bolis S, Marozzi A, Rossini F, et al. High dose intravenous immunoglobulin (IVIgG) in Evans' syndrome. Allergol Immunopathol (Madr) 1991;19(5): 186.

71. Hilgartner MW, Bussel J. Use of intravenous gamma globulin for the treatment of autoimmune neutropenia of childhood and autoimmune hemolytic anemia. Am J Med 1987;83(4A): 25–9.

72. Mitchell CA, Van der Weyden MB, Firkin BG. High dose intravenous gammaglobulin in Coombs positive hemolytic anemia. Aust N Z J Med 1987;17(3):290–4.

73. Petrides PE, Hiller E. Autoimmune hemolytic anemia combined with idiopathic thrombocytopenia (Evans syndrome). Sustained remission in a patient following high-dose intravenous gamma-globulin therapy. Clin Investig 1992;70(1):38–9.

74. Ritch PS, Anderson T. Reversal of autoimmune hemolytic anemia associated with chronic lymphocytic leukemia following high-dose immunoglobulin. Cancer 1987; 60(11):2637–40.

75. Roldan R, Roman J, Lopez D, et al. Treatment of hemolytic anemia and severe thrombocytopenia with high-dose methylprednisolone and intravenous immunoglobulins in SLE [letter]. Scand J Rheumatol 1994;23(4):218–9.

76. Flores G, Cunningham-Rundles C, Newland AC, Bussel JB. Efficacy of intravenous immunoglobulin in the treatment of autoimmune hemolytic anemia: results in 73 patients. Am J Hematol 1993;44(4):237–42.

77. Telen MJ, Rao N. Recent advances in immunohematology. Curr Opin Hematol 1994;1(2):143–50.

78. Blanchette VS, Kirby MA, Turner C. Role of intravenous immunoglobulin G in autoimmune hematologic disorders. Semin Hematol 1992;29(3 Suppl 2): 72–82.

79. Nugent DJ. IVIG in the treatment of children with acute and chronic idiopathic thrombocytopenic purpura and the autoimmune cytopenias. Clin Rev Allergy 1992;10(1–2):59–71.

80. Smiley JD, Talbert MG. Southwestern Internal Medicine Conference: high-dose intravenous gamma globulin therapy: how does it work? Am J Med Sci 1995;309(5):295–303.

81. Wordell CJ. Use of intravenous immune globulin therapy: an overview. DICP 1991;25(7–8):805–17.

82. Dietrich G, Pereira P, Algiman M, et al. A monoclonal anti-idiotypic antibody against the antigen-combining site of anti-factor VIII autoantibodies defines an idiotope that is recognized by normal human polyspecific immunoglobulins for therapeutic use (IVIg). J Autoimmun 1990;3(5):547–57.

83. Rossi F, Dietrich G, Kazatchkine MD. Antiidiotypic suppression of autoantibodies with normal polyspecific immunoglobulins. Res Immunol 1989;140(1):19–31.

84. Roux KH, Tankersley DL. A view of the human idiotypic repertoire. Electron microscopic and immunologic analyses of spontaneous idiotype-anti-idiotype dimers in pooled human IgG. J Immunol 1990;144(4):1387–95.

85. Andersson JP, Andersson UG. Human intravenous immunoglobulin modulates monokine production in vitro. Immunology 1990;71(3):372–6.

86. Andersson UG, Bjork L, Skansen-Saphir U, Andersson JP. Down-regulation of cytokine production and interleukin-2 receptor expression by pooled human IgG. Immunology 1993;79(2): 211–6.

87. Aukrust P, Froland SS, Liabakk NB, et al. Release of cytokines, soluble cytokine receptors, and interleukin-1 receptor antagonist after intravenous immunoglobulin administration in vivo. Blood 1994;84(7):2136–43.

88. Shimozato T, Iwata M, Kawada H, Tamura N. Human immunoglobulin preparation for intravenous use induces elevation of cellular cyclic adenosine 3′:5′-monophosphate levels, resulting in suppression of tumour necrosis factor alpha and interleukin-1 production. Immunology 1991;72(4): 497–501.

89. Dwyer JM. Manipulating the immune system with immune globulin. N Engl J Med 1992;326(2):107–16.

90. Macey MG, Newland AC. CD4 and CD8 subpopulation changes during high dose intravenous immunoglobulin treatment. Br J Haematol 1990;76(4):513–20.

91. Pogliani EM, Della VA, Casaroli I, et al. Lymphocyte subsets in patients with idiopathic thrombocytopenic purpura during high-dose gamma globulin therapy. Allergol Immunopathol (Madr) 1991;19(3):113–6.

92. Siragam V, Crow AR, Brinc D, et al. Intravenous immunoglobulin ameliorates ITP via activating Fc gamma receptors on dendritic cells. Nat Med 2006;12(6):688–92.

93. Bowdler AJ. The role of the spleen and splenectomy in autoimmune hemolytic disease. Semin Hematol 1976;13(4): 335–48.

94. Ruben FL, Hankins WA, Zeigler Z, et al. Antibody responses to meningococcal polysaccharide vaccine in adults without a spleen. Am J Med 1984;76(1): 115–21.

95. Katkhouda N, Mavor E. Laparoscopic splenectomy. Surg Clin North Am 2000;80(4):1285–97.

96. Targarona EM, Espert JJ, Bombuy E, et al. Complications of laparoscopic splenectomy [In Process Citation]. Arch Surg 2000;135(10):1137–40.

97. Bisharat N, Omari H, Lavi I, Raz R. Risk of infection and death among post-splenectomy patients. J Infect 2001; 43(3):182–6.

98. Cervera H, Jara LJ, Pizarro S, et al. Danazol for systemic lupus erythematosus with refractory autoimmune thrombocytopenia or Evans' syndrome. J Rheumatol 1995; 22(10):1867–71.

99. Pignon JM, Poirson E, Rochant H. Danazol in autoimmune haemolytic anaemia. Br J Haematol 1993;83(2): 343–5.

100. Schreiber AD, Chien P, Tomaski A, Cines DB. Effect of danazol in immune thrombocytopenic purpura. N Engl J Med 1987;316(9):503–8.

101. Bussone G, Ribeiro E, Dechartres A, et al. Efficacy and safety of rituximab in adults' warm antibody autoimmune haemolytic anemia: retrospective analysis of 27 cases. Am J Hematol 2009;84(3): 153–7.

102. Coiffier B. Hepatitis B virus reactivation in patients receiving chemotherapy for cancer treatment: role of lamivudine prophylaxis. Cancer Invest 2006; 24(5):548–52.

103. Carson KR, Evens AM, Richey EA, et al. Progressive multifocal leukoencephalopathy following rituximab therapy in HIV negative patients: a report of 57 cases from the Research on Adverse Drug Event and

Reports (RADAR) project. Blood. 2009;113(20):4834–40.

104. Sokol RJ, Hewitt S, Stamps BK. Autoimmune hemolysis: mixed warm and cold antibody type. Acta Haematol 1983;69(4):266–74.

105. Heddle NM. Acute paroxysmal cold hemoglobinuria. Transfus Med Rev 1989;3(3):219–29.

106. Roelcke D, Pruzanski W, Ebert W, et al. A new human monoclonal cold agglutinin Sa recognizing terminal N-acetylneuraminyl groups on the cell surface. Blood 1980;55(4):677–81.

107. Roelcke D. The Lud cold agglutinin: a further antibody recognizing N-acetylneuraminic acid-determined antigens not fully expressed at birth. Vox Sang 1981;41(5–6):316–8.

108. Roelcke D. A further cold agglutinin, F1, recognizing a N-acetylneuraminic acid-determined antigen. Vox Sang 1981;41(2):98–101.

109. Silberstein LE. Natural and pathologic human autoimmune responses to carbohydrate antigens on red blood cells. Springer Semin Immunopathol 1993; 15(2–3):139–53.

110. Berentsen S, Ulvestad E, Gjertsen BT, et al. Rituximab for primary chronic cold agglutinin disease: a prospective study of 37 courses of therapy in 27 patients. Blood 2004;103(8):2925–8.

111. Berentsen S, Beiske K, Tjonnfjord GE. Primary chronic cold agglutinin disease: an update on pathogenesis, clinical features and therapy. Hematology 2007;12(5):361–70.

112. Sokol RJ, Hewitt S, Stamps BK, Hitchen PA. Autoimmune haemolysis in childhood and adolescence. Acta Haematol 1984;72(4):245–57.

113. Kurlander RJ, Rosse WF, Logue GL. Quantitative influence of antibody and complement coating of red cells on monocyte-mediated cell lysis. J Clin Invest 1978;61(5):1309–19.

114. Gelfand EW, Abramson N, Segel GB, Nathan DG. Buffy-coat observations and red-cell antibodies in acquired hemolytic anemia. N Engl J Med 1971;284(22):1250–2.

115. Dacie JV, Lewis SM. Practical Haematology. 5th ed. Edinburgh: Churchill Livingstone; 1975.

116. Wolach B, Heddle N, Barr RD, et al. Transient Donath–Landsteiner haemolytic anaemia. Br J Haematol 1981;48(3):425–34.

117. Nordhagen R, Stensvold K, Winsnes A, et al. Paroxysmal cold haemoglobinuria. The most frequent acute autoimmune haemolytic anaemia in children? Acta Paediatr Scand 1984;73(2):258–62.

118. Linden JV, Wagner K, Voytovich AE, Sheehan J. Transfusion errors in New York State: an analysis of 10 years' experience. Transfusion 2000;40(10):1207–13.

119. Sazama K. Reports of 355 transfusion-associated deaths: 1976 through 1985. Transfusion 1990;30(7):583–90.

120. Beauregard P, Blajchman MA. Hemolytic and pseudo–hemolytic transfusion reactions: an overview of the hemolytic transfusion reactions and the clinical conditions that mimic them. Transfus Med Rev 1994;8(3):184–99.

121. Pineda AA, Brzica Jr SM, Taswell HF. Hemolytic transfusion reaction. Recent experience in a large blood bank. Mayo Clin Proc 1978;53(6):378–90.

122. van der Meulen JA, McNabb TC, Haeffner-Cavaillon N, et al. The Fc gamma receptor on human placental plasma membrane. I. Studies on the binding of homologous and heterologous immunoglobulin G1. J Immunol 1980;124(2):500–7.

123. Lee SI, Heiner DC, Wara D. Development of serum IgG subclass levels in children. Monogr Allergy 1986;19:108–21.

124. Kumpel BM. Lessons learnt from many years of experience using anti-D in humans for prevention of RhD immunization and haemolytic disease of the fetus and newborn. Clin Exp Immunol 2008;154(1):1–5.

125. Roberts IA. The changing face of haemolytic disease of the newborn. Early Hum Dev 2008;84(8):515–23.

126. Fung Kee FK, Eason E, Crane J, et al. Prevention of Rh alloimmunization. J Obstet Gynaecol Can 2003;25(9):765–73.

127. Judd WJ, Luban NL, Ness PM, et al. Prenatal and perinatal immunohematology: recommendations for serologic management of the fetus, newborn infant, and obstetric patient. Transfusion 1990;30(2):175–83.

128. Frigoletto FD, Greene MF, Benacerraf BR, et al. Ultrasonographic fetal surveillance in the management of the isoimmunized pregnancy. N Engl J Med 1986;315(7):430–2.

129. Nicolaides KH, Rodeck CH. Rhesus disease: the model for fetal therapy. Br J Hosp Med 1985;34(3):141–8.

130. Morris ED, Murray J, Ruthven CR. Liquor bilirubin levels in normal pregnancy: a basis for accurate prediction of haemolytic disease. Br Med J 1967;2(548):352–4.

131. Weiner CP. Human fetal bilirubin levels and fetal hemolytic disease. Am J Obstet Gynecol 1992;166(5):1449-54.

132. Mari G, Deter RL, Carpenter RL, et al. Noninvasive diagnosis by Doppler ultrasonography of fetal anemia due to maternal red-cell alloimmunization. Collaborative Group for Doppler Assessment of the Blood Velocity in Anemic Fetuses. N Engl J Med 2000; 342(1):9–14.

133. Bullock R, Martin WL, Coomarasamy A, Kilby MD. Prediction of fetal anemia in pregnancies with red-cell alloimmunization: comparison of middle cerebral artery peak systolic velocity and amniotic fluid OD450. Ultrasound Obstet Gynecol 2005; 25(4):331–4.

134. Rubo J, Wahn V. High-dose intravenous gammaglobulin in rhesus-haemolytic disease. Lancet 1991;337(8746): 914.

135. Arndt PA, Garratty G. The changing spectrum of drug-induced immune hemolytic anemia. Semin Hematol 2005;42(3):137–44.

136. Florendo NT, MacFarland D, Painter M, Muirhead EE. Streptomycin-specific antibody coincident with a developing warm autoantibody. Transfusion 1980;20(6):662–8.

137. Hart MN, Mesara BW. Phenacetin antibody cross-reactive with autoimmune erythrocyte antibody. Am J Clin Pathol 1969;52(6):695–701.

138. Petz LD. Drug-induced autoimmune hemolytic anemia. Transfus Med Rev 1993;7(4):242–54.

139. Wright MS. Drug-induced hemolytic anemias: increasing complications to therapeutic interventions. Clin Lab Sci 1999;12(2):115–8.

140. Kirtland III HH, Mohler DN, Horwitz DA. Methyldopa inhibition of suppressor-lymphocyte function: a proposed cause of autoimmune hemolytic anemia. N Engl J Med 1980;302(15):825–32.

141. Worlledge SM. The interpretation of a positive direct antiglobulin test. Br J Haematol 1978;39(2):157–62.

142. Kelton JG. Impaired reticuloendothelial function in patients treated with methyldopa. N Engl J Med 1985; 313(10):596–600.

143. Hunter E, Raik E, Gordon S, Taylor KB. Incidence of positive Coombs' test, LE cells and antinuclear factor in patients on alpha-methyldopa ('Aldomet') therapy. Med J Aust 1971;2(16): 810–2.

144. Bakemeier RF, Leddy JP. Erythrocyte autoantibody associated with alpha-methyldopa: heterogeneity of structure and specificity. Blood 1968;32(1): 1–14.

145. LoBuglio AF, Jandl JH. The nature of the alpha-methyldopa red-cell antibody. N Engl J Med 1967;276(12): 658–65.

146. Devereux S, Fisher DM, Roter BL, Hegde UM. Factor VIII inhibitor and raised platelet IgG levels associated with methyldopa therapy. Br J Haematol 1983;54(3):485–8.

147. Kerr RO, Cardamone J, Dalmasso AP, Kaplan ME. Two mechanisms of erythrocyte destruction in penicillin-induced hemolytic anemia. N Engl J Med 1972;287(26):1322–5.

148. Levine BB, Fellner MJ, Levytska V, et al. Benzylpenicilloyl-specific serum

antibodies to penicillin in man. II. Sensitivity of the hemagglutination assay method, molecular classes of the antibodies detected, and antibody titers of randomly selected patients. J Immunol 1966;96(4):719–26.

149. Spath P, Garratty G, Petz L. Studies on the immune response to penicillin and cephalothin in humans. I. Optimal conditions for titration of hemagglutinating penicillin and cephalothin antibodies. J Immunol 1971;107(3):854–9.

150. Garratty G, Arndt PA. Positive direct antiglobulin tests and haemolytic anaemia following therapy with beta-lactamase inhibitor containing drugs may be associated with nonimmunologic adsorption of protein onto red blood cells. Br J Haematol 1998;100(4):777–83.

151. Moore SB, Taswell HF, Pineda AA, Sonnenberg CL. Delayed hemolytic transfusion reactions. Evidence of the need for an improved pretransfusion compatibility test. Am J Clin Pathol 1980;74(1):94–7.

152. Pineda AA, Taswell HF, Brzica SM Jr. Transfusion reaction. An immunologic hazard of blood transfusion. Transfusion 1978;18(1):1–7.

153. Mollison PL. Blood Transfusion in Clinical Medicine. Oxford, England: Blackwell; 1993.

154. Cooper RA, Bunn HF. Hemolytic anemia. In: Braunwald E, Fauci AS, Isselbacher KJ, et al, editors. Harrison's Online. 12th ed. New York, NY, USA: McGraw-Hill; 1991. pp. 1531–7.

155. Moake JL, Rudy CK, Troll JH, et al. Unusually large plasma factor VIII:von Willebrand factor multimers in chronic relapsing thrombotic thrombocytopenic purpura. N Engl J Med 1982;307(23): 1432–5.

156. Levy GG, Nichols WC, Lian EC, et al. Mutations in a member of the ADAMTS gene family cause thrombotic thrombocytopenic purpura. Nature 2001;413(6855):488–94.

157. Moore JC, Hayward CP, Warkentin TE, Kelton JG. Decreased von Willebrand factor protease activity associated with thrombocytopenic disorders. Blood 2001;98(6):1842–6.

158. Rock G, Shumak KH, Sutton DM, et al. Cryosupernatant as replacement fluid for plasma exchange in thrombotic thrombocytopenic purpura. Members of the Canadian Apheresis Group. Br J Haematol 1996;94(2):383–6.

159. Rock GA, Shumak KH, Buskard NA, et al. Comparison of plasma exchange with plasma infusion in the treatment of thrombotic thrombocytopenic purpura. Canadian Apheresis Study Group. N Engl J Med 1991;325(6):393–7.

160. Novitzky N, Jacobs P, Rosenstrauch W. The treatment of thrombotic thrombocytopenic purpura: plasma infusion or exchange? Br J Haematol 1994;87(2):317–20.

161. Swisher KK, Terrell DR, Vesely SK, et al. Clinical outcomes after platelet transfusions in patients with thrombotic thrombocytopenic purpura. Transfusion 2009;49(5):873–87.

162. Bell WR, Braine HG, Ness PM, Kickler TS. Improved survival in thrombotic thrombocytopenic purpura-hemolytic uremic syndrome. Clinical experience in 108 patients. N Engl J Med 1991;325(6): 398–403.

163. Elliott MA, Heit JA, Pruthi RK, et al. Rituximab for refractory and or relapsing thrombotic thrombocytopenic purpura related to immune-mediated severe ADAMTS13-deficiency: a report of four cases and a systematic review of the literature. Eur J Haematol 2009; 83(4):365–72.

164. McCrae KR, Sadler J, Cines DB. Thrombotic thrombocytopenic purpura and the hemolytic uremic syndrome. In: Hoffman R, Benz EJ, Shattil SJ, et al, editors. Hematology: Basic Principles and Practice. 3rd ed. Churchill Livingstone; 2009. p. 2009–112.

165. Brodsky RA. How I treat paroxysmal nocturnal hemoglobinuria. Blood 2009;113(26):6522–7.

166. Ferguson MA. Colworth Medal Lecture. Glycosyl-phosphatidylinositol membrane anchors: the tale of a tail. Biochem Soc Trans 1992;20(2):243–56.

167. Hillmen P, Richards SJ. Implications of recent insights into the pathophysiology of paroxysmal nocturnal haemoglobinuria. Br J Haematol 2000;108(3):470–9.

168. Parker C, Omine M, Richards S, et al. Diagnosis and management of paroxysmal nocturnal hemoglobinuria. Blood 2005;106(12):3699–709.

169. Saso R, Marsh J, Cevreska L, et al. Bone marrow transplants for paroxysmal nocturnal haemoglobinuria. Br J Haematol 1999;104(2):392–6.

170. Brodsky RA, Young NS, Antonioli E, et al. Multicenter phase 3 study of the complement inhibitor eculizumab for the treatment of patients with paroxysmal nocturnal hemoglobinuria. Blood 2008;111(4):1840–7.

171. Hillmen P, Young NS, Schubert J, et al. The complement inhibitor eculizumab in paroxysmal nocturnal hemoglobinuria. N Engl J Med 2006;355(12):1233–43.

172. Schrier SL. Extrinsic Nonimmune Hemolytic Anemias. In: Hoffman R, Benz Jr EJ, Shattil SJ, et al, editors. Hematology: Basic Principles and Practice. 3rd ed. New York: Churchill Livingstone; 2000. p. 630–8.

CHAPTER 11

Iron deficiency anemia, anemia of chronic disorders and iron overload

MJ Pippard

Chapter contents

Introduction

Disturbances of iron metabolism are among the commonest disorders affecting human populations. This high frequency reflects the combination of an essential requirement for iron by all living organisms, with a relatively precarious human iron balance. Iron in heme is maintained in the reduced ferrous state (Fe^{2+}) for oxygen transport by hemoglobin and for storage and use of oxygen in muscles by myoglobin. It is also essential for a wide range of cellular heme and iron-sulfur proteins that are responsible for electron transport and energy generation in mitochondrial respiration and the citric acid cycle, and for ribonucleotide reductase, responsible for DNA synthesis.[1] To be available for absorption, dietary iron needs to be in a soluble form, but in an oxygen-rich environment it is readily converted to insoluble ferric (Fe^{3+}) hydroxide ('rust'),[2] or bound as insoluble ferric iron complexes, particularly in a predominantly vegetarian diet. This places an upper limit on the capacity of dietary iron to meet increased iron needs, whether physiologic or due to blood loss. As a result, iron deficiency anemia affects, at a conservative estimate, at least 500 million of the world's population,[3] and this takes no account of the additional, greater numbers of people who will have borderline iron status with depleted iron stores.[4,5] In this context it is perhaps not surprising that humans conserve iron rigorously, with no mechanism for active iron excretion.[6]

The lack of an active excretory mechanism for iron means that if the normal regulation of iron status through control of iron absorption breaks down, or there is a non-physiologic parenteral source of iron, such as red cell transfusion in chronic anemias, iron overload results. Such iron loading disorders are less common than iron deficiency, affecting perhaps 5 million of the world's population. However, they are potentially fatal: the very feature that makes iron essential to living organisms – its ability to undergo reversible oxidation-reduction between Fe^{2+} and Fe^{3+} – is capable of generating tissue damaging oxygen free radicals. Normally, the tight binding of ferric iron by the plasma iron transport protein, transferrin, and the intracellular iron storage protein, ferritin, limit this potential toxicity while maintaining the iron in a soluble and relatively available state. However, these protective mechanisms are overwhelmed in disorders that are associated with a parenchymal iron loading, leading to damage to liver, heart and endocrine glands.

Spectrum of pathology related to disorders of iron metabolism

Iron deficiency

A persistent negative iron balance leads eventually to exhaustion of iron stores, the development of iron deficient erythropoiesis and eventually anemia. Lack of iron thus has major direct effects on the bone marrow and blood, though other tissues are also affected by the impaired iron supply. This chapter reviews these changes and their accompanying diagnostic features.

Iron maldistribution

Anemia secondary to a variety of inflammatory illnesses is the commonest form of anemia encountered in hospital practice. Here, the main disturbance of iron metabolism is retention of iron by macrophages of the reticuloendothelial system, with no change in the total amount of body iron. However, the block on iron release leads to a reduction in transferrin iron supplying erythropoiesis, one of several factors contributing to the pathophysiology of the anemia of chronic disorders. Diagnosis is thus likely to depend upon assessment of the pattern of changes in iron metabolism, and the hematologist may be involved in excluding more specific causes for anemia, including iron deficiency.

Impaired iron supply to the erythron may accompany rare inherited causes of iron mal-distribution that limit iron release from cells (e.g. a 'loss of function' mutation affecting ferroportin or aceruloplasminemia), as will be discussed in a later section. In addition, impaired iron supply to the erythron may occur in association with acquired causes of localized tissue iron overload, for example in pulmonary hemosiderosis, and with renal tubular iron loading in paroxysmal nocturnal hemoglobinuria.

Iron overload

Iron accumulating within macrophages is relatively non-toxic, these cells being specialized to deal with the high throughput of iron derived from hemoglobin in senescent red cells. By contrast, iron loading of parenchymal cells is associated with saturation of the plasma transferrin, the appearance of more labile and toxic non-transferrin-bound iron in the plasma,[7] accumulation of iron in hepatocytes, cardiac myocytes and endocrine cells, and increased degradation of ferritin to insoluble hemosiderin within cellular lysosomes:[8] the end result is the pattern of organ damage that is characteristic of hemochromatosis. There are no clear direct effects on bone marrow function, but iron-induced liver damage and cirrhosis may have indirect effects on blood cells (e.g. red cell macrocytosis, or cytopenias related to hypersplenism). By contrast, disturbed bone marrow function with massive ineffective erythropoiesis (e.g. in the β-thalassemia intermedia syndromes and some patients with sideroblastic or congenital dyserythropoietic anemias – see Chapters 9, 14, and 15), is definitely associated with inappropriately increased iron absorption and eventual iron overload. The hematologist is likely to be involved in the diagnosis and treatment of iron overload, including phlebotomy in hereditary hemochromatosis and iron chelation in iron-loading anemias.

Major pathways of iron exchange

These were delineated many years ago by use of ferrokinetic studies, following the tissue uptake of ^{59}Fe after its intravenous injection bound to plasma transferrin.[9] The pathways (Fig. 11.1) are dominated (80–90% of plasma iron turnover) by the supply of plasma iron, bound to the circulating transport protein, transferrin, to bone marrow erythroid precursors for hemoglobin synthesis. At the end of their life span, red cells are phagocytosed by tissue macrophages. Heme oxygenase releases the iron from heme for recycling back to plasma transferrin, or alternatively diversion to intracellular ferritin, a protein cage made up of 24 H- (Heavy) and L- (Light) subunits which can store up to 4500 atoms of iron. A smaller uptake by the liver hepatocytes is the main alternative site of transferrin iron uptake (approximately 10%), and reflects expression of transferrin receptors on hepatocytes as well as erythroblasts. Whereas macrophages gain nearly all their iron in the unidirectional flow from senescent red cells, hepatocytes are able to take up iron in a variety of forms (see below) as well as to release the iron in times of increased need. This makes the liver the major 'buffer' within the system, and the prime target for iron loading and damage in iron overload conditions. There is very limited exchange of iron with the exterior. Obligatory losses (skin and gastrointestinal mucosal cell loss) of approximately 1 mg/day in males (rather more in women of child-bearing age with the

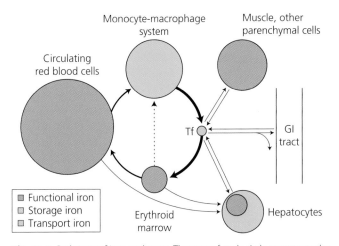

Monocyte-macrophage system

Muscle, other parenchymal cells

Circulating red blood cells

Tf

GI tract

☐ Functional iron
☐ Storage iron
☐ Transport iron

Erythroid marrow

Hepatocytes

Fig. 11.1 Pathways of iron exchange. The area of each circle represents the normal amount of iron within a compartment, and the width of the arrows represents the size of the iron fluxes between compartments. Iron supplied to and recycled from erythropoiesis dominates internal iron exchange. The dotted line represents iron released from the normal 'wastage' of erythroblasts which die during maturation. Tf, transferrin. *(After Brittenham GM. The red cell cycle. In: Brock JH, Halliday JW, Pippard MJ, Powell LW, editors. Iron metabolism in health and disease. London: Saunders; 1994. p. 31–62, with permission from Elsevier).*

additional losses of menstruation, pregnancy and lactation)[10] are normally balanced by absorption of a similar amount from the diet.

Over recent years, understanding of the processes of cellular iron uptake through transferrin receptors, and regulation of intracellular iron homeostasis, has greatly increased. The discovery of the genetic basis of HFE-related hemochromatosis in the mid 1990s, combined with the use of molecular genetic studies of animal models with altered iron metabolism or erythropoiesis, led to rapid advances, with identification of additional proteins involved in regulating iron absorption and internal exchange.[11] An understanding of these molecular processes underpins discussion of the pathophysiology of the iron disorders and their diagnosis.

Molecular mechanisms in iron metabolism

Cellular uptake of iron from transferrin

Cell surface expression of the classical transferrin receptor (TfR1) is greatest on rapidly dividing cells such as erythroid precursors, though it is also required for normal development of lymphoid cells and neuroepithelial differentiation in the developing nervous system. The receptor has a greater affinity for fully saturated, diferric, transferrin than for monoferric transferrin,[12] and does not bind apotransferrin at the neutral pH of plasma. These affinities in part account for the importance of measuring the transferrin saturation as a vital part of a screen for the risk of an iron loading condition,[13] and the fact that transferrin saturation is a better guide to iron supply to the tissues in iron deficiency than the serum iron value.[14] At a high transferrin saturation most plasma iron is present as diferric transferrin, and iron uptake via transferrin receptors is enhanced. By contrast, the increased concentrations of serum transferrin which are found in iron deficiency mean that the small amount of iron present is in the form of monoferric transferrin, with its reduced rate of uptake by transferrin receptors.

After receptor-mediated endocytosis of the transferrin/receptor complex (Fig. 11.2), acidification of the endosome releases the iron from the transferrin, which at low pH even after releasing its iron still has a high affinity for the receptor.[15] The apotransferrin recycles with the receptor back to the cell membrane, where it dissociates and is released into the plasma to continue its role in iron delivery to the tissues. The iron is reduced to Fe^{2+} by a ferrireductase, STEAP3,[16] before being transported into the cytosol from the endosome by divalent metal transporter, DMT1 (previously known as NRAMP2, or DCT1).[17]

Regulation of cellular iron homeostasis

The intracellular iron content is finely regulated at the level of translation of the mRNA of several key iron-related proteins.[18] Two iron-regulatory proteins (IRP1, coded on chromosome 9, and IRP2, coded on chromosome 15), are able to bind to sequences which form stem loop structures called iron responsive elements (IREs) in the untranslated regions of mRNAs for transferrin receptor and both H- and L-subunits of ferritin (Fig. 11.3). When IRP1 contains an iron-sulfur (4Fe-4S) cluster it has a low affinity for the IRE (and functions as cytoplasmic aconitase), while IRP2 is unstable in the presence of iron. However, when intracellular 'labile' (metabolically active) iron is at a low level, IRP binding to IREs that are present in the 3′ untranslated region of the mRNA for transferrin receptor protects the message from cytoplasmic degradation and allows its translation: at the same time, binding of IRP to the single stem loop in the 5′ untranslated region of the ferritin mRNA inhibits ferritin protein synthesis. The relative rates of synthesis of the two proteins are reversed in conditions of iron excess, and this reciprocal relationship serves to stabilize the intracellular labile iron content. Other iron related proteins also have IRE structures in their mRNAs.[19] Those with 5′ IREs include the cellular iron exporter protein, ferroportin, (see below) and erythroid delta-aminolevulinic acid synthase (ALAS). IRP binding to the latter enables heme synthesis to be matched to the iron supply: the initial part of the heme synthetic pathway is switched off when the cell is deficient in iron. At least one isoform of DMT1 has an IRE in its 3′ untranslated mRNA, and IRP binding may stabilize its mRNA in an iron depleted cell, leading to increased expression and enhanced iron uptake.

Iron entering the cell cytosol becomes available for a variety of functional iron compounds or can be taken up by the iron storage protein, ferritin (Fig. 11.2). However, control of these intracellular movements is only just beginning to be explored. The H-subunits of ferritin have an intrinsic ferroxidase activity which is important for their storage function. Mitochondrial iron importers (mitoferrin-1 and -2) have been shown to be essential for heme and iron-sulfur cluster synthesis in the mitochondria of a variety of cells. Mitoferrin-1, itself stabilized by a mitochondrial ATP binding cassette transporter protein,[20] is essential for iron utilization by the mitochondria of erythroid cells.[21] The amount of mitoferrin may thus regulate the delivery of iron for incorporation into protoporphyrin by the enzyme ferrochelatase in the final step of heme synthesis.

Disturbances of intracellular iron distribution resulting from abnormal mitochondrial iron homeostasis are

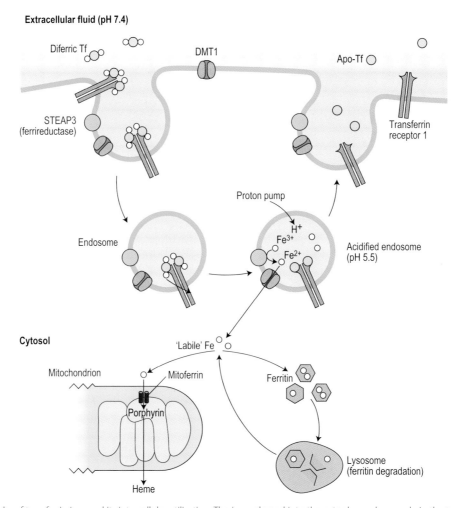

Extracellular fluid (pH 7.4)

Fig. 11.2 Cellular uptake of transferrin iron and its intracellular utilization. The iron released into the cytoplasm plays a role in the translational regulation of transferrin receptor, ferritin and erythroid ALA-synthase (see Fig. 11.3). Heme synthesis dominates in erythroid cells, whereas ferritin metabolism is crucial in iron storage cells (macrophages and hepatocytes) Ferritin is constantly catabolized and the iron is either released back to the cytosol or remains in lysosomes as insoluble hemosiderin.

associated with a number of inherited diseases. For example, mutations in erythroid ALAS are responsible for X-linked sideroblastic anemia, with iron accumulation within mitochondria related to impaired protoporphyrin synthesis.[22] Mutations in two other mitochondrial proteins give rise to mitochondrial iron accumulation, and decreased cytosolic iron with defects in iron-sulfur cluster formation and heme synthesis. Mutations in the gene for ATP-binding cassette 7 (ABCB7) underlie the sideroblastic anemia with spinocerebellar ataxia that is linked to Xq13 (see Chapter 14).[23] Autosomal recessive inheritance of increased numbers of trinucleotide repeats in the gene coding for the mitochondrial iron chaperone, frataxin, is accompanied by the neurological and cardiac problems of Friedreich's ataxia and by up-regulation of the mitochondrial iron importer, mitoferrin, with mitochondrial iron loading.[24]

Regulation of iron uptake in specific tissues

Superimposed upon the general mechanisms of the regulation of cellular iron uptake described above are more specific mechanisms related to the different functions of 'iron user'

cells (mainly in the erythron, but to a lesser extent all other tissues, to support their need for 'functional' iron compounds), and the 'iron donor' cells that are involved in recycling iron to plasma transferrin or intracellular ferritin (the macrophages and hepatocytes) or in iron absorption (duodenal mucosal cells).

Developmental (transcriptional) regulation of iron uptake in the erythron

Committed erythroid progenitors express erythropoietin receptors maximally at the late BFU-E and CFU-E stages, declining from the proerythroblast stage. Erythropoietin prevents apoptosis of these progenitors and allows their proliferation. It also activates IRP and thus up-regulates synthesis of transferrin receptors[25] which reach a peak in the basophilic erythroblasts. Uptake of iron thus precedes the onset of maximum heme synthesis in later polychromatic erythroblasts.[26] Any iron not subsequently used appears in cytoplasmic ferritin and siderotic granules (giving rise to normal sideroblasts on Perls' staining of marrow smears, or to Pappenheimer bodies in mature red cells on Romanowsky

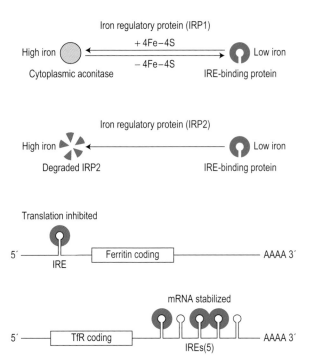

Fig. 11.3 Coordinate regulation of synthesis of ferritin and transferrin receptor-1 (TfR1) by the interaction of iron binding proteins (IRPs) with mRNA iron responsive elements (IRE). When cytoplasmic iron (see Fig. 11.2) is low, IRPs bind to IRE stem-loop structures to inhibit ferritin translation but to increase translation of TfR1 by preventing degradation of its mRNA. When iron levels are high, IRP1 functions as a cytoplasmic aconitase and no longer binds to IREs and IRP2 is degraded: this allows increased ferritin synthesis but reduces TfR1 synthesis.

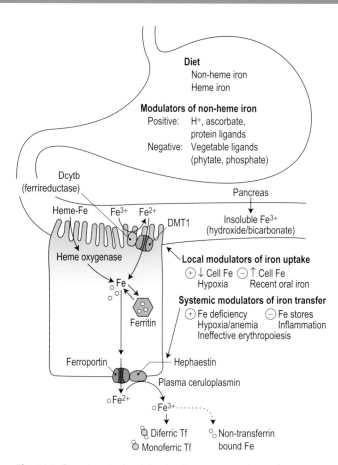

Fig. 11.4 Gastrointestinal and duodenal enterocyte pathways for iron absorption. Iron taken up at the enterocyte brush border may be transferred to the plasma via ferroportin or incorporated into ferritin to be shed into the lumen of the gut at the end of the enterocyte's life span. DMT1, divalent metal transporter 1; Tf, transferrin.

staining of peripheral blood films). These are more prominent where transferrin saturation, and thus the proportion of diferric transferrin, which has a high affinity for the receptor (see above), is increased, and are absent when a low saturation gives rise to iron-deficient erythropoiesis.

Hepatocyte iron uptake

The hepatocyte is able to take up iron in many forms, including transferrin- and non-transferrin-bound iron, hemoglobin–haptoglobin and heme–hemopexin complexes (which provide a potential direct shunt from the erythron to the hepatocyte in conditions associated with hemolysis or ineffective erythropoiesis), and any tissue ferritin which has been released into the circulation as the result of cell damage. The hepatocyte has a low level of expression of classical transferrin receptors (TfR1), but expresses a homolog, transferrin receptor 2 (TfR2).[27,28] This differs from TfR1 in having no 3′ IRE in its mRNA, and it is thus not down-regulated in the presence of iron overload.[29] Homozygous inheritance of a mutation in the TfR2 gene underlies some cases of hemochromatosis, implicating this receptor in the pathway that regulates iron absorption in relation to iron stores (see below).[30] Iron uptake by hepatocytes from transferrin may occur by the receptor-mediated endocytosis described above or, following release of the iron at the hepatocyte surface, by the route taken by non-transferrin-bound iron.[15] Although the detailed mechanisms of iron uptake (and release) by hepatocytes remain somewhat uncertain, it is clear that the

liver may continue to take in iron from various sources, even when there are already increased iron stores, and it is thus highly vulnerable to damage in iron-loading disorders.

Macrophage iron uptake

The phagocytic cells of the reticuloendothelial system normally recycle approximately 20 mg iron a day from hemoglobin in senescent red cells and the normal small proportion of ineffective erythropoiesis.[9,26] Although they express transferrin receptors, these are at a low level, and do not account for a significant proportion of the plasma iron turnover derived from transferrin. Increased uptake of iron from lactoferrin produced by neutrophils is no longer thought to be a significant source of the increased macrophage storage iron that is seen with inflammation.[31]

Uptake of iron by duodenal mucosal cells

Duodenal mucosal cells are specialized to take up soluble iron at their apical brush border and to transfer this across their basolateral membrane to circulating plasma transferrin (Fig. 11.4). Stomach acid has an important role in the solubilization of non-heme iron, and the detailed make-up of the diet influences its availability for absorption. For example, phytates and phosphates in vegetarian diets inhibit non-heme iron absorption by forming insoluble complexes, whereas ascorbate and meat protein digestion products form soluble complexes and enhance absorption. Heme iron from animal products is also relatively well absorbed.

Reduction from Fe^{3+} to Fe^{2+} is an essential initial step in the uptake of dietary non-heme iron.[32] It is mediated by a heme-containing ferrireductase, duodenal cytochrome b (Dcytb) which is expressed in the apical brush border membrane of duodenal enterocytes and induced by iron deficiency.[33] Ascorbate could have a role as an electron donor in this process, contributing to its ability to promote the availability of iron for absorption. An apical mucosal iron transporter, DMT1, then transfers the Fe^{2+} into the enterocyte.[34] Alternative splicing generates two isoforms of intestinal DMT1, only one of which has a 3′ IRE that could potentially be regulated by the IRE/IBP mechanism: the presence of further isoforms containing an additional 5′ exon may be required for up-regulation in iron deficiency.[35] Dietary heme is taken up at the apical surface by a separate ill-understood mechanism, and the iron released by intracellular heme oxygenase is thought to join the same metabolic pool as that derived from non-heme iron.[36] Once inside the cell, the iron may either be incorporated into ferritin stores (to be shed with the enterocyte into the gut lumen at the end of the cell's life span) or transferred across the basolateral membrane by another iron transporter protein, ferroportin (also known as Ireg1).[37]

Duodenal enterocytes also express TfRs at their basolateral membrane, and iron uptake by this route during their maturation from duodenal crypt cells into absorptive enterocytes may contribute to modulation of the expression of transporter proteins through IRE/IBP mechanisms or through transcriptional regulation.[38] The observation that a large oral dose of iron may result in a 'mucosal block' to absorption of a subsequent oral dose has been attributed to a rapid and selective down-regulation of Dcytb and DMT1 with no effect on the mRNA of basolateral iron transport molecules.[39]

Iron release from 'donor' cells

As well as being found in the basolateral membrane of the duodenal enterocyte, ferroportin is also found in macrophages and hepatocytes.[40] Ferroportin transports reduced (Fe^{2+}) iron and is coupled with the copper oxidases, plasma ceruloplasmin and its membrane bound homolog, hephaestin:[41] the iron released as Fe^{3+} is taken up by plasma transferrin. A ceruloplasmin defect impairs macrophage and hepatocyte iron release,[42] giving rise to liver iron overload that is resistant to phlebotomy.[43] Transferrin is not essential for release of iron at the plasma membrane, since its absence in rare cases of congenital atransferrinemia does not prevent increased iron uptake from the duodenum and subsequent development of liver parenchymal iron overload.[44]

Regulation of iron absorption and internal iron exchange

Iron absorption in health and disease

Iron absorption is normally extremely sensitive to changes in body iron status, and both heme and non-heme iron absorption show an inverse relationship to iron stores.[45] However, pathological disturbances also influence iron absorption (Fig. 11.4). Inflammatory disease reduces absorption contributing to the impaired iron supply which is characteristic of the anemia of chronic disorders.[46] It has also long been recognized that grossly expanded erythropoiesis, particularly when the latter is ineffective as, for example, in the β-thalassemia disorders, can be associated with a marked increase in iron absorption, even in the face of pre-existing iron overload and an increased transferrin saturation.[47,48] Hypoxia is known to potentiate mucosal iron uptake in animal studies,[49] and in normal humans, stimulation of erythropoiesis by injection of recombinant erythropoietin markedly enhanced non-heme iron absorption.[50] Iron absorption studies carried out sequentially during treatment with erythropoietin and phlebotomy of iron-loaded patients with chronic renal failure suggested that anemic hypoxia enhanced mucosal iron uptake, while reduction in iron stores and increased erythropoiesis independently increased the transfer of iron to the plasma.[51] The concept of 'iron store' and 'erythroid' regulators of iron absorption gained currency, but their mechanisms remained obscure.[52] It is now known that hepcidin, a 25 amino-acid peptide hormone derived from a propeptide produced by the liver,[53] plays a key role in mediating these effects.

Role of hepcidin

In 2001 it was reported that expression of hepcidin was increased in iron loaded mice,[54] and that mice in which *HAMP*, coding for hepcidin, had been knocked out developed hepatic but not macrophage iron overload.[55] This pattern of disturbed iron metabolism in hepcidin deficient mice mirrors that seen in human hemochromatosis[56] and it became clear that the various types of hemochromatosis (see Table 11.3, below) are associated with inappropriately low production of hepcidin except in rare cases with a ferroportin mutation that prevents a response to hepcidin. Conversely, hepcidin over-expression in mice led to iron deficiency,[57] including in mice with inactivation of *TMPRSS6* (coding for matriptase-2, a liver transmembrane serine protease).[58,59] A human inherited iron-refractory iron deficiency anemia (IRIDA) was then shown to be associated with over-expression of hepcidin resulting from recessive inheritance of inactivating mutations of *TMPRSS6*.[60,61]

It is now clear that hepcidin is the major physiological regulator of iron absorption and internal iron exchange (Fig. 11.5), and that inappropriate hepcidin production underlies much iron pathophysiology.[11] Hepcidin binds to ferroportin at the 'donor' cell surface and promotes the transporter's internalization followed by ubiquitin-mediated lysosomal degradation.[62,63,64] Hepcidin-induced degradation of ferroportin prevents iron release to circulating plasma transferrin and leads to reduced iron absorption, a block on the release of iron derived from senescent red cells within macrophages, and reduced serum iron concentration. It is therefore a negative regulator of iron release from cells. Hepcidin is excreted rapidly into the urine consistent with its regulation at the level of production. Decreased hepcidin production is seen with hypoxia[65] and in association with ineffective erythropoiesis,[66] as well as in iron deficiency. Conversely increased

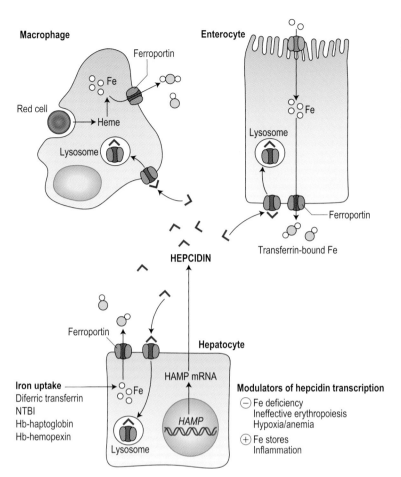

Fig. 11.5 Central role of hepcidin in iron metabolism. Hepcidin produced by hepatocytes down-regulates iron export to circulating transferrin from iron 'donor' cells (hepatocytes, macrophages and duodenal enterocytes) by promoting the internalization and lysosomal degradation of ferroportin. Hepatocytes take up iron in a number of forms, whereas enterocytes obtain their iron predominantly from the gut lumen (see Fig. 11.4) and macrophages are specialized to deal with the high throughput of iron from senescent red cells.

hepcidin production, occurs with inflammation[65] as well as with increased iron stores.

Regulation of hepcidin production

Uncovering the genetic basis of the various types of hemochromatosis (see Table 11.3, below) and of IRIDA stimulated exploration of signal pathways that act on the liver to regulate hepcidin production.[67] Iron status signals via the bone morphogenetic protein (BMP) pathway (Fig. 11.6).[68,69] Hemojuvelin (HJV), mutated in most cases of juvenile hemochromatosis, is a glycosylphosphoinositol (GPI)-linked cell surface protein which acts as a co-receptor for BMP6 (a key endogenous regulator of hepcidin synthesis).[69] It is thought that cell surface HFE (commonly mutated in adult hemochromatosis) and TfR2 (mutated in other cases of hemochromatosis) associates with HJV on the cell surface to allow signaling via BMP receptors and a SMAD pathway to the hepcidin promoter. It is possible that the link to iron status may be provided by competitive interactions between HFE and diferric transferrin for binding to TfR1: only the HFE remaining would then be available to associate with TfR2, the complex being stabilized by diferric transferrin.[70] A physiological increase in diferric transferrin would signal increased hepcidin transcription, reducing iron absorption and release from macrophages, while pathological disruption of HFE, HJV or TfR2 (in hemochromatosis) would be

accompanied by reduced hepcidin synthesis and increased iron absorption. Negative regulation of hepcidin production by matriptase-2 (TMPRSS6)[71] is mediated by proteolysis of membrane HJV,[72] and its absence accounts for the overexpression of hepcidin in familial iron-refractory iron deficiency anemia.

The increase in hepcidin in response to inflammation is predominantly mediated by interleukin-6 (IL-6)[73] and activation of signal transduction via STAT3.[74] Suppression of hepcidin production in association with ineffective erythropoiesis in thalassemia major occurs independently of iron stores.[75] A number of potential mechanisms for the 'erythroid regulator' are emerging. Erythropoietin can directly down-regulate hepcidin production through the erythropoietin receptor and C/EBPα transcription factor,[76,77] but this cannot account for a dependence of the erythroid regulator on the presence of an expanded erythroid marrow. Growth differentiation factor 15 (a member of the transforming growth factor β family) is up-regulated in serum from patients with thalassemia and congenital dyserythropoietic anemia type 1, and suppresses hepcidin production *in vitro*.[78,79] Its release from apoptotic erythroblasts would explain the greater iron loading in anemias with expanded erythroid marrow due to ineffective erythropoiesis rather than hemolysis. A further candidate molecule derived from erythroblasts is 'twisted gastrulation' which has been shown to interfere with BMP signaling via its receptor[80] and would

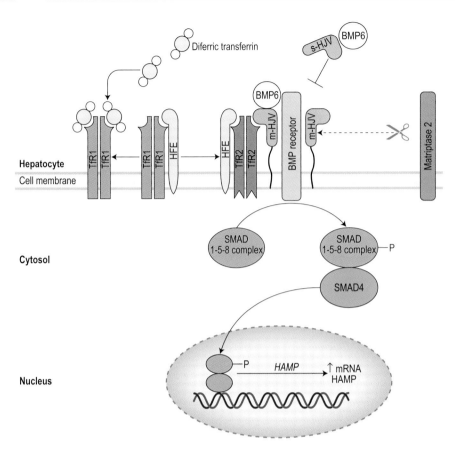

Fig. 11.6 Proposed mechanisms for regulation by iron of hepcidin production. Bone morphogenetic protein 6 (BMP6) activates transcription of the *HAMP* gene via a SMAD pathway. The receptor for BMP6 requires HFE, transferrin receptor 2 (TfR2), and membrane-bound hemojuvelin (m-HJV) as co-receptors. Diferric transferrin up-regulates the pathway by competing with HFE to bind to transferrin receptor 1 (TfR1) so that when iron is present HFE is available to associate with TfR2. Proteolysis of m-HJV by matriptase-2, and furin-mediated secretion of soluble HJV (s-HJV), which competes with m-HJV for BMP6, provide negative regulation of the pathway. Production of s-HJV is increased with iron deficiency and hypoxia.

thus suppress hepcidin synthesis. Finally, hypoxia may inhibit hepcidin production through involvement of the hypoxia inducible factor (HIF)/von Hippel–Lindau pathway. HIF-1α, induced by hypoxia and stabilized by iron deficiency, up-regulates furin-mediated cleavage of HJV to produce a soluble form of HJV: it is likely that this competes with membrane HJV for the co-receptors for BMP, thus down-regulating hepcidin production.[81]

Assessment of iron status

There is no single measure of iron status that is applicable in every situation. Combinations of measures of iron stores (macrophage and hepatocyte), iron supply to the tissues, and functional hemoglobin iron are often needed to arrive at a clear assessment of iron status.[82] The measures used are summarized in Table 11.1. All are subject to potential confounding factors.

Serum transferrin receptors

Serum transferrin receptors are truncated soluble receptors that are shed into the circulation mainly from the erythroblasts in the marrow.[83] The measurement reflects both the iron status of individual eythroblasts and the total mass of the erythron.[84] It is likely to be of most value in distinguishing iron deficiency from the anemia of chronic disorders.[85]

Serum ferritin

Serum ferritin is apoferritin made up from glycosylated ferritin light chains, the release of which from cells reflects current ferritin protein synthesis.[86] It is thus related to the intracellular labile iron that determines IRP affinity for the IRE, and only indirectly to iron stores through the release of ferritin iron either within the cytosol or through lysosomal degradation.[87] Ferritin protein synthesis also increases in response to inflammatory cytokines, behaving as an acute phase protein independently of iron stores. Damage to ferritin-rich tissues can release iron-containing ferritin into the circulation giving high ferritin values, e.g. in hepatitis, splenic infarction, or bone marrow infarction in sickle cell disease. Its use as a guide to the presence of increased iron stores is thus limited,[88] though a low serum ferritin is a clear indication that iron stores are absent. The dependence of ferritin protein synthesis on translational regulation by the IRP/IRE mechanism is illustrated by the rare hereditary hyperferritinemia/cataract syndrome, where autosomal dominant mutations in critical parts of the IRE stem loop are accompanied by uncontrolled synthesis of ferritin light chain: high serum ferritin values are seen with the development of cataracts, but there is no iron overload and transferrin saturations are not increased.[89] Other uncommon autosomal dominant causes of a high serum ferritin but normal transferrin saturation include loss of function 'ferroportin disease' and a benign hyperferritinemia associated with a point mutation in the coding sequence of L-ferritin.[90]

Table 11.1 Laboratory assessment of body iron status and confounding factors

Measurement	Representative reference range (adults)	Confounding factors	Diagnostic use
Functional iron			
Hemoglobin concentration Males Females	 13–18 g/dl 12–16 g/dl	Other causes for anemia besides iron deficiency; a reciprocal relationship with iron stores should be expected in all anemias except in iron deficiency anemia	Assess severity of IDA; response to a therapeutic trial of iron confirms IDA. Not applicable to assessment of iron overload
Red cell indices MCV MCH	 80–94 fl 27–32 pg	May be reduced in other disorders of hemoglobin synthesis (e.g. thalassemia, sideroblastic anemias) in addition to iron deficiency	
Tissue iron supply			
Serum iron	10–30 µmol/l	Labile measures: normal short-term fluctuations mean that a single value may not reflect iron supply over a longer period	Raised saturation of TIBC used to assess risk of tissue iron loading (e.g. in hemochromatosis or iron-loading anemias)
Saturation of TIBC	16–50%		
Serum transferrin receptor	2.8–8.5 mg/l	Directly related to extent of erythroid activity as well as inversely related to iron supply to cells	Decreased saturation of TIBC, reduced red cell ferritin, increased zinc protoporphyrin, and increased serum transferrin receptors indicate impaired iron supply to the erythroid marrow
Red cell zinc protoporphyrin	<80 µmol/mol Hb (<70 µg/dl red cells)	Stable measures: reduced iron supply at time of red cell formation leads to increases in free protoporphyrin and hypochromic red cells, and reduced red cell ferritin. However, values may not reflect current iron supply	One or more of these measurements may be helpful in conjunction with a measure of iron stores in distinguishing iron deficiency from anemia of chronic disorders
Red cell ferritin (basic)	3–40 ag/cell		
% hypochromic red cells	<10%	May be increased by other causes of impaired iron incorporation into heme (e.g. lead poisoning, aluminum toxicity in chronic renal failure, sideroblastic anemias)	
Iron stores			
Serum ferritin	15–300 µg/l	Increased as an acute phase protein and by release of tissue ferritins after organ damage Decreased by ascorbate deficiency	Serum ferritin is of value throughout the range of iron stores
Tissue biopsy iron Liver (chemical assay)	 3–33 µmol/g dry wt	Potential for sampling error on needle biopsy, especially when this is <0.5 mg, or liver is nodular	Liver biopsy remains the 'gold standard' in iron overload
Bone marrow (Perls' stain)		Qualitative assessment – needs specific assessment of macrophage iron	Bone marrow iron may be graded as absent, normal or increased and is most commonly used to differentiate ACD from IDA

ACD, anemia of chronic disorders; IDA, iron deficiency anemia; MCV, mean corpuscular volume; MCH, mean corpuscular hemoglobin; TIBC, total iron binding capacity.

The reciprocal relationship between the synthesis of transferrin receptors and ferritin within cells that is mediated by the IRE/IBP mechanism (Fig. 11.3) has its counterpart in values for serum transferrin receptors (increased) and serum ferritin (reduced) during the development of iron deficiency. The sensitivity of these measures for assessing iron status is increased by expressing them as a ratio.[91,92]

Tissue biopsy

Bone marrow biopsy is used to examine macrophage iron stores. It is primarily used for supporting a diagnosis of the anemia of chronic disorders rather than iron deficiency. Bone marrow biopsy touch preparations may give results comparable to aspirates.[93] Positive identification of the absence of iron stores may be inaccurate[94] unless careful examination of macrophages is made.

Liver biopsy provides the opportunity for histological examination of increased hepatocyte iron and any fibrotic or cirrhotic changes. The periportal distribution of iron accumulation in hemochromatosis may reflect selective expression of ferroportin in periportal hepatocytes and its degradation when hepcidin production is low.[64] In addition, chemical iron determination allows a quantitative assessment of the degree of iron loading. Quantitative phlebotomy in patients with thalassemia major who had undergone curative allogeneic bone marrow transplantation has confirmed that the liver iron concentration is a reliable indicator of total body iron stores in secondary iron overload resulting from red cell transfusions.[95] Magnetic resonance quantitative measurements (particularly T2*) of liver (and cardiac) iron[96] may reduce the future need for liver biopsy in iron overload disorders.

Potential clinical use of hepcidin assay

Difficulties in measuring urinary and serum hepcidin with lack of standardization[97] have so far restricted investigation of potential diagnostic uses. Plasma hepcidin concentrations are highly correlated with serum ferritin values in normal men,[98] and identification of inappropriately low hepcidin levels for existing iron stores might be diagnostically helpful in predicting the severity of the clinical course in iron loading disorders. However, like many other measures of iron status, confounding by the effects of inflammation is likely to make interpretation difficult. The possibility that hepcidin measurement might help to identify patients with anemia of chronic disease who also have an element of iron deficiency requires investigation.[99]

Iron deficiency

Iron supply to the erythron may be impaired as a result of an overall deficiency of body iron (absolute iron deficiency), or as a result of a demand outstripping supply (functional iron deficiency). Absolute iron deficiency develops when the ability of the diet and iron absorption to keep pace with iron requirements or losses is exceeded. The identification of iron deficiency anemia is not usually difficult, and the main clinical diagnostic task is to determine the cause of the negative iron balance.

Causes of iron deficiency

Iron deficiency anemia is extremely common[3] particularly among women of child-bearing age and pre-school children (who have increased physiological requirements for iron and whose intake is more likely to fall below the reference nutrient intake). In the UK in 2000–2001 the mean daily intake was 14.0 mg for men, and 11.6 mg for women,[100] and can be compared with the estimated average requirements of 6.7 mg for men and 11.4 mg for the majority of premenopausal women.[101]

The combination of a diet with poorly available iron and physiological increased iron requirements is probably the commonest cause of iron deficiency on a world scale. However, diet alone is very seldom the cause of iron deficiency in men or post-menopausal women in whom pathological blood loss should be suspected. Blood loss of more than about 6 ml (3 mg iron)/day, added to obligatory losses of about 1 mg/day through shedding of skin and intestinal cells, is likely to exceed the maximum iron absorptive capacity, hookworm infestation being a major cause in many parts of the world. In women of reproductive age, menstruation adds an average of 20 mg/month, and menorrhagia is a likely cause of anemia. In men or postmenopausal women, occult gastrointestinal blood loss must be considered, and in these patients, as well as younger women who have symptoms suggestive of gastrointestinal disease, endoscopic and/or radiological investigation of the gut is likely to be required.[102] This should be considered whether or not fecal occult blood tests are positive, since such bleeding may be intermittent. Less commonly, malabsorption of iron may be responsible for negative iron balance. Iron deficiency is a predictable complication after gastrectomy, where loss of the stomach acid and more rapid transit past the duodenal absorptive area of the gut, combine to reduce dietary iron availability. Celiac disease may present with isolated iron deficiency and features of hyposplenism on the blood film. Autoimmune gastritis, often without cobalamin deficiency, and *Helicobacter pylori* infection may account for many patients whose iron deficiency is otherwise unexplained.[103] The causes of iron deficiency are summarized in Table 11.2.

There remain a minority of patients in whom the cause remains uncertain. In older patients, bleeding from angiodysplastic lesions in the gut may be suspected, but careful follow-up is required since re-investigation may be needed if there are new symptoms or worsening of the negative iron balance. One of the rare genetic defects affecting iron metabolism may be suspected: iron-refractory iron deficiency anemia has already been discussed as a disorder with inappropriately high hepcidin production caused by inactivating mutation of the TMPRSS6 gene; three patients with autosomal recessive inheritance of mutations in DMT1 had an iron deficiency anemia but this was associated with increased transferrin saturation and hepatic iron loading.[104]

Clinical features of iron deficiency anemia

The symptoms of iron deficiency anemia are nonspecific, and where the anemia has developed over a prolonged period of negative iron balance the patient may be well adapted even at low concentrations of hemoglobin. Tiredness and shortness of breath are common complaints, while in the elderly with pre-existing cardiovascular pathology, angina or heart failure may develop. Other symptoms may be related to effects of iron deficiency on epithelial tissues or the gastrointestinal tract. For example, a sore mouth may be due to glossitis and/or angular cheilosis, and brittle nails may reflect the atrophic skin and nail changes, though frank koilonychia is now uncommon. Difficulty in swallowing may be related to an esophageal or pharyngeal web: this is still seen occasionally, particularly in middle-aged women with a history of chronic iron deficiency, and is a premalignant condition. Pica is sometimes a feature, and where this

Table 11.2 Causes of iron deficiency

Increased physiological requirements	
Growth	Pre-term and low birthweight
	Pre-school children
	Adolescents
Reproduction	Menstruation
	Pregnancy
	Lactation
Dietary insufficiency or poor bioavailability	
	Early introduction of cow's milk (low iron content) in infancy
	Vegetarian diet (insoluble phytate iron complexes)
	Antacids/protein pump inhibitors
	Clay eating (pica)
Blood loss	
Gastrointestinal	Epistaxes
	Varices
	Erosive gastritis
	Peptic ulcer
	Aspirin or other NSAIDS
	Carcinoma of stomach, colon
	Meckel's diverticulum
	Angiodysplasia
	Inflammatory bowel disease
	Diverticulosis
	Hemorrhoids
Pulmonary	Hemoptysis
	Pulmonary hemosiderosis
Genitourinary	Menorrhagia
	Post-menopausal bleeding
	Parturition
	Hematuria (e.g. renal or bladder origin)
	Hemoglobinuria (e.g. paroxysmal nocturnal hemoglobinuria)
Other blood loss	Trauma
	Widespread bleeding disorder
	Self-inflicted
Malabsorption	
	Post gastrectomy
	Autoimmune gastritis
	Helicobacter pylori infection
	Chronic systemic inflammatory disease
	Gluten-induced enteropathy (celiac disease)
Genetic	Congenital iron-refractory iron deficiency anemia (IRIDA)

involves ingestion of clay or chalk this may be the cause rather than the result of iron deficiency, through the formation of insoluble iron complexes in the gut lumen.

Development and pathological effects of iron deficiency

The development of iron deficiency can be considered in three stages[105] corresponding to the sequential involvement of storage iron, iron supply to the tissues, and the functional compartment of hemoglobin iron.

Exhaustion of iron stores

The first response to a negative iron balance is the mobilization of any iron stores from macrophages and hepatocytes, and an up-regulation of iron absorption. Assessment of iron stores will show declining values (Table 11.1), but there is no good evidence that depletion of iron stores has any harmful effects apart from reducing the ability to respond to increased demands for iron whether these are physiologic (e.g. pregnancy) or pathologic (e.g. hemorrhage). Erythropoiesis remains unaffected at this stage.

Iron-deficient erythropoiesis

A continued negative iron balance after iron stores are exhausted, leads to a decline in serum iron concentration and transferrin saturation to below the value of 16% found necessary to support normal erythropoieses.[14] The reduced iron supply to the erythron leads to up-regulation of transferrin receptors on the erythroblasts, with a rise in serum transferrin receptor concentration (Table 11.1). Other measures also begin to reflect the impaired iron supply, with increase in red cell protoporphyrin, and detection of poorly hemoglobinized reticulocytes and hypochromic red cells.[82,106,107] At this stage the hemoglobin concentration, mean red cell volume (MCV) and mean corpuscular hemoglobin (MCH) may still be in the reference range, though the blood film may show occasional hypochromic red cells.

Iron deficiency anemia

Further depletion of body iron leads to the development of iron deficiency anemia. The hemoglobin concentration drops below the threshold for definition of anemia (13.0 g/dl in men and 12.0 g/dl in women), and the red cell MCV and MCH are reduced. On the blood film, the red cells become more obviously hypochromic and variable in size, and poikilocytosis may be marked often with elongated 'pencil' forms (Fig. 11.7). Target cells may be visible. Reticulocytes are not increased appropriately for the degree of anemia, though serum erythropoietin concentrations are markedly raised. Platelet counts are usually increased, but there are case reports of associated thrombocytopenia.[108] The serum transferrin saturation is likely to be very low: this effect is exacerbated by a rising serum transferrin concentration – transcriptional regulation of transferrin synthesis by the liver is inhibited by iron excess and stimulated by its absence.[109]

A bone marrow examination is rarely needed to confirm the diagnosis. Marrow sideroblasts disappear early in the development of iron deficient erythropoiesis.[14] Erythroblasts show delayed hemoglobinization with a ragged, vacuolated cytoplasm, and relatively pyknotic nucleus for the stage of hemoglobinization. The white cell series is usually normal. Absence of stainable marrow iron stores in a randomly selected population of 38-year-old women could be predicted by a serum ferritin concentration of <16 μg/l (specificity 98%; sensitivity 75%).[110]

Mechanism of iron deficiency anemia

Impaired heme synthesis within individual erythroid precursors clearly accounts for many of the marrow and peripheral

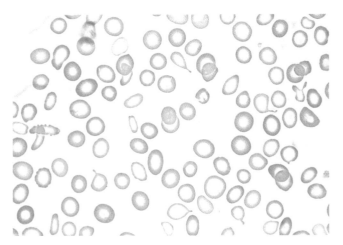

Fig. 11.7 Peripheral blood film from an iron-deficient pre-school child. (Hb of 5.5. g/dl and MCV of 50 fl). Microcytes and poikilocytes are prominent, as well as poor hemoglobinization of the red cells. ×1000.

blood findings, but not why the anemia is hypoproliferative, with an inappropriately low reticulocyte count despite raised erythropoietin concentrations. Studies in iron deficient rats[111] suggest that iron deficiency produces a maturation defect between CFU-E and early normoblasts.

Non-hematological effects of iron deficiency

These are less well defined than the effects on the erythron, and it has been difficult to disentangle the effects of anemia from those of tissue iron deficiency: anemia and depletion of tissue iron-containing enzymes usually develop in parallel.

The epithelial abnormalities described above are poorly correlated with tissue enzyme levels[112] and may respond slowly or not at all to iron therapy. Gastric atrophy and esophageal webs are also associated with circulating parietal cell antibodies, achlorhydria and an increased risk of pernicious anemia,[113] suggesting additional predisposing genetic factors.

Iron deficiency may impair immune function, with reduced T-cell and neutrophil function, while there are inconsistent data on whether iron supplements may increase the severity of some infections (e.g. malaria).[31,114] It remains uncertain whether iron has any significant effects in protecting against or potentiating the risk of infection. However, the links between immunity and iron metabolism have been re-emphasized by the discovery of the central role of hepcidin which down-regulates iron supply in response to infection and inflammation.

Work performance, aerobic capacity and endurance capacity is impaired in the presence of iron deficiency.[115] The effects can be attributed to anemia, though additional effects of tissue iron depletion on muscle oxidative metabolism and function are possible.

Iron deficiency anemia in children has been associated with impaired cognitive, motor and behavioral development, but separation from confounding socioeconomic disadvantage has been difficult.[116] Iron is taken up from transferrin by brain capillary endothelial cells, transferred by less certain mechanisms to the different brain cells.[117] It accumulates throughout childhood reaching highest concentrations in the basal ganglia. Since iron deficiency is common in pre-school children even in developed nations, there remains a need to determine whether it causes any psychomotor impairment and whether this is reversible.

Diagnosis of iron deficiency

The identification of a microcytic hypochromic anemia in a patient with a good reason for iron deficiency (e.g. menorrhagia) may require no further immediate investigation, diagnosis being confirmed by the correction of the hematological abnormalities with iron therapy. Lack of response to iron therapy is most likely to be due to a failure to take the treatment, or to continued occult blood loss. The diagnosis should be reviewed to make sure that other causes of microcytic anemia (e.g. defects of globin chain synthesis, severe and chronic underlying inflammatory disease or sideroblastic anemia) have been excluded: low serum ferritin combined with anemia will confirm the presence of depleted total body iron. However, because the serum ferritin is an acute phase protein, it may be within the reference range in the presence of an inflammatory disorder, even when there is coexistent depletion of iron stores (see discussion of the diagnosis of anemia of chronic disorders). Mild iron deficiency anemia may still have a red cell MCV within the reference range, and here the main differential diagnosis is with the anemia of chronic disease.

Treatment of iron deficiency

Treatment is usually readily achieved with an oral preparation of a simple iron salt, preferably ferrous sulphate (200 mg three times daily provides 180 mg elemental iron per day). Adverse effects such as nausea, epigastric pain, diarrhea and constipation are related to the amount of available iron, and can usually be ameliorated by reducing the dose of ferrous sulphate, switching to ferrous gluconate (which contains only 35 mg iron in each 300 mg tablet), and/or taking the iron with food. Although these measures reduce the amount of iron available to be absorbed, the speed of regeneration of the hemoglobin concentration is not usually critical. Slow release preparations should be avoided – they are an expensive way of avoiding adverse gastrointestinal effects by giving iron which is less available (it tends to be carried past the main absorptive site in the duodenum).

Parenteral iron (e.g. IV iron sucrose, Venofer®, or iron dextran, CosmoFer®) should be restricted to patients with proven iron deficiency who cannot tolerate even small doses of oral iron, or in whom continuing blood loss is so great that the oral therapy cannot keep pace. Adverse effects include anaphylaxis, and fever and arthropathy may occur particularly when large doses are given intravenously: this underscores the preference for oral iron therapy whenever possible.

Functional iron deficiency

Pathophysiology

A functional iron deficiency develops when the demands of the erythron for iron outstrip the ability to deliver iron to the marrow. For example, this balance is disturbed in thalassemia intermedia syndromes, when blood supply to the expanded marrow may be insufficient, even with increased plasma transferrin saturation, to satisfy the demands of the erythoblasts.[118] When erythropoietin therapy for the anemia of chronic renal disease was introduced, it was noted that even in patients with adequate or increased amounts of storage iron from previous red cell transfusions, the stimulation of erythropoiesis was typically accompanied by a drop in transferrin saturation[119] and the appearance of hypochromic red cells.[107] The impaired iron supply limited the hemoglobin response to erythropoietin, an effect which could be corrected by iron therapy.

Treatment

During erythropoietin therapy for the anemia of renal disease, the emphasis has moved away from avoiding iron therapy and its associated risk of iatrogenic iron overload.[120] The aim now is to maintain the iron supply (assessed by transferrin saturation or the percentage of hypochromic red cells), and thus the response to erythropoietin, through regular small doses of intravenous iron (e.g. 100 mg iron sucrose each month), provided the serum ferritin does not exceed 500–1000 μg/l.[121]

The pathophysiology of the anemia of renal failure has much in common with the anemia of chronic disorders, considered in the following section.

Anemia of chronic disorders

A normochromic normocytic anemia with an inappropriately low reticulocyte response develops in patients with a variety of inflammatory disorders provided these last more than a few days. Where the inflammatory stimulus is prolonged the anemia may become more microcytic. The severity of the hypoproliferative anemia is proportional to that of the underlying disorder, which may be infection, malignancy or an autoimmune disease such as rheumatoid arthritis. Inflammatory stimulation of the synthesis of acute phase proteins is reflected in an increase in plasma viscosity or erythrocyte sedimentation rate, and may be obvious on a blood film by the presence of increased formation of red cell rouleaux. The pathogenesis of the anemia is multifactorial: it involves the activation of cellular immunity and the production of a range of inflammatory cytokines by monocytes/macrophages, T lymphocytes and hepatocytes,[122] and is accompanied by an alteration in the handling of iron by macrophages (and other iron-donating cells) that is mediated by hepcidin and results in characteristic changes in measures of iron status.

Pathogenesis

Impaired production of erythropoietin

Patients with the anemia of chronic disorders generally have lower serum concentrations of erythropoietin compared with patients with other causes for anemia.[123,124] However, this is not a universal finding, and patients with juvenile chronic arthritis may retain a normal erythopoietin drive to the marrow:[125] this may account for the more profound red cell microcytosis often encountered in these patients, in whom limitations on the iron supply to the erythron appear to play a more dominant role. Pro-inflammatory cytokines interleukin-1 (IL1) and tumor necrosis factor-alpha (TNFα) are the likely mediators of reduced erythropoietin production by the kidney in response to anemic hypoxia.[122]

Inhibition of erythropoiesis

The inflammatory cytokines IL1 and TNFα also inhibit the growth of erythroid progenitors,[122] particularly CFU-E. These cytokine effects, mediated by promotion of apoptosis,[126] require the presence of marrow stromal cells (mainly macrophages), which are stimulated by IL1 to release interferon-γ (IFNγ), and by TNFα to release IFNβ.[127,128] The suppressive effect of IL1 and IFNγ could be reversed by high doses of exogenous erythropoietin, but the effects of TNFα may be more resistant to erythropoietin. Hepcidin has now also been found to inhibit erythroid colony growth.[129] The effects of reduced erythropoietin production and inhibition of eythropoiesis are thus likely to be the main cause of the hypoproliferative nature of the anemia in inflammatory disorders.

Decreased red cell survival

Activation of macrophages and enhanced erythophagocytosis is responsible for a modest reduction in red cell survival in inflammation.[130] Although the reduction in red cell survival would not, on its own, be sufficient to produce significant anemia, it compounds the impaired erythroid response (see above) mediated via inflammatory cytokines.

Reduction in iron supply to the erythroid marrow

Inflammation, and the anemia of chronic disorders, is associated with reduced serum iron concentrations and retention of iron within macrophages, as the result of increased hepcidin production induced by interleukin-6 (IL6).[65,73] In addition, the inflammatory cytokines IL1 and TNFα stimulate ferritin synthesis within macrophages and hepatocytes,[131,132] through an effect on transcription and translation of the mRNA which is independent of the IRP/IRE regulatory mechanism. Ferritin thus behaves as an acute phase protein providing a repository for the iron 'blocked' within macrophages. The plasma concentration of transferrin also tends to be reduced, and the reduction of transferrin saturation is thus often less severe than in iron deficiency anemias. The end result of these changes is the redistribution of iron from circulating red cells to macrophage iron stores (Fig. 11.8). Despite increased marrow iron staining and raised serum ferritin values, there is a modestly reduced iron supply to the erythroblasts. The finding that serum concentrations of transferrin receptor are not generally increased in the anemia of chronic disorders (unlike iron deficiency)[85] may relate to cytokine-induced inhibition of receptor synthesis. Alternatively, cytokine-induced inhibition of erythropoiesis may lead to a balanced decrease in both erythropoiesis and iron supply, so that the iron requirements of individual erythroblasts continue to be met and there is no activation of transferrin receptor synthesis through the IRP/IRE regulatory mechanism. In patients with inflammatory disorders who develop more severe red cell microcytosis there may be either more severe impairment of iron supply to the erythron, or

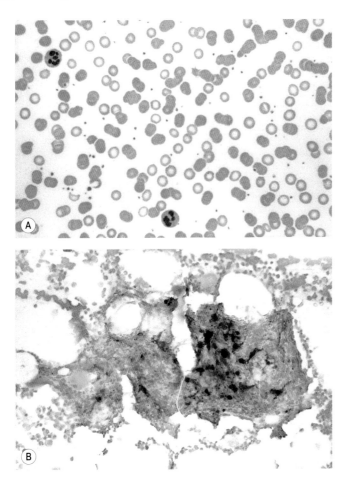

Fig. 11.8 (A, B) Peripheral blood film (A) and bone marrow aspirate stained for iron (B) from a 63-year-old lady with active rheumatoid arthritis (Hb 7.2 g/dl, MCV 66 fl). Marked hypochromia and rouleaux of the red cells (ESR 110 mm/h) was accompanied by plentiful marrow iron stores. These are the features of a block in macrophage iron release in a severe case of the anemia of chronic disorder. *(From Pippard MJ, Weatherall DJ 1984 Iron absorption in non-transfused iron loading anaemias: prediction of risk for iron loading, and response to iron chelation treatment, in thalassaemia intermedia and congenital sideroblastic anaemias. Haematologia 17:407–14).*

the suppression of erythropoiesis may be less marked. Both these factors appear to play a part in the microcytic anemia of juvenile chronic arthritis where abnormal cytokine production is dominated by an increase in IL6,[125] which stimulates hepcidin production but has little inhibitory effect on erythropoietin production or the response of the erythron. This suggests that differences in the amount and pattern of cytokine expression between different inflammatory disorders or between individual patients may account for variation in the effects on iron metabolism and erythropoiesis, and the corresponding degree of anemia and red cell microcytosis.

Diagnosis

The finding of a mild to moderate normochromic anemia in association with an obvious underlying disorder usually makes the clinical diagnosis of the anemia of chronic disorders, and the pattern of disturbance of the measures of iron status usually helps to confirm the diagnosis. Difficulty may arise when there is a possibility of iron deficiency coexisting

with the anemia of chronic disorders. Here the inflammatory increase in ferritin synthesis by macrophages and hepatocytes (see above) can lead to serum ferritin values which are within the normal reference range, even where iron stores are absent. Interpretation must take into account that values up to 70 µg/l may still be associated with absent iron stores where there is an acute phase response.[133] Furthermore these values must be considered in relation to the accompanying anemia, since there may still be inadequate iron stores to permit full regeneration of the hemoglobin once the inflammatory stimulus is removed. An increase in serum transferrin receptor concentration considered on its own may not reliably indicate a coincidental absolute iron deficiency where erythropoiesis is maintained despite a hepcidin-induced reduction in iron supply to the erythron, e.g. in juvenile chronic arthritis.[125] Under these circumstances the transferrin receptor/log ferritin ratio may yield a better distinction between anemia of chronic disorders alone and combined with iron deficiency (Fig. 11.9).[92,134] However, bone marrow examination, and Perls' stain for hemosiderin iron, may still be the simplest way to be certain whether there are iron stores present.

Treatment

The main approach is to treat the underlying inflammatory disorder: in many cases it is the underlying disease that gives rise to the main symptoms rather than the accompanying, generally modest, anemia. It may be possible to target one or more of the inflammatory cytokines: for example in rheumatoid arthritis an antibody to TNFα (infliximab) reversed excessive apoptosis among marrow erythroid progenitors and partially corrected the anemia.[135]

Where the underlying disease is intractable and the anemia is impairing quality of life (e.g. in association with cancer, where patients undergoing chemotherapy are especially at risk), red cell transfusion may help. Erythropoietic stimulating agents (ESAs) have been trialled in an attempt to obtain a more sustained rise in hemoglobin and avoid the need for, and potential complications of, transfusion. However, the outcomes of these trials have been disappointing: significant improvement in quality of life has not been shown consistently and there are concerns about increased venous thromboembolic disease and mortality in ESA-treated patients with a range of solid tumors.[136] Erythropoietin-induced down-regulation of hepcidin synthesis[76,77] might also be expected to improve iron supply to the erythron, but a hemoglobin rise is achieved more quickly if parenteral iron is given with the ESA.[137] Intravenous iron supplementation alone is likely to have limited benefit as it bypasses only one of the several restrictions on erythropoiesis in inflammatory disease, i.e. the hepcidin-induced limitation on iron supply. The possibility that iron chelators might be used to treat the anemia by 'shuttling' iron out of macrophage iron stores has been raised,[138] but has not been taken further.

Iron overload

Iron overload may be primary, resulting from a genetically determined increase in iron absorption, or secondary to a disturbance of erythropoiesis or other diseases (Table 11.3). The distinction is not always clear-cut. For example,

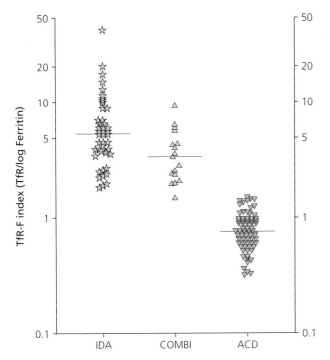

coinheritance of the C282Y mutation of the *HFE* gene (see below) may contribute to iron loading in diseases such as porphyria cutanea tarda,[139] and an unidentified genetic component may be required to allow the dietary iron loading in sub-Saharan iron overload.[140] However, the severe secondary iron overload that accompanies some genetic or acquired anemias is either the result of regular transfusion of red cells or a marked increase in iron absorption mediated by ineffective erythropoiesis: an additional contribution from a hemochromatosis gene is not required.

Iron overload disorders – definitions and pathophysiology

Severe iron overload (Table 11.3), whether primary (due to an inherited disorder of iron metabolism) or secondary (most commonly to disorders with expanded ineffective erythropoiesis), is arbitrarily defined as greater than 5 g excess iron.[141] The phenotype of hemochromatosis is the combination of such iron overload with iron-induced tissue damage. Hereditary hemochromatosis now encompasses several genotypes that result in excessive iron absorption with eventual parenchymal iron overload.[142] *HFE* mutations are common in populations of northern European origin,[143] while the other mutations are rare (Table 11.3). These genetic changes all involve disruption of the hepcidin/ferroportin axis (Fig. 11.5): mutations of *HAMP* directly prevent hepcidin production; mutations of *HFE*, *TFR2* and *HJV* disrupt

the signaling pathway that up-regulates hepcidin production in response to iron (Fig. 11.6), and 'gain of function' mutations of ferroportin are insensitive to hepcidin.

In patients receiving multiple red cell transfusions, or parenteral iron therapy, the iron is first released within macrophages (where it is relatively non-toxic), but subsequently undergoes redistribution to parenchymal tissues. The redistribution is likely to occur more quickly with low levels of hepcidin production when erythropoiesis is less well-suppressed, for example at times before red cell transfusion is due. The constant low levels of hepcidin in less anemic patients with ineffective erythropoiesis who do not require regular red cell transfusion lead to excessive iron absorption and parenchymal iron loading similar to that seen in hereditary hemochromatosis.

Primary iron overload

HFE-related (Type 1) hereditary hemochromatosis

Genetics. The disorder is inherited as an autosomal recessive: the *HFE* gene is located on the short arm of chromosome 6 and codes for an HLA-class-1-like protein.[144] In populations of northern European origin nearly all patients with hereditary hemochromatosis are homozygous for a point mutation responsible for a cysteine to tyrosine substitution at amino acid 282 (C282Y). Around 9% of people in the UK carry the C282Y mutation, but this becomes less frequent on moving south through Europe, being only 0.5% in Italy.[145] Mild increases in body iron are seen in less than a quarter of heterozygotes, but they are not at risk of clinically important iron overload.[146] A second mutation, substituting a histidine with aspartic acid at amino acid 63 (H63D), is more common in the general population and has a less defined role in predisposing towards iron loading: 4% of patients with hemochromatosis were found to be compound heterozygotes (C282Y/H63D), though most individuals with this genotype are not iron loaded.

Clinical features. A sustained positive iron balance leads to progressive accumulation of iron, and presentation, usually in the 4th or 5th decade, with evidence of iron-induced organ damage. A variety of clinical presentations mean that a high degree of clinical suspicion is necessary. Weakness and fatigue are prominent, while arthralgia, and impotence in males are common.[147,148] Arthritis particularly affects the second and third metacarpal-phalangeal joints, and a destructive arthropathy of the hip and knee joints may also occur. Late onset diabetes, abnormal liver function tests or skin pigmentation may all trigger suspicion. In younger patients cardiac failure and arrhythmias are more common at presentation, perhaps the result of more rapid accumulation of iron. Abdominal pain may result from hepatic enlargement or hepatocellular carcinoma.

Diagnosis. An increase in transferrin saturation is the first biochemical abnormality in the development of iron overload, and a fasting saturation of greater than 55% (men and post-menopausal women) or 50% (pre-menopausal women) suggests a risk of increased parenchymal iron uptake: a parallel measurement of serum ferritin allows an estimate of the current accumulation of excess iron stores. Genetic testing, initially for the common mutations of *HFE*, allows consideration of liver biopsy to be restricted to: 1)

Table 11.3 Causes of iron overload

Condition	Features of iron overload	Prevalence of iron overload
Primary iron overload		
Disordered hepcidin/ferroportin regulatory axis with parenchymal iron loading		
• Type 1 hemochromatosis (HFE-related)	Autosomal recessive. Adult onset. *HFE* mutations. Hepcidin inappropriately low.	Common in those of northern European origin.
• Type 2 hemochromatosis (juvenile)	Autosomal recessive. Presentation in 2nd or 3rd decade of life. Type 2a *HJV* mutations. Hepcidin low. Type 2b *HAMP* mutations. Hepcidin absent.	Rare
• Type 3 hemochromatosis	Autosomal recessive. Adult onset. *TFR2* mutations. Hepcidin low.	Rare – small proportion of adult hemochromatosis.
• Type 4 hemochromatosis (ferroportin 'gain of function')	Autosomal dominant SLC40A1 'gain of function' mutations Hepcidin insensitivity – levels high	Rare
Impaired cellular iron export with macrophage and parenchymal iron loading		
Type 4 'hemochromatosis' (ferroportin disease)	Autosomal dominant. SLC40A1 'loss of function' mutations. Mainly macrophage iron accumulation with low risk of damage. Hepcidin high.	Uncommon
Aceruloplasminemia	Autosomal recessive. *CP* mutations with loss of plasma ferroxidase. Brain and liver iron accumulation and damage.	Rare
Impaired iron utilization by the erythron with parenchymal iron loading		
• Congenital atransferrinemia	Autosomal recessive. *TF* mutations. Microcytic anemia with hepatocyte iron loading.	Very rare
• DMT1 mutations	Autosomal recessive *SLC11A2* mutations. Microcytic anemia with hepatocyte iron loading.	Very rare
Neonatal hemochromatosis	Fatal liver damage with iron loading. Mechanisms unknown. Possible autosomal recessive component.	Rare
Secondary iron overload		
Iron-loading anemias		
• Massive ineffective erythropoiesis (severe β-thalassemia syndromes, sideroblastic anemias, congenital dyserythropoietic anemias)	Increased iron absorption and/or blood transfusion. Hepcidin low.	Common, as a result of thalassemia, in those of Mediterranean, Middle-Eastern, and Asian origin. Other causes rare.
• Refractory hypoplastic anemias (e.g. chronic renal failure, pure red cell aplasia, aplastic and myelodysplastic syndromes)	Blood transfusion. Hepcidin variable.	Relatively common where adequate transfusion services available.
• Severe chronic hemolytic anemias (e.g. pyruvate kinase deficiency, congenital spherocytosis, sickle cell disease)	Mainly blood transfusion.	Rare as causes of severe iron overload.
Sub-Saharan dietary iron overload	Increase in both dietary iron and iron absorption. Macrophage and parenchymal iron loading.	Common in sub-Saharan Africa
Causes of modest iron overload		
• Chronic liver disease (alcoholic cirrhosis, portocaval anastamosis)	Increased iron absorption.	Common
• Metabolic syndrome	Mainly macrophage iron loading.	Relatively common
• Porphyria cutanea tarda	Increased iron absorption. Increased frequency of HFE mutations.	Relatively uncommon
Local iron overload		
• Lung (idiopathic pulmonary hemosiderosis)	Pulmonary hemorrhage.	Rare
• Renal (e.g. paroxysmal nocturnal hemoglobinuria)	Hemoglobinuria with renal tubular hemosiderosis.	Rare

those patients with a raised ferritin as well as transferrin saturation but who lack pathogenic mutations (where the question is whether there is an alternative explanation, e.g. hepatitis C, alcoholic or fatty liver); 2) patients with homozygous C282Y or C282Y/H63D, who have a serum ferritin >1000 µg/l, or abnormal liver function tests (where the question is whether fibrosis has progressed to cirrhosis, with the need to monitor for potential complications of the latter). Where patients have raised fasting transferrin saturation, but no evidence of increased iron stores (i.e. normal serum ferritin), the measures of iron status should be repeated at annual intervals: regular phlebotomy can then be started if the serum ferritin becomes elevated. Patients with pathogenic mutations and a raised serum ferritin, but to a level of <1000 µg/l and with no evidence of liver damage, do not require a diagnostic liver biopsy.[149] Quantitative phlebotomy – estimating the total amount of iron removed (at approximately 200 mg/unit of blood) before iron stores are exhausted, provides both treatment and confirmation of the diagnosis of iron overload.

Treatment. Removal of the excess iron by regular phlebotomy cannot reverse established cirrhosis and does not help the arthropathy, but even in those with established disease there is a reduction in mortality from cardiac and hepatic failure. Hepatocellular carcinoma is a major cause of death in those with cirrhosis, and regular monitoring with serum α-fetoprotein and liver ultrasound imaging may allow prompt intervention.

Patients diagnosed and treated before cirrhosis has developed have a normal life expectancy.[147] Phlebotomy at a rate of 450 ml/week is usually well tolerated, and continuation until iron stores are exhausted (serum ferritin <20 µg/l) allows calculation of the total iron load. Weekly phlebotomy may need to be continued for many months or years, since the excess iron is usually greater than 10 g in those with established tissue damage. The rate of phlebotomy may need to be reduced if the hemoglobin drops below 12 g/l. Thereafter current practice is to carry out phlebotomy at less frequent intervals (usually 2–6 times each year) to maintain the serum ferritin below 50 µg/l. However, this target is arbitrary, and some relaxation may allow the frequency of phlebotomy to be further reduced: iron absorption is still regulated by iron stores in hemochromatosis, albeit at a higher level, and maintenance of very low iron stores will increase the rate at which iron re-accumulates.[150]

Screening. Counseling and testing (phenotypic and genotypic) should be offered to siblings and parents, and considered for partners and children, of probands. Siblings in particular are at high (1 in 4) risk of having also inherited the hemochromatosis genes.

Population screening for HFE mutations remains controversial, since although there are clear benefits in early identification of those at risk, many of the approximately 1 in 200 people of northern European origin who have a hemochromatosis genotype will never develop the phenotype of severe iron loading and symptomatic disease[151,152] In the clinic it is currently difficult to predict which C282Y homozygote patients have already reached a stable relatively low level of iron accumulation and do not require phlebotomy treatment,[153] though elderly patients with serum ferritin values well below 1000 µg/l are most unlikely to progress. Phenotypic expression of the disease is likely to be dependent on an interaction with other genetic modifiers (e.g. *cis* and *trans*-acting polymorphisms that may impact on hepcidin expression[154]) and with physiological and environmental factors (e.g. symptomatic iron overload is less frequent in women before the menopause, while a high alcohol intake, enhancing the bioavailability of dietary iron,[155] is common in men with symptomatic disease).

Non HFE-related hereditary hemochromatosis

The following types of hereditary hemochromatosis are all rare, but extended genetic testing may be needed if a typical clinical picture cannot be explained by HFE mutations.

Type 2 hemochromatosis (juvenile hemochromatosis) is a more severe form of iron overload which presents before the age of 30 years with cardiomyopathy and gonadal failure.[156] The majority of cases (type 2a) are due to autosomal recessive inheritance of mutations of the gene coding for hemojuvelin (*HJV*), but in a minority (type 2b) it is the hepcidin gene itself (*HAMP*) that is mutated.[157]

Type 3 hemochromatosis has a similar clinical picture to HFE-related hemochromatosis. It results from autosomal recessive inheritance of mutations of the gene coding for transferrin receptor 2 (*TFR2*).[157]

Type 4 hemochromatosis arises from one of two broad types of mutation of the ferroportin gene, both inherited as autosomal dominants.[11] Mutations that prevent ferroportin regulation by hepcidin give rise to 'gain of function' and the typical clinical picture of hemochromatosis with parenchymal iron loading. By contrast, 'loss of function' mutations give rise to 'ferroportin disease', characterized by iron accumulation in macrophages, a high serum ferritin, and a low tolerance of phlebotomy. It is thus mainly a disorder of iron maldistribution rather than typical hemochromatosis.

Iron loading in other inherited disorders of iron metabolism

Other rare autosomal recessive disorders of iron supply, cellular iron uptake or iron release from cells give rise to a combination of iron loading with impaired utilization of iron.

Hereditary atransferrinemia is a very rare disorder characterized by severe microcytic anemia and parenchymal liver iron overload.[158] It illustrates the essential role for transferrin in delivering iron to the erythron, and the lack of dependence on transferrin for iron release to plasma and uptake by the liver. Increased iron absorption may reflect the absence of diferric transferrin from the signaling pathway that up-regulates hepcidin production in response to iron (Fig. 11.6).

Divalent metal transporter-1 (DMT1) defects, also exceedingly rare, give rise to a microcytic hypochromic anemia consistent with the role of the transporter in uptake of transferrin-bound iron by the erythron (Fig. 11.2). Accompanying hepatic iron overload implies an excessive iron absorption by a route that bypasses DMT1 for intestinal mucosal uptake.[104]

Aceruloplasminemia is characterized by iron accumulation in liver, spleen and brain with neurodegeneration.[158,159] Hepatic iron loading resistant to phlebotomy[43] and reduced serum iron with microcytic hypochromic anemia[159] are consistent with the ferroxidase role of ceruloplasmin in promoting cellular iron efflux via ferroportin.

Neonatal hemochromatosis

This is a rare severe form of hemochromatosis, characterized by perinatal liver failure, widespread tissue iron loading and high mortality.[160] In some cases it may be related to maternal infection, but others show features consistent with autosomal recessive inheritance of unknown basis.

Secondary iron overload

Parenteral iron loading

In transfusion-dependent anemias, each unit of red cells delivers approximately 200 mg iron. In congenital anemias such as β-thalassemia major, this can add up to 100 g iron by the end of the second decade of life, by which time most patients will have died from the toxic effects of the excess iron.[161] These include cardiac arrhythmias and heart failure, diabetes and failure of puberty, and cirrhosis. The rate of iron loading through regular transfusions is considerably greater than the maximum possible through increased iron absorption, and pathologic changes may therefore occur somewhat earlier than where the latter route predominates.[162]

Increased dietary iron intake

Increased oral intake of iron does not normally result in significant iron loading.[163] In sub-Saharan iron overload a combination of unusually high dietary iron bioavailability with an underlying (unknown) genetic defect is required to produce the disorder.[140] A ferroportin polymorphism common in African people is associated with higher serum ferritin concentrations, but there is no increased prevalence in affected families.[164]

Increased iron absorption

In patients with iron loading anemias associated with massive erythroid expansion (e.g. the β-thalassemia intermedia syndromes,[47] congenital dyserythropoietic anemias[165]) the rate of iron loading is directly related to the degree of erythroid expansion (Fig. 11.10).[162] For a given degree of erythroid expansion increased absorption is more pronounced with dyserythropoiesis than hemolysis.[48] However, even in HbH disease, where the defect is primarily hemolytic, iron overload from excessive iron absorption can be a problem.[166] The risk of iron loading via the gastrointestinal route may be concealed in some patients in whom a mild and asymptomatic anemia coexists with a marked expansion of dyserythropoietic marrow. Such patients may be at particular risk of misguided oral iron therapy,[167] and liver biopsy may be needed to determine the true extent of iron loading.

Mild degrees of iron excess are seen in some cases of chronic liver disease, and the metabolic syndrome (associated with diabetes, hypertension, hypertriglyceridemia, and obesity) can be a cause of high serum ferritin, though usually

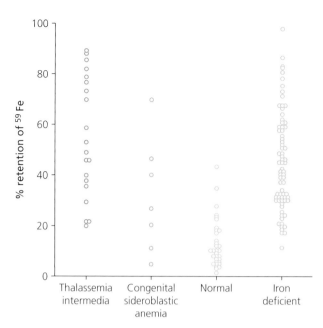

Fig. 11.10 Iron absorption from a test dose of 5 mg ^{59}Fe ferrous sulphate measured by whole body counting. Patients with massive ineffective erythropoiesis had iron retention similar to that of patients with iron deficiency, despite the fact that they had already accumulated substantial amounts of excess iron. *(From Pippard MJ, Weatherall DJ. Iron absorption in non-transfused iron loading anaemias: prediction of risk for iron loading, and response to iron chelation treatment, in thalassaemia intermedia and congenital sideroblastic anaemias. Haematologia 1984;17:407–14).*

with only modest increase in iron stores and no increase in transferrin saturation.[168,90]

Pathogenesis of iron-induced damage

Changes of liver fibrosis are seen very early in the development of iron overload in transfusion-dependent thalassemia.[169] In the liver, lipid peroxidation by iron-catalyzed hydroxyl radicals[170] results in impairment of membrane-dependent functions of mitochondria, including mitochondrial respiration, and damage to lysosomes resulting in their increased fragility. In iron overload, the lysosomal uptake of ferritin results in partial ferritin degradation to insoluble hemosiderin, and this may also increase the lysosomal fragility.[8] Pathologic fibrogenesis is mediated by the activation and proliferation of hepatic stellate cells, probably as the result of iron-induced oxidative stress. The degree of damage in various organs is not always clearly correlated with their iron content. In particular, the heart may show functional impairment despite relatively low and patchy iron deposition.

Treatment

Management of secondary iron overload in the iron-loading anemias is mainly dependent on the use of iron chelation therapy. It is the metabolically active labile iron within cells which is both the main catalyst for free radical formation and the major source of chelatable iron.[171] Deferoxamine is the most longstanding iron chelating agent in clinical use and has to be given as a continuous infusion on a regular daily basis to produce effective iron removal. Nevertheless, when used conscientiously in this way, maintenance of serum ferritin below 2500 µg/l prevents cardiac complications of iron overload,[172] and allows improved pubertal growth and prolonged survival. Its main disadvantage is the need for parenteral administration, and there are now two alternative oral chelators that have had significant clinical exposure, deferiprone and deferasirox.[173,174] The sites of action of the chelators may differ and this has provided a rationale for combined therapies where the iron overload is particularly severe.[175]

References

1. Dallman PR, Beutler E, Finch CA. Annotation: effects of iron deficiency exclusive of anaemia. British Journal of Haematology 1978;40:179–84.

2. Aisen P. Iron metabolism: an evolutionary perspective. In: Brock JH, Halliday JW, Pippard MJ, Powell LW, editors. Iron metabolism in health and disease. London: Saunders; 1994. p. 1–30.

3. DeMaeyer E, Adiels-Tegman M. The prevalence of anaemia in the world. Rapport Trimestriel de Statistiques Sanitaires Mondiales 1985;38: 302–16.

4. Cook JD, Finch CA, Smith NJ. Evaluation of the iron status of a population. Blood 1976;48:449–55.

5. Expert Scientific Working Group. Summary of a report on assessment of the iron nutritional status of the United States population. American Journal of Clinical Nutrition 1985;42:1318–30.

6. McCance RA, Widdowson EM. Absorption and excretion of iron. Lancet 1937;ii:680–4.

7. Esposito BP, Breur W, Sirankapracha P, et al. Labile plasma iron in iron overload: redox activity and susceptibility to chelation. Blood 2003;102:2670–7.

8. Selden C, Owen M, Hopkins JM, Peters TJ. Studies on the concentration and intracellular localization of iron proteins in liver biopsy specimens from patients with iron overload with special reference to their role in lysosomal disruption. British Journal of Haematology 1980;44:593–603.

9. Finch CA, Duebelbeiss K, Cook JD, et al. Ferrokinetics in man. Medicine 1970;49:17–53.

10. Green R, Charlton R, Seftel H, et al. Body iron excretion in man: a collaborative study. American Journal of Medicine 1968;45:336–53.

11. Andrews NC. Forging a field: the golden age of iron biology. Blood 2008;112: 219–30.

12. Huebers H, Csiba E, Huebers E, Finch CA. Competitive advantage of diferric transferrin in delivering iron to reticulocytes. Proceedings of the National Academy of Sciences, USA 1983;80: 300–4.

13. Edwards CQ, Kushner JP. Screening for hemochromatosis. New England Journal of Medicine 1993;328:1616–20.

14. Bainton DF, Finch CA. The diagnosis of iron deficiency anemia. American Journal of Medicine 1964;37:62–70.

15. Baker E, Morgan EH. Iron transport. In: Brock JH, Halliday JW, Pippard MJ, Powell LW, editors. Iron metabolism in health and disease. London: Saunders; 1994. p. 63–95.

16. Ohgami RS, Campagna DR, Greer EL, et al. Identification of a ferrireductase required for efficient transferrin-dependent iron uptake in erythroid cells. Nature Genetics 2005;37: 1264–9.

17. Fleming MD, Romano MA, Su MA, et al. Nramp2 is mutated in the anemic Belgrade (b) rat: evidence of a role for Nramp2 in endosomal iron transport. Proceedings of the National Academy of Sciences, USA 1998;95:1148–53.

18. Kuhn LC. Molecular regulation of iron proteins. Baillière's Clinical Haematology 1994;7:763–85.

19. Cairo G, Peitrangelo A. Iron regulatory proteins in pathobiology. Biochemistry Journal 2000;352:241–50.

20. Chen W, Paradkar PN, Li L, et al. Abcb10 physically interacts with mitoferrin-1 (Slc25a37) to enhance its stability and function in the erythroid mitochondria. Proceedings of the National Academy of Sciences, USA 2009;106:16263–38.

21. Shaw GC, Cope JJ, Li L, et al. Mitoferrin is essential for erythroid iron assimilation. Nature 2006;440:96–100.

22. May A, Bishop DF. The molecular biology and pyridoxine responsiveness of X-linked sideroblastic anaemia. Haematologica 1998;83:56–70.

23. Bekri S, Kispal G, Lange H, et al. Human ABC7 transporter: gene structure and mutation causing X-linked sideroblastic anemia with ataxia with disruption of cystosolic iron-sulfur protein maturation. Blood 2000;96:3256–64.

24. Huang ML, Becker EM, Whitnall M, et al. Elucidation of the mechanism of mitochondrial iron loading in Friedreich's ataxia by analysis of a mouse mutant. Proceedings of the National Academy of Sciences, USA 2009;106:16381–6.

25. Weiss G, Houston T, Kastner S, et al. Regulation of cellular iron metabolism by erythropoietin: activation of iron-regulatory protein and upregulation of transferrin receptor expression in erythroid cells. Blood 1997;89: 680–7.

26. Brittenham GM. The red cell cycle. In: Brock JH, Halliday JW, Pippard MJ, Powell LW, editors. Iron metabolism in health and disease. London: Saunders; 1994. p. 31–62.

27. Kawabata H, Yang R, Hirama T, et al. Molecular cloning of transferrin receptor 2. A new member of the transferrin receptor-like family. Journal of Biological Chemistry 1999;274:20826–32.

28. West AP Jr, Bennett MJ, Sellers VM, et al. Comparison of the interactions of transferrin receptor and transferrin receptor 2 with transferrin and the hereditary hemochromatosis protein HFE. Journal of Biological Chemistry 2000;275:38135–8.

29. Fleming RE, Migas MC, Holden CC, et al. Transferrin receptor 2: continued expression in mouse liver in the face of iron overload and in hereditary hemochromatosis. Proceedings of the National Academy of Sciences, USA 2000;97:2214–9.

30. Camaschella C, Roetto A, Cali A, et al. The gene TFR2 is mutated in a new type of haemochromatosis mapping to 7q22. Nature Genetics 2000;25:14–5.

31. Brock JH. Iron in infection, immunity, inflammation and neoplasia. In: Brock JH, Halliday JW, Pippard MJ, Powell LW, editors. Iron metabolism in health and disease. Saunders; 1994. p. 353–89.

32. Raja KB, Simpson RJ, Peters TJ. Investigation of a role for reduction in ferric iron uptake by mouse duodenum. Biochimica et Biophysica Acta 1992;1135:141–6.

33. McKie AT, Barrow D, Latunde-Dada GO, et al. An iron-regulated ferric reductase associated with the absorption of dietary iron. Science 2001;291:1755–9.

34. Gunshin H, Mackenzie B, Berger UV, et al. Cloning and characterization of a mammalian proton-coupled metal-ion transporter. Nature 1997;388:482–8.

35. Hubert N, Hentze MW. Previously uncharacterised isoforms of divalent metal transporter (DMT)-1: implications for regulation and cellular function. Proceedings of the National Academy of Sciences, USA 2002;99:12345–50.

36. Uzel C, Conrad ME. Absorption of heme iron. Seminars in Hematology 1998;35:27–34.

37. McKie AT, Marciani P, Rolfs A, et al. A novel duodenal iron-regulated transporter, IREG1, implicated in the basolateral transfer of iron to the circulation. Molecular Cell 2000;5: 299–309.

38. Zoller H, Theurl I, Koch R, et al. Mechanisms of iron mediated regulation of the duodenal iron transporters divalent metal transporter 1 and ferroportin 1. Blood Cells, Molecules , and Diseases 2002;29:488–97.

39. Frazer DM, Wilkins SJ, Becker EM, et al. A rapid decrease in the expression of DMT1 and Dcytb, but not Ireg1 or hephaestin explains the mucosal block phenomenon of iron absorption. Gut 2003;52:340–6.

40. Fleming MD. The regulation of hepcidin and its effects on systemic and cellular iron metabolism Hematology. American Society of Hematology Education Program; 2009. p. 151–8.

41. Vulpe CD, Kuo YM, Murphy TL, et al. Hephaestin, a ceruloplasmin homologue implicated in intestinal iron transport, is defective in the sla mouse. Nature Genetics 1999;21:195–9.

42. Harris ZL, Durley AP, Man TK, Gitlin JD. Targeted gene disruption reveals an essential role for ceruloplasmin in cellular iron efflux. Proceedings of the National Academy of Sciences, USA 1999;96:10812–7.

43. Hellman NE, Schaefer M, Gehrke S, et al. Hepatic iron overload in aceruloplasminaemia. Gut 2000; 47:858–60.

44. Beutler E, Gelbart T, Lee P, et al. Molecular characterization of a case of atransferrinemia. Blood 2000;96:4071–4.

45. Lynch SR, Skikne BS, Cook JD. Food iron absorption in idiopathic hemochromatosis. Blood 1989;74: 2187–93.

46. Weber J, Were JM, Julius HW, Marx JJ. Decreased iron absorption in patients with active rheumatoid arthritis, with and without iron deficiency. Annals of the Rheumatic Diseases 1988;47:404–9.

47. Pippard MJ, Callender ST, Warner GT, Weatherall DJ. Iron absorption and loading in beta-thalassaemia intermedia. Lancet 1979;2:819–21.

48. Pootrakul P, Kitcharoen K, Yansukon, et al. The effect of erythroid hyperplasia on iron balance. Blood 1988;71:1124–9.

49. Raja KB, Simpson RJ, Pippard MJ, Peters TJ. In vivo studies on the relationship between intestinal iron (Fe^{3+}) absorption, hypoxia and erythropoiesis in the mouse. British Journal of Haematology 1988; 68:373–8.

50. Skikne BS, Cook JD. Effect of enhanced erythropoiesis on iron absorption. Journal of Laboratory and Clinical Medicine 1992;120:746–51.

51. Hughes RT, Smith T, Hesp R, et al. Regulation of iron absorption in iron loaded subjects with end stage renal disease: effects of treatment with recombinant human erythropoietin and reduction of iron stores. British Journal of Haematology 1992;82:445–54.

52. Finch CA. Regulators of iron balance in humans. Blood 1994;84:1697–702.

53. Park CH, Valore EV, Waring AJ, Ganz T. Hepcidin, a urinary antimicrobial peptide synthesized in the liver. Journal of Biological Chemistry 2001;276: 7806–10.

54. Pigeon C, Ilyin G, Courselaud B, et al. A new mouse liver-specific gene, encoding a protein homologous to human antimicrobial peptide hepcidin, is overexpressed during iron overload. Journal of Biological Chemistry 2001;276:7811–9.

55. Nicolas G, Bennoun M, Devaux I, et al. Lack of hepcidin gene expression and severe tissue iron overload in upstream stimulatory factor 2 (USF2) knockout mice. Proceedings of the National Academy of Sciences, USA 2001;98:8780–5.

56. Fillet G, Beguin Y, Baldelli L. Model of reticuloendothelial iron metabolism in humans: abnormal behaviour in idiopathic hemochromatosis and in inflammation. Blood 1989;74: 844–51.

57. Nicolas G, Bennoun M, Porteu A, et al. Severe iron deficiency anemia in transgenic mice expressing liver hepcidin. Proceedings of the National Academy of Sciences, USA 2002;99:4596–601.

58. Du X, She E, Gelbart T, et al. The serine protease TMPRSS6 is required to sense iron deficiency. Science 2008;320: 1088–92.

59. Folgueras AR, de Lara FM, Pendas AM, et al. Membrane-bound serine protease matriptase-2 (Tmprss6) is an essential regulator of iron homeostasis. Blood 2008;112:2539–45.

60. Finberg KE, Heeney MM, Campagna DR, et al. Mutations in TMPRSS6 cause iron-refractory iron deficiency anemia (IRIDA). Nature Genetics 2008;40: 569–71.

61. Ramsay AJ, Hooper JD, Folgueras AR, et al. Matriptase-2 (TMPRSS6): a proteolytic regulator of iron homeostasis. Haematologica 2009;94:840–9.

62. Nemeth E, Tuttle MS, Powelson J, et al. Hepcidin regulates cellular iron efflux by binding to ferroportin and inducing its internalization. Science 2004;306: 2090–3.

63. De Domenico I, Ward DM, Langelier C, et al. The molecular mechanism of hepcidin-mediated ferroportin down-regulation. Molecular Biology of the Cell 2007;18:2569–78.

64. Ramey G, Deschemin J-C, Durel B, et al. Hepcidin targets ferroportin for degradation in hepatocytes. Haematologica 2009;95:501–4.

65. Nicolas G, Chauvet C, Viatte L, et al. The gene encoding the iron regulatory peptide hepcidin is regulated by anemia, hypoxia, and inflammation. Journal of Clinical Investigation 2002;110:1037–44.

66. Origa R, Galanello R, Ganz T, et al. Liver iron concentrations and urinary hepcidin in β-thalassemia. Haematologica 2007;92:583–8.

67. Camaschella C, Silvestri L. New and old players in the hepcidin pathway. Haematologica 2008;98:1441–4.

68. Babitt JL, Huang FW, Xia Y, et al. Modulation of bone morphogenetic protein signaling in vivo regulates systemic iron balance. Journal of Clinical Investigation 2007;117:1933–99.

69. Andriopoulos B, Corradini E, Xia Y, et al. BMP6 is a key endogenous regulator of hepcidin expression and iron metabolism. Nature Genetics 2009;41: 482–7.

70. Fleming MD. The regulation of hepcidin and its effects on systemic and cellular iron metabolism. Hematology: American Society of Hematology Education Program; 2008. p. 151–8.

71. Finberg KE, Whittlesey RL, Fleming MD, Andrews NC. Down-regulation of Bmp/Smad signaling by Tmprss6 is required for maintenance of systemic iron homeostasis. Blood 2010;115:3817–26.

72. Silvestri L, Pagani A, Nai A, et al. The serine protease matriptase-2 (TMPRSS6) inhibits hepcidin activation by cleaving membrane hemojuvelin. Cell Metabolism 2008;8:502–11.

73. Nemeth E, Rivera S Gabayan V, et al. IL-6 mediates hypoferremia of inflammation by inducing the synthesis of the iron regulatory hormone hepcidin. Journal of Clinical Investigation 2004;113:1271–6.

74. Wrighting DM, Andrews NC. Interleukin-6 induces hepcidin expression through STAT3. Blood 2006;108:3204–9.

75. Kattamis A, Papassotiriou I, Palaiologou D, et al. The effects of erythropoietic activity and iron burden on hepcidin expression in patients with thalassemia major. Haematologica 2006;91: 809–12.

76. Ashby DR, Gale DP, Busbridge M, et al. Erythropoietin administration in humans causes a marked and prolonged reduction in circulating hepcidin. Haematologica 2010;95:505–8.

77. Pinto JP, Ribeiro S, Pontes H, et al. Erythropoietin mediates hepcidin expression in hepatocytes through EPOR signaling and regulation of C/EBPα. Blood 2008;111(12):5727–33.

78. Tanno T, Bhanu NV, Oneal PA, et al. High levels of GDF15 in thalassemia suppress expression of the iron regulatory protein hepcidin. Nature Medicine 2007;13:1096–101.

79. Tamary H, Shalev H, Perez-Avraham G, et al. Elevated growth differentiation

factor 15 expression in patients with congenital dyserythropoietic anemia type 1. Blood 2008;112:5241–4.

80. Tanno T, Porayette P, Sripichai O, et al. Identification of TWSG1 as a second novel erythroid regulator of hepcidin expression in murine and human cells. Blood 2009;114:181–6.

81. Silvestri L, Pagani A, Camaschella C. Furin-mediated release of soluble hemojuvelin: a new link between hypoxia and iron homeostasis. Blood 2008;111:924–31.

82. Worwood M. Laboratory determination of iron status. In: Brock JH, Halliday JW, Pippard MJ, Powell LW, editors. Iron metabolism in health and disease. London: Saunders; 1994. p. 449–76.

83. Cook JD. The measurement of serum transferrin receptor. American Journal of Medical Sciences 1999;318:269–76.

84. Cazzola M, Beguin Y. New tools for clinical evaluation of erythron function in man. British Journal of Haematology 1992;80:278–84.

85. Ferguson BJ, Skikne BS, Simpson KM, et al. Serum transferrin receptor distinguishes the anemia of chronic disease from iron deficiency anemia. Journal of Laboratory and Clinical Medicine 1992;19:385–90.

86. Worwood M. Serum ferritin. Clinical Science 1986;70:215–20.

87. De Domenico I, Ward DM, Kaplan J. Specific iron chelators determine the route of ferritin degradation. Blood 2009;114:4546–51.

88. Worwood M, Cragg SJ, Jacobs A, et al. Binding of serum ferritin to concanavalin A: patients with homozygous β thalassaemia and transfusional iron overload. British Journal of Haematology 1980;46:409–16.

89. Cazzola M, Bergamaschi G, Tonon L, et al. Hereditary hyperferritinemia-cataract syndrome: relationship between phenotypes and specific mutations in the iron-responsive element of ferritin light-chain mRNA. Blood 1997;90:814–21.

90. Camaschella C, Poggiali E. Towards explaining 'unexplained hyperferritinemia'. Haematologica 2009;94:307–9.

91. Skikne BS, Flowers CH, Cook JD. Serum transferrin receptor: a quantitative measure of tissue iron deficiency. Blood 1990;75:1870–6.

92. Punnonen K, Irjala K, Rajamaki A. Serum transferrin receptor and its ratio to serum ferritin in the diagnosis of iron deficiency. Blood 1997;89:1052–7.

93. Pasquale D, Chikkappa G. Bone marrow biopsy imprints (touch preparations) for assessment of iron stores. American Journal of Hematology 1995;48:201–2.

94. Barron BA, Hoyer JD, Tefferi A. A bone marrow report of absent stainable iron is not diagnostic of iron deficiency. Annals of Hematology 2001;80:166–9.

95. Angelucci E, Brittenham GM, McLaren CE, et al. Hepatic iron concentration and total body iron stores in thalassemia major. New England Journal of Medicine 2000;343:327–31.

96. Anderson LJ, Holden S, Davis B, et al. Cardiovascular T2-star (T2*) magnetic resonance for the early diagnosis of myocardial iron overload. European Heart Journal 2001;22:2171–9.

97. Kroot JJ, Kemna EH, Bansal SS, et al. Results of the first international round robin for the quantification of urinary and plasma hepcidin assays: need for standardization. Haematologica 2009;94:1631–3.

98. Roe MA, Collings R, Dainty JR. Plasma hepcidin concentrations significantly predict interindividual variation in iron absorption in health men. American Journal of Clinical Nutrition 2009;89:1088–91.

99. Theurl I, Aigner E, Theurl M, et al. Regulation of iron homeostasis in anemia of chronic disease and iron deficiency anemia: diagnostic and therapeutic implications. Blood 2009;113:5277–86.

100. Henderson L, Irving K, Gregory J, et al. The National Diet and Nutrition Survey: adults aged 19 to 64 years. Volume 3: Vitamin and mineral intake and urinary analytes. London: HMSO; 2003.

101. Department of Health. Dietary reference values for food energy and nutrients for the United Kingdom. London: HMSO; 1989.

102. Rockey DC, Cello JP. Evaluation of the gastrointestinal tract in patients with iron-deficiency anemia. New England Journal of Medicine 1993;329:1691–5.

103. Hershko C, Hoffbrand AV, Keret D. Role of autoimmune gastritis, *Helicobacter pylori* and celiac disease in refractory or unexplained iron deficiency anemia. Haematologica 2005;90:585–95.

104. Iolascon A, De Falco L, Beaumont C. Molecular basis of inherited microcytic anemia due to defects in iron acquisition or heme synthesis. Haematologica 2009;94:395–408.

105. Charlton RW, Bothwell TH. Definition, prevalence and prevention of iron deficiency. Clinics in Haematology 1982;11:309–25.

106. Brugnara C. Reticulocyte cellular indices: a new approach in the diagnosis of anemias and monitoring of erythropoietic function. Critical Reviews in Clinical Laboratory Sciences 2000;37:93–130.

107. MacDougall IC, Cavill I, Hulme B, et al. Detection of functional iron deficiency during erythropoietin treatment: a new approach. British Medical Journal 1992;304:225–6.

108. Berger M, Brass LF. Severe thrombocytopenia in iron deficiency anemia. American Journal of Hematology 1987;24:425–8.

109. McKnight GS, Lee DC, Hemmaplardh D, et al. Transferrin gene expression. Effects of nutritional iron deficiency. Journal of Biological Chemistry 1983;255:144–7.

110. Hallberg L, Bengtsson C, Lapidus, et al. Screening for iron deficiency: an analysis based on bone marrow examinations and serum ferritin determinations in a population sample of women. British Journal of Haematology 1993;85:787–98.

111. Kimura H, Finch CA, Adamson JW. Hematopoiesis in the rat: quantitation of hematopoietic progenitors and the response to iron deficiency anemia. Journal of Cell Physiology 1986;126:298–306.

112. Jacobs A. Iron-containing enzymes in the buccal epithelium. Lancet 1961;ii:1331–3.

113. Jacobs A, Kilpatrick GS. The Paterson–Kelly syndrome. British Medical Journal 1964;2:79–82.

114. Prentice AM. Iron metabolism, malaria, and other infections: what is all the fuss about? Journal of Nutrition 2008;138:2537–41.

115. Haas JD, Brownlie T. Iron deficiency and reduced work capacity: a critical review of the research to determine a causal relationship. Journal of Nutrition 2001;131:676S–88S.

116. Grantham-Mcgregor S, Ani C. A review of studies on the effect of iron deficiency on cognitive development in children. Journal of Nutrition 2001;131:649S–66S.

117. Moos T, Rosengren Nielson T, Skjorringe T, Morgan EH. Iron trafficking inside the brain. Journal of Neurochemistry 2007;103:1730–40.

118. Pootrakul P, Wattanasaree J, Anuwatanakulchai M, Wasi P. Increased red blood cell protoporphyrin in thalassemia: a result of relative iron deficiency. American Journal of Clinical Pathology 1984;82:289–93.

119. Eschbach JW, Egrie JC, Downing MR, et al. Correction of the anemia of end-stage renal disease with recombinant human erythropoietin: results of a combined Phase I and II clinical trial. New England Journal of Medicine 1987;316:73–8.

120. Gokal R, Millard PR, Weatherall DJ, et al. Iron metabolism in haemodialysis patients. Quarterly Journal of Medicine 1979;48:369–91.

121. Drueke TB, Barany P, Cazzola M, et al. Management of iron deficiency in renal anemia: guidelines for the optimal therapeutic approach in erythropoietin-treated patients. Clinical Nephrology 1997;48:1–8.

122. Weiss G, Goodnough LT. Anemia of chronic disease. New England Journal of Medicine 2005;352:1011–23.

123. Baer AN, Dessypris EN, Goldwasser E, Krantz SB. Blunted erythropoietin response to anaemia in rheumatoid arthritis. British Journal of Haematology 1987;66:559–64.

124. Miller CB, Jones RJ, Piantadosi S, et al. Decreased erythropoietin response in patients with the anemia of cancer. New England Journal of Medicine 1990;322:1689–92.

125. Cazzola M, Ponchio L, de Benedetti F, et al. Defective iron supply for erythropoiesis and adequate endogenous erythropoietin production in the anemia associated with systemic-onset juvenile chronic arthritis. Blood 1996;87: 4824–30.

126. Selleri C, Sato T, Anderson S, et al. Interferon-gamma and tumor necrosis factor-alpha suppress both early and late stages of hematopoiesis and induce programmed cell death. Journal of Cell Physiology 1995;165:538–46.

127. Means RT, Krantz SB. Inhibition of human erythroid colony formation by IFN-gamma can be corrected by human recombinant erythropoietin. Blood 1991;78:2564–70.

128. Means RT, Krantz SB. Inhibition of human erythroid colony-forming units by tumor necrosis factor requires beta interferon. Journal of Clinical Investigation 1993;91:416–9.

129. Dallalio G, Law E, Means RT. Hepcidin inhibits in vitro erythroid colony formation at reduced erythropoietin concentrations. Blood 2006;107: 2702–4.

130. Dinant HJ, De Maat CEM. Erythropoiesis and mean red cell lifespan in normal subjects and in patients with the anaemia of active rheumatoid arthritis. British Journal of Haematology 1992;39:437–44.

131. Konijn AM, Carmel N, Levy R, Hershko C. Ferritin synthesis in inflammation II. Mechanism of increased ferritin synthesis. British Journal of Haematology 1981;49:361–70.

132. Rogers JT, Bridges KR, Durmowicz GP, et al. Translational control during the acute phase response. Ferritin synthesis in response to interleukin-1. Journal of Biological Chemistry 1990;265:14572–8.

133. Coenen JLLM, van Dieijen-Visser MP, van Pelt J. Measurements of serum ferritin used to predict concentrations of iron in bone marrow in anemia of chronic disease. Cinical Chemistry 1991;37:560–3.

134. Punnonen K, Kaipiainen-Seppanen O, Riittinen L, et al. Evaluation of iron status in anemic patients with rheumatoid arthritis using an automated immunoturbidimetric assay for transferrin receptor. Clinical Chemistry and Laboratory Medicine 2000;38: 1297–300.

135. Papadaki HA, Kritikos HD, Valatas V, et al. Anemia of chronic disease in rheumatoid arthritis is associated with increased apoptosis of bone marrow erythroid cells: improvement following anti-tumor necrosis factor-α antibody therapy. Blood 2002;100:474–82.

136. Bennett CL, Silver SM, Djulbegovic B, et al. Venous thromboembolism and mortality associated with recombinant erythropoietin and darbepoetin administration for the treatment of cancer-associated anemia. Journal of the American Medical Association 2008;299:914–24.

137. Adamson JW. The anemia of inflammation/malignancy: mechanisms and management. Hematology: American Society of Hematology Educational Program; 2008. p. 159–65.

138. Vreugdenhill G, Swaak AJG, De Jeu-Jaspars C, van Eijk HG. Correlation of iron exchange between the oral iron chelator 1,2-dimethyl-3-hydroxypyrid-4-one(L1) and transferrin and possible antianaemic effects of L1 in rheumatoid arthritis. Annals of the Rheumatic Diseases 1990;49:956–7.

139. Roberts AG, Whatley SD, Morgan RR, et al. Increased frequency of the haemochromatosis Cys282Tyr mutation in sporadic porphyria cutanea tarda. Lancet 1997;349:321–3.

140. Gordeuk V, Mukiibi J, Hasstedt SJ, et al. Iron overload in Africa. Interaction between a gene and dietary iron content. New England Journal of Medicine 1992;326:95–100.

141. Pippard MJ. Secondary iron overload. In: Brock JH, Halliday JW, Pippard MJ, Powell LW, editors. Iron metabolism in health and disease. London: Saunders; 1994. p. 271–309.

142. Pietrangelo A. Hereditary hemochromatosis – a new look at an old disease. New England Journal of Medicine 2004;350:2383–97.

143. Adams PC, Reboussin DM, Barton JC. Hemochromatosis and iron-overload screening in a racially diverse population. New England Journal of Medicine 2005;352:1769–678.

144. Feder JN, Gnirke A, Thomas W, et al. A novel MHC class I-like gene is mutated in patients with hereditary haemochromatosis. Nature Genetics 1996;13:399–408.

145. Merryweather-Clarke AT, Pointon JJ, Shearman JD, Robson KJ. Global prevalence of putative haemochromatosis mutations. Journal of Medical Genetics 1997;34:275–8.

146. Bulaj ZJ, Griffen LM, Jorde LB, et al. Clinical and biochemical abnormalities in people heterozygous for hemochromatosis. New England Journal of Medicine 1996;335:1799–805.

147. Niederau C, Fischer R, Purschel A, et al. Long-term survival and causes of death in patients with hereditary hemochromatosis. Gastroenterology 1991;110:1107–19.

148. Adams PC, Deugnier Y, Moirand R, Brissot P. The relationship between iron overload, clinical symptoms, and age in 410 patients with genetic hemochromatosis. Hepatology 1997; 25:162–6.

149. Dooley J, Worwood M. Genetic haemochromatosis. Guidelines on diagnosis and therapy compiled on behalf of the British Committee for Standards in Haematology. Abingdon: Darwin Medical Communications; 2000.

150. Piperno A, Girelli, Nemeth E, et al. Blunted hepcidin response to oral iron challenge in HFE-related hemochromatosis. Blood 2007;110: 4096–100.

151. Jackson HA, Carter K, Darke C, et al. HFE mutations, iron deficiency and overload in 10,500 blood donors. British Journal of Haematology 2001;114: 474–84.

152. Beutler E, Felitti VJ, Koziol JA, et al. Penetrance of 845G –> A (C282Y) HFE hereditary haemochromatosis mutation in the USA. Lancet 2002;359:211–8.

153. Adams PC, Barton JC. How I treat hemochromatosis. Blood 2010;116: 317–25.

154. Bayele HK, Srai SKS. Genetic variation in hepcidin expression and its implications for phenotypic differences in iron metabolism. Haematologica 2009;94:1185–8.

155. Charlton RW, Jacobs P, Seftel H, Bothwell TH. Effect of alcohol on iron absorption. British Medical Journal 1964;2:1427–9.

156. Kelly AL, Rhodes DA, Roland JM, et al. Hereditary juvenile haemochromatosis: a genetically heterogenous life-threatening iron-storage disease. Quarterly Journal of Medicine 1998;91:607–18.

157. Camaschella C. Understanding iron homeostasis through genetic analysis of hemochromatosis and related disorders. Blood 2005;106:3710–7.

158. Jeong SY, David S. Glycophosphotidylinositol-anchored ceruloplasmin is required for iron efflux from cells in the central nervous system. Journal of Biological Chemistry 2003;278:27144–8.

159. Bosio S, De Gobbi M, Roetto A, et al. Anemia and iron overload due to compound heterozygosity for novel ceruloplasmin mutations. Blood 2002;100:2246–8.

160. Kelly AL, Lunt PW, Rodrigues F, et al. Classification and genetic features of neonatal haemochromatosis: a study of 27 affected pedigrees and molecular

analysis of genes implicated in iron metabolism. Journal of Medical Genetics 2001;38:599–610.

161. Modell B. Advances in the use of iron-chelating agents for the treatment of iron overload. Progress in Hematology 1979;11:267–312.

162. Pippard MJ, Weatherall DJ. Iron absorption in non-transfused iron loading anaemias: prediction of risk for iron loading, and response to iron chelation treatment, in β thalassaemia intermedia and congenital sideroblastic anaemias. Haematologia 1984;17: 407–14.

163. Sayers MH, English G, Finch C. Capacity of the store-regulator in maintaining iron balance. American Journal of Hematology 1994;47:194–7.

164. McNamara L, Gordeuk VR, MacPhail AP. Ferroportin (Q248H) mutations in African families with dietary iron overload. Journal of Gastroenterology and Hepatology 2005;20:1855–8.

165. Wickramasinghe SN, Thein SL, Srichairatanakool S, Porter JB. Determinants of iron status and bilirubin levels in congenital dyserythropoietic anaemia type I. British Journal of Haematology 1999;107:522–5.

166. Chen FE, Ooi C, Ha SY, et al. Genetic and clinical features of hemoglobin H disease in Chinese patients. New England Journal of Medicine 2000; 343:544–50.

167. Peto TEA, Pippard MJ, Weatherall DJ. Iron overload in mild sideroblastic anaemias. Lancet 1983;i:375–8.

168. Moirand R, Moertaji AM, Loreal O, et al. A new syndrome of liver iron overload with normal transferrrin saturation. Lancet 1997;349:95–7.

169. Iancu TC, Neustein HB, Landing BH. The liver in thalassaemia major: ultrastructural observation. In: Iron Metabolism. Ciba Foundation Symposium 51. North Holland: Elsevier; 1977. p. 293–309.

170. McCord JM. Iron, free radicals, and oxidative injury. Seminars in Hematology 1998;35:5–12.

171. Pippard MJ, Callender ST, Finch CA. Ferrioxamine excretion in iron-loaded man. Blood 1982;60:288–94.

172. Olivieri NF, Nathan DG, MacMillan JH, et al. Survival in medically treated patients with homozygous α-thalassemia. New England Journal of Medicine 1994;331:574–8.

173. Maggio A. Light and shadows in the iron chelation treatment of haematological diseases. British Journal of Haematology 2007;138:407–21.

174. Cappellini MD, Porter JD, El-Beshlawy A, et al. Tailoring iron chelation by iron intake and serum ferritin: the prospective EPIC study of deferasirox in 1744 patients with transfusion-dependent anemias. Haematologica 2010;95: 557–66.

175. Angelucci E, Barosi G, Camaschella C, et al. Italian Society of Hematology practice guidelines for the management of iron overload in thalassemia major and related disorders. Haematologica 2008;93:741–52.

Macrocytic anemia

R Green

Chapter contents

Macrocytic anemias fall into two categories: those associated with megaloblastic hemopoiesis and those associated with normoblastic hemopoiesis.[1-3] The most common causes of megaloblastic hemopoiesis are vitamin B$_{12}$ or folate deficiency. Disruption of vitamin B$_{12}$ or folate metabolic pathways may also cause this type of disturbed hemopoiesis as may vitamin B$_{12}$ or folate-independent mechanisms that interfere with DNA synthesis.

Megaloblastic hemopoiesis

Paul Ehrlich first used the term megaloblast in 1880 to describe a morphologically abnormal erythroblast seen in the bone marrow of patients with untreated pernicious anemia. It was subsequently found that megaloblasts occur in many other conditions (see Boxes 12.1 and 12.2). Megaloblastic erythropoiesis is characterized by three features: 1) erythroblasts that are larger than normal at all stages of maturation; 2) a dissociation between cytoplasmic and nuclear maturation leading to early and late polychromatic erythroblasts with well-hemoglobinized (i.e. polychromatic) cytoplasm having nuclei containing considerably less mature and more open appearing chromatin than their normal counterparts (Figs 12.1 and 12.2); and 3) the generation of larger than normal macrocytes typically oval in shape (Fig. 12.3). In megaloblastic erythropoiesis there is also an increased relative number of early and late polychromatic erythroblasts with dysplastic features (see Chapter 5), an increased number of basophilic erythropoietic cells relative to more mature erythroblasts (Fig. 12.4) and erythroid hyperplasia, giving the overall appearance of a maturation arrest of the bone marrow. The severity of each of these morphologic abnormalities increases with increasing severity of the anemia.

Megaloblastic erythropoiesis is substantially ineffective and the extent of ineffectiveness is generally proportional to the extent of the anemia. The ineffectiveness of megaloblastic erythropoiesis results from an abnormality of the red cell precursors during the S-phase of the cell cycle, which leads to apoptosis with consequent phagocytosis by bone marrow macrophages of a substantial proportion of the early and late polychromatic megaloblasts.[4] The biochemical lesion is believed to occur during the S-phase of the cell cycle, uniformly throughout the maturational sequence among precursors undergoing mitosis. Hence, vitamin B$_{12}$-deficient or folate-deficient early polychromatic megaloblasts appear morphologically to become arrested at all stages of the cell cycle.

Usually patients with megaloblastic erythropoiesis also show morphologic abnormalities ('megaloblastic changes') in cells of the granulocyte series. The two most striking abnormalities are the formation of giant metamyelocytes in the marrow (Fig. 12.5) and the presence of hypersegmented neutrophil granulocytes in the blood (Fig. 12.6). The giant metamyelocytes are 17–30 μm or more in diameter and usually have long horseshoe-shaped nuclei, sometimes with one or more bud-like protuberances. In addition, these cells may contain cytoplasmic vacuoles, nuclear perforations or unevenly stained chromatin. Giant metamyelocytes have DNA contents in the entire range between the diploid (2c) and tetraploid (4c) values. This seems to result from abnormal development in promyelocytes and myelocytes that have been arrested or retarded during their progress through

©2011 Elsevier Ltd
DOI: 10.1016/B978-0-7020-3147-2.00012-2

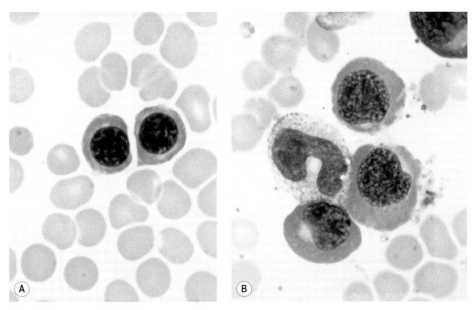

Fig. 12.1 (A, B) Differences between megaloblastic and normoblastic erythropoiesis as seen in bone marrow smears. (A) Two early polychromatic normoblasts from a healthy adult. (B) Three early polychromatic megaloblasts (and one giant neutrophil metamyelocyte) from a patient with severe pernicious anemia. May–Grünwald–Giemsa stain. ×1000.

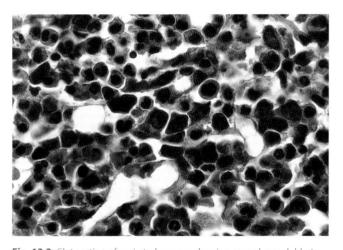

Fig. 12.2 Clot section of aspirated marrow showing several megaloblasts. These have relatively little condensed chromatin and contain several nucleoli some of which abut on the nuclear membrane. H&E stain. ×400.

the cell cycle, in much the same way as occurs in the erythroid series. Most of these defective giant cells may be phagocytosed by bone marrow macrophages but a few undergo nuclear segmentation and develop into giant polymorphonuclear leukocytes known as 'macropolycytes' (Fig. 12.7); these have hyperdiploid DNA contents. By contrast, hypersegmented neutrophils have diploid DNA contents and are presumed to be derived from relatively normal-looking metamyelocytes with diploid DNA contents. In either case, the underlying problem appears to be a qualitative defect in DNA synthesis.

Megakaryocytes are usually normal or decreased in number and occasionally display markedly hyperlobated nuclei with corresponding hyperdiploid DNA content.

Vitamin B$_{12}$-related and folate-related causes of megaloblastic anemia

The vitamin B$_{12}$- and folate-related causes of macrocytosis with megaloblastic erythropoiesis are given in Box 12.1.

Vitamin B$_{12}$

The vitamin B$_{12}$ molecule consists of two parts aligned at right angles to each other: 1) a planar corrin nucleus (containing four pyrrole rings); and 2) the ribonucleotide of 5,6-dimethylbenzimidazole. A cobalt atom is located at the center of the corrin nucleus and is coordinately bonded to the four pyrrole rings and below the pyrrole plane, to one of the nitrogen atoms of the ribonucleotide as well as to an upper ligand above the pyrrole plane such as methyl, deoxyadenosyl, cyano or hydroxo. The two naturally occurring B$_{12}$ coenzymes contain the methyl or deoxyadenosyl group and are known as methylcobalamin and deoxyadenosylcobalamin, respectively. In nature, vitamin B$_{12}$ is synthesized exclusively by prokaryotic microorganisms. Synthesis by bacteria resident in the gut serves as the main source of B$_{12}$ in ruminant herbivores and in others through deliberate or incidental coprophagia. Other animals and man obtain B$_{12}$ by consuming foods of animal origin, including dairy products. Vegetables and fruits are devoid of vitamin B$_{12}$ except through contamination by bacteria. A mixed diet contains about 5–30 μg vitamin B$_{12}$ per day and 1–3 μg of this are absorbed. The vitamin in food is largely protein-bound and is released from its bound state within the stomach by the action of the proteolytic enzyme pepsin. Most of the released B$_{12}$ rapidly attaches to a B$_{12}$-binding protein found in saliva and gastric juice known as R-binder, a haptocorrin-like binder. Subsequently, B$_{12}$ is released from the R-binder in the jejunum as a result of the alkaline pH and degradation by pancreatic trypsin. The released B$_{12}$ then combines with intrinsic factor,

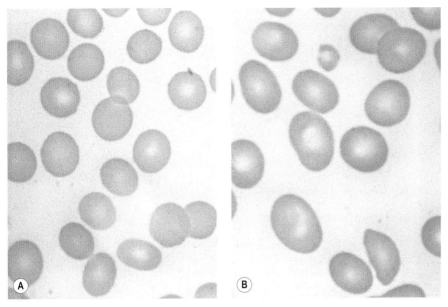

Fig. 12.3 (A, B) Red cells from a healthy adult (A) and from a case of severe pernicious anemia (B). The pernicious anemia patient's red cells are macrocytic and oval in shape (oval macrocytes). May–Grünwald–Giemsa stain. ×1000.

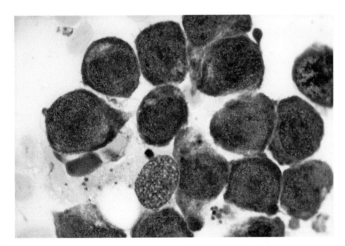

Fig. 12.4 Bone marrow smear from a patient with severe pernicious anemia showing a marked increase in the proportion of basophilic erythroblasts. May–Grünwald–Giemsa stain. ×1000.

a glycoprotein secreted by the parietal cells of the fundus and body of the stomach (Fig. 12.8). The vitamin B_{12}-intrinsic factor complex, which is resistant to digestion, passes down to the distal portion of the ileum where absorption takes place via a specific receptor, termed cubam, on the brush border of the mucosal cells. This receptor is coded for by two genes, cubilin and amnionless.[5] There is a mucosal delay of a few hours before the absorbed vitamin B_{12} enters the portal blood. Most of the newly absorbed vitamin B_{12} in portal blood and 20–30% of total circulating B_{12} is attached to a specific B_{12} binding protein known as transcobalamin (TC) (previously transcobalamin II) although most of the vitamin B_{12} in the blood is bound to haptocorrin (previously transcobalamin I).

Vitamin B_{12} is found mainly in the liver, the hepatic stores being 2–5 mg. The absorption of 1–3 μg vitamin B_{12} per day balances an inevitable daily loss of the same magnitude. Loss occurs largely in the urine and feces via desquamation of epithelial cells and in the bile. There is an enterohepatic circulation of vitamin B_{12}:[6] about 3–6 μg is excreted daily into the intestinal tract, mainly in the bile, of which all but about 1 μg is reabsorbed in the terminal ileum. If intrinsic factor is absent or ileal absorption is defective, there is failure to conserve vitamin B_{12} secreted in the bile.[7]

The biochemical mechanisms by which vitamin B_{12} deficiency leads to its main clinical consequences of anemia, peripheral neuropathy and subacute combined degeneration of the spinal cord remain uncertain.[2] Only two reactions are known to require vitamin B_{12} in man. These are: 1) the isomerization of methylmalonyl coenzyme A to succinyl coenzyme A, which occurs in the mitochondria and is dependent on deoxyadenosylcobalamin; and 2) the cytosolic methylation of homocysteine to methionine, which requires the enzyme homocysteine-methionine methyl transferase (methionine synthase), the methyl donor 5-methyltetrahydrofolate (methyl-THF) and the coenzyme methylcobalamin. During the latter reaction the methyl-THF is converted to THF and impairment of this reaction in bone marrow cells results in defective methylation of deoxyuridylate to thymidylate due to a decreased availability of 5,10-methylenetetrahydrofolate (5,10-methylene-THF) (Fig. 12.9). Defective thymidylate synthesis is thought to lead to defective DNA synthesis, caused by misincorporation of uracil into DNA and, consequently, to the development of megaloblastic hematopoiesis and anemia.[2] The mechanism by which impairment of the transferase reaction results in decreased levels of 5,10-methylene-THF is still controversial. Some have suggested that this impairment results in 'trapping' of intracellular folates in the form of 5-methyl-THF which cannot be converted to 5,10-methylene-THF.[8,9] Others

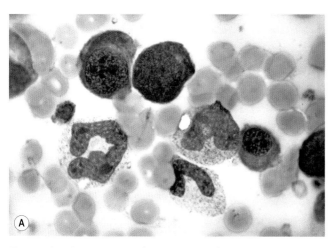
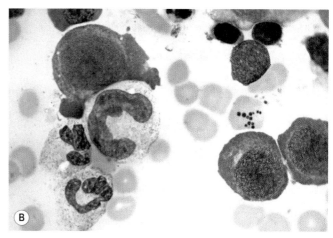

Fig. 12.5 (A, B) Marrow smear from a patient with pernicious anemia. (A) Giant metamyelocyte, normal-sized neutrophil band form and neutrophil myelocyte with a slightly indented nucleus. The nucleus of the giant metamyelocyte has a bud-like protrusion along its length. (B) Giant metamyelocyte adjacent to two normal-sized neutrophil granulocytes. May–Grünwald–Giemsa stain. ×1000.

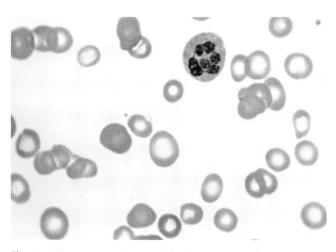

Fig. 12.6 Hypersegmented neutrophil and macrocytes in the blood smear of a patient with pernicious anemia. May–Grünwald–Giemsa stain. ×1000.

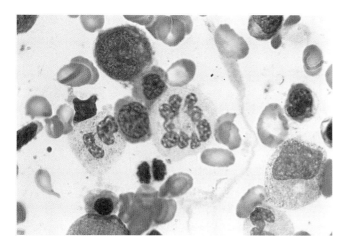

Fig. 12.7 Hypersegmented macropolycyte and a normal-sized neutrophil with two nuclear segments from the bone marrow smear of a patient with pernicious anemia. The nuclear and cytoplasmic areas of the macropolycyte are similar to those of the giant metamyelocytes in Fig. 12.5. May–Grünwald–Giemsa stain. ×1000.

Box 12.1 Vitamin B_{12}-related and folate-related causes of macrocytosis with megaloblastic erythropoiesis

Vitamin B_{12}-related

(a) Inadequate dietary intake: veganism

(b) Gastric lesions: pernicious anemia, total or partial gastrectomy, congenital intrinsic factor deficiency, congenitally abnormal intrinsic factor

(c) Intestinal lesions: stagnant loop syndrome, ileal resection, Crohn's disease, chronic tropical sprue, fish tapeworm, selective malabsorption with proteinuria (Imerslund–Gräsbeck syndrome)

(d) Other causes of malabsorption of vitamin B_{12}: food cobalamin malabsorption, some drugs, chronic pancreatitis, Zollinger–Ellison syndrome, HIV infection, irradiation, graft versus host disease, etc.

(e) Acquired abnormality of cobalamin metabolism: nitrous oxide toxicity

(f) Inherited abnormalities of cobalamin transport and metabolism

Folate-related

(a) Inadequate dietary intake

(b) Malabsorption: celiac disease, jejunal resection, tropical sprue

(c) Increased requirement or loss: pregnancy, prematurity, hemolytic anemia, malignant disease, chronic inflammatory disease, long-term dialysis, congestive heart failure, liver disease

(d) Acquired abnormality of folate metabolism: dihydrofolate reductase inhibitors

(e) Complex mechanism: anti-convulsant therapy, ethanol abuse, oral contraceptive drugs

(f) Congenital disorders of folate absorption and metabolism

---

have considered that the important consequence of the impairment of the transferase reaction is the failure of methionine synthesis which in turn results in a reduced availability of formate and inadequate formylation of tetrahydrofolate, formyltetrahydrofolate being the necessary substrate for polyglutamate synthesis, required for 5, 10-metheylene-THF-polyglutamate formation (Fig. 12.9).[10]

The biochemical mechanism underlying the neurologic damage induced by vitamin B_{12} deficiency is unclear.[2,11,12] The balance of evidence suggests that the neurologic damage

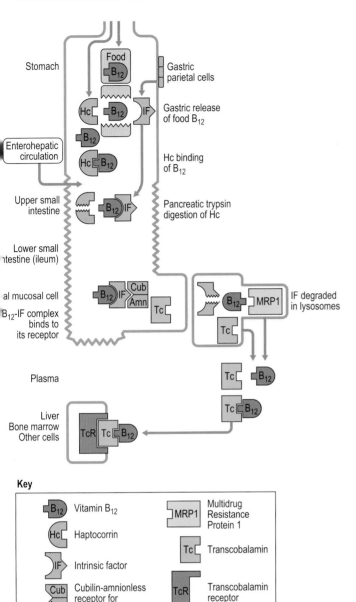

Key

B_{12}	Vitamin B_{12}	MRP1	Multidrug Resistance Protein 1
Hc	Haptocorrin	Tc	Transcobalamin
IF	Intrinsic factor		
Cub / Amn	Cubilin-amnionless receptor for IF-B_{12} complex	TcR	Transcobalamin receptor

Fig. 12.8 Diagram showing vitamin B_{12} absorption, cellular uptake and enterohepatic recirculation. (Adapted from Hoffbrand AV, Green R in Hoffbrand AV, Catovsky D, Tuddenham EGD, Eds. Postgraduate Hematology 5th Edition, Oxford, Blackwell Ltd).

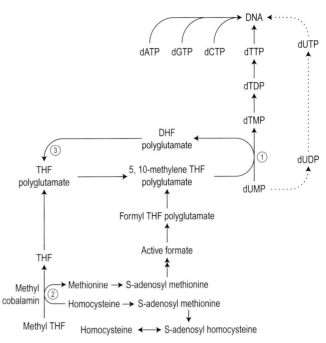

Fig. 12.9 Biochemical pathways involved in vitamin B_{12} and folate deficiency. The interrupted lines show how uracil is misincorporated into DNA as a consequence of impaired methylation of deoxyuridine monophosphate (dUMP) to deoxythymidine monophosphate (dTMP). dUDP, deoxyuridine diphosphate; dUTP, deoxyuridine triphosphate; dTDP, deoxythymidine diphosphate; dTTP, deoxythymidine triphosphate; THF, tetrahydrofolate; DHF, dihydrofolate; 1, thymidylate synthase; 2, homocysteine methyltransferase (methionine synthase); 3, dihydrofolate reductase.

may result from a failure to methylate basic proteins in myelin sheaths secondary to a failure of the synthesis of S-adenosylmethionine from methionine as a consequence of the decreased methylcobalamin-dependent conversion of homocysteine to methionine (Fig. 12.9).[5] The clinicopathologic features of subacute combined degeneration of the cord and the peripheral neuropathy caused by vitamin B_{12} deficiency are described in the section on pernicious anemia. These neurologic abnormalities have also developed in patients with vitamin B_{12} deficiency due to veganism, partial or total gastrectomy, abnormal overgrowth of small intestinal bacterial flora, ileal resection and the Imerslund–Gräsbeck syndrome. A severe peripheral neuropathy has also been reported in inadequately-treated patients with congenital transcobalamin II deficiency.

Causes of vitamin B_{12} deficiency (Box 12.1)

- **Inadequate dietary intake**

Veganism.[13,14] As vitamin B_{12} is not found in vegetables or fruit, strict vegetarians (vegans – i.e. those who do not eat meat or fish and little or no milk, milk products or eggs) have a very low to apparently absent dietary intake of this vitamin. The largest group of vegans is found amongst the Hindus. Although the majority of vegans have low serum vitamin B_{12} levels, most vegans have normal hematological values, including mean cell volumes (MCV), and appear to be in good health. It appears that the enterohepatic circulation of vitamin B_{12} enables avid conservation of the very small quantities of vitamin B_{12} absorbed from the diet and likely derived through microbial contamination of food to ensure adequate supplies of the vitamin to marrow and other cells despite the extremely low vitamin B_{12} stores. However, some vegans with a low serum B_{12} level develop a megaloblastic anemia which responds to treatment with either oral or parenteral vitamin B_{12} and a few suffer from vitamin B_{12} neuropathy. Breast-fed infants of vegan mothers may develop vitamin B_{12} deficiency during the first year of life.[15] People on a predominantly vegetarian diet who consume some dairy products may also develop low serum B_{12} levels and it is possible that some of them have an additional acquired defect in the ability to release B_{12} from food (see below).

- **Gastric lesions**

Pernicious anemia.[3] In this condition impaired vitamin B_{12} absorption and vitamin B_{12} deficiency result from a marked reduction in the secretion of intrinsic factor secondary to gastric atrophy caused by autoimmune destruction of gastric parietal cells. The vitamin B_{12} deficiency may lead to anemia, neurologic damage or both. Though the disease is common in people of Northern European origin, it also occurs in Africans, Asians, Chinese and other races. The diagnosis may be missed or delayed in these ethnic groups because of masking of the hematological features of macrocytosis by coexistent thalassemia or iron deficiency. Pernicious anemia is uncommon before the age of 30 years and the incidence increases with advancing age, most affected individuals being 50–70 years old. According to the older literature, the overall prevalence in the UK is about 1 per 1000 of the general population, but rises to 1% after the age of 60 years. A study among the multiethnic population of Los Angeles, California, aged 60 years or over showed that the prevalence of mild cobalamin deficiency due to undiagnosed pernicious anemia was at least 2.7% in women and 1.4% in men; the prevalence was 4.3% in black women and 4.0% in white women.[16] The male:female ratio in pernicious anemia is about 1 : 1.5. A family history of pernicious anemia is present in about 20% of patients. Autoimmune diseases (thyroid diseases, vitiligo, hypoparathyroidism and hypofunction of the adrenal glands) are more common in patients with pernicious anemia and their relatives than in the general population, and patients show a slightly higher than normal incidence of the blood group A. Pernicious anemia patients have an increased incidence of adenocarcinoma of the non-cardia portion of the stomach, and surprisingly, also have an increased risk of esophageal squamous cell carcinoma.[17] There is a more substantial increase in gastric carcinoid tumors but these tend to be of the benign type.[18]

The above data indicate that there is a genetic predisposition to the development of gastric atrophy and that autoimmune mechanisms are involved. However, the absence of intrinsic factor and parietal cell antibodies in some cases of pernicious anemia suggests that these antibodies may be a consequence rather than the cause of the damage to the gastric mucosa. Studies of a murine model of autoimmune chronic atrophic gastritis suggest that cell-mediated rather than humoral immunity may be involved.[19] Indeed, the gastric mucosa in pernicious anemia shows infiltration with plasma cells and lymphocytes, with an excess of CD4[+] cells. These histological changes revert to a more normal appearance and both acid and intrinsic factor (IF) secretion increase following steroid administration.

When pernicious anemia was first recognized over a century ago, the disease was diagnosed at an advanced stage, usually with severe megaloblastic anemia, other cytopenias and progressive neurologic abnormalities. Today, with the availability of automated full blood counts (including MCV), automated serum B_{12} and folate and red cell folate assays as well as assays for metabolites that rise in B_{12} deficiency, particularly methylmalonic acid, B_{12} deficiency is usually diagnosed at an early stage. In one study, 44% of B_{12}-responsive patients had hematocrit values within the normal range and 36% had MCVs within the normal range.[20] In developing countries patients still present with severe megaloblastic anemia.

Symptoms and signs. Symptoms are of slow onset and may include tiredness, weakness, dyspnea, a sore tongue and gastrointestinal disturbances (anorexia, nausea, vomiting, dyspepsia, constipation, diarrhea) and loss of weight. There may be slight jaundice, a low-grade pyrexia and slight enlargement of the spleen. Neurologic symptoms, which affect only some patients, usually begin in the lower limbs and are symmetrical. The most frequent of these are paresthesiae in the extremities, difficulty in walking and muscle weakness. Others include poor vision, stiffness of the limbs, impotence and in advanced cases, impairment of bladder and rectal control. Neurologic signs include sensory loss (particularly loss of position and vibration senses) which is worse in the legs, ataxia, positive Romberg sign, impairment of memory and, less commonly, the features of spastic paraplegia. The severity of neurologic impairment correlates inversely with the hematocrit;[21] about a quarter of cases with B_{12} neuropathy are not anemic and a slightly lower proportion do not have a high MCV.[22]

Laboratory investigations and treatment. Patients diagnosed at the earliest stages have a hemoglobin level and MCV within the reference range. Those diagnosed slightly later first present with an increased red cell distribution width (RDW) followed by a high MCV (macrocytosis) and high mean cell hemoglobin (MCH) and still with a hemoglobin level within the reference range. Later, there is both macrocytosis and mild to severe anemia, depending on the duration and severity of the deficiency. In anemic patients, the reduction of the red cell count is more marked than that of the hemoglobin level. Usually some of the macrocytes are oval in shape (see Fig. 12.3). With increasing anemia, the red cells also show an increasing degree of anisocytosis and poikilocytosis. The poikilocytes include tear-drop-shaped and irregularly-shaped cells as well as small red cell fragments (schistocytes). There is a rough inverse correlation between the degree of anemia and the MCV; unusually mild degrees of macrocytosis for the extent of anemia are found when there are many small red cell fragments (usually in patients with Hb less than 7 g/dl) and in patients with coexistent iron deficiency, chronic disorder or thalassemia syndrome.[23] The circulating neutrophil granulocytes of most cases show a tendency towards hypersegmentation of their nuclei (Fig. 12.6), more than 3% of the neutrophils containing five or more nuclear segments, although hypersegmentation may not be present in early stages of B_{12} deficiency.[24] There may be mild neutropenia or thrombocytopenia, particularly in severely anemic patients.

The bone marrow is hypercellular and in severely anemic patients there may be an almost complete replacement of fat cells by hemopoietic cells. Hemopoiesis is megaloblastic in type. The myeloid/erythroid (M/E) ratio is usually reduced due to erythroid hyperplasia. The quantity of stainable iron in the marrow fragments is usually normal or increased. There are abnormal sideroblasts but few, if any, ringed sideroblasts.

Serum bilirubin level of the unconjugated type may be slightly elevated and the serum lactate dehydrogenase is usually increased, often dramatically. The serum iron is high but falls within 48 h of a single injection of vitamin B_{12}. The serum vitamin B_{12} level is below the normal reference range in 95–97% of cases. However, a low serum vitamin B_{12} level should be considered as presumptive rather than definitive evidence of vitamin B_{12} deficiency as low levels are also seen in about one-third of patients with folate deficiency; this is especially the case in countries not practising folic acid fortification. Furthermore, low vitamin B_{12} levels may be found in normal individuals, particularly in pregnant women or in the elderly, sometimes without any hematologic, neurologic or even biochemical disturbances attributable to a deficiency of this vitamin. Red cell folate levels are low in the majority of patients with pernicious anemia and normal in the remainder. The serum folate level is low in 10% of cases presumably because of secondary intestinal malabsorption of folate resulting from intestinal megaloblastosis caused by B_{12} deficiency and may be high in 20–30%, resulting from the methyl-folate trap, discussed above (Fig. 12.9). Parietal cell antibodies, directed against the α and β subunits of the proton pump (H^+, K^+ ATPase) of the gastric parietal cell,[19] are found in the serum in about 85% of patients and IgG anti-intrinsic factor antibodies in 55%. The gastric juice contains an IgA antibody against intrinsic factor in about 60% of cases.

Because of the impairment of the mitochondrial adenosylcobalamin-dependent conversion of methylmalonyl CoA to succinyl CoA, plasma methylmalonic acid (MMA) levels are increased in vitamin B_{12} deficiency (but not in folate deficiency). In addition, the impairment of the methylation of homocysteine, which is dependent both on methylcobalamin and methyl-THF, leads to an increase in plasma homocysteine (HCYS) levels in either vitamin B_{12} or folate deficiency. Nearly all clinically confirmed cases of vitamin B_{12} deficiency have increased levels of plasma MMA or HCYS or both.[25] Whereas increased MMA levels are highly specific for vitamin B_{12} deficiency, increased HCYS levels are less specific, being found in patients with impaired renal function, hypothyroidism, B_6 deficiency, alcoholism and some inborn errors of homocysteine metabolism.[26]

Vitamin B_{12} absorption tests, such as the Schilling test (now unavailable), showed impaired absorption of an orally-administered physiologic dose of radiolabeled vitamin B_{12}; the impaired absorption was improved by the simultaneous oral administration of intrinsic factor. Newer methods, replacing the Schilling test, are now under development. The definitive diagnosis of pernicious anemia requires the presence of circulating antibodies to intrinsic factor. Intrinsic factor antibodies, though insensitive, are highly specific, being virtually confined to pernicious anemia. Demonstration of impairment of intrinsic factor production was achieved indirectly by performing a Schilling test, with and without intrinsic factor.[3,5,27] There is gastric achlorhydria with raised levels of serum gastrin. Although the diagnosis of pernicious anemia cannot be sustained in the absence of achlorhydria, gastric aspiration is rarely performed nowadays. Therefore the presence of achlorhydria is established indirectly by demonstrating elevated levels of gastrin or pepsinogen in the blood. However, severe achlorhydria caused by simple atrophic gastritis is not uncommon in elderly subjects with adequate intrinsic factor secretion. Parietal cell antibodies are also not specific for pernicious anemia, being found in a small percentage of healthy individuals (2% of those less than 30 years of age and 16% of those greater than 60 years) and in a higher proportion of individuals with various disorders such as myxedema, Graves' disease, iron deficiency anemia and gastritis without pernicious anemia. Because of the present difficulty of arriving at a definitive diagnosis of pernicious

anemia, the diagnosis must often be presumptive, after exclusion of other causes of megaloblastic hemopoesis or neurological abnormalities. Frequently, management of such patients is empirical and because vitamin B_{12} treatment is inexpensive and safe, it is instituted without a definitive diagnosis. Ideally, if there is no objective improvement in the patients condition, then B_{12} treatment should be withdrawn. If efficacious, then it is important to maintain treatment, even if symptoms have not returned.

Patients with pernicious anemia may be initially treated with six intramuscular injections, each of 1 mg hydroxocobalamin, over 2–12 weeks to replenish body stores of vitamin B_{12}. This should be followed by 1 mg hydroxocobalamin intramuscularly every 3 months, throughout life. In the USA, cyanocobalamin is the form of B_{12} used. As it is not retained as well as hydroxocobalamin, it should be given monthly for maintenance. High dose daily oral B_{12} may be used as an alternative since there is passive absorption of B_{12}.[28,29] Though inefficient (1% of the dose given is absorbed), doses of 1–2 mg daily suffice to maintain adequate vitmain B_{12} levels. Hematologic abnormalities are rapidly and completely reversed by vitamin B_{12} therapy. Neurologic symptoms of recent onset may improve considerably over 6–12 months.

Total or partial gastrectomy.[30,31] Total gastrectomy results in the removal of the intrinsic factor-secreting cells and therefore inevitably leads to vitamin B_{12} depletion and eventually to megaloblastic anemia due to vitamin B_{12} deficiency. This anemia appears 2–10 years after the operation depending on the size of the B_{12} store and the extent of gastric resection. These factors determine the time taken for normal vitamin B_{12} stores to be depleted after the abrupt cessation or drastic diminution of vitamin B_{12} absorption. It is best to commence regular B_{12} therapy soon after the gastrectomy. The probability of developing vitamin B_{12} deficiency is a function of the amount of stomach resected. In most cases, the vitamin B_{12} deficiency appears to result from a combination of the loss of intrinsic factor-secreting mucosa at operation and the subsequent atrophy of the remainder of the gastric mucosa. The deficiency may also result from a failure to release vitamin B_{12} from food due to a deficiency of acid and gastric pepsin (see below). In a few cases, and particularly when blind loops have been created (as happens following a Polya type gastrectomy), the vitamin B_{12} deficiency may be the consequence of the development of an abnormal intestinal bacterial flora. The frequency with which gastrectomy is now carried out has markedly reduced since the advent of successful medical treatments for peptic ulceration and *Helicobacter pylori* infection. However, the widespread use of H blockers and proton pump inhibitors to reduce acid secretion has contributed to food B_{12} malabsorption (see below). In addition, the obesity epidemic in Western countries has led to a growth in the practice of gastric reduction surgery which may be complicated by nutrient, including vitamin B_{12} malabsorption.[32] This malabsorption is caused by both a failure to digest and release food B_{12} and a diminution in intrinsic factor production. The clinical picture in such patients is further complicated by multiple nutrient deficiencies including that of copper, which can produce a myeloneuropathy resembling that seen in vitamin B_{12} deficient myelopathy as well as anemia, which may be macrocytic.[33]

Congenital intrinsic factor deficiency or mutation.[34–36] Patients with this rare group of disorders present with megaloblastic anemia in childhood and usually during the first 3 years of life. The syndromes are characterized by the total absence of intrinsic factor or the production of a mutant intrinsic factor molecule which binds but fails to promote vitamin B_{12} absorption, However, in contrast to pernicious anemia, hydrochloric acid and pepsin are present in gastric juice, there is a normal-looking gastric mucosa, and parietal cell and intrinsic factor antibodies are absent. Inheritance is autosomal recessive and heterozygotes appear clinically normal.

- **Intestinal lesions**

Abnormal intestinal microbial flora.[37] Vitamin B_{12} deficiency may develop in conditions in which there is small intestinal stasis. Such conditions include multiple jejunal diverticula, small-intestinal strictures, intestinal involvement in systemic sclerosis, and stagnant intestinal loops resulting either from gastrointestinal surgery or from fistulae complicating regional iletis or tuberculosis. Intestinal stasis results in increased number of bacteria (e.g. enterobacteria, bacteroides, streptococci, lactobacilli and Gram-positive anaerobes) in the upper small intestine. These bacteria consume and even convert vitamin B_{12} from ingested food into inactive cobinamides and other vitamin B_{12} analogues and thus decrease the availability of vitamin B_{12} for absorption at the terminal ileum.[38,39] Patients with vitamin B_{12} deficiency due to the presence of abnormal intestinal bacterial flora show a substantial improvement in absorption soon after a course of a broad-spectrum antibiotics such as tetracycline.

Ileal resection and inflammatory bowel disease (including Crohn's disease and chronic tropical sprue). Because vitamin B_{12} is absorbed in the terminal ileum, deficiency may result from diseases affecting the lower part of the ileum (e.g. Crohn's disease, chronic tropical sprue) or resection of more than about 60 cm of the terminal ileum.[40] The extent of impairment of B_{12} absorption is proportional to the extent of resection. Megaloblastic anemia is present in 60–90% of patients with tropical sprue. About 90% of patients with this disease malabsorb vitamin B_{12} and many also malabsorb folate. The absorption of vitamin B_{12} frequently returns to normal after a course of broad-spectrum antibiotics and in the early stages of the disease may improve following therapy with folic acid.

Infestation with the fish tapeworm (Diphyllobothrium latum).[41,42] Infestation with this tapeworm is seen in people living around the freshwater lakes of Northern Europe including Finland, the Baltic states, Switzerland, Germany and Russia, as well as Japan and North America. However, megaloblastic anemia caused by this tapeworm is more or less confined to Finland, the Baltic states and Russia. Infestation occurs by eating raw or partly cooked fish containing a larval form of the worm. The adult tapeworm may grow to a length of 10 m and is found attached by its head to the mucosa of the ileum. Only a few per cent of infested humans develop megaloblastic hemopoiesis or neurologic abnormalities due to vitamin B_{12} deficiency. The tapeworm causes these effects by depriving the host of vitamin B_{12} in the intestinal lumen derived either from ingested food or from bile. Although most fish tapeworms are attached to the distal half of the small intestine, the worms of anemic individuals are attached more proximally and it appears that parasites with a high attachment extract vitamin B_{12} before it reaches the absorptive site in the ileum. Vitamin B_{12} deficiency due to infestation with the fish tapeworm is becoming less common because of pollution of the lakes and a consequent reduction in the population of potentially infective fish. Whereas in the past about 20% of Finns harbored the fish tapeworm this figure had come down to about 2% in 1977.[43]

Selective malabsorption of vitamin B_{12} with or without proteinuria (Imerslund–Gräsbeck syndrome, autosomal recessive megaloblastic anemia MGA1).[44,45] This disorder is inherited as an autosomal recessive and patients present with megaloblastic anemia between the ages of 1 and 15 years, but usually before the age of 2. Vitamin B_{12} deficiency results from a failure of the terminal ileum to absorb vitamin B_{12} from the vitamin B_{12}–intrinsic factor complex. The defect of absorption only affects vitamin B_{12}, the absorption of other substances being entirely normal. The gastric juice contains normal quantities of intrinsic factor and the histology of the stomach and terminal ileum is normal. Over 90% of cases have proteinuria (0.2–1 g protein/l urine) but there are usually no other defects of renal function. Renal biopsy has shown no consistent pattern of abnormality. The anemia is corrected by parenteral vitamin B_{12} but the mild proteinuria persists. The molecular defect underlying this disorder is now known. Two genes code proteins that comprise the vitamin B_{12}–intrinsic factor complex.[46,47] The first, cubulin (CUBN), is defective in the MGA1 described in Finland. The other, amnionless (AMN), results in a milder phenotype and is the type described in Norwegian patients. In some parts of the world, MGA1 is the most common cause of vitamin B_{12} deficiency in infancy.

Other causes of malabsorption of vitamin B_{12}, usually without megaloblastic anemia. In several of the situations discussed in the following section, the malabsorption of vitamin B_{12} is either not sufficiently severe or does not continue for a sufficiently long period to cause the development of megaloblastic anemia.

Malabsorption of food cobalamin.[48–50] There is now growing evidence that many patients with a low serum vitamin B_{12} level fail to adequately release the vitamin from its protein-bound state in food as a consequence of impaired secretion of acid and pepsin by the stomach (Fig. 12.8). Such patients usually have no hematologic or obvious neurologic abnormality. However, some cases have abnormal homocysteine and methylmalonic acid levels, or show neuroelectrophysiologic abnormalities. A few patients may display mild hematologic abnormalities or neurologic dysfunction. In an occasional case the gastric dysfunction has progressed to involve intrinsic factor secretion and pernicious anemia has developed. It is not clear whether these conditions are causally related; however, their co-occurrence may be purely coincidental. In food cobalamin malabsorption, conventional vitamin B_{12} absorption tests such as the Schilling test gave a normal result but a modification of the test employing protein-bound instead of free radiolabeled vitamin B_{12} gave an abnormal result. In these tests, the vitamin was usually bound *in vitro* to egg or chicken serum. Conditions associated with food cobalamin malabsorption include non-specific gastritis, *H. pylori* gastritis, partial gastrectomy, vagotomy, gastric bypass surgery for treatment of obesity, bacterial overgrowth in the stomach, alcohol abuse and the use of acid suppressing drugs. The latter include cimetidine, omeprazole, ranitidine and gelusil.[51] About 45% of unexplained low serum vitamin B_{12} levels, in patients who have not been subjected to gastric surgery, may be caused by malabsorption of food cobalamin. Patients with food cobalamin malabsorption respond to vitamin B_{12} given orally.

Drugs. Malabsorption of vitamin B_{12} has been demonstrated in patients receiving aminosalicylates, neomycin, colchicine, slow-release potassium chloride, metformin, phenformin, colestyramine and large doses of vitamin C. Rarely, megaloblastic anemia has developed following prolonged treatment with aminosalicylates or metformin. With most of the other drugs, the duration of use is not long enough to result in depletion of vitamin B_{12} stores.

Chronic pancreatitis. Vitamin B_{12} malabsorption, rarely with megaloblastic anemia, has also been described in severe pancreatic disease. Here, the impaired secretion of trypsin by the diseased pancreas causes reduced degradation of vitamin B_{12}–R binder complexes and, consequently, reduced availability of the vitamin for binding to intrinsic factor.

Zollinger–Ellison syndrome. The vitamin B_{12} malabsorption that occurs in this syndrome may be caused by inactivation of pancreatic trypsin by low pH, leading to impaired release of the vitamin from salivary and gastric R binder.

HIV infection. Low serum vitamin B_{12} levels and abnormal vitamin B_{12} absorption results have been reported in the later stages of HIV infection but only a few patients show evidence of tissue B_{12} deficiency such as elevated plasma methylmalonic acid or homocysteine levels. Rarely there is a hematologic response to parenteral vitamin B_{12} therapy. The low serum vitamin B_{12} levels frequently appear to be due to reduced levels of haptocomin.[52]

Other causes. Impaired absorption of vitamin B_{12} has been reported in about 30% of cases of gluten-sensitive enteropathy, after total body irradiation, after ileal irradiation (e.g. during radiotherapy to the cervix), in graft-versus-host disease, lymphoma involving the ileum, tuberculous enteritis, in giardiasis and in folate, protein, riboflavin or pyridoxine deficiency.

• *Acquired abnormality of cobalamin metabolism*

Inactivation of vitamin B_{12} by nitrous oxide.[53,54] The continuous exposure of patients to a mixture of 50% N_2O and 50% O_2 for 5–6 days or more (once used in the management of severe tetanus) may cause bone marrow aplasia with severe megaloblastic changes in the residual hemopoietic cells.[55] Continuous exposure for 5–24 h (e.g. during the post-operative ventilation of patients who have undergone cardiac bypass surgery) often induced mildly megaloblastic erythropoiesis.[56] It is also possible that the intermittent use of nitrous oxide over long periods (e.g. Entonox – a mixture of equal parts of N_2O and O_2 – inhaled for 15–20 min two or three times a day to facilitate physiotherapy) may induce megaloblastic changes.[57] Furthermore, neuropathy resembling that seen in vitamin B_{12} deficiency has been described in dentists repeatedly exposed to N_2O over a long period.[58] Vitamin B_{12} deficient or depleted individuals are particularly susceptible to the effects of N_2O.[59] These effects seem to result from the irreversible oxidation of methylcobalamin by N_2O and its consequent inactivation.

• *Inherited abnormalities of cobalamin transport and metabolism*

Congenital transcobalamin deficiency.[60–62] A few children have been reported in whom a megaloblastic anemia resulted from the complete absence of transcobalamin (TC). Transcobalamin is concerned with the active transport of vitamin B_{12} into all cell types following absorption from the vitamin-B_{12}–intrinsic factor complex in the terminal ileum. Most patients present with severe megaloblastic anemia, leukopenia, thrombocytopenia and failure to thrive within a few weeks of birth. Neurologic damage is usually seen only when vitamin B_{12} therapy is delayed. Inheritance is autosomal recessive. Some patients have additional features such as marked hypogammaglobulinemia, granulocyte dysfunction, bizarre red cell morphology or erythroid hypoplasia. Since most of the vitamin B_{12} in serum is bound to haptocorrin, the serum vitamin B_{12} level in affected infants may be deceptively normal before maternally-derived vitamin B_{12} is depleted. By contrast, the unsaturated vitamin B_{12}-binding capacity of the serum, which is normally largely dependent on the presence of apotranscobalamin, is greatly reduced (normal range, 1000 ± 200 pg/ml). Homocysteine and methylmalonic acid levels are elevated in the plasma.[63] There is also impaired absorption of vitamin B_{12} which is not corrected by the administration of intrinsic factor.[64] The anemia responds to the regular injection of 1000 μg vitamin B_{12} two or three times a week. These massive doses probably work, despite the absence of the specific transport protein, by causing free vitamin B_{12} to enter cells by passive diffusion. Mutations in TC have also been described in which the TC is functionally abnormal.[65] Megaloblastic anemia responsive to parenteral vitamin B_{12} despite high serum cobalamin levels has been described. The cause was ascribed to homozygosity for a congenitally abnormal TC molecule. The abnormal TC bound vitamin B_{12} but the TC–B_{12} complex did not bind to the TC receptor.[65] In another patient, pancytopenia at the age of 6 weeks appeared to be due to compound heterozygosity for absent TC and for the functionally abnormal TC variant.[66]

Several single nucleotide polymorphisms (SNP) in the TC gene have also been identified which code for variants in the protein. Recently, it has been reported that these SNP, which occur in high frequency in some populations, appear to have functional consequences including, in the case of the most common SNP (776C>G), higher levels of methylmalonic acid and lower levels of holo TC in the plasma of individuals homozygous for the GG variant.[67] The functional importance of such SNP may have significance with respect to differential susceptibility of individuals to the development of vitamin B_{12} deficiency and its consequences. The human transcobalamin receptor has been cloned and its gene sequence determined.[68] It has been identified as CD320.

Methylmalonic acidurias.[35,69] These rare congenital disorders result from an impairment of the conversion of methylmalonyl CoA to succinyl CoA, a reaction which is dependent both on adenosylcobalamin and on the apoenzyme methylmalonyl CoA mutase. Affected children have severe metabolic acidosis with high concentrations of methylmalonic acid in the urine, blood and CSF. The underlying defect lies in various mutations in either: 1) the methylmalonyl CoA mutase apoenzyme, which may either be lacking (mut°) or defective (mut⁻), and in either case the disorder is unresponsive to vitamin B_{12}; or, 2) a defect in formation of adenosylcobalamin (CblA, CblB, CblH), in which case the disorder may be responsive to large doses of vitamin B_{12}. Two groups of patients with adenosylcobalamin deficiency exist, (a) CblA (or CblH which is an interallelic variant of CblA) in which there is a failure to reduce vitamin B_{12} from the cob(III)alamin to the cob(I)alamin form, and, (b) CblB in which there is a failure to convert cob(I)alamin to adenosylcobalamin. Cases with a mutation in methylmalonyl CoA mutase are treated by restricting the intake of amino acids that are degraded through the propionate pathway but several develop multiple organ failure including infarction of the basal ganglia, pancreatitis, nephritis and cardiomyopathy and do not survive long.

Combined deficiency of adenosylcobalamin and methylcobalamin.[35,63,69] Affected patients have both methylmalonic aciduria due to a failure to synthesize adenosylcobalamin, and homocystinuria and hypomethioninemia due to a failure to synthesize methylcobalamin. Three groups of disorders with different primary defects are recognized, namely CblC, CblD and CblF disease. CblC disease is the most common and most cases present in infancy with lethargy, feeding difficulties and failure to thrive. Others present in childhood or adolescence with neurologic symptoms such as spasticity, psychosis or a retinopathy with perimacular pigmentation. In most cases, there is megaloblastic anemia and there may be macrocytosis, hypersegmented neutrophils and in some cases thrombocytopenia.

Methylcobalamin deficiency. In this deficiency, defective methylcobalamin synthesis leads to homocystinuria and hypomethioninemia in the absence of methylmalonic aciduria. Two groups of disorders exist, CblE disease and CblG disease. CblG disease is caused by impaired methylation of cob(I)alamin caused by mutations in the apoenzyme methionine synthase with which cob(I)alamin is associated. CblE disease is caused by mutations in a reductase which is required for the reduction of cobalamin to cob(I)alamin prior to its methylation. The diagnosis is often made before the age of 2 years but has sometimes been made in adults. Clinical features include megaloblastic anemia, and various neurologic disturbances. The hematologic and biochemical abnormalities are reversed by parenteral vitamin B_{12} or hydroxocobalamin administered frequently but the neurologic deficits tend to show only a partial correction. In CblF, there is a defect in the ability to release vitamin B_{12} from lysosomes.[63]

Folates

The folates are a family of compounds derived from the biologically inactive parent compound pteroyl monoglutamic acid (folic acid). Most intracellular folates are pteroyl polyglutamates with a total of 3–7 (usually 4, 5 or 6) glutamic acid residues linked together by γ-carboxy peptide bonds. By contrast most of the extracellular folates are monoglutamates. Naturally occurring intracellular and extracellular folates are also in the reduced di- or tetrahydrofolate form and, in addition, contain a single carbon unit in various states of reduction (e.g. methyl, formyl, methylene, methenyl).

Folates are present in a wide variety of animal and vegetable foods; particularly high concentrations are found in yeast, spinach, Brussels sprouts and liver. The folate content of an average diet is greatly influenced by the method of preparation of food and by whether or not there is fortification of the diet with folic acid, as is the case in the USA as well as more than 50 other countries where folic acid fortification has been introduced for the prevention of neural tube defects. Folic acid fortification has not been introduced in European countries. Folates are rapidly destroyed by heat and 30–90% may be lost during cooking. About 80% of a 200 µg dose of ³H-pteroylglutamic acid is absorbed; less folate is absorbed from dietary polyglutamates than monoglutamates. The amount of folate absorbed by an adult is 100–200 µg per day. Prior to absorption, dietary pteroyl polyglutamates are first hydrolysed into monoglutamates by deconjugating enzymes in the gut known as folate conjugases. In the enterocyte, folate monoglutamates are converted into 5-methyltetrahydrofolate before transfer to portal blood. The jejunum and upper part of the ileum absorb folate more actively than the remainder of the small intestine. A high-affinity folate transporter has been identified that uses a proton-coupled system to facilitate folate absorption.[70]

The total folate content of the human body is about 6–10 mg, most of which is found in the liver. Absorbed folate is balanced by an equal loss of folate in sweat, desquamated cells (e.g. skin cells) and urine. Because of the relatively large daily requirement, folate stores may become depleted and folate deficiency develop within 3–4 months of taking a folate-depleted diet.

Folate coenzymes are involved in the transfer of single carbon units in a number of reactions. 5,10-methylenetetrahydrofolate is required for the methylation of deoxyuridylate to thymidylate. 10-formyltetrahydrofolate and 5,10-methenyltetrahydrofolate are involved in the supply of carbons 2 and 8 of the purine ring, respectively. 5-methyltetrahydrofolate participates in methionine synthesis. Other folate-dependent reactions in humans include the conversion of serine to glycine and the degradation of histidine through formiminoglutamic acid to glutamic acid.

Folate deficiency causes megaloblastic hemopoiesis but only rarely leads to neurologic damage. A very few folate-responsive patients with subacute combined degeneration of the cord have been reported in whom cobalamin deficiency seemed to have been excluded. The hematological changes are attributed to impaired DNA synthesis secondary to defective methylation of deoxyuridylate to thymidylate. However, studies of DNA synthesis have suggested that most folate- (or vitamin B_{12}) deficient human marrow cells elongate daughter DNA strands at a normal rate. Still, defective methylation of deoxyuridylate in folate deficiency results in an increase in the intracellular pool of deoxyuridine triphosphate and, consequently, to misincorporation of uracil into DNA[71] and this appears to be the biochemical basis of the megaloblastic change.

Folate and neural tube defects

There is an important but incompletely understood association between folate and neural tube defects. When folic acid

(4 mg/day orally) is given before conception and during the first trimester of pregnancy to women with a previous infant with a neural tube defect, the probability of recurrence of such a defect in the subsequent pregnancy is markedly reduced.[72] A lower dose of folate (400 μg/day) has been recommended to reduce the risk of the first occurrence of a neural tube defect.[73] However, at the time of writing, folic acid fortification of the diet has not been introduced in the UK or elsewhere in Europe. Folic acid fortification of cereals and grains was mandated in the USA in 1998 and in Canada in 1999. In addition, there is an increased incidence of neural tube defects and other congenital malformations in the babies of women receiving drugs known to interfere with folate metabolism including anticonvulsant drugs such as sodium valproate, carbamazepine, phenytoin and primidone.[74]

Causes of folate deficiency (Box 12.1)

- ### *Inadequate dietary intake*

Megaloblastic anemia due to a dietary folate deficiency tends to occur in the poor, the neglected elderly, the mentally disturbed, chronic alcoholics, and infants fed almost exclusively on goat's milk (which only contains 12% of the folate in cow's milk). 'Goat's milk anemia' has been reported in various countries including Germany, Italy, New Zealand and the USA. Inadequate folate intake contributes to the development of folate deficiency after gastric surgery, in patients with prolonged severe illnesses and in patients with epilepsy receiving anti-convulsant drugs. In countries where folic acid fortification has been implemented, the prevalence of low plasma folate has dropped from 22% in the population to 1.7%.[75]

Malabsorption. Diseases such as gluten-sensitive enteropathy and tropical sprue, which affect the upper part of the small intestine, often cause anemia due to malabsorption of folate. Reduced absorption of folate is also seen after partial gastrectomy or jejunal resection and when Crohn's disease affects the upper small intestine. In addition, it has been reported in patients taking salazopyrine (asulphidine) for inflammatory bowel disease.

Increased requirements or loss. An increased requirement of folate due to increased nucleic acid turnover may lead to folate deficiency, particularly in those taking suboptimal quantities of folate in their diet. An increased requirement occurs in pregnancy because of the needs of the growing fetus,[76] in chronic hemolytic anemias due to compensatory erythroid hyperplasia, and in premature infants because of the rapid growth during the first 2–3 months. There is also an increased folate requirement in various malignant diseases (leukemia, lymphoma, myeloproliferative neoplasms, myeloma, carcinoma), presumably due to increased proliferation of neoplastic cells. The folate requirement of the newborn on a weight for weight basis is ten-fold that of an adult and premature babies may develop megaloblastic anemia at 4–6 weeks of age.

Before the use of folate supplements during pregnancy, megaloblastic anemia was found in the latter part of pregnancy in only 2.8% of women in the UK.[77] However, examination of the bone marrow revealed that megaloblastic hemopoiesis was much more common, being present in 25% and in over 50%, respectively, of women in the UK

and in South India. With the increasing awareness of the importance of adequate folate intake pre-conceptually and during pregnancy, the incidence of megaloblastic anemia of pregnancy in the developed world is now quite low. Megaloblastic anemia is particularly common in twin pregnancies and is most likely to present after the 36th week of gestation, around the time of delivery or early in the postpartum period. Folic acid fortification has mitigated folate deficiency in pregnancy where this practice has been instituted.

Patients with chronic inflammation such as those with tuberculosis or severe rheumatoid arthritis tend to become folate-deficient, probably because of a combination of: 1) inadequate intake (as the result of a poor appetite) and, 2) an increased requirement to support the increased formation of chronic inflammatory cells. In psoriasis and exfoliative dermatitis there may also be increased loss of folate via desquamation of skin cells.

Some folate is lost during long-term hemodialysis or peritoneal dialysis as folates are only loosely bound to plasma proteins. This loss is modest but may aggravate negative folate balance caused by other mechanisms. There is a substantial increase in the urinary loss of folate (to >100 μg/day) in some patients with congestive heart failure or liver disease that has been attributed to hepatocellular damage.

- ### *Acquired abnormality of folate metabolism*

Therapy with dihydrofolate reductase inhibitors.[78,79] The enzyme dihydrofolate reductase, which is present in most mammalian cells, catalyses the reduction of dihydrofolate to tetrahydrofolate as well as the reduction of pteroyl glutamic acid to dihydrofolate. The dihydrofolate is derived from the 5,10-methylenetetrahydrofolate-dependent methylation of deoxyuridylate to thymidylate in which the folate is oxidized to dihydrofolate. The administration of dihydrofolate reductase inhibitors (such as methotrexate, pyrimethamine and triamterene) appears to cause megaloblastic hemopoiesis by impairing the regeneration of 5,10-methylenetetrahydrofolate from dihydrofolate and thus reducing the rate of methylation of deoxyuridylate. Trimethoprim, which is present in co-trimoxazole (Septrin or Septra), is a weak inhibitor of mammalian dihydrofolate reductase: when used in conventional dosage it causes megaloblastic hemopoiesis only in patients with a preexisting impairment of the methylation of deoxyuridylate due, for example, to a mild degree of vitamin B_{12} or folate deficiency. When necessary, as in the use of high dose or intrathecal methotrexate, the hematologic effects of dihydrofolate reductase inhibitors may be reversed by using folinic acid (5-formyl tetrahydrofolate)

- ### *Complex or unknown mechanism*

Anti-convulsant therapy and ethanol abuse. Most patients with macrocytosis associated with anti-convulsant therapy[79,80] or chronic alcoholism[3,79,81–83] do not suffer from folate deficiency (see below). In those who do, the deficiency seems to be caused mainly by an inadequate diet. Although the data are conflicting, malabsorption of folate has been described both in treated epileptics and in chronic alcoholics, and may contribute to the development of folate deficiency. Differential susceptibility of individuals to these agents may reside in differences in polymorphisms of the enzymes involved in folate metabolism. This has been incompletely investigated.

Oral contraceptive drugs. Folate-responsive megaloblastic anemia has been reported in only a few women on the contraceptive pill in whom other causes of folate deficiency appeared to have been excluded. The evidence that the pill has a significant effect on folate status is weak and controversial. Some data suggest that the pill may cause impaired folate absorption and increased urinary folate loss.

- *Congenital disorders of folate absorption and metabolism*[35,84]

A number of patients with hereditary folate malabsorption have been reported, in whom there appears to be an abnormality in a transport system specific for folic acid. The molecular basis of this disorder has recently been identified as a defect in the proton-coupled folate transporter.[70] The condition presents in the first few months of life with megaloblastic anemia (and other hematologic abnormalities such as macrocytosis, leukopenia and, occasionally, thrombocytopenia), vomiting, diarrhea, mouth ulcers, recurrent infections, failure to thrive and neurologic abnormalities. The neurologic abnormalities can be attributed to defective transport of folic acid across the choroid plexus. Neurologic abnormalities include hypotonia, seizures, mental retardation and ataxia. Folate levels in serum, red cells and cerebrospinal fluid (CSF) are very low. The hematologic abnormalities and gastrointestinal symptoms respond to high doses of folic acid, or preferably reduced folate such as folinic acid given orally or smaller doses parenterally, and in some cases seizures improve.

The most frequent inherited disorder of folate metabolism is methylene tetrahydrofolate reductase (MTHFR) deficiency. Patients may present at any time from infancy to childhood. Symptoms vary markedly in different cases and some infants are severely ill with seizures, abnormalities of gait, breathing disorders and coma. Megaloblastic anemia or other hematologic abnormalities are usually absent. Serum, red cell and CSF folate levels are reduced, plasma homocysteine levels are increased, plasma methionine levels are normal or reduced and there is homocystinuria. Arterial and venous thrombosis may occur and histopathologic features resembling subacute combined degeneration of the cord have been found at autopsy.

Rare cases of megaloblastic hemopoiesis with normal or high serum folate levels have been caused by glutamate formiminotransferase deficiency or cyclodeaminase deficiency (there is increased formiminoglutamic acid in blood and urine after histidine loading), dihydrofolate reductase deficiency, methionine synthase deficiency or deficiency of other enzymes involved in folate metabolism. Mental retardation has developed in some cases. In addition to the mutations in the above enzymes involved in folate metabolism, there is increasing recognition that SNP of the enzymes result in functional modification of those enzymes. The most interesting of these are the polymorphisms of MTHFR, some of which show high allelic frequency in some populations. These have been implicated as a risk factor for increased incidence of neural tube defects, hyperhomocysteinemia and possibly an increased risk of venous thrombosis.

> **Box 12.2** Vitamin-B_{12}-independent and folate-independent causes of macrocytosis with megaloblastic erythropoiesis
>
> **Abnormalities of nucleic acid synthesis**
>
> (a) Therapy with anti-purines (e.g. mercaptopurine, thioguanine, azathioprine), anti-pyrimidines (e.g. fluorouracil, azauridine, cytarabine), hydroxyurea, cyclophosphamide, procarbazine, aciclovir. Arsenic poisoning.
>
> (b) Orotic aciduria, Lesch–Nyhan syndrome
>
> **Uncertain etiology**
>
> (a) Anti-convulsant therapy,[†] chronic alcoholism[†]
>
> (b) Myelodysplastic syndromes, erythroleukemia
>
> (c) Congenital dyserythropoietic anemia, types I and III
>
> (d) Thiamine-responsive anemia
>
> ---
>
> [†]See also Box 12.1.

Vitamin B_{12}-independent and folate-independent causes of megaloblastic erythropoiesis (Box 12.2)

Abnormalities of nucleic acid synthesis

Drug-induced impairment of DNA synthesis[78]

A number of drugs that interfere with DNA synthesis cause macrocytosis with megaloblastic erythropoiesis. These include mercaptopurine, thioguanine, azathioprine, fluorouracil (which inhibits thymidylate synthase), the pyrimidine analog cytarabine (which inhibits DNA polymerase), and hydroxyurea (which inhibits ribonucleotide reductase). Other drugs which cause megaloblastic changes include zidovudine, cyclophosphamide, procarbazine and aciclovir. Arsenic poisoning also causes macrocytosis.

Orotic aciduria[85,86]

This is a rare inherited disorder of pyrimidine synthesis characterized by severe megaloblastic anemia, failure to thrive, the excretion of large quantities (0.5–1.5 g/d) of orotic acid in the urine and impaired cellular (but not humoral) immunity. The disorder is caused by a greatly reduced activity of two enzymes, orotidylic pyrophosphorylase and orotidylic decarboxylase, which are involved in the conversion of orotic acid to uridine monophosphate, a precursor of the pyrimidine bases of DNA. Affected patients appear to be homozygous for an autosomal recessive gene and present between the ages of 3 months and 7 years. The serum vitamin B_{12} and red cell folate levels are normal and there is no response to vitamin B_{12} or folate therapy. The anemia and the failure of growth and development both respond well to daily administration of 1–1.5 g uridine.

Lesch–Nyhan syndrome[87]

This sex-linked inherited syndrome is characterized by mental retardation, choreoathetosis, self-mutilation (especially biting of the lips and fingers) and gout. It is caused by a deficiency of the enzyme hypoxanthine phosphoribosyltransferase, which is involved in purine synthesis. Some cases have megaloblastic anemia that is responsive to adenine. Affected children with the Lesch–Nyhan syndrome may also have an increased susceptibility to infection due to defective function of B-lymphocytes. Evidence of B-cell dysfunction includes a reduced number of B-cells, decreased IgG levels, reduced isoagglutinin titers and an impaired response to pokeweed mitogen.

Uncertain etiology

Anti-convulsant therapy[3]

Some patients who develop megaloblastic erythropoiesis as a consequence of treatment with phenytoin (either on its own or in combination with other anticonvulsant drugs) do not suffer from folate deficiency or an impairment of methylation of deoxyuridylate due to any other cause. The cause of the megaloblastic change is obscure.

Chronic alcoholism[3]

A proportion of chronic alcoholics display megaloblastic erythropoiesis, usually of a mild degree, in the absence of evidence of folate deficiency such as a low serum, red cell or hepatic folate level or an abnormality in the methylation of deoxyuridylate as judged by the deoxyuridine suppression test. In addition to megaloblasts, the bone marrow often shows vacuolation of proerythroblasts and ringed sideroblasts. All these abnormalities, which are rapidly reversed on stopping alcohol consumption, presumably result from a direct toxic effect of ethanol or its metabolites on erythropoietic cells. There is some evidence to support the hypothesis that the bone marrow damage is at least partly caused by acetaldehyde generated locally by the metabolism of ethanol by bone marrow macrophages.[88] Chronic alcohol consumption causes red cell macrocytosis without megaloblastic changes in the bone marrow.

Myelodysplastic syndromes and erythroleukemia

The megaloblastic erythropoiesis seen in these disorders is not primarily caused by vitamin B_{12} or folate deficiency. However, it may occasionally be complicated by folate deficiency as a result of an increased requirement for folate.

Thiamine-responsive anemia[89,90]

This rare autosomal recessive disorder is characterized by megaloblastic anemia (rarely sideroblastic erythropoiesis) (Fig. 12.10), mild thrombocytopenia and leukopenia, sensorineural deafness and diabetes mellitus. The megaloblastic anemia in this disorder is refractory to vitamin B_{12}, folate and pyridoxine therapy. The anemia, but not the progressive deafness, responds to oral administration of large doses (20–100 mg/day) of thiamine. In some cases, thiamine also improves the diabetes. Patients do not show any of the clinical features of the syndrome produced by dietary deficiency of thiamine (beriberi) and appear not to be deficient in this vitamin. The disease gene has been localized to chromosome 1q23.2–23.3 and it was considered that the gene product may be a thiamine transporter.[90,91] The precise underlying defect in this disorder is now known to result from a block in the synthesis of the ribose portion of nucleic acids caused by disruption of the thiamine-

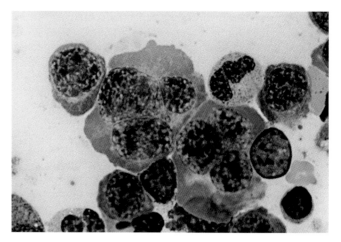

Fig. 12.10 Marrow smear from a child with thiamine-responsive anemia showing megaloblastic change and two multinucleate megaloblasts. May–Grünwald–Giemsa stain. ×1000.

Box 12.3 Causes of macrocytosis with normoblastic erythropoiesis

Normal neonates (physiologic)
Chronic alcoholism[†]
Chronic liver disease[†]
Hemolytic anemia[†]
Hypothyroidism
Therapy with anti-convulsant drugs[†]
Normal pregnancy
Chronic pulmonary disease (with hypoxia)
Heavy smoking
Myelodysplastic syndromes
Hypoplastic and aplastic anemia

[†]Some cases show megaloblastic erythropoiesis.

---

dependent transketolase enzyme that is involved in the pentose cycle.[92]

Macrocytosis with normoblastic erythropoiesis[3]

The conditions in which at least a proportion of the patients with macrocytosis have normoblastic erythropoiesis are listed in Box 12.3. Chronic alcohol abuse is a very common cause of macrocytosis (usually without anemia). The extent of alcohol consumption that induces macrocytosis varies considerably in different individuals; only about 35% of subjects who consume 100–800 g (mean 380 g) alcohol per day (equivalent to an average of a bottle of spirits per day) develop MCV above the normal range.[83] Alcohol-induced macrocytosis is associated with normoblastic erythropoiesis in about 70% of cases and in these the macrocytosis is independent of folate deficiency or an impairment of the

5,10-methylenetetrahydrofolate-dependent methylation of deoxyuridylate. Similarly, phenytoin-induced macrocytosis is occasionally associated with normoblastic erythropoiesis, usually with no evidence of impairment of methylation of deoxyuridylate. The mechanism underlying the macrocytosis in both these conditions is uncertain but may be an impairment of cell proliferation by a direct effect of alcohol or the drug or their metabolites on erythroblasts. The macrocytosis seen in non-folate-deficient patients with hemolytic anemia results from various erythropoietin-induced alterations in the kinetics of erythropoiesis; the reticulocytes produced by patients with stimulated erythropoiesis are considerably larger than normal reticulocytes and mature into rounded macrocytes.

About 25% of patients with hypothyroidism (without associated pernicious anemia) have macrocytic red cells; the macrocytosis seems to result from a deficiency of thyroid hormones. Patients with hypothyroidism may also have acanthocytes in their blood films (Fig. 12.11). The MCV of hypothyroid patients falls when they become euthyroid.[93] Patients with hypothyroidism also have elevated levels of homocysteine which fall upon treatment with thyroid hormone.[94]

In pregnancy, there is a slight and progressive increase in the MCV even in the absence of folate deficiency; occasionally the MCV may rise above the reference range for adults.[95]

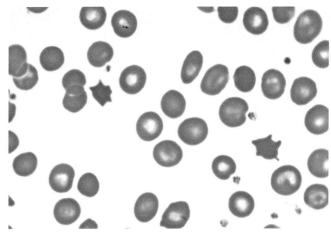

Fig. 12.11 Photomicrograph of a blood film of a 70-year-old man with severe hypothyroidism (Hb 9.1 g/dl; MCV 95 fl). In addition to macrocytes, two acanthocytes are seen. May–Grünwald–Giemsa stain. × 1000.

Another cause of macrocytosis with normoblastic erythropoiesis is chronic pulmonary disease.[96] Here, the macrocytosis is sometimes associated with true polycythemia secondary to a reduced PO_2 in arterial blood and has been attributed to a swelling of red cells.

References

1. Wickramasinghe SN. Morphology, biology and biochemistry of cobalamin- and folate-deficient bone marrow cells. Baillières Clin Haematol 1995;8:441–59.

2. Wickramasinghe SN. The wide spectrum and unresolved issues of megaloblastic anemia. Semin Hematol 1999;36:3–18.

3. Chanarin I. The Megaloblastic Anaemias. 3rd ed. Oxford: Blackwell Scientific Publications; 1990.

4. Koury MJ, Horne DW, Brown ZA, et al. Apoptosis of late-stage erythroblasts in megaloblastic anemia: association with DNA damage and macrocyte production. Blood 1997;89:4617–23.

5. Green R, Miller JW. Vitamin B_{12}. In: Zempleni J, Rucker RB, editors. Handbook of Vitamins. Boca Raton, FL: Taylor and Francis; 2007. p. 413–57.

6. Green R, Jacobsen DW, van Tonder SV, Kew MC, Metz J. Enterohepatic circulation of cobalamin in the nonhuman primate. Gastroenterology 1981;81:773–6.

7. Green R, Jacobsen DW, Van Tonder SV, et al. Absorption of biliary cobalamin in baboons following total gastrectomy. J Lab Clin Med 1982;100:771–7.

8. Herbert V, Zalusky R. Interrelations of vitamin B_{12} and folic acid metabolism: folic acid clearance studies. J Clin Invest 1962;41:1263–76.

9. Noronha J, Silverman, M. On folic acid, vitamin B_{12}, methionine and formiminoglutamic acid metabolism. In: Heinrich H, editor. Vitamin B_{12} and intrinsic factor. Stuttgart: Enke; 1962. p. 728–36.

10. Chanarin I, Deacon R, Lumb M, Perry J. Vitamin B_{12} regulates folate metabolism by the supply of formate. Lancet 1980;2:505–7.

11. Scott JM, Dinn JJ, Wilson P, Weir DG. Pathogenesis of subacute combined degeneration: a result of methyl group deficiency. Lancet 1981;2:334–7.

12. Weir DG, Scott JM. The biochemical basis of the neuropathy in cobalamin deficiency. Baillières Clin Haematol 1995;8:479–97.

13. Matthews JH, Wood JK. Megaloblastic anaemia in vegetarian Asians. Clin Lab Haematol 1984;6:1–7.

14. Campbell M, Lofters WS, Gibbs WN. Rastafarianism and the vegans syndrome. Br Med J (Clin Res Ed) 1982;285:1617–8.

15. Monagle PT, Tauro GP. Infantile megaloblastosis secondary to maternal vitamin B_{12} deficiency. Clin Lab Haematol 1997;19:23–5.

16. Carmel R. Prevalence of undiagnosed pernicious anemia in the elderly. Arch Intern Med 1996;156:1097–100.

17. Ye W, Nyren O. Risk of cancers of the oesophagus and stomach by histology or subsite in patients hospitalised for pernicious anaemia. Gut 2003;52:938–41.

18. Kokkola A, Sjoblom SM, Haapiainen R, et al. The risk of gastric carcinoma and carcinoid tumours in patients with pernicious anaemia. A prospective follow-up study. Scand J Gastroenterol 1998;33:88–92.

19. Glesson PA, Toh, BH. Molecular targets in pernicious anaemia. Immunology Today 1991;12:233–8.

20. Stabler SP, Allen RH, Savage DG, Lindenbaum J. Clinical spectrum and diagnosis of cobalamin deficiency. Blood 1990;76:871–81.

21. Healton EB, Savage DG, Brust JC, et al. Neurologic aspects of cobalamin deficiency. Medicine (Baltimore) 1991;70:229–45.

22. Lindenbaum J, Healton EB, Savage DG, et al. Neuropsychiatric disorders caused by cobalamin deficiency in the absence of anemia or macrocytosis. N Engl J Med 1988;318:1720–8.

23. Spivak JL. Masked megaloblastic anemia. Arch Intern Med 1982;142:2111–4.

24. Carmel R, Green R, Jacobsen DW, Qian GD. Neutrophil nuclear segmentation in mild cobalamin deficiency: relation to metabolic tests of cobalamin status and observations on ethnic differences in neutrophil segmentation. Am J Clin Pathol 1996;106:57–63.

25. Savage DG, Lindenbaum J, Stabler SP, Allen RH. Sensitivity of serum

methylmalonic acid and total homocysteine determinations for diagnosing cobalamin and folate deficiencies. Am J Med 1994;96:239–46.

26. Green R. Metabolite assays in cobalamin and folate deficiency. Baillières Clin Haematol 1995;8:533–66.

27. Schilling RF. A new test for intrinsic factor activity. J Lab Clin Med 1953;42:946.

28. Kuzminski AM, Del Giacco EJ, Allen RH, et al. Effective treatment of cobalamin deficiency with oral cobalamin. Blood 1998;92:1191–8.

29. Eussen SJ, de Groot LC, Clarke R, et al. Oral cyanocobalamin supplementation in older people with vitamin B_{12} deficiency: a dose-finding trial. Arch Intern Med 2005;165:1167–72.

30. Deller DJ, Witts LJ. Changes in the blood after partial gastrectomy with special reference to vitamin B_{12}. I. Serum vitamin B_{12}, haemoglobin, serum iron, and bone marrow. Q J Med 1962;31:71–88.

31. Johnson HD, Hoffbrand AV. The influence of extent of resection, type of anastomosis, and ulcer site on the haematological side-effects of gastrectomy. Br J Surg 1970;57:33–7.

32. MacLean LD, Rhode BM, Shizgal HM. Nutrition following gastric operations for morbid obesity. Ann Surg 1983;198:347–55.

33. Juhasz-Pocsine K, Rudnicki SA, Archer RL, Harik SI. Neurologic complications of gastric bypass surgery for morbid obesity. Neurology 2007;68:1843–50.

34. McIntyre OR, Sullivan LW, Jeffries GH, Silver RH. Pernicious anemia in childhood. N Engl J Med 1965;272:981–6.

35. Rosenblatt DS, Whitehead VM. Cobalamin and folate deficiency: acquired and hereditary disorders in children. Semin Hematol 1999;36:19–34.

36. Katz M, Mehlman CS, Allen RH. Isolation and characterization of an abnormal human intrinsic factor. J Clin Invest 1974;53:1274–83.

37. Donaldson RM Jr. Small bowel bacterial overgrowth. Adv Intern Med 1970;16:191–212.

38. Brandt LJ, Bernstein LH, Wagle A. Production of vitamin B_{12} analogues in patients with small-bowel bacterial overgrowth. Ann Intern Med 1977;87:546–51.

39. Allen RH, Stabler SP. Identification and quantitation of cobalamin and cobalamin analogues in human feces. Am J Clin Nutr 2008;87:1324–35.

40. Thompson WG, Wrathell E. The relation between ileal resection and vitamin B_{12} absorption. Can J Surg 1977;20:461–4.

41. Von Bondsdorff B. Diphyllobothriasis in Man. London: Academic Press; 1977.

42. [No authors listed] Anaemia and the fish-tapeworm. Lancet 1977;1:292.

43. Saarni M, Palva I, Ahrenberg P. Finns and the fish tapeworm. Lancet 1977;1:806.

44. Grasbeck R. Familial selective vitamin B_{12} malabsorption. N Engl J Med 1972;287:358.

45. Altay C, Cetin M, Gumruk F, et al. Familial selective vitamin B_{12} malabsorption (Imerslund–Grasbeck syndrome) in a pool of Turkish patients. Pediatr Hematol Oncol 1995;12:19–28.

46. Fyfe JC, Madsen M, Hojrup P, et al. The functional cobalamin (vitamin B_{12})-intrinsic factor receptor is a novel complex of cubilin and amnionless. Blood 2004;103:1573–9.

47. He Q, Madsen M, Kilkenney A, et al. Amnionless function is required for cubilin brush-border expression and intrinsic factor-cobalamin (vitamin B_{12}) absorption in vivo. Blood 2005;106:1447–53.

48. Carmel R, Sinow RM, Karnaze DS. Atypical cobalamin deficiency. Subtle biochemical evidence of deficiency is commonly demonstrable in patients without megaloblastic anemia and is often associated with protein-bound cobalamin malabsorption. J Lab Clin Med 1987;109:454–63.

49. Carmel R, Sinow RM, Siegel ME, Samloff IM. Food cobalamin malabsorption occurs frequently in patients with unexplained low serum cobalamin levels. Arch Intern Med 1988;148:1715–9.

50. Carmel R. Malabsorption of food cobalamin. Baillières Clin Haematol 1995;8:639–55.

51. McColl KE. Effect of proton pump inhibitors on vitamins and iron. Am J Gastroenterol 2009;104(Suppl. 2):S5–9.

52. Remacha AF, Cadafalch J. Cobalamin deficiency in patients infected with the human immunodeficiency virus. Semin Hematol 1999;36:75–87.

53. Chanarin I. Cobalamins and nitrous oxide: a review. J Clin Pathol 1980;33:909–16.

54. Chanarin I. The effects of nitrous oxide on cobalamins, folates and on related events. In: Goldberg L, editor. CRC Critical Reviews on Toxicology. Florida: CRC Press; 1982:179–213.

55. Lassen HC, Henriksen E, Neukirch F, Kristensen HS. Treatment of tetanus; severe bone-marrow depression after prolonged nitrous-oxide anaesthesia. Lancet 1956;270:527–30.

56. Amess JA, Burman JF, Rees GM, et al. Megaloblastic haemopoiesis in patients receiving nitrous oxide. Lancet 1978;2:339–42.

57. Nunn JF, Sharer NM, Gorchein A, et al. Megaloblastic haemopoiesis after multiple short-term exposure to nitrous oxide. Lancet 1982;1:1379–81.

58. Layzer RB. Myeloneuropathy after prolonged exposure to nitrous oxide. Lancet 1978;2:1227–30.

59. Schilling RF. Is nitrous oxide a dangerous anesthetic for vitamin B_{12}-deficient subjects? JAMA 1986;255:1605–6.

60. Burman JF, Mollin DL, Sourial NA, Sladden RA. Inherited lack of transcobalamin II in serum and megaloblastic anaemia: a further patient. Br J Haematol 1979;43:27–38.

61. Hall CA. The neurologic aspects of transcobalamin II deficiency. Br J Haematol 1992;80:117–20.

62. Kaikov Y, Wadsworth LD, Hall CA, Rogers PC. Transcobalamin II deficiency: case report and review of the literature. Eur J Pediatr 1991;150:841–3.

63. Carmel R, Green R, Rosenblatt DS, Watkins D. Update on cobalamin, folate, and homocysteine. Hematology Am Soc Hematol Educ Program 2003:62–81.

64. Barshop BA, Wolff J, Nyhan WL, et al. Transcobalamin II deficiency presenting with methylmalonic aciduria and homocystinuria and abnormal absorption of cobalamin. Am J Med Genet 1990;35:222–8.

65. Haurani FI, Hall CA, Rubin R. Megaloblastic anemia as a result of an abnormal transcobalamin II (Cardeza). J Clin Invest 1979;64:1253–9.

66. Seligman PA, Steiner LL, Allen RH. Studies of a patient with megaloblastic anemia and an abnormal transcobalamin II. N Engl J Med 1980;303:1209–12.

67. Miller JW, Ramos MI, Garrod MG, et al. Transcobalamin II 775G>C polymorphism and indices of vitamin B_{12} status in healthy older adults. Blood 2002;100:718–20.

68. Jiang W, Sequeira JM, Nakayama Y, et al. Characterization of the promoter region of TCblR/CD320 gene, the receptor for cellular uptake of transcobalamin-bound cobalamin. Gene 2010;466:49–55.

69. Linnell JC, Bhatt HR. Inherited errors of cobalamin metabolism and their management. Baillières Clin Haematol 1995;8:567–601.

70. Qiu A, Jansen M, Sakaris A, et al. Identification of an intestinal folate transporter and the molecular basis for hereditary folate malabsorption. Cell 2006;127:917–28.

71. Blount BC, Mack MM, Wehr CM, et al. Folate deficiency causes uracil misincorporation into human DNA and chromosome breakage: implications for cancer and neuronal damage. Proc Natl Acad Sci USA 1997;94:3290–5.

72. [No authors listed] Prevention of neural tube defects: results of the Medical Research Council Vitamin Study. MRC Vitamin Study Research Group. Lancet 1991;338:131–7.

73. Report from an Expert Advisory Group. (1992) on folic acid and the prevention of neural tube defects. London: Department of Health; Scottish Office Home and Health Department; Welsh Office; Department of Health and Social Services, Northern Ireland, 1992.

74. Christensen B, Rosenblatt DS. Effects of folate deficiency on embryonic development. Baillières Clin Haematol 1995;8:617–37.

75. Jacques PF, Selhub J, Bostom AG, et al. The effect of folic acid fortification on plasma folate and total homocysteine concentrations. N Engl J Med 1999;340:1449–54.

76. Chanarin I, Rothman D, Ward A, Perry J. Folate status and requirement in pregnancy. Br Med J 1968;2:390–4.

77. Giles C. An account of 335 cases of megaloblastic anaemia of pregnancy and the puerperium. J Clin Pathol 1966;19:1–11.

78. Scott JM, Weir DG. Drug-induced megaloblastic change. Clin Haematol 1980;9:587–606.

79. Wickramasinghe SN. The deoxyuridine suppression test: a review of its clinical and research applications. Clin Lab Haematol 1981;3:1–18.

80. Reynolds EH, Laundy M. Haematological effects of anticonvulsant treatment. Lancet 1978;2:682.

81. Wu A, Chanarin I, Levi AJ. Macrocytosis of chronic alcoholism. Lancet 1974;1:829–31.

82. Unger KW, Johnson D Jr. Red blood cell mean corpuscular volume: a potential indicator of alcohol usage in a working population. Am J Med Sci 1974;267:281–9.

83. Wickramasinghe SN, Corridan B, Hasan R, Marjot DH. Correlations between acetaldehyde-modified haemoglobin, carbohydrate-deficient transferrin (CDT) and haematological abnormalities in chronic alcoholism. Alcohol Alcohol 1994;29:415–23.

84. Zittoun J. Congenital errors of folate metabolism. Baillières Clin Haematol 1995;8:603–16.

85. Smith LH Jr. Pyrimidine metabolism in man. N Engl J Med 1973;288:764–71.

86. Rajantie J. Orotic aciduria in lysinuric protein intolerance: dependence on the urea cycle intermediates. Pediatr Res 1981;15:115–9.

87. van der Zee SP, Lommen EJ, Trijbels JM, Schretlen ED. The influence of adenine on the clinical features and purine metabolism in the Lesch–Nyhan syndrome. Acta Paediatr Scand 1970;59:259–64.

88. Wickramasinghe SN, Hasan R. Possible role of macrophages in the pathogenesis of ethanol-induced bone marrow damage. Br J Haematol 1993;83:574–9.

89. Haworth C, Evans DI, Mitra J, Wickramasinghe SN. Thiamine responsive anaemia: a study of two further cases. Br J Haematol 1982;50:549–61.

90. Fleming JC, Tartaglini E, Steinkamp MP, et al. The gene mutated in thiamine-responsive anaemia with diabetes and deafness (TRMA) encodes a functional thiamine transporter. Nat Genet 1999;22:305–8.

91. Diaz GA, Banikazemi M, Oishi K, et al. Mutations in a new gene encoding a thiamine transporter cause thiamine-responsive megaloblastic anaemia syndrome. Nat Genet 1999;22:309–12.

92. Boros LG, Steinkamp MP, Fleming JC, et al. Defective RNA ribose synthesis in fibroblasts from patients with thiamine-responsive megaloblastic anemia (TRMA). Blood 2003;102:3556–61.

93. Horton L, Coburn RJ, England JM, Himsworth RL. The haematology of hypothyroidism. Q J Med 1976;45:101–23.

94. Hussein WI, Green R, Jacobsen DW, Faiman C. Normalization of hyperhomocysteinemia with L-thyroxine in hypothyroidism. Ann Intern Med 1999;131:348–51.

95. Chanarin I, McFadyen IR, Kyle R. The physiological macrocytosis of pregnancy. Br J Obstet Gynaecol 1977;84:504–8.

96. Freedman BJ, Penington DG. Erythrocytosis in emphysema. Br J Haematol 1963;9:425–30.

Recommended reading

Bhatt HR, James VHT, Besser GM, et al. Advances in Thomas Addison's diseases, Vols 1 and 2. Journal of Endocrinology, Bristol; 1994;69–80.

Wickramasinghe SN, editor. Megaloblastic anaemia. Baillière's Clinical Haematology Vol 8/No 3. London: Baillière Tindall; 1995;657–78.

Carmel R, editor. Beyond megaloblastic anemia: new paradigms of cobalamin and folate deficiency. Seminars in Hematology, Vol 36/No 1. Philadelphia: WB Saunders; 1999;1–2.

CHAPTER 13

Aplastic anemia and pure red cell aplasia

EC Gordon-Smith

Acquired aplastic anemia

Acquired aplastic anemia (AA) is an uncommon disorder which in Europe and the United States affects about 2 per million of the population per annum; in other parts of the world including South-East Asia the incidence may be 2–3 times higher.[1] Any age may be affected; there are two peaks, one occurring in adolescents and young adults, a second occurring after the age of 60, this bimodal distribution being most marked in white males.[2,3,4] Male : female ratio is about equal but there may be a preponderance of males in the younger or adolescent age group.[4]

Definition and differential diagnosis

AA is defined by peripheral blood pancytopenia with a hypocellular bone marrow in which normal hemopoiesis is replaced to a greater or lesser extent by fat cells in the absence of genetic, malignant or predictable myelosuppres-sive causes. Remaining hemopoietic precursors and circulating blood cells are morphologically normal or show only minor abnormalities. The exclusions in the definition emphasize that other diseases may produce a similar morphological picture and these need to be excluded in coming to a diagnosis (Table 13.1). Hypoplastic myelodysplastic syndrome (MDS) may be particularly difficult to distinguish; the distinction may not be critical since there is considerable overlap in the pathogenesis and management of both conditions.

Hairy cell leukemia (HCL) is occasionally misdiagnosed as AA. The bone marrow aspirate in HCL is often aparticulate and dilute, hairy cells may be scanty and the marrow trephine appears to show hypocellularity, but the reticulin is increased and the hemopoietic tissue is not replaced by fat cells but by the abundant cytoplasm of hairy cells. Confusion may be compounded by inappropriate treatment of HCL with anti-thymocyte globulin (ATG). ATG may lead to a temporary response in HCL.[5] Immunophenotyping will detect the HCL.

©2011 Elsevier Ltd
DOI: 10.1016/B978-0-7020-3147-2.00013-4

Table 13.1 Differential diagnosis of acquired aplastic anemia (AA)

Pathophysiology	Examples	Differential features
Inherited AA	Fanconi anemia	Chromosome fragility Dysmorphism Family history
	Dyskeratosis congenita	Nail/skin changes Leukoplakia X-linked, family history Short telomere syndromes
Malignant AA	Hypoplastic MDS	Blood cell morphology Cytogenetics
	Acute leukemia (presenting as AA)	Spontaneous remission followed by leukemic relapse
Toxic AA	Irradiation Chemotherapy Benzene	History of exposure
Immune mediated	Autoimmune pancytopenia Large granular lymphocytosis Acute graft-versus-host disease	Multiple autoantibodies Immunophenotype Post-transplant

Table 13.2 Drugs implicated in aplastic anemia

Drug group	Examples	References

Antibiotics	Chloramphenicol
	Sulfonamides
	  Sulfsalazine
	  Co-trimoxazole
		6, 9

Anti-inflammatory agents	Gold salts Indomethacin, sulindac Diclofenac	6, 10, 11
Thyrostatic drugs	Carbimazole Thiouracils	7
Anti-convulsants	Felbamate Carbamazepine Hydantoins	8

Anti-diabetic agents	Sulfonylureas
	  Chlorpropamide
	  Tolbutamide
		6

Anti-platelet drugs	Ticlopidine Clopidogrel	
Occupational/Domestic substances	Benzene Hexachlorocyclohexane (Lindane)	12–14 14

Etiology

In about one quarter to one third of the patients with AA suspicion may be directed to a particular agent, usually a drug or virus as the precipitating cause. In the great majority of patients no etiologic agent can be identified.

Drugs

The list of drugs which have been recorded as precipitating aplastic anemia is long,[6] but mostly only single or a few cases have been reported for each drug and the evidence against many of the drugs is slim. Some of the more commonly implicated drugs[7–11] are listed in Table 13.2. A difficulty in determining the role of drug exposure is the delay between exposure and the identification of marrow damage. Typically there is a delay of 2–3 months between marrow injury and the onset of pancytopenia. AA may develop only after prolonged or repeated exposure to the drug. The association can only be made if it is certain the patient was exposed to the drug and that the causation had been noted before.

Industrial/domestic chemicals

Benzene is myelotoxic.[12–14] Exposure to sufficient levels leads inevitably to marrow damage but there seems to be wide variation in the dose required to induce toxicity between individuals There is good epidemiologic evidence that chronic exposure to benzene causes AA, often progressing to MDS and acute leukemia. Some chemicals which have been implicated as a cause of AA are shown in Table 13.2. DDT has been implicated but considering its previously very widespread use and the paucity of reported cases it seems that this compound has little or no hematologic toxicity and that reports may well be confounded by the solvents, including benzene, in the preparation of DDT for spraying.

Viruses

Hepatitis. Hepatitis is a precursor of aplastic anemia in about 5–10% of cases in the West, perhaps double that in the Far East.[12] In the majority of cases no specific virus can be identified and the association is based on clinical grounds and the presence of abnormal liver function tests. The delay between the clinical hepatitis and the onset of pancytopenia is of the order of 6–12 weeks, a similar period to that between drug exposure and aplasia. There is some suggestion that chloramphenicol administration followed by hepatitis is particularly likely to be associated with aplastic anemia.[15] Further evidence to support the association is the finding that in one series over a quarter of patients who underwent orthotopic liver transplant for fulminant liver failure following viral hepatitis developed aplastic anemia whereas patients transplanted for other reasons had no marrow failure.[16] The prognosis in these patients relates to the severity of the marrow depression and not the supposed viral agent. The patients respond equally well to immunosuppressive therapy or stem cell transplantation as others with the same degree of marrow failure. Occasionally familial AA may be precipitated in siblings by hepatitis.[17]

Parvovirus. Parvovirus B19 infection in non-immune individuals may lead to a transient pure red cell aplasia of clinical importance to people with hemolytic anemia (see below). The virus specifically infects the erythroid precursors and does not normally produce true aplastic anemia.

Epstein–Barr virus. EBV infection is commonly accompanied by neutropenia or thrombocytopenia probably of an immune origin. Rarely there may be true marrow aplasia which behaves like other cases of acquired disease,[18] though within this group there are some patients who develop pancytopenia with marrow aplasia in whom there is spontaneous recovery in 4–6 weeks.

Pathophysiology

Normal hemopoiesis takes place in the specialized environment of the bone marrow where pluripotent hemopoietic stem cells (HSC) give rise to lineage specific committed progenitors which produce the mature cells for the circulation. There is an intimate relationship between the HSC and the cells of the microenvironment of the marrow, including osteoblasts, which is epitomized in the concept of the stem cell niche. The quiescent stem cell is protected within the niche; mobilized stem cells are able to repopulate the niche even after extensive trafficking. It is in this environment that self-renewal can take place. Differentiation and maturation are controlled by specific cytokines and growth factors which act on specific lineages. Self-renewal occurs close to endosteal surfaces. Maturation increases towards the central arteriole (see Chapters 2–4).

The stem cell in aplastic anemia

There are qualitative and quantitative abnormalities of hemopoietic stem cells in AA.[19–23] Short-term colony assays of committed progenitor cells – colony-forming units (CFU-C, CFU-E), burst-forming units (BFU-E) – are markedly reduced in AA and remain low even after recovery.[19–21] Committed progenitors, identified by long-term culture initiating cells (LTCIC) are also reduced and have a poorer proliferative potential than normal stem cells, with poorer survival of colony forming cells in long-term bone marrow culture.

The microenvironment in aplastic anemia

Long-term cultures depend upon a viable and confluent stroma for proper growth. Cross-over experiments have shown that stroma grown from aplastic anemia marrow can support colony-forming cells from normal marrow but that colony forming cells (CD34[+]) from aplastic marrow will not grow on either normal or aplastic marrow suggesting that the stroma is not at fault in the pathogenesis of AA.[19,20] It is not always possible to grow stroma from AA and there may be a degree of heterogeneity in the pathophysiology.

Hemopoietic growth factor production is normal in AA.[24,25] Erythropoietin (Epo), thrombopoietin (Tpo) and granulocyte colony stimulating factor (G-CSF) levels are increased though the concentration of circulating G-CSF is low in both normals and patients with AA. These observations might explain why Epo is ineffective in the treatment of AA whereas G-CSF may have a part to play in direct stimulation of bone marrow stem cells. A possible role for thrombopoietin receptor agonists in promoting platelet production in AA has yet to be determined.

It is clear that the stem cell in aplastic anemia is damaged but the precise nature of that damage and the subsequent changes which may lead to the evolution of abnormal clones are not fully understood.[26,27] The observation that there is shortening of the telomeres in the myeloid series in acquired aplastic anemia[28,29] and that marked shortening of telomeres is a feature of dyskeratosis congenita and other inherited types of aplastic anemia[30,31] has suggested that damage to telomeres or the mechanisms which control their regeneration are consequences in the pathogenesis of aplastic anemia[26,27] which may account for the increased risk of MDS and acute leukemias in both inherited and acquired syndromes.[32]

Autoimmune basis of aplastic anemia

AA has been considered a probable autoimmune disorder since the introduction of anti-thymocyte globulin (ATG) for successful immunosuppressive treatment of the disease.[33] The process is thought to be mediated by CD8[+] T-cells. Oligoclones of expanded CD8[+] CD28[−] cells, directed against as yet unidentified antigens, recognize and induce apoptosis in autologous myeloid cells.[34] In some instances the T-cells clones have been found to disappear on recovery. There is also some evidence that Tregs, which control auto-reactive T-cells, are reduced in AA,[35] which may result in the dysregulation of autoimmunity.

Hematology

The peripheral blood film shows pancytopenia without gross morphological abnormalities in the remaining cells. There may be some macrocytosis of remaining red cells usually with an absolute reticulocytopenia. A relative reticulocytosis should always raise the possibility of associated paroxysmal nocturnal hemoglobinuria (PNH). Granulocytes often show increased staining of granules, the so-called toxic granulation of neutropenia. The neutrophil alkaline phosphatase score is increased (it falls if PNH develops). Monocytes may be reduced in proportion to the granulocytes. Platelets are reduced and of small and uniform size. There is usually a variable reduction in the lymphocyte count, but sometimes the count is normal or even increased so that the total white cell count may be normal. Abnormal cells are not seen. The bone marrow aspirate is normally easily obtained, typically with many fragments which have a lacy, empty appearance (Fig. 13.1A). The cell trails are hypocellular with a relative increase in lymphocytes and plasma cells and other non-hemopoietic forms. There may be a minor degree of dyserythropoiesis but in general remaining hemopoietic precursors are normal in appearance. Lymphocytes and plasma cells may appear to be increased but this is because of the

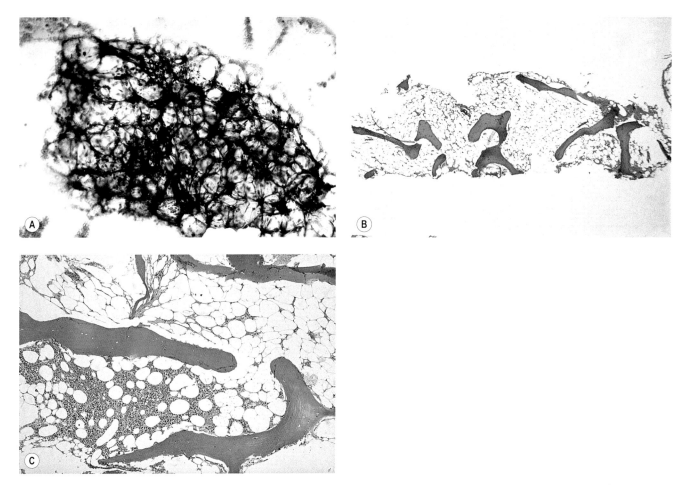

Fig. 13.1 (A–C) (A) Fragment from a bone marrow aspirate of a patient with severe aplastic anemia showing typical 'lacy' appearance of the fragment which contains a little or no hemopoietic cells. May–Grünwald–Giemsa. (B) Trephine biopsy from a patient with severe aplastic anemia showing the disappearance of hemopoietic cells between the trabeculae and replacement by fat cells. Hematoxylin-Eosin stain. ×100. (C) Trephine biopsy from a patient with severe aplastic anemia showing a residual island of apparently normal hemopoiesis in an otherwise fatty marrow. Hematoxylin-Eosin stain. ×200.

lack of hemopoietic cells and there is no consistent increase in lymphocytes or in any subset in the marrow taken from patients with aplastic anemia. In the early stages of aplastic anemia, macrophages appear active with increased intracellular iron and erythrophagocytsis may be prominent. In a proportion of cases the hypocellularity of the marrow is patchy with areas of cellular marrow remaining. The bone marrow aspirate under these circumstances may be misleadingly cellular. A trephine biopsy (sometimes more than one) is necessary to assess cellularity properly.

The trephine shows the fat replacement of marrow with or without the remaining islands of cellularity (Fig. 13.1B, C). The presence or absence of cellular 'hot pockets'[36] does not correlate with the severity of the peripheral blood pancytopenia and the apparent cellularity of a trephine specimen may not be reflected in the blood count. Non-hematopoietic cells remain, sometimes giving the impression of a chronic inflammatory infiltrate. Reticulin fibers are scanty, commensurate with the degree of hypocellularity. The architecture of the bone marrow remains essentially normal in distinction from the abnormal distribution of hemopoiesis in MDS.

Cytogenetic studies on bone marrow are required at presentation of patients with aplastic anemia, mainly to exclude hypoplastic MDS. Typically chromosome configuration and number are normal in aplastic anemia but it is now clear that in a number of cases there may be evidence for a clone of cytogenetically abnormal cells to be present at presentation which may be stable or transient but does not seem to affect response to treatment.[37] However, in some series the development of trisomy 8 was associated with a good response to immunosuppression whereas monosomy 7 carried a poor prognosis with high probability of transforming to MDS or acute leukemia.[38,39]

Clinical presentation

The clinical features derive from the decrease in peripheral blood cells and are non-specific. The patient may be feeling completely well at the time when easy bruising or petechiae appear or may have a more or less prolonged period of feeling tired from anemia. Infection may be the presenting feature but this seems to be less common in acquired aplastic anemia than bleeding manifestations. The spleen, liver and lymph nodes are not enlarged and jaundice is only a feature in those patients with post-hepatitic aplasia who have a prolonged cholestatic phase after the infection.

At presentation it is necessary to take a detailed drug, occupational and symptomatic history to try to establish an etiological agent so that this may be avoided in the future. Unfortunately, even if such an occupational or other exposure is suspected there is no way of proving the suspicion.

Classification of aplastic anemia

A classification of the severity of the marrow damage in AA was devised in the 1970s to allow the comparison of the effectiveness of different treatments in this disease without a gross imbalance in the severity of the different groups.[40] The original classification was based on observations of survival curves of collective series of drug-induced aplastic anemia which showed that there appeared to be two populations, one with a median survival of a few months and a 1-year survival of <10%, another which had a more prolonged survival, even though the patients remained with a degree of pancytopenia. Studies of these patients' peripheral blood and bone marrow allowed prognostic features to be devised which identified the severe aplastic anemia (SAA) and the non-severe aplastic anemia (NSAA). It is clear that the degree of marrow damage is not a double population but a spectrum and improving support and treatments have led to modification of the classification into three groups, very severe aplastic anemia (VSAA), having been added[41] (Table 13.3). The classification includes an assessment of the degree of hypocellularity of the marrow based on the trephine biopsy findings. This is the most subjective of the measurements, particularly as the cellularity may vary quite considerably in different samples and indeed in the same sample, the so called 'hot pockets'.

Clinical course

The clinical course is modified by the transfusion support and antibiotic therapy which the patient receives. There are some events which may interrupt the clinical course apart from catastrophes associated with the low platelet count and neutropenia. The proliferative capacity of the marrow is greatly reduced but the marrow also appears to be unstable in that abnormal clones of cells – PNH, myelodysplastic or leukemic – may appear during the disease, sometimes all three in the same individual. In patients who have a remission or partial response about 25–40% will develop a clonal disorder or relapse within 5–10 years though this is not necessarily associated with a poor prognosis.[42,43] The degree of aplasia may vary and the course of the disease is not always predictable. Aplastic anemia may present in pregnancy or responsive disease relapse at that time.[44] Management is mainly supportive. Recovery is by no means certain after delivery and immunosuppression is often required.

Some, perhaps most, patients present with a degree of pancytopenia which stabilizes over a long period of time (months or years). In general the greater the degree of pancytopenia the worse the prognosis as indicated in the grading of severity in Table 13.3. Patients with lesser degrees of pancytopenia, particularly those with a relative preservation of granulocytes, have a better prognosis, but clearly this is not a stepwise progression but a continuous spectrum.

A minority of patients present with minor degrees of pancytopenia or deficiency in only one cell line, but over the succeeding months or years the aplasia gradually becomes more profound. This is most usually observed in patients who present with amegakaryocytic thrombocytopenia which progresses over a period of years to true aplastic anemia.

Clonal evolution in aquired aplastic anemia

The pathophysiology of AA needs to take into account the observation of the frequent emergence of abnormal clones of cells in the aplastic hemopoiesis.[42,43] The most common event is for paroxysmal nocturnal hemoglobinuria (PNH) clones to emerge, sometimes more than one clone in a single individual. The frequency and diversity of the somatic mutations which lead to PNH suggest that such clones occur in normal marrow but are not expressed because normal hemopoiesis swamps the progeny of the clone. Indeed, clones with the PNH genotype and phenotype are found in normal individuals.[45] When the marrow is damaged in AA the PNH clone may have a growth advantage and may come to dominate hemopoiesis or at least provide a substantial part of it. Since the PNH phenotype lacks a range of surface proteins normally attached by the phosphatidyl inositol glycan (PIG) anchor, it is tempting to surmise that the target for immune attack lies within these proteins or the anchor itself and that absence of the proteins in the PNH clone allows the PNH precursor cell to escape the autoimmune suppression. (The intimate relationship between AA and PNH is discussed in detail in Chapter 20.) The same may be true of other cytogenetic abnormalities which are common in MDS or acute leukemia. While progression to MDS, or less commonly AML, may occur, hemopoiesis in some AA patients produces clones with abnormal cytogenetics which are commonly seen in MDS, but in the aplastic setting may be transient or stable without progressing to a more malignant phase.

Treatment of aplastic anemia

The choice of treatment for AA depends upon a number of factors, the age of the patient, the severity of the bone marrow

Table 13.3 Gradation of severity of acquired aplastic anemia[40,41]

Grade of severity	Definition	
	Peripheral blood	***Bone marrow**
VSAA	Neutrophils <0.2×10⁹/l Platelets < 20×10⁹/l Reticulocytes <20×10⁹/l Transfusion dependent	<25% normal cellularity. Moderately hypocellular <30%. Remaining cells hemopoietic.
SAA	Neutrophils <0.5 but >0.2×10⁹/l Otherwise as for VSAA	As for VSAA
NSAA	Neutrophils <1.5 but >0.5×10⁹/l Platelets <100 >20×10⁹/l Reticulocytes <60 but >20×10⁹/l	Hypocellular

NSAA: non severe aplastic anemia; SAA: severe aplastic anemia; VSAA, very severe aplastic anemia.

*The bone marrow in aplastic anemia is often patchy in cellularity and the assessment of cellularity, even with a good trephine, may be difficult.

damage, the availability of suitable donor and the general health of the patient. Whichever mode of treatment is eventually advanced the most important aspect is to be able to provide comprehensive support for the patient with blood products and infection control. The two main treatment modalities are immunosuppression and stem cell transplantation, each of which has its own advantages and disadvantages. Guidelines for the management of both adults[46] and children[47,48] have been produced.

Immunosuppression

Immunosuppression with anti-thymocyte globulin (ATG) was introduced in 1977.[33] Subsequent trials confirmed the effectiveness of this form of treatment. Overall, between 75% and 80% of the patients achieve remission, defined as freedom from transfusion, following a first course of treatment with ATG.[46] Younger age, absolute reticulocyte count and absolute lymphocyte count may be predictors of response.[49] There are differences in response rate between different ATG preparations.[50] The addition of ciclosporin after the ATG treatment improves the speed of response and perhaps the frequency.[51,52] A proportion of responders remain dependent on continued ciclosporin administration, often at a low dose.

ATG is given through a central venous line to avoid problems with phlebitis. Fever, rigors and general lethargy are common in the first 2 days of treatment, the subsequent days usually remaining trouble-free. Some 7–10 days post-infusion serum sickness, with rash, joint pain and fever, may occur, modified by giving corticosteroids in moderate dosage, 1 mg/kg/day, increasing if necessary if serum sickness occurs. As support improved, so the survival improved for those who did not show a response to the first course of ATG. Subsequent courses also produce remission as defined by freedom from transfusion and some patients have received multiple courses with success in patients who have shown some response to the previous treatments.[53] The main causes of failure of support measures are refractoriness to platelet transfusions and antibiotic resistant infections, especially fungal.

Growth factors

The effect of G-CSF on neutrophil production in AA has been extensively investigated. A dose of 5–10 mg/kg daily by subcutaneous injection raises the neutrophil count in most patients except those with VSAA. However, there has not been clear evidence of adding G-CSF to the immunosuppressive regimen.[54]

Cyclophosphamide

Interest was raised in the use of high dose cyclophosphamide as immunosuppression for patients who failed to respond to ALG[55] as well as first line therapy.[56] Responses were seen in seven out of 10 patients and there was no evidence of clonal evolution in a 10-year follow up. The time to response and the period of severe pancytopenia were prolonged. However, a randomized controlled trial of cyclophosphamide compared with ATG showed that the toxicity of the cyclophosphamide outweighed the potential benefit.[57]

Anabolic steroids

Anabolic steroids, particularly oxymetholone, were the only form of bone marrow stimulation before the introduction of immunosuppression and cytokines. Responses are undoubtedly achieved in NSAA though control trials have failed to demonstrate a benefit in SAA. Nevertheless, anabolic steroids do have a place in the management of AA, though side-effects, virilization and hepatotoxicity make them difficult to manage.

In summary, immunosuppression with ATG and ciclosporin is the first treatment option for patients with all degrees of severity of AA who do not have an HLA matched sibling donor, for patients with NSAA irrespective of donor availability, for patients over 30 with a donor who have SAA or NSAA (but not VSAA) and for patients with systemic disease which makes stem cell transplantation high risk.[46] The response should be assessed at 4 months. If there is no response or partial response, a second course of ATG should be given to patients without a sibling donor. For those with a donor, a decision may have to be made to proceed with a stem cell transplantation.

Stem cell transplantation

HLA matched sibling transplants

Transplant for AA using bone marrow from HLA-matched sibling donors was introduced by E. Donnell Thomas and colleagues in Seattle in 1969. An early trial demonstrated superiority of this transplantation compared with support and anabolic steroids,[58] the only non-transplant treatment then available. Subsequent experience worldwide recorded by the European Bone Marrow Transplant (EBMT) Group and the International Bone Marrow Transplant Registry (IBMTR), as well as the continuing reports from Seattle, indicated that some 70–80% of patients survive with grafts.[59-61] These results are overall similar to treatment with ATG in terms of survival but transplantation has an advantage in children and young adults and in patients with VSAA. The majority of successfully transplanted patients show some degree of stable mixed chimaerism in the hemopoiesis and some recover full autologous marrow function.[62] About 15% have chronic graft-versus-host disease and late relapse may occur but the risk of clonal evolution is small compared with the 40% post-ATG.

Matched unrelated donor and cord blood transplants

The results of transplantation using alternative donors to HLA matched siblings have improved markedly over the past decade since heavy myeloablative conditioning regimens were supplanted by non-myeloablative protocols involving fludarabine[63] or low dose irradiation.[64] Using these non-myeloablative regimens has produced 2-year survival of 73%, children and younger patients responding well with considerable deterioration in results with each decade of age. The use of stem cells derived from umbilical cord blood has improved donor availability for a children with a number of diseases including acquired aplastic anemia.[65] For adults the main difficulty is failure to obtain sufficient stem cells to establish the graft. Attempts to improve results using double cord transplants are at an experimental stage.[66]

Conclusion: Aplastic anemia

There have been considerable advances over the past 20 years in understanding the pathogenesis of AA. The nature of the autoimmune processes underlying the stem cell damage is clearer but the target for the immune remains elusive. Improvements in management have derived in no small part from better support from blood transfusion and antibiotic selection as well as better understanding of transplant conditioning.

Pure red cell aplasia

As the name implies, pure red cell aplasia (PRCA) encompasses a variety of disorders characterized by an isolated failure of red cell production in the bone marrow with preservation of proliferation and differentiation in other lineages. The failure to produce reticulocytes and hence red cells may be inherited or acquired. The main causes of PRCA are given in Table 13.4. DBA may be inherited as an autosomal dominant condition (the main group), autosomal recessive (rare) or sporadic. A number of different genes have been identified so far, all of which are involved in ribosomal biogenesis or function. DBA presents mainly in infancy or early childhood and has to be differentiated from acquired PRCA in children.[67,68]

Acquired PRCA

Acquired PRCA is a rare disorder characterized by anemia with absent reticulocytes and absent or reduced erythroid precursors in the marrow. The marrow is otherwise normal; in some cases there may be an increase in megakaryocytes and modest rise in circulating platelets. Acquired PRCA may be an acute self-limiting condition seen almost exclusively in children or a chronic disorder, mainly arising in adult life.

Transient erythroblastopenia of childhood

Acute, self-limiting transient erythroblastopenic anemia (TEC) in infants and children was first described in Sweden.[69] The incidence in Sweden was about 4.3/100 000/year.[70] TEC usually presents around 2 years of age[71] but may occur in infants[72,73] or older children. Children usually present with pallor and symptoms of anemia but in some cases anemia may be an incidental finding. Rarely there may be reversible neurologic signs or symptoms.[74]

Investigations. The main requirement is to exclude Diamond-Blackfan anemia (DBA) (Table 13.5). TEC presents with a normocytic, normochromic anemia with a reticulocytopenia (<2%). Patients may present later, in the early recovery phase, when the reticulocyte count is beginning to recover. In about half the patients the platelet count is raised >400×10^9/l.[71] Absolute neutropenia is not uncommon at some stage during the illness. In the prospective study about 30% had neutrophils <1.0×10^9/l and three out of 50 had <0.5×10^9/l.[71] The proportion of fetal hemoglobin (HbF) may be slightly elevated for age but mostly is normal and raised HbF does not reflect recovery. Markers of hemolysis are not present. The bone marrow typically shows maturation arrest at the pronormoblast stage but complete absence of erythroid precursors may occur.[75] The myeloid:erythroid ratio is markedly raised. There is usually age-appropriate lymphocyte predominance in the marrow but abnormal clones or morphological anomalies are not present though a population of lymphocytes with a common or pre-B cell ALL phenotype in otherwise typical TEC has been described.[76]

Etiology and pathogenesis. The etiology of TEC is unclear. The anemia may develop following a virus-like illness and a number of viruses have been implicated including parvovirus B19 but information from prospective studies has failed to show any definite association of TEC with any particular virus.[77] Red cell aplasia following parvovirus infection mostly occurs in the immunocompromised patient.[78] The mechanism of erythropoietic suppression is also not clear

Table 13.4 Classification of pure red cell aplasia (PRCA)

Etiology	Disorder	Pathology	Pathophysiology	Clinical
Genetic	Diamond–Blackfan anemia	Absent erythropoietic progenitors in marrow	Defective ribosomal biogenesis	Usually presents in infancy. May be steroid responsive
	Congenital dyserythropoietic anemias	Abnormal erythropoiesis with characteristic morphologic changes	Three main CDA types. Ineffective erythropoiesis	Variable anemia. May present in adult. Hyperbilirubinemia may be present (see Chapter 15)
Acquired	Transient erythroblastopenia of childhood	Reticulocytopenia. Normocellular marrow with erythroid hypoplasia	Usually follows non-specific virus infection. Immune mediated	Peak incidence age 2 years. Spontaneous recovery in 4–8 weeks
	Parvovirus B19 aplastic crisis	Reticulocytopenia. Giant pronormoblasts with absent precursors	Mediated by infection with parvovirus B19	Manifest in patients with chronic hemolytic anemia. Recovery with antibody response
	Acquired PRCA	Reticulocytopenic anemia. Red cell precursors absent or rarely show maturation arrest	Autoimmune. Most commonly antibody mediated. Rarely lymphocyte cytotoxicity	Primary spontaneous or with thymoma Secondary with autoimmune disease or lymphoma

Table 13.5 Differential diagnosis of Diamond–Blackfan anemia (DBA) and transient erythroblastopenia of childhood (TEC)

	DBA	TEC
Red cell aplasia	Present	Present
Neutropenia	No	Present in about 50%
Age	Usually <1 year	Usually >1 year
Inheritance	Sporadic and dominant defects of ribosome biogenesis	Acquired
Red cells	Macrocytic	Normocytic
HbF	Elevated	Normal
Erythrocyte adenosine deaminase (eADA)	Elevated	Normal
Recovery	Steroid dependent or absent	Spontaneous at 4–8 weeks

DBA, Diamond–Blackfan anemia; TEC, transient erythroblastopenia of childhood

but perhaps involves post infective mechanisms. Immune pathways are thought to play a role including IgG and IgM mediated pathways and cellular inhibition.[79] There may be a genetic background to some cases of TEC. A number of case reports document TEC occurring in siblings[80] though this in itself would not distinguish environmental factors from inherited.[81] A study of affected siblings and their families in Sweden demonstrated a linkage between TEC and the chromosome 19q13.2 in which the DBA affected gene *RPS19* is located but did not show any anomaly of that gene in TEC.[82]

Clinical course and management. Spontaneous recovery is the rule. Reticulocytes reach a maximum usually about 4 weeks after presentation and hemoglobin reaches pre-anemic levels by about 8 weeks. Occasionally the anemia and symptoms require red cell transfusion support. Any neurological signs or symptoms also resolve. There is no place for treatment with steroids or other immunosuppressive agents.

Parvovirus B19 infection

Infection with parvovirus B19 is very common, about 80% of the population having IgG antibodies to the virus by the age of 50 years. The virus shows tropism to rapidly dividing cells which express the P blood group antigen globoside (Gb4) which is found on most red cells precursors but also on a variety of other cells including platelets and tissues from the heart, lung, liver, kidney and endothelium.[83,84] Infection during pregnancy has serious consequences on the fetus but in other immunocompetent individuals rarely produces clinically important disease. The main exception is in people with chronic hemolytic anemia. The virus enters the red cell precursors and inhibits proliferation. Erythropoiesis is switched off for up to 7 days until the IgM specific antibody response neutralizes the virus. With a normal red cell life span of 120 days the inhibition is too short to produce a meaningful drop in hemoglobin though reticulocytopenia does occur. In patients with chronic hemolytic anemia with short red cell life the inhibition is sufficient to cause an acute, reticulocytopenic anemia, the so called 'aplastic crisis'. Once the normal immune response has occurred the patients are unlikely to have a relapse.

In patients with inherited or acquired immunodeficiency, infection of red cell precursors continues and red cell aplasia persists. This may occur in severe combined immune deficiencies, HIV infection, transplant patients on immunosuppression, acute leukemias, systemic lupus and other causes of immunosuppression.[78,84] In many instances the red cell aplasia will resolve in response to intravenous immunoglobulin containing IgG anti parvovirus antibody.[85]

Diagnosis. In the setting of an aplastic crisis in a patient with chronic hemolytic anemia the diagnosis is relatively straightforward. The reticulocytopenia together with absent or only IgM antibodies to parvovirus suggest the diagnosis without the need for bone marrow examination. Recovery occurs once IgM antibodies develop. In the immunocompromised patient the diagnosis requires bone marrow examination in patients who develop reticulocytopenic anemia. The bone marrow appearance is characteristic. The marrow is usually hypercellular with giant multinucleate pronormoblasts with intranuclear inclusions with a clear halo ("lantern" cells). Late normoblasts are absent. The pronormoblasts may show cytoplasmic reactivity to anti-parvovirus antibodies.[84] In doubtful cases it may be necessary to identify parvovirus infection by PCR.[86,87]

Chronic, acquired PRCA

PRCA in adults and older children is almost always an autoimmune disease though humoral inhibitors of erythropoiesis are rarely demonstrated. As with other immune cytopenias, the condition may be primary or secondary, associated with other autoimmune disorders or lymphoproliferative disease (Table 13.6). A particular association is with thymoma. Rarely PRCA is drug induced.

Primary PRCA

Primary PRCA is rare. The majority of cases seem to be antibody mediated despite the lack of specific antibody detection. The immune reaction is against red cell precursors in the marrow: part of the difficulty of demonstrating antibody inhibitors arises from the lack of reliable *in vitro* assays to measure inhibitor activity.[88] At least some cases may have resulted from erythropoietic suppression by an undetected clone of NK or T-cell large granular lymphocytes (LGL). This association would be present particularly in patients with PRCA with raised rheumatoid factor antibodies and probably many cases attributed to CLL. The LGL cells may be present in peripheral blood and bone marrow and may be identified by immunophenotyping as well as morphology. However, in many instances the LGL clone can be identified only by T-cell receptor (TCR) gene rearrangement using PCR but only if CD3 positive clones are involved. The association with LGL clones may explain why some patients are refractory to immunosuppression with corticosteroids and ciclosporin but do respond to alemtuzumab.[89,90]

Table 13.6 Classification of persistent pure red cell aplasia

Etiology	Class	Disorders/examples	References
Primary			See text
Secondary	Autoimmune disorders	SLE	106, 107
		Rheumatoid arthritis	108
		Sjögren's syndrome	109
		Hypogammaglobulinemia	See text
		Erythropoietin antibodies	
	Lymphoproliferative disease	Large granular lymphocytosis	89, 102
		Chronic lymphocytic leukemia	98
		Non-Hodgkin lymphoma	100
	Infections	Hepatitis	See text
		Parvovirus B19	
		EBV	
		HIV	
	Drugs	D-penicillamine	See text
		Phenytoin	
		Azathioprine	
		Isoniazid	
		Oxcarbazepine	
	Thymoma	Thymic hyperplasia	See text
		Malignant thymoma	
	Allogeneic stem cell transplants	ABO mismatched transplants	110

SLE, systemic lupus erythematosus.

Secondary PRCA

The main groups of diseases which are associated with PRCA are shown in Table 13.6. In nearly all instances the aplasia is immune mediated.

PRCA and thymoma. Some 5–10% of cases of PRCA are associated with thymoma; less than 5% of thymoma patients develop PRCA though there are variations in reported series.[91,92] Presentation of PRCA may lead to the identification of the thymoma or may follow many years after resection of a tumor. The aplasia does not necessarily respond to removal of the thymoma – immunosuppressive treatment is usually required. Several histologic types of thymoma have been associated with PRCA, not just lymphocytic.[90] Other paraneoplastic features of thymoma, including, most commonly, myasthenia gravis, may occur together or sequentially with PRCA.

Drug-induced PRCA. A number of drugs have been associated with PRCA[93,94] (Table 13.6). Azathioprine-induced anemia is well recognized.[95] The drug is used in nephrology often together with erythropoietin in renal transplant patients. The use of alpha erythropoietins, particularly given subcutaneously, has been responsible for severe immune mediated PRCA with antibodies developing to both the synthetic and endogenous growth factor.[96,97]

Viruses and PRCA

PRCA has been associated with a number of virus infections in addition to parvovirus B19. The association with HIV infection is complex because the immune suppression produced by the HIV infection may lead to infection by parvovirus and induction of red cell aplasia. In addition, some of the drugs used to manage HIV infection may themselves be the trigger for PRCA.

PRCA and lymphoproliferative disease

PRCA is a well recognized association with lymphoproliferative diseases, particularly CLL.[98] There has been some indication that sometimes the autoimmune complications of CLL may be triggered by treatment with single agent fludarabine or chlorambucil though this seems less likely when cyclophosphamide is also given, at least as far as autoimmune hemolytic anemia is concerned.[99] Other lymphoproliferative disorders have also been described with PRCA including small cell lymphocytic lymphoma,[100] Hodgkin lymphoma[101] and LGL lymphocytosis.[89,102,103]

Treatment of pure red cell aplasia

Immunosuppression is the mainstay of therapy for PCRA.[104] Corticosteroids are the traditional first line but ciclosporin is at least as effective in achieving remission and has fewer side-effects.[104] Withdrawal of putative agents, drugs or erythropoietin, is essential. Treatment is effective for almost all etiologies except severe post stem cell transplant aplasia. Rituximab has been successful in a number of cases mainly associated with B-cell proliferations[105] and alemtuzumab may be effective in presumed T-cell association. In practice management requires identification and treatment of any underlying disorder together with immunosuppression starting with corticosteroids and/or ciclosporin with monoclonal antibodies tried in patients who fail to respond.

References

1. Gordon-Smith EC, Issaragrisil S. Epidemiology of aplastic anaemia. Baillière's Clinical Haematology 1992;5:475–91.

2. Szklo M, Sensenbrenner L, Markowitz J, et al. Incidence of aplastic anemia in metropolitan Baltimore: a population based study. Blood 1985;66:115–9.

3. Linet MS, McCaffrey LD, Morgan WF, et al. Incidence of aplastic anemia in a three county area of South Carolina. Cancer Res 1986;46:426–9.

4. Mary JY, Baumelou E, Guiguet M, the French Cooperative Group for Epidemiological Study of Aplastic Anemia in France: a prospective multicentre study. Blood 1990;75:1646–53.

5. Fujiwara S. Miyake H. Nosaka K, et al. Hairy cell leukemia responsive to anti-thymocyte globulin used as immunosuppressive therapy for aplastic anemia. International Journal of Hematology 2009;90:471–5.

6. Kaufman DW, Kelly JP, Jurgelon JM, et al. Drugs in the aetiology of agranulocytosis and aplastic anaemia. European Journal of Haematology Supplementum 1996;60:23–30.

7. Thomas D, Moisidis A, Tsiakalos A, et al. Antithyroid drug-induced aplastic anemia. Thyroid 2008;18:1043–8.

8. Toledano R, Gil-Nagel A. Adverse effects of antiepileptic drugs. Seminars in Neurology 2008;28:317–27.

9. Kaufman DW, Kelly JP, Levy M, Shapiro S. The drug etiology of agranulocytosis and aplastic anemia. Monographs in Epidemiology and Biostatistics, vol 18. New York: Oxford University Press; 1991. Chapter 11, Antiinfective drugs, p. 204–16.

10. Inman WHW. Study of fatal bone marrow suppression with special reference to phenylbutazone and oxyphenbutazone. Br Med J 1977;i:1500–5.

11. Anonymous. The International Agranulocytosis and Aplastic Anemia Study. Risks of agranulocytosis and aplastic anemia. A first report of their relation to drug use with special reference to analgesics. JAMA 1986;256;1749–57.

12. Issaragrisil S, Kaufman DW, Anderson T, et al. The epidemiology of aplastic anemia in Thailand. Blood 2006;107:1299–307.

13. Smith MT. Overview of benzene-induced aplastic anaemia. European Journal of Haematology Supplementum 1996;60:107–10.

14. Muir KR, Chilvers CE, Harriss C, et al. The role of occupational and environmental exposures in the aetiology of acquired severe aplastic anaemia: a case control investigation. British Journal of Haematology 2003;123:906–14.

15. Hagler L, Pastore RA, Bergin JJ, et al. Aplastic anemia following viral hepatitis: report of two fatal cases and review of the literature. Medicine (Baltimore) 1975;54:139–64.

16. Tzakis AG, Arditi M, Whitington PF, et al. Aplastic anemia complicating orthotopic liver transplantation for non-A, non-B hepatitis. N Engl J Med 1988;319;393–6.

17. Breakey VR, Meyn S, Ng V, et al. Hepatitis-associated aplastic anemia presenting as a familial bone marrow failure syndrome. Journal of Pediatric Hematology/Oncology 2009;31:884–7.

18. Lazarus KH, Baehner RL. Aplastic anemia complicating infectious mononucleosis: a case report and review of the literature. Pediatrics 1981;67:907–10.

19. Marsh JCW, Chang J, Testa NG, et al. In vitro assessment of marrow 'stem cell' and stromal function in aplastic anaemia. Brit J Haematol 1991;78:258–67.

20. Maciewski JP, Anderson S, Katevas P, et al. Phenotypic and functional analysis of bone marrow progenitor cell compartment in bone marrow failure. British Journal of Haematology 1994;87:227–34.

21. Scopes J, Daly S, Atkinson R, et al. Aplastic anaemia: evidence for dysfunctional bone marrow progenitor cells and the corrective effect of granulocyte colony stimulating factor. Blood 1996;87:3179–85.

22. Marsh JCW, Testa NG. Stem cell defect in aplastic anemia. In: Schrezenmeier H, Bacigalupo A, editors. Aplastic Anemia. Pathophysiology and Treatment. Cambridge: Cambridge University Press; 2000. p. 1–20.

23. Maciejewski JP, Selleri C, Sata T, et al. A severe and consistent deficit in marrow and circulating primitive hematopoietic cells (long-term culture-initiating cells) in acquired aplastic anemia. Blood 1996;88:1983–91.

24. Gurion R, Gafter-Gvili A, Paul M, et al. Hematopoietic growth factors in aplastic anemia patients treated with immunosuppressive therapy-systematic review and meta-analysis. Haematologica 2009;94:712–9.

25. Kojima S. Cytokine abnormalities in aplastic anemia in Aplastic Anemia. In: Schrezenmeier H, Bacigalupo A, editors. Pathophysiology and Treatment. Cambridge: Cambridge University Press; 2000. p. 21–40.

26. Young NS, Bacigalupo A, Marsh JC, Aplastic anemia: pathophysiology and treatment. Biology of Blood and Marrow Transplantation 2010;16(1 Suppl):S119–25.

27. Young NS, Calado RT, Scheinberg P. Current concepts in the pathophysiology and treatment of aplastic anemia. Blood 2006;108:2509–19.

28. Ball SE, Gibson FM, Rizzo S, et al. Progressive telomere shortening in aplastic anemia. Blood 1998;91:3582–92.

29. Brummendorf TH, Maciejewski JP, Young NS, Lansdorp PL. Telomere length in leukocyte subpopulations of patients with aplastic anemia. Blood 2001;97:895–900.

30. Savage SA, Alter BP. The role of telomere biology in bone marrow failure and other disorders. Mechanisms of Ageing and Development 2008;129:35–47.

31. Savage SA, Alter BP. The role of telomere biology in bone marrow failure and other disorders. Mechanisms of Ageing and Development 2008;129:35–47.

32. Calado RT, Young NS. Telomere diseases. New England Journal of Medicine 2009;361:2353–65.

33. Speck B, Gluckman E, Haak HL, van Rood JJ. Treatment of aplastic anaemia by antilymphocyte globulin with and without allogeneic bone-marrow infusions. Lancet 1977;2:1145–8.

34. Young NS, Scheinberg P, Calado RT. Aplastic anemia. Current Opinion in Hematology 2008;15:162–8.

35. Solomou EE, Rezvani K, Mielke S, et al. Deficient CD4þ CD25þ FOXP3þ T regulatory cells in acquired aplastic anemia. Blood 2007;110:1603–6.

36. Kansu E, Erslev AJ. Aplastic anemia with 'hot pockets'. Scand J Haematol 1976;17:326–34.

37. Gupta V, Brooker C, Tooze JA, et al. Clinical relevance of cytogenetics abnormalities in adult patients with acquired aplastic anaemia. British Journal of Haematology 2006;134:95–9.

38. Maciejewski JP, Selleri C. Evolution of clonal cytogenetic abnormalities in aplastic anemia. Leuk Lymphoma 2004;45:433–40.

39. Maciejewski JP, Risitano AM, Sloand EM, et al. Distinct clinical outcomes for cytogenetic abnormalities evolving from aplastic anemia. Blood 2002;99:3129–35.

40. Camitta BM, Rappeport JM, Parkman R, et al. Selection of patients for bone marrow transplantation in severe aplastic anemia. Blood 1975;45:355–63.

41. Bacigalupo A, Bruno B, Sarocco P, et al. Antithymocyte globulin, cyclosporin, prednisolone and granulocyte-colony stimulating factor for severe aplastic anaemia: an update of the GITMO/EBMT study on 100 patients. Blood 2000;95:1931–4.

42. de Planque MM, Bacigalupo A, Wursch A, et al. Long-term follow-up of severe aplastic anaemia patients treated with antithymocyte globulin. Severe Aplastic

Anaemia Working Party of the European Cooperative Group for Bone Marrow Transplantation (EBMT). British Journal of Haematology 1989;73:121–6.

43. Socie G, Rosenfeld S, Frickhofen N, et al. Late clonal diseases of treated aplastic anemia. Seminars in Hematology 2000;37:91–101.

44. Tichelli A, Socie G, Marsh J, et al. European Group for Blood and Marrow Transplantation Severe Aplastic Anaemia Working Party. Outcome of pregnancy and disease course among women with aplastic anemia treated with immunosuppression. Annals of Internal Medicine 2002;137:164–72.

45. Araten DJ, Nafa K, Pakdeesuwan K, Luzzatto L. Clonal populations of haematopoietic cells with paroxysmal nocturnal hemoglobinuria genotype and phenotype are present in normal individuals. Proceedings of the National Academy of Sciences of the United States of America 1992;96;5209–14.

46. Marsh JC, Ball SE, Cavenagh J, et al. Guidelines for the diagnosis and management of aplastic anaemia. British Committee for Standards in Haematology. British Journal of Haematology 2009;147:43–70.

47. Davies JK, Guinan EC. An update on the management of severe idiopathic aplastic anaemia in children. British Journal of Haematology 2007;136:549–56.

48. Locasciulli A, Oneto R, Bacigalupo A, et al. Outcome of patients with acquired aplastic anaemia given first line bone marrow transplantation or immunosuppression treatment in the last decade: a report from the European Group for Blood and Marrow Transplantation (EBMT). Haematologica 2007;91:11–1.

49. Scheinberg P, Wu CO, Nunez O, Young NS. Predicting response to immunosuppressive therapy and survival in severe aplastic anaemia. British Journal of Haematology 2009;144: 206–16.

50. Scheinberg P, Wu CO, Scheinberg P, et al. A randomized trial of horse versus rabbit antithymocyte globulin in severe acquired aplastic anemia. Blood 2010; Suppl 1:American Society of Hematology, Abstracts LBA-4

51. Bacigalupo A, Brand R, Oneto R, et al. Treatment of acquired severe aplastic anaemia: bone marrow transplantation compared with immunosuppressive therapy – the European Group for Blood and Marrow Transplantation Experience. Seminars in Hematology 2000;37:69–80.

52. Frickhofen N, Heimpel H, Kaltwasser JP, Schrezenmeier H, for the German Aplastic Anaemia Study Group. Antithymocyte globulin with or without cyclosporin A: 11-year follow-up of a randomised trial comparing treatments of aplastic anaemia. Blood 2003;101:1236–124.

53. Gupta V, Gordon-Smith E, Cook G, et al. A third course of anti-thymocyte globulin in aplastic anaemia is only beneficial in previous responders. British Journal of Haematology 2005;128: 110–11.

54. Gluckman E, Rokicka-Milewska R, Hann I, et al. Results and follow-up of a phase III randomized study of recombinant human-granulocyte stimulating factor as support for immunosuppressive therapy in patients with severe aplastic anaemia. Br J Haematol 2002;119:1075–82.

55. Brodsky R, Chen A, Brodsky I, Jones R. High-dose cyclophosphamide as salvage therapy for severe aplastic anaemia. Experimental Hematology 2004;32: 435–40.

56. Brodsky RA, Sensenbrenner LL, Douglas-Smith B, et al. Durable treatment-free remission after high dose cyclophosphamide therapy for previously untreated severe aplastic anemia. Annals of Internal Medicine 2001;135:477–48.

57. Tisdale JF, Maciejewski JP, Nunez O, et al. Late complications following treatment for severe aplastic anemia (SAA) with high-dose cyclophosphamide (Cy): follow-up of a randomized trial. Blood 2002;100:4668–70.

58. Camiia BM, Thomas ED, Nathan DG, et al. Severe aplastic anemia: a prospective study of the effect of early marrow transplantation on acute mortality. Blood 1976;48; 63–70.

59. Ades L, Mary JY, Robin M, et al. Long-term outcome after bone marrow transplantation for severe aplastic anaemia. Blood 2004;103:2490–249.

60. Champlin RE, Perez WS, Passweg J, et al. Bone marrow transplantation for severe aplastic anemia: a randomised controlled study of conditioning regimens. Blood 2007;109:4582–5.

61. Myers KC, Davies SM. Haemopoietic stem cell trans-plantation for bone marrow failure syndromes in children. Biology of Blood and Marrow Transplantation 2009;15:279–29.

62. McCann S, Passweg J, Bacigalupo A, et al. The influence of cyclosporin alone, or cyclosporin and methotrexate, on the incidence of mixed haematopoietic chimaerism following allogeneic sibling bone marrow transplantation for severe aplastic anaemia. Bone Marrow Transplantation 2007;39:109–11.

63. Bacigalupo A, Locatelli F, Lanino E, et al. Fludarabine, cyclophosphamide and ATG for alternative donor transplants in acquired severe aplastic anaemia – a report of the EBMT SAA Working Party. Bone Marrow Transplantation 2005;41:45–50.

64. Deeg HJ, O'Donnell M, Tolar J, et al. Optimization of conditioning for marrow transplantation from unrelated donors for patients with aplastic anemia after failure of immunosuppressive therapy. Blood 2006;108:1485–91.

65. Ruggeri A, de Latour RP, Rocha V, et al. Double cord blood transplantation in patients with high risk bone marrow failure syndromes. British Journal of Haematology 2008;143:404–8.

66. Smith AR, Wagner JE. Alternative haematopoietic stem cell sources for transplantation: place of umbilical cord blood. British Journal of Haematology 2009;147:246–61.

67. Vlachos A, Ball S, Dahl N, et al. Diagnosing and treating Diamond–Blackfan anaemia: results of an international clinical consensus conference. British Journal of Hamatology 2008;142:859–76.

68. Skeppner G, Forestier E, Henter JI, Wranne L. Transient red cell aplasia in siblings: a common environmental or a common hereditary factor? Acta Paediatrica 1998;87:43–7.

69. Wranne L. Transient erythroblastopenia in infancy and childhood. Scandinavian Journal of Haematology 1970;7:76–81.

70. Skeppner G, Wranne L. Transient erythroblastopenia of childhood in Sweden: incidence and findings at the time of diagnosis. Acta Paediatrica 1993;82:574–8.

71. Cherrick I, Karayalcin G, Lanzkowski C. Transient erythroblastopenia of childhood. Prospective study of fifty patients. American Journal of Pediatric Hematology/Oncology 1994;16:320–4.

72. Ware RE, Kinney TR. Transient erythroblastopenia of childhood in the first year of life. American Journal of Hematoloy 1991;37:156–8.

73. Miller R, Burman B. Transient erythroblastopenia of childhood in infants <6 months of age. American Journal of Pediatric Hematology/Oncology 1994;16:246–8.

74. Michelson AD, Marshall PC. Transient neurological disorder associated with transient erythroblastopenia of childhood. American Journal of Pediatric Hematology/Oncology 1987;9:161–3.

75. Fisch P, Handgretinger R, Schaefer H-E. Pure red cell aplasia. Review. British Journal of Haematology 2000;111: 1010–22.

76. Foot AB, Potter MN, Ropner JE, et al. Transient erythroblastopenia of childhood with CD10, TdT, and cytoplasmic mu lymphocyte positivity in bone marrow. Journal of Clinical Pathology 1990;43:857–9.

77. Skeppner G, Kreuger A, Elinder G. Transient erythroblastopenia of childhood: Prospective study of 10 patients with special reference to viral infections. Journal of Pediatric Hematology/Oncology 2002;24: 294–8.

78. Geetha D, Zachary JB, Baldado HM, et al. Pure red cell aplasia caused by parvovirus B19 infection in solid organ transplant recipients: a case report and

review of literature. Clinical Transplantation 2000;14:586–91.

79. Freedman MH. Pure red cell aplasia in childhood and adolescence: pathogenesis and approaches to diagnosis. British Journal of Haematology 1993;85: 246–53.

80. Shaw J, Meeder R. Transient erythroblastopenia of childhood in siblings: case report and review of the literature. Journal of Pediatric Hematology/Oncology 2007;29;659–60.

81. Skeppner G, Forestier E, Henter JI, Wranne L. Transient red cell aplasia in siblings: a common environmental or a common hereditary factor? Acta Paediatrica 1998;87:43–7.

82. Gustavsson P, Klar J, Matsson H, et al. Familial transient erythroblastopenia of childhood is associated with the chromosome 19q13.2 region but not caused by mutations in coding sequences of the ribosomal protein S19 (RPS19) gene. British Journal of Haematology 2002;119:261–4.

83. Young NS, Brown KE. Parvovirus B19. New England Journal of Medicine 2004;350:586–97.

84. Florea AV, Ionescu DN, Melhem MF. Parvovirus B19 infection in the immunocompromised host. Archives of Pathology and Laboratory Medicine 2007;131:799–804.

85. Mouthon L, Guillevin L, Tellier Z. Intravenous immunoglobulins in autoimmune- or parvovirus B19-mediated pure red-cell aplasia. Autoimmunity Reviews 2005;4:264–9.

86. Koch WC, Adler SP. Detection of human parvovirus B19 DNA by using polymerase chain reaction. Journal of Clinical Microbiology 1990;28:65–9.

87. Kleinman SH, Glynn SA, Lee TH, et al. A linked donor-recipient study to evaluate parvovirus B19 transmission by blood component transfusion. National Heart, Lung, and Blood Institute Retrovirus Epidemiology Donor Study-II (NHLBI REDS-II). Blood 2009;114: 3677–83.

88. McKoy JM, Stonecash RE, Cournoyer D, et al. Epoetin-associated pure red cell aplasia: past, present, and future considerations. Transfusion 2008;48:1754–62.

89. Go RS, Li CY, Tefferi A, Phyliky RL. Acquired pure red cell aplasia associated with lymphoproliferative disease of

granular T lymphocytes. Blood 2001;98:483–5.

90. Dungarwalla M, Marsh JC, Tooze JA, et al. Lack of clinical efficacy of rituximab in the treatment of autoimmune neutropenia and pure red cell aplasia: implications for their pathophysiology. Annals of Hematology 2007;86:191–7.

91. Kuo T, Shih L. Histologic types of thymoma associated with pure red cell aplasia: a study of five cases including a composite tumor or organoid thymoma associated with an unusual lipofibroadenoma. International Journal of Surgical Pathology 2001;9:29–35.

92. Thompson CA, Steensma DP. Pure red cell aplasia associated with thymoma: clinical insights from a 50-year single-institution experience. British Journal of Haematology 2006;135:405–7.

93. Bunn HF. Drug-induced autoimmune red-cell aplasia. New England Journal of Medicine 2002;346:522–3.

94. Smalling R, Foote M, Molineux G, et al. Drug-induced and antibody-mediated pure red cell aplasia: a review of literature and current knowledge. Biotechnology Annual Review 2004;10:237–50.

95. Agrawal A, Parrott NR, Riad HN, Augustine T. Azathioprine-induced pure red cell aplasia: case report and review. Transplantation Proceedings 2004;36: 2689–91.

96. Schellekens H. Immunologic mechanisms of EPO-associated pure red cell aplasia. Baillière's Best Practice in Clinical Haematology 2005;18: 473–80.

97. Casadevall N, Nataf J, Viron B, et al. Pure red-cell aplasia and antierythropoietin antibodies in patients treated with recombinant erythropoietin. N Engl J Med 2002;346:469–75.

98. Diehl LF, Ketchum LH. Autoimmune disease and chronic lymphocytic leukemia: autoimmune hemolytic anemia, pure red cell aplasia, and autoimmune thrombocytopenia. Seminars in Oncology 1998;25: 80–97.

99. Dearden C, Wade R, Else M, et al. The prognostic significance of a positive direct antiglobulin test in chronic lymphocytic leukemia: a beneficial effect of the combination of fludarabine and cyclophosphamide on the incidence of

hemolytic anemia. Blood 2008;111: 1820–6.

100. Cobcroft R. Pure red cell aplasia associated with small cell lymphocytic lymphoma. British Journal of Haematology 2001;113:260.

101. Mohri H, Harano H, Okubo T. Concomitant association of myasthenia gravis and pure red cell aplasia after chemotherapy for Hodgkin's disease. American Journal of Hematology 1997;54:343.

102. Go RS, Lust JA, Phyliky RL. Aplastic anemia and pure red cell aplasia associated with large granular lymphocyte leukemia. Seminars in Hematology 2003;40:196–200.

103. Lacy MQ, Kurtin PJ, Tefferi A. Pure red cell aplasia: association with large granular lymphocyte leukemia and the prognostic value of cytogenetic abnormalities. Blood 1996;87:3000–6.

104. Sawada K, Fujishima N, Hirokawa M. Acquired pure red cell aplasia: updated review of treatment. British Journal of Haematology 2008;142:505–14.

105. Ghazal H. Successful treatment of pure red cell aplasia with rituximab in patients with chronic lymphocytic leukemia. Blood 2002;99:1092–4.

106. Kiely PD, McGuckin CP, Collins DA, et al. Erythrocyte aplasia and systemic lupus erythematosus. Lupus 1995;4: 407–11.

107. Habib GS, Saliba WR, Froom P. Pure red cell aplasia and lupus. Seminars in Arthritis and Rheumatism 2002;31: 279–83.

108. Fujii T, Yajima T, Kameda H, et al. Successful treatment with cyclosporin A of pure red cell aplasia associated with rheumatoid arthritis. Journal of Rheumatology 1996;23:1803–5.

109. Cavazzana I, Ceribelli A, Franceschini F, Cattaneo R. Unusual association between pure red cell aplasia and primary Sjögren's syndrome: a case report. Clinical and Experimental Rheumatology 2007;25:309–11.

110. Damodar S, George B, Mammen J, et al. Pre-transplant reduction of isohaemagglutinin titres by donor group plasma infusion does not reduce the incidence of pure red cell aplasia in major ABO-mismatched transplants. Bone Marrow Transplantation 2005;36:233–5.

Sideroblastic anemia

A May

Sideroblastic anemias (SAs) are heterogeneous disorders characterized by accumulation of iron in the mitochondria of developing erythroblasts and varying degrees of red cell hypochromia. The abnormal, perinuclear mitochondria are visualized after Perls' staining of bone marrow smears for iron. These are seen as a complete or partial ring of Prussian blue staining siderotic granules, in a substantial proportion of erythroblasts (Fig. 14.1).[1,2] Recent studies further associate this excess iron with mitochondrial ferritin.[3] SAs are inherited or acquired. The acquired forms may be secondary and reversible, or primary in nature.[4]

Hereditary sideroblastic anemia

Hereditary SAs (HSAs) are very rare and all patterns of inheritance have been observed (Table 14.1). The anemia may be isolated or syndromic, and severity varies markedly. Some patients die in infancy or childhood; others have a normal life span. Although several genetic defects are now implicated a significant proportion of cases remain unexplained.[5] The diagnosis is often achievable from clinical presentation and cell morphology but genetic diagnosis clarifies treatment options. This helps generate confident management plans which will avoid secondary complications and allows risk assessment for recurrence within families.

X-linked inheritance

ALA synthase 2 defect

The common form of X-linked SA (XLSA) is caused by mutations in the erythroid-specific, 5'-aminolevulinate synthase gene (*ALAS2*) at Xp11.21. Within the mitochondrial matrix, ALAS2 homodimer uses co-factor pyridoxal phosphate to catalyze the first step of heme synthesis.[6] Decreased ALAS2 activity leads to decreased protoporphyrin production and decreased heme. Iron continues to enter the erythroblast unchecked, accumulates in the mitochondria and becomes most visible in the late erythroblasts on staining.

In male patients the severity of the anemia is variable. It is microcytic-hypochromic and may respond to pyridoxine treatment (Fig. 14.1A, B).[7,8] Female carriers have the potential to produce two RBC populations, one microcytic-hypochromic and one normal, depending on which erythroblast X-chromosome is active (Fig. 14.1C). Carriers are usually unaffected but some are anemic due to skewed X chromosome inactivation against that carrying the normal allele, accounting for almost one third of probands.[9,10] Anemic carriers of mild or moderately severe mutations have the same presentation as male hemizygotes (Fig. 14.2). Patients can present at any age with symptoms of anemia or iron overload.[4,11]

Physical examination is unremarkable although mild hepatosplenomegaly may be present. Red cell size and hemoglobin content are broadly distributed and variable proportions of microcytic-hypochromic and normocytic-normochromic cells are seen on the blood film (Fig. 14.1A,B). Anisocytosis, poikilocytosis, elliptocytosis and target cells may be present. An occasional cell with basophilic stippling or Pappenheimer bodies and an occasional late erythroblast may be seen; the numbers of these increase after splenectomy. White cell and platelet counts are normal.

In the bone marrow erythropoiesis is expanded but ineffective; iron overload from increased dietary iron absorption

©2011 Elsevier Ltd
DOI: 10.1016/B978-0-7020-3147-2.00014-6

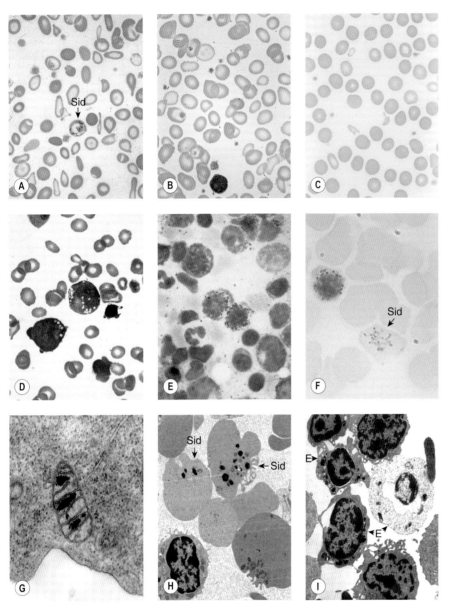

Fig. 14.1 (A–I) Morphology of blood (A, B, C) and bone marrow cells (D–I) in sideroblastic anemia: (A) pyridoxine-responsive XLSA. Note the siderocyte (Sid; arrow). (B) pyridoxine-refractory XLSA; (C) female XLSA heterozygote; (D) vacuolated myeloid cells in Pearson's syndrome; (E) Perls' stain of RARS showing ring sideroblasts; (F) Perls' stain of congenital SA of unknown cause showing ring sideroblast and siderocyte (arrow); (G) electron microscopy showing mitochondrial iron in RARS erythroblast; (H) electron microscopy of siderocyte; (I) group of ring sideroblasts in RARS (arrows). RARS: refractory anemia with ring sideroblasts. Sid: siderocyte. E: erythroblast.

may develop. Transferrin saturation is usually increased; even mildly anemic patients may present with secondary iron overload in the absence of blood transfusion.[12] Total erythrocyte protoporphyrin (TEP) is low/normal. Severe anemia requiring regular blood transfusions is a rare occurrence. Phlebotomy has been successful for preventing iron overload, reversing iron overload and maintaining normal iron levels in pyridoxine-responsive patients (see below). This may additionally improve the hemoglobin level.[13] Iron chelation may be required for correcting iron overload. Splenectomy is not recommended because this has led to thrombotic complications.[4]

At least 120 cases from 70–80 families are reported (January 2011). More than 50 different mutations are involved, scattered across seven exons encoding the catalytic and C-terminal domains.[4,5] Missense mutations predominate; null mutations, or those predicted to be very severe, are found only in female heterozygotes. *ALAS2* variations causing anemia in one member of a family may occasionally be silent in another.[14]

Pyridoxal phosphate (vitamin B_6) is required for ALAS2 activity and stability. Many patients respond partially to pharmacologic doses of oral pyridoxine but some do not or barely do so.[13] Responsive patients remain on maintenance doses of about 25–200 mg oral pyridoxine/day for life.[4] Complete correction of hematological changes with pyridoxine, although rare, has been reported.[15] Pyridoxine responsiveness is most associated with mutations involving amino acids fairly close to the pyridoxal phosphate binding site that cause partial loss of enzyme function or stability.[16,17] Refractoriness is associated with mutations that cause irreversible disruption of activity or cause loss of *in vivo* activity through faulty interaction with components required for intramitochondrial processing.[18] Iron overload, or its complications, also contribute to pyridoxine refractoriness. There may be some response to folate due to secondary deficiency.

Not all *ALAS2* mutations cause SA. Mutations leading to deletion or substitution of the C-terminal 19 amino acids generate truncated ALAS2 protein of increased activity and

Table 14.1 Characteristic features of different types of hereditary sideroblastic anemia†

Chromosomal location	Gene	Defective protein	Protein location	Protein function	Main clinical outcomes	Usual age of onset	Severity of anemia	MCV**	TEP
Xp11.21	ALAS2	ALA synthase 2	Mitochondrial matrix	Heme synthesis	Anemia	Any	Variable	M: low F: low/high	N/↓ N
Xq13.3	ABCB7	ABCB7 transporter	Mitochondrial inner membrane	Transport precursor for cytoplasmic Fe-S cluster biogenesis	Ataxia, anemia	Childhood	Moderate/mild	M: low F: none described	↑
1q23.3	SLC19A2	Thiamine transporter, THTR1	Plasma membrane	High affinity thiamine transport	Diabetes, deafness, megaloblastic anemia	Childhood	Variable	Normal/high	N
3p22.1	SLC25A38	Putative glycine transporter	Mitochondrial inner membrane	Presumed mitochondrial glycine import	Anemia	Infancy/childhood	Severe	Low	N
12p11.21	YARS2	Mitochondrial tyrosyl-tRNA synthetase	Mitochondrial matrix	Aminoacylation of mitochondrial tRNATyr	Mitochondrial myopathy, anaemia, lactic acidosis	Infancy/childhood	Variable	Normal/high***	?
12q24.33	PUS1	Mitochondrial pseudouridine synthase 1	Mitochondrial matrix	Mitochondrial tRNA modification	Mitochondrial myopathy, anemia, lactic acidosis	Childhood/early adolescence	Variable	Normal	?
14q32	GLRX5	Glutaredoxin 5	Mitochondrial matrix	Mitochondrial and cytoplasmic Fe-S cluster biogenesis	Anemia	Middle age*	Moderate	Low	?
mit DNA	del mit DNA	Indirectly affects respiratory chain components	Specifically affects mitochondrial proteins	ATP production electron transport	Megaloblastic anemia, mitochondrial myopathy, pancreatic exocrine dysfunction, lactic acidosis	Infancy	Severe	Normal/high	↑

N = normal; TEP = total erythrocyte protoporphyrin.

†Please note this table does not include information on non-anemic carriers of HAS.

*Only one case described (January 2011).

**All have broad distribution of cell size reflected in a raised Red Cell Distribution Width (RDW).

***Personal communication from Dr Juliana Teo.

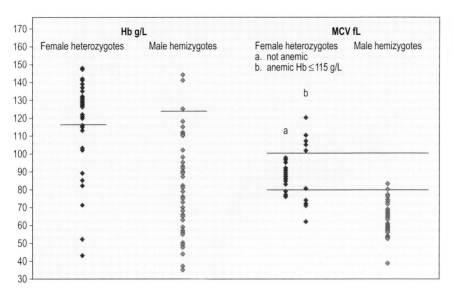

Fig. 14.2 Hemoglobin levels and red cell size (MCV) in documented hemizygotes and heterozygotes of *ALAS2*-associated XLSA.

cause X-linked, dominant erythropoietic protoporphyria, not anemia.[19]

Female carriers of severe/null mutations that prevent erythrocyte production go undetected unless they become anemic because of either skewed but incomplete X-chromosome inactivation against the normal allele or some mechanism selecting against cells expressing the normal allele. In these cases red cells produced by residual effective erythropoiesis from expression of normal *ALAS2* are *macrocytic*, the number of ring sideroblasts may be very low and the cause of the ineffective erythropoiesis may go unsuspected or misdiagnosed (Fig. 14.2).[10,20]

ABCB7 defect

A second XLSA is associated with slow/non-progressive, cerebellar ataxia (XLSA/A). This is usually diagnosed in infants and young children who present with delayed walking ability.[21] There is mild to moderate microcytic-hypochromic anemia (Hb 8–15 g/dl) with red cell appearances indistinguishable to those of ALAS2 deficiency. However, in contrast, there are features of iron deficiency (normal/decreased serum iron, normal/low transferrin iron saturation, increased serum transferrin receptor concentration and variably increased TEP predominantly of the zinc form) rather than iron overload.[22–24] Elevated serum ferritin did, however, develop in two patients, despite low/normal transferrin saturations, so monitoring iron levels is warranted.[24] Ferrokinetic studies have not been reported and bone marrow reports do not give a consistent picture. Down-regulation of *ABCB7* in non-erythroid cells decreases cell proliferation;[25] erythroid hypoplasia may play a role therefore in the anemia. Rational management and treatment of the unusual distribution of iron in these patients awaits a better understanding of the molecular aetiology.

Brain magnetic resonance imaging (MRI) shows selective cerebellar atrophy (Fig. 14.3A). Dysmetria, finger-nose and heel-shin ataxia, dysarthria, intention tremor and diminished deep tendon reflexes are usually present to varying degrees. Nystagmus, strabismus and abnormal plantar responses may or may not be present. Early difficulty in sitting and walking is often followed by some improvement over time. Intelligence is normal and there is no sensory loss.[21,26]

The defect lies in *ABCB7* at Xq13.3 encoding an ATP-dependent 'half-transporter' consisting of N-terminal transmembrane transporter and C-terminal ATPase domains. Within the inner mitochondrial membrane, ABCB7 homodimer exports some component essential for cytoplasmic Fe-S cluster formation.[27] Four separate families with 12 affected patients have been reported. In each of the three families studied a different missense mutation was detected (I400M, V411L, E433K) affecting a different amino acid within the transmembrane transport domain. Yeast cells lacking homologous Atm1p, show reduced cytoplasmic Fe-S cluster generation, normal mitochondrion Fe-S, and mitochondrial iron overload. This phenotype was partially reversed by the intracellular expression of human ABCB7 but less so by the E433K mutant, implicating loss of cytoplasmic Fe-S cluster generation in the XLSA/A syndrome.[23]

Cellular iron homeostasis in humans is regulated at the translational level through the interaction of two iron regulatory proteins (IRP1 and IRP2) with mRNA hairpin-like secondary structure elements known as iron response elements (IRE). IRP1 is formed by loss of Fe-S from cytoplasmic (c-) aconitase. ALAS2 mRNA has a 5' IRE and protein levels are controlled at the translation stage by iron.[28] Low cytoplasm Fe-S decreases ALAS2 activity through conversion of c-aconitase (4Fe-4S) to IRP1 that binds to the 5' IRE and blocks translation. This explains microcytic-hypochromic anemia and mitochondrial iron loading with ABCB7 deficiency; however, additionally, excess mitochondrial iron is somehow not available to ferrochelatase that uses zinc instead to form zinc-protoporphyrin.

Most female XLSA/A heterozygotes have two RBC populations in their peripheral blood and a bimodal red-cell-size distribution. Some have raised total erythrocyte protoporphyrin, but none has yet been reported with anemia or cerebellar ataxia.

Autosomal recessive sideroblastic anemia

Putative deficit of mitochondrial glycine import

Mutations in *SLC25A38* at 3p22.1 cause non-syndromic HSA with more than 30 probands (January 2011) from more

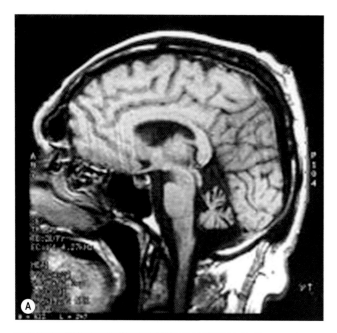

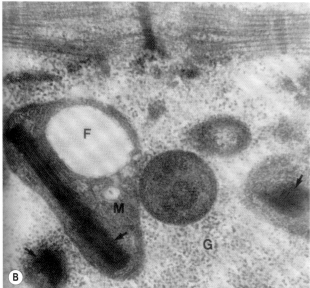

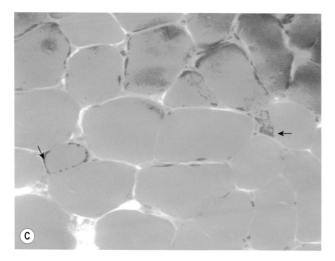

Fig. 14.3 (A–C) Syndromic sideroblastic anaemia: (A) MRI scan of the brain of a patient with XLSA/A showing cerebellar atrophy.[26] (B, C) Mitochondrial inclusions and ragged red fibers in a muscle biopsy of a patient with myopathy with lactic acidosis and sideroblastic anemia.[32,34] *(These figures are reproduced by permission of (A) BMJ Publishing Group Ltd @ 2001, license number 2382030149869, (B) John Wiley and Sons Inc. @ 2005, license number 2382570556744 and (C) BMJ Publishing Group Ltd @ 2007, license number 2382021149604.)*

than 25 families[29] (author's unpublished data). This gene, expressed highly in erythroblasts encodes a putative transporter of glycine, located on the mitochondrial inner membrane. ALAS2 has a high K_M for its substrate glycine and maximal activity requires millimolar concentrations. Decreased glycine supply within the erythroblast mitochondrion leads to decreased ALAS2 activity and decreased heme. Iron uptake, normally inhibited by heme, continues and excess accumulates.

Homozygosity or compound heterozygosity for nonsense, frameshift, splice site and chain termination mutations as well as missense mutations are implicated. These result in severe microcytic-hypochromic anemia of early onset. Erythrocyte protoporphyrin levels are normal and there is evidence of iron loading. The anemia is pyridoxine-refractory and patients usually require regular blood transfusions. No other tissue appears to be affected and some cases have been cured by bone marrow transplantation. Carriers are unaffected.

Glutaredoxin 5 defect

Glutaredoxin 5 (GLRX5) is one of two mitochondrial glutaredoxins. GLRX5 is involved in transport of assembled Fe-S clusters from the scaffold protein (ISCU) to both mitochondrial and cytoplasmic Fe-S destinations.[27]

One *GLRX5* mutation has been reported to cause HSA in a single patient.[30] The patient presented in middle age with iron overload, diabetes, darkened skin and a microcytic-hypochromic anemia (Hb 8.9 g/dL, MCV 59 fl, MCH 16 pg) unresponsive to folate and pyridoxine. Blood transfusions were required but with subsequent iron chelation the patient became transfusion independent (Hb 11.3 g/dl, MCV 64 fl, MCH 22 pg). In peripheral blood mononuclear cells, a splice-site mutation in its homozygous form decreased GLRX5 mRNA, decreased both cytoplasm and mitochondrial Fe-S cluster proteins and increased IRP1 activity. In erythroblasts this would decrease ALAS2 activity and decrease heme as occurs in the GLRX5-deficient zebrafish.[31] No other tissue appears to be affected.

Pseudouridine synthase 1 defect

Several families (6 families, 11 cases (January 2011)) have been described carrying missense (x1) or nonsense (x2) mutations in *PUS1* at 12q24.33.[5,32–34] This gene encodes pseudouridine synthase 1 required to modify mitochondrial tRNA uridine ensuring accurate translation of mitochondrial mRNA. Patients present in infancy, childhood or early teenage years with hypotonia, fatigue, weakness, exercise intolerance, lactic acidosis and SA (known as myopathy with lactic acidosis and sideroblastic anemia or MLASA). The myopathy usually progresses, with distal muscle wasting particularly affecting the hands. Pallor, short stature, micro-cephaly, a short philtrum and a slow gait are usually apparent. Marked growth failure, cognitive and behavior problems have also been described. Severity varies among family members.

The red blood cells show great variation in size with fairly normocytic mean values (MCV 71–100 fl); the severity of the anemia varies from mild/moderate (Hb 7–10 g/dl) to transfusion-dependent. There is iron deposition in mito-chondria of erythroblasts. Muscle biopsy may show paracrys-talline inclusions within the mitochondria ragged red fibers and/or decreased staining for cytochrome oxidase (Fig. 14.3B, C); complex I and IV activities may be decreased.

Mitochondrial tyrosyl-tRNA synthetase defect

A second gene affecting mitochondrial protein synthesis is now also implicated in the MLASA syndrome. Three cases from two unrelated families without *PUS1* mutations were found to be homozygous for the same mutation in the *YARS2* gene that encoded a functionally abnormal mito-chondrial tyrosyl-tRNA synthetase. Decreased activities of skeletal muscle respiratory chain (RC) complexes I, III and IV and specific reduction of mitochondrial-DNA encoded RC subunit synthesis in myotubes generated by transdifferentia-tion of patient-derived fibroblasts were demonstrated. Out-comes differed between the families but were more severe than that from defective PUS1, with earlier onset of both anaemia (10 weeks, infancy, 7 yr) and the chronic lactic acidosis (3 months, infancy, early childhood). The two most severely affected became dependent on regular blood trans-fusion in infancy, suffered great difficulty with walking and swallowing and one succumbed to respiratory failure at 17 yr; cognition and IQ are not affected.[35]

Defective high-affinity thiamine transporter THTR-1

Most cases of thiamine-responsive megaloblastic anemia (TRMA) are associated with sideroblastic erythropoiesis. TRMA typically presents in infancy or childhood as vitamin B_{12}/folate-refractory megaloblastic anemia, sensorineural deafness and diabetes mellitus.[36] Additional complications vary including mild leukopenia, thrombocytopenia, nystag-mus, optic atrophy, retinitis pigmentosa, short stature, stroke, cardiac anomalies. More recently, patients lacking one of the usual triad of symptoms have been diagnosed.[37]

TRMA is caused by homozygosity or compound heterozy-gosity for loss of function or missense mutations in *SLC19A2* on 1q 23.3, encoding the high-affinity, plasma-membrane, thiamine transporter THTR-1.[38,39] More than 20 mutations have been described. Passive thiamine transport and/or co-expression of THTR-2 maintain cell viability. Pharmaco-logic doses of thiamine (usually 20–75 mg/day orally) correct the anemia and decrease or delay the need for insulin but achieve little or no improvement in hearing. Follow-up studies have now been reported with unexplained differ-ences in long-term outcomes regarding maintenance of response to thiamine.[37,40]

Thiamine (vitamin B_1) is important in glucose metabolism and energy production. It is required for thiamine pyro-phosphate (TPP), a co-factor of several enzyme reactions

including three within the mitochondrion (alpha keto-glutarate dehydrogenase, pyruvate dehydrogenase, branched-chain keto acid dehydrogenase), the cytoplasmic enzyme transketolase and the peroxisomal enzyme 2-hydroxyphytanoyl-CoA lyase. Decreased production of ribose and nucleotides through diminished transketolase activity is thought to be the cause of the megaloblastosis. An adverse effect on production of succinyl Co-A, the substrate of the ALAS2 reaction, may be the cause of the SA.

Additional modes of inheritance not yet explained

There remain families with HSA where the mode of inherit-ance and/or pathogenesis remain unresolved. For instance, in one pedigree there was moderately severe microcytic-normocytic anemia, autosomal dominant inheritance of red cell dimorphism and increased total erythrocyte protopor-phyrin and in which two family members had ring sideroblasts. In another pedigree there was maternally inherited mild SA, normocytic-macrocytic RBC and increased free erythrocyte protoporphyrin.[41,42]

Mitochondrial inheritance

Pearson's syndrome is a rare, often fatal disorder of infancy characterized by macrocytic anemia, pancreatic exocrine dys-function and lactic acidosis.[43,44] Patients present with failure to thrive and persistent diarrhea. Neutropenia and thrombo-cytopenia may be present, and hepatic and renal functions may be impaired. It is caused by one of more than 19 dele-tion mutations in mitochondrial DNA of varying sizes including the common 4977bp lying between positions 5500 and 16000bp. Loss of genes encoding mitochondria-specific tRNA disrupts mitochondrial biogenesis and func-tion and the degree to which a tissue is affected depends on the proportion of mitochondrial DNA that is the deleted form. All hemopoietic lineages can be affected and promi-nent vacuoles in both myeloid and erythroid cells are seen on bone marrow smears (Fig. 14.1D). Erythropoiesis is meg-aloblastic with a high percentage of ring sideroblasts. Het-eroplasmy renders maternal inheritance difficult to determine and most cases are described as of 'sporadic' occurrence. Treatment is supportive and although prognosis is poor some patients survive to develop Kearns–Sayre syndrome, a mitochondrial encephalomyopathy.[45]

Acquired sideroblastic anemia

Acquired SAs are the most common types subdivided into:

1. Reversible types secondary to hypothermia, nutritional deficiency or ingestion of certain substances.
2. Primary or idiopathic acquired SA (a myelodysplastic syndrome; see also Chapter 20).

Secondary acquired sideroblastic anemia

Drugs and toxic agents reported to cause sideroblastic eryth-ropoiesis include alcohol, isoniazid, progesterone, D,L-penicillamine, chloramphenicol and zinc supplement excess

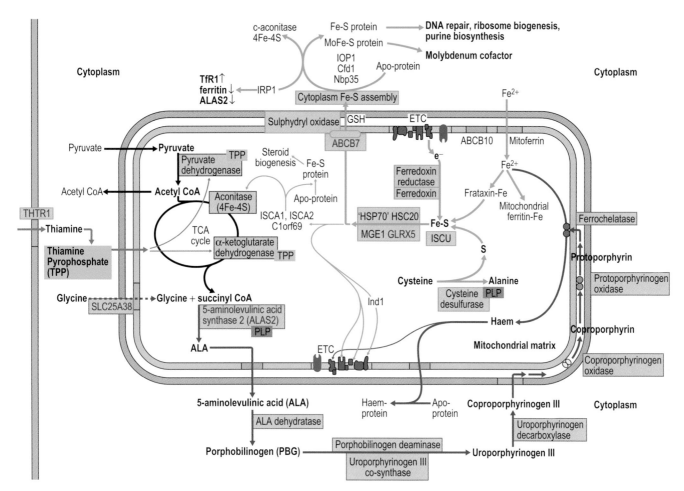

Fig. 14.4 Interrelationship between pathways of mitochondrial metabolism involved in hereditary sideroblastic anemia. Red text: proteins known to be affected; blue arrow: heme synthesis pathway; green arrow: Fe-S cluster biogenesis.

that antagonizes copper absorption. Copper deficiency in parenteral food and through trientene chelation also causes SA.[4] Lead poisoning may lead to SA.[46] Hemodialysis-induced pyridoxine deficiency can precipitate SA even without ALAS2 mutation.[47] The resultant red cell and bone marrow appearances depend on the pathways affected; a hemolytic component may be involved causing reticulocytosis, a feature which is unusual in primary SA.

Primary acquired sideroblastic anemia

Primary acquired SA, referred to as refractory anemia with ring sideroblasts (RARS), is a myelodysplastic syndrome (MDS). It affects mainly elderly people or people of late middle age and is characterized by ineffective hemopoiesis, peripheral blood cytopenias and an increased risk of developing leukemia.[48–50] Patients present with progressive anemia and associated symptoms such as breathlessness, fatigue and pallor. Organomegaly is not usually present except in cases of iron overload.

The blood count shows normocytic or macrocytic anemia refractory to treatment with vitamin B_{12} or folate, normal neutrophils and platelets. The red cell size distribution is increased but reticulocyte numbers remain normal or only slightly increased. Red cell anisocytosis may be marked and some hypochromia is usually present giving rise to a dimorphic appearance of the red cells in some patients.

The bone marrow shows erythroid hyperplasia with ineffective dyserythropoiesis such as increased proportion of early erythroblasts. Abnormalities in other cell lineages are absent and blast cells remain below 5%. More than 15% erythroblasts are ring sideroblasts (providing the patient is not iron deficient) occurring at all stages of erythroid differentiation (Fig. 14.1E).

There is no association with any particular cytogenetic change except for rearrangements involving Xq13.[50] Prognosis is good if there is no karyotypic abnormality, trilineage dysplasia or transfusion dependence. Life expectancy of patients over 70 years may not be reduced. The overall risk of transformation to leukemia is between 5% and 10% at 10 years from diagnosis in those with a normal karyotype who are not dependent on blood transfusion.

Treatment consists of alleviation of symptoms of anemia and avoidance or treatment of iron overload resulting from blood transfusion. More vigorous interventions may play a role when shown to be efficacious and safe.[52,53] Regular monitoring of the blood count and iron stores is required.

The cause is unknown. It appears to be a clonal disorder arising from a hemopoietic stem cell abnormality that is yet to be defined. Whether the mitochondrial iron overload is caused by the mutation causing the clonal proliferation, is due to a somatic mutation in the cell triggered by subsequent mutation to proliferate or occurs entirely as a secondary phenomenon remains to be seen. Characteristic metabolic changes are beginning to be identified confirming RARS as a distinct MDS category.[54,55] Mitochondrial ferritin is upregulated even at the earliest stage of differentiation. Genes encoding heme synthesis enzymes are up-regulated and *ABCB7* down-regulated.

Some RARS patients have an associated thrombocytosis ($>450 \times 10^9$/l). These have been included in the WHO Classification as MDS/myeloproliferative neoplasms in the entity 'RARS associated with marked thrombocytosis' (RARS-T). An association between acquisition of *JAK2* V617F and the development of thrombocytosis suggests 'transformation' from RARS.[55]

Differential diagnosis of primary sideroblastic anemia

The diagnosis of sideroblastic anemia relies on the visual observation firstly of peripheral blood red cell hypochromia and then of ring sideroblasts in the marrow after staining for iron using a Perls' Prussian blue reaction (Fig. 14.1F). Electron microscopy may be required to confirm the subcellular location of the iron in difficult or unusual cases (Fig. 14.1G-I). For syndromic cases, histochemical staining of sections from biopsied muscle and measurement of respiratory complex activity by assay or by staining are often required and brain MRI is essential for some. There is considerable overlap of peripheral blood morphology and bone marrow features between different SA types. Sex, age of onset, severity of anemia, MCV, TEP, the ratio of zinc:free erythrocyte protoporphyrin (EPP) and presence of additional syndrome-associated pathology are therefore additional important differentiating features (Table 14.1). Almost half inherited or congenital SA remain unexplained and further genetic causes remain to be found. With their high rate of heme synthesis, erythroid cells are particularly sensitive to defects of mitochondrial iron metabolism. The genes identified in SA affect mitochondrial proteins directly or indirectly (Fig. 14.4, Table 14.1) and the syndromic cases highlight the importance of pathways of iron homeostasis to other conditions.

Acknowledgments

The chapter structure and a few sentences remain those of Professor SN Wickramasinghe, a source of great inspiration who sadly could not contribute more. Thanks to Ruth Pitman and Kevin Barnes for the electron microscopic images in Fig. 14.1, and to Dr Edward Fitzsimons for Fig. 14.1D. I would also like to thank Dr Briedgeen Kerr for her help in researching the data for Figure 14.2 and for her permission to use it here in this way. Thanks also to Professors Massimo Zeviani and Simon Hammans for agreeing to my use of their published images and to Dr Juliana Teo and Professor John Christodoulou for permission to refer to their unpublished data.

References

1. Bessis MC, Breton-Gorius J. Ferritin and ferruginous micelles in normal erythroblasts and hypochromic hypersideremic anemias. Blood 1959;14:423–32.

2. Wickramasinghe SN, Fulker MJ, Losowsky MS, Hall R. Microspectrophotometric and electron microscopic studies of bone marrow in hereditary sideroblastic anaemia. Acta Haematol 1971;45:236–44.

3. Cazzola M, Invernizzi R, Bergamaschi G. Mitochondrial ferritin expression in erythroid cells from patients with SA. Blood 2003;101:1996–2000.

4. Bottomley SS. Sideroblastic anemias. In: Greer JP, Foerster J, Rodgers GM, et al, editors. Wintrobe's Clinical Hematology, 12th ed. Philadelphia: Lippincott Williams & Wilkins; 2008. p. 835–55.

5. Bergmann AK, Campagna DR, McLoughlin EM, et al. Systematic molecular genetic analysis of congenital sideroblastic anemia: evidence for genetic heterogeneity and identification of novel mutations. Pediatr Blood Cancer 2010;54:273–8.

6. Ferreira GC, Gong J. 5-Aminolevulinate synthase and the first step of heme biosynthesis. J Bioenerg Biomembr 1995;27:151–9.

7. Harris JW, Whittington RM, Weisman R Jr, Horrigan DL. Pyridoxine responsive anemia in the human adult. Proc Soc Exp Biol Med 1956;91:427–32.

8. May A, Bishop DF. The molecular biology and pyridoxine responsiveness of X-linked sideroblastic anaemia. Haematologica 1998;83:56–70.

9. Cazzola M, May A, Bergamaschi G, et al. Familial-skewed X-chromosome inactivation as a predisposing factor for late-onset X-linked sideroblastic anemia in carrier females. Blood 2000;96:4363–5.

10. Aivado M, Gatterman N, Rong A, et al. X-linked sideroblastic anemia associated with a novel ALAS2 mutation and unfortunate skewed X-chromosome inactivation patterns. Blood Cells Mol Dis 2006;37:40–5.

11. Anderson KE, Sassa S, Bishop DF, Desnick RJ. Disorders of heme biosynthesis: X-linked sideroblastic anemia and the porphyrias. In: Scriver CR, Beaudet AL, Sly WS, et al, editors. The Metabolic and Molecular Bases of Inherited Disease. Vol 2. 8th ed. New York, NY: McGraw-Hill; 2001. p. 2991–3062.

12. Peto TE, Pippard MJ, Weatherall DJ. Iron overload in mild sideroblastic anaemias. Lancet 1983;1(8321):375–8.

13. Cotter PD, May A, Li L, et al. Four new mutations in the erythroid-specific 5-aminolevulinate synthase (ALAS2) gene causing X-linked sideroblastic anemia: increased pyridoxine responsiveness after removal of iron overload by phlebotomy and coinheritance of hereditary hemochromatosis. Blood 1999;93:1757–69.

14. Cazzola M, May A, Bergamaschi G, et al. Absent phenotypic expression of X-linked sideroblastic anemia in one of 2 brothers with a novel ALAS2 mutation. Blood 2002;100:4236–8.

15. Cotter PD, May A, Fitzsimons EJ, et al. Late-onset X-linked sideroblastic anemia. Missense mutations in the erythroid δ-aminolevulinate synthase (ALAS2) gene in two pyridoxine-responsive patients initially diagnosed with acquired refractory anemia and ringed sideroblasts. J Clin Invest 1995;96:2090–6.

16. Shoolingin-Jordan PM, Al-Daihan S, Alexeev D, et al. 5-Aminolevulinic acid synthase: mechanism, mutations and medicine. Biochim Biophys Acta 2003;1647:361–6.

17. Astner I, Schulze JO, van den Hevel J, et al. Crystal structure of 5-aminolevulinate synthase, the first enzyme of heme biosynthesis,

and its link to XLSA in humans. EMBO J 2005;24:3166–77.

18. Furuyama K, Fujita H, Nagai T, et al. Pyridoxine refractory X-linked sideroblastic anemia caused by a point mutation in the erythroid 5-aminolevulinate synthase gene. Blood 1997;90:822–30.

19. Whatley SD, Ducamp S, Gouya L, et al. C-terminal deletions in the ALAS2 gene lead to gain of function and cause a previously undefined type of human porphyria, X-linked dominant protoporphyria, without anemia or iron overload. Am J Hum Genet, 2008;83: 408–14.

20. Cortesao E, Vidan J, Pereira J, et al. Onset of X-linked sideroblastic anemia in the fourth decade. Haematologica 2004; 89:1261–3.

21. Pagon RA, Bird TD, Detter JC, Pierce I. Hereditary sideroblastic anaemia and ataxia: an X linked recessive disorder. J Med Genet 1985;22:267–73.

22. Allikmets R, Raskind WH, Hutchinson A, et al. Mutation of a putative mitochondrial iron transporter gene (ABCB7) in X-linked sideroblastic anemia and ataxia (XLSA/A). Hum Mol Genet 1999;8:743–9.

23. Bekri S, Kispal G, Lange H, et al. Human ABC7 transporter: gene structure and mutation causing X-linked sideroblastic anemia with ataxia with disruption of cytosolic iron-sulfur protein maturation. Blood 2000;96:3256–64.

24. Maguire A, Hellier K, Hammans S, May A. X-linked cerebellar ataxia and sideroblastic anaemia associated with a missense mutation in the ABC7 gene predicting V411L. Br J Haematol 2001;115:910–7.

25. Cavadini P, Biasiotto G, Poli M, et al. RNA silencing of the mitochondrial ABCB7 transporter in HeLa cells causes an iron-deficient phenotype with mitochondrial iron overload. Blood 2007;109:3552–9.

26. Hellier KD, Hatchwell E, Duncombe AS, et al. X-linked sideroblastic anaemia with ataxia: another mitochondrial disease? J Neurol Neurosurg Psychiatry 2001;70: 65–9.

27. Lill R. Function and biogenesis of iron-sulphur proteins. Nature 2009; 460:831–8.

28. Dandekar T, Stripecke R, Gray NK, et al. Identification of a novel iron-responsive element in murine and human erythroid δ-aminolevulinic acid synthase mRNA. EMBO J 1991;10:1903–9.

29. Guernsey DL, Jiang H, Campagna DR, et al. Mutations in mitochondrial carrier family gene SLC25A38 cause nonsyndromic autosomal recessive congenital sideroblastic anemia. Nat Genet 2009;41:651–3.

30. Camaschella C, Campanella A, De Falco L, et al. The human counterpart of zebrafish shiraz shows sideroblastic-like microcytic anemia and iron overload. Blood 2007;110:1353–8.

31. Wingert RA, Galloway JL, Barut B, et al. Deficiency of glutaredoxin 5 reveals Fe-S clusters are required for vertebrate haem synthesis. Nature 2005;436:1035–39.

32. Inbal A, Avissar N, Shaklai M, et al. Myopathy, lactic acidosis, and sideroblastic anemia: a new syndrome. Am J Med Genet 1995;55:372–8.

33. Casas KA, Fischel-Ghodsian N. Mitochondrial myopathy and sideroblastic anaemia. Am J Med Genet 2004;125A: 201–4.

34. Fernandez-Vizarra E, Berardinelli A, Valente L, et al. Nonsense mutation in pseudouridylate synthase 1 (PUS1) in two brothers affected by myopathy, lactic acidosis and sideroblastic anaemia (MLASA). J Med Genet 2007;44:173–80.

35. Riley LG, Cooper S, Hickey P, et al. Mutation of the mitochondrial tyrosyl-tRNA synthetase gene, YARS2, causes myopathy, lactic acidosis, and sideroblastic anemia-MLASA syndrome. Am J Hum Genet 2010;87:52–9.

36. Rogers LE, Porter S, Sidbury Jr JB. Thiamine-responsive megaloblastic anemia. J Pediatr 1969;74:494–504.

37. Bergmann AK, Sahai I, Falcone JF, et al. Thiamine-responsive megaloblastic anemia: identification of novel heterozygotes and mutation update. J Pediatr 2009;155:888–92.

38. Fleming JC, Tartaglini E, Steinkamp MP, et al. The gene mutated in thiamine-responsive anemia with diabetes and deafness (TRMA) encodes a functional thiamine transporter. Nat Genet 1999; 22:305–8.

39. Neufeld EJ, Fleming JC, Tartaglini E, Steinkamp MP. Thiamine-responsive megaloblastic anemia syndrome: a disorder of high-affinity thiamine transport. Blood Cells Mol Dis 2001;27: 135–8.

40. Ricketts CJ, Minton JA, Samuel J, et al. Thiamine-responsive megaloblastic anaemia syndrome: long-term follow-up and mutation analysis of seven families. Acta Paediatr 2006;95:99–104.

41. van Waveren Hogervorst GD, van Roermund HPC, Snijders PJ. Hereditary sideroblastic anaemia and autosomal inheritance of erythrocyte dimorphism in a Dutch family. Eur J Haematol 1987; 38:405–9.

42. Tuckfield A, Ratnaike S, Hussein S, Metz J. A novel form of hereditary sideroblastic anaemia with macrocytosis. Br J Haematol 1997;97:279–85.

43. Pearson HA, Lobel JS, Kocoshis SA, et al. A new syndrome of refractory sideroblastic anemia with vacuolization of marrow precursors and exocrine pancreatic dysfunction. J Pediatr 1979; 95:976–84.

44. Rotig A, Cormier V, Blanche S, et al. Pearson's marrow-pancreas syndrome: a multisystem mitochondrial disorder in infancy. J Clin Invest 1990;86: 1601–8.

45. McShane MA, Hammans SR, Sweeney M, et al. Pearson syndrome and mitochondrial encephalomyopathy in a patient with a deletion of mtDNA. Am J Hum Genet 1991;48:39–42.

46. Domingo-Claros A, Alonso E, Banda Ed Ede L. Schizophrenia and refractory anaemia with ring sideroblasts. Br J Haematol 2004;125:543.

47. Gill H, Yip T, Lo W-K. Anemia in a patient newly transferred from peritoneal dialysis to hemodialysis. Am J Kid Dis 2010;56:xxxvii–ix.

48. Vardiman JW, Harris NL, Brunning RD. The World Health Organization (WHO) classification of the myeloid neoplasms. Blood 2002;100:2292–302.

49. Cazzola M, Malcovati L. Myelodysplastic syndromes – coping with ineffective hematopoiesis. New Engl J Med 2005;352(6):536–8.

50. Malcovati L, Germing U, Kuendgen A, et al. Time-dependent prognostic scoring system for predicting survival and leukemic evolution in myelodysplastic syndromes. J Clin Oncol 2007;25: 3503–10.

51. Dewald GW, Brecher M, Travis LB, Stupca PJ. Twenty-six patients with hematologic disorders and X chromosome abnormalities. Frequent idic(X)(q13) chromosomes and Xq13 anomalies associated with pathologic ringed sideroblasts. Cancer Genet Cytogenet 1989;42:173–85.

52. Bowen D, Culligan D, Jowitt S, et al. Guidelines for the diagnosis and therapy of adult myelodysplastic syndromes. Br J Haematol 2003;120:187–200.

53. Hellström-Lindberg E, Malcovati L. Supportive care, growth factors, and new therapies in myelodysplastic syndromes. Blood Rev 2008;22:75–91.

54. Boultwood J, Pellagatti A, Nikpour M, et al. The role of the iron transporter ABCB7 in refractory anemia with ring sideroblasts. PLoS One 2008;3: e1970.

55. Malcovati L, Della Porta MG, Pietra D, et al. Molecular and clinical features of refractory anemia with ringed sideroblasts associated with marked thrombocytosis. Blood 2009;114:3538–45.

CHAPTER 15

Congenital dyserythropoietic anemias

R Renella, GW Hall, DJP Ferguson, WG Wood

Dedicated to SN Wickramasinghe, from whose chapter in the previous edition the present one is derived.

Chapter contents

The congenital dyserythropoietic anemias (CDAs) are a heterogeneous group of rare inherited anemias, without additional cytopenias and with no tendency to neoplastic transformation.[1,2] The cause of the peripheral anemia is a block in erythroid maturation, associated with a variable degree of erythroid dysplasia (dyserythropoiesis) in the bone marrow. The ineffectiveness of erythropoiesis results in a suboptimal reticulocyte response for the degree of anemia despite the presence of marked erythroid hyperplasia. Based largely on the nature of the dysplastic changes seen by light and electron microscopy, the CDAs have been divided into three major types, designated CDA types 1, 2 and 3 (Table 15.1), and other forms designated CDA groups IV–VII (see Table 15.2 below).[3,4]

Congenital dyserythropoietic anemia, type 1 (CDA-1)

CDA-1 has a variable presentation, as it can become apparent during the neonatal period or indeed at any time during the first five decades of life. It may also present *in utero*, with manifestations of fetal anemia requiring antenatal transfusions.[5–7] However, patients usually have a mild to moderate anemia and may show jaundice, hepatosplenomegaly and cholelithiasis. A few are nevertheless severely anemic and transfusion-dependent. There is an increased tendency for some patients to develop marked iron overload despite a limited number of transfusions and lack of transfusion dependence (Fig. 15.1). Some cases have congenital abnormalities such as syndactyly, aberrations of the bones of the hands and feet (absence or hypoplasia of some phalanges, additional phalanges), dysplastic nails, short stature and abnormal pigmentation of areas of the skin (Fig. 15.2).

The disorder is inherited in an autosomal recessive manner. The disease gene was identified and localized to chromosome 15q15.1–15.3 in a highly inbred group of Israeli Bedouins.[8] The *CDAN1* gene has been highly conserved during evolution, has no known orthologues and the codanin-1 protein contains no recognizable motifs to provide clues as to its function. Over 20 mutations of *CDAN1* have been described. The majority are missense mutations. Null mutations also occur, but to date no patients have been found who are either homozygous or compound heterzygous for these null mutations, suggesting such a combination is likely to be lethal. Incomplete sequencing may explain CDA-1 patients without *CDAN1* mutations, but there is also likely to be genetic heterogeneity in this disorder.[9]

The average hemoglobin (Hb) is 9.0 g/dl (range 6.0–12.6 g/dl), and the mean cell volume (MCV) increased in 75% of cases. The peripheral blood film shows macrocytes and basophilic stippling (Fig. 15.3) and the reticulocyte count is normal or only minimally raised. There is megaloblastic erythroid hyperplasia in the bone marrow (Fig. 15.4). Some of the more mature basophilic erythroblasts and many of the early and late polychromatic erythroblasts show dyserythropoietic features. The characteristic morphological abnormality is internuclear bridging, where chromatin strands connect pairs of almost completely separated polychromatic erythroblasts (0.6–2.8 strands per 100 erythroblasts) (Fig.15.5A, B). There is also an increase in the percentage of binucleate polychromatic erythroblasts, which

DOI: 10.1016/B978-0-7020-3147-2.00015-8

Table 15.1 Summary of clinical and molecular features of CDA 1-3

Type	BM morphology	Symptoms and signs	Inheritance and molecular	Epidemiology	Age at presentation	Specific therapy
CDA-1	Erythroid hyperplasia, megaloblastic appearance, internuclear chromatin bridges in polychromatophilic erythroblasts.	Anemia (most cases during neonatal period). Iron overload. Splenomegaly and hepatomegaly. Rare: extramedullary hematopoiesis.	Autosomal recessive. Gene: *CDAN1* (15q15). Other unknown locus**	Founder effects (Israel and Switzerland). Cases from central Europe, Arabic Countries, India, Japan, China.	*In utero* (hydrops fetalis), neonatal, childhood or early adulthood.	IFN-α (HSCT)
CDA-2	Erythroid hyperplasia with binuclearity, late orthochromatic cytoplasm with highly condensed nuclei, pseudo-Gaucher cells.	Anemia and jaundice. Gallstones (60%) Cholecystectomy (30%) Splenomegaly (usually by adulthood). Iron overload. Rare: paravertebral hematopoiesis. Aplastic crisis (parvovirus B19).	Autosomal recessive. Gene: *CDAN2* (20p11.23). Other unknown locus**	Most frequent. Founder effect (Southern Italy). Cases mostly European (incl. Eastern and Mediterranean basin).	Majority are diagnosed age 5–30 (average 18–20 years).	Splenectomy (HSCT)
CDA-3	Erythroid hyperplasia with multinuclearity (up to 12 nuclei per cell). Nuclear lobulation and karyorrhexis.	Mild anemia. No iron overload.	Autosomal dominant. (familial cases). Locus 15q22 Autosomal recessive (sporadic cases).	Rarest form. Founder effect (Sweden, Argentina, USA).	N/A	N/A (HSCT?)

**Evidence for genetic heterogeneity in CDA-1/2. BM, bone marrow; HSCT, hemopoietic stem cell transplant.

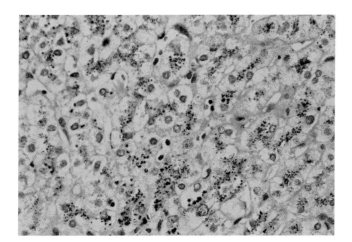

Fig. 15.1 Needle biopsy of the liver of a 40-year-old patient with CDA-1 who had received few transfusions, showing grade 4/4 iron overload. Perls' stain. ×100.

account for 3.5–7.0% of all erythroblasts. The latter may contain nuclei of different size and show partial fusion of the two nuclear masses; the two nuclei within the same cell may display different staining characteristics (Fig. 15.6). The most striking abnormality, seen on electron microscopy (EM), is the presence of nuclei with a spongy (or 'Swiss-cheese') appearance in a high proportion (up to 60%) of the mononucleate early and late polychromatic erythroblasts. These nuclei have multiple rounded electron-lucent areas within abnormally electron-dense heterochromatin (Fig. 15.7). Nuclei with a spongy appearance may also contain nuclear-membrane-lined cytoplasmic intrusions,

sometimes with cytoplasmic organelles (Fig. 15.7B). An abnormally low percentage of mononucleate early polychromatic erythroblasts synthesize DNA; the non-DNA-synthesizing cells have DNA contents between 2c and 8c (1c = the haploid DNA content, i.e. the DNA content of a spermatozoon) and appear to be derived from the maturation of cells whose progress in the cell cycle has been arrested. These morphologically abnormal cells are destroyed *in situ*, resulting in ineffective erythropoiesis.[10]

All CDA-1 patients with confirmed mutations in *CDAN1* have responded to α-interferon, with an increase in Hb, reduction in MCV, decrease in the proportion of erythroblasts with the 'Swiss-cheese' ultrastructural abnormality and a decrease in ineffective erythropoiesis.[11,12] Currently, the first step of therapy for eligible CDA-1 patients (EM positive, awaiting/positive *CDAN1* sequencing) should be with α-interferon. Some patients show a hematological response to splenectomy. The only available curative treatment for genetic conditions of hematopoiesis is hemopoietic stem cell transplantation (HSCT) which has been used with some success in patients with CDA-1, CDA-2 and a variant case.[13–16] Transplantation has been limited to severe cases where splenectomy was ineffective, transfusion needs exceeded tolerance levels for iron overload, and a HLA-identical donor was available.

Congenital dyserythropoietic anemia, type 2 (CDA-2)

CDA-2, previously referred to as *h*ereditary *e*rythroblastic *m*ultinuclearity with *p*ositive *a*cidified *s*erum test (HEMPAS),

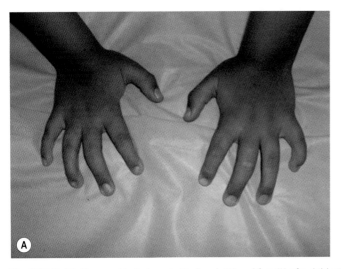
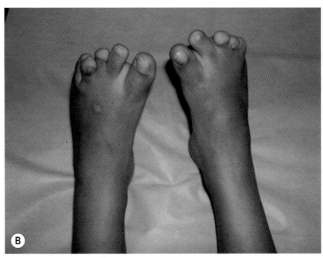

Fig. 15.2 (A, B) Dysmorphic features in the hands (A) and feet (B) of a child with CDA-1. *(Courtesy of Dr Aurora Feliu-Torres, Buenos Aires, Argentina.)*

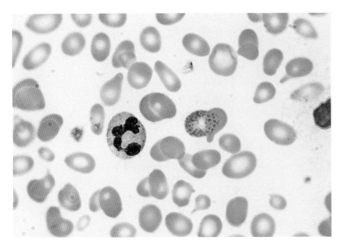

Fig. 15.3 Blood film of a case of CDA-1, showing oval macrocytes, moderate anisopoikilocytosis including tear drop-shaped cells and a coarsely-stippled red cell. May–Grünwald–Giemsa stain. × 1000.

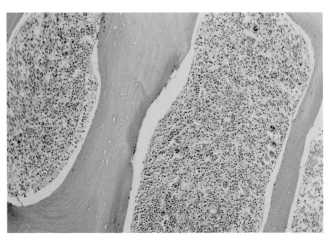

Fig. 15.4 Trephine biopsy of bone marrow from a patient with CDA-1, showing an intensely hypercellular marrow with complete replacement of fat cells by hemopoietic (largely erythropoietic) cells. Hematoxylin and eosin. × 200.

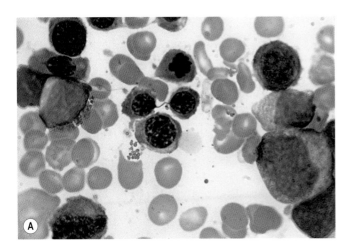
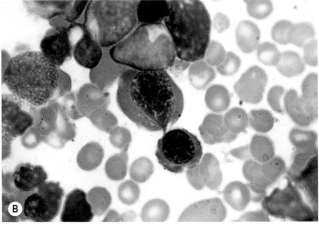

Fig. 15.5 (A, B) Internuclear chromatin strands joining incompletely separated erythroblasts in a marrow smear from a case of CDA-1. × 1000. In (A) the chromatin strand connects two nuclei of equal size (May–Grünwald–Giemsa stain) and in (B) nuclei of unequal size.

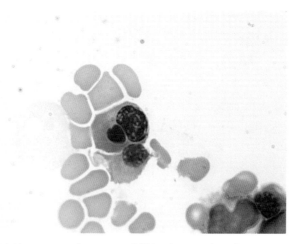

Fig. 15.6 Marrow smear from a case of CDA-1 showing a binucleate erythroblast in which the two nuclei have stained differently. The other two erythroblasts in the photomicrograph are joined by an internuclear chromatin strand that has been stretched during the preparation of the smear. May–Grünwald–Giemsa stain. ×1000.

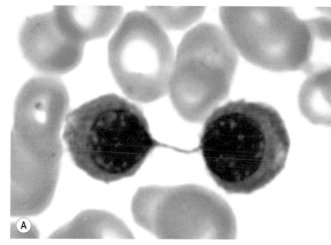

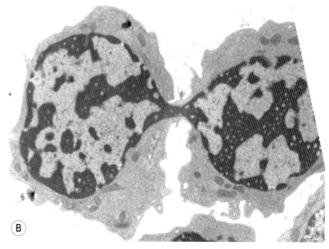

Fig. 15.7 (A, B) Erythroblasts from a case of CDA-1, showing internuclear bridges. (A) May–Grünwald–Giemsa stain. ×1000. (B) Electron micrograph showing the internuclear bridging and the spongy ('Swiss cheese') nuclear appearance.

is the most common type of CDA. Many of the reported cases were of southern Italian ancestry, but cases have also been reported from northwestern Europe and North Africa. Clinical features include mild to moderate anemia, mild jaundice, splenomegaly in 65% of cases, cholelithiasis and a tendency to develop iron-overload. Patients usually present between the ages of 1 month and 25 years, but there is frequently a delay in establishing the diagnosis.[17]

The disorder is inherited in an autosomal recessive manner, and the disease gene localizes to chromosome 20p11. The gene, CDAN2, encodes for the SEC23B protein, a component of the COP-II coat protein complex, which plays a role in vesicular transport from the endoplasmic reticulum to the Golgi apparatus. More than 25 mutations have been described, both missense and null alleles. Two specific missense mutations constitute nearly half of all the mutant alleles.[18] However, there is evidence that an additional locus could be involved in CDA-2.[19]

The average Hb is 8 g/dl. The red cells are normochromic and normocytic and show moderate anisocytosis, poikilocytosis and basophilic stippling. The reticulocyte count is either normal or minimally raised. Some cases present with minimal anemia, while occasional patients are transfusion-dependent, even without the co-inheritance of a β-thalassemia trait. The bone marrow shows normoblastic erythroid hyperplasia. A few of the basophilic erythropoietic cells and early polychromatic erythroblasts and 10–35% of the late erythroblasts are binucleate; the nuclei are usually of equal size (Fig. 15.8). In addition, a small proportion of the erythroblasts are trinucleate or multinucleate. Many of the mononucleate and binucleate late erythroblasts have orthochromatic cytoplasm and highly-condensed, apparently structureless nuclei. The anemia results from ineffective erythropoiesis. A high rate of phagocytosis of mononucleate and binucleate late erythroblasts by bone marrow macrophages is seen on bone marrow examination. Electron microscopy reveals a characteristic double membrane (consisting of smooth endoplasmic reticulum) aligned parallel to and at a distance of 40–60 nm from the cell membrane

in a substantial proportion of the late erythroblasts (Fig. 15.9A, B). These double membranes are referred to as peripheral cisternae. Bone marrow macrophages are often laden with lipid and appear as pseudo-Gaucher cells (Fig. 15.9C).

The red cells give a positive acidified serum lysis test (Ham test) with about 30% of fresh ABO-compatible normal sera but not with the patient's own serum. The reactive sera contain an antibody that combines specifically with an antigen on the CDA-2 red cells. This IgM antibody can be removed by absorption with red cells of patients with CDA-2, but not with red cells of patients with paroxysmal nocturnal hemoglobinuria (PNH). Due to the problems in performing this test in routine laboratories because of the difficulty in obtaining appropriate control antisera, finding an alternative test has become a priority.[20] The anion transport protein (band 3) of the red cell membrane is underglycosylated in CDA-2 and, consequently, is migrates faster than normal on SDS polyacrylamide gel electrophoresis (SDS-PAGE). This technique has progressively replaced the Ham test. If results are suggestive for CDA-2 in SDS-PAGE, genetic analysis of CDAN2 is

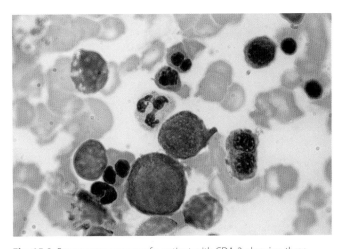

Fig. 15.8 Bone marrow smear of a patient with CDA-2, showing three binucleate late polychromatic erythroblasts and one binucleate early polychromatic erythroblast. The two nuclei of one of the late erythroblasts are stuck together and each shows a bud-like protrusion. May–Grünwald–Giemsa stain. ×1000.

warranted. Specific therapy for CDA-2 is not yet available, and supportive care constitutes the best standard practice, although splenectomy results in a substantial increase in Hb in some cases but without effect on iron overloading. Studies identifying the criteria for splenectomy in patients with CDA-2 need to be performed. HSCT has been attempted with some success in a very limited number of selected patients with CDA-2 (see discussion of HCST for CDA-1).

Congenital dyserythropoietic anemia, type 3 (CDA-3)

CDA-3 is the rarest of the three classical types of CDA. Familial cases have been described in Sweden, Argentina and the USA. The largest is a five-generation family from the Væsterbotten district of Sweden, whose ancestry can be traced back to the 19th century. It contains more than 30 cases inherited in an autosomal dominant manner.[21] CDA-3 is not as severe

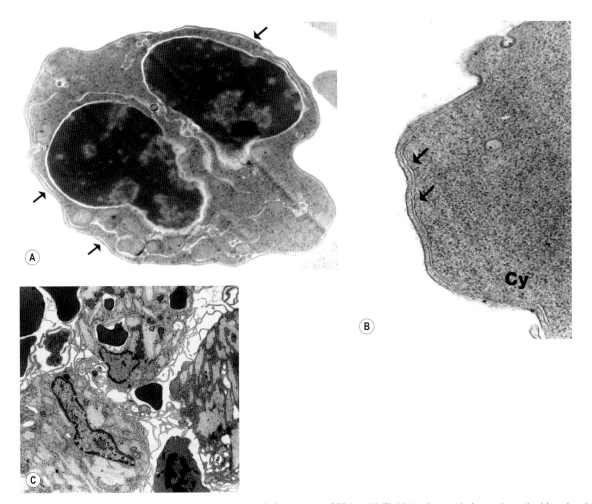

Fig. 15.9 (A–C) Electron micrographs of bone marrow cells from a case of CDA-2. (A) (B) A binucleate polychromatic erythroblast showing the characteristic double membrane running parallel to the cell membrane (arrows). (C) Cluster of three pseudo-Gaucher cells, each with several large electron-lucent secondary lysosomes containing lipid. Uranyl acetate and lead citrate. (A) × 14 500; (B) × 17 700; (C) × 4800.

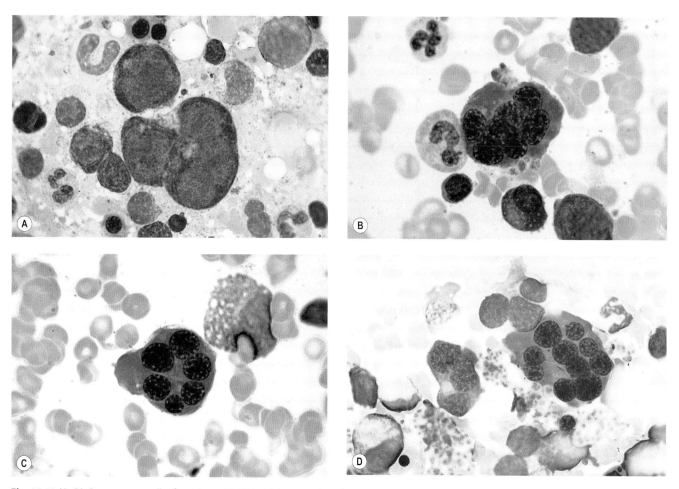

Fig. 15.10 (A–D) Bone marrow cells of a patient with CDA-3. (A) Tetranucleate basophilic erythropoietic cell near two mononucleate basophilic erythropoietic cells. (B)–(D) Giant multinucleate polychromatic erythroblasts. The cell in (D) contains 10 nuclei. May–Grünwald–Giemsa stain. ×1000.

as the other types and the anemia is mild. Patients present with ocular abnormalities (angioid streaks with macular degeneration), do not have iron overload (probably due to predominant intravascular hemolysis with hemosiderinuria) and do not have splenomegaly (except the Argentinian family). In the Swedish family there is an increased tendency to develop monoclonal gammopathy and multiple myeloma while sporadic cases have developed lymphoma.[21,22] Sporadic cases do not have autosomal dominant inheritance as parents and relatives were entirely normal; they may represent *de novo* mutations or demonstrate genetic heterogeneity. The clinical features of the sporadic cases are also extremely variable.

In CDA-3, Hb levels are usually between 7 and 14 g/dl, the MCV is usually raised or normal and the granulocyte and platelet counts are normal. The blood film shows macrocytes (and, sometimes, occasional giant erythrocytes), poikilocytosis, fragmented red cells and basophilic stippling. The reticulocyte count is normal or slightly raised. The acidified serum lysis test is negative. The bone marrow shows marked erythroid hyperplasia and megaloblastic erythropoiesis in the absence of vitamin B$_{12}$ or folate deficiency. Large uninucleate erythroblasts with enlarged lobulated nuclei and many giant multinucleate erythroblasts with up to 12 nuclei per cell are commonly present. The tendency to multinuclearity

begins in the basophilic erythropoietic cells but is most marked in the early and late polychromatic erythroblasts. Over 35% of all erythroblasts may be binucleate or multinucleate (Fig. 15.10) and the latter may have total DNA contents up to 40c. Sometimes the two nuclei of a binucleate cell or two or more of the nuclei within a multinucleate cell are joined together either by a narrow strand of chromatin or over a wide area of nuclear contact. The giant mononucleate erythroblasts have DNA contents of up to 20c. Other abnormalities affecting erythroblasts include coarse basophilic stippling of the cytoplasm and karyorrhexis. Electron microscopy studies show a variety of nonspecific abnormalities including differences in the ultrastructural appearances of different nuclei within the same multinucleate cell (Fig. 15.11). In addition, in some patients occasional erythroblast sections contain stellate or branching intracytoplasmic inclusions composed of precipitated β-globin chains (Fig. 15.12). The anemia results largely from ineffective erythropoiesis; both mononucleate and multinucleate cells may be seen within bone marrow macrophages.

Specific therapy for CDA-3 is not available and supportive care constitutes best standard practice. Hematopoietic stem cell transplantation for CDA-3 has not been attempted, possibly due to the moderate symptoms presented by patients with CDA-3.

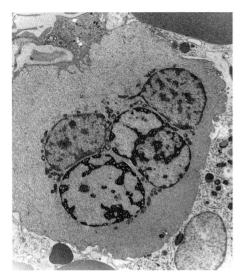

Fig. 15.11 Electron micrograph of a giant multinucleate erythroblast from a case with the sporadic form of CDA-3. Note the different ultrastructural appearances of the different nuclei within the same cell. Uranyl acetate and lead citrate. × 3500.

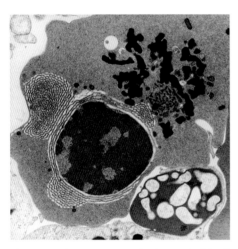

Fig. 15.12 Electron micrograph of an erythroblast from a patient with the sporadic form of CDA-3, showing branching intracytoplasmic inclusions and extensive reduplication of the nuclear membrane. *(From British Journal of Haematology 65: 250–251.)*

Other types of congenital dyserythropoietic anemia

Approximately 40% of cases of CDA diagnosed in the UK are of types other than types 1, 2 and 3. A tentative classification of other forms of CDA has been attempted (Table 15.2).[3] Examples of these atypical cases are illustrated in Figs 15.13–15.16. It is not clear how many of these are distinct clinical or hematological entities. Sequencing of *CDAN1* and *CDAN2* genes will determine whether atypical cases are allele specific phenotypes of the known genes.

Now that two of the genes responsible for CDA are known it should be possible to determine whether or not the diseases represent defects in different genes of a common metabolic pathway whose perturbation leads to the dyserythropoietic and karyorrhectic abnormalities. If so, it may

Table 15.2 Wickramasinghe's CDA variants group classification

For sake of clarity, groups of variants are indicated with Roman numerals, while major types are in Arabic numerals. To be considered a variant, at least three families must have been described with the features. First outlined by Sunitha Wickramasinghe *(Wickramasinghe 2000).*[3]

	Features	Inheritance
Group CDA-IV	Severe transfusion-dependent normoblastic anemia with hypercellular marrow but absence of other features of CDA-1/2/3. If anemia is only moderate, then CDA-IVb.	Not clear
Group CDA-V	Mild normo/macrocytic anemia without medullary hyperplasia and erythroid dysplasia, but unconjugated hyperbilirubinemia. Has been reported in the literature as 'primary shunt hyperbilirubinemia'	Autosomal recessive/ dominant
Group CDA-VI	Mild anemia with important macrocytosis (MCV 120–130 fl) and marked megaloblastoid hypercellular erythropoiesis. Orotic aciduria and thiamine-responsive anemia should be excluded.	Not clear
Group CDA-VII	As CDA-IV, but marked irregular nuclear shapes and with cytoplasmic globin-like inclusions (not reactive to α nor β antibodies). β thalassemia has to be excluded.	Not clear
Group CDA-VIII*	CDA with prominent post-splenectomy erythroblastemia (10–40 × 10⁹ erythroblast/ml) but no resolution of a moderate anemia. Marrow showed irregular nuclei (clover-leaf forms) and karyorrhexis.	Not clear
Different variants	Reports of cases where classification and further delineation not possible. Many will possibly be classified within the spectrum of the major types when comprehensive molecular testing becomes available.	

*Previously identified as CDA with prominent post-splenectomy erythroblastemia.

indicate a novel pathway crucial to erythropoiesis. Alternatively, it may be that the dysmorphic similarities are coincidental and that the various CDA subtypes are molecularly unrelated to each other.

Diagnosis of congenital dyserythropoietic anemia

The possibility of CDA should be considered whenever there is a suboptimal absolute reticulocyte count for the degree of

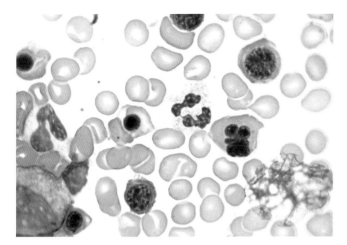

Fig. 15.13 Erythroblasts from a marrow smear from an atypical case of CDA group-IV. One of the erythroblasts has a lobulated nucleus. May–Grünwald–Giemsa stain. ×1000.

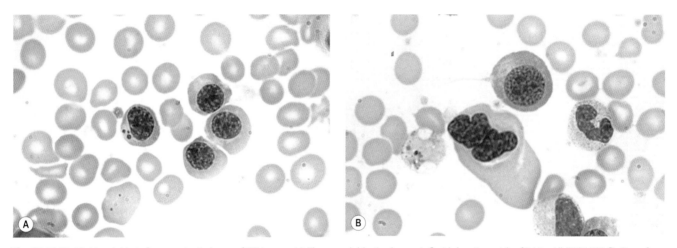

Fig. 15.14 (A, B) Megaloblasts from an atypical case of CDA group-VI. The megaloblastic change is florid despite an Hb of 14.5 g/dl (MCV 125 fl). One of the megaloblasts and a polychromatic macrocyte in (A) contain Howell–Jolly bodies and the binucleate megaloblast in (B) has irregular nuclear outlines. May–Grünwald–Giemsa stain. ×1000.

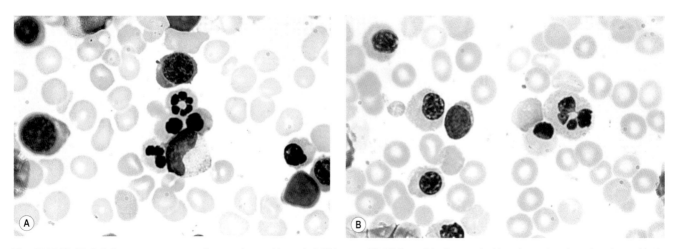

Fig. 15.15 (A, B) Cells from marrow smears of two patients with atypical CDA group-VII. (A) One of the late erythroblasts has a ring-shaped nucleus with six nuclear segments and another has a nucleus with three segments. (B) One of the erythroblasts has four nuclear masses joined by fine chromatin strands. ×1000.

anemia, unexplained hyperbilirubinemia or unexplained iron overload. Acquired dyserythropoiesis and causes of congenital dyserythropoiesis of known etiology (conventionally not included under the heading CDA) must be excluded. Causes of acquired dyserythropoiesis are given in Chapters 5, 14 and 20. The diagnosis of specific types or groups of CDA depends on the demonstration of their characteristic features and especially on the light and electron microscope appearances of the bone marrow erythroblasts, and should follow Fig. 15.17.

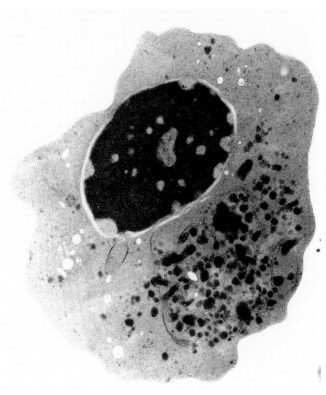

Fig. 15.16 Electron micrograph of an erythroblast from a patient with atypical CDA group-VII, showing multiple electron-dense foci of precipitated non-globin protein. Much of this material appears to be enclosed within a double membrane. Uranyl acetate and lead citrate.

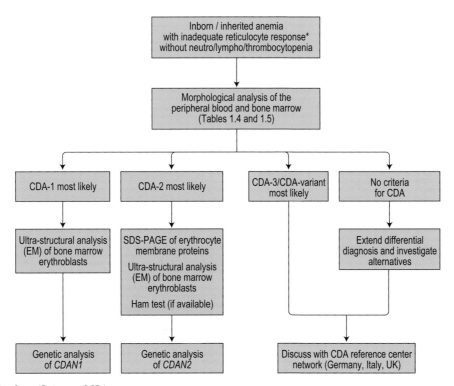

Fig 15.17 The diagnosis of specific types of CDA.

References

1. Renella R, Wood WG. The congenital dyserythropoietic anemias. Hematol Oncol Clin North Am 2009;23:283–306.

2. Wickramasinghe SN. Congenital dyserythropoietic anaemias: clinical features, haematological morphology and new biochemical data. Blood Rev 1998;12:178–200.

3. Wickramasinghe SN. Congenital dyserythropoietic anemias. Curr Opin Hematol 2000;7:71–8.

4. Heimpel H, Wendt F. Congenital dyserythropoietic anemia with karyorrhexis and multinuclearity of erythroblasts. Helv Med Acta 1968;34:103–15.

5. Heimpel H, Schwarz K, Ebnother M, et al. Congenital dyserythropoietic anemia type I (CDA I): molecular genetics, clinical appearance, and prognosis based on long-term observation. Blood 2006;107:334–40.

6. Shalev H, Kapelushnik J, Moser A, et al. A comprehensive study of the neonatal manifestations of congenital dyserythropoietic anemia type I. J Pediatr Hematol Oncol 2004;26:746–8.

7. Shalev H, Kapleushnik Y, Haeskelzon L, et al. Clinical and laboratory manifestations of congenital dyserythropoietic anemia type I in young adults. Eur J Haematol 2002;68:170–4.

8. Dgany O, Avidan N, Delaunay J, et al. Congenital dyserythropoietic anemia type I is caused by mutations in codanin-1. Am J Hum Genet 2002;71:1467–74.

9. Ahmed MR, Chehal A, Zahed L, et al. Linkage and mutational analysis of the CDAN1 gene reveals genetic heterogeneity in congenital dyserythropoietic anemia type I. Blood 2006;107:4968–9.

10. Wickramasinghe SN, Pippard MJ. Studies of erythroblast function in congenital dyserythropoietic anaemia, type I: evidence of impaired DNA, RNA, and protein synthesis and unbalanced globin chain synthesis in ultrastructurally abnormal cells. J Clin Pathol 1986;39:881–90.

11. Lavabre-Bertrand T, Blanc P, Navarro R, et al. alpha-Interferon therapy for congenital dyserythropoiesis type I. Br J Haematol 1995;89:929–32.

12. Lavabre-Bertrand T, Ramos J, Delfour C, et al. Long-term alpha interferon treatment is effective on anaemia and significantly reduces iron overload in congenital dyserythropoiesis type I. Eur J Haematol 2004;73:380–3.

13. Remacha AF, Badell I, Pujol-Moix N, et al. Hydrops fetalis-associated congenital dyserythropoietic anemia treated with intrauterine transfusions and bone marrow transplantation. Blood 2002;100:356–8.

14. Ayas M, al-Jefri A, Baothman A, et al. Transfusion-dependent congenital dyserythropoietic anemia type I successfully treated with allogeneic stem cell transplantation. Bone Marrow Transplant 2002;29:681–2.

15. Iolascon A, Sabato V, de Mattia D, Locatelli F. Bone marrow transplantation in a case of severe, type II congenital dyserythropoietic anaemia (CDA II). Bone Marrow Transplant 2001;27:213–15.

16. Ariffin WA, Karnaneedi S, Choo KE, Normah J. Congenital dyserythropoietic anaemia: report of three cases. J Paediatr Child Health 1996;32:191–3.

17. Heimpel H, Anselstetter V, Chrobak L, et al. Congenital dyserythropoietic anemia type II: epidemiology, clinical appearance, and prognosis based on long-term observation. Blood 2003;102:4576–81.

18. Schwarz K, Iolascon A, Verissimo F, et al. Mutations affecting the secretory COPII coat component SEC23B cause congenital dyserythropoietic anemia type II. Nat Genet 2009;41:936–40.

19. Iolascon A, De Mattia D, Perrotta S, et al. Genetic heterogeneity of congenital dyserythropoietic anemia type II. Blood 1998;92:2593–4.

20. Denecke J, Marquardt T. Congenital dyserythropoietic anemia type II (CDAII/HEMPAS): Where are we now? Biochim Biophys Acta. 2008.

21. Sandstrom H, Wahlin A. Congenital dyserythropoietic anemia type III. Haematologica 2000;85:753–7.

22. McCluggage WG, Hull D, Mayne E, et al. Malignant lymphoma in congenital dyserythropoietic anaemia type III. J Clin Pathol 1996;49:599–602.

Section D

Disorders affecting the leukocyte lineages

CHAPTER 16

Abnormalities in leukocyte morphology and number

G Zini

Many diseases are associated with changes in the morphology, function and/or concentration of one or more types of circulating leukocytes. Although such changes are often non-specific they may provide diagnostic clues in both hereditary and acquired disorders. The term *leukopenia* is applied to a decrease in the concentration of circulating white blood cells (WBC) below the reference range. The terms granulocytopenia, neutropenia, eosinopenia, basopenia, lymphopenia and monocytopenia are used to describe reductions in the concentrations of various WBC subpopulations. An increase in the concentration of circulating leukocytes above the reference range for the age of an individual is termed *leukocytosis*. This can be due to an increase in one or more leukocyte subpopulations normally present in blood or to the appearance of immature leukocytes in the circulation, or both. Increases in the neutrophils, eosinophils, basophils,

monocytes or lymphocytes are described as neutrophil leukocytosis (neutrophilia), eosinophil leukocytosis (eosinophilia), basophil leukocytosis (basophilia), monocytosis and lymphocytosis, respectively.

Neutrophils

In the peripheral blood (PB) of healthy white adults the mean neutrophil count is 4.4 (4.3–4.6) $\times$ 10^9/l,[1,2] while in healthy black adults it is 3.6 (3.3–3.9) $\times$ 10^9/l.[3]

Neutropenia

Neutropenia is defined as the absolute neutrophil count (ANC) in PB lower than 1.5 $\times$ 10^9/l. Referring to white

DOI: 10.1016/B978-0-7020-3147-2.00016-X

Infections
>   Bacterial: brucellosis, Gram-negative septicemia, typhoid and
>   paratyphoid fevers, tuberculosis, tularemia
>   Viral: CMV, HIV, EBV, HCV, measles, mumps, rubella, influenza, HIV,
>   parvovirus, dengue, yellow fever, varicella, smallpox
>   Rickettsial: typhus

Drugs (see Box 16.2), alcohol and other chemicals

Ionizing radiation

Hypersplenism

Leukemia

Myelodysplastic syndromes

Aplastic anemia and paroxysmal nocturnal hemoglobinuria

Bone marrow infiltration by tumors

Myelofibrosis

Megaloblastic anemia

Anaphylactic shock

Immune neutropenia

Amidopyrine-induced agranulocytosis

Systemic lupus erythematosus (SLE)

Rheumatoid arthritis, scleroderma

Autoimmune neutropenia

Neonatal alloimmune neutropenia

Hemophagocytic syndromes

Dialysis neutropenia

Chronic idiopathic neutropenia

Cyclical neutropenia

Familial benign chronic neutropenia

Severe congenital neutropenia

Congenital aleukia

Other rare neutropenic syndromes

Miscellaneous: hyperthyroidism, hypopituitarism, Addison's disease,
Kawasaki disease, copper deficiency, starvation, anorexia nervosa

Pseudoneutropenia

population, a useful classification in predicting risk infection indicates neutropenia as mild, moderate or severe according to the ANC value of $1.0-1.5 \times 10^9/l$, $0.5-1.5 \times 10^9/l$ or less than $0.5 \times 10^9/l$ respectively. Neutropenia may arise from various disorders of bone marrow (BM) function resulting in a decreased rate of release of neutrophils from the BM into the circulation. It is a common manifestation in several BM failures, such as aplasia, leukemia or myelodysplasia (see Chapters 13, 18, 20 for details). The conditions that may be associated with a neutropenia are listed in Box 16.1. Clinically neutropenia is considered as acute when it occurs over hours to a few days, usually developing from rapid neutrophil use/destruction or from impaired production. Neutropenia is considered chronic, when it lasts months to years, usually arising from reduced production or excessive splenic sequestration. Neutropenia can be caused by an intrinsic defect in BM myeloid cells, the *congenital and idiopathic neutropenias*, or by factors extrinsic to BM, the *acquired neutropenias*.

Congenital and idiopathic neutropenias

Severe congenital neutropenia (Kostmann's disease). Kostmann disease[4] is a rare autosomal recessive disorder of neutrophil number. The ANC is characteristically less than $0.2 \times 10^9/l$. Severe persistent neutropenia results in an increased susceptibility to bacterial infections. Granulocyte colony-stimulating factor (G-CSF) receptors are expressed on myeloid cells in slightly increased numbers, while the binding affinity for G-CSF to its receptor is normal. The *neutrophil elastase* gene mutations (*ELA2*) have been found in a subgroup of patients with Kostmann disease, although these mutations are also found in some healthy family members.[5] Autosomal recessive inheritance[6] of homozygous hematopoietic cell-specific protein-1 (HS1)-associated protein X-1 (HAX-1) mutations appear to lead to the increased apoptosis of myeloid precursors observed in patients with severe congenital neutropenia.[7] HAX-1 functions include signal transduction, cytoskeletal control and regulation of apoptosis and it is reported to play a role in suppression of apoptosis in lymphocytes and neurons, resulting in prolonged survival of these cells.[8] While the *G-CSF receptor* gene mutations have not been detected at birth, patients with Kostmann disease who develop leukemia have been found to have acquired these mutations.[9] Point mutations in the gene for the G-CSF receptor *CSF3R* have been implicated in the progression of severe congenital neutropenia to leukemia. These mutations lead to the production of truncated CSF3R receptors determining hyper-responsive forms (G-CSFR-hyper) with increased proliferation and highly decreased maturation of myeloid cells.[10,11]

Congenital aleukia (reticular dysgenesis). Reticular dysgenesis[12] is a rare inherited disorder characterized by the failure of hematopoietic stem cells committed to myeloid and lymphoid development. Red blood cell count (RBC) is normal, while platelet count may be decreased. There are no lymphocytes in the thymus, which is hypoplastic, and there is complete absence of peripheral lymphoid tissues. Allogenic BM transplant (BMT) remains the sole therapeutic option.[13]

Benign chronic neutropenias

Familial benign chronic neutropenia. This disorder,[14,15] inherited as an autosomal dominant trait, is characterized by chronic moderate to severe neutropenia, monocytosis, lymphocytosis and occasionally moderate eosinophilia. Patients with mild or moderate neutropenia are asymptomatic. The BM is normocellular and usually shows few neutrophil precursors beyond the myelocyte stage. Patients have a reduced reserve myeloid pool in the BM, which makes G-CSF therapy not appropriate.[16]

Non-familial benign chronic neutropenia. Cases of chronic benign neutropenia without any identified familial pattern are grouped in this category. In several patients, the presence of autoantibodies suggests the immune aetiology.[17] Even though neutropenia is usually severe in patients with *chronic benign neutropenia of infancy and childhood*, the risk of infection is very low. BM is hypercellular and the granulopoietic differentiation is present until the stage of band form. A reduced neutrophil chemotaxis from BM to PB is a possible explanation. In situations causing acute stress such as infection or cortisol administration, the number of circulating neutrophils increases.[18] G-CSF therapy in the forms with a benign course is not indicated.

Familial cyclic neutropenia. This is a rare disorder,[19–21] in which neutropenia of 4–10 days duration occurs at intervals of 15–35 days (average 21 days). Most cases present in infancy or childhood with periodic bouts of fever, malaise, headache, sore throat, oral ulceration, skin infections or, occasionally, infections of the lungs and other organs. Neutropenia results from cyclic changes in neutrophil granulocytopoiesis. Cyclic neutropenia has been transferred by BM transplantation to a histocompatible sibling with acute lymphoblastic leukemia.[22] In about 25% of patients, the condition is inherited as a dominant trait with point mutations involving the neutrophil elastase gene *ELA-2* on chromosome 19p13.3. Sporadic, not familial, as well as acquired cases associated with large granular lymphocyte (LGL) expansion are reported in the literature.[23,24]

Chronic idiopathic neutropenia of adult. This is a cytokine-mediated syndrome characterized by varying degrees of neutropenia associated with a low number of lineage-specific CD34+ cells and increased production of inhibitors of hematopoiesis (including tumor growth factor (TGF)-β1 and tumor necrosis factor (TNF)-α) and lymphopenia due to selective loss of primed/memory T-cells and natural killer (NK) cells. Other symptoms, reported in about 50% of patients, include splenomegaly, osteopenia and/or osteoporosis. The presence of features of chronic antigenic stimulation and increased concentrations of a variety of macrophage-derived pro-inflammatory cytokines[25] are suggestive of the existence of an unrecognized low-grade chronic inflammatory process, which may be involved in the pathogenesis of the disorder. Neutropenia in these patients is probably resulting from a combination of at least three factors:[26] reduced production of BM neutrophils, enhanced neutrophil extravasation and increased sequestration and/or extravasation of neutrophils into the spleen.

Neutropenia in patients with congenital immune defects

Neutropenia can be associated with congenital immunologic defects and patients with combined defects are at very high risk of infection. Neutropenia is reported in about one fourth of patients with *Bruton agammaglobulinemia* (X-linked hypogammaglobulinemia),[27] in about 50% of patients with *dysgammaglobulinemia,*[28] and in several patients with *hyper IgM syndrome* or with isolated *IgA syndrome*.[29] Treatment with intravenous infusion of immunoglobulin is required, possibly associated with G-CSF.

Neutropenia in patients with congenital chromosomal abnormalities

Shwachman–Diamond syndrome. Shwachman–Diamond[30] syndrome is a rare autosomal recessive disorder characterized by pancreatic exocrine insufficiency, metaphyseal chondrodysplasia, mental retardation, thrombocytopenia and defective neutrophil motility. The mutations involve a single gene, the *Shwachman-Bodian-Diamond-Syndrome* (*SBDS*) gene on chromosome 7q11. Neutropenia is determined by an increased apoptosis of myeloid precursors caused by the SBDS. About 20% of patients evolve into acute leukemia.

Chediak–Higashi syndrome. Chediak–Higashi[31] syndrome is a rare autosomal recessive disorder characterized by recurrent infections, albinism, and by the presence of a reduced number of granules and/or formation of some abnormally large granules (by progressive fusion of normally formed granules) in most granule-containing cells.

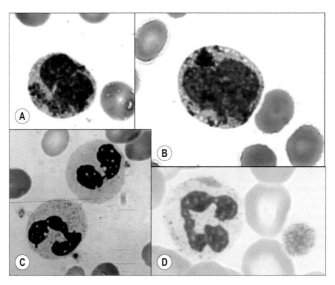

Fig. 16.1 (A–D) (A, B) Cells from a peripheral blood smear of a patient with the Chediak–Higashi syndrome showing the presence of giant granules within the neutrophil series. May–Grünwald–Giemsa stain. (C) Peripheral blood neutrophil (up) showing the Pelger–Huët anomaly (bilobed nucleus). May–Grünwald–Giemsa stain. (D) May–Hegglin anomaly: giant platelet (left), neutrophil wih grayish-blue cytoplasmic inclusion (right). May–Grünwald–Giemsa stain.

The giant granules present in neutrophils are peroxidase-positive and represent primary granules that have fused together. The abnormal granule fusion and function is determined by mutations of the *CHS1* gene coding for the lysosomal trafficking regulator (LYST) protein on chromosome 1q42. Neutropenia is present in about 75% of patients. BMT provides a supportive cure for hematological signs but it does not prevent the neurologic deterioration.[32] The affected cells include the neutrophils, eosinophils, lymphocytes, monocytes, melanocytes, Schwann cells of peripheral nerves, fibroblasts, vascular endothelial cells, renal tubular cells, and the parenchymal cells of the adrenal and pituitary glands. There is a deficiency of platelet dense granules, leading to easy bruising and bleeding. The large granules in leukocytes vary from a pale slate-gray to a dark reddish colour (Romanowsky stain) (Fig. 16.1A,B). There is a marked reduction in circulating NK cells.[33] The leukocyte abnormalities are associated with recurrent infections. Some affected children, particularly those who live beyond early childhood, develop a terminal accelerated phase characterized by a lymphoma-like picture with lymphadenopathy, hepatosplenomegaly, neuropathy, widespread infiltration of tissues by non-clonal lymphatic and histiocytic cells, and pancytopenia. Death results from the complications of pancytopenia.

WHIM syndrome. Wart, hypogammaglobulinemia, infection and myelokathexis (WHIM) syndrome is a rare congenital autosomal dominant disorder determined by mutation in the gene coding for the neutrophil chemokine receptor CXCR.[34] It is characterized by chronic non-cyclic neutropenia and increased susceptibility to bacterial and viral infections, especially from common serotype human papilloma virus, resulting in warts on the hands and feet starting in childhood. There is myeloid hyperplasia with degenerating granulocytes in the BM (myelokathexis).

Glycogen storage disease type 1b. It is a rare congenital autosomal recessive condition, determined by mutations on chromosome 11q23. These mutations cause glycogen accumulation in tissues due to deficiency of intracellular enzymes, which normally catalyze reactions that convert glycogen compounds to glucose. Severe neutropenia with consequent high risk of infections is present only in the type 1b and is determined by a disturbed myeloid maturation.[35]

Other rare conditions

Other metabolic congenital disorders complicated by moderate to severe neutropenia are *propionic acidemia*, *methylmalonic acidemia* and *isovaleric acidemia*. Neutropenia is a feature of a number of other rare syndromes:

- *cartilage–hair hypoplasia*,[36] an autosomal recessive disorder caused by mutations at chromosome 9p13, presenting with dwarfism, abnormally fine and sparse hair, hyperextensible joints and lymphopenia
- *Barth syndrome*, an X-linked recessive cardioskeletal myopathy
- *dyskeratosis congenita* (*Zinsser–Cole–Engman syndrome*), a multi-organ syndrome
- *'Lazy' leukocyte syndrome*,[37] in which recurrent mouth and ear infections are associated with an impairment of the release of neutrophils from the BM, normal neutrophil morphology, and an impaired response to chemotactic stimuli.

Congenital dysgranulopoietic neutropenia. Congenital dysgranulopoietic neutropenia[38,39] is characterized by ineffective myelopoiesis and morphological abnormalities in the neutrophilic series. The term has been used to describe a disorder affecting six unrelated children presenting recurrent severe bacterial infections since birth, marked neutropenia, impaired neutrophil migration, normal numbers of BM colony-forming cells, normal or slightly increased colony-stimulating activity in the serum, and prominent morphologic and ultrastructural abnormalities in granulopoietic cells beginning from the neutrophil promyelocyte/myelocyte stage. The abnormalities of these cells included numerous autophagic vacuoles, abnormally electron-lucent primary granules, myelinization of primary granules, granule fusion, absence or marked decrease of secondary granules, and maturation of the cytoplasm ahead of the nucleus. Stem cell involvement in the pathogenesis of this disorder is postulated.[40]

Acquired neutropenias

Immune neutropenia. Immune neutropenia is caused by the presence of specific antineutrophil antibodies: neutrophils are destroyed either by splenic sequestration or by complement-mediated lysis.

Neonatal alloimmune neutropenia. In this syndrome, neutrophils and neutrophil precursors of the fetus are destroyed by the transplacental passage of maternal IgG alloantibodies formed against HLA or neutrophil-specific antigens (NA1 and NA2) present on fetal as well as on paternal neutrophils but not on maternal ones.[41,42] The incidence is estimated at 1 in 500 live births. Most patients recover spontaneously usually within 2 months, depending on

the life span of the maternal immunoglobulins. The neutropenia is occasionally severe and may cause life-threatening neonatal infections. Such patients respond well to intravenous immunoglobulins and G-CSF. The antibodies against neutrophil-specific antigens transferred to the fetus by the transplacental passage may be present either because the mother is affected by an autoimmune disease or as consequence of maternal sensibilization against the antigens of the fetal neutrophils of paternal origin. Despite a very low number of ANC, there is usually a spontaneous resolution within a few months. Supportive treatment with antibiotics is required in presence of infections, such as onphalitis or cellulitis.

Autoimmune neutropenia. Autoimmune neutropenia as a consequence of antineutrophil antibodies is a common finding associated with various *collagen-vascular disorders*, including rheumatoid arthritis (30% of patients with Felty's syndrome), *Systemic lupus erythematodes* (SLE, 50% of patients), Sjögrens syndrome, scleroderma, polymyositis and polymyalgia rheumatica. It has also been described in association with *autoimmune hemolytic anemia, immune thrombocytopenic purpura* or both. In adults, autoimmune neutropenia is less likely to resolve spontaneously as compared to infants and children. In a subset of patients who have antibodies against the granulocyte precursors, the clinical course is more aggressive.[43] Severe autoimmune neutropenias respond to treatment with metothrexate, steroids, G-CSF and granulocyte-macrophage colony stimulating factor (GM-CSF). *Chronic autoimmune neutropenia*[44,45] is usually a relatively mild disease not associated with any other autoimmune disorders and characterized by recurrent infections, particularly of the oropharynx and skin. In some patients, the antineutrophil antibody has the specificity anti-NA2 or pan-Fcγ RIII (CD16, NA1/NA2). Some patients requiring treatment have responded to G-CSF. The *LGL leukemia* is often associated with neutropenia (see Chapter 28).

Infections associated with neutropenia. Infections are the most common cause of acquired neutropenia with different pathogenetic mechanisms (Box 16.1). In particular, some viruses (EBV, HAV, HBV, HCV and HIV) induce a severe and prolonged neutropenia by direct damage of the granulocytic precursors.[46,47] Fungal, rickettsial and protozoal infections damage the BM endothelial cells causing vasculitis and severe cytopenias.[48] Bacterial septicemia, in particular with Gram-negative agents, may induce neutropenia through an endotoxin-induced shift of neutrophils from the circulating to the marginated cell pools, a reduced survival time of circulating granulocytes (due either to destruction of cells within the circulation or to an accelerated rate of egress of cells from the blood), and a BM failure to adequately increase the rate of effective granulocytopoiesis. In certain circumstances, infection may be associated both with a failure adequately to increase effective granulocytopoiesis and with an exhaustion of the marrow granulocyte pool so that neutropenia is seen together with a left shift. This is particularly common in very severe bacterial infections and in bacterial infections in neonates and alcoholics (who have a reduced BM granulocyte pool). In several infections associated with spleen enlargement, such as typhoid fever, malaria and kala-azar, neutropenia results from splenic trapping and destruction of neutrophils in the spleen. In most of the latter cases, neutropenia does not require treatment, which should be focused on the underlying disease.

Drug-induced neutropenia. Neutropenia is the most common drug-induced blood dyscrasia.[49,50] Some drugs (e.g. alkylating agents or antifolate drugs), certain chemicals (e.g. benzene) and irradiation induce neutropenia in all affected individuals in a dose-dependent manner. Other drugs cause neutropenia only occasionally and this phenomenon is usually at least partly based on a genetic polymorphism of drug metabolism. Drugs of the latter category may either cause neutropenia as part of an aplastic anemia (AA) or induce a selective neutropenia. Furthermore, several of the drugs causing AA in susceptible individuals initially cause a neutropenia that subsequently progresses to AA. The agranulocytosis induced by amidopyrin[51] (and possibly also by other drugs) is often attributed to the destruction of circulating neutrophils and neutrophil precursors by drug-related immune mechanisms. There is also evidence that some drug metabolites may directly damage neutrophils and their precursors through the myeloperoxidase (MPO) system.[52] Drugs that may occasionally cause selective neutropenia are listed in Box 16.2. The relatively high-risk drugs include amidopyrine and the antithyroid drugs. Some of the listed drugs usually induce a mild to moderate neutropenia that is asymptomatic and does not progress despite continuation

of the drug. Other drugs usually cause a complete or almost complete absence of neutrophils (agranulocytosis).

Idiosyncratic drug-induced agranulocytosis (incidence 2.4–15.4 cases per million) results in a life-threatening clinical syndrome[53] characterized by fever, sweating, vomiting, sore throat, dysphagia due to necrotic ulceration of the mouth and pharynx, extreme prostration and, frequently, death from overwhelming infection. At autopsy, necrotic ulcers are found in the mucous membranes of the entire alimentary tract as well as in the vagina. The prognosis is considerably improved if the offending drug is stopped and infection is adequately controlled by antibiotic therapy. To date, drug-induced agranulocytosis remains a serious adverse event due to the high frequency of sepsis with severe deep infections (such as pneumonia), septicemia, and septic shock in about two-thirds of all patients. Old age (>65 years), septicemia or shock, metabolic disorders such as renal failure, and a neutrophil count below $0.1 \times 10^9/l$ are poor prognostic factors. Drugs or their metabolites might induce neutropenia by one or both of the following mechanisms: direct toxic effect on myeloid precursors or marrow environmental, dose-dependent inhibition of granulopoiesis, and immune-mediated destruction of granulocytes or their precursors. The classic example of a drug that causes agranulocytosis by a toxic effect on the BM is chlorpromazine, which causes a transient and moderate neutropenia in one-third of treated individuals. It causes agranulocytosis in about 1 in 1200 individuals, usually after a cumulative dose of 10–20 g over 20–30 days. Chlorpromazine appears to cause agranulocytosis by inhibiting DNA synthesis and cell proliferation in the granulocyte precursors of susceptible individuals. At the time of the agranulocytosis, the BM shows few or no neutrophil granulocytopoietic cells. The susceptibility of occasional individuals to develop agranulocytosis following therapy with chlorpromazine or other sulphur-containing drugs such as carbimazole or metiamide may depend on their genetically determined ability to oxidize the drug to highly-reactive myelotoxic metabolites (sulphoxides) more rapidly than most individuals.[54] It is likely that many other drugs that cause neutropenia do so by directly or indirectly impairing biochemical processes within granulocytopoietic cells or by causing some form of immune destruction of the cells. The best understood example of a drug that causes agranulocytosis by destroying circulating neutrophils is amidopyrine. Individuals with amidopyrine-induced agranulocytosis have a history of previous exposure to the drug and may, after recovery from the initial agranulocytosis, show a recurrence of agranulocytosis within 12 h of a test dose. The serum of such individuals contains an antibody that causes agglutination of neutrophils followed by an acute neutropenia in the presence of the drug. It has been suggested that the antibody may be directed against complexes between drug metabolites and cellular components. The BM shows increased granulocytopoietic activity and a depletion of the more mature precursors. The dynamics of drug-induced neutropenia vary depending on the underlying mechanism: it has rapid onset in the immune-mediated mechanism, especially if the patient was previously exposed, while it is delayed when drugs exert direct marrow toxicity. Recombinant human G-CSF is indicated in patients who do not improve their ANC levels after the drug discontinuation.

Box 16.2 Main drugs which may cause neutropenia

Analgesic drugs: amidopyrine, dipyrone

Antibacterial drugs: cephalosporins, chloramphenicol, clindamycin, co-trimoxazole (sulphamethoxazole-trimethoprim), other sulphonamides, doxycycline, dapsone, gentamicin, isoniazid, lincomycin, metronidazole, nitrofurantoin, penicillins, rifampicin, streptomycin, tetracycline, vancomycin

Anticoagulant drugs: dicoumarol, phenindione

Anticonvulsant drugs: carbamazepine, ethosuximide, phenytoin, primidone, sodium valproate, troxidone (trimethadione)

Antidiabetic drugs: chlorpropamide, tolbutamide

Antihistamines: brompheniramine, chlorphenamine, mepyramine, promethazine, trimeprazine

Anti-inflammatory drugs: celecoxib, fenoprofen, ibuprofen, indometacin, oxyphenbutazone, penicillamine, phenylbutazone, sodium aurothiomalate

Antimalarial drugs: amodiaquine, dapsone, hydroxychloroquine, pamaquin pyrimethamine, quinine

Antithyroid drugs: carbimazole, methimazole, methylthiouracil, potassium perchlorate, propylthiouracil

Anxiolytic, antipsychotic and antidepressant drugs: amitriptyline, chlordiazepoxide, chlorpromazine, clozapine, diazepam, imipramine, meprobamate, mianserin, prochlorperazine, promazine, thioridazine, trifluoperazine, trimeprazine

Cardiovascular drugs: captopril, diazoxide, hydralazine, methyldopa, pindolol, procainamide, propranolol, quinidine

Diuretics: bendroflumethiazide, bumetanide, chlorothiazide, chlorthalidone, hydrochlorothiazide, spironolactone

Miscellaneous: allopurinol, arsenicals, cimetidine, colchicine, griseofulvin, levamisole, levodopa

Miscellaneous neutropenias

Neutropenia and nutritional deficiencies. Vitamin B_{12}, folic acid or copper deficiency can result in suppressed or ineffective granulopoiesis. In various series, neutropenia associated with a large number of degenerated dysmorphic myeloid cells in the marrow was seen in 17–49% of cases, suggesting abnormal release and/or maturation failure.[55] In PB, hyper-segmented granulocytes with more than five nuclear lobes are the morphologic hallmark of megaloblastic granulopoiesis. Replenishment of nutrients generally corrects the neutropenia. Starvation, anorexia or cachexia may also induce neutropenia.

Dialysis neutropenia. Dialysis neutropenia[56] is the result of pulmonary sequestration of neutrophils after complement activation by the dialyzer membrane. Increased expression of neutrophil adhesion receptors, such as CD11b/CD18, suggests that neutrophil adhesion to the capillary endothelium is a possible mechanism. An alternative hypothesis is that the complement fragment C5a modulates neutrophil mechanical properties via the cytoskeleton – largely filamentous actin (F-actin) – stiffening them and thereby slowing their passage through the pulmonary capillaries. Acute cardiopulmonary failure may occur. After some hours, neutropenia is usually reversed and a rebound neutrophilia occurs.

Neutropenia and bone marrow infiltration. Replacement of normal BM elements by leukemic or tumor cells results in cytopenias, including neutropenia. Leukoerythroblastic blood smears are often noted when neoplastic BM infiltration occurs. Other conditions causing BM cavity compromise, such as osteopetrosis, can also result in neutropenia.

Pseudoneutropenia. A false reduced neutrophil count provided by routine hematology analyzers is mainly caused by *in vitro* agglutination of neutrophils,[57] usually EDTA-dependent. This artifact is completely solved after addition of kanamycin in the tube.[58] The presence of paraproteinemia, a prolonged storage after the withdrawal and the asymmetric distribution of circulating neutrophils to the marginate pool are reported too as possible causes of pseudoneutropenia.

Neutrophilia

Neutrophilia is defined as an increased absolute neutrophil count (ANC) in PB above 2SD of the mean value for healthy individuals, i.e. above $9.5 \times 10^9/l$. Some of the causes of a neutrophil leukocytosis are listed in Box 16.3. Physiologic neutrophilia is seen in pregnancy, labor, and newborns. Neutrophilia can result from altered rates of neutrophil release from the BM, changes in margination and egress from the blood or both. *Shift neutrophilia (pseudoneutrophilia)* results from a shift of cells from marginal to the circulating granulocyte pool without any quantitative change in the total blood granulocyte pool (TBGP), while in *true neutrophilia* TBGP is increased. Both pools are approximately equal in size and are in constant equilibrium.[59] Strenuous exercise, electric shocks, emotional states, vomiting, convulsions, paroxysmal tachycardia and epinephrine injection are the most frequent causes of shift neutrophilia. In the true neutrophilia, an increased rate of release of neutrophils from the BM into the blood occurs acutely as a result of the emptying of the BM granulocyte pool into the blood or more slowly in

---

> **Box 16.3** Main causes of neutrophilia
>
> Physiologic: neonates, exercise, emotion, pregnancy, parturition, lactation
>
> Acute infections
>
> > Bacterial: various pyogenic cocci, *Escherichia coli*, *Pseudomonas aeruginosa*, *Corynebacterium diphtheriae*, *Francisella tularensis*
> >
> > Spirochaetal: syphilis, Weil's disease
> >
> > Rickettsial: typhus, Rocky Mountain spotted fever
> >
> > Chlamydial: psittacosis
> >
> > Viral: rabies, poliomyelitis, smallpox, herpes simplex infection, herpes zoster, chickenpox
> >
> > Protozoal: *Pneumocystis carinii* infection
> >
> > Mycotic: actinomycosis, coccidioidomycosis
> >
> > Helminthic: liver fluke, filariasis
>
> Acute inflammation not caused by infections: surgical operations, burns, infarcts, hepatic necrosis, crush injuries, rheumatoid arthritis, rheumatic fever, vasculitis, myositis, pancreatitis, hypersensitivity reactions, etc.
>
> Endocrine/metabolic: Cushing's syndrome, thyrotoxicosis, uremia, diabetic acidosis, gout
>
> Acute hemorrhage and acute hemolysis
>
> Myeloproliferative neoplasms and myelodysplastic/myeloproliferative neoplasms
>
> Malignant diseases: carcinoma, lymphoma, other solid tumors
>
> Drugs: adrenaline, corticosteroids, lithium
>
> Hereditary neutrophilia
>
> Miscellaneous: convulsions, paroxysmal tachycardia, electric shock, vomiting, after splenectomy, postneutropenic rebound neutrophilia, cigarette smoking

---

association with an increased rate of granulocytopoiesis. The first of these mechanisms is responsible for the initial acute neutrophilia in response to bacterial endotoxins, corticosteroids and etiocholanolone. The second mechanism operates when there is a sustained neutrophil leukocytosis, in conditions such as infections, inflammation and malignant diseases. The level of neutrophilia is the result of the balance between the production rate and the death rate of neutrophils.

Neutrophilia in acute infection or inflammation

During an average acute infection the ANC rises to levels of $15–25 \times 10^9/l$. In certain infections such as pneumococcal pneumonia or childhood infections, ANC ranges from 20 to $40 \times 10^9/l$ (but may reach levels $>80 \times 10^9/l$), while the eosinophil and basophil counts are reduced. The most common cause of neutrophil leukocytosis is an acute infection with a pyogenic organism. However, neutrophil leukocytosis also occurs in infections with certain non-pyogenic organisms (e.g. in poliomyelitis, herpes zoster, typhus). Tuberculosis does not usually cause a neutrophil leukocytosis but it may occur when there is rapid local spread of tubercle bacilli as in tuberculosis meningitis. Severe infections may be accompanied by a left-shifted differential count and toxic granulation or Döhle bodies within neutrophils. Young children may respond to acute infections with a lymphocytosis rather than a neutrophil leukocytosis. A persistent chronic neutrophilia is associated with inflammatory non-infectious conditions such as obstructive bronchopneumonia, burns, postoperative states, acute myocardial infarction, acute attack of gout, acute glomerulonephritis, rheumatic fever, collagen vascular diseases, hypersensitivity reaction, auto-inflammatory syndromes, and cigarette smoking.[60] The neutrophilic activation is mediated by circulating cytokines, such as TNF-α, interleukin (IL)-1β, IL-6 and IL-8. A *leukemoid reaction* is defined by a WBC count more than 50×10^9/l and it resembles leukemia but arises from other causes such as infection or cancer.

Neutrophilia and cancer

Neutrophilia can occur in association with rapidly growing metastatic lung and gastrointestinal neoplasms. This process is thought to be due to superinfections, high levels of TNF-α or to direct BM stimulation by neutrophilic growth factors produced by cancer cells in some tumor types such as squamous cell cancers of the head and neck.[61] In some patients with carcinoma or sarcoma, the increase of neutrophil granulocytopoiesis results from the production of proteins, which stimulate the growth of CFU-GM.[62] In Cushing's syndrome, pheochromocytoma and in other catecholamine-secreting tumors, neutrophilia is associated with ectopic secretion of adrenocorticotropic hormone or corticotropin-releasing hormone.[63] The high ANC in clonal hematological malignancies is mainly determined by an impairment of apoptosis with an abnormally long survival time in the blood.

Miscellaneous neutrophilias

Drug-related neutrophilia. Drugs very rarely induce neutrophilia, except for glucocorticoids, catecholamine, etiocholanolone and lithium. Neutrophilia seen in patients on long-term corticosteroid therapy is associated with a normal rate of release of neutrophils from the BM into the blood, a decreased rate of egress from the blood into the tissues as well as a decreased rate of apoptosis, due to drug-induced reduction of adhesion molecules on neutrophils and endothelial cells.[64] Moreover neutrophilia can result from poisoning with lead, mercury, digitalis, camphor, antipyrine, phenacetin, quinidine, pyrogallol, turpentine, arsphenamine and insect venoms.

Hereditary chronic neutrophilia. Familial cases of hereditary neutrophilia mimicking a myeloproliferative disorder are reported in the literature. An activating mutation in the CSF3R gene favors dimerization of the G-CSF receptor transmembrane domain, strongly promoting activation and hypersensitivity for proliferation and differentiation.[65]

Neutrophilia in acute hemorrhage is probably related to the release of adrenal corticosteroids and/or epinephrine secondary to pain.

Qualitative and morphological abnormalities

Qualitative and/or morphologic abnormalities of leukocytes may be hereditary or acquired, permanent or transient.

Inherited abnormalities

Pelger–Huët anomaly is a benign, dominantly inherited anomaly of granulocytes[66] marked by failure of normal nuclear lobe development during terminal differentiation,

due to mutations in the *lamin B receptor* (*LBR*) gene.[67] The incidence at birth in different studies ranges from as high as 1 in 1000, to 1 in 4000, 6000 or even in 10 000 persons. *Pelger–Huët anomaly* does not impair neutrophil function and is readily identified by two morphologic hallmarks: the bilobated 'pince-nez' nuclei and the excessively coarse clumping of nuclear chromatin. Heterozygotes have bilobed nuclei in 69–93% of neutrophils (Fig. 16.1C); cells with three lobes are <10% while only rare neutrophils have four lobes. Some individuals display eosinophils with round condensed nuclei and excessively coarse clumping of nuclear chromatin in lymphocytes and monocytes. In homozygote states, round or oval unsegmented nuclei are present in >95% of neutrophils.

May–Hegglin anomaly. Macrothrombocytopenia with leukocyte inclusions (May–Hegglin anomaly, MHA) is a rare autosomal dominant disorder characterized by thrombocytopenia, giant platelets, and Döhle body-like inclusions in leukocytes. The *MHA* gene has been localized to a 13.6-cM region on chromosome 22.[68] The cytoplasmic inclusions are 2–5 μm in diameter, appear grayish-blue when stained by a Romanowsky method (Fig. 16.1D) and are composed of stacks of rough endoplasmic reticulum, similar to Döhle bodies but larger.

Alder–Reilly anomaly is associated with the genetic mucopolysaccharidoses (lack of lysosomal enzymes necessary to break down mucopolysaccharides) except Morquio syndrome and is characterized by the presence of dense azurophilic granules, resembling toxic granulation in all leukocytes including neutrophils. It apparently does not interfere with the leukocyte function. Associations with a mutation of the MPO structural gene[69] and with a myelodysplastic syndrome (MDS)[70] have been reported in the literature.

Jordans' anomaly (familial vacuolization of leukocytes) is characterized by the presence of fatty inclusions in all neutrophils and most monocytes and lymphocytes (Fig. 16.2A). These inclusions measure from 2 to 5 μm and appear as unstained vacuoles in panoptical stains while they strongly stain with Sudan II and Nile blue sulphate. This anomaly has only been reported in a few families.[71,72]

Hereditary hypersegmentation of neutrophils is a rare condition inherited in an autosomal dominant character.[73] The proportion of neutrophils with five or more lobes exceeds a tenth and one-third in heterozygotes and homozygotes, respectively.

Hereditary giant neutrophilia is a rare and asymptomatic autosomal dominant anomaly, in which a fraction of neutrophils (1–2%) is nearly double in size and has 6–10 nuclear lobes, in the absence of chromatin abnormalities, dysplastic features and circulating precursors.[74]

Myeloperoxidase deficiency (Alius–Grignaschi anomaly). First described in 1969, MPO deficiency is a benign autosomal recessive disorder that leads to absence of this enzyme in neutrophils and monocytes, but not in eosinophils. After the introduction of automated differential counting based on cytochemical reactions for MPO (Fig. 16.2B, D), this condition has a reported incidence of 1 in 2000 and became the most common disorder of the neutrophil function, as complete (Fig. 16.2C) or partial deficiency. In a recent report, a significantly higher occurrence of severe infections and chronic inflammatory processes was noted among MPO-deficient patients.[75]

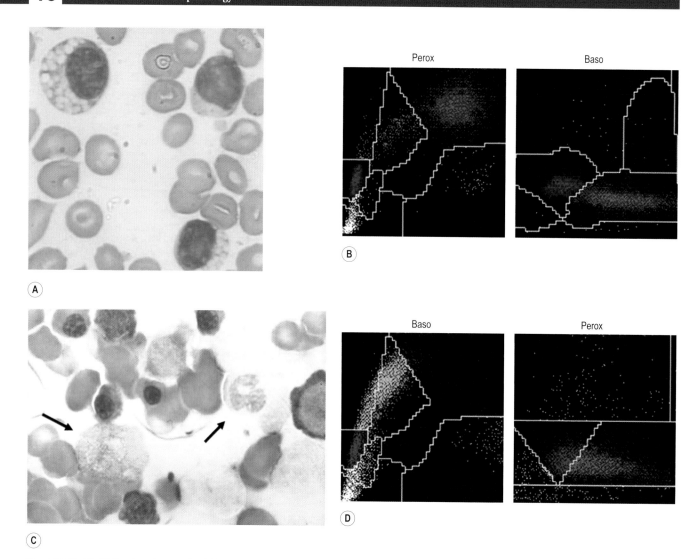

Fig. 16.2 (A–D) (A) Two lymphocytes (up left and down right) in a peripheral blood smear of a patient with Jordans' anomaly with unstained vacuoles of fatty inclusions. May–Grünwald–Giemsa stain. (B) Peripheral blood analysis in a normal patient, obtained by the automated ADVIA2120 hematology analyzer, based on automated peroxidase staining and volume analysis. Neutrophils (pink cloud) are normally located according to their volume (*y* axis) and their normal MPO content (*x* axis) in the perox cytogram; neutrophil nuclei (pink) are normally located in the baso cytogram according to their volume (*y* axis) and their nuclear density (*x* axis). (C) Marrow smear of a patient with MPO deficiency: one negative neutrophil (right arrow) and one positive eosinophil (left arrow) (cytochemical MPO staining). (D) Peripheral blood analysis in a patient with MPO partial deficiency, obtained by the automated ADVIA2120 hematology analyzer, based on automated peroxidase staining and volume analysis. Neutrophils (few pink dots and green cloud) are abnormally located in the monocyte region, according to their volume (*y* axis) and their very low MPO content (*x* axis) in the perox cytogram, while eosinophils (yellow dots) are normally displayed; in the baso cytogram, neutrophil nuclei (pink) are normally located according to their volume (*y* axis) and their normal nuclear density (*x* axis).

Specific granule deficiency. Neutrophil-specific granule deficiency (SGD) is a rare congenital disorder,[76] presenting with increased susceptibility to pyogenic infections. Neutrophils have bilobated nuclei and contain more primary than secondary (specific) granules. Leukocyte alkaline phosphatase activity is reduced. Lactoferrin deficiency[77] in these patients is confined to myeloid cells and is secondary to a deficiency of RNA transcripts.

Chronic granulomatous disease of childhood. Chronic granulomatous disease (CGD) is a congenital disorder, mostly with X-linked inheritance[78] and comprises a rare group of genetic disorders, in which neutrophils, monocytes and eosinophils can ingest but cannot kill catalase-positive bacteria and fungi due to a deficiency of NDPH oxidase or to an abnormality in its activation.

Acquired abnormalities

Left shift indicates the presence in the PB of an increased proportion of neutrophils at a slightly earlier stage of maturation than usual (band forms and neutrophils with only two nuclear segments), with occasional circulating myeloid precursors. Infections, toxic conditions or other severe illnesses, such as hypoxia and shock, can cause a left shift.

Hypersegmentation or *right shift* indicates the presence of abnormally increased nuclear lobulation of neutrophils with

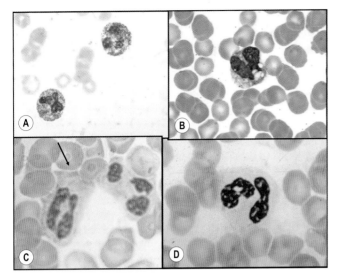

Fig. 16.3 (A–D) (A) Two neutrophils with toxic granulations from peripheral blood of a patient with infection. May–Grünwald–Giemsa stain. (B) One neutrophil with vacuolization from peripheral blood of a patient with acute infection. May–Grünwald–Giemsa stain. (C) One neutrophil with an elongated peripheral Döhle body (arrow) from peripheral blood of a healthy pregnant woman. May–Grünwald–Giemsa stain. (D) Hypogranular neutrophil with dysplastic nucleus (acquired anomaly) from peripheral blood of a patient with a myelodysplastic syndrome. May–Grünwald–Giemsa stain.

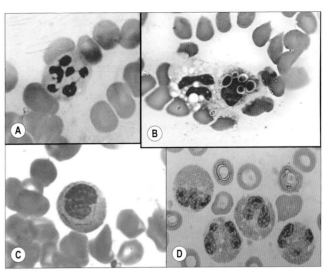

Fig. 16.4 (A–D) (A) Macropolycyte from peripheral blood of a patient with vitamin B_{12} deficiency. May–Grünwald–Giemsa stain. (B) Neutrophil (right) with ingested spore in the peripheral blood of a patient with systemic candidiasis. May–Grünwald–Giemsa stain. (C) Neutrophil with three elongated needle shaped Auer rods from peripheral blood of a patient with acute promyelocytic leukemia in treatment with ATRA (all-trans retinoic acid). May–Grünwald–Giemsa stain. (D) Four morphologically normal eosinophils from peripheral blood of a patient with dermatitis. May–Grünwald–Giemsa stain.

four, five or more nuclear segments. It is one of the first hematologic abnormalities seen in vitamin B_{12} or folate deficiency. Normal mature circulating neutrophils have an average of three lobes and always fewer than five lobes. More than three cells having five lobes or a single cell with six lobes found in the course of a 100 cell differential is evidence of hypersegmentation.

Toxic granulations (Fig. 16.3A) are purple or dark-blue staining azurophilic granules in the cytoplasm of neutrophils, bands and metamyelocytes resulting from an abnormality in the maturation of the primary granules with a consequent retention of their azurophilic property,[79] while *toxic vacuolizations* (Fig. 16.3B) are vacuoles representing phagocytosis and depletion of toxic granules. Both are seen in severe infections and in other toxic conditions.

Döhle bodies are single or multiple blue or grayish-blue cytoplasmic inclusions, representing free ribosomes or rough endoplasmic reticulum,[80] usually situated at the periphery and protruding beyond the normal contour of the cell (Fig. 16.3C). They are associated with myeloid 'left shifts' and are found in normal pregnancy, in various infections, in patients with various neoplasms and after severe burns.

Macropolycytes are very large polymorphonuclear leukocytes, with a diameter >16 μm, often showing hypersegmented nuclei with 6–14 nuclear segments (Fig. 16.4A). They may be found in the blood in vitamin B_{12} or folate deficiency and in infections, myeloproliferative disorders and drug-induced BM damage. The macropolycytes seen in vitamin B_{12} deficiency have tetraploid or hypotetraploid DNA contents and appear to result from nuclear segmentation in giant metamyelocytes that are not phagocytized by BM macrophages. The occurrence of macropolycytes has been reported as an inherited condition in a single family.

Hypogranular neutrophils (acquired 'specific granule' deficiency) are found especially in MDS (Fig. 16.3D) but may also be seen in other conditions such as Ph-negative chronic myeloid leukemia (CML), chronic myelomonocytic leukemia (CMML) and acute myeloid leukemia (AML). In addition, they may be found in neonates and in patients with burns.

Pseudo Pelger–Huët anomaly. The morphological abnormalities similar to the hereditary form are commonly seen in MDS, in AML, in chronic myeloproliferative disorders and, more rarely, chronic lymphatic leukemia. The acquired Pelger–Huët anomaly develops transiently in patients treated with paclitaxel and docetaxel[81] and the anomaly has also been found in patients with severe hematological toxicity caused by valproic acid.[82] It may also be seen after mononucleosis.

Acquired myeloperoxidase deficiency may occur in AML, MDS and myeloproliferative disorders as well as in Hodgkin's disease, lead poisoning and pregnancy.

Botryoid nuclei are small, moderately pyknotic nuclear segments which are clustered like grapes on a stem, observed in over 50% of neutrophils in patients with heat stroke.[83]

Intracellular organisms. Ingested microrganisms, such as bacteria *Rickettsiae*, fungi (Fig. 16.4B), etc., may be rarely seen in the cytoplasm of neutrophils and sometimes of monocytes.

Auer rods are pink or red-stained needle-shaped structures seen in the cytoplasm of myeloid cells, containing agglomeration of azurophilic granules containing enzymes such as acid phosphatase, MPO and esterase, and may represent abnormal derivatives of cytoplasmic granules. Auer rods can be seen in myeloid neoplasms ranging from AML to MDS, but not in normal or non-neoplastic reactive states (Fig. 16.4C).

Eosinophils

Eosinophils are quite rare in PB, while tissues of the pulmonary and gastrointestinal systems are their normal environment. In healthy adults the reference interval of eosinophils in PB is $0.02-0.5 \pm 2SD \times 10^9/l$.[2] The number is physiologically slightly increased in newborns and in the presence of environmental stimuli (mainly allergens), while it may be decreased in normal pregnancy and during labor.

Eosinopenia

Eosinopenia is defined as a reduction of circulating eosinophils $<0.01 \times 10^9/l$. Idiopathic eosinopenia appears to be a very rare event or syndrome. Eosinopenia in acute stress is mediated by adrenal glucocorticosteroids and epinephrine, while in acute inflammatory states it is not dependent upon the endocrine mechanisms. Eosinopenia has also been reported in Cushing's syndrome, acromegaly, systemic lupus erythematosus (SLE) and AA.

Drug-induced eosinopenia

Eosinopenia develops promptly after the administration of corticotropin, corticosteroids, epinephrine or histamine, but disappears within hours unless repeated doses are given.[84] In patients treated by corticosteroids, eosinopenia appears to result both from an impairment of the release of eosinophils from the BM and from the increased margination (or sequestration) of blood eosinophils. β-blockers inhibit adrenaline-induced eosinopenia and favor an increase in the number of circulating eosinophils.

Eosinopenia of acute infection or inflammation

The response to acute inflammation involves a rapid and persistent decrease in the numbers of circulating eosinophils, as a consequence of release of small amounts of the chemotactic factors into the circulation.[85,86]

Eosinophilia

Eosinophilia (Fig. 16.4D) is commonly seen in a wide spectrum of allergic responses, medication usage, and many skin diseases such as dermatitis, parasitic infestations, some autoimmune disorders and malignancy (Box 16.4). Eosinophilia is defined as an increase of circulating eosinophils $>0.6 \times 10^9/l$, although an increase in eosinophils (with or without concurrent peripheral eosinophilia) can be observed in body fluids, such as CSF and urine, and in many tissues, such as skin, lung, heart, liver, intestine, bladder, BM, muscle or nerve. Eosinophilia may be defined as mild, moderate or severe when the number of circulating eosinophils is $0.6-1.5 \times 10^9/l$, $1.5-5.0 \times 10^9/l$ or $>5 \times 10^9/l$, respectively. IL-5, IL-3 and GM-CSF are the primary stimuli for eosinophil production. High eosinophilia persistent for >6 months carries significant risk of end-organ damage. According to the 2008 WHO classification, *primary eosinophilia* include *chronic eosinophilic leukemia not otherwise specified* and *neoplasms associated with rearrangements of with PDGFRA, PDGFRAB or FGFR1 genes*[87] (see Chapter 25). *Secondary eosinophilia* is a reactive phenomenon driven by eosinophilopoietic cytokines released by non-myeloid cells and is usually solved after specific treatment of the underlying condition.

Eosinophilia and asthma

An increased number of eosinophils is observed in patients with asthma, both atopic and non-atopic. A hallmark of allergic disease is eosinophil infiltration of the tissues. Selective traffic of eosinophils into allergic tissues is caused by high levels of IL-5, CCR3 (CD193) binding chemokines and of the adhesion molecules P-selectin and vascular cells

---

Box 16.4 Main causes of eosinophilia

Parasitic infestations

Metazoan infestations: ancylostomiasis (hookworm infestation), angiostrongyliasis, ascariasis, clonorchiasis, cysticercosis, echinococcosis (hydatid cyst), fascioliasis, fasciolopsiasis, filariasis, gnathostomiasis, loiasis, onchocerciasis, paragonimiasis, schistosomiasis, strongyloidiasis, toxocariasis, trichinellosis, visceral larva migrans (toxocariasis)

Arthropod infestations: scabies

Certain fungal and bacterial infections: allergic pulmonary aspergillosis, chronic tuberculosis (occasionally), coccidioidomycosis, disseminated histoplasmosis, *Pneumocystis pneumoniae* infection, scarlet fever

Allergic disorders: bronchial asthma, atopic eczema, hay fever, allergic vasculitis, Stevens–Johnson syndrome, drug sensitivity (gold, sulphonamides, penicillin)

Graft-versus-host reaction

Skin diseases: pemphigus, bullous pemphigoid, eczema, psoriasis, herpes gestationis, subcutaneous eosinophilic angiolymphoid hyperplasia with eosinophilia, eosinophilic lymphofolliculosis (Kimura's disease), granulomatous dermatitis with eosinophilia (Well's disease), diffuse fasciitis with eosinophilia (Schulman's syndrome)

Postinfection rebound eosinophilia

Reactive 'pulmonary' eosinophilia

Löffler's syndrome (pulmonary infiltration with eosinophilia), tropical pulmonary eosinophilia

Idiopathic hypereosinophilic syndrome

Leukemias, myeloproliferative neoplasms, myeloid and lymphoid neoplasms with abnormalities of *PDGFRA, PDGFB* or *FGFR1*

Other malignant diseases: *Mycosis fungoides*, Sézary syndrome, Hodgkin's disease, other lymphomas (T-cell), angioimmunoblastic lymphadenopathy, carcinoma (usually with metastasis), multiple myeloma, heavy chain disease

Connective tissue disorders

Churg–Strauss syndrome and systemic necrotizing vasculitis (variants of polyarteritis nodosa), systemic sclerosis, rheumatoid arthritis

Thrombocytopenia with absent radii

Certain disorders of neutrophils: Job's syndrome, severe congenital neutropenia, familial benign chronic neutropenia, cyclical neutropenia

Wiskott–Aldrich syndrome

Cyclical eosinophilia with angioedema

Hereditary eosinophilia

Miscellaneous: ulcerative colitis, Crohn's disease, eosinophilic gastroenteritis, Goodpasture's syndrome, pancreatitis, chronic active hepatitis, after splenectomy, after irradiation of intra-abdominal tumors

adhesion molecule-1. The T-helper 2 (Th2) allergen specific lymphocytes take a relevant part in this process. Eosinophil-mediated damage to the respiratory epithelium is a major pathogenetic mechanism in asthma,[88] playing an important role in the maintenance of bronchial inflammation and also in tissue injury.

Eosinophilic gastrointestinal disorders

In patients with gastrointestinal disorders, eosinophilia is associated with various abnormal gastrointestinal symptoms and with the presence of eosinophilic infiltration in one or more areas of the gastrointestinal tract, in the absence of any other identified cause of eosinophilia.

Eosinophils and parasitic infestations

An IL-5 and Th2 mediated eosinophilia is a common feature in parasitic infestations, such as *Trichinella spiralis, Nippostrongylus brasiliensis, Fasciola epatica* and *Schistosoma mansoni*. A tropical syndrome characterized by eosinophilia, lymph node enlargement and pulmonary symptoms has been described under the name *tropical eosinophilia*. Although microfilariae are absent from the blood, this syndrome is caused by occult filariasis, while the microfilariae are destroyed in the tissues by an immune mechanism.

Eosinophilia in tumors

The eosinophilia associated with malignant tumors may be caused by a tumor-derived glycoprotein, which stimulates eosinophil granulocytopoiesis.[89] Lung tumors release a factor chemotactic for eosinophils, which resembles eosinophil chemotactic factor for anaphylaxis (ECF-A). In Hodgkin's lymphoma, eosinophilic proliferation is caused by IL-5 produced by tumor cells.

Miscellaneous

Allergic granulomatosis (Churg–Strauss syndrome) is a systemic vasculitis probably of multi-factorial origin, characterized by eosinophilia, asthma, fever and vasculitis of various organ systems. Up to 50% of patients have circulating protoplasmic-staining (perinuclear), antineutrophil cytoplasmic antibodies (p-ANCA).

Eosinophilia-myalgia syndrome is associated with L-tryptophan ingestion and is characterized by eosinophilia and interstitial infiltrates on the chest.

Atopic dermatitis is an inflammatory, chronic skin disease characterized by eosinophilia, pruritus, eczematous lesions, xerosis and lichenification.

Qualitative and morphological abnormalities

Pelger or pseudo-Pelger anomalies can be detected in eosinophils too, in the same disorders as in neutrophils.

Eosinophilic peroxidase deficiency is a very rare familial disorder, not correlated with any particular disease, characterized by the presence of morphologically normal eosinophils, partially or totally lacking the dimethylaminoazobenzene-positive specific granules.[90] *Pseudoeosinopenia* is the characteristics of these individuals, when differential count is

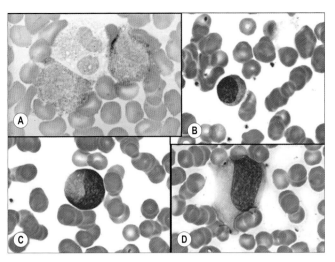

Fig. 16.5 (A–D) (A) Peripheral blood smear of a patient with eosinophilic peroxidase deficiency: one negative eosinophil and two positive neutrophils (cytochemical MPX staining). (B–D) Three atypical lymphocytes reactive-type from peripheral blood of a patient with infectious mononucleosis. May–Grünwald–Giemsa stain.

performed with analyzers based on cytochemical reactions for MPO (Fig. 16.5A).

Basophils

Basophils are the least frequent leukocytes. In healthy adults the reference intervals of basophils in PB is $0.02–0.1 \times 10^9/l$.[2]

Basopenia

Basopenia[91] is defined as a basophil count less than $0.01 \times 10^9/l$ and may be found in patients with acute hypersensitivity reactions, autoimmune urticaria, acute stress, hyperthyroidism, Cushing's syndrome and pregnancy as well as in response to the administration of progesterone, corticosteroids or corticotrophin. The blood basophil count falls on the day of ovulation.

Basophilia

A reactive basophil leukocytosis may occur in hypersensitivity reactions, hypothyroidism, ulcerative colitis, smallpox, chickenpox and the idiopathic hypereosinophilic syndrome as well as after exposure to ionic radiations. Basophil leukocytosis also occurs in mastocytosis, CML, polycythemia vera, essential thrombocythemia, myelofibrosis, basophilic leukemia, eosinophilic leukemia, and Ph-positive acute leukemia. In CML, a further and considerable increase in both immature and mature basophils may precede transformation of the disease to a more malignant phase (see Chapter 24). Basophilia is also reported after splenectomy.

Monocytes

Monocytes are the largest leukocytes. In healthy adults, the reference interval for monocytes in the PB is $0.2–1.0 \times 10^9/l$.[2]

Physiologic

Infants

Certain bacterial infections

Tuberculosis, brucellosis, secondary syphilis, subacute bacterial endocarditis, typhoid, recovery from many acute infections

Certain protozoal infections

Leishmaniasis (visceral and cutaneous), malaria, trypanosomiasis

Certain rickettsial infections

Typhus, Rocky Mountain spotted fever

Myelodysplastic syndromes

Acute monoblastics and myelomonocytic leukemias

Myeloproliferative neoplasms and myelodysplastic/myeloproliferative neoplasms

Other malignant diseases: Hodgkin's disease, other lymphomas, carcinoma, multiple myeloma, malignant histiocytosis

Miscellaneous: cyclical neutropenia, chronic idiopathic neutropenia, recovery from drug-induced neutropenia, ulcerative colitis, regional enteritis, sarcoidosis, connective tissue disease, post-splenectomy, lipid storage diseases

In newborns, the levels are physiologically increased, while in the elderly monocyte levels are decreased.

Monocytopenia

Monocytopenia is defined as level of PB monocytes $<0.2 \times 10^9/l$. Early monocytopenia after chemotherapy is a risk factor for neutropenia. Monocytopenia is seen in cases of *aplastic anemia*.[92] *Cyclic neutropenia* is notable for intermittent periods of monocytopenia. Transient, significant monocytopenia occurs during the first 30 min of *hemodialysis*: monocyte counts return to normal within hours after the procedure ends without any rebound monocytosis.[93] Monocytopenia also occurs in *severe thermal injuries*, in *acquired immunodeficiency syndrome* and in *hairy cell leukemia*.

Monocytosis

Monocytosis is defined by the presence of circulating monocytes $\geq 1.0 \times 10^9/l$. The various causes are listed in Box 16.5. The spleen is a site for storage and rapid deployment of monocytes and splenic monocytes are a resource that the body exploits to regulate inflammation.[94] Monocytosis occurs as a compensatory event in association with congenital as well as drug-induced *neutropenia*. It represents a benign non-prognostic epiphenomenon in *lymphomas* and other *solid tumors*, without any predictive significance for metastasis. In patients with vascular disorders, increasing monocytosis correlates with an increased risk of heart attack.

Lymphocytes

In healthy adults, the reference intervals of PB lymphocytes are $1.0-3.0 \times 10^9/l$.[2] About 3% of circulating lymphocytes are LGL, which are NK or CD8$^+$ T-cells.

Lymphopenia

Lymphopenia is defined by the presence of less than $1 \times 10^9/l$ lymphocytes in PB. Since most circulating lymphocytes are CD4$^+$ (helper), in most cases lymphopenia depends on depletion of CD4$^+$ T-lymphocytes.

Congenital lymphopenias

DiGeorge syndrome is a rare congenital disorder where symptoms vary greatly between individuals, but commonly include a history of recurrent infection, heart defects and characteristic facial features. Often the parathyroid glands may have failed to develop, leading to low serum levels of calcium, resulting in tetany and seizures. The thymus may also be underdeveloped or absent, resulting in a pure deficiency of T-lymphocytes (CD3$^+$ $<0.5 \times 10^9/l$). The heterogeneity in the symptoms is related to the amount of genetic material lost in the chromosomal 22 deletion. Although 90% of cases have been attributed to a 22q11.2 deletion, other chromosome defects (e.g. chromosome 10 or 18) have been identified. Therapy is aimed at correcting the defects in the affected organs or tissues.[95]

MHC class 1 or class 2 deficiencies are rare inherited disorders involving a deficiency of class I and II major histocompatibility complexes. Lymphopenia, hypogammaglobulinemia and lack of immune response can result in serious infections. In MHC class 1 deficiency, infections are mainly caused by pyogenic bacteria and *Pneumocystis jerovici* (*carinii*), while in MHC class 2 deficiency malabsorption induced by *Candida albicans* or *Cryptosporidium parvum* is commonly reported.

Ataxia telangiectasia is an autosomal recessive disorder of chromosome 11q involved in DNA repair processes, characterized by cortical cerebellar degeneration, thymus hypoplasia, lymphopenia and hypogammaglobulinemia. Prognosis is very poor.

Severe combined immunodeficiency (SCID) is a life-threatening syndrome of recurrent infections, diarrhea, dermatitis, and failure to thrive. It is caused by a variety of mutations that interfere with the differentiation or function of T-cells, B-cells, and occasionally NK cells. The most common autosomal recessive form is due to absence of the enzyme ADA (adenosine deaminase), while the X-linked form is due to the absence of a cell-surface receptor protein γ_c, which is a component of the receptor for IL-2, IL-4 and IL-7. The latter patients have low levels of T-lymphocytes but normal to elevated numbers of virgin B-lymphocytes. Clinically, most patients present before age 3 months with unusually severe and frequent infections by common or opportunistic pathogens. Presently, hematopoietic stem cell gene therapy represents a therapeutic opportunity.[96]

Acquired lymphopenias

Drug-induced lymphopenia is a common adverse event, in particular during the treatment of malignancies and autoimmune diseases. Most cytotoxic and immunosuppressive drugs affect CD4$^+$ T-cells more profoundly. Since their regeneration seems to be slower than that of CD8$^+$ T cells, the frequent occurrence of CD4$^+$ lymphopenia may merely reflect this phenomenon. Critically low numbers of CD4$^+$ cells, irrespective of the cause, predispose to opportunistic

Physiologic: infants and young children

Certain viral infections: infectious mononucleosis, cytomegalovirus infection, infectious hepatitis, chickenpox, smallpox, measles, rubella, mumps, influenza, primary HIV infection

Pertussis, brucellosis, tuberculosis, secondary and congenital syphilis

Chronic lymphoproliferative disorders, lymphomas

Post-splenectomy

infections as in HIV infection. There is no such critically low value for CD8$^+$ cells, and their essential role in various pathological conditions is as yet to be established. Temporary lymphopenia develops after the administration of corticosteroids that induce lymphocyte apoptosis. In addition, lymphopenia, probably due to elevated plasma cortisol levels, is seen following surgery or trauma and in many acute illnesses, such as most infections (including malaria), burns and heart failure. Psoralene and PUVA treatment induce lymphopenia through cutaneous vascularization.

Miscellaneous lymphopenias

CD4$^+$ lymphocytes are selectively destroyed in HIV-1 and HIV-2 infections. Lymphopenia also occurs in malaria and tuberculosis. Other causes of lymphopenia include Cushing's syndrome, uremia, SLE, advanced carcinoma and Hodgkin's disease, AA, agranulocytosis, MDS, alcohol abuse, anorexia nervosa and graft-versus-host disease.

Lymphocytosis

In adults, lymphocytosis is defined by an increased absolute number of circulating lymphocytes more than 4×10^9/l. The various causes of lymphocytosis are listed in Box 16.6. For details of lymphocytosis due to chronic lymphoid leukemias and lymphomas see Chapters 28 and 29.

X-linked lymphoproliferative syndrome (Duncan's syndrome). This is an X-linked recessive condition[97] in which there is a mutation in the gene encoding SLAM (signaling-lymphocyte activation molecule) associated protein, located on Xq25. In affected boys, primary EBV infection causes a life-threatening illness, with fulminant hepatitis, hemophagocytic syndrome and 50% mortality. Some patients subsequently develop AA, acquired hypogammaglobulinemia, or lymphoproliferative disorders including B-cell lymphoma (diffuse large B-cell lymphoma or Burkitt-like lymphoma). AA may respond to corticosteroids, anti-thymocyte globulin or immunosuppression followed by syngeneic BMT and appears to have an immunologic basis.

Lymphocytosis and infections

Tuberculosis, syphilis and *brucellosis* may be associated with an increase in both lymphocytes and granulocytes, while the only acute bacterial infection frequently associated with a lymphocytosis is whooping cough (*pertussis*).[98] In some children with this disorder, the lymphocyte count may exceed 50×10^9/l, which is caused by the lymphocytosis-promoting factor (LPF), a protein toxin from *Bordetella pertussis*. Lymphocytosis around $20–30 \times 10^9$/l (but sometimes up to 100 $\times 10^9$/l), may be found in several viral infections. The most common is Epstein–Barr virus (EBV) that induces the presence of a polyclonal population of CD8$^+$, NK and T-$\gamma\delta$ circulating lymphocytes, while CD4$^+$ subpopulation is normal. Large, atypical, reactive type lymphocytes are commonly detected in PB. *Infectious mononucleosis*[99] is a clinical syndrome resulting from an acute self-limiting primary infection by EBV, characterized by fever, pharyngitis, the presence of increased numbers of highly atypical lymphocytes in PB, and the production of heterophile antibodies. EBV infects and replicates in the B-lymphocytes and epithelial cells of the pharynx and also in a small proportion of T-cells: all three cell types have the specific receptor for EBV, namely CD21 (C3d receptor). Morphologic features of atypical lymphocytes include large size, irregular shape, increased cytoplasmic basophilia, and diffuse chromatin pattern, prominent nucleoli and a scalloped margin at points of contact with other cells (Fig.16.5B, C, D). The atypical lymphocytes are not the virus-infected B-lymphocytes, but T-lymphocytes with CD8$^+$ cytotoxic/suppressor phenotype. These cells may contain tartrate-resistant acid phosphatase and may show block-positivity when stained by the periodic acid-Schiff (PAS) method. Hematological complications include autoimmune hemolytic anemia due to a cold antibody with anti-I specificity, thrombocytopenia due to peripheral destruction of platelets, and rarely granulocytopenia or AA, the latter occurring several weeks after infectious mononucleosis. Another rare complication is severe pancytopenia secondary to hemophagocytosis. When infectious mononucleosis is associated with a hemophagocytic syndrome (see Chapter 5) the BM shows increased numbers of promonocytes and phagocytic histiocytes. BM aplasia is a rare complication while disseminated intravascular coagulation has been observed in association with the hemophagocytic syndrome. Changes very similar to those of infectious mononucleosis may be seen in *cytomegalovirus infection* (CMV), while lesser changes may be seen in *toxoplasmosis, malaria, herpes simplex, varicella zoster, rubella* or other viral infections such as *infectious hepatitis* or *HIV infection* (see Chapter 5).

References

1. Cronkite EP, Fliedner TM. Granulocytopoiesis. N Engl J Med 1964; 270:1347–51.

2. Dacie JV, Lewis SM. Practical Haematology. Ninth Edition. Edinburgh: Churchill Livingstone; 2001.

3. Reed WW, Diehl L. Leukopenia, neutropenia, and reduced hemoglobin levels in healthy American blacks. Arch Intern Med 1991;151:501–5.

4. Kostmann R. Infantile genetic agranulocytosis (agranulocytosis infantilis hereditaria): a new recessive lethal disease in man. Acta Pediatr Scand 1956;45:1–18

5. Dror Y, Sung L. Update on childhood neutropenia: molecular and clinical advances. Hematol Oncol Clin North Am 2004;18:1439–58.

6. Ward AC, Dale DC. Genetic and molecular diagnosis of severe congenital neutropenia. Current Opinion in Hematology 2009;16:9–13.

7. Germeshausen M, Grudzien M, Zeidler C, et al. Novel HAX1 mutations in patients

with severe congenital neutropenia reveal isoform-dependent genotype-phenotype associations. Blood 2008;111:4954–7.

8. Chao JR, Parganas E, Boyd K, et al. Hax1-mediated processing of HtrA2 by Parl allows survival of lymphocytes and neurons. Nature 2008;452:98–102.

9. Weinblatt ME, Scimeca P, James-Herry A, et al. Transformation of congenital neutropenia into monosomy 7 and acute nonlymphoblastic leukemia in a child treated with granulocyte colony-stimulating factor. J Pediatr 1995; 126:263–5.

10. Germeshausen M, Ballmaier M, Welte K. Incidence of *CSF3R* mutations in severe congenital neutropenia and relevance for leukemogenesis: results of a long-term survey. Blood 2007;109:93–9.

11. Beel K, Vanderberghe P. G-CSF receptor (CSF3R) mutations in X-linked neutropenia evolving to acute myeloid leukemia or myelodysplasia. Haematologica 2009;94:1449–52.

12. De Vaal OM, Seynhaeve V. Reticular dysgenesis. Lancet 1959;11:1123.

13. Emile JF, Geissmann F, de la Calle O, et al. Langerhans cell deficiency in reticular dysgenesis. Blood 2000;96:58–62.

14. Cutting HO, Lang JE. Familial benign chronic neutropenia. Annals of Internal Medicine 1964;61:876.

15. Busch FH. Familial benign chronic neutropenia in a Danish family. Ugeskrift for Laeger 1990;152:2565–6.

16. Joyce RA, Boggs DR, Chervenick PA. Neutrophil kinetics in hereditary and congenital neutropenias. N Engl J Med 1976;295:1385–90.

17. Bux J, Kissei K, Nowak K, et al. Autoimmune neutropenia: clinical and laboratory studies in 143 patients. Ann Hematol 1991;63:249–52.

18. Jonsson OG, Buchanan GR. Chronic neutropenia during childhood: a 13-year experience in a single institution. Am J Dis Child 1991;145:232–5.

19. Reimann HA, De Berardinis CT. Periodic (cyclic) neutropenia, an entity. Blood 1949;4:1109.

20. von Schulthess GK, Fehr J, Dahinden C. Cyclic neutropenia: amplification of granulocyte oscillations by lithium and long-term suppression of cycling by plasmapheresis. Blood 1983;62:320–6.

21. Dale DC, Hammond WP IV. Cyclic neutropenia: a clinical review. Blood Reviews 1988;2:178.

22. Krance RA, Spruce WE, Forman SJ, et al. Human cyclic neutropenia transferred by allogeneic bone marrow grafting. Blood 1982;60:1263–6.

23. Morley AA, Carew JP, Baikie AG Familial cyclical neutropenia. Brit J Haemat 1967;13:719–38.

24. Loughran TP, Clark EA, Price TH, et al. Adult onset cyclic neutropenia is associated with increased large granular lymphocyte. Blood 1986;68:1082–7.

25. Papadaki HA, Coulocheri S, George D, Eliopoulos GD. Patients with chronic idiopathic neutropenia of adults have increased serum concentrations of inflammatory cytokines and chemokines. Am J Hematol 2000;65:271–7.

26. Papadaki HA, Palmblad J, Eliopoulos GD. Non-immune chronic idiopathic neutropenia of adult: an overview. Eur J Haematol (2001) 2001;67:35–44.

27. Bruton OC. Agammaglobulinemia. Pediatrics 1952;9:722–8.

28. Kozlowski C, Evans DI. Neutropenia associated with X-linked agammaglobulinaemia. J Clin Pathol 1991;44:388–90.

29. Ng RP, Prankerd TA. IgA deficiency and neutropenia. Br Med J 1976;1:563.

30. Shwachman H, Diamond L, Oski F, et al. The syndrome of pancreatic insufficiency and bone marrow dysfunction. J Pediatr 1964;65:645–63.

31. Root RK, Rosenthal AS, Bales DJ. Abnormal bactericidal, metabolic, and lysosomal functions of Chediak-Higashi syndrome leukocytes. J Clin Invest 1972;51:649–65.

32. Tardieu M, Lacroix C, Neven B. Progressive neurologic dysfunctions 20 years after allogeneic bone marrow transplantation for Chediak-Higashi syndrome. Blood 2005;106:40–2.

33. Virelizier J-L, Lagrue A, Durandy A, et al. Reversal of natural killer defect in a patient with Chediak–Higashi syndrome after bone marrow transplantation. New England Journal of Medicine 1982;306: 1055–6.

34. Hernandez PA, Gorlin, RJ, Gelb B, et al. WHIM syndrome, an autosomal dominant disorder: clinical, hematological, and molecular studies. Am J Med Genet 2000;91:368–76.

35. Schaub J, Heyne K. Glycogen storage disease type Ib. Eur J Pediatr 1983;140: 283–8.

36. Lux SE, Johnston RB Jr, August CS, et al. Chronic neutropenia and abnormal cellular immunity in cartilage-hair hypoplasia. New England Journal of Medicine 1970;282:231–6.

37. Miller ME, Oski FA, Harris MB. Lazy-leucocyte syndrome. A new disorder of neutrophil function. Lancet 1971;i: 665–9.

38. Parmley RT, Crist WM, Ragab AH, et al. Congenital dysgranulopoietic neutropenia: clinical, serologic, ultrastructural, and in vitro proliferative characteristics. Blood 1980;56:465–75.

39. Lightsey AL, Parmley RT, Marsh WL, et al. Severe congenital neutropenia with unique features of dysgranulopoiesis. Am JHematol 1985;18:59–71.

40. Olcay L, Yetgin S, Erdemli E, et al. Congenital dysgranulopoietic neutropenia. Pediatr Blood Cancer 2008;50:115–9.

41. Maheshwari A, Christensen RD, Calhoun DA. Immune-mediated neutropenia in the neonate. Acta Paediatr Suppl 2002;91: 98–103.

42. Verheugt FW, van Noord-Bokhorst JC, von dem Borne AEG, et al. A family with allo-immune neonatal neutropenia: group-specific pathogenicity of maternal antibodies. Vox Sanguinis 1979;36:1–8.

43. Capsoni F, Sarzi-Puttini P, Zanella A. Primary and secondary autoimmune neutropenia. Arthritis Res Ther 2005; 7:208–14.

44. Boxer LA, Greenberg MS, Boxer GJ, Stossel TP. Autoimmune neutropenia. New England Journal of Medicine 1975; 293:748–53.

45. Verheugt FWA, von dem Borne AEG Kr, van Noord-Bokhorst JC, Engelfriet CP. Autoimmune granulocytopenia: the detection of granulocyte antibodies with the immunofluorescence test. British Journal of Haematology 1978;39:339–50.

46. Lee WM. Hepatitis B Virus infection. NEJM 1997;337:1733–45.

47. Levine AM, Karim R, Mack V, et al. Neutropenia in human immunodeficiency virus. Infection Arch Intern Med 2006; 166:405–10.

48. Cines DB, Lyss AP, Bina M, et al. Fc and C3 Receptors induced by herpes simplex virus on cultured human endothelial cells. J Clin Invest 1982;69:123–8.

49. van der Klauw MM, Goudsmit R, Halie MR, et al. A population-based case-cohort study of drug-associated agranulocytosis. Arch Intern Med 1999;159:369–74.

50. Van der Klauw MM, Goudsmit R, Halie MR, et al. Agranulocytosis induced by nonchemotherapy drugs. Ann Int Med 2008;148:320–1.

51. Dameshek W, Colmes A. The effect of drugs in the production of agranulocytosis with particular reference to amidopyrine hypersensitivity. J Cl Inv 1936;15:85.

52. Uetrecht JP. Reactive metabolites and agranulocytosis. Eur J Haemat 1996; 57(suppl):83–8.

53. Andrès E, Zimmer J, Affenberger S, et al. Idiosyncratic drug-induced agranulocytosis: update of an old disorder. Eur J of Int Med 2006;17(8): 529–35.

54. Pisciotta AV. Immune and toxic mechanisms in drug-induced agranulocytosis. Sem in Hemat 1973; 10:279–310.

55. M. Crist WM, Parmley RT, Holbrook CT, et al. Dysgranulopoietic neutropenia and abnormal monocytes in childhood vitamin B12 deficiency. Am J Hematol 1980;9:89–107.

56. Tabor B, Geissler B, Odell R, et al. Dialysis neutropenia: the role of the cytoskeleton. Kidney International 1998;53:783–9.

57. Glasser L. Pseudo-neutropenia secondary to leukoagglutination. Am J Hematol 2005;80:147.

58. Hoffmann JJ. EDTA-induced pseudo-neutropenia resolved with kanamycin. Cl Lab Haemat 2001;23:193–6.

59. von Vietinghoff S, Ley K. Homeostatic regulation of blood neutrophil counts. J Immunology 2008;181:5183–8.

60. Galeazzi M, Gasbarrini G, Ghirardello A, et al. Autoinflammatory syndromes. Clin Exp Rheumatol 2006;24:79–85.

61. Hocking W, Goodman J, Golde D. Granulocytosis associated with tumor cell production of colony-stimulating activity. Blood 1983;61:600–3.

62. Kimura N, Niho Y, Yanase T. A high level of colony-stimulating activity in a lung cancer patient with extensive leucocytosis, and the establishment of a CSA producing cell line (KONT). Scand J Haemat 1982;28:417–24.

63. Sawka AM, Kudva YC, Singh R, et al. Persistent neutrophilia as a preceding symptom of pheochromocytoma. J Clin Endocrinol Metab 2005;90:2472–3.

64. Ngakawa M, Terashima T, D'yachkova Y, et al. Glucocorticoid-induced granulocytosis: contribution of marrow release and demargination of intravascular granulocytes. Circulation 1998;98: 2307–13.

65. Plo I, Zhang Y, Le Couédic JP, Nakatake M, et al. An activating mutation in the CSF3R gene induces a hereditary chronic neutrophilia. J Exp Med 2009;206:1701–7.

66. Cunningham JM, Patnaik MM, Hammerschmidt DE, et al. Historical perspective and clinical implications of the Pelger–Huet cell. Am J Hematol 2009;84:116–9.

67. Cohen TV, Klarmann KD, Sakchaisri K, et al. The lamin B receptor under transcriptional control of C/EBPepsilon is required for morphological but not functional maturation of neutrophils. Hum Mol Genet. 2008;17:2921–33.

68. Martignetti JA,.Heath KE, Harris J, et al. The gene for May–Hegglin anomaly localizes to a <1-mb region on chromosome 22q12.3-13.1. Am J Hum Genet 2000;66:1449–54.

69. Presentey B. Alder anomaly accompanied by a mutation of the myeloperoxidase structural gene. Acta Haematol 1986; 75:157–9159.

70. Ghandi MK, Howard MR, Hamilton PJ. The Alder–Reilly anomaly in association with the myelodysplastic syndrome. Clin Lab Haematol 1996;18:39–40.

71. Rozenszajn L, Klajman A, Yaffe D, Efrati P. Jordans' anomaly in white blood cells. Blood 1966;28:258.

72. Piva E, Pajola R, Binotto G, et al. Jordans' anomaly in a new neutral lipid storage

disease. Am J Hematol 2009;84:254–5.

73. Undritz VE. Eine neue Sippe mit erblich-konstitutionellen Hochsegmentierung der Neutrophilenkerne Undritz. Schweizerische Medizinische Wochenschrift 1964;94:1365.

74. Davidson WM, Milner RDG, Lawler SD, et al. Giant neutrophil leucocytes: an inherited anomaly. Br J Haematol 1960; 6:339–43.

75. Kutter D, Devaquet P, Vanderstocken G, et al. Consequences of total and subtotal myeloperoxidase deficiency: risk or benefit ? Acta Haemat 2000;104:10–5.

76. Ambruso DR, Sasada M, Nishiyama H, et al. Defective bactericidal activity and absence of specific granules in neutrophils from a patient with recurrent bacterial infections. J Clin Immunol 1894;4:23–6.

77. Breton-Gorius J, Mason DY, Buriot D, et al. Lactoferrin deficiency as a consequence of a lack of specific granules in neutrophils from a patient with recurrent infections. Detection by immunoperoxidase staining for lactoferrin and cytochemical electron microscopy. Am J Pathol 1980;99:413–6.

78. Di Matteo G, Giordani L, Finocchi A, et al. Molecular characterization of a large cohort of patients with chronic granulomatous disease and identification of novel CYBB mutations: an Italian multicenter study. Mol Immunol 2009; 46:1935–41.

79. Schofield KP, Stone PC, Beddall AC, Stuart J. Quantitative cytochemistry of the toxic granulation blood neutrophil. British Journal of Haematology 1983; 53:15–22.

80. Itoga T, Laszlo J. Döhle bodies and other granulocytic alterations during chemotherapy with cyclophosphamide. Blood 1962;20:668–74.

81. Juneja SK, Matthews JP, Luzinat R, et al. Association of acquired Pelger–Huët anomaly with taxoid therapy. Br J Haemat 1996;93:139–41.

82. Ganick DJ, Sunder T, Finley JL. Severe hematologic toxicity of valproic acid. A report of four patients. Am J Ped Hematol Oncol 1990;12:80–5.

83. Hernandez JA, Aldred SW, Bruce JR, et al. 'Botryoid' nuclei in neutrophils of patients with heatstroke. Lancet 1980;ii:642–3.

84. Krause JR, Boggs DR. Search for eosinopenia in hospitalized patients with normal blood leukocyte concentration. Am J Hematol 2006;24:55–63.

85. Bass DA, Gonwa TA, Szejda P. Eosinopenia of acute infection. J Clin Invest 1980;65:1265–71.

86. Gleich GG. Mechanisms of eosinophil-associated inflammation. J Allergy Clin Immun 2000;105:651–63.

87. Tefferi A. Modern diagnosis and treatment of primary eosinophilia. Acta Haematol 2005;114:52–60.

88. Wardlaw AJ. Eosinophil trafficking in asthma. Clin Med 2001 May–Jun;1(3): 214–8.

89. Slungaard A, Ascensao J, Zanjani E, Jacob HS. Pulmonary carcinoma with eosinophilia. Demonstration of a tumor-derived eosinophilopoietic factor. New England Journal of Medicine 1983;309:778–81.

90. Cappelletti P, Doretto P, Signori D, et al. Eosinophilic peroxidase deficiency. Cytochemical and ultrastructural characterization of 21 new cases. Am J Clin Pathol 1992;98:615–22.

91. Dvorak HF, Dvorak AM. Basophil leukocytes: structure, function and role in disease. Clinics in Haematology 1975; 4:651–83.

92. Twomey JJ, Douglass CC, Sharkey O Jr. The monocytopenia of aplastic anemia. Blood 1973;41:187–95.

93. Nockher WA, Wieme J Jr, Scherberich JE. Haemodialysis monocytopenia: differential sequestration kinetics of CD14+CD16+ and CD14++ blood monocyte subsets. Clin Exp Immunol 2001;123:49–55.

94. Swirski FK,Nahrendorf M, Etzrodt M, et al. Identification of splenic reservoir monocytes and their deployment to inflammatory sites. Science 2009;325: 612–6.

95. Minier F, Carles D, Pelluard F, et al. DiGeorge syndrome, a review of 52 patients. Arch Pediatr 2005;12:254–7.

96. Aiuti A, Brigida I, Ferrua F, et al. Hematopoietic stem cell gene therapy for adenosine deaminase deficient-SCID. Immunol Res 2009;44:150–9.

97. Sullivan JL. The abnormal gene in X-linked lymphoproliferative syndrome. Curr Opin Imm 1999;11:431–4.

98. Horwitz MS, Moore GT. Acute infectious lymphocytosis: an etiologic and epidemiologic study of outbreak. N Engl J Med 1968;279:399–404.

99. Okano M. Haematological associations of Epstein–Barr virus infection. Baillière's Clinical Haematology 2000;13:199–214.

CHAPTER 17

Disorders of phagocyte function

G Bouma, AJ Thrasher

Chapter Contents

Introduction

Metchnikoff in the 19th century identified phagocytes as an essential and primary component in the elimination of a harmful agent, and predicted that defects in phagocyte function would predispose the host to microbial invasion.[1] Subsequently, patients with decreased phagocyte counts or compromised phagocytic function (for either inherited or acquired reasons) have been shown to suffer recurrent and often fatal infections. The cells implicated in these disorders arise primarily from the myeloid lineage, namely eosinophils, neutrophils, monocytes, macrophages and dendritic cells. During an infection and the subsequent inflammatory reaction, phagocyte production and activation is initiated by enhanced proliferation and maturation of phagocyte precursors in the bone marrow (BM), which are then released into the circulation at an accelerated rate (Fig. 17.1A). Competent phagocytic cells (Fig. 17.1B) activate specific adhesive receptors which aid in rolling and firm adhesion to the endothelium. In response to gradients of chemokinetic and chemotactic molecules, the phagocytes traverse the vascular endothelial wall and migrate towards the site of infection. Interactions between the phagocyte and microbe precede engulfment, degranulation and activation of the respiratory burst, which in combination result in microbial killing primarily within the phagocytic vacuole. Defects in any part of this complex process manifest as immunodeficiency of phagocyte function, highlighted in Fig. 17.1. Primary defects of phagocytes are the result of genetic mutations (Table 17.1), many of which have been identified very recently, and the results of which affect adhesion, migration, respiratory burst activity and degranulation.

Disorders of phagocyte maturation

Severe congenital neutropenia (SCN) is a heterogeneous disease with different forms of inheritance. Patients present with life-threatening infections due to very low circulating neutrophil counts and are usually diagnosed at birth or soon thereafter.[2] Although SCN was originally described as Kostmann syndrome,[3] this form is now recognized as a discrete genetic disorder. Studies of BM of SCN patients indicate a relatively selective defect of neutrophil formation and a maturational arrest at the promyelocytic stage (Fig. 17.1A). Cyclic neutropenia, in contrast, is characterized by regular and consistent oscillations of neutrophil count, usually with a periodicity of 21 days, which clinically manifests as fever, mouth ulcers and infection at the nadir (which lasts from 3 to 6 days) of the neutrophil count.[4,5] Over 90% of patients with either disorder respond to granulocyte-colony stimulating factor (G-CSF) therapy,[6,7] although refractory cases and those complicated by hematologic malignancy may be rescued by hematopoietic stem cell transplantation. Initially approximately 10% of patients with SCN were thought to develop acute myeloid leukemia or myelodysplasia, often accompanied by monosomy 7 and cytogenetic abnormalities including trisomy 21.[8–10] More recent data, however, from the Severe Chronic Neutropenia International Registry (http://depts.washington.edu/registry/), indicate that the incidence is significantly higher than previously recognized with a cumulative incidence of 21%.[6,11,12] It is thought that an association exists between G-CSF therapy, acquired mutations of the G-CSF receptor and the risk of leukemia,[6,10,13,14] but proving such an association is hampered by the fact that almost all patients are on G-CSF treatment.

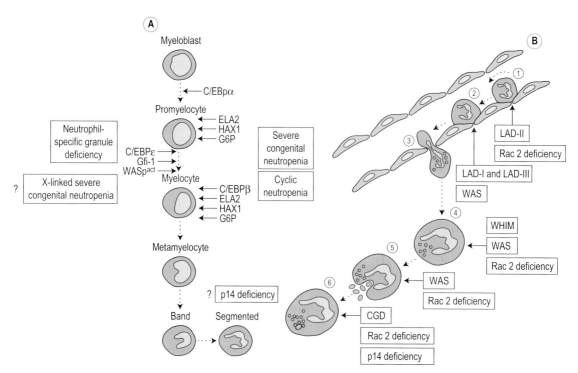

Fig. 17.1 (A, B) Schematic drawings of myelopoiesis (A) and phagocyte functions (B). Myelopoiesis (A) proceeds by commitment of myeloid precursors and subsequent differentiation into granulocytes and monocytes (dotted arrows). Various transcription factors have been shown to be involved in key stages of myeloid development, including members of the CCAAT/enhancer binding protein (C/EBP) including α, β and γ (solid arrows). Recently, two patients with neutrophil specific granule deficiency have been shown to have mutations in C/EBPε. Severe congenital neutropenia is thought to result from maturational arrest at the promyelocytic or myelocyte stage and in many cases is due to mutations in the *ELA2* or *HAX1* genes. The mechanism for neutropenia and monocytopenia in X-linked congenital neutropenia and for neutropenia in p14 deficiency is at present unknown. The initiation of inflammation (B; dotted arrows) begins with phagocyte activation by rolling (1), adhesion (2), and transmigration (3) of the endothelium; chemotactic migration to the site of infection (4), followed by bacterial phagocytosis (5) degranulation and intracellular killing (6). Phagocyte deficiencies can affect any part of this process as indicated by solid arrows. CGD, chronic granulomatous disease; LAD, leukocyte adhesion deficiency; WAS, Wiskott–Aldrich syndrome; WHIM, warts, hypogammaglobulinemia, infections and myelokathexis.

Most frequently, SCN follows an autosomal dominant inheritance, or arises sporadically. Occasionally, SCN may arise as an autosomal recessive disorder, indicating that there is genetic heterogeneity. Similarly, cyclic neutropenia usually follows an autosomal dominant or sporadic pattern of inheritance. The underlying genetic lesions that account for the majority of cases of SCN or cyclic neutropenia have recently been identified. Detailed studies of families with autosomal dominant cyclic neutropenia identified a genetic lesion mapping to a region on chromosome 19p13.3 containing the genes for three neutrophil serine proteases, azurcidin, proteinase 3 and neutrophil elastase (encoded by the *ELA2* gene). It was subsequently determined that mutations in *ELA2* (which is synthesized at the promyelocytic stage of neutrophil development; Fig. 17.1A), were responsible for this form of cyclic neutropenia.[15] Furthermore, because many of the hematological features of cyclic neutropenia are shared with SCN, it was later determined that heterozygous mutations in the same gene account for about 50% of autosomal dominant SCN.[15–19] At least 52 different mutations have been described, but there does not seem to be a clear association between particular *ELA2* mutations and the clinical form of neutropenia (cyclic vs. SCN), although the diversity of mutations in SCN appears to be wider than in cyclic neutropenia. The most common type of mutation in cyclic neutropenia disrupts the normal splice donor site at the end of the fourth exon, causing an in frame deletion of 10 amino acids and is seldom seen in SCN.[20] In SCN many mutations are located in the fifth exon and it appears that the G185R mutation is associated with a particularly severe phenotype.[16,20]

Neutrophil elastase is a monomeric, 218-amino acid (25 kDa), chymotryptic serine protease synthesized by promyelocytes and promonocytes during the early stages of primary granule production, and is formed as a proenzyme during differentiation before final storage in azurophilic granules in its active state.[21] It has activity against many proteins including matrix components and clotting factors, and is effectively neutralized by a number of endogenous inhibitors including the serpins α$_1$-antitrypsin and monocyte/neutrophil elastase inhibitor (MNEI; gene symbol ELANH2) and the non-serpin, elfin. The mechanism by which elastase defects results in neutropenia remains uncertain. One possibility is that haploinsufficiency of enzymatic activity causes reduced survival or increased apoptosis of myeloid precursors because of disturbances in the hematopoietic microenvironment. Evidence against this is provided by the observation that no consistent effect of elastase mutants was found on proteolytic activity, substrate specificity or serpin inhibition,[22] suggesting loss of function is not the primary mechanism responsible for neutropenia. Furthermore, elastase null mutant mice generated by gene targeting are not

Table 17.1 Phagocyte immunodeficiency diseases

Disease	Genetic defect	Phenotypic defect
Disorders of phagocyte maturation		
Severe congenital neutropenia	AD or sporadic ELA2 mutation HAX1 mutation Gfi-1 mutation	Severe neutropenia. Developmental arrest of myeloid precursors usually at promyelocytic stage. Increased apoptosis
Cyclic neutropenia	AD or sporadic ELA2 mutation	Fluctuations between normal granulocyte counts and severe neutropenia with 21-day periodicity. Increased apoptosis in myeloid precursors
X-linked neutropenia	X-linked activating WAS mutation	Neutropenia and monocytopenia, and lymphocyte abnormalities
Neutrophil specific granule deficiency	AR C/EBPε mutation	Absent secondary and tertiary granule proteins. Primary granules lack defensins
Glucose-6-phosphatase deficiency	AR G6PC3 mutation	Loss of glucose-6-phosphatase activity. Increased susceptibility to apoptosis
p14 deficiency	AR p14 (MAPBPIP) mutation	Defective lysosome function. Neutropenia, hypoglammaglobulinemia, short stature and hypopigmentation
Deficiencies of adhesion and migration		
LAD-I	AR ITGB2 mutation	High peripheral neutrophil counts and inability to make pus. Lack or reduction of CD18 expression
LAD-II	AR GDP-fucose transporter mutation	Granulocytes unable to bind to selectins on endothelium. Congenital disorder of fucosylation
LAD-III	AR RASGRP2 mutation FERMT3 mutation	High peripheral neutrophil counts and severe bleeding tendency. Defective integrin activation
WHIM	AD or AR CXCR4 mutation	Warts, hypoglammaglobulinemia, infections and myelokathexis
Phagocyte signalling abnormalities		
WAS	X-linked WAS mutation	Dysfunctional actin polymerization in hematopoietic cells. Defects of cell activation, adhesion, migration and phagocytosis
Rac2 deficiency	AD Rac2 mutation	Abnormal granulocyte chemotaxis, respiratory burst and degranulation. High peripheral neutrophil counts
Deficiencies of the phagocyte respiratory burst		
CGD	X-linked gp91phox mutation AR p47phox, p22phox, p40phox and p67phox mutations	Phagocytes unable to produce superoxide

AD, autosomal dominant; AR, autosomal recessive; C/EBP, CGD, chronic granulomatous disease; CXCR4, CXC-containing chemokine receptor-4; CCAAT/enhancer binding protein; ELA2, elastase 2; FERMT3, fermitin family homolog 3; G6PC3, glucose-6-phosphate catalytic subunit 3; Gfi-1, growth factor independent-1 transcription repressor; HAX1, HCLS1-associated protein X-1; ITGB2, integrin beta-2; LAD, leukocyte adhesion deficiency; MAPBPIP, MAPBP-interacting protein; Rac2, Ras-related C3 botulinum toxin substrate 2; RASGRP2, RAS guanyl releasing protein-2; WAS, Wiskott–Aldrich syndrome; WHIM, warts, hypoglammaglobulinemia, infections and myelokathexis.

neutropenic.[23] More recent studies suggest that elastase mutants elicit the unfolded protein response (UPR), which ultimately leads to apoptosis of granulocytic precursors. UPR is triggered by accumulation of misfolded proteins in the endoplasmic reticulum and consists of three major mechanisms. First global protein synthesis is attenuated. Second transcription of endoplasmic reticulum resident proteins involved in normal protein folding, such as the chaperone binding immunoglobulin protein (BiP), is induced. And third, endoplasmic reticulum-associated protein degradation (ERAD) of misfolded proteins is triggered. However, if the endoplasmic reticulum stress is severe, the UPR triggers apoptosis.[24] Two recent studies provide evidence for a role of UPR in the pathogenesis of SCN. Several ELA2 mutants showed insufficient intracellular trafficking and accumulation of cytoplasmic elastase and cells expressing mutant elastase proteins demonstrated up-regulation of BiP and increased apoptosis, suggesting UPR activation.[25] Similarly, the second study confirmed increased BiP expression in cells expressing mutant elastase, but also in granulocytic precursors isolated from patients with SCN.[26]

While *ELA2* mutations account for about 50% of SCN cases, the original pedigree described by Kostmann[3] do not carry mutations in the *ELA2* gene.[27] Recently three patients belonging to the original 'Kostmann family' were found to carry mutations in the *HAX1* gene.[28] *HAX1* mutations are found in about a third of SCN patients and so far nine mutations have been described with the W44X mutation comprising 72% of cases.[28–30] HAX1 protein is a mitochondrial molecule regulating the mitochondrial membrane potential and failure to maintain the mitochondrial membrane potential due to loss of HAX1 function result in accelerated spontaneous and induced apoptosis of neutrophils.[28]

A family with X-linked congenital neutropenia and monocytopenia was shown to have a mutation in the gene encoding the Wiskott–Aldrich syndrome (WAS) protein (WASp, see later).[31] To date three distinct mutations in the *WAS* gene have been described to yield this X-linked neutropenia.[31–33] These patients are quite distinct from those with WAS phenotypically, with normal or near normal platelet counts and platelet volumes, and none of the typical immunologic abnormalities. It appears that WASp is rendered constitutively active by a genetic mutation in the conserved GTPase-binding domain (based on the ability of mutant protein to enhance Arp2/3-mediated actin polymerization), and within the autoinhibitory hydrophobic core. Mutations resulting in typical or attenuated WASp almost invariably occur outside this region. The mechanism by which constitutively active WASp leads to neutropenia and monocytopenia remains unclear, but it is thought that enhanced and delocalized actin polymerization disrupts normal mitosis and leads to decreased cell proliferation and increased apoptosis of granulocyte precursor cells.[34]

During hematopoiesis, cellular proliferation, differentiation and survival are largely dependent on the regulation of gene expression by the actions of transcription factors. Members of the CCAAT/enhancer binding protein (C/EBP) family of transcription factors are key regulators of cellular differentiation and function in many tissues. Six homologous members of this family have been identified (C/EBPα, β, γ, δ, ε and ξ), each existing as distinct isoforms.[35] All members have been shown to possess an activation domain, a DNA-binding basic region and are able to homodimerize and heterodimerize with each other through a leucine-rich dimerization domain, termed the leucine zipper, which determines specificity of dimer formation. C/EBPα, β, δ and ε are all expressed during hematopoiesis (Fig. 17.1A); however, C/EBPε, the newest member of the family, is expressed exclusively in cells of myeloid and T-cell lineages.[36] Targeted disruption of the C/EBPε gene in mice results in defects of granulopoiesis, neutrophil phagocytosis and bacterial killing, migration, and impaired cytokine production after an inflammatory challenge.[37,38] In addition, there is accelerated apoptosis in maturing granulocytic cells.[39] Neutrophil-specific granule deficiency (SGD) is a very rare congenital disorder, possibly inherited in an autosomal recessive fashion that is characterized by a lack of specific (secondary) granule proteins such as lactoferrin, transcobalamin, collagenase, gelatinase B (tertiary granules), abnormalities of migration, disaggregation and bactericidal

activity, and atypical bilobed nuclei. Primary granules are markedly depleted of defensins although expression of myeloperoxidase and lysozyme is unaffected.[40] Eosinophils also lack eosinophilic-specific granules and are undetectable by Giemsa–Wright staining. Despite the lack of lactoferrin in neutrophils, saliva from patients contains normal levels suggesting a specific defect of myeloid granulopoiesis. Given the striking similarity between SGD and mutant mice generated by targeting of the C/EBPε gene it is unsurprising that mutations have now been found in at least two patients.[41,42] Recently a heterozygous mutation in a third patient has been revealed, although this mutation resulted in enhanced expression of C/EBPε and another myeloid transcription factor PU.1.[43] Interestingly, this SGD patient had reduced levels of the transcription factor growth factor indepence-1 (Gfi-1), which could explain the increased expression of C/EBPε and PU.1, as the expression of these are repressed by Gfi-1. Gfi-1 is a zinc-fingered transcription factor, which functions downstream of C/EBPε and PU.1, and gene targeted Gfi-1$^{-/-}$ mice lack mature circulating neutrophils.[44] Mutations in the human *Gfi-1* gene cause severe neutropenia and result in loss of repression of ELA2 and C/EBPε expression, which may impair the proliferation and survival of immature granulocytes.[45,46]

Most recently, mutations in the *G6PC3* gene encoding the glucose-6-phosphatase were found to give rise to SCN. Linkage analysis of two families revealed a mutation in the *G6PC3* gene that abolished its enzymatic activity and result in increased susceptibility to apoptosis.[47] Screening of a larger cohort of patients identified seven unrelated SCN patients with mutations in the same gene and it was found that myeloid progenitor cells showed enlarged rough endoplasmatic reticulum and increased BiP levels,[47] suggesting involvement of UPR as has been hypothesized for SCN caused by *ELA2* mutations.

Low neutrophil counts but intact neutrophil maturation in the BM were found in four patients from one family with recurrent *Streptococcus pneumoniae* infection as well as hypogammaglobulinemia, short stature and hypopigmented skin.[48] A mutation in the endosomal adaptor protein 14 (p14) was found to be the cause, resulting in decreased protein expression and subsequently defective lysosome function and delayed killing.[48] Although this may explain their immunodeficiency, it is still unclear why these patients are neutropenic.

Deficiencies of adhesion and migration

Leukocyte adhesion disorders arise from defects in cell aggregation and adhesion to extracellular matrix and vascular endothelium. Integrins form a large family of molecules involved in intercellular and cell-substratum adhesion. Each is a heterodimer of non-covalently linked α and β chains. The members of a particular family share a common β chain, but each possess a unique α chain. The best known of the integrins are from the $β_2$ family, and expression of these are confined primarily to monocytes, neutrophils, and activated lymphocytes. These are known as lymphocyte-function-associated antigen (LFA-1 or CD11a/CD18), complement receptor-3 (CR3, Mac-1 or CD11b/CD18), p150, 95 (or CD11c/CD18), and $αvβ_2$ or (CD11d/CD18). All $β_2$

integrins are constitutively represented on the plasma membrane of the leukocyte, and are both quantitatively and functionally up-regulated by activation of the cell. The counter-receptors for leukocyte β_2 integrin molecules are members of the immunoglobulin gene superfamily, intercellular adhesion molecule-1 (ICAM-1) and ICAM-2, which are expressed on endothelial cells. Resting leukocytes (particularly B lymphocytes and cells of the monocyte–macrophage lineage) themselves express a third ligand for LFA-1, ICAM-3, which is constitutively expressed, and which may be important for interleukocyte signaling. Three distinct human disorders of leukocyte adhesion have been recognized (leukocyte adhesion deficiency type 1 [LAD-I], LAD type 2 [LAD-II] and LAD type 3 [LAD-III]) (Fig. 17.1B). LAD-I is a rare inherited disease characterized in its severe form by delayed separation of the umbilical cord, recurrent life-threatening bacterial (usually with *Staphylococcus aureus* and Gram-negative enteric organisms) and fungal infections, gingivitis, delayed wound healing, and chronic leukocytosis. Patients are neutrophilic in the absence of infection with marked granulocytosis during acute infection. The absence of pus formation at sites of infection is one of the hallmarks of LAD-I.[49,50] Lymphocytes, monocytes and granulocytes show defects of adhesion to endothelial cells, cell migration, cell-mediated cytolysis and antigen presentation. Surprisingly, patients are not overtly susceptible to viral infection. LAD-I is an autosomal recessive disorder caused by mutations in the *ITGB2* gene encoding CD18 which is located on chromosome 21.[49,51] Patients with LAD-I are therefore deficient in their cell-surface expression of the glycoprotein β_2-integrin subunit (CD18). Most mutations in the *ITGB2* gene are heterogeneous and found in a highly conserved ~240-residue domain.[51] The degree of deficiency of the molecule usually correlates well with the severity of the clinical condition. Patients suffering from the severe form of the disease (less than 1% normal cell surface expression of CD18) die in childhood unless treated by hematopoietic stem cell transplantation, whereas those with moderate disease (2–5% expression) can survive into adulthood. Recently, gene therapy has successfully been used to correct a natural model of LAD-I in dogs,[52] which may provide an alternative to stem cell transplantation for patients for whom no suitable donor can be found.

LAD-II has been described in only a few patients.[53–55] It results from a general defect in fucose metabolism leading to an absence of sialyl-Lewis X (SLeX) and other fucosylated ligands for selectins, which are a group of cell-adhesion molecules expressed on endothelial cells, and mediate rolling along the endothelium before firm attachment is achieved. The phenotype of the immunodeficiency is similar to that of LAD-I, but less severe. Additional features include severe mental retardation and short stature suggesting that these molecules are also important in development. LAD-II is now known to belong to a growing group of congenital disorders of glycosylation (CDG), in which glycosylation of proteins is defective due to molecular lesions in genes required for the assembly of lipid-linked oligosaccharides, their transfer to nascent proteins (CDG-I), or the processing of protein-bound glycans (CDG-II). Missense genetic mutations in patients with LAD-II (also known as CDG-IIc) have been identified in a highly conserved GDP-fucose transporter, which explains the observed defect of GDP-fucose import into the Golgi apparatus where fucosylation takes place.[56–58] Fucosylation of fibroblasts from LAD-II patients grown *in vitro* can be corrected by fucose addition to culture medium.[59] Similarly, oral fucose treatment of LAD-II patients can restore selectin ligands and improve the immunodeficiency, suggesting that the defective transporter has partial activity, or that less efficient independent pathways exist.[58,59]

LAD-III was initially described as a variant of LAD-I, and presents with similar, but less severe, symptoms to LAD-I and an additional severe bleeding tendency, similar to Glanzmann thrombasthenia.[60] Patients have normal β_1, β_2 and β_3-integrin expression, but defective integrin activation through 'inside-out' signaling pathways.[61,62] Two genes have been implicated in LAD-III. First, mutations in the *RASGRP2* gene, which encodes for calcium- and diacylglycerol-regulated guanine exchange factor (CalDAG-GEFI), were identified in patients with LAD-III[63] and mice lacking CalDAG-GEFI exhibited similar leukocyte defects.[64] However, not all cases showed mutations in the *RASGRP2* gene suggesting genetic heterogeneity among patients. Recently another gene has been implicated in LAD-III. Mutations in *FERMT3*, encoding the hematopoietic-restricted kindlin-3 protein, were found in LAD-III patients.[65–67] Kindlin-3 protein expression was lost in these patients and transfecting affected cells with *kindlin3* cDNA restored integrin-mediated adhesion and migration defects.[65]

Myelokathexis is a rare cause of severe chronic neutropenia and is characterized by degenerative changes and hypersegmentation in mature neutrophils which are also functionally abnormal.[68] In the BM, there is relative granulocytic hyperplasia with cytoplasmic vacuolation, nuclear hypersegmentation, and pyknotic nuclear lobes connected by thin filaments. Some evidence points to an intrinsic acceleration of apoptosis in neutrophil precursors.[69] In association with *w*arts, *h*ypogammaglobulinemia, and recurrent respiratory tract *i*nfections, *m*yelokathexis forms part of the WHIM syndrome, which is usually inherited in an autosomal dominant fashion, although an autosomal recessive inheritance can also be observed. Most patients carry heterozygous mutations in the gene encoding the chemokine receptor CXCR4 and typically these mutations result in expression of a truncated form of CXCR4 with a loss of the last 10–19 amino acids of its cytoplasmic tail.[70–72] Truncation of its intracellular tail reduces the ability of CXCR4 to be internalized upon ligand binding (desensitization) and consequently lymphocyte and granulocyte migration in response to CXCL12, the functional ligand of CXCR4, is increased.[70,72,73] Normal expression of CXCR4 on neutrophils is down-regulated when the cells mature and re-expressed on senescent cells, which then home to the BM to die.[74] Alterations in this pathway due to WHIM-causing mutations are likely the cause of mature neutrophil retention in the BM of WHIM patients.

Phagocyte signaling abnormalities

Many aspects of phagocyte function depend on the ability to modulate shape and therefore dynamically organize the actin cytoskeleton. Two inherited disorders are known to produce abnormalities of these processes. The Wiskott–Aldrich syndrome (WAS) is a rare inherited X-linked recessive disease characterized by immune dysregulation (deficiency and autoimmunity) and microthrombocytopenia.[75,76] In its less severe form, known as X-linked thrombocytopenia (XLT) or attenuated WAS, mutations in the same gene produce the characteristic platelet abnormality but minimal immunologic disturbance. In the absence of hematopoietic stem cell transplantation, many patients with WAS die in childhood and early adulthood from hemorrhage, infection or lymphoid malignancy.

The WAS gene encodes a 502 amino acid proline-rich intracellular protein (WASp) expressed exclusively in hematopoietic cells, which belongs to a family of more widely expressed proteins involved in transduction of signals from receptors on the cell surface to the actin cytoskeleton. The Rho family GTPases (Cdc42, Rac and Rho) regulate many aspects of cell function including cytoskeletal rearrangement, progression through cell cycle, and vesicle trafficking.[77,78] WASp binds to the GTP-bound form of Cdc42 *in vitro*, less well to GTP-bound Rac, but not to Rho, and clusters physically with polymerized actin.[79] These findings and others have led to the suggestion that WASp is a direct effector for Cdc42, although its multi-domain structure undoubtedly supports a multifunctional role in the regulated assembly of cytoskeletal complexes. Cdc42 induces the formation of distinct actin-filament-containing protrusions known as filopodia in fibroblast and monocytic cell lines. In contrast, growth-factor-induced activation of the related GTP-binding protein Rac leads to accumulation of an actin network at the cell periphery producing lamellipodia and membrane ruffling. Cdc42 and Rac have also been shown to participate in the establishment of cell-substratum focal adhesion complexes distinct from Rho-induced focal adhesions. For WASp, the interaction with Cdc42/Rac has been shown to be mediated through a Cdc42/Rac interactive binding (CRIB) motif (or GTPase-binding domain, GBD), which is found in many downstream effectors of Cdc42 and Rac. In addition, the C-terminal portion of WASp has been shown to interact directly with the actin-related protein (Arp)2/3 complex, indicating the critical regulatory role for WASp in the nucleation and branching of actin filaments.[80] In its inactive state, WASp is thought to block the Arp2/3-binding site by intramolecular interactions between the C-terminus and the GBD.[81] WASp therefore acts as a regulated scaffold for the organized recruitment of signaling molecules and effector proteins at sites of new actin polymerization. In the absence of WASp, macrophages and dendritic cells have now been shown to have marked abnormalities of chemotaxis, chemokinesis, adhesion and phagocytosis of both opsonized particles and apoptotic cells.[82–86] Neutrophils appear to demonstrate normal chemotaxis *in vitro*, but under conditions of physiologic shear flow display defective 'outside-in' integrin signaling.[82,87]

In neutrophils, the GTPase Rac has been shown to be critical for activity of the NADPH oxidase, through interaction with p67[phox] (see below).[88] Both Rac1 and Rac2 are highly homologous although Rac2 accounts for >96% of the Rac protein expressed in neutrophils. A single male infant has been described with a point mutation in one allele of the *Rac2* gene.[89,90] This results in an inability of the mutant protein to bind GTP, and dominant inhibition of the normal protein.[91] Clinically, this patient suffered from recurrent infections, poor wound healing and absence of pus in infected areas. His peripheral neutrophil count was also high, and when tested *in vitro* neutrophils exhibited decreased chemotaxis, polarization, azurophilic granule secretion and superoxide anion production.

Deficiencies of the phagocyte respiratory burst

Chronic granulomatous disease (CGD) is a rare but important genetic disorder caused by defects in the enzyme responsible for the oxidative or 'respiratory' burst in all phagocytes.[92,93] Failure to produce a respiratory burst results in characteristic susceptibility to severe and recurrent infections by catalase-positive organisms, *Staphylococcus aureus*, *Burkholderia cepacia*, *Aspergillus* species and *Serratia marcescens*, and also a tendency to develop granulomatous inflammation, particulary affecting hollow organs. The phagocytic NADPH-oxidase (NOX-2, a member of a family of 7 mammalian isoforms) catalyses the transmembrane passage of electrons from NADPH to molecular oxygen, and in doing so regulates phagosomal pH and ionic composition.[93] This is critical for activation of proteolytic enzymes as they are discharged into the phagocytic vacuole. Previous suggestions that a cascade of free radical reactions resulting from production of superoxide radical were important for direct microbicidal activity are probably incorrect as in transgenic mice lacking the major neutrophil proteases microbial killing was abolished despite a normal oxidative burst.[93] The NADPH-oxidase consists of a membrane-bound flavocytochrome b_{558} and four cytosolic factors, p47[phox], p67[phox], p40[phox] and p21rac2, which translocate to the membrane on activation of the cell (the suffix *phox* represents phagocyte oxidase).[93] Activation is initiated classically by opsonized particles, but also by many soluble inflammatory mediators and through toll-like receptor-signaling pathways. The redox center of the oxidase is the flavocytochrome b_{558}, which consists of two proteins with apparent molecular weights of 23 kDa (p22[phox], α subunit) and 76–92 kDa (gp91[phox], β subunit) respectively, and are arranged as a 1:1 heterodimer. Both p22[phox] and gp91[phox] are missing in cells derived from most CGD patients with a molecular lesion of either subunit, indicating that mutual interaction is necessary for assembly of the mature complex.[94] The flavocytochrome b_{558} almost certainly comprises the complete electron transporting system and forms the membrane docking site for the cytosolic components. In resting neutrophils, the plasma membrane is devoid of flavocytochrome b_{558}, which resides almost exclusively in specialized light density intracellular vesicles and within the membranes of specific granules. When the cell is activated the plasma membrane invaginates to form the phagocytic vacuole with which vesicles containing flavocytochrome b_{558} fuse. The cytosolic components form an activation complex which translocates to the membrane to associate with the flavocytochrome b_{558}. Assembly of the complete NADPH-oxidase complex may induce conformational changes in flavocytochrome b_{558} which permit binding of the substrate NADPH, and which are energetically favorable for electron transport.[95]

The majority of CGD patients follow an X-linked recessive inheritance (67%; X91[0] CGD) and are genetically heterogeneous, while the remaining cases are autosomal recessive and are equally distributed among females and males.[96]

Autosomal recessive CGD is most commonly caused by lack of p47^{phox} (A47^{0}CGD), which usually follows a slightly milder clinical course than X-linked CGD.[96] A GT dinucleotide deletion at a GTGT repeat at the beginning of the second exon is found in the majority of mutant alleles, resulting in a chain terminator at amino acid residue 51, which has been found to arise from recombination events (probably partial) between highly homologous pseudogenes, which contain the GT deletion.[97–99] Deficiency of p67^{phox} and p22^{phox} is much less common. Interestingly, a patient was recently described with mutations in p40^{phox}, who showed a substantial defect in superoxide release during phagocytosis, but unaffected superoxide production in response to phorbol ester.[100] Treatment for CGD is dependent on prophylaxis against both bacterial and fungal infection with antibiotics. Stem cell transplantation may also be curative, and is a reasonable option particularly if an HLA-matched sibling donor is available. As CGD is a disorder of hematopoietic cells, gene therapy is an alternative attractive option for treatment. Gene therapy of X-linked CGD was described recently in two adults and although effective in clearing life-threatening infection, retrovirus-induced insertional mutagenesis induced myelodysplastic complications.[101] These studies demonstrate proof of principle of the gene therapy approach, and are soon to be followed by newer trial of more sophisticated gene delivery systems.

Extrinsic disorders of phagocytosis

Once localized to the area of inflammation, phagocytic cells directly attack invading microorganisms. They do this by internalization of particles into phagocytic vacuoles, or phagosomes. On the cell surface, leukocytes express carbohydrate mannosyl–fucosyl receptors that can bind non-encapsulated microbes carrying these surface sugars in the absence of opsonization, in addition to high-affinity receptors for IgG and complement, FcR and CR1/CR3, respectively, which cooperate with each other to bind to their corresponding ligands. Opsonization of particles with IgG and fragments of complement, in particular C3 breakdown products such as C3bi, renders them much more susceptible to phagocytosis. Deficiency of these components results in susceptibility to infection by organisms whose main route of destruction is by phagocytosis, in particular, pyogenic bacteria. Mannose-binding lectin (MBL) is a soluble defense collagen (related to C1q, and pulmonary surfactant protein (SP-A)) which can activate complement independently of the classical and alternative pathways.[102] In addition, it acts as an opsonin of mannose-rich pathogens, and has been shown to directly enhance FcR-mediated phagocytosis by both monocytes and macrophages.[102] These ligands are elements of innate immunity which may be particularly important as a first line of defense before the generation of cellular immunity and high-affinity specific antibodies, and may be functionally most important in children between the ages of 6 months (at a time when maternal antibody levels have waned) and 2 years (before which time the generation of anticarbohydrate IgG is inefficient). Genetically determined MBL deficiency is associated with increased susceptibility and severity of infection, although absence of MBL may also be entirely without clinical phenotype.[103]

References

1. Yang KD, Quie PG, Hill HR. Phagocytic system. In: Ochs HD, Smith CIE, Puck JM, editors. Primary Immunodeficiency Diseases. A Molecular and Genetic Approach. New York: Oxford University Press; 1999. p. 82–96.

2. Welte K, Zeidler C, Dale DC. Severe congenital neutropenia. Semin Hematol 2006;43:189–95.

3. Kostmann R. Infantile genetic agranulocytosis; agranulocytosis infantilis hereditaria. Acta Paediatr 1956;45(Suppl.):1–78.

4. Haurie C, Dale DC, Mackey MC. Cyclical neutropenia and other periodic hematological disorders: a review of mechanisms and mathematical models. Blood 1998;92:2629–40.

5. Dale DC, Hammond WPT. Cyclic neutropenia: a clinical review. Blood Rev 1988;2:178–85.

6. Rosenberg PS, Alter BP, Bolyard AA, et al; Severe Chronic Neutropenia International Registry. The incidence of leukemia and mortality from sepsis in patients with severe congenital neutropenia receiving long-term G-CSF therapy. Blood 2006;107:4628–35.

7. Dale DC, Bonilla MA, Davis MW, et al. A randomized controlled phase III trial of recombinant human granulocyte colony-stimulating factor (filgrastim) for treatment of severe chronic neutropenia. Blood 1993;81:2496–502.

8. Freedman MH, Bonilla MA, Fier C, et al. Myelodysplasia syndrome and acute myeloid leukemia in patients with congenital neutropenia receiving G-CSF therapy. Blood 2000;96:429–36.

9. Tschan CA, Pilz C, Zeidler C, et al. Time course of increasing numbers of mutations in the granulocyte colony-stimulating factor receptor gene in a patient with congenital neutropenia who developed leukemia. Blood 2001;97:1882–4.

10. Cassinat B, Bellanne-Chantelot C, Notz-Carrere A, et al. Screening for G-CSF receptor mutations in patients with secondary myeloid or lymphoid transformation of severe congenital neutropenia. A report from the French neutropenia register. Leukemia 2004;18:1553–5.

11. Dale DC, Bolyard AA, Schwinzer BG, et al. The Severe Chronic Neutropenia International Registry: 10-Year Follow-up Report. Support Cancer Ther 2006;3:220–31.

12. Freedman MH, Alter BP. Risk of myelodysplastic syndrome and acute myeloid leukemia in congenital neutropenias. Semin Hematol 2002;39:128–33.

13. Tidow N, Pilz C, Kasper B, Welte K. Frequency of point mutations in the gene for the G-CSF receptor in patients with chronic neutropenia undergoing G-CSF therapy. Stem Cells 1997;1(Suppl. 15):113–9; discussion 120.

14. Dong F, Brynes RK, Tidow N, et al. Mutations in the gene for the granulocyte colony-stimulating-factor receptor in patients with acute myeloid leukemia preceded by severe congenital neutropenia. N Engl J Med 1995;333:487–93.

15. Horwitz M, Benson KF, Person RE, et al. Mutations in ELA2, encoding neutrophil elastase, define a 21-day biological clock in cyclic haematopoiesis. Nat Genet 1999;23:433–6.

16. Bellanne-Chantelot C, Clauin S, Leblanc T, et al. Mutations in the ELA2 gene correlate with more severe expression of neutropenia: a study of 81 patients from the French Neutropenia Register. Blood 2004;103:4119–25.

17. Zeidler C, Germeshausen M, Klein C, Welte K. Clinical implications of ELA2-, HAX1-, and G-CSF-receptor (CSF3R) mutations in severe congenital neutropenia. Br J Haematol 2009; 144:459–67.

18. Dale DC, Person RE, Bolyard AA, et al. Mutations in the gene encoding neutrophil elastase in congenital and cyclic neutropenia. Blood 2000;96: 2317–22.

19. Ancliff PJ, Gale RE, Liesner R, et al. Mutations in the ELA2 gene encoding neutrophil elastase are present in most patients with sporadic severe congenital neutropenia but only in some patients with the familial form of the disease. Blood 2001;98:2645–50.

20. Horwitz MS, Duan Z, Korkmaz B, et al. Neutrophil elastase in cyclic and severe congenital neutropenia. Blood 2007;109:1817–24.

21. Bode W, Meyer E Jr, Powers JC. Human leukocyte and porcine pancreatic elastase: X-ray crystal structures, mechanism, substrate specificity, and mechanism-based inhibitors. Biochemistry 1989;28:1951–63.

22. Li FQ, Horwitz M. Characterization of mutant neutrophil elastase in severe congenital neutropenia. J Biol Chem 2001;276:14230–41.

23. Belaaouaj A, McCarthy R, Baumann M, et al. Mice lacking neutrophil elastase reveal impaired host defense against gram negative bacterial sepsis. Nat Med 1998;4:615–8.

24. Ron D, Walter P. Signal integration in the endoplasmic reticulum unfolded protein response. Nat Rev Mol Cell Biol 2007;8:519–29.

25. Kollner I, Sodeik B, Schreek S, et al. Mutations in neutrophil elastase causing congenital neutropenia lead to cytoplasmic protein accumulation and induction of the unfolded protein response. Blood 2006;108:493–500.

26. Grenda DS, Murakami M, Ghatak J, et al. Mutations of the ELA2 gene found in patients with severe congenital neutropenia induce the unfolded protein response and cellular apoptosis. Blood 2007;110:4179–87.

27. Melin M, Entesarian M, Carlsson G, et al. Assignment of the gene locus for severe congenital neutropenia to chromosome 1q22 in the original Kostmann family from Northern Sweden. Biochem Biophys Res Commun 2007;353: 571–5.

28. Klein C, Grudzien M, Appaswamy G, et al. HAX1 deficiency causes autosomal recessive severe congenital neutropenia (Kostmann disease). Nat Genet 2007; 39:86–92.

29. Germeshausen M, Grudzien M, Zeidler C, et al. Novel HAX1 mutations in patients with severe congenital neutropenia reveal isoform-dependent genotype-phenotype associations. Blood 2008;111:4954–7.

30. Smith BN, Ancliff PJ, Pizzey A, et al. Homozygous HAX1 mutations in severe congenital neutropenia patients with sporadic disease: a novel mutation in two unrelated British kindreds. Br J Haematol 2009;144:762–70.

31. Devriendt K, Kim AS, Mathijs G, et al. Constitutively activating mutation in WASP causes X-linked severe congenital neutropenia. Nat Genet 2001;27:313–17.

32. Ancliff PJ, Blundell MP, Cory GO, et al. Two novel activating mutations in the Wiskott–Aldrich syndrome protein result in congenital neutropenia. Blood 2006; 108:2182–9.

33. Beel K, Cotter MM, Blatny J, et al. A large kindred with X-linked neutropenia with an I294T mutation of the Wiskott-Aldrich syndrome gene. Br J Haematol 2009;144:120–6.

34. Moulding DA, Blundell MP, Spiller DG, et al. Unregulated actin polymerization by WASp causes defects of mitosis and cytokinesis in X-linked neutropenia. J Exp Med 2007;204:2213–24.

35. Lekstrom-Himes J, Xanthopoulos KG. Biological role of the CCAAT/enhancer-binding protein family of transcription factors. J Biol Chem 1998;273:28545–8.

36. Antonson P, Stellan B, Yamanaka R, Xanthopoulos KG. A novel human CCAAT/enhancer binding protein gene, C/EBPepsilon, is expressed in cells of lymphoid and myeloid lineages and is localized on chromosome 14q11.2 close to the T-cell receptor alpha/delta locus. Genomics 1996;35:30–8.

37. Yamanaka R, Barlow C, Lekstrom-Himes J, et al. Impaired granulopoiesis, myelodysplasia, and early lethality in CCAAT/enhancer binding protein epsilon-deficient mice. Proc Natl Acad Sci USA 1997;94:13187–92.

38. Lekstrom-Himes J, Xanthopoulos KG. CCAAT/enhancer binding protein epsilon is critical for effective neutrophil-mediated response to inflammatory challenge. Blood 1999;93:3096–105.

39. Verbeek W, Wachter M, Lekstrom-Himes J, Koeffler HP. C/EBPepsilon −/− mice: increased rate of myeloid proliferation and apoptosis. Leukemia 2001;15: 103–11.

40. Gombart AF, Koeffler HP. Neutrophil specific granule deficiency and mutations in the gene encoding transcription factor C/EBP(epsilon). Curr Opin Hematol 2002;9:36–42.

41. Gombart AF, Shiohara M, Kwok SH, et al. Neutrophil-specific granule deficiency: homozygous recessive inheritance of a frameshift mutation in the gene encoding transcription factor CCAAT/enhancer binding protein-epsilon. Blood 2001;97:2561–7.

42. Lekstrom-Himes JA, Dorman SE, Kopar P, et al. Neutrophil-specific granule deficiency results from a novel mutation with loss of function of the transcription factor CCAAT/enhancer binding protein epsilon. J Exp Med 1999;189: 1847–52.

43. Khanna-Gupta A, Sun H, Zibello T, et al. Growth factor independence-1 (Gfi-1) plays a role in mediating specific granule deficiency (SGD) in a patient lacking a gene-inactivating mutation in the C/EBPepsilon gene. Blood 2007;109: 4181–90.

44. Hock H, Hamblen MJ, Rooke HM, et al. Intrinsic requirement for zinc finger transcription factor Gfi-1 in neutrophil differentiation. Immunity 2003;18: 109–20.

45. Person RE, Li FQ, Duan Z, et al. Mutations in proto-oncogene GFI1 cause human neutropenia and target ELA2. Nat Genet 2003;34:308–12.

46. Zhuang D, Qiu Y, Kogan SC, Dong F. Increased CCAAT enhancer-binding protein epsilon (C/EBPepsilon) expression and premature apoptosis in myeloid cells expressing Gfi-1 N382S mutant associated with severe congenital neutropenia. J Biol Chem 2006;281: 10745–51.

47. Boztug K, Appaswamy G, Ashikov A, et al. A syndrome with congenital neutropenia and mutations in G6PC3. N Engl J Med 2009;360:32–43.

48. Bohn G, Allroth A, Brandes G, et al. A novel human primary immunodeficiency syndrome caused by deficiency of the endosomal adaptor protein p14. Nat Med 2007;13:38–45.

49. Anderson DC, Springer TA. Leukocyte adhesion deficiency: an inherited defect in the Mac-1, LFA-1, and p150,95 glycoproteins. Annu Rev Med 1987; 38:175–94.

50. Etzioni A, Doerschuk CM, Harlan JM. Of man and mouse: leukocyte and endothelial adhesion molecule deficiencies. Blood 1999;94:3281–8.

51. Hogg N, Bates PA. Genetic analysis of integrin function in man: LAD-1 and other syndromes. Matrix Biol 2000; 19:211–22.

52. Bauer TR, Allen Jr JM, Hai M, et al. Successful treatment of canine leukocyte adhesion deficiency by foamy virus vectors. Nat Med 2008;14:93–7.

53. Etzioni A, Frydman M, Pollack S, et al. Brief report: recurrent severe infections caused by a novel leukocyte adhesion

deficiency. N Engl J Med 1992;327: 1789–92.

54. Marquardt T, Brune T, Luhn K, et al. Leukocyte adhesion deficiency II syndrome, a generalized defect in fucose metabolism. J Pediatr 1999;134:681–8.

55. Hidalgo A, Ma S, Peired AJ, et al. Insights into leukocyte adhesion deficiency type 2 from a novel mutation in the GDP-fucose transporter gene. Blood 2003;101: 1705–12.

56. Lubke T, Marquardt T. von Figura K, Korner C. A new type of carbohydrate-deficient glycoprotein syndrome due to a decreased import of GDP-fucose into the golgi. J Biol Chem 1999;274:25986–9.

57. Lubke T, Marquardt T, Etzioni A, et al. Complementation cloning identifies CDG-IIc, a new type of congenital disorders of glycosylation, as a GDP-fucose transporter deficiency. Nat Genet 2001;28:73–6.

58. Luhn K, Wild MK, Eckhardt M, et al. The gene defective in leukocyte adhesion deficiency II encodes a putative GDP-fucose transporter. Nat Genet 2001; 28:69–72.

59. Marquardt T, Luhn K, Srikrishna G, et al. Correction of leukocyte adhesion deficiency type II with oral fucose. Blood 1999;94:3976–85.

60. Kuijpers TW, Van Lier RA, Hamann D, et al. Leukocyte adhesion deficiency type 1 (LAD-1)/variant. A novel immunodeficiency syndrome characterized by dysfunctional beta2 integrins. J Clin Invest 1997;100: 1725–33.

61. McDowall A, Inwald D, Leitinger B, et al. A novel form of integrin dysfunction involving beta1, beta2, and beta3 integrins. J Clin Invest 2003;111: 51–60.

62. Kinashi T, Aker M, Sokolovsky-Eisenberg M, et al. LAD-III, a leukocyte adhesion deficiency syndrome associated with defective Rap1 activation and impaired stabilization of integrin bonds. Blood 2004;103:1033–6.

63. Pasvolsky R, Feigelson SW, Kilic SS, et al. A LAD-III syndrome is associated with defective expression of the Rap-1 activator CalDAG-GEFI in lymphocytes, neutrophils, and platelets. J Exp Med 2007;204:1571–82.

64. Bergmeier W, Goerge T, Wang HW, et al. Mice lacking the signaling molecule CalDAG-GEFI represent a model for leukocyte adhesion deficiency type III. J Clin Invest 2007;117:1699–707.

65. Svensson L, Howarth K, McDowall A, et al. Leukocyte adhesion deficiency-III is caused by mutations in KINDLIN3 affecting integrin activation. Nat Med 2009;15:306–12.

66. Kuijpers TW, van de Vijver E, Weterman MA, et al. LAD-1/variant syndrome is caused by mutations in FERMT3. Blood 2009;113:4740–6.

67. Mory A, Feigelson SW, Yarali N, et al. Kindlin-3: a new gene involved in the pathogenesis of LAD-III. Blood 2008; 112:2591.

68. Bassan R, Viero P, Minetti B, et al. Myelokathexis: a rare form of chronic benign granulocytopenia. Br J Haematol 1984;58:115–17.

69. Aprikyan AA, Liles WC, Rodger E, et al. Impaired survival of bone marrow hematopoietic progenitor cells in cyclic neutropenia. Blood 2001;97:147–53.

70. Hernandez PA, Gorlin RJ, Lukens JN, et al. Mutations in the chemokine receptor gene CXCR4 are associated with WHIM syndrome, a combined immunodeficiency disease. Nat Genet 2003;34:70–4.

71. Tassone L, Notarangelo LD, Bonomi V, et al. Clinical and genetic diagnosis of warts, hypogammaglobulinemia, infections, and myelokathexis syndrome in 10 patients. J Allergy Clin Immunol 2009;123:1170–3, 1173: e1171–e1173.

72. Balabanian K, Lagane B, Pablos JL, et al. WHIM syndromes with different genetic anomalies are accounted for by impaired CXCR4 desensitization to CXCL12. Blood 2005;105:2449–57.

73. Gulino AV, Moratto D, Sozzani S, et al. Altered leukocyte response to CXCL12 in patients with warts hypogammaglobulinemia, infections, myelokathexis (WHIM) syndrome. Blood 2004;104:444–52.

74. Martin C, Burdon PC, Bridger G, et al. Chemokines acting via CXCR2 and CXCR4 control the release of neutrophils from the bone marrow and their return following senescence. Immunity 2003; 19:583–93.

75. Thrasher AJ. WASp in immune-system organization and function. Nat Rev Immunol 2002;2:635–46.

76. Bouma G, Burns SO, Thrasher AJ. Wiskott–Aldrich syndrome: immunodeficiency resulting from defective cell migration and impaired immunostimulatory activation. Immunobiology 2009;214:778–90.

77. Mackay DJ, Hall A. Rho GTPases. J Biol Chem 1998;273:20685–8.

78. Worthylake RA, Burridge K. Leukocyte transendothelial migration: orchestrating the underlying molecular machinery. Curr.Opin.Cell Biol 2001;13:569–77.

79. Aspenstrom P, Lindberg U, Hall A. Two GTPases, Cdc42 and Rac, bind directly to a protein implicated in the immunodeficiency disorder Wiskott–Aldrich syndrome. Curr Biol 1996;6: 70–5.

80. Machesky LM, Insall RH. Scar1 and the related Wiskott–Aldrich syndrome protein, WASP, regulate the actin cytoskeleton through the Arp2/3 complex. Curr Biol 1998;8:1347–56.

81. Kim AS, Kakalis LT, Abdul-Manan N, et al. Autoinhibition and activation

mechanisms of the Wiskott–Aldrich syndrome protein. Nature 2000;404: 151–8.

82. Zicha D, Allen WE, Brickell PM, et al. Chemotaxis of macrophages is abolished in the Wiskott–Aldrich syndrome. Br. J. Haematol 1998;101:659–65.

83. Linder S, Nelson D, Weiss M, Aepfelbacher M. Wiskott–Aldrich syndrome protein regulates podosomes in primary human macrophages. Proc Natl Acad Sci USA 1999;96:9648–53.

84. Lorenzi R, Brickell PM, Katz DR, et al. Wiskott–Aldrich syndrome protein is necessary for efficient IgG-mediated phagocytosis. Blood 2000;95:2943–6.

85. Leverrier Y, Lorenzi R, Blundell MP, et al. Cutting edge: the Wiskott–Aldrich syndrome protein is required for efficient phagocytosis of apoptotic cells. Journal of Immunology 2001;166:4831–4.

86. Burns S, Thrasher AJ, Blundell MP, et al. Configuration of human dendritic cell cytoskeleton by Rho GTPases, the WAS protein, and differentiation. Blood 2001;98:1142–9.

87. Zhang H, Schaff UY, Green CE, et al. Impaired integrin-dependent function in Wiskott–Aldrich syndrome protein-deficient murine and human neutrophils. Immunity 2006;25:285–95.

88. Segal AW, Abo A. The biochemical basis of the NADPH oxidase of phagocytes. Trends Biochem Sci 1993;18:43–7.

89. Williams DA, Tao W, Yang F, et al. Dominant negative mutation of the hematopoietic-specific Rho GTPase, Rac2, is associated with a human phagocyte immunodeficiency. Blood 2000;96: 1646–54.

90. Ambruso DR, Knall C, Abell AN, et al. Human neutrophil immunodeficiency syndrome is associated with an inhibitory Rac2 mutation. Proc Natl Acad Sci USA 2000;97:4654–9.

91. Gu Y, Jia B, Yang FC, et al. Biochemical and biological characterization of a human Rac2 GTPase mutant associated with phagocytic immunodeficiency. J Biol Chem 2001;276:15929–38.

92. Goldblatt D, Thrasher AJ. Chronic granulomatous disease. Clin Exp Immunol 2000;122:1–9.

93. Segal AW. How neutrophils kill microbes. Annu Rev Immunol 2005;23:197–223.

94. Parkos CA, Dinauer MC, Jesaitis AJ, et al. Absence of both the 91kD and 22kD subunits of human neutrophil cytochrome b in two genetic forms of chronic granulomatous disease. Blood 1989;73:1416–20.

95. Bedard K, Krause KH. The NOX family of ROS-generating NADPH oxidases: physiology and pathophysiology. Physiol Rev 2007;87:245–313.

96. van den Berg JM, van Koppen E, Ahlin A, et al. Chronic granulomatous disease: the European experience. PLoS One 2009;4: e5234.

97. Gorlach A, Lee PL, Roesler J, et al. A p47-phox pseudogene carries the most common mutation causing p47-phox-deficient chronic granulomatous disease. J Clin Invest 1997;100:1907–18.

98. Roesler J, Curnutte JT, Rae J, et al. Recombination events between the p47-phox gene and its highly homologous pseudogenes are the main cause of autosomal recessive chronic granulomatous disease. Blood 2000; 95:2150–6.

99. Vazquez N, Lehrnbecher T, Chen R, et al. Mutational analysis of patients with p47-phox-deficient chronic granulomatous disease: the significance of recombination events between the p47-phox gene (NCF1) and its highly homologous pseudogenes. Exp Hematol 2001;29:234–43.

100. Matute JD, Arias AA, Wright NA, et al. A new genetic subgroup of chronic granulomatous disease with autosomal recessive mutations in p40phox and selective defects in neutrophil NADPH oxidase activity. Blood 2009;114: 3309–15.

101. Ott MG, Schmidt M, Schwarzwaelder K, et al. Correction of X-linked chronic granulomatous disease by gene therapy, augmented by insertional activation of MDS1-EVI1, PRDM16 or SETBP1. Nat Med 2006;12:401–9.

102. Jack DL, Klein NJ, Turner MW. Mannose-binding lectin: targeting the microbial world for complement attack and opsonophagocytosis. Immunol Rev 2001;180:86–99.

103. Dahl M, Tybjaerg-Hansen A, Schnohr P, Nordestgaard BG. A population-based study of morbidity and mortality in mannose-binding lectin deficiency. J Exp Med 2004;199:1391–9.

CHAPTER 18

Acute myeloid leukemias

SD Boyd, DA Arber

Chapter Contents

Introduction

The acute myeloid leukemias (AML) are malignancies of immature precursors of the non-lymphoid hematopoietic lineages, involving the bone marrow (BM), peripheral blood (PB), and possibly other tissues. Taken together, this heterogeneous group of neoplasms has an estimated incidence between 1.6 and 3.7 per 100 000 population per year in the US and Western Europe.[1–3] Yearly incidence rates appear to increase with patient age, and the median age at diagnosis is 65.[2] AML is the predominant form of acute leukemia in adults, but accounts for only 15–20% of acute leukemias in pediatric patients.[4] Environmental exposures or therapies that damage DNA, and a number of clinical syndromes

affecting DNA repair pathways or tumor suppressor genes lead to increased risk of AML. Intensive study has revealed many somatic genetic lesions that appear to contribute to the development of AML. Approximately 20% of cases show recurrent cytogenetic abnormalities, while fewer than 10% of cases have a normal karyotype and fail to show mutations in genes such as *FMS-like tyrosine kinase 3 (FLT3)*, *nucleophosmin (NPM1)*, *CCAAT/enhancer-binding protein alpha (CEBPA)* and *myeloid/lymphoid or mixed lineage leukemia (MLL)* that are commonly altered in AML.[5,6] High-resolution studies of genomic copy number alterations in AML with comparison to normal somatic cell DNA from the affected patients, as well as initial full-genome sequencing efforts have given indications that there may be additional recurrent genetic lesions in this malignancy, as well as many other mutations

DOI: 10.1016/B978-0-7020-3147-2.00018-3

that may be very rare, pathogenic only in concert with numerous other mutations, or entirely unrelated to pathogenesis.[7–9] Prognosis of patients with AML shows a striking relationship with the cytogenetic and other mutational features of the malignant blasts, with the implication that a complete diagnostic report for AML should contain this information, despite the logistical challenges of combining data from several laboratory disciplines into a unified synopsis.

Classification systems

The rapid evolution of classification schemes for AML has resulted from several successive waves of new technology entering the clinical hematology laboratory and being validated in clinical trials. The French-American-British (FAB) classification of 1976 and its later modifications primarily relied upon morphologic examination, cytochemical tests, and limited immunophenotyping to establish lineage-related classification of myeloid blasts. In the years that followed, additional data including recognition of common cytogenetic abnormalities, clinical history and correlation with clinical outcomes led to the World Health Organization (WHO) classification scheme in 2001, with distinct AML categories defined by: 1) recurrent cytogenetic abnormalities; 2) presence of myelodysplastic changes; 3) history of methylating agent or topoisomerase 2 inhibitor chemotherapy drug exposure, or 4) a 'not otherwise specified' category encapsulating the FAB morphologic/cytochemical classification.[10] The defining BM blast percentage for AML was decreased from 30% to 20% at this time, largely because myelodysplastic syndrome (MDS) patients with over 20% blasts had been found to have a poor prognosis very similar to those with AML.[11] The transition from FAB to WHO 2001 was a pragmatic effort to generate a clinically useful classification system providing prognostic information relevant to the therapeutic options available, while incorporating cytogenetic findings likely related to disease pathogenesis, and still retaining familiar entities defined by their morphology and antigen expression. Incorporating the response to therapy as part of the basis for the classification scheme may necessitate future revisions if new therapies with distinctive properties come into wide use. For the practicing hematopathologist, knowledge of the preceding classification systems is essential, given that long-running clinical trials often refer to the older systems, and reports with the correct current classification and parallel classification by the older terminology are appreciated by clinicians and trial researchers.

A revised WHO classification was published in 2008 (Table 18.1), and builds on the insights of the 2001 system with an increased number of recurrent cytogenetic abnormalities, and the creation of provisional categories for AML cases with mutations in the *NPM1* or *CEBPA* genes.[6] The key role of cytogenetic data is further increased by the stipulation that cases with the t(8;21)(q22;q22), inv(16)(p13.1q22), t(16;16)(p13.1;q22), or t(15;17)(q22;q12) need not have >20% blasts to be diagnosed as AML. Additional weight is given to cytogenetic abnormalities in the AML with myelodysplasia-related changes category, where specific MDS-associated cytogenetic findings can take the place of

Table 18.1 World Health Organization classification of acute myeloid leukemia (AML) and related precursor neoplasms

AML with recurrent genetic abnormalities
AML with t(8;21)(q22;q22); (*RUNX1-RUNX1T1*)
AML with inv(16)(p13.1q22) or t(16;16)(p13.1;q22); (*CBFB-MYH11*)
Acute promyelocytic leukemia (APL) with t(15;17)(q22;q12); (*PML-RARA*)
AML with t(9;11)(p22;q23); (*MLLT3-MLL*)
AML with t(6;9)(p23;q34); (*DEK-NUP214*)
AML with inv(3)(q21q26.2) or t(3;3)(q21;q26.1); (*RPN1-EVI1*)
AML (megakaryoblastic) with t(1;22)(p13;q13); (*RBM15-MKL1*)
AML with mutated NPM1 (provisional)
AML with mutated CEBPA (provisional)
AML with myelodysplasia-related changes
Therapy-related myeloid neoplasms
Acute myeloid leukemia, not otherwise specified (NOS)
AML with minimal differentiation
AML without maturation
AML with maturation
Acute myelomonocytic leukemia
Acute monoblastic and monocytic leukemia
Acute erythroid leukemia
   Pure erythroid leukemia
   Erythroleukemia, erythroid/myeloid
Acute megakaryoblastic leukemia
Acute basophilic leukemia
Acute panmyelosis with myelofibrosis
Myeloid sarcoma
Myeloid proliferations related to Down syndrome
   Transient abnormal myelopoiesis
   Myeloid leukemia associated with Down syndrome
Blastic plasmacytoid dendritic cell neoplasm

morphologic evidence of myelodysplasia. Two entities found in patients with Down syndrome are now classified separately, and the therapy-related AML category has been simplified to a single entity for patients with history of exposure to any of a broad range of cytotoxic drugs or ionizing radiation therapy. Adjustments to the criteria for AML with myelodysplasia-related changes, and the addition of blastic plasmacytoid dendritic cell neoplasm as an AML-related precursor neoplasm are the other significant changes from the WHO 2001 scheme.[6] In the sections that follow, we will use the WHO 2008 framework to organize discussion of these malignancies, after a brief review of the clinical features and laboratory methods required for their analysis.

Methods for diagnosis and classification

Clinical history

Clinical history submitted for patients with AML may include a variety of nonspecific findings such as fatigue, bruising, fever, flu-like symptoms or unexpected infections, typically related to the decreased red cell and platelet counts and loss of normal leukocytes that result from extensive BM infiltration by malignant blasts. Disseminated intravascular coagulopathy (DIC) is a feared presentation of acute promyelocytic leukemia (APL), but can also be seen in other subcategories of AML. Cases with very high blast counts may manifest leukostasis with impaired oxygenation of blood in the lungs and subsequent hypoxia, or leukoblastic emboli.

Hepatosplenomegaly is relatively common, and other findings and complaints can include bone pain; skin, gum or other tissue masses (notably in AML cases with monocytic differentiation); and rarely, central nervous system (CNS) involvement.

Peripheral blood and bone marrow cell count and morphology

Complete blood counts and morphologic review of PB smears usually reveal multiple abnormalities in AML patients. Reduced counts of red cells, platelets and the normal leukocytes are commonly seen, but the white blood cell count (WBC) is most often elevated due to circulating blasts. Patients usually present before the WBC count rises above 50×10^9 cells per liter, but a minority of patients have WBC counts over 100×10^9 cells per liter, and occasional cases show WBC counts as low as 1×10^9 cells per liter with few circulating blasts. BM evaluation should be performed from aspirate smears of adequate quality reviewed in conjunction with bone marrow trephine biopsy (BMTB) sections. With the exception of a few cytogenetically-defined subcategories, blasts in the PB or BM must be ≥20% of total nucleated cells for a diagnosis of AML, based on a 200-cell count in the blood or a 500-cell count in the BM. The presence of Auer rods (linear filaments of primary granules) (Fig. 18.1) is the only definitive morphologic finding sufficient to distinguish myeloid blasts from lymphoid ones, but other features typical of myeloid blasts include larger blast size, fine chromatin, multiple often easily visualized nucleoli and cytoplasmic granulation. Blasts of some cases of AML (corresponding to those formerly classified in the FAB M0 and M1 categories) may be morphologically similar to lymphoblasts, small to medium in size with few nucleoli and minimal amounts of agranular cytoplasm, while others (corresponding to monoblasts and promyelocytes in the FAB M4 and M5 categories) show monocytic differentiation, being large in size with round to delicately folded or convoluted nuclei, fine lacy chromatin, visible nucleoli and basophilic cytoplasm with absent to minimal granulation. A background of

dysplasia in other BM myeloid lineages may also provide evidence that blasts are more likely to be of myeloid type. In some subcategories of AML, modifications of the blast count are part of the WHO 2008 classification: promonocytes are considered as blasts in AML cases with myelomonocytic , monoblastic or monocytic differentiation; the abnormal promyelocytes in APL are considered blasts; and in AML not otherwise specified erythroid/myeloid erythroleukemia cases, the blast percentage is calculated from non-erythroid BM nucleated cells.[6] Patients with myeloid sarcomas are considered to have AML regardless of PB or BM blast counts.

Immunophenotyping

Flow cytometry (FCM) is the preferred method of characterizing surface and internal antigen expression in leukemia cases, as modern flow cytometers and fluorescent antibodies enable four or more antigens to be measured simultaneously on each cell assayed, together with forward and side light scatter properties that correlate with cell size and internal complexity or granularity. Given the large number of different antigens that may be expressed by AML or other leukemic blasts, panels of antibodies used for diagnosis can be extensive, and are usually designed with one common antibody (typically binding the leukocyte marker CD45) present in all tubes used for staining cells, so that cell populations defined by CD45 expression and forward or side light scatter can be uniformly compared across all antibody stains in the panel. Myeloid surface antigens include CD13, CD33, CD117 (for more immature precursors), and CD15 (for more mature cells), while monocytic markers include CD14 and CD64. Megakaryocytic lineage is suggested by the platelet antigens CD41a and CD61, while erythroid markers include CD71, glycophorin and hemoglobin A. Surface expression of CD34 is a broad marker of immaturity seen in myeloid and lymphoid lineage blasts. Internal antigens helpful for characterizing myeloid blasts include myeloperoxidase (MPO) and TdT, which, as its role in lymphoid biology would suggest, is usually negative in AML but can be expressed aberrantly in a subset of cases. Many AML cases can be demonstrated to express antigens of other hematopoietic lineages: for example, t(8;21)-containing cases often show expression of the B cell antigens CD19, Pax5 or cytoplasmic CD79a; and T cell markers CD2 or CD7 are not uncommon in several subtypes of AML.[12] The aberrant expression of such markers typically does not warrant a diagnosis of biphenotypic or mixed phenotype acute leukemia (see Chapter 19), but may increase the sensitivity and specificity of detecting residual or recurrent disease following therapy.

Cytochemistry

A key part of lineage determination in the FAB classification scheme, cytochemical testing on air-dried blood or BM aspirate smear slides is performed to a more limited degree in most modern laboratories, with the result that many leukemias may not be fully evaluated by FAB criteria under current protocols.[13] Cytochemical stains for myeloperoxidase (MPO) and the somewhat less specific Sudan Black B (SBB) are used to identify myeloid lineage, although these

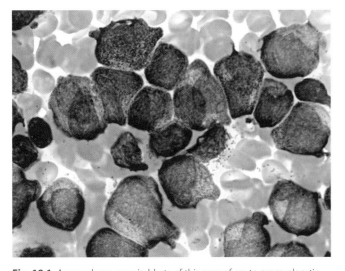

Fig. 18.1 Auer rods are seen in blasts of this case of acute promyelocytic leukemia.

stains are negative in very early myeloblasts and monoblasts, as well as in erythroid and megakaryocytic blasts. SBB has the advantage of being usable even when the air-dried smears have not been recently prepared. The nonspecific esterase (NSE) activity that characterizes monocytes and monoblasts can be detected by reactivity with alpha naphthyl butyrate esterase, or sodium fluoride-inhibited reactivity with alpha naphthyl acetate esterase. Naphthol-ASD-chloroacetate esterase (CAE) activity is specific for neutrophil and mast cell lineages. Using these stains, AML with minimal differentiation cases are defined by having less than 3% of blasts positive for MPO, SBB or CAE, and lacking NSE activity; the designation of these cases as acute myeloid leukemias relies on immunophenotypic detection of expression of some combination of CD13, CD117 or CD33 and lack of lymphoid differentiation markers. AML without maturation is distinguished from AML with minimal differentiation by having >3% MPO or SBB-positive blasts, or the presence or Auer rods (which should also stain for both MPO and SBB). Monoblasts and promonocytes seen in the acute myelomonocytic or acute monoblastic or monocytic leukemia categories show blast-equivalent cells with NSE reactivity but usually no MPO or SBB reactivity. Acute megakaryoblastic leukemias may show NaF-resistant NSE activity for alpha naphthyl acetate, but are MPO and SBB negative.

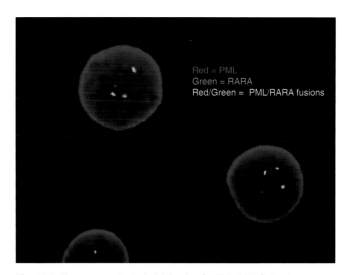

Red = PML
Green = RARA
Red/Green = PML/RARA fusions

Fig. 18.2 Fluorescence *in situ* hybridization for *PML-RARA* fusion in acute promyelocytic leukemia with t(15;17) translocation. The red *PML* probe and the green *RARA* probe spatially overlap in each of the two fusion chromosomes resulting from the translocation; the remaining normal copies of chromosome 15 and of chromosome 17 each show only a single probe. *(Photo courtesy of Dr Athena Cherry and C. Dana Bangs, Department of Pathology, Stanford University.)*

Cytogenetics and molecular testing

Conventional karyotype analysis, fluorescence *in situ* hybridization (FISH) assays for detecting translocations, and molecular biology tests for point mutations or other small genetic lesions have become an integral part of evaluating and sub-classifying acute myeloid leukemias, and can guide therapy, most notably for APL carrying t(15;17) that respond to all-trans retinoic acid (ATRA) treatment (Fig. 18.2). Cytogenetic and molecular testing additionally impacts therapeutic decision-making for patients with favorable cytogenetic or gene mutation-containing leukemias such as cases with low WBC counts and t(8;21), inv(16), t(16;16), or *NPM1* mutation without cytogenetic abnormalities and without *FLT3*-internal tandem duplication, in which allogeneic stem cell transplant does not appear to confer increased survival.[14,15] The key cytogenetic and mutational lesions in AML will be discussed in greater detail in the following sections dealing with each classification category.

Acute myeloid leukemia with recurrent genetic abnormalities

These leukemias feature balanced translocations or inversions, or belong to new provisional categories defined by mutation of the *NPM1* or *CEPBA* genes. These cytogenetic or mutationally-defined features have been associated with prognostic significance in clinical trials (Table 18.2). Most cases with recurrent translocations or inversions have some characteristic morphologic, immunophenotypic or clinical features.[16-19] If the classic t(8;21), inv(16), t(16;16), or t(15;17) translocations are present, 20% blood or BM blasts are not required for diagnosis. It should be noted that AML in patients with a history of chemotherapy or radiation

Table 18.2 AML with recurrent genetic abnormalities: prognostic correlations

AML with t(8;21)(q22;q22); (*RUNX1-RUNX1T1*)	Good prognosis
AML with inv(16)(p13.1q22) or t(16;16) (p13.1;q22); (*CBFB-MYH11*)	Good prognosis
Acute promyelocytic leukemia (APL) with t(15;17)(q22;q12); (*PML-RARA*)	Good prognosis
AML with t(9;11)(p22;q23); (*MLLT3-MLL*)	Intermediate prognosis; better than AML with other 11q23 translocations
AML with t(6;9)(p23;q34); (*DEK-NUP214*)	Poor prognosis, similar to AML with myelodysplasia-related changes
AML with inv(3)(q21q26.2) or t(3;3) (q21;q26.1); (*RPN1-EVI1*)	Poor prognosis
AML (megakaryoblastic) with t(1;22) (p13;q13); (*RBM15-MKL1*)	Probably good prognosis with intensive AML chemotherapy
AML with mutated NPM1 (provisional)	Good prognosis
AML with mutated CEBPA (provisional)	Good prognosis

therapy should be classified in the therapy-related AML category regardless of other findings. Multilineage dysplasia is commonly seen in the recurrent translocation/inversion cases with inv(3), t(3;3), or t(6;9), but the cytogenetic findings take priority for classification of these entities. Since the latter chromosomal changes were found also in patients clinically presenting as MDS, cases with inv(3), t(3;3), or t(6;9) can be classified as AML only when ≥20% blasts are present.

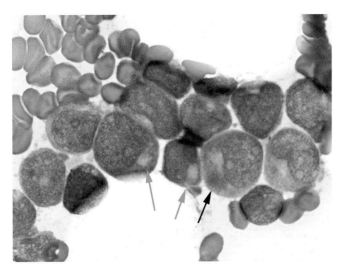

Fig. 18.3 AML t(8;21)(q22;q22); (*RUNX1-RUNX1T1*) morphology. Green arrows indicate prominent perinuclear hofs. Black arrow shows a salmon-colored granule.

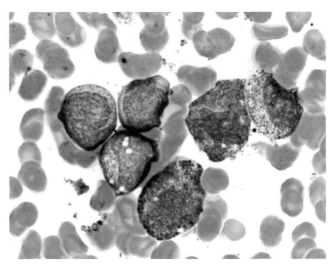

Fig. 18.4 AML with inv(16)(p13.1q22) (*CBFB-MYH11*) morphology. Abnormal eosinophil precursors with atypical granules are prominent.

AML with t(8;21)(q22;q22); (*RUNX1-RUNX1T1*)

Cases with the t(8;21) (q22;q22) translocation most commonly present in younger patients, and comprise 5–10% of AML diagnoses. Morphologic features are typically consistent with the former FAB M2 category ('with maturation') with blasts displaying ample cytoplasm with abundant granules and some blasts containing Auer rods (Fig. 18.3). Telltale features suggesting this diagnosis include prominent perinuclear hofs, the presence of larger pink granules among the more typical darker cytoplasmic granules, and frequent aberrant expression of B-cell antigens such as CD19, Pax5, or cytoplasmic CD79a. Other morphologic findings that can be seen are Auer rods in more mature granulocytes, abnormal very large granules in blasts, and varying degrees of dyspoietic morphology in granulocytes, including Pelger–Huetoid bilobed neutrophils. CD34 (often overexpressed) and myeloid antigens CD13, CD33 and MPO are usually positive by FCM, although CD33 may be weak. The *RUNX1* gene (synonyms: *AML1*, *CBFA*) encodes the core binding factor alpha protein (CBFA), one component of a heterodimeric hematopoietic transcription factor; the abnormal fusion to the *RUNX1T1* gene (synonym: *ETO*, for eight-twenty-one) likely impairs or misdirects gene-regulatory activity.[20] Prognosis for these cases is good with modern therapies, although high presenting WBC counts (>20 × 10^9 cells per liter) and *KIT* mutations (see below) lead to an intermediate prognosis.

AML with inv(16)(p13.1q22) or t(16;16)(p13.1;q22); (*CBFB-MYH11*)

The inv(16) or t(16;16) cases are also predominantly diagnosed in younger patients and account for 5–10% of all AML. Lesions affecting 16p13.1 involve the gene for the second half of the core binding factor (CBF) transcription factor (*CBFB* core-binding factor beta) fused to a smooth muscle myosin heavy chain gene (*MYH11*), possibly indicating an underlying biological basis for the good prognosis and younger demographic that these cases share with t(8;21)

AML.[21] Clinically, these leukemias show a high rate of extramedullary disease, approaching 50% of cases. The morphologic features of inv(16) or t(16;16) AML are highly distinctive, with most but not all cases showing granulocytic or monocytic blasts (often consistent with FAB M4 criteria) accompanied by abnormal eosinophil precursors in the BM (Fig. 18.4). The eosinophil precursors at the promyelocyte and myelocyte-equivalent stages show occasional to numerous large purple or basophilic granules of variable shape, intermixed with eosinophilic granules. FCM often documents several blast populations with myeloid or monocytic marker expression, and frequent (but nonspecific) aberrant expression of the T-cell marker CD2. FISH or real-time PCR (RT-PCR) testing is more sensitive than conventional karyotyping for detection of the inv(16)(p13.1q22) abnormality.

Acute promyelocytic leukemia (APL) with t(15;17)(q22;q12); (*PML-RARA*)

The dangerous prospect of DIC in patients with APL, the responsiveness of cases with the t(15;17)(q22;q12) translocation to all-trans retinoic acid (ATRA), and the good overall prognosis if acute life-threatening bleeding or clotting events are avoided make it imperative for the pathologist to recognize the morphologic features of these leukemias, and ensure that prompt confirmatory molecular testing is performed. Frequently, treatment with ATRA is initiated even before cytogenetic confirmation of the diagnosis is obtained. The disease may appear throughout adult life but is most common in the middle-aged. Roughly two-thirds of cases present with low WBC counts and show classic 'hypergranular' morphology, with abnormal promyelocytes displaying bilobed nuclei, dense granulation with large granules ranging in color from pink to violet, and frequent Auer rods (Fig. 18.5). Some cells may contain numerous and overlapping Auer rods. The 'microgranular' morphologic variant often has higher WBC counts but relatively sparse granulation of the blasts, with fewer cells containing Auer rods. The presence of bilobed nuclei is consistent and may be the best morphologic clue to

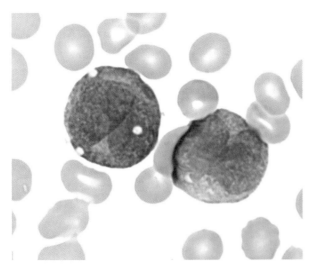

Fig. 18.5 Acute promyelocytic leukemia morphology. This case showed a t(15;17)(q22;q12) *PML-RARA* translocation. The bilobed nuclear morphology is characteristic. See also Fig. 18.1.

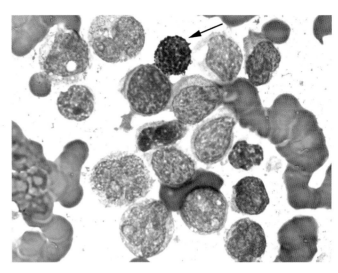

Fig. 18.6 Morphology of AML with t(6;9)(p23;q34); (*DEK-NUP214*). Basophilia is frequently seen (black arrow).

the diagnosis in the microgranular variant.[22-24] FCM of hyper-granular cases usually highlights blasts and promyelocytes with a broad range of side-scatter of light, staining negative for CD34 and HLA-DR, with bright CD33, variable CD13, and strong MPO. Microgranular cases are more often positive for CD34 (at least in a fraction of blasts), more likely to show aberrant expression of CD2, and unfortunately can occasionally express the monocytic marker CD64, necessitating careful review of morphology and cytogenetic correlation to distinguish these cases from monocytic AML with folded nuclei and monocytic FCM immunophenotype. APL cases are usually negative for adhesion molecules CD11b and CD11c that are most often strongly expressed in AML with monocytic differentiation. Cytochemical stains for MPO or SBB are strongly positive in both variant and classic cases. The aberrant RARA (retinoic acid receptor alpha) fusion protein generated by the t(15;17)(q22;q12) translocation appears to prevent normal myeloid maturation, and is targeted by ATRA therapy, leading to progressive granulocytic differentiation and eventual cell death. Several less common variant translocations with the 17q12 RARA gene have been reported in AML cases with APL-like morphology and immunophenotype, including the ATRA-resistant t(11;17)(q23;q12) *ZBTB16-RARA* and t(17;17)(q11.2;q12) *STAT5B-RARA* cases, as well as likely ATRA-responsive t(11;17)(q13;q12) *NUMA1-RARA* and t(5;17)(q35;q12) *NPM1-RARA*.[25] These variant translocations appear to correlate with morphologic differences, such as in t(11;17)(q23;q12) *ZBTB16-RARA* cases featuring non-bilobed nuclei, no Auer rods and Pelgeroid neutrophils. The WHO 2008 classification indicates that cases with *RARA* translocations other than the classic t(15;17)(q22;q12) should be diagnosed as 'AML with a variant *RARA* translocation'.

AML with t(9;11)(p22;q23); (*MLLT3-MLL*)

The WHO 2008 classification splits t(9;11)(p22;q23); (*MLLT3-MLL*) cases out from the former WHO 2001 category featuring a variety of 11q23 translocations of the *MLL* gene, to reflect the intermediate prognosis of *MLLT3-MLL* cases compared to the poor prognosis of the other 11q23 entities.[26,27] The t(9;11) translocation is usually seen in pediatric patients, and blasts show monocytic or myelomonocytic morphology (FAB M5 or M4). As with other monocytic AML cases, there can be extramedullary disease including involvement of gums, skin and other tissues. The product of the *MLL* gene has been shown to have histone methyltransferase activity and likely plays a role in gene regulation by acting with other chromatin remodeling proteins. The numerous variant translocation partners reported for this gene in AML suggest that there are various ways of preventing normal MLL function, or misdirecting its activity, that can contribute to leukemogenesis.

AML with t(6;9)(p23;q34); (*DEK-NUP214*)

t(6;9) AML is an uncommon variety that can affect a wide age range of patients, and is most distinctive for the presence of BM or blood basophilia (>2% basophils), seen in approximately half of cases (Fig. 18.6).[18,28] WBC counts are typically low in the peripheral blood in adult patients (median value 12×10^9 cells per liter), anemia and thrombocytopenia are common, and myelodysplasia can be seen in all lineages. Patients occasionally present before the blast count has risen to 20%, in which case careful monitoring is recommended. No distinctive morphologic features have been reported for the blasts, which can be myeloid or monocytic, with unremarkable myeloid or monocytoid FCM immunophenotype and cytochemistry.[18] The t(6;9) is most commonly the sole detectable cytogenetic abnormality in these cases, and is given priority for classification over any findings of myelodysplasia. The effects of the fusion of the chromatin-associated protein DEK and the nuclear pore protein NUP214 on the cell have not been elucidated, but could involve derangement of gene expression or nuclear transport, among other possibilities. The prognosis of these cases is generally poor.

Fig. 18.7 (A, B) AML with inv(3)(q21q26.2) (*RPN1-EVI1*) morphology. The small and atypical megakaryocytes are often accompanied by other dysplastic findings in erythroid precursors and granulocytes. Panel (A) shows a bone marrow biopsy. Panel (B) shows the morphology of the bone marrow aspirate smear.

AML with inv(3)(q21q26.2) or t(3;3)(q21;q26.1); (*RPN1-EVI1*)

AML with inv(3) or t(3;3) is relatively rare (1–2% of AML cases), and is primarily a disease of adults. It is commonly found in association with myelodysplastic findings in granulocytes and platelets, with lesser dyspoiesis of the erythroid lineage. PB platelet counts are often within the normal range, or increased. Patients may present before the blast count exceeds 20%. The most striking morphologic feature in the BM is the presence of monolobated or hypolobated megakaryocytes that may be increased in number (Fig. 18.7).[16,17,29] Blasts are myeloid, monocytic or megakaryoblastic with an unremarkable myeloid blast immunophenotype, including possible expression of CD41 and CD61 in megakaryoblastic cases. The *EVI1* (*ecotropic virus integration-1*) gene is an oncogene with zinc finger protein homology, proposed to have transcriptional repression activity via recruitment of histone deacetylases to chromatin.[30] Fusion to the gene for proteasome component *RPN1* may serve primarily to drive high expression of EVI1. Some patients with chronic myelogenous leukemia (CML) develop inv(3) or t(3;3) chromosomal abnormalities, often as their disease accelerates or enters blast crisis, but such cases with documented t(9;22) translocations should be treated as CML rather than AML with inv(3) or t(3;3). Prognosis is usually poor in all AML cases with these chromosome 3 abnormalities.

AML (megakaryoblastic) with t(1;22)(p13;q13); (*RBM15-MKL1*)

This is very rare form of infant leukemia usually seen in patients without Down syndrome. It is commonly associated with hepatosplenomegaly or other organomegaly. The blasts show megakaryocytic differentiation similar to those of the FAB M7 type, and are medium-sized or larger, with rounded nuclei containing fine reticular chromatin, visible nucleoli, agranular basophilic cytoplasm, and occasional cytoplasmic blebbing (Fig. 18.8).[31–33] The FCM immunophenotype commonly shows blasts lacking CD45, CD34 and HLA-DR but expressing myeloid markers CD13 and CD33 as well as megakaryocyte antigens CD41, CD61 and possibly CD42. Overt multilineage dysplastic features are not usually present in the BM, although micromegakaryocytes are common. As with other megakaryoblastic leukemias, BM collagen fibrosis is typically present and may result in aspirates with falsely low blast counts, necessitating correlation with BMTB. The fusion partners in the translocation are *RBM15*, a gene encoding a protein with RNA-binding motifs, and *MKL1*, a transcriptional coactivator of serum response factor (SRF).[34] Prognosis for these patients appears to be relatively good, although the number of patients reported in the literature is low.[35]

Acute myeloid leukemia with gene mutations

Many gene mutations have been detected in AML blasts, but a handful of specific mutations appear to occur most frequently or be most potently selected in the process of leukemogenesis.[5] Mutations in the tyrosine kinase receptor genes *FLT3* (FMS-like tyrosine kinase 3) and *KIT* are relatively common. *FLT3* mutations are found in up to one-third of the 40–50% of adult AML cases that have a normal karyotype, and take the form of internal tandem duplications (ITD) and point mutations of the kinase domain (TKD) that correlate with a poor prognosis.[36] *FLT3* mutation is also seen in AML with recurrent cytogenetic abnormalities and worsens prognosis, although the mutations are uncommon in the context of t(8;21), inv(16) and 11q23 translocations, and may not worsen the already bad prognosis of t(6;9) and inv(3) cases. *KIT* mutations are most common in the core binding factor translocation categories t(8;21) and inv(16), and herald a poorer prognosis.[37]

The 2008 WHO classification creates two new provisional diagnostic entities, defined by mutation in *nucleophosmin* (*NPM1*) or *CCAAT/enhancer binding protein-alpha* (*CEBPA*). These mutations are most often detected in AML with

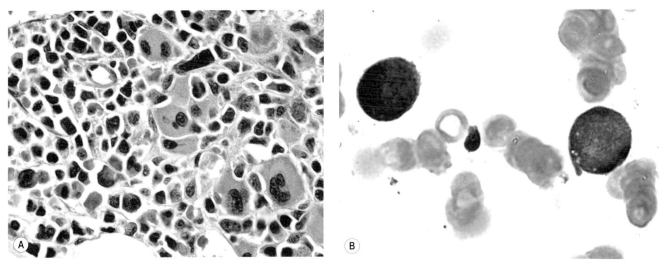

Fig. 18.8 (A, B) AML with t(1;22) p13;q13); (*RBM15-MKL1*). The morphology is that of a megakaryoblastic acute myeloid leukemia. Panel (A) shows the bone marrow biopsy. Panel (B) shows blasts in peripheral blood.

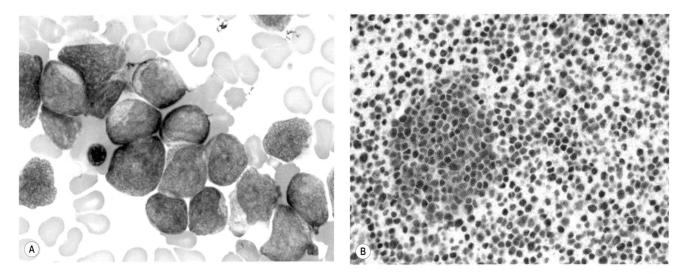

Fig. 18.9 (A, B) (A) AML without maturation, with NPM1 and FLT3-ITD mutation and cup-like nuclear invaginations. (B) Bone marrow trephine biopsy of AML with NPM1 mutation showing infiltrates of blasts with cytoplasmic expression of NPM1 protein. Nuclear-only expression is seen with the areas of normal hematopoiesis.

normal cytogenetics. In the absence of *FLT3*-ITD, mutation of *NPM1* or *CEBPA* indicates a favorable prognosis for the patient's disease.

AML with mutated *NPM1*

The *NPM1* gene at 5q35 encodes a nuclear shuttling protein reported to have roles in ribosome and centrosome biology as well as regulation of other cellular systems such as the *ARF-TP53* tumor suppressor pathway. *NPM1*-mutated AML cases are more common in adults than children (approximately 30% of adult cases and 5% of pediatric ones) and in women compared to men.[38] Most have a normal karyotype, and there is little overlap with cases having recurrent translocations, partial tandem duplication of MLL, or mutations in *CEPBA*. About half of adult normal karyotype AML cases have mutated *NPM1*; about 40% of these (20% of normal

karyotype cases) have both *NPM1* and *FLT3*-ITD mutations. Morphologically, most *NPM1*-mutant cases are myelomonocytic or monocytic without myelodysplastic findings, but other morphologies including AML without maturation (Fig. 18.9A), AML with maturation and erythroleukemia, as well as small numbers of cases with myelodysplasia have also been reported. The blast immunophenotype is typical for myelomonocytic or monocytic AML, but consistent lack of expression of CD34 is a hallmark regardless of blast morphology. A useful immunohistochemical surrogate for mutation in *NPM1* is detection of aberrant cytoplasmic localization of the protein (Fig. 18.9B). Mutations of the gene are typically detected by PCR-based methods, with the most common being tetranucleotide insertions in exon 12 that change the reading frame, ablate a nuclear localization signal and create a spurious nuclear export signal, contributing to the cytoplasmic accumulation of the protein.[39]

Isolated *NPM1* mutation in normal karyotype AML confers a good prognosis, and even cases with coexisting *FLT3*-ITD mutation appear to benefit, compared to those with *FLT3*-ITD alone; however, *NPM1* mutations should always be studied in conjunction with *FLT3* mutations. The significance of *NPM1* mutation in the context of myelodysplasia-related findings, or additional chromosomal abnormalities is less clear.

AML with mutated *CEBPA*

The *CEBPA* gene at 19q31.1 is a tumor suppressor and transcription factor implicated in the differentiation of many disparate cell lineages, including granulocytes.[40] There is evidence that the t(8;21) RUNX1-RUNX1T1 fusion product may act by repressing expression of *CEBPA*. *CEBPA* mutations are detected in approximately 10% of all AML cases, and 15–18% of cases with normal karyotype, with no apparent association with patient age or sex. There is little overlap with cases having *NPM1* mutation, while *FLT3*-ITD mutations occur in approximately 25% of *CEBPA*-mutant cases. Taken together, the clinical features of *CEBPA*-mutant AML suggest relative preservation of erythropoiesis, worse thrombocytopenia, higher blast count in the blood, and less frequent extramedullary disease than AML without *CEBPA* mutation. Blast morphology is most often consistent with FAB M1 (without maturation) and M2 (with maturation), with rarer examples having myelomonocytic or monocytic morphology. Immunophenotype is typical for myeloid blasts, and CD34 and HLA-DR are most often positive. A high percentage of cases show aberrant expression of the T-cell marker CD7. Gene sequencing is needed for full evaluation, given that over 100 distinct mutations have been reported throughout the gene, with 5′ exons often showing frame-shifting insertions or deletions producing truncated dominant-negative protein products, while 3′ exons more commonly have frame-preserving small insertions or deletions.[41,42] The prognosis of isolated *CEBPA*-mutant AML with normal karyotype is favorable; consensus about the effect of this mutation in the context of *FLT3*-ITD or other cytogenetic abnormalities has not yet been reached.

Acute myeloid leukemia with myelodysplasia-related changes (AML-MRC)

AML-MRC is characterized by a myeloid blast count ≥20% in the blood or bone marrow of a patient with any or all of the following: 1) prior history of MDS or myelodysplastic/myeloproliferative neoplasm; 2) characteristic myelodysplasia-associated cytogenetic abnormalities; 3) multilineage dysplasia in at least 50% of cells in two cell lineages. The kind of data supporting the AML-MRC diagnosis should be included in the bottom line of the pathology report. There should be no history of cytotoxic chemotherapy or radiation treatment (which would warrant classification as therapy-related AML) and no evidence for 'AML with recurrent genetic abnormality' cytogenetic abnormalities, which take diagnostic precedence. This diagnosis is more common in older patients and very rare in the pediatric population, but with the new cytogenetic criteria introduced

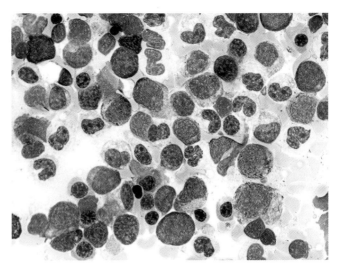

Fig. 18.10 AML with myelodysplasia-related changes. Blasts and dysplastic precursors of all three hematopoietic lineages were present in this case.

in the WHO 2008 classification, the rate of diagnosis in children will likely increase. The clinical features of the case may be dominated by severe cytopenias. For establishing morphologic multilineage dysplasia, the following findings should be documented: neutrophils with hypogranular cytoplasm, hyposegmented nuclei, or bizarre nuclear segmentation patterns; erythroid precursors with megaloblastoid changes (with delayed nuclear maturation relative to cytoplasmic hemoglobinization), multiple nuclei, irregular nuclear contours, nuclear fragments, or the presence of ring sideroblasts, cytoplasmic inclusions, or periodic acid-Schiff (PAS) staining vacuoles; and megakaryocytes with micromegakaryocyte morphology, hyposegmented nuclei, or widely-separated nuclear lobes (Fig. 18.10).[43] Blast morphology is variable, but blast with features of AML with maturation and acute myelomonocytic leukemia are most common. Some cases are designated as hypocellular AML, if BM cellularity is less than 30%, or less than 20% in patients over 60 years of age; these cases often represent progression of hypocellular MDS. Immunophenotyping is of limited utility for diagnosis, as the blasts show typical myeloid marker expression and common non-specific aberrancies such as expression of CD7 or TdT. The defining cytogenetic abnormalities for AML-MRC are similar to those defining MDS and listed in Table 20.5. Many of these are monosomies or chromosome arm losses, but a number of balanced translocations can also be used to support the diagnosis once a prior history of chemotherapy or radiation exposure is ruled out. Strikingly, up to half of cases with these defining cytogenetic abnormalities do not show sufficient morphologic evidence to meet the criteria for multilineage dysplasia. It appears from clinical trials that the AML-MRC-defining cytogenetic abnormalities portend a worse prognosis than do isolated morphologic findings of multilineage dysplasia. The presence of mutations in other significant AML-associated genes such as *FLT3*, *NPM1* and *CEBPA* should be evaluated and noted in the report in cases with normal cytogenetics but multilineage dysplasia. Prognosis in AML-MRC is poor, and appears worse still for patients with characteristic monosomies or expression of the *EVI1* gene.[43–45]

Therapy-related myeloid neoplasms

The previous, 2001 WHO classification included categories for AML arising following alkylating agent therapy (usually 5–7 years after treatment, with a period of MDS seen) or topoisomerase II inhibitor therapy (usually 1–3 years after treatment). In the 2008 WHO classification, a single category of therapy-related AML (t-AML) is used to encompass these entities as well as AML arising following other cytotoxic drug treatments including fludarabine and anti-tubulin drugs, as well as ionizing radiation if used on large fields containing active bone marrow. These cases together comprise approximately 15% of AML diagnoses, and most show multilineage dysplasia, often with myelodysplasia-associated chromosome abnormalities such as loss of part or all of chromosomes 5 or 7, a complex karyotype, or, in patients with a history of topoisomerase II inhibitor treatment, translocations involving 11q23.[46,47] A variety of myeloid blast morphologies can be seen, with monoblastic and myelomonocytic cytology being most common. Immunophenotype is not specific for t-AML and is usually consistent with the blast morphology. Prognosis is poor, but appears to be influenced by the underlying cytogenetic abnormalities as well as the initial malignancy for which the patient was treated.

Acute myeloid leukemia, not otherwise specified (AML, NOS)

This category now represents a diagnosis of exclusion, for those leukemias that do not meet the criteria for the other genetically-defined, myelodysplasia-associated, or therapy-related types. The subtypes within AML, NOS are defined by blast morphology, immunophenotype and cytochemical staining, and largely follow the former FAB categories. The shift from the FAB classification to the WHO 2001 and 2008 schemes warrants caution in reading the older medical literature, since many leukemias that would have been classified as particular FAB entities are currently classified in the various new categories. Blood or BM blasts must be ≥20% of nucleated cells for this category, with the exception of erythroblastic leukemias where modified counting rules are employed.

AML with minimal differentiation

This relatively rare AML variety corresponds in part with FAB M0 AML and is most common in infants and the elderly. Blasts are usually medium-sized, with dispersed or partially condensed chromatin, inconspicuous nucleoli, and minimal agranular basophilic cytoplasm without Auer rods. Some cases have smaller blasts with more condensed chromatin, morphologically indistinguishable from lymphoblasts. With these findings, the differential diagnosis includes lymphoblastic leukemias, megakaryoblastic AML, acute leukemias of ambiguous lineage, and blastic lymphomas. The immunophenotype reveals the myeloid nature of the blasts, with any or all of CD13, CD117 and CD33 seen, but no evidence of later differentiation markers of myeloid (CD11b, CD15, CD65) or monocytic (CD14, CD64) lineage, or of lymphoid markers apart from TdT. CD34, CD38 and HLA-DR are often positive. FCM may detect small numbers of blasts with

cytoplasmic MPO antigen present, but by definition for this category <3% of blasts may show cytochemical staining for MPO, SBB or CAE. Occasional weak nonspecific staining for NSE is seen but is distinct from monocytic staining. Many cases formerly classified as AML FAB-M0 now fall into the AML with myelodysplasia-related changes category.

AML without maturation

AML without maturation corresponds in part with FAB M1 AML and is defined by cases where blasts are ≥90% of non-erythroid cells, and there is minimal differentiation to more mature granulocyte forms. Older epidemiologic data indicate that 5–10% of all AML cases meet these criteria. Blast morphology can be similar to that of AML with minimal differentiation, or can show basophilic cytoplasmic granulation or even Auer rods, but by definition at least 3% of blasts must show cytochemical staining for MPO or SBB. Immunophenotype shows cytoplasmic staining for MPO, as well as surface expression of any or all of the myeloid markers CD13, CD33, CD117, or more rarely, CD11b. CD34 and HLA-DR are most often positive, and there is usually no staining for mature granulocyte markers CD15 or CD65 or monocyte markers CD14 and CD64. Aberrant expression of less-specific lymphoid markers such as CD7 is not infrequent, but more specific cytoplasmic lymphoid markers such as cCD3, cCD79a and cCD22 are not seen. Many cases of FAB M1 AML are now classified as AML with *NPM1* mutation (with or without concurrent *FLT3* mutation); these are associated with some specific features, including a high absolute blast count and cup-like nuclear invaginations in the blasts, lack of CD34 or HLA-DR expression, and normal karyotype (Fig. 18.9A). A second group of reclassified cases comprises those with myelodysplasia-related changes. The less common AML with *CEBPA* mutation category has a predominance of cases with FAB M1 morphology immunophenotype and cytochemistry.

AML with maturation

This group corresponds in part with FAB M2 AML and is distinguished from AML without maturation by the presence of maturing granulocytes making up more than 10% of non-erythroid BM nucleated cells, with <20% monocytic lineage cells present, and myeloblasts comprising 20–89% of non-erythroid cells. Blasts commonly show cytoplasmic granules, and Auer rods are often seen. Cytochemistry and immunophenotype show typical myeloid reactivity and antigen expression, including more mature markers such as CD11b, CD15 or CD65, usually without expression of monocytic markers CD14 and CD64. Current classification puts many cases with FAB M2 findings into categories based on recurrent genetic abnormalities or myelodysplasia-related changes.

Acute myelomonocytic leukemia (AMML)

These cases correspond in part with FAB M4 AML and are separated from AML without maturation or AML with maturation by the requirement for more than 20% monocyte lineage cells and more than 20% maturing granulocyte lineage cells among non-erythroid BM nucleated cells. Myeloblasts, monoblasts and promonocytes must comprise 20%

or more of total nucleated cells in blood or BM. The FCM immunophenotype of blasts shows typical myeloid and monocytic patterns. Diagnostic challenges can include distinguishing AMML from chronic myelomonocytic leukemia (CMML), which requires the pathologist to distinguish between promonocytes, with their less mature chromatin, subtle nucleoli, and delicate nuclear folds, and the more mature atypical monocytes in CMML, which have greater chromatin condensation and nuclear convolution or folding. Definitive diagnosis in such cases requires correlation with the BM, where more immature forms may be more obvious. Post-chemotherapy recovering BM specimens may also show many immature monocyte lineage cells, making it difficult to assess for residual disease in patients with a history of AML with monocytic or myelomonocytic features. In such cases, if there is no telltale immunophenotypic aberrancy, resampling the BM after additional recovery time may help resolve the conundrum. Many cases formerly diagnosed as FAB M4 are now found to be AML with *NPM1* mutation or AML with myelodysplasia-related changes in the WHO 2008 scheme.

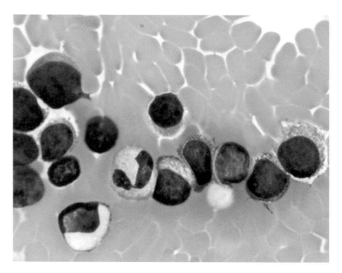

Fig. 18.11 AML-NOS: acute erythroid leukemia (pure erythroid leukemia) morphology.

Acute monoblastic and monocytic leukemia

In these cases, which correspond in part with FAB M5a and M5b AML, monoblasts, promonocytes and monocytes comprise at least 80% of non-erythroid nucleated BM cells, while maturing neutrophil lineage cells must be <20%. In monoblastic cases, monoblasts make up at least 80% of the monocytic cells, whereas acute monocytic cases have a majority of promonocytes. Clinically, there is a tendency towards extramedullary disease, particularly involving the skin, gums or CNS. Monoblasts are typically relatively large blasts with rounded nuclear contours, fine lacy chromatin with visible nucleoli, and ample variably basophilic cytoplasm that may be agranular or contain MPO-negative fine basophilic granules. Auer rods are not seen in monoblasts. MPO cytochemistry is usually negative, and NSE is positive. Promonocytes are considered blast-equivalents, and often have less basophilic, finely granulated cytoplasm and show characteristic delicate nuclear folds not seen in monoblasts. Cytoplasmic vacuoles can be seen in both monoblasts and promonocytes. The blast immunophenotype in these cases often lacks CD34, but includes HLA-DR and myeloid antigens such as CD13, CD15, CD65, or CD33, which is often bright. Several or many monocytic markers including CD4, CD11b, CD11c, CD14, CD36, CD64, CD163 or lysozyme may be expressed. Many AML cases with features of the FAB M5 category contain translocations involving *MLL* at 11q23. If a case shows the t(9;11)(p22;q23); (*MLLT3-MLL*), it should be classified as AML with recurring genetic abnormality; other 11q23 cases, if not in a patient with a history of cytotoxic therapy, can be classified as AML, NOS, with the chromosomal abnormality noted in the report. If hemophagocytosis is seen in cases with maturation or with monocytic or myelomonocytic features, it may indicate the presence of the relatively uncommon t(8;16)(p11.2;p13.3) translocation, which does not define an AML with recurrent genetic abnormalities category but is frequently associated with hemophagocytosis.[48]

Acute erythroid leukemia

Erythroid precursors and/or blasts are the predominant cell type of this leukemia, which partially corresponds to FAB M6, is relatively rare (<5% of AML) and is found mainly in adults. In the more common erythroid/myeloid variant, erythroid precursors represent at least 50% of total BM nucleated cells, and myeloblasts are at least 20% of the remaining non-erythroid nucleated cells. The less common pure erythroid leukemia is diagnosed when at least 80% of BM nucleated cells are undifferentiated or proerythroblastic cells, without evidence for a significant myeloblast population among non-erythroid nucleated cells (Fig. 18.11).[49] The erythroid/myeloid variant usually presents with pancytopenia and circulating nucleated red cells, while the BM erythroid precursors can be strikingly abnormal, with megaloblastoid changes, fragmented or multiple nuclei, and blocky cytoplasmic PAS staining. Dysplastic features are common in megakaryocytes as well, and many cases meet the morphologic criteria of AML with myelodysplasia-related changes and should be classified as such. The myeloid blasts typically show a lack of maturation by morphology and immunophenotype. FCM of erythroblasts in these cases often shows a population lacking CD34 and HLA-DR, without myeloid antigens, and expressing aberrant dim CD71 (transferrin receptor), glycophorin, and possibly hemoglobin A. The proerythroblasts and early basophilic erythroblasts of pure erythroid leukemia show a similar immunophenotype. Expression of megakaryocytic markers such as CD41 or CD61 may complicate distinguishing erythroleukemia cases from acute megakaryoblastic leukemias. A variety of non-neoplastic causes of dyserythropoiesis and erythroid hyperplasia must be ruled out, including vitamin B_{12} or folate deficiency, drug effects, heavy metal poisoning, and congenital dyserythropoietic disorders.

Acute megakaryoblastic leukemia

Most AML cases with megakaryoblasts, corresponding to AML FAB M7, now meet the 2008 WHO criteria for AML with t(1;22), AML with myelodysplasia-related changes, or the Down syndrome-associated disorders discussed below. The small number of remaining cases may, like other megakaryoblastic leukemias, demonstrate extensive marrow fibrosis limiting marrow aspiration. The blasts are relatively large with dense smooth chromatin, variable nucleoli, and scant to moderate amounts of cytoplasm. The cytoplasmic membrane may show irregular contours, and some examples show membrane protrusions or blebs. A spectrum of morphologies toward micromegakaryocytes is sometimes seen. FCM often reveals blasts lacking CD34, HLA-DR and CD45, variable expression of myeloid markers such as CD13 or CD33, and frequent expression of megakaryocyte antigens CD41 or CD61. At least 50% of blasts must show evidence of megakaryocytic differentiation. Ultrastructural analysis and ultracytochemistry can be diagnostic if demarcation membranes or bulls-eye granules are visualized, or if peroxidase activity is visualized in the nuclear membrane and endoplasmic reticulum but not the Golgi body or granules.[50,51] Prognosis in both adults and children is poor.

Acute basophilic leukemia

This is a vanishingly rare leukemia showing blasts with aberrant basophilic differentiation and occasional involvement of skin, bones or other tissues, sometimes with symptoms of hyperhistaminemia. Reported immunophenotypes show lack of CD117, with variable CD34 and HLA-DR, and frequent expression of CD13 or CD33 with CD123, CD22 and CD11b. Cytochemistry is negative for MPO or SBB reactivity. One report using electron microscopy methods suggests that this may be an under-recognized entity.[52,53] Acute basophilic leukemia may be difficult to distinguish from another rare entity, acute mast cell leukemia, which is described in Chapter 26.

Acute panmyelosis with myelofibrosis (APMF)

Another very rare disease, acute panmyelosis, must, by definition, present *de novo* rather than evolving from another condition. Acute panmyelosis with myelofibrosis (APMF) features pancytopenia, myelofibrosis, a proliferation of all myeloid lineages (panmyelosis) and increased blasts.[54,55] There is usually prominent reticulin fibrosis, with fewer cases showing collagen fibrosis. Megakaryocytic dysplasia is often seen, but there must be insufficient evidence to diagnosis AML with myelodysplasia-related changes in order to consider this diagnosis. Myelodysplastic syndrome with fibrosis must also be ruled out, based on the blast count. The presence of dysplastic features and a lack of splenomegaly distinguish this entity from most myeloproliferative neoplasms. APMF typically differs from acute megakaryoblastic leukemia by showing expression of CD34 on blasts and by the panmyeloid proliferation seen amid the marrow fibrosis. The prognosis is typically poor.

Myeloid sarcoma

Mass involvement of a tissue site by myeloid blasts defines myeloid sarcoma. These lesions can present in isolation, or may accompany blood or BM myeloid diseases including MDS, myeloproliferative neoplasms, or myelodysplastic/myeloproliferative varieties. In any case, myeloid sarcoma is equivalent to a diagnosis of AML regardless of blast counts in blood or BM. The subcategories of myeloid sarcoma in the WHO 2001 classification have now been consolidated into a single category. Pediatric cases are less likely than adult cases to present without blood or BM leukemia, but are more likely to show 11q23 or (8;21) translocations, although the source of tissue for karyotypic analysis may be a possible confounder of these data, given that most adult samples are biopsied tissues, whereas pediatric samples are typically from BM blast populations. Inclusion of this entity in the differential diagnosis for tissue masses is critical, as many of the most helpful immunohistochemical stains may not be part of routine panels used to evaluate suspected lymphomas or small round blue cell tumors. Immunostains for myeloperoxidase, CD33, CD68, CD4, CD163, CD34, CD117, CD43, LAT and CD61 can help to evaluate suspected cases, although CD34 is commonly negative on the monocytic leukemic blasts that are a frequent cause of these lesions.[56] CD68 is the most commonly positive marker in myeloid sarcomas overall, but is not particularly specific. In the unlikely circumstance that a portion of the specimen has not already been formalin-fixed at the time of morphologic review, FCM and cytochemical stains can greatly assist diagnosis.

Myeloid proliferations related to Down syndrome

Down syndrome patients show a 10 to 100-fold increase in leukemia incidence compared to the rest of the population. Two unique entities with megakaryoblastic morphology have been reported in the early years of life, and are given separate status in the 2008 WHO classification.

Transient abnormal myelopoiesis (TAM)

Roughly one-tenth of patients with Down syndrome are born with clinical findings of acute megakaryoblastic leukemia, but in approximately 75% of cases the disease undergoes a mysterious spontaneous remission within a few months.[57,58] Despite this favorable behavior, some cases cause life-threatening complications such as cardiac or respiratory compromise, hyperviscosity, hepatic or renal dysfunction (particularly hepatic fibrosis), splenic necrosis or disseminated intravascular coagulopathy. The blasts have morphology consistent with the former FAB M7 megakaryoblastic category, and most often express CD34, CD4, typical myeloid markers such as CD13, CD33 and CD117, megakaryocytic markers CD41, CD42, CD61, or CD71, and aberrant CD7 and CD56, without expression of myeloperoxidase, glycophorin, HLA-DR or monocytic markers CD14 or CD64. An unusual genetic feature of these cases beyond the patient's trisomy 21 is the frequent mutation of the *GATA1* transcription factor gene.[59] There is little consensus about optimal therapeutic strategies for this usually transient condition.

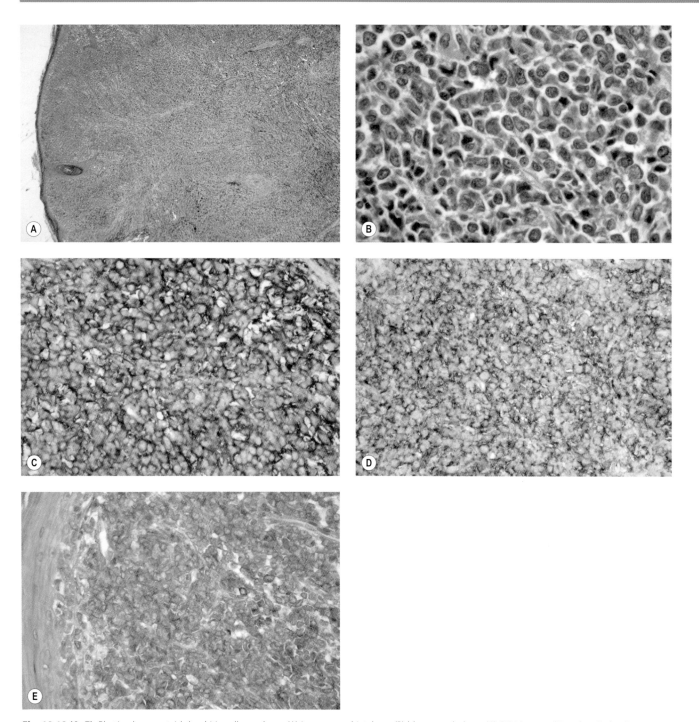

Fig. 18.12 (A–E) Blastic plasmacytoid dendritic cell neoplasm. (A) Low-power histology; (B) blast morphology; (C) CD4 immunohistochemical stain; (D) CD56 immunohistochemical stain; (E) CD123 immunohistochemical stain. *(Photos courtesy of Dr Roger Warnke, Department of Pathology, Stanford University.)*

Myeloid leukemia associated with Down syndrome

In 20–30% of Down syndrome patients who develop transient abnormal myelopoiesis, the transient disease is followed within 1–3 years by a recurrent and non-remitting AML. PB cytopenias and BM myelodysplastic features often precede the development of ≥20% blasts in the blood or BM, but no distinction is made between MDS and AML in this context. The BM may show extensive fibrosis. Extramedullary disease, particularly in the liver and spleen, is common. The blast immunophenotype is similar to that seen in TAM, except that about half of cases have CD34-negative blasts, and a third of cases fail to express CD41 and CD56. In addition to trisomy 21, these leukemias share the *GATA1* mutations seen in TAM, and have a relatively high rate of complete or partial trisomy 8 and trisomy 1.[59] The prognosis is very good compared to other childhood cases of AML. If an older Down syndrome child develops AML without *GATA1* mutation, the leukemia should be classified as a conventional, non-Down syndrome case would be.

Blastic plasmacytoid dendritic cell (BPDC) neoplasm

This rare entity, formerly referred to as blastic NK lymphoma or agranular CD4[+] CD56[+] hepatodermic neoplasm, is an aggressive malignancy often presenting in the skin with frequent BM and systemic leukemic involvement.[60–62] The closeness of its relationship to other acute myeloid leukemias in the 2008 WHO classification is debatable; indeed, the underlying developmental pathways and physiology of plasmacytoid dendritic cells are subjects of current research.[63] It appears that the plasmacytoid dendritic cells seen in the T-cell zones of lymphoid tissues are the predominant source of type I interferon in response to viral infections. Apparently reactive proliferations of plasmacytoid dendritic cells can be seen in association with CMML, hyaline vascular Castleman's disease, viral infections and granulomatous lymphadenitis, and can usually be distinguished from BPDC neoplasm by their normal morphology and lack of CD56 expression. The violaceous nodules formed by the neoplasm in the skin typically show sparing of the epidermis and infiltration of the dermis and subcutaneous fat. Most patients also show BM involvement ranging from sparse to full infiltration. In approximately 65% of cases, circulating tumor cells in the blood are seen. Roughly half of cases have disease in the lymph nodes and a third have disease in the spleen. The tumor cells are medium-sized blasts with irregular nuclear contours, smooth chromatin, one to several visible nucleoli, and scant agranular blue-gray cytoplasm sometimes containing microvacuoles (Fig. 18.12A, B). The blastic cells are negative for CD34 and CD117, but express CD4 (Fig.18.12C), CD56 (Fig.18.12D), TCL1, CD43, CD45RA, CD68 (as small cytoplasmic dots), the plasmacytoid dendritic cell marker CD123 (the IL-3 receptor alpha chain, Fig.18.12E), BDCA-2 (CD303), CLA (cutaneous lymphocyte-associated antigen), the interferon-alpha induced MxA (myxovirus-resistance protein A), CD2-AP (CD2 adapter protein) and, in about one-third of cases, TdT.[64,65] Expression of CD34, CD117, CD14, CD13 or lysozyme argues against BPDC, and would favor a diagnosis of AML. Cytogenetic analysis usually shows a complex karyotype with loss of 5q, 12p, 6q, and deletions of chromosomes 13, 9 and 15 being relatively common abnormalities. If one of the recurrent genetic abnormalities of AML in the 2008 WHO classification is detected, then the case should be classified as AML. Similarly, cytochemical stains for MPO or NSE should be negative, and prompt classification as AML if positive. The prognosis of the disease is poor, with median survival of approximately 1 year.

References

1. Bhayat F, Das-Gupta E, Smith C, et al. The incidence of and mortality from leukaemias in the UK: a general population-based study. BMC Cancer 2009;9:252.

2. Deschler B, Lubbert M. Acute myeloid leukemia: epidemiology and etiology. Cancer 2006 Nov 1;107(9):2099–107.

3. Yamamoto JF, Goodman MT. Patterns of leukemia incidence in the United States by subtype and demographic characteristics, 1997–2002. Cancer Causes Control 2008 May;19(4):379–90.

4. Aquino VM. Acute myelogenous leukemia. Curr Probl Pediatr Adolesc Health Care 2002 Feb;32(2):50–8.

5. Mrozek K, Marcucci G, Paschka P, et al. Clinical relevance of mutations and gene-expression changes in adult acute myeloid leukemia with normal cytogenetics: are we ready for a prognostically prioritized molecular classification? Blood 2007 Jan 15;109(2): 431–48.

6. Swerdlow SH, Campo E, Harris NL, et al., editors. WHO Classification of Tumours of Haematopoietic and Lymphoid Tissues. 4th ed. Lyon: IARC; 2008.

7. Ley TJ, Mardis ER, Ding L, et al. DNA sequencing of a cytogenetically normal acute myeloid leukaemia genome. Nature 2008 Nov 6;456(7218):66–72.

8. Mardis ER, Ding L, Dooling DJ, et al. Recurring mutations found by sequencing an acute myeloid leukemia genome. N Engl J Med 2009 Sep 10;361(11): 1058–66.

9. Walter MJ, Payton JE, Ries RE, et al. Acquired copy number alterations in adult acute myeloid leukemia genomes. Proc Natl Acad Sci USA 2009 Aug 4;106(31): 12950–5.

10. Jaffe ES, Harris NL, Stein H, Vardiman JW. World Health Organization Classification of Tumours: Pathology and Genetics of Tumours of Haematopoietic and Lymphoid Tissues. Lyon, France: IARC Press; 2001.

11. Greenberg P, Cox C, LeBeau MM, et al. International scoring system for evaluating prognosis in myelodysplastic syndromes. Blood 1997 Mar 15;89(6):2079–88.

12. Khalidi HS, Medeiros LJ, Chang KL, et al. The immunophenotype of adult acute myeloid leukemia: High frequency of lymphoid antigen expression and comparison of immunophenotype, French-American-British classification, and karyotypic abnormalities. American Journal of Clinical Pathology 1998;109: 211–20.

13. Bennett JM, Catovsky D, Daniel MT, et al. Proposals for the classification of the acute leukaemias. French-American-British (FAB) co-operative group. Br J Haematol 1976 Aug;33(4):451–8.

14. de Labarthe A, Pautas C, Thomas X, et al. Allogeneic stem cell transplantation in second rather than first complete remission in selected patients with good-risk acute myeloid leukemia. Bone Marrow Transplant 2005 Apr;35(8): 767–73.

15. Schlenk RF, Dohner K, Krauter J, et al. Mutations and treatment outcome in cytogenetically normal acute myeloid leukemia. New England Journal of Medicine 2008;358(18): 1909–18.

16. Bitter MA, Neilly ME, Le Beau MM, et al. Rearrangements of chromosome 3 involving bands 3q21 and 3q26 are associated with normal or elevated platelet counts in acute nonlymphocytic leukemia. Blood 1985 Dec;66(6): 1362–70.

17. Secker-Walker LM, Mehta A, Bain B. Abnormalities of 3q21 and 3q26 in myeloid malignancy: a United Kingdom Cancer Cytogenetic Group study. Br J Haematol 1995 Oct;91(2):490–501.

18. Slovak ML, Gundacker H, Bloomfield CD, et al. A retrospective study of 69 patients with t(6;9)(p23;q34) AML emphasizes the need for a prospective, multicenter initiative for rare 'poor prognosis' myeloid

malignancies. Leukemia 2006 Jul; 20(7):1295–7.

19. Arber DA, Carter NH, Ikle D, Slovak ML. Value of combined morphologic, cytochemical, and immunophenotypic features in predicting recurrent cytogenetic abnormalities in acute myeloid leukemia. Hum Pathol 2003 May;34(5):479–83.

20. Downing JR. The AML1-ETO chimaeric transcription factor in acute myeloid leukaemia: biology and clinical significance. British Journal of Haematology 1999;106:296–308.

21. Byrd JC, Mrozek K, Dodge RK, et al. Pretreatment cytogenetic abnormalities are predictive of induction success, cumulative incidence of relapse, and overall survival in adult patients with de novo acute myeloid leukemia: results from Cancer and Leukemia Group B (CALGB 8461). Blood 2002 Dec 15;100(13):4325–36.

22. Golomb HM, Rowley JD, Vardiman JW, et al. 'Microgranular' acute promyelocytic leukemia: a distinct clinical, ultrastructural, and cytogenetic entity. Blood 1980;55(2):253–9.

23. McKenna RW, Parkin J, Bloomfield CD, et al. Acute promyelocytic leukaemia: a study of 39 cases with identification of a hyperbasophilic microgranular variant. British Journal of Haematology 1982; 50:201–14.

24. Neame PB, Soamboonsrup P, Leber B, et al. Morphology of acute promyelocytic leukemia with cytogenetic or molecular evidence for the diagnosis: charaterization of additional microgranular variants. American Journal of Hematology 1997; 6:131–42.

25. Redner RL. Variations on a theme: the alternate translocations in APL. Leukemia 2002 Oct;16(10):1927–32.

26. Rubnitz JE, Raimondi SC, Tong X, et al. Favorable impact of the t(9;11) in childhood acute myeloid leukemia. Journal of Clinical Oncology 2002;20(9): 2302–9.

27. Mrozek K, Heinonen K, Lawrence D, et al. Adult patients with de novo acute myeloid leukemia and t(9;11)(p22;q23) have a superior outcome to patients with other translocations involving band 11q23: a Cancer and Leukemia Group B study. Blood 1997;90(11):4532–8.

28. Pearson MG, Vardiman JW, Le Beau MM, et al. Increased numbers of marrow basophils may be associated with a t(6;9) in ANLL. Am J Hematol 1985 Apr;18(4): 393–403.

29. Sweet DL, Golomb HM, Rowley JD, Vardiman JW. Acute myelogenous leukemia and thrombocythemia associated with an abnormality of chromosome no. 3. Cancer Genetics and Cytogenetics 1979;1(1):33–7.

30. Cattaneo F, Nucifora G. EVI1 recruits the histone methyltransferase SUV39H1 for transcription repression. J Cell Biochem 2008 Oct 1;105(2):344–52.

31. Carroll A, Civin C, Schneider N, et al. The t(1;22) (p13;q13) is nonrandom and restricted to infants with acute megakaryoblastic leukemia: a Pediatric Oncology Group Study. Blood 1991;78(3): 748–52.

32. Chan WC, Carroll A, Alvarado CS, et al. Acute megakaryoblastic leukemia in infants with t(1;22)(p13;q13) abnormality. American Journal of Clinical Pathology 1992;98(2):214–21.

33. Lion T, Haas OA, Harbott J, et al. The translocation t(1;22)(p13;q13) is a nonrandom marker specifically associated with acute megakaryocytic leukemia in young children. Blood 1992;79(12): 3325–30.

34. Cen B, Selvaraj A, Prywes R. Myocardin/ MKL family of SRF coactivators: key regulators of immediate early and muscle specific gene expression. J Cell Biochem 2004 Sep 1;93(1):74–82.

35. Duchayne E, Fenneteau O, Pages MP, et al. Acute megakaryoblastic leukaemia: a national clinical and biological study of 53 adult and childhood cases by the Groupe Francais d'Hematologie Cellulaire (GFHC). Leuk Lymphoma 2003 Jan; 44(1):49–58.

36. Kottaridis PD, Gale RE, Linch DC. Flt3 mutations and leukaemia. Br J Haematol 2003 Aug;122(4):523–38.

37. Paschka P, Marcucci G, Ruppert AS, et al. Adverse prognostic significance of KIT mutations in adult acute myeloid leukemia with inv(16) and t(8;21): a Cancer and Leukemia Group B Study. J Clin Oncol 2006;24(24):3904–11.

38. Falini B, Nicoletti I, Martelli MF, Mecucci C. Acute myeloid leukemia carrying cytoplasmic/mutated nucleophosmin (NPMc+ AML): biologic and clinical features. Blood 2007;109(3):874–85.

39. Bolli N, Nicoletti I, De Marco MF, et al. Born to be exported: COOH-terminal nuclear export signals of different strength ensure cytoplasmic accumulation of nucleophosmin leukemic mutants. Cancer Research 2007;67(13):6230–7.

40. Koschmieder S, Halmos B, Levantini E, Tenen DG. Dysregulation of the C/ EBPalpha differentiation pathway in human cancer. Journal of Clinical Oncology 2009;27(4):619–28.

41. Ahn JY, Seo K, Weinberg O, et al. A comparison of two methods for screening CEBPA mutations in patients with acute myeloid leukemia. JMolDiagn 2009; 11(4):319–23.

42. Ho PA, Alonzo TA, Gerbing RB, et al. Prevalence and prognostic implications of CEBPA mutations in pediatric acute myeloid leukemia (AML): a report from the Children's Oncology Group. Blood 2009;113(26):6558–66.

43. Arber DA, Stein AS, Carter NH, et al. Prognostic impact of acute myeloid leukemia classification. Importance of detection of recurring cytogenetic abnormalities and multilineage dysplasia on survival. Am J Clin Pathol 2003 May; 119(5):672–80.

44. Lugthart S, van Drunen E, van Norden Y, et al. High EVI1 levels predict adverse outcome in acute myeloid leukemia: prevalence of EVI1 overexpression and chromosome 3q26 abnormalities underestimated. Blood 2008;111(8): 4329–37.

45. Breems DA, van Putten WL, De Greef GE, et al. Monosomal karyotype in acute myeloid leukemia: a better indicator of poor prognosis than a complex karyotype. Journal of Clinical Oncology 2008;26(29): 4791–7.

46. Rund D, Ben-Yehuda D. Therapy-related leukemia and myelodysplasia: evolving concepts of pathogenesis and treatment. Hematology 2004 Jun;9(3):179–87.

47. Rund D, Krichevsky S, Bar-Cohen S, et al. Therapy-related leukemia: clinical characteristics and analysis of new molecular risk factors in 96 adult patients. Leukemia 2005 Nov;19(11):1919–28.

48. Haferlach T, Kohlmann A, Klein HU, et al. AML with translocation t(8;16)(p11;p13) demonstrates unique cytomorphological, cytogenetic, molecular and prognostic features. Leukemia 2009;23(5):934–43.

49. Garand R, Duchayne E, Blanchard D, et al. Minimally differentiated erythroleukaemia (AML M6 'variant'): a rare subset of AML distinct from AML M6. British Journal of Haematology 1995;90:868–75.

50. Eguchi M, Ozawa T, Sakakibara H, et al. Ultrastructural and ultracytochemical differences between megakaryoblastic leukemia in children and adults. Analysis of 49 patients. Cancer 1992 Jul 15;70(2): 451–8.

51. Zipursky A, Christensen H, De Harven E. Ultrastructural studies of the megakaryoblastic leukemias of Down syndrome. Leuk Lymphoma 1995 Jul; 18(3–4):341–7.

52. Peterson LC, Parkin JL, Arthur DC, Brunning RD. Acute basophilic leukemia. A clinical, morphologic, and cytogenetic study of eight cases. American Journal of Clinical Pathology 1991;96(2):160–70.

53. Shvidel L, Shaft D, Stark B, et al. Acute basophilic leukaemia: eight unsuspected new cases diagnosed by electron microscopy. Br J Haematol 2003;120(5): 774–81.

54. Bearman RM, Pangalis GA, Rappaport H. Acute ('malignant') myelosclerosis. Cancer 1979;43(1):279–93.

55. Sultan C, Sigaux F, Imbert M, Reyes F. Acute myelodysplasia with myelofibrosis: a report of eight cases. BrJ Haematol 1981;49(1):11–16.

56. Pileri SA, Ascani S, Cox MC, et al. Myeloid sarcoma: clinico-pathologic, phenotypic and cytogenetic analysis of 92 adult patients. Leukemia 2007;21(2): 340–50.

57. Massey GV, Zipursky A, Chang MN, et al. A prospective study of the natural history of transient leukemia (TL) in neonates with Down syndrome (DS): Children's Oncology Group (COG) study POG–9481. Blood 2006;107(12):4606–13.

58. Ganick DJ. Hematological changes in Down's syndrome. Crit Rev Oncol Hematol 1986;6(1):55–69.

59. Pine SR, Guo Q, Yin C, et al. Incidence and clinical implications of GATA1 mutations in newborns with Down syndrome. Blood 2007;110(6):2128–31.

60. Brody JP, Allen S, Schulman P, et al. Acute agranular CD4-positive natural killer cell leukemia. Comprehensive clinicopathologic studies including virologic and in vitro culture with inducing agents. Cancer 1995 May 15; 75(10):2474–83.

61. Feuillard J, Jacob MC, Valensi F, et al. Clinical and biologic features of CD4(+) CD56(+) malignancies. Blood 2002 Mar 1;99(5):1556–63.

62. DiGiuseppe JA, Louie DC, Williams JE, et al. Blastic natural killer cell leukemia/ lymphoma: a clinicopathologic study. American Journal of Surgical Pathology 1997;21(10):1223–30.

63. Herling M, Jones D. CD4+/CD56+ hematodermic tumor: the features of an evolving entity and its relationship to dendritic cells. Am J Clin Pathol 2007 May;127(5):687–700.

64. Pilichowska ME, Fleming MD, Pinkus JL, Pinkus GS. CD4+/CD56+ hematodermic neoplasm ('blastic natural killer cell lymphoma'): neoplastic cells express the immature dendritic cell marker BDCA-2 and produce interferon. Am J Clin Pathol 2007 Sep;128(3):445–53.

65. Marafioti T, Paterson JC, Ballabio E, et al. Novel markers of normal and neoplastic human plasmacytoid dendritic cells. Blood 2008 Apr 1;111(7):3778–92.

CHAPTER 19

Acute lymphoblastic leukemia/lymphoma and mixed phenotype acute leukemias

A Porwit, M-C Béné

Chapter Contents

Introduction

Acute leukemias are clonal malignant diseases of early hematopoietic progenitor cells. The lymphoblastic forms (acute lyphoblastic leukemia, ALL) are characterized by homogeneous blast cell populations. The accurate diagnosis and classification of acute lymphoblastic and mixed phenotype acute leukemias requires multiple diagnostic techniques[1] including:

- microscopy (morphology, cytochemistry and histology)
- immunophenotyping (flow cytometry and/or immunohistochemistry)
- genetics (metaphase karyotyping, fluorescence in situ hybridization (FISH))
- and/or molecular genetics.

All of these techniques are complementary in the diagnostic process. The diagnosis is primarily based on examination of peripheral blood (PB) and bone marrow (BM), but the disease may involve lymph nodes, central nervous system (CSN), skin, testes and other soft tissues. ALL may occur at any age but approximately 85% of patients with ALL are under the age of 15 years.

Acute lymphoblastic leukemia/lymphoma

Clinical presentation

Symptoms may be of abrupt onset, or more insidiously, occurring over a period of weeks or even months. Patients usually present clinical signs of BM failure. Tiredness and pallor are induced by anemia. Infections are linked to the underlying neutropenia. Purpura, bruising or gum bleeding are related to thrombocytopenia. Fever may be present, and half of affected children have bony pain. Differential diagnosis will include infections, immune diseases, macrophage disorders, congenital BM diseases, aplastic anemia and secondary infiltration of other tumors.[2] Less commonly, lymphadenopathy, splenic or liver involvement, the symptoms associated with a mediastinal mass or CNS disease may be the presenting features of ALL. Rarely, testicular or other tumor-forming presentation may be the first sign of the disease.

Most patients present with anemia and/or thrombocytopenia. Approximately 25% of patients have a leukocyte count of $<5 \times 10^9$/l, 50% between 5 and 50×10^9/l, and 25% $>50 \times 10^9$/l. Leukocyte counts $>100 \times 10^9$/l may lead to leukostasis and should be treated as a medical emergency.[3]

©2011 Elsevier Ltd
DOI: 10.1016/B978-0-7020-3147-2.00019-5

High blast counts are more commonly found in T-ALL patients.

At the time of diagnosis the BM is usually hypercellular, with replacement of normal hematopoiesis by the blast cells. Rare patients present marrow hypoplasia, before developing a typical leukemic picture.[4] Such patients may improve spontaneously or respond transiently to aplasia-directed immunosuppressive treatment before leukemia becomes apparent.

The term lymphoblastic lymphoma (LBL) is used when the disease is confined to an extramedullary infiltrate with no or minimal involvement of PB and BM. Patients with T-LBL constitute above 90% of LBL cases and usually present with signs associated with a mediastinal mass.[5] Patients with B-LBL often present skin or head and neck lesions and are usually asymptomatic.

Classification

The French-American-British (FAB) classification of acute lymphoblastic leukemia introduced in 1976 was based on morphology alone and recognized three types of blast cells in ALL, namely: small homogeneous blasts with round nuclei and scanty cytoplasm (L1), larger blasts with irregular nuclei, prominent nucleoli and more abundant cytoplasm (L2) and basophilic cells with prominent cytoplasmic vacuoles (L3).[6] The L3 type included most cases previously termed B-ALL and expressing surface-immunoglobulin (SIg). However, some other types of ALL, particularly those with t(1;19), could also present with this cytology. The morphological FAB classification did not have any clinical significance.

The WHO classification in 2001 largely adopted the 1994 revised European–American classification of lymphoid neoplasms (REAL).[7] Thus, the WHO classification recognized precursor T- and B-cell neoplasms corresponding to ALL, but excluded cases with the t(8;14)(q24;q32), (and the rarer variants with t(2;8)(p12;q24) and t(8;22)(q24;q11)), which have undergone immunoglobulin gene rearrangement and express surface immunoglobulins. These cases correspond to leukemic presentation of Burkitt's lymphoma, which in the WHO system was classified with mature B-cell neoplasms. Such cases, if present with peripheral blood involvement, were termed Burkitt cell leukemia.

In the WHO 2008 classification, B-cell lymphoblastic leukemia/lymphomas are defined as neoplasms of precursor cells committed to B-lineage.[1] They include B-ALL and B-LBL and are further subdivided by the presence or absence of specific recurring cytogenetic abnormalities (Table 19.1). The following cytogenetic entities have been recognized in B-lymphoblastic leukemia/lymphoma: t(9;22)(q34;q11), t(1;19)(q23;p13), t(12;21)(p12;q22), t(various;11q23 rearranged), hyperdiploid ALL, hypodiploid ALL and B-lymphoblastic leukemia/lymphoma not otherwise specified (NOS). T-lymphoblastic leukemia/lymphomas are defined as neoplasms of precursor cells committed to the T-lineage and include T-ALL and T-LBL.

Cytology, cytochemistry and histopathology

The morphology of lymphoid blasts should be evaluated on well-prepared May–Grünewald–Giemsa or Romanowsky-

Table 19.1 WHO 2008 classification of precursor lymphoid neoplasms

B lymphoblastic leukemia/lymphoma
B lymphoblastic leukemia/lymphoma, NOS
B lymphoblastic leukemia/lymphoma with recurrent genetic abnormalities:
   B lymphoblastic leukemia/lymphoma with t(9;22)(q34;q11.2); BCR-ABL1
   B lymphoblastic leukemia/lymphoma with t(v;11q23), MLL rearranged
   B lymphoblastic leukemia/lymphoma with t(12;21)(p13;q22); TEL-AML1 (ETV6-RUNX1)
   B lymphoblastic leukemia/lymphoma with hyperdiploidy
   B lymphoblastic leukemia/lymphoma with hypodiploidy
   B lymphoblastic leukemia/lymphoma with t(5;14)(q31;q32); (IL3-IGH)
   B lymphoblastic leukemia/lymphoma with t(1;19)(q23;p13.3); E2A-PBX1 (TCF3-PBX1)
T lymphoblastic leukemia/lymphoma

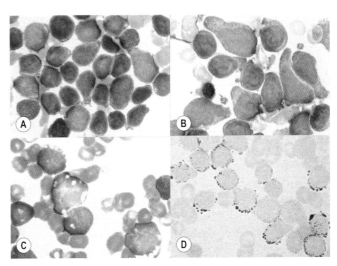

Fig. 19.1 (A–D) (A–C) May–Grünwald–Giemsa stain showing lymphoblasts with variable morphology. (D) Periodic acid Schiff reaction showing typical blocks and granules in a clear cytoplasmic background.

stained smears of PB or BM. Cytological appearance is variable (Fig. 19.1). In most cases, the blasts are small to medium-sized with round nuclei and fine but densely packed homogeneous chromatin. Nucleoli are small and usually single or absent. In some patients, blasts can have rather condensed chromatin making distinction from chronic lymphocytic leukemia difficult. The cytoplasm is scanty and weakly basophilic. Cytoplasmic vacuoles may be present. In 10–15% of cases, blasts are larger, with irregular nuclei showing clefting or indentation. Nucleoli are more prominent, often large and occasionally multiple. The cytoplasm is relatively abundant and may be finely reticulated. Basophilia is variable. Scanty azurophil granules are rarely present and usually readily distinguished from granules in myeloid precursors but sometimes similar to those of large granular lymphocytes. A 'hand-mirror' variant has been described but is probably of no clinical significance.[8]

There are no discriminant diagnostic cytochemical stains that distinguish ALL. Lymphoblasts are negative when stained for myeloperoxidase. Very rarely, coarse granular or

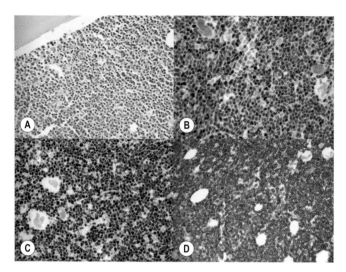

Fig. 19.2 (A–D) Bone marrow biopsy findings in ALL. (A) Giemsa stain; (B) nuclear reaction with antibodies to TdT; (C) nuclear PAX5 stain in B-precursor ALL; (D) cytoplasmic CD3 stain in T-ALL.

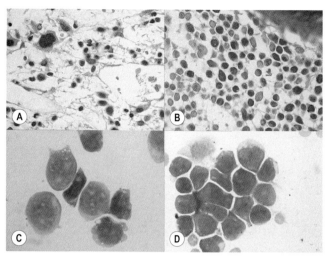

Fig. 19.3 (A–D) (A) Hematoxilin-eosin stain of bone marrow biopsy from a 14-year old girl with pancytopenia showing hypocellularity, stromal edema and mild fibrosis. (B) Same patient 11 weeks later showing typical picture of ALL. (C) Cerebrospinal fluid cytospin from a patient with CNS relapse of T-ALL (D) Cytospin of vitreous fluid showing blasts from a child with ALL involving the iris.

globular positivity with Sudan Black B may be present. T-lineage ALL frequently shows localized or polar staining of acid phosphatase, but these appearances are not specific. The periodic acid-Schiff (PAS) reaction is useful in identifying lymphoblasts, which usually show fine granules or blocks of positivity (Fig. 19.1). These are found in up to 95% of cases, although they may be very rare, occurring in less than 1% of blasts. The distinctive feature of positivity in lymphoblasts is the absence of any diffuse PAS cytoplasmic staining, which is present in myeloid lineage cells. Lymphoblasts show a clear-glass cytoplasm in which positive granules and blocks are sharply defined. Neutrophils stain strongly and serve as an internal control for the quality of the PAS stain.

Marrow trephine biopsies usually show maximal cellularity due to the diffuse invasion of sinuses by blast cells (Fig. 19.2A). The lymphoblastic population is usually homogeneous. In the majority of cases, the cells are small with scanty cytoplasm. Nuclei show finely stippled chromatin, often with peripheral condensation. Nucleoli are small and seldom multiple. A minority of cases show larger cells with irregular nuclei and increased cytoplasm. T-lineage ALL may show some degree of nuclear irregularity, and the nuclei may be small and hyperchromatic. Varying degrees of reticulin fibrosis (reversible on successful treatment) may be present in more than half the cases, which can lead to 'dry-tap' aspirations of BM. This is more common in B-lineage compared to T-lineage ALL and has been shown to be of poor prognostic significance.[9] Areas of marrow necrosis, usually patchy, but occasionally extensive, may be present, and can delay diagnosis if no circulating blasts are present. Cases presenting as aplastic anemia (Fig. 19.3A, B) may show a degree of reticulin fibrosis not generally seen in true aplasia, and are usually of common-B-lineage ALL phenotype. If no material has been submitted for flow cytometry, immunophenotyping can be performed on bone marrow biopsy using antibodies to terminal deoxynucleotidyl transferase (TdT), PAX-5 to show B-cell lineage and CD3 to show T-cell lineage (Fig. 19.2B, C, D).

At both presentation or relapse, almost any organ system can be infiltrated by leukemia (Fig. 19.3D). The CNS (Fig. 19.3C) and the testis (Fig. 19.4) are favored sites of relapse.

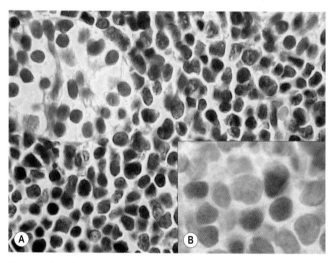

Fig. 19.4 (A, B) (A) Hematoxilin-eosin stain of a section from testis involved by ALL. A seminiferous tubule is at top left. (B) Nuclear positivity for TdT in infiltrating blasts.

Immunophenotypic diagnosis

Similar to morphology, the immunophenotypic study of suspected acute leukemia cases is an essential component of diagnosis, allowing further definition of the lineage and maturation stage of blast cells. Immunophenotyping results by flow cytometry can be obtained within a few hours after sampling and are very important in the first stages of therapy initiation. Even if the initial (cytologic) investigations strongly suggest a diagnosis of ALL, a comprehensive immunophenotyping should be carried out, including non-lymphoid lineage markers to exclude undifferentiated acute myeloid leukemia or mixed phenotype acute leukemia (MPAL). Multiparameter flow cytometry on whole BM or PB has now become the standard procedure. A sound strategy

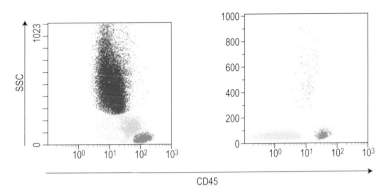

Fig. 19.5 Typical scattergrams after CD45 labeling. On the left panel: granulocytes (red), monocytes (green), lymphocytes(magenta) clearly delineate the blast area of immature cells (cyan) in a normal bone marrow. On the right panel typical of a B-precursor acute lymphoblastic leukemia sample, a few lymphocytes remain but monocytes and granulocytes are nearly absent. The population of blasts (cyan) displays a typical low SSC and low CD45 expression.

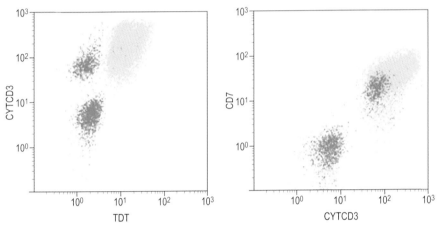

Fig. 19.6 Example of typical flow cytometry findings in T-ALL. Combined scattergrams of lymphocytes (magenta) and blasts (cyan). Blast co-express cytoplasmic CD3, CD7 and TdT. T-lymphocytes co-express cytoplasmic CD3 and CD7 but lack TdT. B-lymphocytes lack all markers and appear as a second cyan cluster.

should make use of CD45-gating combined with the side scatter (SSC) signal of flow cytometry, which allows to better identify the blast population. In most ALL cases, blasts display low CD45 expression and low SSC characteristics (Fig. 19.5). There is currently no recommended set of immunophenotyping combinations, but a mandatory panel of markers has been proposed by the European Leukemia Net (www.leukemia-net.org). The best orientation combination towards B-lineage, T-lineage or myeloid lineage leukemia relies on the intracytoplasmic detection of relevant antigens. Concomitant labeling, after permeabilization, for cytoplasmic CD79a, CD3 and myeloperoxidase will usually display positivity for only one of these markers, therefore pointing at the relevant lineage. However, in some cases of T-ALL/LBL a weak expression of cytoplasmic CD79a has been reported.[10,11] Nuclear labeling for TdT may further differentiate between precursor (positive) and mature (negative) lymphoproliferations (Fig. 19.6). This step should be followed or accompanied by extensive cell surface marker investigation.

B-cell lymphoblastic leukemia/ lymphoma (B-LBL)

The maturation steps of normal B-precursor cells in the bone marrow have been well characterized immunophenotypically, mostly through extensive analyses of leukemias. The initial step of stem-cell committment towards the B-lineage is characterized by the surface expression of CD19 and intracytoplasmic expression of CD79, which will be ultimately used to carry the B-cell receptor (or surface immunoglobulin, SIg) towards the cell membrane. This is followed by transient expression of CD22 in the cytoplasm and acquisition of CD20 and CD21. An ectopeptidase expressed on most childhood ALLs and thus initially dubbed common-acute lymphoblastic leukemia antigen or cALLA (CD10) is then present transiently. During these steps, the immunoglobulin heavy (IgH) chain genes begin rearranging in order to customize the future variable (V) domain of the IgH. Once a functional rearrangement has been acquired, the new gene is transcribed together with the adjacent constant domains of the μ-chain (IgM heavy chain) and translates in cytoplasmic μ-chains characteristic of the pre-B stage. A transient pre-BCR can then be detected on the surface of the cell, and rearrangement of Ig light chains genes begin until a functional VJ rearrangement gives rise to a potential new variable light chain domain. Both heavy and light chains are then translated and the cell expresses whole immunoglobulins with the newly defined specificity, together with surface CD79. A peculiar long transcript allows such cells to co-express μ and δ-chains of the same specificity as surface IgM and IgD. These naive cells are dubbed 'μδ'. According to that scheme, the European Group for Immunophenotyping of Leukemia (EGIL) proposed in 1995, to classify B-lineage ALL according to the order of appearance of CD10, cμ and sIg, into four classes dubbed B-I (or pro-pro-B), B-II (pro-B or common-B), B-III (or pre-B) and B-IV (or mature B)[12] (Table 19.2). The latter can be identified either by the presence of surface μ-chains or cytoplasmic expession of a light chain (either κ or λ, defining the proliferating clone). Besides these classification markers, B-lineage ALLs often retain expression of the stem-cell marker CD34 and HLA-DR (Fig. 19.7). They may also express the activation markers CD38 and CD71, and co-expression of the myeloid markers CD33, CD13, CD15 of CD65 may be seen. CD10-negative B-I and B-III cases have been shown to have a worse prognosis than B-II ALL. Co-expression of myeloid antigens was previously considered of poor prognosis probably due to overrepresentation of cases with t(9;22). Myeloid markers remain a good indicator of cytogenetic anomalies and are potentially useful in studies of minimal residual disease (MRD) (see below). Investigation for the expression of targets to therapeutic monoclonal antibodies is strongly recommended before initiating such treatment schedules.

T-cell lymphoblastic leukemia/lymphoma (T-LBL)

The maturation of T-cells is initiated in the bone marrow but undergoes its terminal and most crucial stages in the thymus. Committed T-lineage progenitors also begin expressing in their cytoplasm the CD3 complex, later to be used to carry the rearranged T-cell receptor on the cell surface. The expression of CD3 is usually investigated using antibodies directed to the epsilon chain of the CD3 complex. While still in the bone marrow, T-lineage cells first express CD7. However, this molecule may also be displayed on cells engaged in myeloid differentiation. It seems that microenvironmental signals can revert the differentiation of early progenitors (usually co-expressing CD34 and HLA-Class II) towards T-lineage or myeloid lineage, indicating some residual plasticity of these cells. Shortly after CD7 expression, CD5 and CD2 appear on the cell surface signing the end of medullary maturation and migration of the cells towards the thymic epithelium. In normal T-cell differentiation, cortical thymocytes begin transiently expressing CD1a and rearranging the T-cell receptor (TCR). This series of rearrangements will first involve the γ (G) chain of the γδ (D) receptor, and then, in case of failure, proceed towards αβ rearrangements. This important feature explains why TCRG and TCRD rearrangements are good clonality markers. After losing CD1a, the maturing T-cells briefly co-express CD4 and CD8. Then they become naive TCR+ T-cells expressing CD3 on the cell surface, together with either CD4 or CD8, depending on the type of MHC molecule (class II or class I) that they will later use for peptide recognition. EGIL also proposed a classification of T-ALL based on this maturation sequence. T-cells with only cytoplasmic CD3 and CD7 are designated as T-I (pro-T) and those that co-express only additional CD5 and/or CD2 are T-II (or early-T). CD1a+ corticothymocyte-like cells are designated T-III (independent of the CD4 or CD8 status) and mature CD1-negative/surface CD3-positive cells are T-IV.[12] The co-expression of myeloid markers is not uncommon on T-ALL of the earliest stages T-I or T-II, and weak expression of CD10 is also not unusual on T-lineage ALL cells (Table 19.2). Investigation for TCR molecules expression on the cell surface is an additional marker of maturity for T-IV, and cytoplasmic expression of TCRB with the 8A3 antibody has been suggested to allow for further classification of T-ALL.[13]

Cytogenetic abnormalities

Various cytogenetic anomalies can be identified in ALL after succesful examination of metaphases or further investigation via fluorescence *in situ* hybridization (FISH) or variant techniques applicable to cells in interphase. Normal karyotypes should also be further explored by such techniques, as some anomalies are not obvious when using chromosomal banding techniques. Table 19.3, which is not exhaustive, summarizes the significance and approximate frequencies of the main chromosomal abnormalities in ALL.

Cytogenetic investigations can also be guided by the immunophenotype.[14] For instance, B-I ALL are frequently associated to the t(4;11) translocation and anomalies of the *MLL* gene can be suspected upon expression of CD15 or CD65. The Philadelphia chromosome or t(9;22) has been reported to be associated to CD34 and CD10 expression with low CD38 and aberrant CD13 and/or CD33 expression. A similar immunophenotype may be indicative also of t(12;21), but these cases are uniformly CD66c negative. Overexpression of the IL-3 receptor (CD123) has been found in many hyperdiploid cases of ALL.[15]

Several chromosomal abnormalities are of prognostic significance in B-LBL (Table 19.3). The t(9;22) carried a poor prognosis in both children and adults until the advent of tyrosine kinase inhibitors (TKI). The t(4;11) carries a poor prognosis, particularly in infants, and overall 11q23 abnormalities involving disruption of the *MLL* gene are of adverse clinical significance in ALL. Adverse prognosis has been linked to resistance to L-asparaginase and glucocorticoids.[16] The t(1;19), initially thought to be adverse, is on current treatment protocols of neutral significance, except for increased risk of CNS relapse.[17,18] The t(12;21) is found in 25–30% of pediatric B-LBL cases and confers a good prognosis.[17]

Ploidy changes are also of prognostic importance, with hypodiploid and near-haploid karyotypes carrying an adverse prognosis.[19] Conversely, hyperdiploidy carries a favorable prognosis.[17] Of note, ploidy can also be explored by flow cytometry using propidium iodide intercalation in permeabilized cells pretreated by RNAse or using image analysis of the DNA staining with cell cycle analysis software.

T-LBL have fewer clinically significant chromosomal groups (Table 19.3). The t(10;14) has been identified as a favorable finding in children. Cases with normal karyotypes fare better than those with any chromosomal abnormality.[16]

Molecular genetics

Genomic alterations are common in ALL. They can result from the translocation of genomic material generating new fusion genes or from mutations. Fusion genes can be translated in mRNA accessible to reverse transcription and further amplification by polymerase chain reaction, using primers of both initial genes. Very recently, monoclonal antibodies

Table 19.2 Immunophenotypic classification of acute lymphoblastic leukemia

Type of leukemia[a]	Antigen expression																		
	CD45	CD19	CD34	CD10	TdT	CD20	cCD79	CD22	cIgM	sCD79	sIg or κ or λ	cCD3	CD7	CD5	CD2	CD1a	CD4	CD8	sCD3
B-I Early-B	±	+	+	−	+	−	+	±	−	−	−	−	−	−	−	−	−	−	−
B-II Common	±	+	±	+	+	±	+	+	−	−	−	−	−	−	−	−	−	−	−
B-III Pre-B	±	+	±	±	+	±	+	+	+	−	−	−	−	−	−	−	−	−	−
B-IV Burkitt	+	+	−	−	−	+	+	+	−	+	+	−	−	−	−	−	−	−	−
T-I Early-T	±	−	±	±	+	−	−[b]	−	−	−	−	+	+	−	−	−	−	−	−
T-II Pro-T	+	−	±	±	+	−	−[b]	−	−	−	−	+	+	+	+	−	±	±	−
T-III Cortical thymic	+	−	±	±	+	−	−[b]	−	−	−	−	+	+	+	+	+	±	±	±
T-IV Mature T	+	−	−	−	±	−	−	−	−	−	−	+	+	+	+	−	±	±	+

[a] According to EGIL.[12] Columns in dark grey are mandatory for lineage assignment and classification. c, cytoplasmic; s, surface.

[b] Rare cases positive

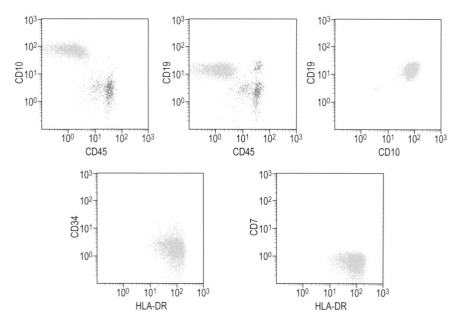

Fig. 19.7 Example of typical flow cytometry findings in B-precursor ALL of EGIL BII category. Negative/dim CD45, bright expression of CD10 and CD19 (top left and middle panel) and coexpression of these antigens on ALL blast cells (cyan, top left panel). The top left and middle panel show blasts (cyan) together with granulocytes (red) which have lost or not yet acquired CD10 and lymphocytes (magenta) where the subset of mature CD19+ B-cells is clearly visible (middle panel). Lower panels show bright expression of HLA-DR, weak expression of CD34 (left panel) and absence of CD7 (right panel).

Table 19.3 Frequency of cytogenetic anomalies in ALL

Anomaly	Frequency in childhood ALL[a]	Frequency in adult ALL[a]	Prognosis
B-precursor ALL			
t(12;21)(p13;q22)	22–25%	1–2%	Favorable
Hyperdiploid	25%	5%	Favorable
t(1;19)(q23;p13)	5%	3%	Favorable
t(9;22)(q23;p11)	2–5%	20%	Unfavorable
Chr.11q23	2%	5%	Unfavorable
Chr.21 internal duplication	2%	2%	Unfavorable
del9p (cryptic)	35%	8%	Unfavorable
t(5;14)(q31;q32)	1%	1%	Not established
T-lineage ALL			
t(1;14)p32q11)	15%	13%	Favorable
t(5;14)(q35;q32)	24%	6%	Favorable
t(10;14)(q24;q11)	8%	10%	Favorable
t(11;14)(p13;q11)	7%	2%	Unfavorable
t(10;11)(p13;q14)	4%	3%	Unfavorable
inv(7,) p15q34/t(7;7)(p15;q34);	5%	5%	Unfavorable
6q23 duplication	8–15%	NA	Unfavorable
6q deletion	6%	11%	Unfavorable
9p deletion	30%	10%	Unfavorable

[a]17,27–29

Table 19.4 Examples of genes frequently involved in molecular anomalies of acute lymphoblastic leukemias

B-cell precursor acute leukemia	T-lineage leukemia
TEL/AML1	TAL1, TAL2,SIL/TAL
E2A/PBX1	LMO1, LMO2
BCR/ABL1	TLX1 (HOX11), TLX3(HOX11L2)
MLL	HOXA
CDKN2A/B	NOTCH1
PAX5	PTEN
FLT3	CALM/AF10
PTPN11	CDKN2A/2B
kRAS or nRAS	NUP/ABL
	RAS

targeting the fusion proteins resulting from chromosomal translocations have opened a new promising field for the identification of molecular anomalies using a bead assay available for semi-quantitative assessment in flow cytometry after preparation of a protein extract of bone marrow cells.[20]

The upcoming technology of gene expression microarrays also allows rapid screening for a multitude of potential mRNA transcripts, and has allowed the identification of new anomalies.[21] Even newer technologies, still at the stage of clinical research, investigate anomalies of DNA methylation, microRNAs (miRNA) or single nucleotide polymorphism (SNP), many of them appearing to be involved in the pathogenesis of ALL. These studies may also have therapeutic relevance if the molecular changes can be targeted.[22] A number of molecular anomalies have been reported in B- and T-lineage ALL with variable, often not yet fully established prognostic value. Those associated to known genes are summarized in Table 19.4.[16,23]

In B-LBL the molecular changes often affect B-cell transcription factors, such as PAX5 (chromosome 9p), IKAROS (chromosome 7p), and E2A (chromosome 19) or EBF1 (chromosome 5). Gene expression profiling studies have identified a subset of B-precursor ALL (10–20%) with expression profiles very similar to the BCR-ABL1 subset and poor prognosis, despite lack of this translocation. These cases tested negative for other well-known abnormalities but had also an increased frequency of abnormalities in B-cell transcription factor genes. Intrachromosomal amplification of chromosome 21 can be found in about 2% of B-LBL cases and have been reported to be associated with poor prognosis. Activating FLT3 mutations have been found in 8% of B-LBL, often associated with MLL rearrangement and hyperdiploidy. Mutations of downstream effector genes of tyrosine kinase receptors such as the SHP-2 protein tyrosine phosphatase encoding gene PTPN11, usually in the absence of TEL/AML1, have been found in 7% of B-LBL. Finally, RAS mutations have been reported at variable frequencies.

In T-LBL, two types of mutations have been reported, namely type A or type B. The former induce maturation arrest at given stages of differentiation while the latter are independent of cell differentiation. Translocations in T-LBLs often involve loci of the TCR genes on chromosomes 7 or 14. Good prognosis has been associated to translocations involving TLX1 (HOX11) but not TLX3 (HOX11L2). Frequently occurring NOTCH1 mutations have also been reported to be favorable as well as the CALM-AF10 gene fusion. Better understanding of these anomalies will potentially lead to targeted therapy.

Minimal residual disease monitoring

Minimal residual disease is defined as the tumor mass still remaining after chemotherapy or hematopoietic stem-cells transplantation (autologous or more frequently allogeneic in ALL). Upon clinical and hematologic (morphologic) remission, it is suspected that some residual, potentially resistant cells remain, liable to generate a relapse upon regrowth. It has been important to establish reliable means to detect such remaining cells, using molecular or immunophenotypic tools.[24] In ALL, molecular studies have been more readily established in comparison to immunophenotypic ones, essentially due to the progress of molecular amplification instruments. The gold standard for molecular MRD monitoring currently relies on real-time quantitative polymerase reaction (RQ-PCR). Through the generation of fluorescent signals proportional to the amount of amplified sequences, RQ-PCR allows to accurately quantify representative material accessible to amplification (Fig. 19.8). This has been successfully applied to the unique rearrangements of IGH or TCR genes characteristic of specific clones, and to specific fusion-genes or mutations. Using RQ-PCR it is necessary to identify and generate patient-specific probes or primers, test them for their efficiency, and compare serial dilutions of the DNA from diagnosis to follow-up BM material. This complex methodology nonetheless may yield sensitivities of 10^{-4} to 10^{-6}.

The recent sophistication of multiparameter flow cytometry instruments, fluorochromes, and software has been responsible for a renewed interest for this methodology, initially applied to track abnormal cytoplasmic CD3$^+$/TdT$^+$ blasts in the early 1980s.[25] In B-lineage ALL, the differential expression of CD19, CD34, CD10, and CD38 on blast cells and hematogones allows for a successful identification of MRD in a large number of cases. Additional markers such as CD123, when present at diagnosis have been reported to be useful and stable in MRD cells after treatment (Fig. 19.9). Aberrant immunophenotypes noted at diagnoses are called leukemia associated immunophenotypic patterns (LAIP), which can be either aberrant co-expression of other lineage markers (notably myeloid) or, more subtly, differences in fluorescence intensity (under- or over-expression) of marker expression, or asynchronous expression of markers normally associated to different maturation stages.

In T-lineage ALL, the most reliable combination remains the co-expression of cytoplasmic CD3 and nuclear TdT, but requires permeabilization and therefore the potential loss of some cells. An additional marker of interest seems to be the aberrant over-expression of CD99. Markers of T-lineage immaturity are especially useful when combined with CD99 or for minimal residual disease assessment of T-III ALL expressing CD1a (Fig. 19.10).

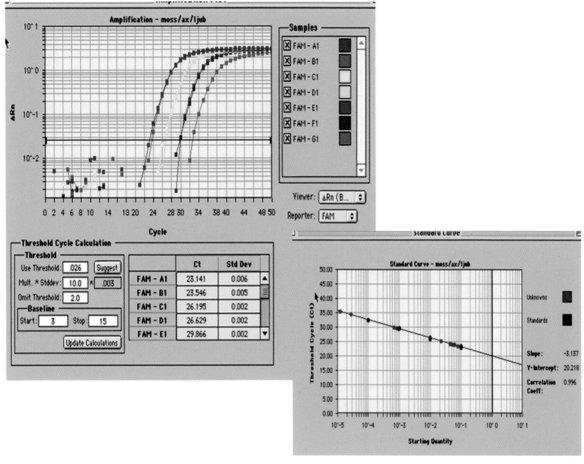

Fig. 19.8 Example of molecular detection of minimal residual disease in B-precursor ALL. RQ-PCR detection of IgH rearrangement at VH4/JH4 is used to determine the copy number of target in tested samples.

Flow cytometry reaches easily the 10^{-3} – 10^{-4} threshold, which has so far been reported of clinical relevance. The development of new instruments, making more rapid screening of larger numbers of cells possible, should soon allow to lower that sensitivity limit.

Of note, both molecular and flow methods can also be applied to PB, usually yielding one log lower cell numbers compared to the bone marrow.[26] MRD studies in blood can certainly be useful in the early stages of therapy for more frequent investigations with less discomfort for the patients.

Mixed phenotype acute leukemias

According to WHO 2008, mixed phenotype acute leukemias (MPAL) belong to acute leukemias of ambiguous lineage that show no clear evidence of differentiation towards one single lineage as summarized in Fig. 19.11. Of note, this figure also takes into account, in this subgroup of ambiguous lineage leukemias, the existence of acute undifferentiated leukemias (AUL) and of other forms of AL difficult to classify such as the rare NK-cell leukemias.

The leukemic blasts of MPAL express antigens of more than one hematopoietic lineage. MPAL can either contain subpopulations of different lineages or one population with antigens of various lineages, or both. The definition and requirements for assigning more than one lineage to a single blast population are presented below under Immunophenotype.

Clinical presentation

There are no characteristic clinical features of these leukemias, which present as other acute leukemias.

Classification

Previously, the term acute biphenotypic leukemia has been applied if a single blast population co-expressed antigens of more than one lineage and the term 'bilineage leukemia' has been applied to leukemias containing separate leukemic populations of more than one lineage. The WHO 2008 classification recognized MPAL with the t(9;22) (q34;q11) *BCR-ABL1* translocation and MPAL with t(v;11q23) *MLL* rearranged as separate entities due to relatively frequent occurrence and characteristic features. Not otherwise specified (NOS) MPAL have been divided depending on their immunophenotype as B/myeloid, T/myeloid and rare types.

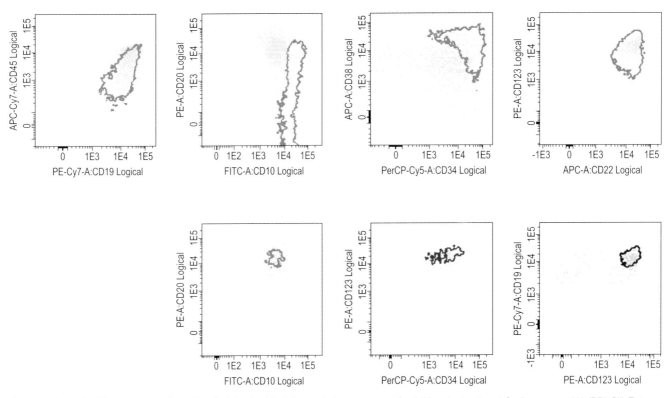

Fig. 19.9 Example of flow cytometry detection of minimal residual disease in bone marrow of a child under treatment for B-precursor ALL (EGIL BII). Top panels show results obtained in a sample taken at 15 days of treatment, MRD level 0.3%. Gate on CD19+ CD45 dim B-precursor cells (cyan) shows that most cells in that area have a pathological overexpression of CD123. Superimposed contours of expression patterns at diagnosis (purple) show that expression of CD20 has increased and expression of CD34, CD38 and CD10 is lower by comparison to diagnosis. Lower panels: analysis of a BM sample taken at day 29 confirms the persistence of a pathological population at a lower level (0.04%). Superimposed contours from day 15 show the same immunophenotype.

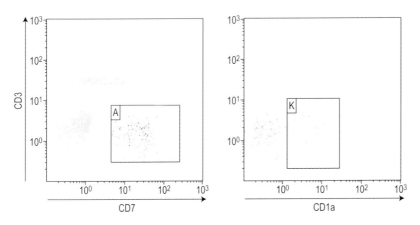

Fig. 19.10 Example of flow cytometry detection of minimal residual disease (at 10^{-4} level) in T-ALL (TIII according to EGIL). CD3$^-$/CD7$^+$ cells in the blast area are first selected (A), then CD1 expression is shown in a subset of these cells (K).

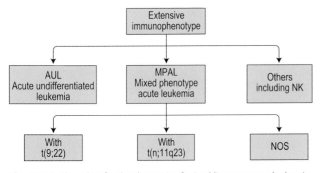

Fig. 19.11 Algorithm for the diagnosis of mixed lineage acute leukemia (MPAL).

Cytology and histopathology

In most cases MPAL are characterized by the presence of blasts with no specific features, most often resembling ALL. In some cases, dimorphic populations are present, one of small lymphoblasts and one of larger myelo- or monoblasts. (Fig. 19.12). Cytochemistry may be of use to show populations positive for myeloperoxidase or nonspecific esterases. Bone marrow biopsies show diffuse infiltrations of blasts. Immunohistochemical stainings for myeloperoxidase and lysozyme may be of help in establishing a diagnosis of MPAL.

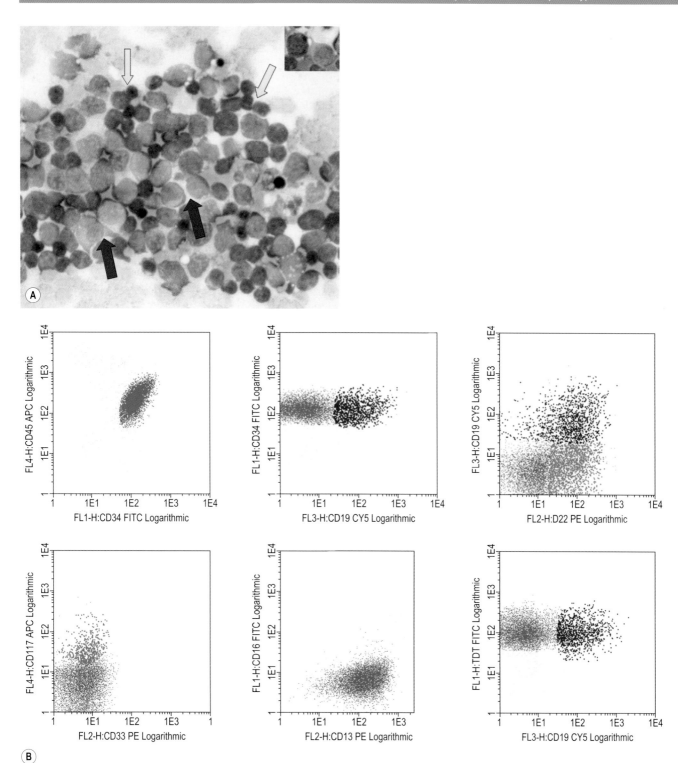

Fig. 19.12 (A, B) Example of MPAL. (A) In MGG stained smear a major population of large blasts (red arrows) and a minor population of small blasts (yellow arrows) could be seen. Insert (right upper corner) shows that some blasts were positive for myeloperoxidase. (B) Flow cytometry findings: blasts were gated on strong expression of CD34 and dim CD45 (upper left plot). Subpopulations of blasts were positive for CD19 and/or CD22 (upper middle and right plot). Most blasts were positive for CD13 and Tdt (lower middle and right plot). A minor subset was positive for CD117 while CD33 was negative (lower left plot). CD10 was negative but a subpopulation was positive for cyt.CD79a.

Immunophenotypic diagnosis of MPAL

The immunophenotypic characteristics allowing the assignment of an acute leukemia to the MPAL group now relies on very strong markers of each lineage. In the initial scoring system published by EGIL in 1995, relevant markers were given respective score points allowing to assign cells with more than two points in more than two lineages to the biphenotypic category of acute leukemias. According to WHO 2008, cells are considered to display myeloid features either if they are positive for intracytoplasmic myeloperoxidase (in cytochemistry or in immunostaining) or display clear signs of monocytic maturation (nonspecific esterase activity in cytochemistry, presence of intracytoplasmic lysozyme and/or surface expression of CD14, CD11c, CD36 or CD64). Engagement in the B-lineage would be considered in two circumstances: 1) if CD19 expression is bright and associated to at least one of the markers CD10, intracytoplasmic CD79a or CD22 (intracytoplasmic or surface); or, 2) if CD19 is dimly expressed but associated with at least two of these additional markers. T-lineage commitment mostly relies on bright expression of intracytoplasmic CD3, explored with strong fluorochromes such as PE or APC. Demonstration of features characteristic to more than one of these three subgroups is significant for MPAL assignment (Figs. 19.11 and 19.12).

Cytogenetics and molecular genetics of MPAL

The two major cytogenetic groups of MPAL depend on the identification of the Philadelphia chromosome and/or *BCR/ABL* as described above, or of anomalies involving the *MLL* gene at 11q23. This can be achieved by classical cytogenetics, FISH or molecular studies. The more recent technology of microarray may help in identifying mRNA transcripts of these fusion genes. The next step would be to identify the molecular anomalies potentially associated to the various subgroups of MPAL as summarized in Fig. 19.11.

References

1. Vardiman JW, Thiele J, Arber DA, et al. The 2008 revision of the World Health Organization (WHO) classification of myeloid neoplasms and acute leukemia: rationale and important changes. Blood 2009;114:937–51.

2. Chessells JM. Pitfalls in the diagnosis of childhood leukaemia. Br J Haematol 2001;114:506–11.

3. Majhail NS, Lichtin AE. Acute leukemia with a very high leukocyte count: confronting a medical emergency. Cleve Clin J Med 2004;71:633–7.

4. Hasle H, Heim S, Schroeder H, et al. Transient pancytopenia preceding acute lymphoblastic leukemia (pre-ALL). Leukemia 1995;9:605–8.

5. Borowitz MJ, Falletta JM. Leukemias and lymphomas of thymic differentiation. Clin Lab Med 1988;8:119-34.

6. Bennett JM, Catovsky D, Daniel MT, et al. Proposals for the classification of the acute leukaemias. French-American-British (FAB) co-operative group. Br J Haematol 1976;33:451–8.

7. Harris NL, Jaffe ES, Diebold J, et al. World Health Organization classification of neoplastic diseases of the hematopoietic and lymphoid tissues: report of the Clinical Advisory Committee meeting – Airlie House, Virginia, November 1997. J Clin Oncol 1999;17:3835–49.

8. Kebriaei P, Anastasi J, Larson RA. Acute lymphoblastic leukaemia: diagnosis and classification. Best Pract Res Clin Haematol 2002;15:597–621.

9. Noren-Nystrom U, Roos G, Bergh A, et al. Bone marrow fibrosis in childhood acute lymphoblastic leukemia correlates to biological factors, treatment response and outcome. Leukemia 2008;22:504-10.

10. Pilozzi E, Pulford K, Jones M, et al. Co-expression of CD79a (JCB117) and CD3 by lymphoblastic lymphoma. J Pathol 1998;186:140–3.

11. Asnafi V, Beldjord K, Garand R, et al. IgH DJ rearrangements within T-ALL correlate with cCD79a expression, an immature/TCRgammadelta phenotype and absence of IL7Ralpha/CD127 expression. Leukemia 2004;18:1997–2001.

12. Bene MC, Castoldi G, Knapp W, et al. Proposals for the immunological classification of acute leukemias. European Group for the Immunological Characterization of Leukemias (EGIL). Leukemia 1995;9:1783–6.

13. Asnafi V, Beldjord K, Boulanger E, et al. Analysis of TCR, pT alpha, and RAG-1 in T-acute lymphoblastic leukemias improves understanding of early human T-lymphoid lineage commitment. Blood 2003;101:2693–703.

14. Hrusak O, Porwit-MacDonald A. Antigen expression patterns reflecting genotype of acute leukemias. Leukemia 2002;16:1233–58.

15. Djokic M, Bjorklund E, Blennow E, et al. Overexpression of CD123 correlates with the hyperdiploid genotype in acute lymphoblastic leukemia. Haematologica 2009;94:1016–19.

16. Meijerink JP, den Boer ML, Pieters R. New genetic abnormalities and treatment response in acute lymphoblastic leukemia. Semin Hematol 2009;46:16–23.

17. Pui CH, Campana D, Pei D, et al. Treating childhood acute lymphoblastic leukemia without cranial irradiation. N Engl J Med 2009;360:2730–41.

18. Garg R, Kantarjian H, Thomas D, et al. Adults with acute lymphoblastic leukemia and translocation (1;19) abnormality have a favorable outcome with hyperfractionated cyclophosphamide, vincristine, doxorubicin, and dexamethasone alternating with methotrexate and high-dose cytarabine chemotherapy. Cancer 2009;115:2147–54.

19. Heerema NA, Nachman JB, Sather HN, et al. Hypodiploidy with less than 45 chromosomes confers adverse risk in childhood acute lymphoblastic leukemia: a report from the children's cancer group. Blood 1999;94:4036–45.

20. Weerkamp F, Dekking E, Ng YY, et al. Flow cytometric immunobead assay for the detection of BCR-ABL fusion proteins in leukemia patients. Leukemia 2009;23:1106–17.

21. Bacher U, Kohlmann A, Haferlach T. Current status of gene expression profiling in the diagnosis and management of acute leukaemia. Br J Haematol 2009;145:555–68.

22. Mullighan CG, Downing JR. Genome-wide profiling of genetic alterations in acute lymphoblastic leukemia: recent insights and future directions. Leukemia 2009;23:1209–18.

23. Harrison CJ. Cytogenetics of paediatric and adolescent acute lymphoblastic leukemia. Br J Haematol 2009;144:147–56.

24. Campana D. Minimal residual disease in acute lymphoblastic leukemia. Semin Hematol 2009;46:100–6.

25. Bradstock KF, Janossy G, Tidman N, et al. Immunological monitoring of residual disease in treated thymic acute lymphoblastic leukaemia. Leuk Res 1981;5:301–9.

26. Coustan-Smith E, Sancho J, Hancock ML, et al. Use of peripheral blood instead of bone marrow to monitor residual disease in children with acute lymphoblastic leukemia. Blood 2002;100:2399–402.

27. Marks DI, Paietta EM, Moorman AV, et al. T-cell acute lymphoblastic leukemia in adults: clinical features, immunophenotype, cytogenetics and outcome from the large randomised prospective trial (UKALL XII/ECOG 2993). Blood 2009 Dec 10;114(25): 5136–45.

28. Moorman AV, Chilton L, Wilkinson J, et al. A population based cytogenetic study of adults with acute lymphoblastic leukaemia (ALL). Blood 2010 Jan 14; 115(2):206–14.

29. Calero Moreno TM, Gustafsson G, Garwicz S, et al. Deletion of the Ink4-locus (the p16ink4a, p14ARF and p15ink4b genes) predicts relapse in children with ALL treated according to the Nordic protocols NOPHO-86 and NOPHO-92. Leukemia 2002;16: 2037–45.

CHAPTER 20

Myelodysplastic syndromes

BS Wilkins, A Porwit

The first report of a patient with myelodysplastic syndrome (MDS) dates from 1900, when Leube described a patient with severe megaloblastic anemia preceding development of overt leukemia.[1] This description was followed by several reports of patients characterized by cytopenia, disturbed maturation of bone marrow (BM) precursors, an increase of blasts and a significant risk of evolving to acute myeloid leukemia (AML).[1] The first international classification of MDS was developed by the French-American-British (FAB) Group[2] (Table 20.1) and extended by the World Health Organization (WHO) 2001 and WHO 2008 (Table 20.2) classifications.[3–5] The diagnosis of MDS is an effort that requires clinical, cytogenetic and pathological expertise, and often also repeated BM studies.

Definition

According to the WHO 2008 classification, MDS may be defined as a group of clonal hematopoeitic stem cell disorders characterized by cytopenia(s), dysplasia in one or more of the major myeloid cell lines, ineffective hematopoiesis and increased risk of AML development.[5] The BM is usually hypercellular. Myelodysplasia, i.e. abnormal maturation in

hematopoiesis, is a hallmark of MDS (Table 20.3). However, myelodysplasia is not definitive evidence of MDS and may be present as a result of various nutritional, toxic, infectious and other factors (Table 20.4). Moreover, a presumptive diagnosis of MDS may be made in a patient with unexplained cytopenia(s) in the absence of overt myelodysplasia if certain defining cytogenetic abnormalities are present (Table 20.5).

Epidemiology

American studies report the median age of MDS patients at diagnosis as 76 years.[6] In Asian countries the median age at diagnosis is 10 years lower.[7] The incidence is higher in men than in women (4.5 vs 2.7 cases/100 000 population/year, respectively). Incidence increases with age with 86% of MDS patients being older than 60 years of age. A prevalence of 1 in 500 in the population over 60 years of age has been suggested.[8] In patients over 85 years, MDS represents about a quarter of all hematologic malignancies. Although studies point towards an increasing incidence, this may at least in part reflect a greater willingness to perform BM investigations in the elderly and increased reporting.[9]

©2011 Elsevier Ltd
DOI: 10.1016/B978-0-7020-3147-2.00020-1

Table 20.1 French-American-British (FAB) group classification of myelodysplastic syndromes[2]

Type	Peripheral blood	Bone marrow
RA	<1% blasts	Dyshemopoiesis in one, two or all three lineages; <5% blasts
RARS	<1% blasts	As RA with ring sideroblasts (RS) comprising >15% erythroblasts
RAEB	<20% blasts	As RA with 5–20% blasts in BM, +/– RS
RAEBt	>30% blasts	As RA with 20–30%* blasts in BM or as RAEB with Auer rods
CMML	As any of the above plus >1 × 10⁹/l monocytes/promonocytes in blood	

*Cases with >30% blasts were classified as acute leukemia.

RA, refractory anemia; RARS, RA with ring sideroblasts; RAEB, RA with excess of blasts; RAEBt, RAEB in transformation; CMML, chronic myelomonocytic leukemia.

Variants that do not fit well into this classification include hypoplastic MDS, fibrotic MDS and juvenile myelomonocytic leukemia.

Etiology of primary MDS is still poorly understood. Certain genetic disorders and exposure to pesticides, organic solvents or ionizing radiation have been implicated as risk factors.[10,11] A large prospective study indicated obesity and smoking as modifiable, although weak, risk factors, while intake of alcohol, meat, fruit and vegetables, and physical activity did not influence the risk of MDS.[12] Secondary MDS, which tends to occur in younger people, develops after exposure to certain chemicals and cytotoxic drugs, especially alkylating agents.[13,14] The younger age at presentation of idiopathic MDS in developing countries suggests a less rigorous control of noxious chemicals in these communities.[15] Childhood MDS is very rare (1.8 cases/1 000 000 population/year).[16] Familial MDS is also very rare and occurs at a younger age.[17]

Classification

The 'minimal' morphologic criteria for MDS diagnosis according to WHO classification is the presence of at least 10% dysplastic forms in at least one hematopoietic lineage (erythroid, granulocytic or megakaryocytic), in an appropriate clinical setting.[4] The FAB classification (Table 20.1) applied the arbitrary limit of 30% blasts for diagnosis of AML, while this limit has been changed to 20% in the WHO classification abolishing the former category of RAEBt. There is still ongoing debate as to how patients with a blast count between 20% and 30% should be classified.[4] Of note, patients with specific translocations such as t(8;21), inv.16 and t(15;17) are classified as AML even if numbers of blasts are below 20%. This rule does not apply to cases of AML with t(9;11)(p22;q23), t(6;9)(p23;q34), inv.3(3)(q21q26.2), t(3;3)(q21;q26.2) and t(1;22)p(13;q13) that are considered as MDS if the number of blasts does not reach 20% within 2 months' follow-up time. Some AML cases may be recognized as myelodysplasia-related, which should be stated in

the report (see Chapter 18). Some of these cases would have been previously diagnosed as RAEB in transformation (RAEBt) and some would have been called AML. It is probable that a large proportion of AML cases in the elderly will fall into AML myelodysplasia-related category.

The 2001 WHO classification took into consideration the extent of dysplasia (unilineage vs multilineage), which has been proven to be of prognostic significance.[18,19] WHO 2008 (Table 20.2) extended the definition of cases with unilineage dysplasia, adding two other categories to refractory anemia (RA): refractory neutropenia (RN) and refractory thrombocytopenia (RT). In WHO 2008, the presence of ring sideroblasts is only of significance in the context of unilineage erythroid dysplasia (RA vs RA with ring sideroblasts, RA-RS). Patients with multilineage dysplasia and less than 5% blasts are diagnosed as refractory cytopenia with multilineage dysplasia (RCMD) independent of the presence of sideroblasts. Refractory anemia with excess of blasts (RAEB) is separated into RAEB I with 5–9% blast cells and RAEB II with 10–19% blast cells in BM smears. WHO 2008 has also stressed the significance of the presence of blasts in peripheral blood (PB), since patients with 2–4% PB blasts and <5% BM blasts are now categorized as RAEB-1.[4] It is important to note that most of these qualitative and quantitative parameters have been derived from blood and aspirated BM appearances. Correlation with their assessment by BM trephine biopsy (BMTB) histology has only a limited evidence base.

Most of the MDS categories in the WHO classification are defined on the basis of morphology, clinical features and peripheral blood cell counts. The only cytogenetically defined category is the MDS associated with isolated del(5q). Introduction of this category made karyotype analysis necessary for definite classification of MDS. Ongoing cytogenetic and molecular studies will probably define more specific MDS subtypes in the near future.

Some examples of MDS do not fit into currently defined categories within the WHO classification and therefore should be categorized as MDS unclassifiable. Especially, patients with hypoplastic MDS and/or MDS with fibrosis, as well as cases with dysplasia and leukocytosis, may be difficult to classify and thus fall into this category.

The revised WHO classification of 2008 has also recognized differences between MDS in adults and in children. The latter usually present with leukopenia and/or thrombocytopenia and less often with anemia. A provisional entity 'refractory cytopenia of childhood' (RCC) has been introduced, which includes childhood presentations with multilineage dysplasia, <2% blasts in PB, <5% blasts in BM and persistent cytopenia. Childhood MDS patients who have increased numbers of blasts should be classified in the same way as adults.[4,5]

Diagnosis

Symptoms of anemia (tiredness, breathlessness and lassitude), thrombocytopenia (bruising or bleeding), or neutropenia (recurrent infections, mouth ulcers) are most common. A large fraction of patients with MDS are asymptomatic and may be diagnosed incidentally when a blood test, performed for an unrelated reason, shows macrocytic anemia. Extramed-

Table 20.2 WHO 2008 classification of myelodysplastic syndromes[4]

Disease	Blood findings	Bone marrow findings
Refractory cytopenia with unilineage dysplasia (RCUD):	Unicytopenia or bicytopenia[1]	Unilineage dysplasia: ≥10% of the cells in one myeloid lineage
[Refractory anemia (RA); refractory neutropenia (RN);	No or rare blasts (<1%)[2]	<5% blasts
Refractory thrombocytopenia (RT)]		<15% of erythroid precursors are ring sideroblasts
Refractory anemia with ring sideroblasts (RARS)	Anemia No blasts	≥15% of erythroid precursors are ring sideroblasts Erythroid dysplasia only <5% blasts
Refractory cytopenia with multilineage dysplasia (RCMD)	Cytopenia(s) No or rare blasts (<1%)[2] No Auer rods <1×10⁹/l monocytes	Dysplasia in ≥10% of the cells in ≥ 2 myeloid lineages (neutrophil and/or erythroid precursors and/or megakaryocytes) <5% blasts in marrow No Auer rods ±15% ring sideroblasts
Refractory anemia with excess blasts-1 (RAEB-1)	Cytopenia(s) <5% blasts[2] No Auer rods <1×10⁹/l monocytes	Unilineage or multilineage dysplasia 5–9% blasts[2] No Auer rods
Refractory anemia with excess blasts-2 (RAEB-2)	Cytopenia(s) 5–19% blasts[3] Auer rods ±[3] <1×10⁹/l monocytes	Unilineage or multilineage dysplasia 10–19% blasts[3] Auer rods ±[3]
Myelodysplastic syndrome – unclassified (MDS-U)	Cytopenias ≤1% blasts[2]	Unequivocal dysplasia in <10% of cells in one or more myeloid lineages when accompanied by a cytogenetic abnormality considered as presumptive evidence for a diagnosis of MDS (see Table 20.6) <5% blasts
MDS associated with isolated del(5q)	Anemia Usually normal or increased platelet count No or rare blasts (<1%)	Normal to increased megakaryocytes with hypolobated nuclei <5% blasts Isolated del(5q) cytogenetic abnormality No Auer rods

[1]Bicytopenia may occasionally be observed. Cases with pancytopenia should be classified as MDS-U.

[2]If the marrow myeloblast percentage is less than 5% but there are 2–4% myeloblasts in the blood, the diagnostic classification is RAEB 1. Cases of RCUD and RCMD with 1% myeloblasts in the blood should be classified as MDS-U.

[3]Cases with Auer rods and <5% myeloblasts in the blood and <10% in the marrow should be classified as RAEB-2.

Although the finding of 5–19% blasts in the blood is, in itself, diagnostic of RAEB-2, cases of RAEB-2 may have less than 5% blasts in the blood if they have Auer rods and/or 10–19% blasts in the marrow. Similarly, cases of RAEB-2 may have less than 10% blasts in the marrow but may be diagnosed by the other two findings, Auer rod+ and/or 5–19% blasts in the blood.

ullary involvement (such as lymphadenopathy and/or splenomegaly) is relatively rare and possibility of MDS/MPN should be first excluded in these patients. Approximately 10% of patients display autoimmune symptoms such as vasculitis, arthritis, polyneuropathy and connective tissue disease-like presentations. The tumor suppressor gene *interferon regulatory factor-1* (*IRF-1*) has been implicated in the pathophysiology of MDS-associated autoimmune deregulation.[20]

A full blood count may reveal anemia, neutropenia, thrombocytopenia or multiple cytopenias. The recommended level for defining anemia is hemoglobin <10 g/l. Neutropenia is defined by absolute neutrophil count <1.8 × 10⁹/l and thrombocytopenia by platelet count <100 × 10⁹/l.

A raised mean cell volume (MCV) is frequently found and may be the only abnormality in the blood count. However, anemia may also be normocytic or microcytic. There is almost always reticulocytopenia. In patients with bone marrow fibrosis, a leukoerythroblastic picture may be found. In cases with del(5q), there may be a slightly elevated platelet count. Other tests are usually normal, but in some patients increased levels of lactate dehydrogenase (LDH) may be present, as a result of increased cell death in BM. High LDH levels carry a poor prognosis. Serum B_{12} levels are usually high, but coincident pernicious anemia has also been reported.[21] A positive direct antiglobulin test, with signs of hemolysis, is found in 8% of patients.[22] Both leukocyte and platelet function tests may be impaired,[23,24] as well as

Table 20.3 Morphologic signs of dysplasia in blood and bone marrow cells in MDS

Lineage	Blood	Bone marrow
Erythropoiesis	Macrocytes Aniso-poikilocytosis Dimorphic picture Polychromasia Punctate basophilia Normoblasts Reticulocytopenia	Erythroid hypercellularity Multinuclearity Dyskaryorrhexis Megaloblasts Cytoplasmic vacuoles Howell–Jolly bodies Ring sideroblasts
Granulopoiesis	Hypogranular neutrophils Unilobed or bilobed neutrophils (Pelger cells) Hypersegmented neutrophils Monocytosis (often with multiple, elongated nuclear lobes) Promonocytes (with fine azurophil granules) Degranulated eosinophils	Hypogranularity of myeloid precursors Increased promonocytes Increased blast cells (type I with scanty agranular cytoplasm and type II with sparse granules)
Thrombopoiesis	Agranular platelets Giant platelets Megakaryocyte fragments	Micromegakaryocytes Large megakaryocytes with single round or oval nucleus Large megakaryocytes with multiple small round nuclei Megakaryoblasts

Table 20.4 Non-clonal causes of dysplasia

Dyserythropoiesis
- Vitamin B_{12} and folic acid deficiency
- Alcohol toxicity
- Methotrexate and other chemotherapy
- Congenital hematological disorders such as congenital dyserythropoietic anemia
- Parvovirus B19 infection may cause erythroblastopenia with giant megaloblastoid erythroblasts
- HIV infection
- Essential element deficiencies
- Exposure to heavy metals, particularly lead or arsenic
- Paroxysmal nocturnal hemoglobinuria
- Autoimmune conditions

Dysgranulopoiesis
- Granulocyte colony-stimulating factor
- Several commonly used drugs and biologic agents (e.g. Bactrim or Mofetil)
- Viral infections (HIV, EBV)
- Chemotherapy/ regenerating bone marrow
- Paraneoplastic conditions (malignancy associated)

Dysmegakaryocytopoiesis
- Infections (HIV)
- Myelofibrosis (paraneoplastic or autoimmune)
- Patients after transplant or chemotherapy

the growth of BM progenitor cells in short-term and long-term cultures.[25] Recent studies stress decreased numbers of early multilineage precursors and erythroid progenitors as characteristics of MDS.[26]

The differential diagnosis includes other causes of macrocytic anemia such as B_{12} or folate deficiency, alcohol toxicity, liver disease, hypothyroidism, hemolytic anemia, other causes of cytopenias such as acute leukemia, aplastic anemia, drug-induced cytopenias, immune thrombocytopenia, and BM infiltration with various tumors.

Diagnosis of MDS depends on BM examination and cytogenetics. However, some patients with persistent mild cytopenia and/or mild dysplasia do not fulfill minimal criteria for MDS and should be followed. For these patients, the terms idiopathic cytopenia of undetermined significance (ICUS) or idiopathic dysplasia of undetermined significance (IDUS) may be applied;[27] some of these patients will, with time, develop MDS.

Blood film examination

Blood films should be prepared fresh since blood samples exposed to anticoagulants are unsatisfactory for accurate morphology. The ability to diagnose MDS depends crucially on optimal staining of PB and BM films. Staining varies enormously between laboratories, so observers should become familiar with their own laboratory's stains. Films sent for a second opinion should be sent unstained. Blood films are most commonly stained using the May–Grünewald–Giemsa or Wright method.[28] It is important that the stain used picks up granularity in neutrophils well and also reveals basophilic stippling in red cells.

Erythrocytes

Anemia is the most common feature of MDS but it is not an obligatory finding. Usually the red cells are large, but they may be of normal size and occasionally are small. Many textbooks list sideroblastic anemia among the causes of a low MCV but this may be misleading, since it only applies to the rare hereditary form. The MDS category of refractory anemia with ring sideroblasts (RA-RS) is associated with a raised or normal MCV. Frequently, red cells in MDS vary in size and shape (aniso-/poikilocytosis). Oval macrocytes are common. When these are accompanied by small hypochromic cells, giving a dimorphic picture, RA-RS should be suspected (Fig. 20.1A). However, small hypochromic red cell fragments may be seen in all forms of MDS. A preponderance of small hypochromic red cells is rarely seen and should suggest acquired hemoglobin H (HbH) disease (Fig. 20.1B). This is a very rare finding in MDS and may be revealed with supravital staining (Fig. 20.1C).[29] Poikilocytosis refers to several types of shape changes: dacrocytes (tear-drop shaped cells), acanthocytes (spur-spike cells), and cell fragments are all frequently seen. MDS is a rare cause of elliptocytosis (small, oval erythrocytes). However, red cell size and shape may be normal. Howell–Jolly bodies are occasionally seen but rather more common is basophilic stippling, which may be fine or coarse (Fig. 20.1D). Fine basophilic stippling confined to large, misshapen, hypochromic cells usually indicates RA-RS.

Table 20.5 Diagnostic and prognostic significance of cytogenetic abnormalities in myelodysplastic syndromes

Cytogenetic finding	Frequency (% of MDS cases according to[53])	Cytogenetic risk[53]	Diagnostic for MDS* according to WHO 2008[5]
Normal karyotype	51.7	Good	No
5q-	11	Good	Yes
-Y	2.8	Good	No
20q-	2	Good	No
+21	1.1	Good	No
12p-	0.6	Good	Yes
#t(1q)	0.6	Good	No
t(7q)	0.6	Good	No
t(17q)	0.5	Good	Yes
-X	0.5	Good	No
9q-	0.5	Good	Yes
-21	0.5	Good	No
t(15q)	0.5	Good	No
15q-	0.4	Good	No
+8	5.3	Intermediate-I	No
11q-	0.9	Intermediate-I	Yes
-7	3.5	Intermediate-II	Yes
Complex = 3 anomalies	2.7	Intermediate-II	Yes
3q abnormality	1.3	Intermediate-II	Yes
7q-	0.9	Intermediate-II	Yes
t(11q23)	0.5	Intermediate-II	Yes
+19	0.4	Intermediate-II	No
Complex>3 anomalies	11.1	Poor	Yes
t(5q)	0.6	Poor	Yes
t(6;9)(p23;q34)	1[5]	Poor	Yes
-13 or del(13q)	3[5]	na	Yes
Idic(X)(q13)	1–2[5]	na	Yes

*In the setting of persistent cytopenia(s) but in absence of definitive morphological features.

#t, translocation; na, not available.

Leukocytes

Neutropenia is very common in MDS. Although it may already be severe at diagnosis, it is frequently mild or may develop later in the course of the disease. Abnormalities in granularity of neutrophils are important features. Classically, there are few if any neutrophil granules (Fig. 20.2A) but sometimes hypergranularity is seen (Fig. 20.2B). The leukocyte alkaline phosphatase (LAP) score may be low.[30] Rarely, giant granules typical of those seen in Chediak–Higashi syndrome have been identified. Auer rods are sometimes seen and, when present, should lead to classification of the disease as RAEB-2, due to their reported negative prognostic significance.[31] Accurate enumeration of blast cells in blood has been stressed in WHO 2008. Cases with 2–4% blast cells in blood are classified as RAEB-1, even if the fraction in BM smears is <5%.[4] Cases with 1% blast cells in blood and <5% in BM are MDS-unclassified.

Abnormal neutrophil nuclear lobation is the other feature to observe. Pseudo-Pelger cells are neutrophils with unilobated or bilobed nuclei with normal condensation of the nuclear chromatin (Fig. 20.2C). It is important to distinguish these cells from myelocytes and metamyelocytes, in which the chromatin remains relatively uncondensed. Frequently, pseudo-Pelger cells display hypogranular cytoplasm and, occasionally, neutrophils with hyperlobated

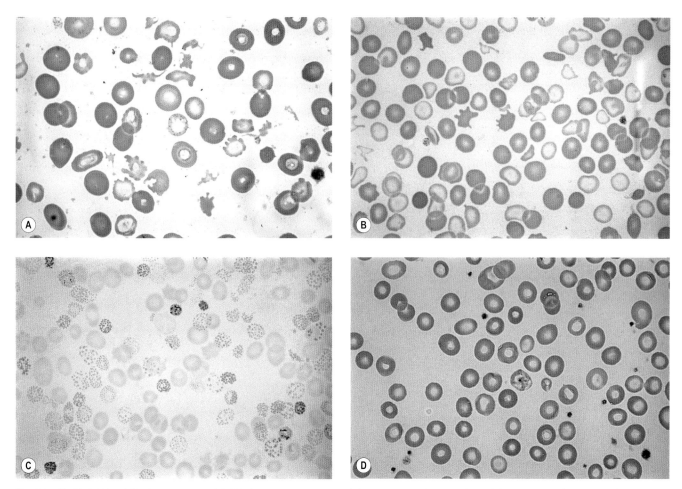

Fig. 20.1 (A–D) (A) Blood film from patient with RARS showing anisocytosis, poikilocytosis, anisochromasia, basophilic stippling and irregularly shaped red cells. (B) Blood film from a patient with acquired HbH disease showing very hypochromic population together with anisocytosis and poikilocytosis and irregularly shaped red cells. (C) Blood film from a patient with acquired HbH disease showing 'golf ball' inclusions when stained with brilliant cresyl blue. (D) Blood film from a patient with RARS showing a Howell–Jolly body in a cell with coarse basophilic stippling.

nuclei are seen. An unusual feature is arachnoid lobation, with the nuclear lobes looking like the segments of a spider's leg.

A relative increase of monocytes can be seen in MDS due to neutropenia while chronic myelomonocytic leukemia (currently classified by the WHO as a myelodysplastic/ myeloproliferative neoplasm, see Chapter 27) is a differential diagnosis in patients with a total monocytosis >1 × 10^9/l. Degranulated eosinophils are sometimes a feature of MDS. Eosinophils with basophilic granules, or vice versa, are sometimes seen. Significant eosinophilia and/or basophilia is seen in approximately 12% of MDS patients and predicts poorer prognosis.[32]

Platelets

Thrombocytopenia is common. Giant platelets or megakaryocyte fragments may circulate in MDS (Fig. 20.2D) and agranular platelets may also be seen.

Thrombocytosis is rare, but occurs in MDS with del(5q). It is important to distinguish myeloproliferative thrombocythemia from the thrombocytosis of MDS. The former should not have dysplastic features, although anemia with ring sideroblasts has been described accompanying marked thrombocytosis, histological BM features resembling essential thrombocythemia and (in most cases) presence of JAK2^{V617F} mutation (see Chapter 27).

Bone marrow examination

Well-prepared, freshly stained BM aspirate films and BMTB sections are the key to accurate diagnosis of MDS. Interpreting BM aspirates in MDS can be difficult and even experts may differ in evaluating borderline dysplasia. Typically, the marrow is hypercellular, but cellularity is better appreciated from BMTB sections than from aspirate films. This is one of the compelling reasons why the two investigations should be seen as complementary. Also, megakaryocyte dysplasia may be easier to evaluate by BM biopsy, especially in cases with fibrosis. A particular value of BMTB is to demonstrate spatial disturbances of hemopoietic tissue and topographic changes (abnormal distribution of precursors, megakaryocytes and blood vessels) within the marrow, which cannot be appreciated in samples obtained by aspiration.

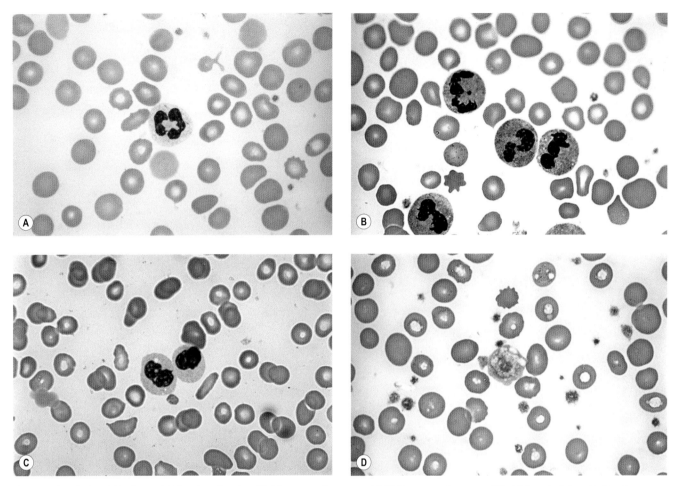

Fig. 20.2 (A–D) Blood film from a MDS patient showing. (A) A hypogranular neutrophil. (B) Hypergranular neutrophils. (C) Pseudo-Pelger–Huët cells. (D) A giant ('balloon-like') platelet.

Bone marrow aspirate

Erythropoiesis

All of the features seen in PB may be present but the BM aspirate gives the opportunity of examining the whole sequence of erythropoiesis. In many cases there is erythroid hyperplasia. Pure red cell aplasia is a rare finding. Frequently, the red cell precursors appear megaloblastic. Multinucleated forms are common and megaloblastic anemia is one of the main differential diagnoses. Mitotic figures are common and there is frequently dyskaryorrhexis (literally, abnormal bursting of a cell nucleus). Pyknosis, nuclear budding and intranuclear bridging are also seen frequently. There is often asynchrony between the maturation of nucleus and cytoplasm, with fully hemoglobinized cells retaining uncondensed nuclear chromatin (Fig. 20.3A).

Sideroblasts are red cell precursors with an accumulation of iron in their mitochondria, which stains blue with Perls stain ('Prussian blue') and appears granular. To be termed ring sideroblasts, the abnormal cells should have at least five siderotic granules in a perinuclear distribution. These granules may surround the entire nucleus, be localized to portions of the perinuclear area or cover at least one-third of the nucleus.[33] Over half of MDS cases have some sideroblasts. Arbitrarily, when ring sideroblasts comprise >15% of the total erythroblast population the disease is designated with ring sideroblasts, (+RS) (Fig. 20.3B).

Granulopoiesis

All of the features seen in peripheral blood may be present in BM smears. Absence of secondary granules may be a feature of all myeloid precursor cells (Fig. 20.4) but primary azurophil granules are usually present in promyelocytes and some myeloblasts. Of interest, it is very unusual for the myeloid cells in MDS not to stain with myeloperoxidase, albeit the staining may be less dense than in controls.

An accurate blast cell count is important prognostically. The FAB group recognized two types of blast cells. Type I blast cells are myeloblasts of variable size, without granules or Auer rods. The nuclear chromatin is uncondensed and there are usually one or two nucleoli. A type II blast cell is usually larger, with rather more cytoplasm, and contains a few azurophil granules. Type II blast cells can be distinguished from promyelocytes, which have a slightly eccentric nucleus with more condensed chromatin and less distinct nucleoli, and have also an obvious Golgi zone. Abnormal promyelocytes may also have excessive granules (more than six) resembling those seen in acute promyelocytic leukemia, although without the bilobed or monocytoid nuclear

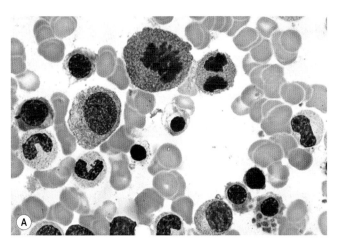

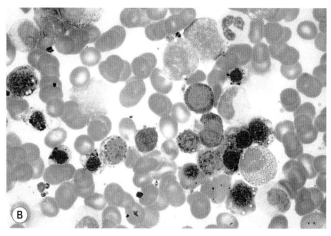

Fig. 20.3 (A–B) (A) Bone marrow film from a patient with RARS showing mitotic figures, and vacuolated and stippled normoblasts. (B) Bone marrow film from a patient with RARS stained with Perls stain showing ring sideroblasts.

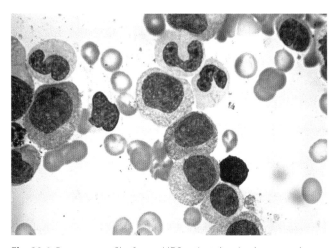

Fig. 20.4 Bone marrow film from a MDS patient showing hypogranular myeloid cells at different stages of maturation.

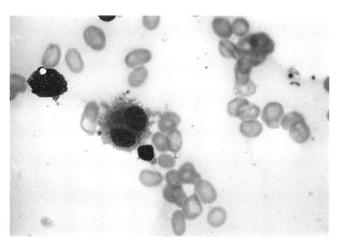

Fig. 20.5 Bone marrow film from a MDS patient showing a micromegakaryocyte.

features of the latter. Goasguen and colleagues[34] later described a type III blast cell with more than 20 azurophil granules but without a visible Golgi zone.

The International Working Group on Morphology of Myelodysplastic Syndrome (IWGM-MDS) agreed on a set of recommendations, including those for the definition and enumeration of blast cells.[33] It has been recommended that agranular or granular blast cells are recognized (replacing the previous type I, II and III blasts) and dysplastic promyelocytes are distinguished from cytologically normal promyelocytes and from granular blast cells. It has been stressed that sufficient cells must be counted (at least 500), to give a precise blast cell percentage, particularly at thresholds that are important for diagnosis or prognosis.[33]

Thrombopoiesis

Usually, numbers of megakaryocytes in MDS correspond to bone marrow cellularity. However, megakaryocytes may also be numerous (often in association with altered histotopography and/or fibrosis) or, less often, decreased in numbers. There are characteristically three types of abnormal

megakaryocytes: micromegakaryocytes (Fig. 20.5), giant megakaryocytes with multiple dispersed nuclei (Fig. 20.6), and moderate-sized megakaryocytes with a single round eccentric nucleus (monolobated megakaryocytes, Fig. 20.7). The latter are characteristic of the MDS with del(5q), but are not specific for this entity.

Bone marrow trephine

General histologic features of myelodysplastic syndromes

In most MDS patients, histologic sections show hypercellularity of hemopoietic tissue, but may also appear normocellular or hypocellular. It is important to remember that the expected range of cellularity is wide in the older age group within which most cases of MDS arise, although cellularity generally decreases as age increases. When relatively young patients present with suspected MDS, what might appear to be increased cellularity should not be overestimated.

Stromal components of the BM usually appear relatively normal in MDS although there may be a slight increase in

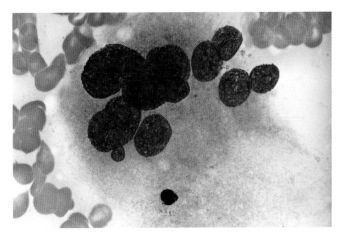

Fig. 20.6 Bone marrow film from a MDS patient showing a giant megakaryocyte with multiple dispersed nuclei.

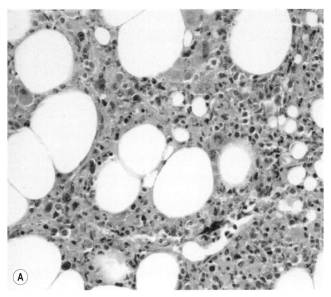

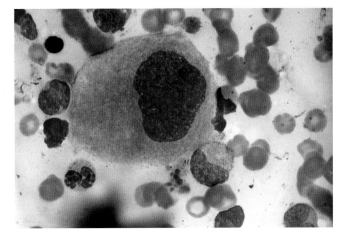

Fig. 20.7 Bone marrow film from a patient with 5q-syndrome showing a mononuclear megakaryocyte.

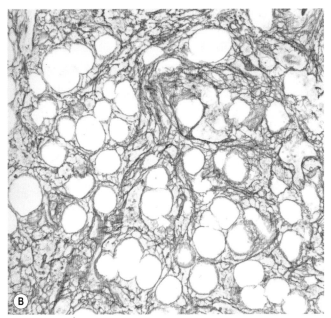

Fig. 20.8 (A–B) Decalcified, paraffin-embedded bone marrow trephine biopsy core from a patient with MDS with fibrosis. (A) Giemsa, objective × 60. (B) Reticulin silver stain confirms an increase of reticulin network corresponding to fibrosis WHO grade 2. Gordon–Sweet stain, objective × 60.

reticulin. Disturbances of trabecular bone remodeling, including new bone formation, are rare. Moderate to severe increases in reticulin, sometimes including collagen formation, is seen in approximately 10–20% of MDS cases and referred to as MDS with fibrosis[35] (Fig. 20.8A, B). Fibrosis may cause difficulties in obtaining representative blast counts from aspirate films and in classification of MDS. It has been shown that patients who have MDS with fibrosis have a worse prognosis than those without.[36] Also, development of fibrosis is regarded as a sign of progress. Fibrosis is often accompanied by increased vascularity.

Assessment of spatial distribution of hemopoiesis in MDS

As mentioned above, BMTB sections have the particular value in MDS, allowing assessment of the spatial distribution of hemopoietic cells. In normal BM, there is a specific topographic distribution of hematopoiesis (described in detail in Chapter 3). Both in primary MDS and in secondary forms of myelodysplasia, this topographic arrangement is disturbed. Displacement of early granulocyte precursors

from trabecular margins is a frequent finding and, accompanying this, scattered metamyelocytes and neutrophil polymorphs may be found immediately adjacent to trabecular margins. The presence of myeloblasts and promyelocytes in groups in the central parts of intertrabecular spaces is less common. Such abnormal localization of immature precursors (ALIP) (Fig. 20.9), which may be reflected by the presence of aggregates (3–5 cells) and/or clusters (>5 cells),[37] is usually seen in the context of an increased blood or BM blast cell count. In cases of MDS with fibrosis, the presence of ALIP will draw attention to increased numbers of blast cells.[38] It should also be noted that ALIP is not a phenomenon specific to MDS. It can be seen in reactive conditions and myeloproliferative neoplasms, and after treatment with G-CSF. Clusters of other hematopoietic cells may mimic

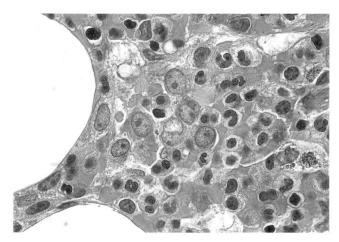

Fig. 20.9 Immature myelomonocytic cells in the center of an intertrabecular space; so-called 'ALIP'. Hematoxylin and eosin-stained section of decalcified, paraffin-embedded bone marrow trephine biopsy core; objective × 100.

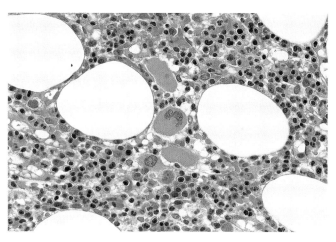

Fig. 20.11 Cluster of atypical, small megakaryocytes in MDS. Hematoxylin and eosin-stained section of decalcified, paraffin-embedded bone marrow trephine biopsy core; objective × 40.

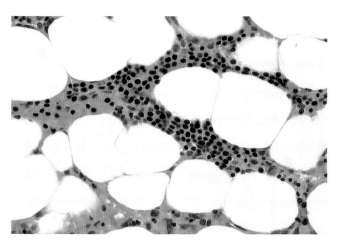

Fig. 20.10 Dyplastic erythropoiesis with irregular clustering of erythroid precursor cells, each cell at a similar (in this example, relatively late) stage of maturation to its neighbors; in normal erythroid cell clusters, a mixture of maturational stages would be present. Hematoxylin and eosin-stained section of decalcified, paraffin-embedded bone marrow trephine biopsy core; objective × 40.

ALIP (e.g. erythropoiesis in B₁₂/folate deficiency, monocytes in chronic myelomonocytic leukemia, large lymphoid cells in lymphoma infiltrates). Immunohistochemical (IHC) stains may be necessary for definite diagnosis.[38]

Spatial disorganization of erythropoiesis is represented by erythroid cell clusters occupying paratrabecular areas of the marrow and also by loss of the normal organization within individual clusters. The clusters are frequently enlarged, with increased numbers of proerythroblasts and early normoblasts. The cells in some clusters may appear synchronous, rather than reflecting a normal spectrum of maturational stages of erythropoiesis (Fig. 20.10). Neighboring clusters may differ markedly from one another, some containing predominantly cells of earlier stages and some predominantly cells showing more advanced maturation. In some patients, erythropoiesis may appear dispersed, with absent or infrequent formation of cell clusters.

Assessment of megakaryocyte morphology and distribution is critical to the interpretation of BMTB histology in MDS.[38,39] Cytologic features are discussed below but spatial distribution of megakaryocytes, as for other hemopoietic lineages, is often highly abnormal. Because of their relatively large size and distinctive morphology, it is usually easy to detect clustering of megakaryocytes (Fig. 20.11) and their displacement from perisinusoidal to paratrabecular locations. Occasional small clusters of 2–3 megakaryocytes may be found in normal or reactive bone marrow but larger groupings are highly atypical and indicate pathology. Paratrabecular location of megakaryocytes has similar significance and is extremely rare in other contexts, unless the BM is severely hypoplastic for unrelated reasons. Even in the latter situation, the possibility of hypoplastic MDS should be considered carefully.

Cytologic features in trephine biopsy sections in MDS

Cytologic features of myelodysplasia in developing hemopoietic cells are best seen in BM aspirate films. In decalcified trephine biopsy sections, it is usually not possible to detect hypogranularity in granulocytic cells. Nuclear abnormalities such as pseudo-Pelger changes can be seen only with difficulty. Failure of nuclear condensation and lobation in terminally differentiated neutrophil polymorphs can be seen in occasional cases. Abnormalities of granulation may be visible in high-quality sections of plastic-embedded trephine biopsies. Since these are generally thinner than those cut from paraffin-embedded specimens (1–2 mm compared with 3–4 mm), familiarity with the normal degree of granularity visible in thin sections is essential. Abnormalities in the proportions of developing granulocytes representing different stages of maturation are more readily appreciable. There are frequently increased promyelocytes and myelocytes accompanied by reduced numbers of metamyelocytes and neutrophils. It is even more difficult in BMTB sections than aspirate films to determine precisely which cells among the immature granulocytes are truly myeloblasts.

In the erythroid series, dysplastic cytology is frequently represented by a megaloblast-like appearance of individual nucleated red cell precursors. As with granulopoiesis, it is usually easy to appreciate the imbalance in relative numbers of cells at different stages of maturation. Increased numbers of dysplastic proerythroblasts and reduced numbers of later cells alter the composition of erythroid nests. Absence of the familiar late normoblasts, abundant in normal BM, is an important clue to the presence of erythroid dysplasia in BMTB sections. The megaloblast-like proerythroblasts may be confused with early myelomonocytic precursors, and may even suggest ALIP. However, Giemsa staining reveals their basophilic cytoplasm (with a perinuclear halo if the tissue has been decalcified), allowing their distinction from other immature hemopoietic cells. Also, nucleoli of proerythroblasts are closely associated with nuclear membrane, while they are usually centrally located in myeloid precursors.

Cells of megakaryocytic lineage demonstrate the most readily appreciable dysplastic cytologic features in BMTB sections. Because megakaryocytes tend to remain adherent to particles in aspirate films, trephine biopsy is often superior for their assessment. Megakaryocyte numbers are frequently increased, with striking spatial abnormalities as described above, and their size is often variable but generally smaller than normal. True micromegakaryocytes, similar in size to promyelocytes, are difficult to see without specific IHC staining, but small megakaryocytes are usually easy to recognize. In addition to their reduced size, these cells typically have reduced numbers of nuclear lobes.

One important aspect of cytology in myelodysplasia, which is often only appreciable in BMTB sections and not in aspirate films, is the increased apoptotic activity that contributes to ineffective hemopoiesis in patients with MDS.[40,41] Apoptotic nuclei, recognizable by their characteristic patterns of nucleic acid condensation, can be seen scattered throughout the hemopoietic tissue and sometimes clustered inside the cytoplasm of stromal macrophages. However, increased apoptotic activity also occurs in other conditions involving increased cell turnover in the BM, including hyperplastic states (e.g. associated with septicemia or in response to malignant disease elsewhere in the body), inflammatory myelopathies such as those associated with HIV infection and systemic lupus erythematosus (SLE), myeloproliferative neoplasms and acute leukemias. Undue significance should not be attributed to finding increased apoptotic activity in BMTB sections if other features of dysplasia are absent or if other features of inflammation are present.

Characteristic features of MDS subtypes

Findings in blood and BM smears diagnostic for various MDS subtypes are summarized in Table 20.2.[4] In patients with refractory cytopenia with unilineage dysplasia, BM is usually hypercellular, but may be normo- or hypocellular. It is important to assess megakaryocyte morphology in trephine sections as well as aspirate films before diagnosis of RA or RN is made for differentiation with RCMD subtype of MDS. At least 30 megakaryocytes should be assessed. In RA, hyperplastic erythropoiesis is prominent. In RN and RT, erythropoiesis may be normal or decreased. Large clusters of normally-maturing erythroid cells may represent the only pathological features in many patients with RARS, in whom

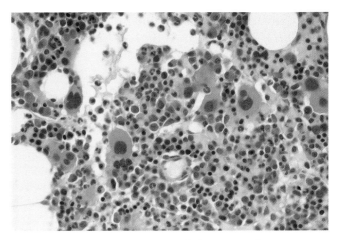

Fig. 20.12 Dysplastic megakaryocytes including mononuclear variants typical of the 5q- syndrome. Hematoxylin and eosin-stained section of decalcified, paraffin-embedded bone marrow trephine biopsy core; objective × 40.

BMTB histology may be otherwise lack dysplastic features in granulopoiesis and megakaryocytes. In MDS with del(5q), erythropoiesis is frequently hypoplastic. Small megakaryocytes with monolobated nuclei are particularly associated with MDS with del(5q) (Fig. 20.12) but may also be present, together with a heterogeneous population of less distinctive dysplastic megakaryocytes, in other forms of myelodysplasia. In RCMD type of MDS, BM is usually hypercellular. Dysplasia may be most prominent in one of the hematopoietic lineages, but it has to be present in at least one more lineage. Before making the RCMD diagnosis, it is important to assess percentage of blast cells in blood and BM films. Ring sideroblasts may be present in RCMD. In MDS of RAEB type, BM is usually also hypercellular, displays multilineage dysplasia and the signs of abnormal spatial distribution of hematopoiesis. ALIP are often present, especially in RAEB-2. The enumeration of blast cells in BMTB may be very important in cases with fibrosis (Fig. 20.8A, B), where their numbers in films may not exceed 5%.

Myelodysplasia in hypoplastic bone marrow

Assessment of myelodysplasia in hypocellular BM specimens poses particular difficulties due to the paucity of hemopoietic tissue available for assessment. Aspiration may have been unsuccessful or may have yielded a suboptimal sample, so that BMTB combined with IHC stains has an important role.[42] The differential diagnosis includes primary MDS, secondary myelodysplasia, and disorders such as hypoplastic/aplastic anemia, paroxysmal nocturnal hemoglobinuria and hypoplastic acute myeloid leukemia.[43] The same criteria should be applied in assessing hemopoietic cell distribution and cytologic features as in normocellular or hypercellular BMTB sections. Even with very little hemopoietic tissue to evaluate, it should be possible to determine whether BMTB sections show: (1) hypoplastic normal hemopoiesis; (2) hypoplastic dysplastic hemopoiesis with evidence of at least partial maturation within each hemopoietic lineage; or (3) hypoplastic acute leukemia with predominance of blast cells and minimal or no evidence of maturation.

Histologic features of secondary myelodysplasia

Dysplastic hemopoiesis may occur in response to a variety of often poorly characterized systemic diseases and toxic insults to the bone marrow. A familiar example is the myelopathy associated with infection by the human immunodeficiency virus (HIV).[44] A similar inflammatory myelopathy can accompany systemic autoimmune conditions, particularly SLE. Hemopoietic recovery following cytotoxic chemotherapy is also often transiently dysplastic,[45] in addition to the predictable megaloblastosis caused by use of folate antagonists.

It is not always possible to determine by BM examination whether dysplasia is primary or secondary but BMTB histology provides important clues to indicate the likelihood of one versus the other. The main features that indicate a secondary origin for myelodysplasia are abnormalities of the BM stroma, reflecting toxic or inflammatory injury of stromal cells, occurring in addition to hemopoietic cell damage. At the least, mildly increased stromal reticulin is usually present. In addition, there is often stromal edema, indicated by separation of hemopoietic cells in the interstitium and widening of sinusoidal lumens (Fig. 20.13), frequently accompanied by interstitial leakage of red blood cells. In more severe injury, gelatinous change occurs; evidence for this may be found in aspirate films as well as in histologic preparations, with irregular masses eosinophilic, periodic acid-Schiff (PAS)-positive material in particles and trails. In histologic sections, distinction between severe edema and gelatinous change can be confirmed by Alcian blue staining; edema fluid remains unstained but, in gelatinous change, the stroma stains turquoise/blue. Stromal injury is occasionally sufficiently severe to cause collagen fibrosis, particularly if necrosis has occurred. Evidence of previous necrosis may be found in the form of dead bone trabeculae or fragments of amorphous debris in the fibrotic stroma showing dystrophic

calcification. Recent severe systemic illness or exposure to cytotoxic agents may leave a distinct cement line within many bone trabeculae, reflecting transient inhibition of normal bone remodeling. Stromal injury may also lead to new bone formation; this is usually only focal and minor in extent but rare patients, for unknown reasons, respond to toxic BM injury with florid neo-osteogenesis.

Other features suggesting a secondary origin for dysplasia are:

- increased phagocytotic activity among stromal macrophages, converting these usually dendritic cells into large forms containing abundant cytoplasmic debris
- the presence of inflammatory cells (particularly plasma cells) in increased numbers in the stroma
- the finding of reactive lymphoid nodules or granulomas.

Assessment of macrophages and plasma cells in the stroma usually requires application of imunohistochemical stains.

If lymphoid nodules are seen, it should be remembered that such aggregates, sometimes with atypical features, might also occur in association with primary MDS. The differential diagnosis must include, in addition, BM involvement by lymphoma provoking secondary myelodysplasia (see Chapter 29). Distinguishing between these alternatives can be extremely difficult and requires integration of all clinical, hematologic, cytogenetic and molecular genetic information available for the individual patient under consideration. Even with such information, it may be necessary to follow the patient's subsequent progress, including repeated biopsy, to establish the nature and clinical significance of such abnormalities.

Use of immunohistochemistry and fluorescent *in situ* hybridization (FISH) in trephine biopsy sections in myelodysplasia

The main application of IHC stains in MDS has been enumeration of CD34[+] hemopoietic stem cells in BMTB sections. The CD34[+] count assessed in this way has prognostic value, with higher counts and clusters being of negative prognostic significance.[36,46] Evaluation of CD34 positivity in BMTB sections must be undertaken with care to exclude capillary endothelial cells. Endothelial cells express this antigen strongly and, particularly when cut in cross-section, cannot always be seen to be associated with a vascular lumen. With experience, hemopoietic cells can be recognized by their characteristic granular IHC staining pattern with monoclonal antibodies reactive with class I CD34 (Fig. 20.14A). Another antigen of help in recognition of ALIP is CD117 (c-kit receptor) (Fig. 20.14B).[47] However, the prognostic significance of enumerating CD117[+] hemopoietic precursors has not yet been established and the staining may be more difficult to interpret than for CD34.

Immunohistochemistry can also be helpful in interpreting BMTB histology in myelodysplastic conditions when cytologic abnormalities cause difficulty in recognizing cells belonging to the various hemopoietic lineages.[38,48,49] Cells of the granulocytic series, at all stages of maturation, can be demonstrated by immunostaining for myeloperoxidase, muramidase (lysozyme) or the CD68 epitope recognized by

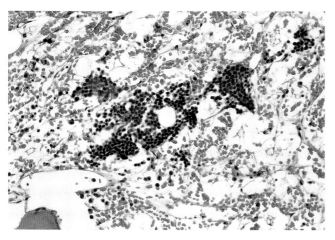

Fig. 20.13 Stromal edema and red cell extravasation, presumed to represent stromal responses to inflammatory or toxic injury. Atypical, cohesive-appearing, 'synchronous' clusters of erythropoietic cells are prominent and other hemopoietic cells are widely separated in the background. Non-nucleated red cells are present throughout the edematous interstitium and a distended sinusoidal lumen can be seen (bottom left) adjacent to the end of a bony trabecula. Hematoxylin and eosin-stained section of decalcified, paraffin-embedded bone marrow trephine biopsy core; objective × 20.

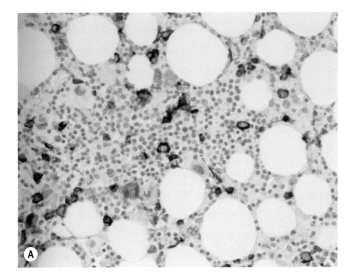

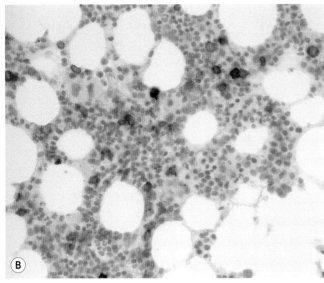

Fig. 20.14 (A–B) (A) Increased numbers and abnormal distribution of CD34⁺ cells visualized by immunohistochemistry in a case of MDS RAEB-I. (B) Increased numbers of CD117 cells shown by immunohistochemistry in the same case; objective × 40.

monoclonal antibody KP1. Use of neutrophil elastase as a target antigen for IHC may be unreliable in MDS if hypogranularity of granulocytes is a feature; otherwise, it can be useful to demonstrate the distribution of promyelocytes and myelocytes. Later granulocytes (metamyelocytes and neutrophil polymorphs) express CD15, CD10 and the calprotectin molecule recognized by monoclonal antibody Mac387. Monocytes and macrophages can be assessed by immunostaining with antibodies to CD14 and CD68R (PG-M1).[49] The use of CD14 is preferred for monocyte recognition since these cells are rarely present in great abundance and CD68R is expressed strongly by the normal population of stromal macrophages.

The identity and distribution of dysplastic erythroid cells can be confirmed by IHC to demonstrate hemoglobin, glycophorin A or C; glycophorin C is expressed slightly earlier in erythropoiesis than glycophorin A. Megakaryocytes are usually easily recognizable from their cytologic features but atypical forms, micromegakaryocytes and megakaryoblasts can be highlighted by immunostaining for CD61 (platelet glycoprotein IIIa) or CD42b (platelet glycoprotein lb). Platelets themselves are visualized with these immunostains; they are not normally shed into marrow stroma in significant quantities and their presence in abundance can be a clue to the occurrence of an inflammatory process causing secondary myelodysplasia.

With increasing understanding of the genetic basis of hemopoietic disorders, including primary MDS, there is a growing interest in demonstrating cytogenetic abnormalities *in situ* in BMTB. Despite the limitations of visualizing signals in sectioned nuclei, in which only part of the chromosomal complement of any cell is represented, methodology has been developed for successful demonstration of numerical chromosomal abnormalities and translocations by FISH in trephine biopsy sections. Application of FISH to the standard assessment of histologic preparations in suspected MDS has, as yet, been limited.[50,51]

Flow cytometry in diagnosis of MDS

Several studies have shown that flow cytometry (FCM) may contribute significantly to diagnosis and prognosis in MDS (reviewed in [52]). Abnormal development of erythroid, myeloid and monocytic cells, identified as phenotypic abnormalities by FCM in MDS correlates with prognostic scoring systems, transfusion dependency, and time to progression to advanced MDS/AML, as well as with outcome after hemopoietic stem cell transplantation. The most widely seen features are:

- within the blast cell compartment: abnormal expression of CD45, CD13, CD33, CD34, CD117, HLA-DR, CD11b, CD7, CD56 (Fig. 20.15), CD19
- within the maturing myeloid compartment: decreased scatter properties, shift to the left with asynchronous marker expression, abnormal patterns of CD13/CD11b (Fig. 20.15) and/or CD13/CD16 expression, and expression of T- and/or B-cell related markers, such as CD7, CD2, CD19 (sc. lineage infidelity)
- within the erythroid compartment: abnormal expression of CD71, CD105, glycophorin A, CD117, CD45
- decreased numbers of B-cell precursors
- abnormal expression of monocyte markers.

Published studies have employed a wide range of methods and reagents. Moreover, BM samples from patients with non-clonal dysplasia have not been sufficiently studied. Therefore, the WHO 2008 recommended that, if three or more phenotypic abnormalities are found involving one or more of the myeloid lineages, the features can be considered as 'suggestive' of MDS.[5] However, in the absence of conclusive morphologic and/or cytogenetic features, flow cytometric abnormalities alone are not diagnostic of MDS. Patients whose cells exhibit aberrant phenotypic features suggesting MDS should be followed carefully to determine whether morphologic features emerge that are sufficient to substantiate the diagnosis. Efforts within the European Leukemia Network (ELNet) to standardize FCM method and reagents for MDS assessment are undertaken to

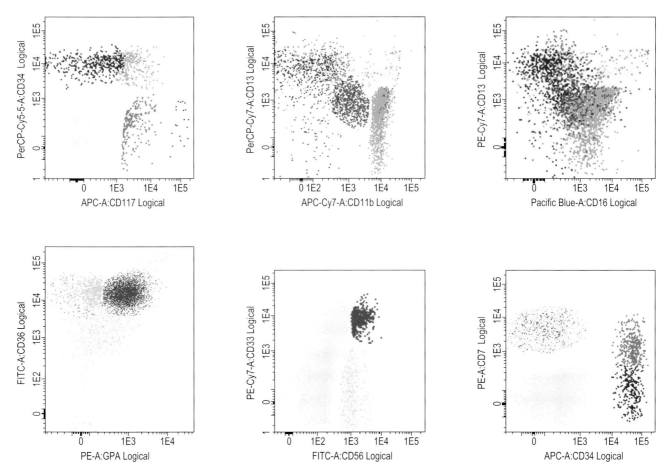

Fig. 20.15 Example of abnormal flow cytometry findings in a case of MDS, RCMD category. Left upper plot shows the presence of a population of CD34⁺ cells (3%), which are in part positive for CD117 (yellow). The CD117⁺/CD34⁺ cells (yellow) show increased expression of CD11b (upper middle plot). A fraction of CD34 cells (65% of CD34⁺ cells, 2% totally) is positive for CD7 (lower right plot). CD34⁺ cells. Upper middle and right plots show that granulopoiesis is left shifted but shows preserved maturation pattern. There is a population of myeloid precursors (CD33⁺) expressing CD56 (lower middle plot). An increased number of erythroid precursors (GPA⁺ CD36⁺) is found (left lower plot).

establish its role and provide robust guidelines for its use in this context.[52]

Genetics

Whenever possible, direct chromosomal analysis of BM cells should be performed in patients with suspected MDS. Clonal cytogenetic abnormalities are found in approximately 50% of patients with primary MDS[53] and more than 90% of patients with secondary MDS.[54] The more advanced the disease, the greater the incidence of karyotypic abnormality. Even when a normal karyotype is found, monosomies and trisomies are sometimes detected by FISH. Cytogenetic abnormalities with prognostic relevance have been identified and incorporated into prognostic scoring (Tables 20.5 and 20.6). However, the prognostic relevance of many cytogenetic changes is still obscure.

By morphology, deletions of 5q are characterized by the presence of atypical megakaryocytes with monolobated nuclei[55] and deletions of 17p by small vacuolated pseudo-Pelger cells.[56] Rearrangements of 3q26 are associated with raised platelet counts and micromegakaryocytes.[57] Isolated del (20q) is found in patients with minimal

Table 20.6 WHO Classification-Based Prognostic Scoring System for MDS*[74,86]

Variable	0	1	2	3
WHO category	RA, RS-RS, 5q-	RCMD	RAEB-1	RAEB-2
Karyotype**	Good	Intermediate	Poor	–
Transfusion requirement#	No	Regular	–	–

*Risk groups were as follows: very low (score 0), low (score 1), intermediate (score 2), high (score 3–4), very high (score 5–6).

**Karyotype: good : normal, del(20q), del (5q), -Y, poor: complex (three or more abnormalities) or anomalies of chromosome 7, intermediate: all other.

#RBC transfusion dependency was defined as having at least one transfusion every 8 weeks over a period of 4 months.

dysplasia and thrombocytopenia, resembling idiopathic thrombocytopenia.[58]

Using array comparative genomic hybridization and single nucleotide polymorphism arrays, chromosomal aberrations undetectable by metaphase karyotype analysis have been found in 20–30% of MDS patients with normal karyotype. The potential clinical significance of these abnormalities was demonstrated by an adverse effect on overall survival.[59,60]

Molecular changes conferring better prognosis in MDS, independent of other risk factors, include recently identified mutations of the *ten-eleven translocation 2* (*TET2*) gene located at 4q24 and found in approximately 20% of patients.[61] Several other gene abnormalities have been reported in MDS, including mutations in genes coding for critical receptor kinases or downstream signaling molecules (*KIT, G-CSFR, PDGFRb,FLT3, FMS, N-RAS, K-RAS, JAK2*) or for certain transcription factors (*RUNX1, CEBPA, PU.1, GATA-1, TP53, MLL*). *RAS* mutations occur in about 10–15% of MDS cases, with *N-RAS* being the most frequently mutated and associated with worse prognosis.[62]

Several studies have attempted to look for critical genes in affected regions in recurring genetic changes in MDS. In MDS with del(5q), the major commonly deleted region (CDR) has been delineated at band 5q31.1. One of the genes in this region is the *RPS14* gene encoding the ribosomal protein S14, a component of the 40S ribosome subunit. Haploinsufficiency of *RPS14* leads to the characteristic 5q- phenotype with impaired expansion of erythroid progenitors and changes in megakaryopoiesis.[63] Two microRNAs (miR), miR-145 and miR-146a are located at chr.5q33 and become haploinsufficient in patients with del(5q) MDS. Interestingly, mice studies have shown that down-regulation of these two miR inappropriately activates innate immune signaling and leads to slight thrombocytosis, as often observed in patients with del(5q) MDS. Moreover, this activation *per se* may increase long-term risk of bone marrow failure and leukemic evolution.[64] The *early-growth response gene 1* (*EGR1*) gene, involved in cellular responses to growth factors, mitogens, and stress stimuli, and the *secreted protein acidic and rich in cysteine* (*SPARC*) gene are other genes, in which abnormalities are implicated in pathogenesis of MDS with del(5q).

CDRs involved in aberrations of chromosome 7 have been less extensively studied. One proposed target is the homeobox (*HOX*) A9 gene, part of a cluster of homeobox genes encoding for DNA-binding transcription factors which have been implicated in differentiation and stem cell commitment in hematopoiesis. Molecular aberrations of the *HOXA9* gene are associated with a poor prognosis in MDS.[62]

Pathogenesis

MDS is considered to be a clonal stem cell disorder and is viewed as the result of the cumulative acquisition of multiple genetic errors occurring over a long period. Some of these abnormalities may be congenital but most are acquired. The acquired genetic abnormalities may be random errors and some environmental insults increase the risk. Chief among these have been exposure to X-irradiation, alkylating agents and benzene and its derivatives. Some individuals may be more prone to acquiring genetic abnormalities in these contexts because they lack effective detoxifying enzymes.[65,66]

Several studies have shown that hematopoietic progenitors in MDS patients are more prone to apoptosis than those of healthy individuals.[67] Dysregulation of proapoptotic pathway components, including tumor necrosis factor

(TNF)-α, Fas-ligand, and/or TNF-related apoptosis-inducing ligand (TRAIL), probably through over-expression of FLICE (caspase8) inhibitory protein (FLIP), have been found. Proapoptotic members of Bcl-2 family, Bax and Bad, are also highly expressed, as well as members of inhibitors of apoptosis (IAP) family (survivin, cIAP, NAIP and XIAP). Constitutive activation of NF-κB has been proposed as another proapoptotic mechanism, since inhibition of NF-κB in CD34$^+$ cells from patients with high-risk MDS resulted in apoptosis.[67] Defects in mitochondrial function may be of importance in patients with RARS, who demonstrate a constitutive leakage of cytochrome C from mitochondria.[68]

In some MDS patients (especially those with hypoplastic MDS), clones carrying a mutation of the X-chromosome gene PIG-A, characteristic of paroxysmal nocturnal hemoglobinuria (PNH) have been found. Such mutations lead to absence of glycosylphosphatidylinositol (GPI) anchor protein expression by hematopoietic cells. Similar to individuals with PNH and aplastic anemia, these MDS patients have an over-representation of the HLA haplotype DR15. They have a lower rate of progression to AML than other MDS patients and may respond well to immunosuppressive therapy.[69,70]

Another subset of MDS patients present oligoclonal expansions of cytotoxic lymphoid cells, which may target hemopoietic cells. Activated T-cells and skewed use of TCR-Vβ have also been shown. Hypothetical models propose immune triggering of the patient's lymphocytes, either by aberrantly expressed oncogenes and fusion gene products in hematopoietic progenitor cells or by super-antigens derived from bacteria or viruses.[20,71]

Clinical course and management

Although MDS in some individuals may follow an indolent course, in most patients the disease will eventually progress. Cytopenias will become worse and BM blast cell counts will increase. In this elderly group, approximately one third will develop acute leukemia, a third will die from the consequences of cytopenias and a third will die from an unrelated cause.[72]

To compare results of treatment in various patient cohorts, clinical studies have widely applied the International Prognostic Scoring System (IPSS), developed 1997 by Greenberg and colleagues. IPSS is based on percentage of BM blast cells, karyotype findings and number of cytopenias.[73] The recently developed WHO-classification-based Prognostic Scoring System (WPSS; Table 20.6) integrates WHO morphological criteria, karyotype and requirements for RBC transfusion to generate an indicator of symptomatic anemia.[74] Applying the WPSS allows stratification of patients into five risk categories (Table 20.6) with significantly different survival outcomes. Other proposed risk models include age and performance status integrated with the number of blast cells, combinations of cytopenias, nature of karyotypic abnormalities and RBC transfusion requirements.[75]

Treatment for MDS is unsatisfactory. The keystone is good supportive care. Even in patients who develop AML, the course may be slow and indolent. Therefore, no attempt at aggressive therapy should be initiated until the pace of the disease is established. Judicious use of red cell transfusions with an aim to maintain a Hb level of 90–100 g/l and use of appropriate antibiotics in case of infections is essential. Some patients will require platelet transfusions. Patients expected to live for a considerable time with regularly repeated red cell transfusions will need to consider iron chelation therapy when the S-ferritin levels exceed 1500 ng/ml.[72]

In patients with MDS with del(5q) the immunomodulatory drug lenalidomide showed 67% major erythroid responses and 45% complete cytogenetic remissions, with median response duration above 2 years.[76,77] Lenalidomide has been shown to up-regulate the tumor suppressor gene *SPARC* and the SPARC protein expression in erythroblasts *in vitro*. Patients with del(5q) MDS are haploinsufficient for *SPARC*, which makes it an interesting target for further investigation. Moreover, lenalidomide inhibits the cell cycle associated phosphatases CDC25C and PPA2, also located at chromosome 5q, which may further explain this drug efficacy in MDS with del(5q). However, due to an unexpectedly high rate of leukemic evolution in lenalidomide-treated patients, there is still a need for long-term studies evaluating the effects of this agent on survival in MDS with del(5q).[78,79] There is some indication that lenalidomide may also be effective in other MDS categories.[80]

Low-dose chemotherapy with cytarabine produces responses in 16% of MDS patients but cytopenias are often prolonged and this treatment has fallen out of favor. The hypomethylating agents 5-azacytidine and decitabine show an overall response rate of 30–50% but the fraction of complete responses is low.[81] A large phase 3 trial compared the outcome of high-risk MDS patients treated with 5-azacytidine, supportive care, and high-dose chemotherapy. 5-Azacytidine has significantly improved the outcome, extending the median survival from 15 to 25 months (hazard ratio 0.58). Hence, 5-azacytidine is currently considered as first-line therapy in high-risk MDS.[82]

High-dose chemotherapy has a dismal record. More than 80% of patients are >60 years of age and many are too frail to withstand the side-effects of this form of therapy. Complete responses occur but seldom last longer than a year. There are very few long-term survivors. Allogeneic stem cell transplantation may be curative and should be considered in younger patients who do not have a low-risk MDS category. Unfortunately, due to their high median age as a group, few MDS patients are suitable for this form of therapy. Decisions to attempt allografting and the type of conditioning (myeloablative or non-myeloablative) should be based on individual risk-assessment.[83]

Immunosuppression with anti-thymocyte globulin, with or without cyclosporine, is effective in younger MDS patients with normal karyotype and without long-standing transfusion requirement.[84] Other experiment treatments include the use of thalidomide, which is believed to exert its effect via the BM stroma, and farnesyl transferase inhibitors, which act by interfering with the *ras* signaling pathway.[85]

References

1. Hellstrom-Lindberg E. Myelodysplastic syndromes: an historical perspective. Hematology Am Soc Hematol Educ Program 2008:42.

2. Bennett JM, Catovsky D, Daniel MT, et al. Proposals for the classification of the myelodysplastic syndromes. Br J Haematol 1982;51:189–99.

3. Harris NL, Jaffe ES, Diebold J, et al. World Health Organization classification of neoplastic diseases of the hematopoietic and lymphoid tissues: report of the Clinical Advisory Committee meeting – Airlie House, Virginia, November 1997. J Clin Oncol 1999;17:3835–49.

4. Vardiman JW, Thiele J, Arber DA, et al. The 2008 revision of the World Health Organization (WHO) classification of myeloid neoplasms and acute leukemia: rationale and important changes. Blood 2009;114:937–51.

5. Swerdlow SH, Campo E, Harris NL, et al. WHO Classification of Tumours of Haematopoietic and Lymphoid Tissues. Lyon: IARC; 2008.

6. Ma X, Does M, Raza A, Mayne ST. Myelodysplastic syndromes: incidence and survival in the United States. Cancer 2007;109:1536–42.

7. Matsuda A, Germing U, Jinnai I, et al. Difference in clinical features between Japanese and German patients with refractory anemia in myelodysplastic syndromes. Blood 2005;106: 2633–40.

8. Williamson PJ, Kruger AR, Reynolds PJ, et al. Establishing the incidence of myelodysplastic syndrome. Br J Haematol 1994;87:743–5.

9. Aul C, Gattermann N, Schneider W. Age-related incidence and other epidemiological aspects of myelodysplastic syndromes. Br J Haematol 1992;82:358–67.

10. Strom SS, Velez-Bravo V, Estey EH. Epidemiology of myelodysplastic syndromes. Semin Hematol 2008;45: 8–13.

11. Rollison DE, Howlader N, Smith MT, et al. Epidemiology of myelodysplastic syndromes and chronic myeloproliferative disorders in the United States, 2001–2004, using data from the NAACCR and SEER programs. Blood 2008;112: 45–52.

12. Ma X, Lim U, Park Y, et al. Obesity, lifestyle factors, and risk of myelodysplastic syndromes in a large US cohort. Am J Epidemiol 2009;169: 1492–9.

13. Natelson EA. Benzene exposure and refractory sideroblastic erythropoiesis: is there an association? Am J Med Sci 2007;334:356–60.

14. Czader M, Orazi A. Therapy-related myeloid neoplasms. Am J Clin Pathol 2009;132:410–25.

15. Gologan R, Georgescu D, Tatic A, et al. Epidemiological data from the registry of patients with myelodysplastic syndrome in a single hospital center of Romania. Leuk Res 2009;33:1556–61.

16. Niemeyer CM, Baumann I. Myelodysplastic syndrome in children and adolescents. Semin Hematol 2008; 45:60–70.

17. Owen C, Barnett M, Fitzgibbon J. Familial myelodysplasia and acute myeloid leukaemia – a review. Br J Haematol 2008;140:123–32.

18. Howe RB, Porwit-MacDonald A, Wanat R, et al. The WHO classification of MDS does make a difference. Blood 2004; 103:3265–70.

19. Germing U, Strupp C, Kuendgen A, et al. Prospective validation of the WHO proposals for the classification of myelodysplastic syndromes. Haematologica 2006;91: 1596–604.

20. Voulgarelis M, Giannouli S, Ritis K, Tzioufas AG. Myelodysplasia-associated autoimmunity: clinical and pathophysiologic concepts. Eur J Clin Invest 2004;34:690–700.

21. Drabick JJ, Davis BJ, Byrd JC. Concurrent pernicious anemia and myelodysplastic syndrome. Ann Hematol 2001;80:243–5.

22. Mufti GJ, Figes A, Hamblin TJ, et al. Immunological abnormalities in myelodysplastic syndromes. I. Serum immunoglobulins and autoantibodies. Br J Haematol 1986;63:143–7.

23. Kohno T, Katamine S, Moriuchi R, et al. Activity of Fgr protein-tyrosine kinase is reduced in neutrophils of patients with myelodysplastic syndromes and chronic myelogenous leukemia. Leuk Res 1996;20:221–7.

24. Mittelman M, Zeidman A. Platelet function in the myelodysplastic syndromes. Int J Hematol 2000;71:95–8.

25. Richert-Boe KE, Bagby GC Jr. In vitro hematopoiesis in myelodysplasia: liquid and soft-gel culture studies. Hematol Oncol Clin North Am 1992;6:543–56.

26. Vercauteren SM, Bashashati A, Wu D, et al. Reduction in multi-lineage and erythroid progenitors distinguishes myelodysplastic syndromes from non-malignant cytopenias. Leuk Res 2009;33:1636–42.

27. Valent P, Horny HP. Minimal diagnostic criteria for myelodysplastic syndromes and separation from ICUS and IDUS: update and open questions. Eur J Clin Invest 2009;39:548–53.

28. Houwen B. Blood film preparation and staining procedures. Clin Lab Med 2002;22:1–14, v.

29. Steensma DP, Gibbons RJ, Higgs DR. Acquired alpha-thalassemia in association with myelodysplastic syndrome and other hematologic malignancies. Blood 2005; 105:443–52.

30. Bendix-Hansen K, Bergmann OJ. Evaluation of neutrophil alkaline phosphatase (NAP) activity in untreated myeloproliferative syndromes and in leukaemoid reactions. Scand J Haematol 1985;35:219–24.

31. Willis MS, McKenna RW, Peterson LC, et al. Low blast count myeloid disorders with Auer rods: a clinicopathologic analysis of 9 cases. Am J Clin Pathol 2005;124:191–8.

32. Matsushima T, Handa H, Yokohama A, et al. Prevalence and clinical characteristics of myelodysplastic syndrome with bone marrow eosinophilia or basophilia. Blood 2003;101:3386–90.

33. Mufti GJ, Bennett JM, Goasguen J, et al. Diagnosis and classification of myelodysplastic syndrome: International Working Group on Morphology of myelodysplastic syndrome (IWGM-MDS) consensus proposals for the definition and enumeration of myeloblasts and ring sideroblasts. Haematologica 2008; 93:1712–17.

34. Goasguen JE, Bennett JM, Cox C, et al. Prognostic implication and characterization of the blast cell population in the myelodysplastic syndrome. Leuk Res 1991;15:1159–65.

35. Lambertenghi-Deliliers G, Orazi A, Luksch R, et al. Myelodysplastic syndrome with increased marrow fibrosis: a distinct clinico-pathological entity. Br J Haematol 1991;78:161–6.

36. Della Porta MG, Malcovati L, Boveri E, et al. Clinical relevance of bone marrow fibrosis and CD34-positive cell clusters in primary myelodysplastic syndromes. J Clin Oncol 2009;27:754–62.

37. Tricot G, de Wolf-Peeters C, Vlietinck R, Verwilghen RL. Bone marrow histology in myelodysplastic syndromes. II. Prognostic value of abnormal localization of immature precursors in MDS. Br J Haematol 1984;58:217–25.

38. Orazi A. Histopathology in the diagnosis and classification of acute myeloid leukemia, myelodysplastic syndromes, and myelodysplastic/myeloproliferative diseases. Pathobiology 2007;74:97–114.

39. Thiele J, Quitmann H, Wagner S, Fischer R. Dysmegakaryopoiesis in myelodysplastic syndromes (MDS): an immunomorphometric study of bone marrow trephine biopsy specimens. J Clin Pathol 1991;44:300–5.

40. Thiele J, Zirbes TK, Wiemers P, et al. Incidence of apoptosis in HIV-myelopathy, myelodysplastic syndromes and non-specific inflammatory lesions of the bone marrow. Histopathology 1997;30: 307–11.

41. Westwood NB, Mufti GJ. Apoptosis in the myelodysplastic syndromes. Curr Hematol Rep 2003;2:186–92.

42. Orazi A, Albitar M, Heerema NA, et al. Hypoplastic myelodysplastic syndromes can be distinguished from acquired aplastic anemia by CD34 and PCNA immunostaining of bone marrow biopsy specimens. Am J Clin Pathol 1997; 107:268–74.

43. Barrett J, Saunthararajah Y, Molldrem J. Myelodysplastic syndrome and aplastic anemia: distinct entities or diseases linked by a common pathophysiology? Semin Hematol 2000;37:15–29.

44. Thiele J, Zirbes TK, Bertsch HP, et al. AIDS-related bone marrow lesions – myelodysplastic features or predominant inflammatory-reactive changes (HIV-myelopathy)? A comparative morphometric study by immunohistochemistry with special emphasis on apoptosis and PCNA-labeling. Anal Cell Pathol 1996;11: 141–57.

45. Wilkins BS, Bostanci AG, Ryan MF, Jones DB. Haemopoietic regrowth after chemotherapy for acute leukaemia: an immunohistochemical study of bone marrow trephine biopsy specimens. J Clin Pathol 1993;46:915–21.

46. Soligo DA, Oriani A, Annaloro C, et al. CD34 immunohistochemistry of bone marrow biopsies: prognostic significance in primary myelodysplastic syndromes. Am J Hematol 1994;46:9–17.

47. Naresh KN, Lampert IA. CD117 Expression as an aid to identify immature myeloid cells and foci of ALIP in bone marrow trephines. Am J Hematol 2006;81:79.

48. Mangi MH, Mufti GJ. Primary myelodysplastic syndromes: diagnostic and prognostic significance of immunohistochemical assessment of bone marrow biopsies. Blood 1992;79: 198–205.

49. Torlakovic EE, Naresh KN, Brunning RD. Bone Marrow Immunohistochemistry. Chicago: American Society for Clinical Pathology Press; 2009.

50. Thiele J, Schmitz B, Fuchs R, et al. Detection of the bcr/abl gene in bone marrow macrophages in CML and alterations during interferon therapy – a fluorescence in situ hybridization study on trephine biopsies. J Pathol 1998; 186:331–5.

51. Wilkins BS, Clark DM. Making the most of bone marrow trephine biopsy. Histopathology 2009;55:631–40.

52. van de Loosdrecht AA, Alhan C, Bene MC, et al. Standardization of flow cytometry in myelodysplastic syndromes: report from the first European Leukemia Net working conference on flow cytometry in myelodysplastic syndromes. Haematologica 2009;94:1124–34.

53. Haase D. Cytogenetic features in myelodysplastic syndromes. Ann Hematol 2008;87:515–26.

54. Smith SM, Le Beau MM, Huo D, et al. Clinical-cytogenetic associations in 306 patients with therapy-related myelodysplasia and myeloid leukemia: the University of Chicago series. Blood 2003;102:43–52.

55. Mahmood T, Robinson WA, Hamstra RD, Wallner SF. Macrocytic anemia, thrombocytosis and nonlobulated megakaryocytes: the 5q-syndrome, a distinct entity. Am J Med 1979;66:946–50.

56. Jary L, Mossafa H, Fourcade C, et al. The 17p-syndrome: a distinct myelodysplastic syndrome entity? Leuk Lymphoma 1997;25:163–8.

57. Secker-Walker LM, Mehta A, Bain B. Abnormalities of 3q21 and 3q26 in myeloid malignancy: a United Kingdom Cancer Cytogenetic Group study. Br J Haematol 1995;91:490–501.

58. Gupta R, Soupir CP, Johari V, Hasserjian RP. Myelodysplastic syndrome with isolated deletion of chromosome 20q: an indolent disease with minimal morphological dysplasia and frequent thrombocytopenic presentation. Br J Haematol 2007;139:265–8.

59. Gondek LP, Tiu R, O'Keefe CL, et al. Chromosomal lesions and uniparental disomy detected by SNP arrays in MDS, MDS/MPD, and MDS-derived AML. Blood 2008;111:1534–42.

60. Starczynowski DT, Vercauteren S, Telenius A, et al. High-resolution whole genome tiling path array CGH analysis of CD34+ cells from patients with low-risk myelodysplastic syndromes reveals cryptic copy number alterations and predicts overall and leukemia-free survival. Blood 2008;112:3412–24.

61. Kosmider O, Gelsi-Boyer V, Cheok M, et al. TET2 mutation is an independent favorable prognostic factor in myelodysplastic syndromes (MDSs). Blood 2009;114:3285–91.

62. Nolte F, Hofmann WK. Myelodysplastic syndromes: molecular pathogenesis and genomic changes. Ann Hematol 2008; 87:777–95.

63. Ebert BL. Deletion 5q in myelodysplastic syndrome: a paradigm for the study of hemizygous deletions in cancer. Leukemia 2009;23:1252–6.

64. Starczynowski DT, Kuchenbauer F, Argiropoulos B, et al. Identification of miR-145 and miR-146a as mediators of the 5q- syndrome phenotype. Nat Med 2010;16:49–58.

65. Sutton JF, Stacey M, Kearns WG, et al. Increased risk for aplastic anemia and myelodysplastic syndrome in individuals lacking glutathione S-transferase genes. Pediatr Blood Cancer 2004;42:122–6.

66. Takeuchi J, Ly H, Yamaguchi H, et al. Identification and functional characterization of novel telomerase variant alleles in Japanese patients with bone-marrow failure syndromes. Blood Cells Mol Dis 2008;40:185–91.

67. Kerbauy DB, Deeg HJ. Apoptosis and antiapoptotic mechanisms in the progression of myelodysplastic syndrome. Exp Hematol 2007;35:1739–46.

68. Tehranchi R, Invernizzi R, Grandien A, et al. Aberrant mitochondrial iron distribution and maturation arrest characterize early erythroid precursors in low-risk myelodysplastic syndromes. Blood 2005;106:247–53.

69. Stern M, Buser AS, Lohri A, et al. Autoimmunity and malignancy in hematology – more than an association. Crit Rev Oncol Hematol 2007;63:100–10.

70. Xiao L, Qiong L, Yan Z, et al. Experimental and clinical characteristics in myelodysplastic syndrome patients with or without HLA-DR15 allele. Hematol Oncol 2010;28(2):98–103.

71. Chamuleau ME, Westers TM, van Dreunen L, et al. Immune mediated autologous cytotoxicity against hematopoietic precursor cells in patients with myelodysplastic syndrome. Haematologica 2009;94:496–506.

72. Jadersten M, Hellstrom-Lindberg E. Myelodysplastic syndromes: biology and treatment. J Intern Med 2009;265:307–28.

73. Greenberg PL. Risk factors and their relationship to prognosis in myelodysplastic syndromes. Leuk Res 1998;22(Suppl. 1):S3–6.

74. Malcovati L, Germing U, Kuendgen A, et al. Time-dependent prognostic scoring system for predicting survival and leukemic evolution in myelodysplastic syndromes. J Clin Oncol 2007;25: 3503–10.

75. Kantarjian H, O'Brien S, Ravandi F, et al. Proposal for a new risk model in myelodysplastic syndrome that accounts for events not considered in the original International Prognostic Scoring System. Cancer 2008;113:1351–61.

76. List A, Kurtin S, Roe DJ, et al. Efficacy of lenalidomide in myelodysplastic syndromes. N Engl J Med 2005;352: 549–57.

77. Ades L, Boehrer S, Prebet T, et al. Efficacy and safety of lenalidomide in intermediate-2 or high-risk myelodysplastic syndromes with 5q deletion: results of a phase 2 study. Blood 2009;113:3947–52.

78. Jadersten M, Saft L, Pellagatti A, et al. Clonal heterogeneity in the 5q- syndrome: p53 expressing progenitors prevail during lenalidomide treatment and expand at disease progression. Haematologica 2009;94:1762–6.

79. Gohring G, Giagounidis A, Busche G, et al. Patients with del(5q) MDS who fail to achieve sustained erythroid or cytogenetic remission after treatment with lenalidomide have an increased risk for clonal evolution and AML progression. Ann Hematol 2010 Apr;89(4):365–74.

80. Raza A, Reeves JA, Feldman EJ, et al. Phase 2 study of lenalidomide in transfusion-dependent, low-risk, and intermediate-1 risk myelodysplastic syndromes with karyotypes other than deletion 5q. Blood 2008;111:86–93.

81. Nimer SD. Myelodysplastic syndromes. Blood 2008;111:4841–51.

82. Fenaux P, Mufti GJ, Hellstrom-Lindberg E, et al. Efficacy of azacitidine compared with that of conventional care regimens in the treatment of higher-risk myelodysplastic syndromes: a randomised, open-label, phase III study. Lancet Oncol 2009;10:223–32.

83. Cutler CS, Lee SJ, Greenberg P, et al. A decision analysis of allogeneic bone marrow transplantation for the myelodysplastic syndromes: delayed transplantation for low-risk myelodysplasia is associated with improved outcome. Blood 2004;104: 579–85.

84. Sloand EM, Wu CO, Greenberg P, Young N, Barrett J. Factors affecting response and survival in patients with myelodysplasia treated with immunosuppressive therapy. J Clin Oncol 2008;26:2505–11.

85. Kasner MT, Luger SM. Update on the therapy for myelodysplastic syndrome. Am J Hematol 2009;84:177–86.

86. Malcovati L, Nimer SD. Myelodysplastic syndromes: diagnosis and staging. Cancer Control 2008;15(Suppl.):4–13.

CHAPTER 21

Molecular studies in myeloproliferative and myelodysplastic/myeloproliferative neoplasms

O Bock, HH Kreipe

Chapter contents

Introduction

Almost 60 years after William Dameshek published his description of myeloproliferative disorders,[1] clinicians, pathologists, and basic scientists have noticed tremendous progress in the field of these diseases. Due to discovery of molecular markers, it is now possible to discriminate between myeloproliferative and reactive states. Targeted therapies for certain subtypes of myeloproliferative diseases have become available.

Discovery of the so-called Philadelphia (Ph$^+$) chromosome in 1960 by Nowell and Hungerford,[2] the subsequent dissection of its molecular structure and of pathways involved in t(9;22) translocation have led to the introduction of imatinib mesylate as the first molecularly targeted therapy in a human malignancy.[3] Until 2005, knowledge of molecular aberrations and genetic defects in the Philadelphia-chromosome negative (Ph$^-$) chronic myeloproliferative disorders (CMPD) was rather sparse. In a minority of cases, chromosomal changes such as trisomies 8 and 9, aberrations of chromosome 1, del(20q) or del(13q) in primary myelofibrosis (PMF) or loss of heterozygosity (LOH) at 9p in polycythemia vera (PV) have been demonstrated.[4,5]

The discovery of the gain-of-function mutation V617F in the tyrosine kinase (TK) Janus kinase 2 (JAK2^{V617F})[6] and other molecular defects in a considerable number of patients with so-called classical Ph$^-$ CMPD resulted in a revision of the WHO classification.[7] To underline the neoplastic nature of these diseases, the WHO classification published in 2008 replaced the term Ph$^-$ CMPD with 'myeloproliferative neoplasm (MPN)'. This new classification has also introduced new standards for diagnostic algorithms including molecular diagnostics (Fig. 21.1). In this chapter, the current knowledge on molecular changes in MPN and myelodysplastic/myeloproliferative neoplasms (MDS/MPN) is summarized. Molecular aspects of MPN with eosinophilia and of systemic mastocytosis are described in Chapters 25 and 26, respectively.

DOI: 10.1016/B978-0-7020-3147-2.00021-3

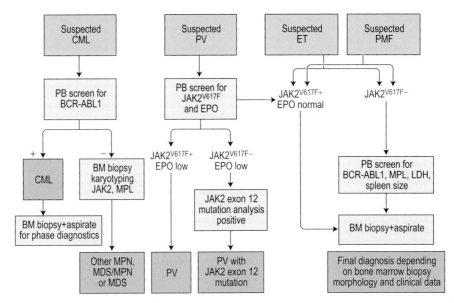

Fig. 21.1 A diagnostic algorithm for MPN. The detection of *BCR-ABL1* (except in instances of very low allele burden) is diagnostic of CML, in the clinical and morphological context of a chronic myeloid neoplasm. When PV is suspected, the presence of a *JAK2* mutation confirms the diagnosis. The JAK2[V617F] mutation is used as a clonal marker in both ET and PMF. However, absence of this mutation does not rule out the MPN diagnosis. In the setting of a chronic myeloid neoplasm associated with bone marrow fibrosis, the presence of the JAK2[V617F] mutation, the MPL mutation or the cytogenetic abnormalities +9 or 13q− is highly suggestive of PMF. Abbreviations: CML, chronic myeloid leukemia; EPO, serum erythropoietin; ET, essential thrombocythemia; MDS, myelodysplastic syndrome; MPN, myeloproliferative neoplasm; PMF, primary myelofibrosis; PV, polycythemia vera. *(Modified from Tefferi A, Skoda R, Vardiman JW. Myeloproliferative neoplasms: contemporary diagnosis using histology and genetics. Nat. Rev. Clin. Oncol. 2009;6:627–637.)*

The Philadelphia chromosome and BCR-ABL in chronic myelogenous leukemia

Chronic myelogenous leukemia (CML) is a clonal stem cell disorder characterized by increased autonomous proliferation of myeloid lineages in the bone marrow (BM). The underlying molecular defect, the balanced reciprocal translocation t(9;22)(q34;q11), was the first chromosomal anomaly consistently present in a human cancer.[8] Translocation t(9;22)(q34;q11.2) results in the Philadelphia chromosome found in 90–95 % of patients.[9,10] This translocation causes a fusion of the *BCR* gene from chromosome 22 with the *ABL1* gene from chromosome 9.[11,12] In 5–10% of patients, a cryptic translocation of 9q34 and 22q11.2 or a variant translocation involving other chromosomes not detectable by conventional karyotype analysis occur. In these patients, the *BCR-ABL1* fusion can be demonstrated by molecular methods such as fluorescent *in situ* hybridization (FISH), reverse transcriptase (RT)-PCR, and Southern blot.[13]

The *BCR-ABL1* fusion results in a deregulated function of the *ABL1* gene.[14] *BCR-ABL1* mRNA encodes for p210 or (rarely) p190 or p230 oncoproteins.[15–19] The binding of ATP to the pockets of p210, p190 or p230 allows phosphorylation of selected tyrosine residues on its substrates. The oncogenic properties of the p210, p190, and p230 proteins rely primarily on the constitutively activated TK.

ABL1 plays a central role in the regulation of the cell cycle, cellular response to genotoxic events, and integrin-signaling pathways.[20] The fusion of BCR with the SH3 domain of ABL1 interrupts the physiologic suppression of the kinase activity, produces the neoplastic phenotype via deregulation of the impact of ABL1 on apoptosis, cell cycle, and cellular adhesion pathways.[21,22] Activation of the RAS pathway results in

an increase of mitotic activity and up-regulation of bcl-2, while activation of 'signal transducers and activators of transcription' (STAT) 1 and STAT5 proteins results in the inhibition of apoptosis.[23–25] Apoptosis inhibition counteracts the protective effect of ABL1 when DNA damage occurs. This results in the accumulation of neoplastic cells and additional genetic changes. Furthermore, BCR-ABL1 negatively influences DNA repair and drives centrosomal hypertrophy, thus increasing the risk of clonal evolution.[26,27] BCR-ABL1 induces abnormalities of cytoskeletal cellular function, phosphorylation of adhesion proteins, the production of an abnormal variant of the β1-integrin, and the phosphorylation of Cdc2-related kinase (Crk)-l resulting in reduced adhesion of the CML cells to BM stroma.[28–30] Interrupted by BCR-ABL1 interaction between hematopoietic progenitor cells and the BM stroma appears to be important for the control of cellular proliferation.

Nowadays, it is generally accepted that CML originates from a single *BCR-ABL1* transformed pluripotent hematopoietic stem cell.[31] This immature precursor and its immature daughter cells appear to be rather resistant to therapy utilizing BCR-ABL1 TK inhibitors. Therefore, this type of anti-neoplastic treatment does not seem to cure the disease.[32]

BCR-ABL1 positive cells or small positive clones have been reported in asymptomatic persons without any signs of CML.[33] Moreover, there are differences in the risk of CML between patients with different HLA-B phenotype.[34] Thus, immunologic factors may also play a role in the evolution of CML, probably restricting the occurrence of CML to subjects with an immunologic failure of resistance against the BCR-ABL1 positive cell population.

Imatinib mesylate and second generation formulas such as nilotinib and dasatinib represent TK inhibitors that have been designed to work against the constitutively activated chimeric BCR-ABL1 protein, which is responsible for the aberrant phenotype of affected cells in CML patients.[35,36]

Karyotyping and conventional cytogenetics accompany the inevitable histopathological evaluation of BM biopsy in the initial diagnostic algorithm in order to demonstrate the presence of the Ph[+] chromosome. Detection of the BCR-ABL1 fusion products by reverse transcriptase (RT)-PCR analysis in patients with CML (and also Ph[+] ALL) has become the golden standard in the diagnostic setting. Standardized real-time quantitative (RQ)-PCR has become the methodology of choice for monitoring molecular response to treatment with TK inhibitors and/or interferon.[37] The achievement of the major molecular response (MMR) is the key issue in evaluating therapy effects. MMR can only be determined by quantitative RT-PCR methodology and was originally defined as the reduction of the BCR-ABL1 fusion transcripts by three logs below a standardized baseline level. The latter was initially introduced as a part of the International Randomized Study of Interferon versus STI571 (IRIS) trial.[38] Since most patients treated with imatinib or other TK inhibitors achieve a complete cytogenetic response (CCyR), the monitoring of minimal residual disease (MRD) by quantification of the BCR-ABL1 transcripts has become increasingly important. It has been shown that CCyR and MMR after 12 months of treatment indicates an improved progression-free survival at 24 months in 100% of the patients treated with imatinib as compared to 95% in the group showing no MMR and 85% in patients who were not in CCyR at 12 months.[38] All patients who achieved CCyR and MMR at 18 months had a 5-year progression-free survival. Moreover, studies in patients followed for several years showed that those achieving MMR early in the first year of treatment had significantly longer CCyR[39].

Despite the improved prognosis of CML patients since start of the imatinib era, a response failure is observed in 25–30% of patients.[40] The individual risk of developing resistance to imatinib is hard to predict and underlying mechanisms are largely unknown. The majority of patients develop de novo mutations in the ABL kinase domain during therapy. Some may even have pre-existing mutations hindering a good response to initial treatment.

A study of lymphoid blast crisis of CML has recently shown that lymphoid blasts but not CML cells express a B-cell specific mutator named AID (antibody diversification enzyme activation-induced deaminase), which promotes genetic instability and somatic hypermutation of tumor suppressor and DNA repair genes.[41] AID may also be responsible for the acquisition of imatinib resistance in CML cells, which justifies testing for the potential targeting of AID and further stresses the need for BCR-ABL1 transcript level monitoring during TK inhibitor treatment.

Due to the clinical importance of MRD, efforts to standardize the methodologies for quantification of BCR-ABL1 transcripts in CML patients are now in progress. Most studies refer to the IRIS trial and the associated International Scale (IS) for BCR-ABL1 transcript quantification,[38] but significant inter-laboratory differences concerning definition of patient molecular status still exist. The increase of BCR-ABL1 transcripts to a level >0.1% on the IS scale can be interpreted as a potential response failure and should lead to a close-meshed monitoring of BCR-ABL1 transcript levels.[42] Successful efforts to standardize methodologies have already been reported.[43] The goal of a recently initiated study is to introduce a conversion factor (CF) allowing the harmonization and comparison of results obtained during molecular monitoring of CML patients before and during therapy.[44] In brief, every participating laboratory generates its own CF, which will allow comparison of BCL-ABL1 transcript levels for upcoming multicenter studies.

Interestingly, there is no concordance between BCR-ABL1 transcript levels in either sorted or unsorted BM aspirate cells and the levels determined in peripheral blood cells, both mononuclear cells and granulocytes. Since drawing blood is less invasive as compared to BM aspiration, it should be considered the standard choice to determine the BCR-ABL1 transcript levels. Apart from BCR-ABL1 levels, other prognostic parameters such as the presence of BM fibrosis[45] or increasing numbers of BM blasts are of importance during clinical follow-up (see Chapter 24 for details).

The Janus kinase 2 in MPN

JAK2[V617F]

The molecular nature of the gain-of-function mutation in JAK2 is a hotspot in exon 14 where the wild-type (WT) guanine (G) is changed to a mutant thymine (T) with consecutive replacement of valine by phenylalanine at position 617 (V617F) in the JH2 pseudokinase.[6,46–48] Even though functional studies are not yet available, it is well accepted that the bulky amino acid phenylalanine changes the conformation of the protein thereby blocking the interaction of the auto-inhibitory JH2 pseudokinase domain with the catalytic domain JH1. This hampers control of catalytic activity and leads to a constitutively activated JAK2 kinase and subsequently, the activation of downstream targets in affected cells.[49]

The effects of mutated JAK2[V617F] show a considerable diversity in various cellular lineages and MPN subtypes affected by this mutation. The JAK2[V617F] clone is autonomous and highly proliferative in vitro, even in the absence of growth factors. All MPN subtypes harboring the JAK2[V617F] show high numbers of endogenous erythroid colonies (EEC) in BM cultures. In addition, the affected lineages are additionally hypersensitive to growth factors such as erythropoietin (EPO), granulocyte-colony stimulating factor (G-CSF) or interleukins. In mouse models, the mutation is powerful enough to mediate a PV-like phenotype and leads to development of myelofibrosis.[47,50,51] Similar findings were demonstrated in MPN patients harboring the JAK2[V617F] mutation, but some of the features observed in the animal model might be due to toxic effects of the JAK2[V617F] overdose. It is of note that strain-specific differences were found in two different mice models showing the JAK2[V617F] mutation. Whereas both the Balb/C and the C57Bl/6 mice showed an increase in hemoglobin and hematocrit, the number of leukocytes and the degree of myelofibrosis were strikingly higher in the Balb/C mice.[50] No thrombocytosis was seen in these models, even though an increase of megakaryocytes in the BM was noted. Direct transfer of knowledge concerning JAK2[V617F] mutation derived from mice models to human MPN appears to be difficult and different phenotypes observed in humans may also develop as a consequence of individual host modifiers.

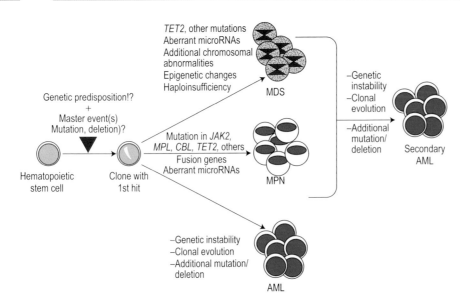

Fig. 21.2 Molecular changes in pathogenesis of myeloproliferative and myeloproliferative/ myelodysplastic neoplasms. *(Modified from Mullighan CG. TET2 mutations in myelodysplasia and myeloid malignancies. Nat. Genet. 2009;41:766–767.)*

Among MPN, PV showed the highest JAK2^{V617F} frequency (~95%) followed by PMF and ET (~50% JAK2^{V617F} mutated cases).[52-55] It is of note that patients with JAK2^{V617F} mutated ET show PV-like features, e.g. elevated hemoglobin and hematocrit levels. Also, it has been suggested that PV patients with a homozygous mutation status (i.e. 50% or more alleles showing the mutant T allele) had a higher risk for development of myelofibrosis.[56-58] However, the mutation *per se* is probably not responsible for myelofibrosis development, since no correlation between the JAK2 status and the clinical course or degree of fibrosis could be demonstrated in PMF.[59,60] A retrospective analysis of 490 MPN patients along with evaluation of follow-up biopsies revealed a correlation between JAK2^{V617F} mutant allele burden and MPN subtypes. In this study, a considerable number of ET cases were characterized by lower allele burden.[61]

Although the discovery of the JAK2^{V617F} mutation was a breakthrough in the field, it became increasingly clear that this molecular defect is not the initiating event in MPN pathogenesis. This is illustrated by X-chromosome inactivation patterns (XCIP) in female ET patients with the JAK2^{V617F} mutation.[62-64] XCIP studies found that the proportion of JAK2^{V617F} positive cells was lower than the total number of clonal cells in a given patient. A higher proportion of cells with the deletion of chromosome 20q in comparison to the percentage of cells with the JAK2^{V617F} mutation was found in patients carrying both anomalies.[64] These studies clearly indicate that the neoplastic hematopoietic stem cell (HSC) must have acquired at least one molecular aberration preceding the JAK2^{V617F} mutation. This master event could be an as yet undiscovered small chromosomal deletion or an insertion spanning only small-size region(s) of a gene, thereby impossible to detect by conventional cytogenetic techniques (Fig. 21.2). This event must lead to a selective advantage of the affected cell, allowing autonomous expansion accompanied by ongoing chromosomal instability and additional molecular defects such as mutations inducing entity-typical phenotypes. In MPN, the mimicry of phenotypes between different entities is not uncommon. This might be a result

of two or more aberrations existing in parallel. It is therefore now widely accepted that JAK2^{V617F} is a secondary mutation leading towards PV or a PV-like clinical appearance, particularly in ET.

JAK2 (K539L and other aberrations in exon 12)

In the diagnostic setting, some patients show high hemoglobin levels, high hematocrit and low serum EPO levels but do not harbor the JAK2^{V617F} mutation. These patients are usually affected by a rather rare molecular defect in exon 12 of the *JAK2* gene. Exon 12 aberrations vary between point mutations leading to the K539L mutation and insertions/ deletions leading to various amino acid substitutions.[65] Two interesting epidemiologic features characterize JAK2 exon 12 aberrations: 1) more women than men were affected when compared to idiopathic erythrocytosis showing the JAK2^{WT}; 2) patients presented at younger age when compared to those with JAK2^{V617F} mutation.[66] However, due to the low frequency of JAK2 exon 12 aberrations and the complexity of testing, this type of molecular analysis should be restricted to patients who are JAK2^{V617F} negative but show clinical parameters strongly suggesting clonal erythropoiesis.

The JAK2^{V617F} mutation in *de novo* acute leukemia and in MPN transformed to acute leukemia

MPN transformation into acute myeloid leukemia (AML) is the major life-threatening event in the course of the disease. The frequency of transformation varies among the MPN subtypes. The general risk for evolving to AML is much higher for patients with PV or PMF than for those having ET. The impact of a history of prior treatment, i.e. with hydroxyurea, is unclear.[67,68] The mechanism of the transforming switch is totally unknown. After discovery of the JAK2^{V617F} mutation, this molecular defect has been suggested to be a powerful co-factor in the process of transformation. A series of studies investigated the occurrence of JAK2^{V617F} in secondary AML developing in patients with a history of MPN and in *de novo* AML or acute lymphoblastic leukemia (ALL). In one study the JAK2^{V617F} mutation was not detected in *de novo* AML M0 – M6-subtype (according to the French-American-British (FAB) classification) but some positive cases of AML M7 were found (2/11, 18%).[69] Another investigation described one case of AML M6 (1/53) positive for JAK2^{V617F} but no positive cases in AML M5 (0/85) or AML M7 (0/14) FAB categories.[70] In one study a frequency of almost 3.0% was reported (3/113 *de novo* AML) with two AML cases showing both the JAK2^{V617F} and t(8;21)(q22;q22). One case assigned to the 'AML without maturation' category had a JAK2 (V607N) mutation.[71] In B- and T-ALL, the JAK2 mutation seems to be extremely rare, except for children with Down syndrome.[72,73]

To investigate the role of JAK2^{V617F} in the transformation of MPN, the mutant allele burden ('gene dosage') has been retrospectively studied in individual patients. It was found that patients with a prior history of MPN and detectable JAK2^{V617F} at diagnosis showed no increase of mutant allele burden during transformation to acute leukemia.[74] The same study demonstrated that both the development of myelofibrosis and leukemic transformation in PV and PMF was found in patients with the JAK2^{WT} status.

It has been noted that in JAK2^{V617F} positive patients, the populations of blasts in transformed MPN are frequently negative for the JAK2 mutation.[63] These findings are in line with the suggestion of the *pre*-JAK2^{V617F} phase, in which clonality has already been achieved by an as yet undefined mechanism (see Fig. 21.2). Thus, JAK2^{V617F}-negative AML developing during course of MPN might arise from the primary clone and could be the key to discovery of the primary master hit. The other scenario could be that, indeed, two separate clones develop independently in an individual patient. Studies of the molecular signatures of JAK2^{V617F}-negative blasts from the AML transformation of MPN could open up relevant insights into the pathogenesis of early MPN development.

Myeloproliferative leukemia virus oncogene (MPL) mutations in MPN

Thrombopoietin (TPO) and its receptor MPL (CD110) are important for hematopoietic stem-cell survival, the differentiation of hematopoietic progenitor cells, and are key regulatory factors in megakaryocyte development and platelet formation.[75] MPL is expressed by hematopoietic tissues, hematopoietic stem cells, erythroid progenitors, megakaryocytes and platelets.[76] Aberrant expression of MPL has been implicated in some hematological malignancies. Earlier studies showed that reduced MPL expression in megakaryocytes from patients with MPN is due to impaired post-translational modifications.[77,78] Reduced platelet MPL expression and weakly labeled megakaryocytes by immunohistochemistry were found to be of diagnostic and prognostic value in MPN.[79–82]

Several studies demonstrated that the megakaryocytic and erythroid lineages co-express MPL and the erythropoi-

etin receptor (EPO-R) as well as transcription factors such as nuclear factor-erythroid derived (NF-E)1 (identical to globin transcription factor (GATA1)) and NF-E2.[83–85] Due to structural homologies between MPL, EPO-R and their ligands, it has been suggested that both megakaryocytic and erythroid lineages arise from a common progenitor.[85] Therefore, abnormal expression and function of MPL or EPO-R could induce proliferation of both megakaryocytic and erythroid lineages.[86] In mice overexpressing the functional MPL receptor, enhanced erythropoiesis and reduced megakaryopoiesis have been demonstrated.[87]

Since the JAK-STAT pathway is constitutively activated in MPN but only half of PMF and ET patients harbor the JAK2^{V617F} mutation, screening for mutations in other cytokine receptors by high throughput DNA sequencing has been performed.[88] Whereas defined regions of the granulocyte-colony stimulating factor receptor (G-CSF-R) and the EPO-R showed no molecular defects, a point mutation W515L in the juxtamembrane domain of MPL (exon 10) was discovered.[88] Cell lines transfected with MPL^{W515L} show cytokine-independent growth and hypersensitivity for TPO. Mouse strains carrying the mutation exhibit high levels of thrombocytosis, massive hepatosplenomegaly and infarctions of the spleen. Analysis of a large cohort (1182 patients) detected a frequency of ~5% MPL^{W515L} in patients with PMF and ET.[89] The latter study revealed another mutation in the *MPL* gene: MPL^{W515K} as well as the occurrence of *MPL* mutations together with JAK2^{V617F} in individual patients.

MPL$^{W515L/K}$ is an activating mutation leading to abnormal cell growth and in the mouse model it causes phenotype mimicking PMF. Similar to the JAK2^{V617F} mutation, single nucleotides are changed (G to T or TG to alanine-alanine (AA)), leading to a substitution of the amino acid tryptophan by leucine or lysine. In JAK2^{V617F} the substitution of the bulky amino acid phenylalanine apparently abrogates the correct interaction of the catalytic JH1 domain with the inhibitory domain JH2, while the change from the rather voluminous tryptophane to the smaller leucine in MPL^{W515L} might effectively interfere with the folding and function of the protein.

In a study of 776 samples from ET patients, the overall frequency of MPL exon 10 mutations was 8.5% in patients with JAK2^{WT}.[90] Patients with the MPL^{W515K} mutation had a higher mutant allele burden than those with MPL^{W515L}. As compared to patients with JAK2^{V617F}, MPL mutated ET patients showed lower hemoglobin levels, higher EPO levels, higher platelets, and endogenous megakaryocyte colony growth but there was no increase in endogenous erythroid colonies and overall lower bone marrow cellularity. MPL mutations lacked prognostic significance with regard to frequency of hemorrhage, thrombosis, development of myelofibrosis, and survival.

One study investigated in a large series of MPN the potential correlation between reduced platelet MPL protein expression and the mutant JAK2^{V617F} allele load in neutrophils.[91] In all MPN subtypes, the higher percentage of mutant JAK2^{V617F} alleles was related to lower MPL expression, which suggests that the presence of JAK2^{V617F} is associated with down-regulation of MPL. In ET cases showing JAK2^{WT}, the MPL expression was significantly higher than in ET with JAK2^{V617F}. PMF patients in this study exhibited the lowest platelet MPL levels followed by PV and ET cases. It has been suggested that JAK2[V617F] may possibly bind MPL in the endoplasmic reticulum (as shown for JAK2[WT] and EPO-R) or impair further processing in the Golgi apparatus, directly inducing down-regulation of MPL. This could also be a counteracting mechanism inhibiting autonomous proliferation mediated by negative regulators such as the adaptor protein Lnk (linker), which normally controls MPL expression.[92]

The axis: growth factor (ligand) – growth factor receptor – intracellular tyrosine kinase seems to involve a large number of players in parallel, making every step in signal transduction rather complicated. Cellular transformation mediated by gain-of-function mutations such as the JAK2[V617F] is dependent on expression of other components such as functional G-CSF-receptor and EPO-R. As shown for JAK2[V617F], a functional EPO-R is necessary not only for JAK2[WT] signaling but also for the mutant form.[93] It is plausible that a composition of molecular aberrations, i.e. concomitant JAK2[V617F] and MPL[W515K/L] mutations in an individual patient could either amplify or abrogate the transforming cellular effects. Thus, the clinical and histological phenotype in MPN could be the result of a mixture of molecular aberrations.

TET2 mutations in MPN and other myeloid malignancies

Soon after the report of Vainchenker et al. at American Society for Hematology Meeting 2008, collaborative studies confirmed that acquired molecular aberrations in the *Ten-Eleven Translocation 2* (*TET2*) gene are frequent in MPN and MDS/MPN.[94,95] These aberrations show considerable variation including frameshifts, nonsense or missense mutations in exon 4 and 12 of the *TET2* gene.[94] The overall *TET2* mutation frequency in MPN is 13% (5% in ET, 16% and 17% in PV and PMF, respectively) and 50% in patients with chronic myelomonocytic leukemia (CMML). *TET2* mutations occur in both JAK2[V617F] and JAK2[WT] cases with frequencies of 17% and 7%, respectively. *TET2* mutations significantly increase with age: mutational frequency is 23% in patients >60 years of age compared to only 4% in younger individuals.[94] In PV and PMF patients, the occurrence of *TET2* mutations did not correlate with any prognostic factor such as survival, rate of transformation to AML or risk of thrombosis. Based on its prevalence in older patients, which often already acquired the JAK2[V617F] mutation, the usefulness of *TET2* as a diagnostic marker appears to be limited. However, another study in patients with PV showed that *TET2* mutations may occur in both JAK2[V617F] and JAK2[WT] clones of an individual patient.[96] An overall frequency of 20% *TET2* mutations was found in a cohort of 61 cases of familial MPN with no age correlation. In this study, sequential occurrence of JAK2[V617F] and subsequently *TET2* mutations in individual patients was reported.[97] Different *TET2* alterations occurred in the same individual suggesting molecular dynamics probably due to genetic instability. *TET2* mutations were also found in other myeloid malignancies with considerably higher mutation frequencies: in *de novo* AML (42%),[98] systemic mastocytosis (29%),[99] MDS with rearranged 4q24 (19%),[100] and in secondary AML (up to 32%).[96] Therefore, alterations in the *TET2* gene appear to be a common event in myeloid malignancies including those showing dysplastic features, chronic myeloproliferation and acute leukemia (see Fig. 21.2). Future studies will show whether the *TET2* gene functions as a tumor suppressor gene or if structurally altered *TET2* contributes to malignant transformation due to its relevant role in normal hematopoietic differentiation. Before discovery of *TET2* alterations, the function of this gene was unclear. Since *TET2* alterations are loss-of-function defects, knock-out and knock-in studies will show the impact of this gene on normal and malignant hematopoiesis.

However, the *TET1* gene, which fusion with the histone methyltransferase MLL has been identified in AML associated with t(10;11)(q22;q23) translocation, was shown to catalyze the reaction from 5-methylcytosine to 5-hydroxymethylcytosine in the DNA suggesting a role for TET proteins in epigenetic regulation.[101]

JAK2[V617F], MPL[W515L/K], BCR-ABL, KIT[D816V]: molecular markers may be combined in an individual patient

Shortly after the JAK2[V617F] mutation and other molecular aberrations were described in MPN, numerous studies reported that various molecular markers in MPN may be combined in an individual patient. The first reported patients with concomitant presence of BCR-ABL and JAK2[V617F] [102] presented typical Philadelphia-positive CML and quickly achieved molecular remission after start of imatinib treatment. However, under imatinib treatment a JAK2[V617F] clone evolved leading to a Philadelphia-negative MPN with myelofibrosis. A retrospective molecular analysis revealed that the JAK2[V617F] positive population with low mutant allele burden was already present at time of CML diagnosis. This case clearly illustrated that different clones may co-exist in MPN and that therapy may create an advantage for one clone, after a competing clone has been successfully repressed.

Besides the combination of BCR-ABL and JAK2[V617F], other molecular marker combinations have been described. These include: JAK2[V617F] and MPL[W515L/K] in MPN and MDS/MPN,[103–107] JAK2[V617F] and KIT[D816V] in systemic mastocytosis with associated non-mast cell hematological disease (SM-AHNMD),[103] *TET2* mutation and JAK2[V617F] in MPN and MDS/MPN.[96,97]

In Philadelphia-negative MPN carrying solely the JAK2[V617F] mutation, megakaryocytes showed variation in their mutant allele burden when this single defect was quantified.[60] Accordingly, various cellular lineages in individuals with combined molecular defects may also show different molecular changes. In a patient with concomitant JAK2[V617F] and MPL[W515L] mutations, CD34-positive cells, granulocytes, and monocytes showed the presence of both mutations. However, T and B lymphocytes carried the MPL[W515L] mutation but were JAK2[WT], whereas the erythropoiesis and the megakaryocytic lineage showed JAK2[V617F] with MPL[WT].[104] These findings strongly argue against a sequential acquisition of molecular defects in various cellular lineages in MPN and favor the hypothesis of parallel proliferation of unrelated hematopoietic stem-cell clones.

Table 21.1 Selected molecular aberrancies in myeloproliferative (MPN) and myelodysplastic/myeloproliferative (MDS/MPN) neoplasms

MPN

Subtype	Chromosomal defect (if demonstrable by conventional methods)	Diagnostic marker	Frequency (if specified)	Methodologies most commonly used
CML	t (9;22) (q34;q11)	Ph$^+$ chromosome, BCR-ABL fusion transcripts, e.g. b2a2/b2a3, b3a2/b3a3, e19a2, others	~100%	Cytogenetics, FISH, nested RT-PCR; real-time RT-PCR
Ph$^-$ MPN PV PMF ET MPN unclassifiable	Aberrations at 9p (i.e. LOH/aUPD)	Point mutation in exon 14 leading to JAK2 (V617F) = substitution of valine by phenylalanine at codon 617	~99% ~50–70% ~50–70% ≥70%	Pyrosequencing, allele-specific real-time PCR, direct sequencing, others
PV Erythrocytosis (reactive state excluded)	Aberrations at 9p (i.e. LOH)	Mutations, deletions, insertions in exon 12 of JAK2 (defects variable – not predictable)	~16 % ~1–2 %	Direct sequencing, pyrosequencing, others
PMF ET		Point mutations in exon 10 of MPL leading to MPL W515L/K	~5–10% ~5–10%	Direct sequencing, allele-specific real-time PCR, pyrosequencing, others
Ph$^-$ MPN	del (20q), del(13q), trisomy 1q, 8	del (20q), del(13q), trisomy 1q, 8	~3%	Real-time copy number assays, FISH, others
Mastocytosis SM SM-AHNMD		Point mutation in exon 17 of KIT leading to KIT D816V = substitution of valine by aspartic acid at codon 816	~100% (may be masked on DNA level; check cDNA)	Direct sequencing, allele-specific real-time PCR, pyrosequencing

MPN with eosinophilia associated with FIP1L1-PDGFRA

CEL	del (4q12)	FIP1L1-PDGFR → may be difficult to detect due to variable fusions	May be masked due to technical limitations	FISH, nested RT-PCR

MDS/MPN

aCML	11q (aUPD)	Mutations in CBL, predominantly involving exon 8 + 9	High when aUPD at 11q is present	Direct sequencing, pyrosequencing, others
CMML	11q (aUPD)			

MPN, MDS, MDS/MPN

Various fusion genes involving receptor or cytoplasmic tyrosine kinases such as PDGFRB, FGFR1, others; deletions/insertions leading to aberrant action of tyrosine kinases; known molecular defects such as JAK2 (V617F) may be combined with others (e.g. MPL W515L/K, KIT D816V)

The casitas B-lineage lymphoma gene (CBL) aberrancies in MPN and other myeloid malignancies

The proto-oncogene *CBL* is a negative regulator of several receptor tyrosine kinase signaling pathways and an adaptor protein in tyrosine-phosphorylation dependent signaling.[108] Ubiquitination of receptor protein-tyrosine kinases (PTKs) terminates signaling by marking active receptors for degradation. CBL is an adaptor protein for receptor PTKs that positively regulates receptor PTK ubiquitination. Ubiquitin-protein ligases, also known as E3s, are the components of ubiquitination pathways that recognize target substrates and promote their ligation to ubiquitin. CBL protein acts as an E3 that can recognize tyrosine-phosphorylated substrates, such as the activated platelet-derived growth factor receptor.[109] It was concluded that CBL functions as an ubiquitin-protein ligase and thus provides a distinct mechanism for substrate targeting in the ubiquitin system (Table 21.1).

The *CBL* gene is located on the 11q23.3 telomeric of the *MLL* gene, which is frequently fused to loci on other chromosomes in translocations causing various types of leukemia. Southern blot analysis in conjunction with FISH in a patient with AML (FAB M1) suggested that the CBL/MLL fusion was the result of an interstitial deletion.[110] Two other studies showed the frequent occurrence of molecular defects other than fusion involving the *CBL* gene.[111,112] Acquired uniparental disomy (aUPD) that leads to loss-of-heterozygosity and can induce the loss-of-function of tumor suppressors or gain-of-function of proto-oncogenes could be demonstrated in the *CBL* gene. aUPD induces a gain-of-function leading to inhibition of the wild-type CBL and prolonged action of tyrosine kinases.[112] In the study by Grand et al., genome-wide SNP screening detected that atypical CML (aCML), CMML and MPN cases with manifest myelofibrosis were most frequently affected by *CBL* mutations.[111] *CBL* mutations were often associated with aUPD at 11q and showed involvement of *CBL* exon 8 and 9 as well as intron regions. These changes span over a region of several hundred base pairs making the diagnostic assay much more difficult by comparison to detection of JAK2[V617F]. Notably, an underlying molecular defect in the *CBL* gene seems to correlate with a shorter overall survival and progression-free survival in MPN patients.[111] Especially in aCML and CMML, *CBL* aberrations offer new insights into the molecular pathology of these MPN subtypes and serve as an important clonal marker allowing exclusion of reactive states in borderline cases.

Summary and future perspectives

Discovery of important mechanisms necessary for proper signal transduction in hematopoiesis, i.e. the induction of signaling by growth factors, receptor activation, recruitment of tyrosine kinases such as JAKs and transmission of signals by effector molecules such as the STATs was indispensable for exploring some of the molecular defects in MPN. However, we have to realize that JAK2[V617F], MPL[W515L/K], *TET2* and other defects might only represent the tip of the iceberg. Even though a constitutively activated kinase is a promising target for up-coming therapies, these therapies will probably not hit the molecular 'master event' responsible for the formation of a pre-malignant clone (Fig. 21.2). Also, we have to consider that in the presence of potentially co-existing clones the successful targeting of the JAK2[V617F] positive clone could lead to a selective growth advantage of another clone (the *pre*-JAK2[V617F] clone or a smaller bystander clone).

The reliable discrimination of the myeloproliferative (neoplastic) from the reactive state by detection of JAK2[V617F],
aberrations in JAK2 (exon 12), MPL[W515L/K] and *TET2* has become a major step in the diagnostic approach. However, we still have to face the diagnostic dilemma that in terms of MPN classification, the detection of the JAK2[V617F] or other molecular defects *per se* is of limited value. Apart from PV, in which JAK2[V617F] in ~99% exerts its effects predominantly on the erythroid lineage, ET and PMF exhibit distinct features that are demonstrated in cases with and without molecular changes. Even though ET showing the JAK2[V617F] could be interpreted as a modified form of PV, true ET clearly shows another course including rare leukemic transformation and virtually no development of myelofibrosis. In a subset of ET cases, the lower mutant allele burden of JAK2[V617F] allows discrimination from the hypercellular, prefibrotic stage of PMF.[61] This finding can be of clinical value as PMF has a high risk for the development of myelofibrosis and the early stage of PMF is sometimes difficult to distinguish from ET by morphological and clinical parameters.

Disease phenotypes in MPN are the result of aberrant molecular signatures and any additional aberration contributes to the overall clinical and histopathological presentation. The varying phenotypes of MPN, even in cases with molecular markers, might also depend on individual host modifiers. Besides the extent of the mutation burden in different lineages, the competition of the JAK2[V617F] positive clone with other bystander clones along with functional negative feedback mechanisms against constitutive signaling might also contribute to differences in the phenotype.

In summary, the investigation of the molecular pathology of MPN and MDS/MPN will be of particular interest in the future allowing: 1) further dissection of aberrant pathways, 2) an increase in the number of the available molecular markers for diagnostic purposes and 3) the discovery and design of effective therapies.

References

1. Dameshek W. Some speculations on the myeloproliferative syndromes. Blood 1951;6:372–5.

2. Nowell PC. Discovery of the Philadelphia chromosome: a personal perspective. J Clin Invest 2007;117:2033–5.

3. Druker BJ, Tamura S, Buchdunger E, et al. Effects of a selective inhibitor of the Abl tyrosine kinase on the growth of BCR-Abl positive cells. Nat Med 1996;2:561–6.

4. Hussein K, Van Dyke DL, Tefferi A. Conventional cytogenetics in myelofibrosis: literature review and discussion. Eur J Haematol 2009;82: 329–38.

5. Kralovics R, Guan Y, Prchal JT. Acquired uniparental disomy of chromosome 9p is a frequent stem cell defect in polycythemia vera. Exp Hematol 2002; 30:229–36.

6. Kralovics R, Passamonti F, Buser AS, et al. A gain-of-function mutation of JAK2 in

myeloproliferative disorders. N Engl J Med 2005;352:1779–90.

7. Swerdlow SH, Campo E, Harris NL, et al. WHO Classification of Tumours of Haematopoietic and Lymphatic Tissues. Lyon: IARC; 2008.

8. Faderl S, Talpaz M, Estrov Z, et al. The biology of chronic myeloid leukemia. N Engl J Med 1999;341:164–72.

9. Nowell PC, Hungerford DA. Chromosome studies in human leukemia. II. Chronic granulocytic leukemia. J Natl Cancer Inst 1961; 27:1013–35.

10. Rowley JD. Letter: A new consistent chromosomal abnormality in chronic myelogenous leukaemia identified by quinacrine fluorescence and Giemsa staining. Nature 1973;243: 290–3.

11. de Klein A, van Kessel AG, Grosveld G, et al. A cellular oncogene is translocated to the Philadelphia chromosome in

chronic myelocytic leukaemia. Nature 1982;300:765–7.

12. Bartram CR, de Klein A, Hagemeijer A, et al. Translocation of c-abl oncogene correlates with the presence of a Philadelphia chromosome in chronic myelocytic leukaemia. Nature 1983; 306:277–80.

13. Dreazen O, Klisak I, Rassool F, et al. The bcr gene is joined to c-abl in Ph1 chromosome negative chronic myelogenous leukemia. Oncogene Res 1988;2:167–75.

14. Muller AJ, Young JC, Pendergast AM, et al. BCR first exon sequences specifically activate the BCR/ABL tyrosine kinase oncogene of Philadelphia chromosome-positive human leukemias. Mol Cell Biol 1991;11:1785–92.

15. Ben-Neriah Y, Daley GQ, Mes-Masson AM, et al. The chronic myelogenous leukemia-specific P210 protein is

the product of the bcr/abl hybrid gene. Science 1986;233: 212–14.

16. Pane F, Intrieri M, Quintarelli C, et al. BCR/ABL genes and leukemic phenotype: from molecular mechanisms to clinical correlations. Oncogene 2002;21: 8652–67.

17. Inokuchi K, Dan K, Takatori M, et al. Myeloproliferative disease in transgenic mice expressing P230 Bcr/Abl: longer disease latency, thrombocytosis, and mild leukocytosis. Blood 2003;102: 320–3.

18. Ohsaka A, Shiina S, Kobayashi M, et al. Philadelphia chromosome-positive chronic myeloid leukemia expressing p190(BCR-ABL). Intern Med 2002; 41:1183–7.

19. Ravandi F, Cortes J, Albitar M, et al. Chronic myelogenous leukaemia with p185(BCR/ABL) expression: characteristics and clinical significance. Br J Haematol 1999;107:581–6.

20. Kawai H, Nie L, Yuan ZM. Inactivation of NF-kappaB-dependent cell survival, a novel mechanism for the proapoptotic function of c-Abl. Mol Cell Biol 2002;22:6079–88.

21. Pluk H, Dorey K, Superti-Furga G. Autoinhibition of c-Abl. Cell 2002;108:247–59.

22. Pendergast AM, Gishizky ML, Havlik MH, Witte ON. SH1 domain autophosphorylation of P210 BCR/ABL is required for transformation but not growth factor independence. Mol Cell Biol 1993;13:1728–36.

23. Bedi A, Zehnbauer BA, Barber JP, et al. Inhibition of apoptosis by BCR-ABL in chronic myeloid leukemia. Blood 1994;83:2038–44.

24. Spiekermann K, Pau M, Schwab R, et al. Constitutive activation of STAT3 and STAT5 is induced by leukemic fusion proteins with protein tyrosine kinase activity and is sufficient for transformation of hematopoietic precursor cells. Exp Hematol 2002; 30:262–71.

25. McCubrey JA, Steelman LS, Abrams SL, et al. Targeting survival cascades induced by activation of Ras/Raf/MEK/ERK, PI3K/PTEN/Akt/mTOR and Jak/STAT pathways for effective leukemia therapy. Leukemia 2008;22:708–22.

26. Deutsch E, Dugray A, AbdulKarim B, et al. BCR-ABL down-regulates the DNA repair protein DNA-PKcs. Blood 2001; 97:2084–90.

27. Koptyra M, Falinski R, Nowicki MO, et al. BCR/ABL kinase induces self-mutagenesis via reactive oxygen species to encode imatinib resistance. Blood 2006;108:319–27.

28. Salgia R, Li JL, Ewaniuk DS, et al. BCR/ABL induces multiple abnormalities of cytoskeletal function. J Clin Invest 1997;100:46–57.

29. Salgia R, Quackenbush E, Lin J, et al. The BCR/ABL oncogene alters the chemotactic response to stromal-derived factor-1alpha. Blood 1999;94:4233–46.

30. Bhatia R, Munthe HA, Forman SJ. Abnormal growth factor modulation of beta1-integrin-mediated adhesion in chronic myelogenous leukaemia haematopoietic progenitors. Br J Haematol 2001;115:845–53.

31. Jorgensen HG, Holyoake TL. Characterization of cancer stem cells in chronic myeloid leukaemia. Biochem Soc Trans 2007;35:1347–51.

32. Bhatia R, Holtz M, Niu N, et al. Persistence of malignant hematopoietic progenitors in chronic myelogenous leukemia patients in complete cytogenetic remission following imatinib mesylate treatment. Blood 2003;101:4701–7.

33. Biernaux C, Loos M, Sels A, et al. Detection of major BCR-ABL gene expression at a very low level in blood cells of some healthy individuals. Blood 1995;86:3118–22.

34. Posthuma EF, Falkenburg JH, Apperley JF, et al. HLA-B8 and HLA-A3 coexpressed with HLA-B8 are associated with a reduced risk of the development of chronic myeloid leukemia. The Chronic Leukemia Working Party of the EBMT. Blood 1999;93:3863–5.

35. Hochhaus A, Kantarjian HM, Baccarani M, et al. Dasatinib induces notable hematologic and cytogenetic responses in chronic-phase chronic myeloid leukemia after failure of imatinib therapy. Blood 2007;109:2303–9.

36. Jabbour E, Cortes JE, Kantarjian H. Optimizing treatment with BCR-Abl tyrosine kinase inhibitors in Philadelphia chromosome-positive chronic myeloid leukemia: focus on dosing schedules. Clin Lymphoma Myeloma 2008; 8(Suppl. 3):S75–81.

37. Branford S, Cross NC, Hochhaus A, et al. Rationale for the recommendations for harmonizing current methodology for detecting BCR-ABL transcripts in patients with chronic myeloid leukaemia. Leukemia 2006;20:1925–30.

38. Hughes TP, Kaeda J, Branford S, et al. Frequency of major molecular responses to imatinib or interferon alfa plus cytarabine in newly diagnosed chronic myeloid leukemia. N Engl J Med 2003; 349:1423–32.

39. Cortes J, Talpaz M, O'Brien S, et al. Molecular responses in patients with chronic myelogenous leukemia in chronic phase treated with imatinib mesylate. Clin Cancer Res 2005;11: 3425–32.

40. Goldman JM. Initial treatment for patients with CML. Hematology Am Soc Hematol Educ Program 2009;453–60.

41. Klemm L, Duy C, Iacobucci I, et al. The B cell mutator AID promotes B

lymphoid blast crisis and drug resistance in chronic myeloid leukemia. Cancer Cell 2009;16:232–45.

42. Hughes TP, Branford S. Measuring minimal residual disease in chronic myeloid leukemia: fluorescence in situ hybridization and polymerase chain reaction. Clin Lymphoma Myeloma 2009;9(Suppl. 3):S266–71.

43. Branford S, Fletcher L, Cross NC, et al. Desirable performance characteristics for BCR-ABL measurement on an international reporting scale to allow consistent interpretation of individual patient response and comparison of response rates between clinical trials. Blood 2008;112:3330–8.

44. Muller MC, Cross NC, Erben P, et al. Harmonization of molecular monitoring of CML therapy in Europe. Leukemia 2009;23:1957–63.

45. Buesche G, Ganser A, Schlegelberger B, et al. Marrow fibrosis and its relevance during imatinib treatment of chronic myeloid leukemia. Leukemia 2007; 21:2420–7.

46. Baxter EJ, Scott LM, Campbell PJ, et al. Acquired mutation of the tyrosine kinase JAK2 in human myeloproliferative disorders. Lancet 2005;365:1054–61.

47. James C, Ugo V, Le Couedic JP, et al. A unique clonal JAK2 mutation leading to constitutive signalling causes polycythaemia vera. Nature 2005;434: 1144–8.

48. Levine RL, Wadleigh M, Cools J, et al. Activating mutation in the tyrosine kinase JAK2 in polycythemia vera, essential thrombocythemia, and myeloid metaplasia with myelofibrosis. Cancer Cell 2005;7:387–97.

49. Kaushansky K. On the molecular origins of the chronic myeloproliferative disorders: it all makes sense. Blood 2005;105:4187–90.

50. Wernig G, Mercher T, Okabe R, et al. Expression of Jak2V617F causes a polycythemia vera-like disease with associated myelofibrosis in a murine bone marrow transplant model. Blood 2006;107:4274–81.

51. Lacout C, Pisani DF, Tulliez M, et al. JAK2V617F expression in murine hematopoietic cells leads to MPD mimicking human PV with secondary myelofibrosis. Blood 2006;108:1652–60.

52. Lippert E, Boissinot M, Kralovics R, et al. The JAK2-V617F mutation is frequently present at diagnosis in patients with essential thrombocythemia and polycythemia vera. Blood 2006; 108:1865–7.

53. Tefferi A, Lasho TL, Schwager SM, et al. The clinical phenotype of wild-type, heterozygous, and homozygous JAK2V617F in polycythemia vera. Cancer 2006;106:631–5.

54. Horn T, Kremer M, Dechow T, et al. Detection of the activating JAK2 V617F

mutation in paraffin-embedded trephine bone marrow biopsies of patients with chronic myeloproliferative diseases. J Mol Diagn 2006;8:299–304.

55. Bock O, Busche G, Koop C, et al. Detection of the single hotspot mutation in the JH2 pseudokinase domain of Janus kinase 2 in bone marrow trephine biopsies derived from chronic myeloproliferative disorders. J Mol Diagn 2006;8:170–7.

56. Antonioli E, Guglielmelli P, Pancrazzi A, et al. Clinical implications of the JAK2 V617F mutation in essential thrombocythemia. Leukemia 2005;19: 1847–9.

57. Wolanskyj AP, Lasho TL, Schwager SM, et al. JAK2 mutation in essential thrombocythaemia: clinical associations and long-term prognostic relevance. Br J Haematol 2005;131:208–13.

58. Campbell PJ, Scott LM, Buck G, et al. Definition of subtypes of essential thrombocythaemia and relation to polycythaemia vera based on JAK2 V617F mutation status: a prospective study. Lancet 2005;366:1945–53.

59. Bock O, Neuse J, Hussein K, et al. Aberrant collagenase expression in chronic idiopathic myelofibrosis is related to the stage of disease but not to the JAK2 mutation status. Am J Pathol 2006;169:471–81.

60. Hussein K, Brakensiek K, Buesche G, et al. Different involvement of the megakaryocytic lineage by the JAK2 V617F mutation in polycythemia vera, essential thrombocythemia and chronic idiopathic myelofibrosis. Ann Hematol 2007;86:245–53.

61. Hussein K, Bock O, Theophile K, et al. JAK2(V617F) allele burden discriminates essential thrombocythemia from a subset of prefibrotic-stage primary myelofibrosis. Exp Hematol 2009;37: 1186–93.

62. Kiladjian JJ, Elkassar N, Cassinat B, et al. Essential thrombocythemias without V617F JAK2 mutation are clonal hematopoietic stem cell disorders. Leukemia 2006;20:1181–3.

63. Kralovics R, Teo SS, Li S, et al. Acquisition of the V617F mutation of JAK2 is a late genetic event in a subset of patients with myeloproliferative disorders. Blood 2006;108:1377–80.

64. Campbell PJ, Baxter EJ, Beer PA, et al. Mutation of JAK2 in the myeloproliferative disorders: timing, clonality studies, cytogenetic associations, and role in leukemic transformation. Blood 2006;108: 3548–55.

65. Scott LM, Tong W, Levine RL, et al. JAK2 exon 12 mutations in polycythemia vera and idiopathic erythrocytosis. N Engl J Med 2007;356:459–68.

66. Schnittger S, Bacher U, Haferlach C, et al. Detection of JAK2 exon 12

mutations in 15 patients with JAK2V617F negative polycythemia vera. Haematologica 2009;94:414–18.

67. Finazzi G, Barbui T. Evidence and expertise in the management of polycythemia vera and essential thrombocythemia. Leukemia 2008;22:1494–502.

68. Huang J, Li CY, Mesa RA, et al. Risk factors for leukemic transformation in patients with primary myelofibrosis. Cancer 2008;112:2726–32.

69. Jelinek J, Oki Y, Gharibyan V, et al. JAK2 mutation 1849G>T is rare in acute leukemias but can be found in CMML, Philadelphia chromosome–negative CML, and megakaryocytic leukemia. Blood 2005;106:3370–3.

70. Frohling S, Lipka DB, Kayser S, et al. Rare occurrence of the JAK2 V617F mutation in AML subtypes M5, M6, and M7. Blood 2006;107:1242–3.

71. Lee JW, Kim YG, Soung YH, et al. The JAK2 V617F mutation in de novo acute myelogenous leukemias. Oncogene 2006;25:1434–6.

72. Levine RL, Loriaux M, Huntly BJ, et al. The JAK2V617F activating mutation occurs in chronic myelomonocytic leukemia and acute myeloid leukemia, but not in acute lymphoblastic leukemia or chronic lymphocytic leukemia. Blood 2005;106:3377–9.

73. Bercovich D, Ganmore I, Scott LM, et al. Mutations of JAK2 in acute lymphoblastic leukaemias associated with Down's syndrome. Lancet 2008;372:1484–92.

74. Mesa RA, Powell H, Lasho T, et al. A longitudinal study of the JAK2(V617F) mutation in myelofibrosis with myeloid metaplasia: analysis at two time points. Haematologica 2006;91:415–16.

75. Kaushansky K. Mpl and the hematopoietic stem cell. Leukemia 2002;16:738–9.

76. Kaushansky K. The role of the MPL receptor in myeloproliferative disorders. Leukemia 1998;12(Suppl. 1):S47–50.

77. Moliterno AR, Spivak JL. Posttranslational processing of the thrombopoietin receptor is impaired in polycythemia vera. Blood 1999;94: 2555–61.

78. Horikawa Y, Matsumura I, Hashimoto K, et al. Markedly reduced expression of platelet c-mpl receptor in essential thrombocythemia. Blood 1997;90: 4031–8.

79. Mesa RA, Hanson CA, Li CY, et al. Diagnostic and prognostic value of bone marrow angiogenesis and megakaryocyte c-Mpl expression in essential thrombocythemia. Blood 2002;99:4131–7.

80. Tefferi A, Yoon SY, Li CY. Immunohistochemical staining for megakaryocyte c-mpl may complement morphologic distinction between

polycythemia vera and secondary erythrocytosis. Blood 2000;96:771–2.

81. Yoon SY, Li CY, Tefferi A. Megakaryocyte c-Mpl expression in chronic myeloproliferative disorders and the myelodysplastic syndrome: immunoperoxidase staining patterns and clinical correlates. Eur J Haematol 2000;65:170–4.

82. Teofili L, Pierconti F, Di FA, et al. The expression pattern of c-mpl in megakaryocytes correlates with thrombotic risk in essential thrombocythemia. Blood 2002;100: 714–17.

83. Martin DI, Zon LI, Mutter G, Orkin SH. Expression of an erythroid transcription factor in megakaryocytic and mast cell lineages. Nature 1990;344:444–7.

84. Vigon I, Mornon JP, Cocault L, et al. Molecular cloning and characterization of MPL, the human homolog of the v-mpl oncogene: identification of a member of the hematopoietic growth factor receptor superfamily. Proc Natl Acad Sci USA 1992;89:5640–4.

85. McDonald TP, Sullivan PS. Megakaryocytic and erythrocytic cell lines share a common precursor cell. Exp Hematol 1993;21:1316–20.

86. Yan XQ, Lacey DL, Saris C, et al. Ectopic overexpression of c-mpl by retroviral-mediated gene transfer suppressed megakaryopoiesis but enhanced erythropoiesis in mice. Exp Hematol 1999;27:1409–17.

87. Kieran MW, Perkins AC, Orkin SH, Zon LI. Thrombopoietin rescues in vitro erythroid colony formation from mouse embryos lacking the erythropoietin receptor. Proc Natl Acad Sci USA 1996;93:9126–31.

88. Pikman Y, Lee BH, Mercher T, et al. MPLW515L is a novel somatic activating mutation in myelofibrosis with myeloid metaplasia. PLoS Med 2006;3:e270.

89. Pardanani AD, Levine RL, Lasho T, et al. MPL515 mutations in myeloproliferative and other myeloid disorders: a study of 1182 patients. Blood 2006;108: 3472–6.

90. Beer PA, Campbell PJ, Scott LM, et al. MPL mutations in myeloproliferative disorders: analysis of the PT-1 cohort. Blood 2008;112:141–9.

91. Moliterno AR, Williams DM, Rogers O, Spivak JL. Molecular mimicry in the chronic myeloproliferative disorders: reciprocity between quantitative JAK2 V617F and Mpl expression. Blood 2006;108:3913–15.

92. Gery S, Gueller S, Chumakova K, et al. Adaptor protein Lnk negatively regulates the mutant MPL, MPLW515L associated with myeloproliferative disorders. Blood 2007;110:3360–4.

93. Lu X, Levine R, Tong W, et al. Expression of a homodimeric type I cytokine receptor is required for JAK2V617F-

mediated transformation. Proc Natl Acad Sci USA 2005;102:18962–7.

94. Tefferi A, Pardanani A, Lim KH, et al. TET2 mutations and their clinical correlates in polycythemia vera, essential thrombocythemia and myelofibrosis. Leukemia 2009;23:905–11.

95. Kosmider O, Gelsi-Boyer V, Ciudad M, et al. TET2 gene mutation is a frequent and adverse event in chronic myelomonocytic leukemia. Haematologica 2009;94:1676–81.

96. Delhommeau F, Dupont S, Della VV, et al. Mutation in TET2 in myeloid cancers. N Engl J Med 2009;360: 2289–301.

97. Saint-Martin C, Leroy G, Delhommeau F, et al. Analysis of the ten-eleven translocation 2 (TET2) gene in familial myeloproliferative neoplasms. Blood 2009;114:1628–32.

98. Abdel-Wahab O, Mullally A, Hedvat C, et al. Genetic characterization of TET1, TET2, and TET3 alterations in myeloid malignancies. Blood 2009;114:144–7.

99. Tefferi A, Levine RL, Lim KH, et al. Frequent TET2 mutations in systemic mastocytosis: clinical, KITD816V and FIP1L1-PDGFRA correlates. Leukemia 2009;23:900–4.

100. Jankowska AM, Szpurka H, Tiu RV, et al. Loss of heterozygosity 4q24 and TET2 mutations associated with myelodysplastic/myeloproliferative neoplasms. Blood 2009;113:6403–10.

101. Tahiliani M, Koh KP, Shen Y, et al. Conversion of 5-methylcytosine to 5-hydroxymethylcytosine in mammalian DNA by MLL partner TET1. Science 2009;324:930–5.

102. Hussein K, Bock O, Theophile K, et al. Chronic myeloproliferative diseases with concurrent BCR-ABL junction and JAK2V617F mutation. Leukemia 2008;22:1059–62.

103. Sotlar K, Bache A, Stellmacher F, et al. Systemic mastocytosis associated with chronic idiopathic myelofibrosis: a distinct subtype of systemic mastocytosis associated with a [corrected] clonal hematological non-mast [corrected] cell lineage disorder carrying the activating point mutations KITD816V and JAK2V617F. J Mol Diagn 2008;10:58–66.

104. Hussein K, Bock O, Theophile K, et al. Biclonal expansion and heterogeneous lineage involvement in a case of chronic myeloproliferative disease with concurrent MPLW515L/JAK2V617F mutation. Blood 2009;113:1391–2.

105. Hussein K, Theophile K, Buhr T, et al. Different lineage involvement in myelodysplastic/myeloproliferative disease with combined MPLW515L and JAK2V617F mutation. Br J Haematol 2009;145:673–5.

106. Pardanani A, Lasho TL, Finke C, et al. Extending Jak2V617F and MplW515 mutation analysis to single hematopoietic colonies and B and T lymphocytes. Stem Cells 2007;25: 2358–62.

107. Lasho TL, Pardanani A, McClure RF, et al. Concurrent MPL515 and JAK2V617F mutations in myelofibrosis: chronology of clonal emergence and changes in mutant allele burden over time. Br J Haematol 2006;135:683–7.

108. Smit L, Borst J. The Cbl family of signal transduction molecules. Crit Rev Oncog 1997;8:359–79.

109. Joazeiro CA, Wing SS, Huang H, et al. The tyrosine kinase negative regulator c-Cbl as a RING-type, E2-dependent ubiquitin-protein ligase. Science 1999;286:309–12.

110. Fu JF, Hsu JJ, Tang TC, Shih LY. Identification of CBL, a proto-oncogene at 11q23.3, as a novel MLL fusion partner in a patient with de novo acute myeloid leukemia. Genes Chromosomes Cancer 2003;37:214–19.

111. Grand FH, Hidalgo-Curtis CE, Ernst T, et al. Frequent CBL mutations associated with 11q acquired uniparental disomy in myeloproliferative neoplasms. Blood 2009;113:6182–92.

112. Sanada M, Suzuki T, Shih LY, et al. Gain-of-function of mutated C-CBL tumour suppressor in myeloid neoplasms. Nature 2009;460:904–8.

113. Tefferi A, Skoda R, Vardiman JW. Myeloproliferative neoplasms: contemporary diagnosis using histology and genetics. Nat Rev Clin Oncol 2009;6:627–37.

114. Mullighan CG. TET2 mutations in myelodysplasia and myeloid malignancies. Nat Genet 2009;41:766–7.

CHAPTER 22

Erythrocytosis and polycythemia

J D van der Walt

Introduction

The term 'erythrocytosis' is derived from Greek words meaning 'too many red cells' and should be distinguished from 'polycythemia', meaning 'too many cells in the blood'.[1] Erythrocytosis has been defined as a greater than two standard deviation-increase from the age-, sex- and race-adjusted norm in hematocrit or hemoglobin level.[2] It is clear, however, that these laboratory parameters may be affected by decreases in plasma volume. Therefore, a clinical diagnosis of 'erythrocytosis' might represent true erythrocytosis, indicating a true increase in red cell mass (RCM), or in fact apparent polycythemia, resulting from either reduced plasma volume (relative polycythemia) or failure to recognize otherwise normal values for hematocrit (*Hct*) or hemoglobin (*Hgb*) level that lie in the extreme right tail of the Gaussian distribution.[3] Hence, for an individual patient, interpretation of laboratory results without knowledge of the personal baseline value remains inaccurate because of the inevitable statistical overlap of extreme values between subjects with and without disease.[3]

The recent development of molecular tests for the $JAK2^{V617F}$ and MPL mutations (see Chapter 21 for details) has allowed the reliable distinction of clonal from non-clonal erythrocytosis and has radically altered the investigation of erythrocytosis. Furthermore the value of aggressive phlebotomy to lower *Hct* levels below 45% in men and 42% in women has not been substantiated.[3] The therapeutic relevance of distinguishing polycythemia vera (PV) from so-called 'essential thrombocythemia (ET) with borderline increased *Hct*' has diminished and has further undermined the value of RCM measurement, which is no longer fundamental to the diagnosis of many patients.[3]

In this chapter, the recent revision of the WHO criteria,[4] which reflects developments in molecular pathogenesis and international consensus on clinico-pathological classification, is used for definition purposes although it is recognized that dissenting views have been published.[5] Erythrocytosis is therefore practically defined according to the thresholds used in the WHO classification,[3,4] i.e.:

- *Hgb* >18.5 g/100 ml in men or 16.5 g/100 ml in women for Caucasians

DOI: 10.1016/B978-0-7020-3147-2.00022-5

- or *Hgb* or *Hct* >99th percentile of method-specific reference range for age, sex and altitude of residence
- or *Hgb* >17 g/100 ml in men or 15 g/100 ml in women for Caucasians (or the equivalent in other races and age groups) if associated with a documented and sustained increase of at least 2 g/100 ml from an individual's baseline value that cannot be attributed to correction of iron deficiency.

The classification of erythrocytosis has recently been the subject of two excellent reviews.[3,6] The term 'idiopathic erythrocytosis' was used by McMullin[6] but has been criticized by Patnaik and Tefferi[3] as an entity, due to misuse of the term for patients who have an inappropriate diagnosis of erythrocytosis or who have been inadequately investigated. Nevertheless, there remain patients who have been fully investigated and who are likely to have abnormalities that have not as yet been defined. These may include defects of the erythropoietin (Epo) signaling pathway or oxygen sensing pathway.[3,6] Therefore, the category 'unclassifiable' is introduced here in accordance with the WHO classification and strictly defined for patients who have been fully investigated and for whom no currently defined cause of the erythrocytosis has been found. Patients who are partially investigated should not be placed in this category. While there are several potential divisions of a classification of patients with proven erythrocytosis, the classification used here (Box 22.1) is adapted from Patnaik and Tefferi.[3]

Box 22.1 Classification of erythrocytosis *(adapted from Patnaik and Tefferi[3])*

1. Congenital erythrocytosis
   a. Associated with reduced P50*
      i. High-oxygen-affinity hemoglobinopathy
      ii. 2,3-Bisphosphoglycerate deficiency
      iii. Methemoglobinemia
   b. Associated with normal P50
      i. VHL mutations including Chuvash erythrocytosis
      ii. PHD2 mutations
      iii. HIF2a mutations
      iv. Epo receptor mutations
2. Acquired erythrocytosis
   a. Primary (clonal)
      i. Polycythemia vera (PV)
   b. Secondary
      i. Hypoxia driven
         1. Chronic lung disease
         2. Right-to-left cardiopulmonary shunts
         3. High-altitude habitat
         4. Tobacco use/carbon monoxide poisoning
         5. Sleep apnea/hypoventilation syndrome
         6. Renal artery stenosis
      ii. Hypoxia independent
         1. Use of androgen preparations/erythropoietin injection
         2. Post-renal transplant
         3. Tumours: cerebellar hemangioblastoma, meningioma, pheochromocytoma, uterine leiomyoma, renal cysts, renal cell carcinoma, parathyroid adenoma, hepatocellular adenoma and carcinoma, etc.
3. Unclassifiable erythrocytosis

*Partial pressure of oxygen at which 50% of *Hgb* is saturated with oxygen.

The pathology of erythrocytosis

The discovery of the *JAK2*[V617F] mutation in 2005[7–10] (see Chapter 21) has profoundly changed both understanding and investigation of the erythrocytoses. Accordingly, modern diagnostic evaluation of a patient with proven erythrocytosis, and for whom no obvious cause is apparent, may begin with screening of the peripheral blood for the *JAK2*[V617F] mutation and serum Epo. A working classification of erythrocytosis into primary, or clonal, i.e. PV, versus secondary has therefore emerged,[6] but the more classical pathogenetic approach is used here.

Congenital erythrocytosis

Associated with reduced P50
High-oxygen-affinity hemoglobinopathy

High-oxygen-affinity hemoglobins release oxygen at a lower rate than normal and thus create relative tissue hypoxia, which might result in compensatory erythrocytosis in approximately one third of affected patients. Affected patients often present with isolated erythrocytosis, in the absence of signs and symptoms of systemic disease.[3] Erythrocytosis is accompanied by chronic hemolysis where the *Hgb* variant is unstable.[6] Bone marrow trephine biopsy (BMTB) investigation shows erythroid hyperplasia but normal megakaryocytes (Fig. 22.1A, B). These patients may have family members who are similarly affected and a family history is therefore essential in the investigation of patients with erythrocytosis. Transmission in affected patients is usually autosomal dominant.

More than 90 mutations have been described and are covered in an exemplary fashion in a web resource: http://globin.bx.psu.edu/hbvar/. Most of the high-oxygen-affinity mutations involve the β-globin chain and $α_1β_2$ contact zones.[11] Serum Epo levels are either normal or elevated and P50 (partial pressure of oxygen at which 50% of *Hgb* is saturated with oxygen) is decreased.[12] Structurally abnormal high-affinity *Hgb* should be suspected[3] if the P50 level is <20 mmHg.

2,3-Bisphosphoglycerate mutase (BPGM) deficiency

BPGM deficiency is a rare cause of erythrocytosis.[13,14] Deficiency of the enzyme results in a high affinity *Hgb* with a left shifted oxygen dissociation curve. This results in a compensatory erythrocytosis. Patients with both autosomal dominant[15] and autosomal recessive inheritance[16] have been described. In a fully penetrant autosomal recessive case, there is an isolated erythrocytosis with normal serum Epo level.[16] Diagnosis is established by showing a low P50, a normal *Hgb* structure and decreased BPGM activity.[3]

Methemoglobinemia

Congenital methemoglobinemias are of three main types:[17,18]

- The autosomal recessive cytochrome b5R deficiency (the most common)

- cytochrome b5 deficiency[19]
- the autosomal dominant hemoglobin M disease.

Methemoglobin causes both an impaired O_2 binding and increased oxygen affinity of the *Hgb*; sometimes resulting in compensatory erythrocytosis.[18]

Methemoglobinemia is clinically suspected when cyanosis is accompanied by normal PaO_2 levels but low saturation per pulse oximeter. Both carboxyhemoglobin and methemoglobin may be measured by modern oximeters.[3]

Associated with normal P50

The involvement of oxygen-sensing pathways in physiologic and pathologic erythropoiesis has recently been reviewed.[20] Red blood cells deliver O_2 from the lungs to the tissues. Better understanding of the physiological regulation of the process has allowed a rational classification of rare cases of congenital erythrocytosis to be developed (Fig. 22.2).[3,6]

A classic physiologic response to hypoxia in humans is the up-regulation of the *Erythropoietin (Epo)* gene, which is the central regulator of red blood cell mass. Reduction of tissue oxygenation triggers increased production of Epo by hypoxia-inducible factor 1 (HIF-1), which is a transcriptional activator composed of an O_2-regulated α subunit and a constitutively expressed β subunit. Hydroxylation of HIF-1α or HIF-2α by the asparaginyl hydroxylase FIH-1 blocks coactivator binding and transactivation. Hydroxylation of HIF-1α or HIF-2α by the prolyl hydroxylase PHD2 is required for binding of the von Hippel–Lindau (VHL) protein, leading to ubiquitination and proteasomal degradation. Mutations in the genes encoding VHL, PHD2, and HIF-2α have all been identified in patients with familial erythrocytosis.[20]

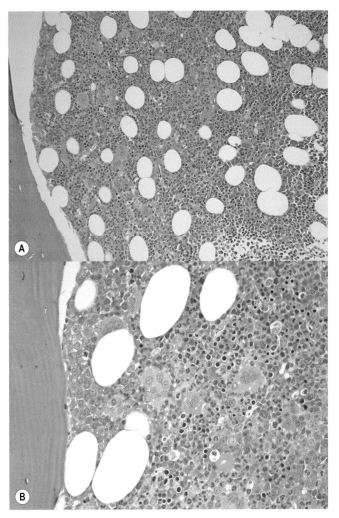

Fig. 22.1 (A–B) Erythrocytosis associated with hemoglobin San Diego. (A) The bone marrow is hypercellular due to erythroid hyperplasia. (B) Megakaryocytes show normal morphology.

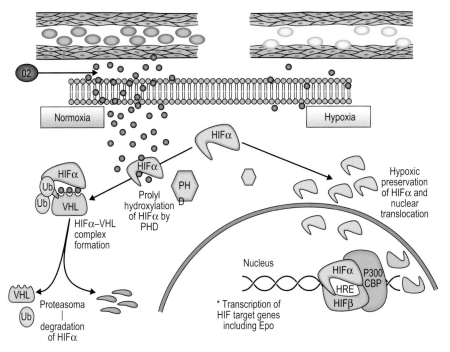

Fig. 22.2 Intracellular oxygen sensing and erythropoietin production. The cellular response to hypoxia is controlled by a family of transcription factors, known as hypoxia-inducible factors (HIFs). In the presence of normoxia, HIFα is rapidly destroyed by a collaborative effect of oxygen, prolyl hydroxylase domain (PHD)-containing enzymes and the von Hippel–Lindau tumor suppressor protein (VHL). Hydroxylated HIFα can bind to VHL, and the HIFα–VHL complex facilitates ubiquitin-mediated proteasomal degradation of HIFα. Under conditions of tissue hypoxia, the proteasomal degradation of HIFα is slowed, resulting in its cytoplasmic accumulation and subsequent translocation to the nucleus, where it dimerizes with HIFβ and enhances the transcription of the *Epo* gene. *(Adapted from Patnaik MM, Tefferi A 2009. The complete evaluation of erythrocytosis: congenital and acquired. Leukemia 23:834–844.)*

VHL mutations including Chuvash erythrocytosis (frequently termed Chuvash polycythemia)

Chuvash erythrocytosis is a rare, autosomal recessive, congenital erythrocytosis, first described in the Chuvash autonomous region in Russia[21] but also occurring in other racial and ethnic groups.[22,23] Affected patients are homozygous for a germline mutation affecting the *VHL* tumor suppressor gene, producing an abnormal VHL protein.[24,25] The mutation in the *VHL* gene disrupts the normal mechanism of hypoxia sensing, ultimately resulting in increased Epo production and erythrocytosis.[6]

In contrast to patients with the VHL disease, an autosomal dominant familial syndrome, patients with Chuvash erythrocytosis do not display an increased predilection for tumors.[3] However, other abnormalities are found.[26] Plasma concentrations of endothelin-1, Epo, plasminogen activator inhibitor-1, transferrin, transferrin receptor, and vascular endothelial growth factor are elevated. Clinical manifestations include increased cardiac valvular abnormalities, hemangiomas, pulmonary arterial hypertension, thrombotic and hemorrhagic events, varicose veins, and shortened life span. In parallel, peripheral blood concentrations of CD4 positive T-helper cells and CD4/CD8 ratio have been found to be lower in the VHL598C>T homozygotes.[26]

Prolyl hydroxlase domain 2 (PHD2) mutations

Under normoxic conditions, PHD2 hydroxylates the α-subunits of HIF proteins, facilitating VHL binding and subsequent ubiquitin-mediated proteasomal degradation of HIF.[3,6] Rare cases of *PHD2* mutations have been described, with the loss of PHD2 function, associated erythrocytosis and normal serum Epo.[3,6] Recently, a novel *PHD2* mutation has been described, associated with both erythrocytosis and recurrent paraganglioma.[27]

Hypoxia inducible factor alpha (HIF2α) mutations

Several erythrocytosis-associated HIF2α mutations have been characterized. All result in impaired degradation and thus aberrant stabilization of HIF2α. However, each exhibits a distinct profile with respect to their effects on PHD2 binding and VHL interaction.[28] Epo levels are usually elevated.[3,6]

Epo receptor (Epo-R) mutations

Epo-R signaling is regulated by the binding of the protein tyrosine phosphatase SHP-1 (or other JAK/STAT regulators) to the distal cytoplasmic region of Epo-R. This interaction results in the down-regulation of the Epo-mediated activation of the JAK2/STAT5 pathway and ultimately production of more red cells.[3,6] *Epo-R* mutations (all in exon 8) that cause erythrocytosis have been reviewed.[29–31] These mutations often result in cytoplasmic truncation of Epo-R, resulting in failure of attachment of SHP-1, ongoing production of red cells and thus erythrocytosis.

Transmission is usually autosomal dominant. Affected patients are usually asymptomatic and display subnormal (or normal) serum Epo level and hypersensitivity of erythroid progenitors to exogenous Epo.[3,6]

Acquired erythrocytosis

Erythrocytosis secondary to hypoxia

Chronic hypoxia leads to physiological secondary erythrocytosis, in order to compensate for the low oxygen concentrations at the pulmonary and/or tissue level. Clinically, interpretation of arterial blood gases, pulmonary function tests and chest radiography is an integral part of the investigation of erythrocytosis.[3] Chronic lung disease, right-to-left cardiopulmonary shunts, high-altitude habitat, tobacco use/carbon monoxide poisoning, sleep apnea/hypoventilation syndrome and renal artery stenosis are all associated with secondary erythrocytosis.[3,6] The bone marrow (BM) morphology is similar to that of patients with congenital erythrocytosis, showing hyperplasia of erythropoiesis and normal megakaryocytes (Fig. 22.1).

Erythrocytosis independent of hypoxia

Erythropoietin and related agents

Epo-stimulating agents (ESAs) were originally designed to replace endogenous Epo in patients with anemia secondary to renal failure. Their use has subsequently been expanded to include patients with anemia of other causes, including cancer patients.[32] Recombinant human Epo and its hyperglycosylated analog darbepoetin alfa and an array of novel ESAs are known to be misused by athletes.[33] Erythrocytosis has also been associated with supraphysiologic doses of anabolic steroids.[34]

Post-renal transplant erythrocytosis

Post-renal transplant erythrocytosis (PTE) affects approximately 10–15% of patients and typically manifests within the first or 2 years following transplantation.[35] The persistent secretion of Epo by the retained diseased native kidney, which is unaffected by feedback inhibition, is believed to play a central role. However, many patients with PTE have a low or normal Epo level and other erythroid growth factors contribute to driving erythropoiesis. The renal angiotensin system is thought to play an important role in PTE. Insulin-like growth factor has been demonstrated to enhance Epo-induced erythropoiesis *in vitro* and circulates in significant amounts in anephric dialysis patients. Adenosine receptors are also present on erythroid cells and stimulate Epo release.[35]

BMTB is most commonly performed in renal failure patients[36] due to cytopenias, pyrexia and suspected malignancies and rarely in cases of PTE, in which erythroid hyperplasia is the expected finding possibly in conjunction with the effects of treatment and chronic disease.

Erythrocytosis secondary to tumors

Several benign and malignant tumors and other lesions have been shown to produce inappropriate Epo. A high expression of *Epo* mRNA in the tumor tissue and the correction of erythrocytosis, together with a fall in the serum Epo levels after the tumor has been removed, is required to establish the association between the tumor and the secondary erythrocytosis.[3]

Uterine leiomyoma are associated with the so-called 'myomatous erythrocytosis syndrome', which is defined by the combination of erythrocytosis, uterine leiomyoma and persistent restoration of normal hematological values after hysterectomy.[37] Vlasveld et al.[37] were able to demonstrate a large gradient between the Epo levels in the uterine vein and artery during hysterectomy, providing direct evidence for *in vivo* Epo production by the uterine leiomyoma.

Renal cell carcinoma has also been associated with Epo production.[38] Burk at al.[39] described a 55-year-old man with clear cell renal carcinoma, pulmonary metastases and erythrocytosis. The increase in RCM was associated with an elevation in erythropoietic stimulatory activity in serum, pleural fluid and tumor-cyst fluid supporting the presence of autonomous tumor secretion of Epo or an Epo-like substance. Erythrocytosis has also been described in cases of tumors arising in polycystic kidneys[40] and renal cysts,[41] as well as in parathyroid adenoma,[42] pheochromocytoma,[43] hepatocellular adenoma[44] and carcinoma,[45] cerebellar hemangioblastoma[46] and meningiomas.[47]

Bone marrow biopsy in erythrocytosis

The histological features of PV are described in detail in the following section. Biopsies of the bone marrow in cases of erythrocytosis lack the findings of panmyelosis and typical megakaryocyte morphology seen in PV. The appearance is of a hyperplastic BM with erythroid hyperplasia. Megakaryocyte morphology is typically normal or reactive (Fig. 21.1). In addition, reactive stromal changes such as perivascular plasmacytosis, eosinophils, cell debris and iron deposits may be seen in cases of erythrocytosis,[48] particularly secondary to smoking, in which bronchopulmonary infection may be a concomitant finding.

Thiele et al.[49] studied BMTB together with clinical data and follow-up of 208 PV patients and 113 secondary polycythemia patients. In only 13 patients (4%) of this cohort, histopathology failed to differentiate clearly between the two diagnoses. Recently, testing for the $JAK2^{V617F}$ mutation has been shown to have a very high sensitivity, specificity and utility for the differential diagnosis between PV and erythrocytosis[50] but BMTB continues to have a role in the diagnosis of erythrocytosis, although it is now more likely to be used in atypical cases.[3]

Polycythemia vera (PV)

Polycythemia vera is a clonal stem cell disease with trilineage myeloid involvement,[4] which in classical cases manifests as panmyeloid proliferation (panmyelosis) in the BM and peripheral erythrocytosis, thrombocytosis and neutrophil leukocytosis.[3,4,6]

Clinical features

The predominant symptoms of PV are related to hypertension or vascular abnormalities associated with increased RCM or to arterial or venous thrombotic episodes such as deep venous thrombosis, myocardial ischemia or cerebrovascular occlusion, portal or splenic vein thrombosis. Headaches, dizziness, visual disturbances, paresthesias, pruritus,

---

Box 22.2 Laboratory abnormalities associated with PV[3]

1. $JAK2^{V617F}$ mutation or
2. Exon 12 mutations of *JAK2*
3. Endogenous erythroid colony growth
4. Low levels of serum erythropoietin
5. Increased baseline phosphorylation of the IGF-1 receptor
6. Increased activity of membrane-associated SH-PTP
7. Constitutive activation of STAT3
8. Up-regulation of negative control elements of the cell cycle (p16/p14)80
9. Increased antiapoptotic proteins (Bcl-xL) in erythroid precursors

---

erythromyalgia and gout are common. Patients may be stratified into low, intermediate (if generic cardiovascular risk factors are present) or high risk categories if age is greater than 60 years or a history of thrombosis is present.[4,51]

Laboratory features

Variations in the classical picture occur and competing classification systems have attempted to separate PV from other forms of MPN for therapeutic purposes. The WHO classification is used here as the basis for classification for the sake of reproducibility. The discovery of the *JAK2* mutations (see Chapter 21) and obsolescence of some laboratory tests has radically changed the approach to diagnosis (see Fig. 21.1 for details). Various other laboratory abnormalities are associated with PV (Box 22.2).

In vitro erythroid colony formation in patients with PV does not require the addition of exogenous Epo, a phenomenon termed 'endogenous erythroid colony growth'. This does not occur in either healthy persons or patients with non-clonal erythrocytosis[3] but the test is not widely available and is not routinely used.[6] The independent clonal proliferation of erythropoiesis in PV is associated with a correspondingly low serum Epo.[6] However, some cases of *JAK2* mutation positive ET may also have lower Epo levels, limiting the utility of the test in borderline cases.[52]

Hemoglobin and hematocrit: the Hct or packed cell volume is a measure of the total number of cells present, of which most are red cells. It is the most accurate way of measuring blood viscosity.[6] In PV viscosity is fundamental to the pathological effects: the greater the viscosity, the greater the sluggishness of the blood flow and thus the greater the severity of complications. A raised Hct is therefore the most important criterion for a diagnosis of PV. The Hb is used as a substitute measure of viscosity but there is not always a direct correlation between the two measurements. Using the Hb as a measure of viscosity may underestimate it, particularly in iron deficient patients.[6]

Red cell mass (RCM): the measurement of RCM is not required in patients who have a raised Hct and a *JAK2* mutation as they satisfy the diagnostic criteria for PV.[4,6] Measuring RCM is an expensive test and its use is now mainly confined to documenting absolute erythrocytosis versus apparent erythrocytosis in investigating rare *JAK2* mutation negative patients who are being investigated for possible PV.[3,6]

Box 22.3 WHO 2008 criteria for the diagnosis of polycythemia vera

Diagnosis requires the presence of both major criteria and one minor criterion or the presence of the first major criterion and two minor criteria.

Major criteria

1. *Hgb* >18.5 g/100 ml in men or 16.5 g/100 ml in women or other evidence of increased red cell volume. (*Hgb* or *Hct* >99th percentile of reference range for age/sex/altitude or *Hgb* >99th percentile of reference range for age/sex/altitude or *Hgb* >17 g/100 ml in men or 15 g/100 ml in women if associated with a documented and sustained increase of at least 2 g/100 ml from an individual's baseline value that is not attributed to correction of IDA, or elevated RCM >25% above mean normal predicted value.)
2. Presence of the *JAK2*^{V617F} or other functionally similar mutations, such as the *JAK2* exon 12 mutation.

Minor criteria

1. BM showing hypercellularity for age with trilineage growth (panmyelosis) and with prominent erythroid and megakaryocytic proliferation.
2. Serum Epo level below the reference range for normal.
3. Endogenous erythroid colony formation *in vitro*.

BM, bone marrow; Epo, erythropoietin; *Hct*, hematocrit; *Hgb*, hemoglobin; IDA, iron deficiency anemia; RCM, red cell mass; WHO, World Health Organization.

World Health Organization 2008 criteria for the diagnosis of PV

Significant changes in the approach to the diagnosis of PV have been brought about by the ability to define clonal erythrocytosis by the detection of *JAK2* mutations, a relatively simple test using polymerase chain reaction (PCR) based techniques.[6] It is also possible to determine whether an individual has a totally mutated *JAK2* or a mixture of wild type and mutated, described as homozygous or heterozygous (see Chapter 21). The WHO criteria for diagnosis of PV are summarized in Box 22.3. In addition to the classical polycythemic phase of PV, the WHO classification recognizes a pre- and a post-polycythemic phase of PV.

Pre-polycythemic PV

Also termed prodromal, latent or evolving PV, this condition, by definition, does not fulfill the criteria for polycythemic PV and may be diagnosed in retrospect or be only suggested in a BMTB report. The presence of marked thrombocytosis and normal or borderline high hemoglobin in the pre-polycythemic phase may lead to confusion with ET.[53] However, BMTB may show the classical features of PV. Recently, Gianelli et al.[54] compared the clinicopathologic and molecular features of 17 patients with evolving PV (e-PV) with those of 14 patients with ET and 19 with classical PV. The results for e-PV were more similar to those for PV than for ET. Patients with e-PV were characterized by an increase in the red cell parameters, splenomegaly and hepatomegaly, together with a hypercellular BM due to increased erythropoiesis and granulopoiesis, associated with megakaryocytic hyperplasia, with pleomorphic aggregates.

Box 22.4 WHO[4] diagnostic criteria for post-polycythemic myelofibrosis

Required criteria

1. Documentation of a previous diagnosis of PV according to WHO criteria (see Box 22.3).
2. Bone marrow fibrosis grade[57,58] 2–3/3 or 3–4/4 (see Chapter 3).

Additional criteria (two required)

1. Anemia or sustained loss of either phlebotomy (in the absence of cytoreductive therapy) or cytoreductive therapy requirement for erythropoiesis.
2. Leukoerythroblastic peripheral blood picture.
3. Increasing splenomegaly defined as either an increase in palpable splenomegaly of ≥5 cm from baseline (distance from the costal margin) or the appearance of newly palpable splenomegaly.
4. Development of ≥1 of 3 constitutional symptoms: >10% weight loss in 6 months, night sweats, unexplained fever (>37.5°C).

The frequency of the *JAK2*^{V617F} mutation was nearly 100% in both e-PV and PV but it was significantly lower in ET (54%).

ePV cases may be placed in the myeloproliferative neoplasm, unclassifiable (MPN, U) category, which should only be used for patients who have had full clinical, laboratory and morphological assessment and who still do not fulfill all the criteria for one of the other MPN diagnoses.[4] Subsequent evolution of clinical, laboratory or morphological findings may allow more precise classification. The concept of a prodromal phase in chronic myeloproliferative neoplasms has recently been reviewed.[55]

Use of MPN, U as a holding category is likely to reduce the number of cases said to have overlapping or transitional features or to have transformed from one disease to another.

Post-polycythemic PV

With progress of PV, erythropoiesis decreases, RCM normalizes and then decreases, and splenomegaly increases.[4] Peripheral blood changes occur and a leukoerythroblastic blood film with poikilocytosis appears. Splenomegaly due to extramedullary hemopoiesis increases. Terminally, blasts may appear and more than 10% blasts in the peripheral blood or BM or the presence of significant myelodysplasia signals progression to an accelerated phase or the development of a myelodysplastic syndrome. The appearance of more than 20% blasts is considered to represent the development of an acute phase, usually acute myeloid leukemia (AML).[4]

The International Working Group for Myelofibrosis Research and Treatment[56] recently proposed standardization criteria for post-polycythemic myelofibrosis (PPMF) and these have been adapted by the WHO[4] (Box 22.4).

Genetics in PV

Cases of PV are by definition Philadelphia chromosome/*BCR-ABL1* negative.[4] Abnormalities of the thrombopoietin receptor (*MPL*) (such as MPL$^{W515K/L}$, MPL^{W515S} and MPL^{S505N}) have been described in 4% of ET and 11% of PMF but not in PV.[62]

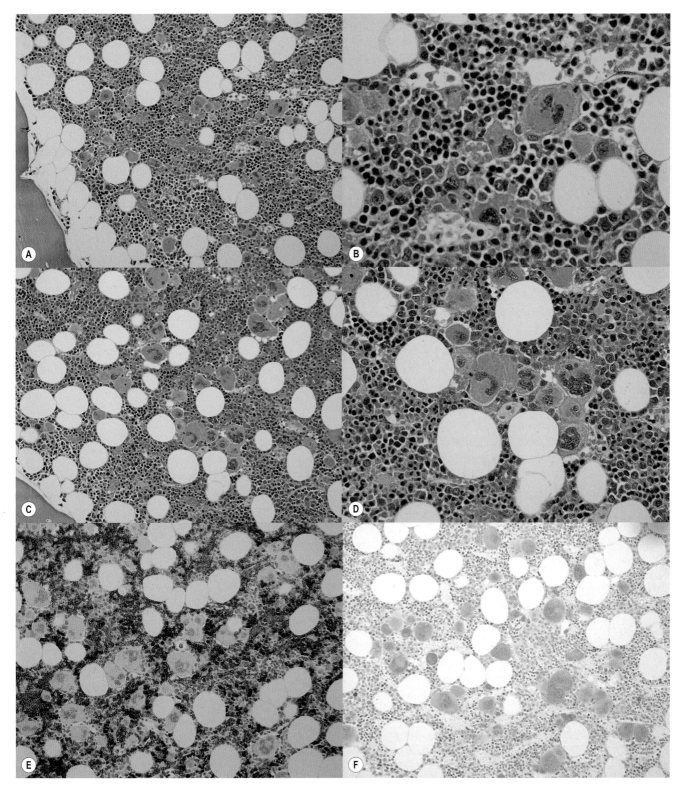

Fig. 22.3 (A–F) Range of morphological changes seen in the polycythemic phase of PV. (A–D) Megakaryocytes are pleomorphic and show variable number and clustering. (E) Erythropoiesis visualized by immunohistochemical staining for glycophorin C. (F) Megakaryocytes visualized by immunohistochemical staining for CD61.

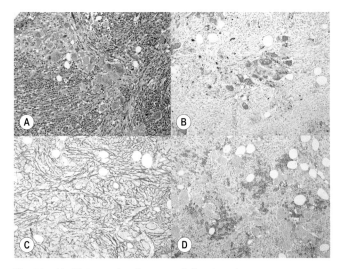

Fig. 22.4 (A–D) Post polycythemic myelofibrosis, early stage.
(A) The reticulin is increased producing a streaming pattern of the cells.
(B) Megakaryocytes visualized by immunohistochemical staining for CD61.
(C) Reticulin staining shows fibrosis grade 2. (D) Erythropoeisis is still present
as visualized by immunohistochemical staining for glycophorin C.

The most important genetic abnormalities in PV are the
$JAK2^{V617F}$ mutation and the functionally similar mutation in
exon 12 of $JAK2$ (see Chapter 21 for details), which are
present in more than 95% of PV cases. However, the $JAK2^{V617F}$
mutation is not specific for PV and is present in other forms
of MPN. This subject has recently been reviewed in depth[59]
and is covered in detail in Chapter 21. At diagnosis, some
20% of patients with PV have cytogenetic abnormalities.[4,60–62]
The commonest recurring abnormalities include +8, +9,
del(20q), del(13q), del(9p) and a combination of +8
and +9.

Evolution to post-PPMF and acceleration are characterized
by increasing cytogenetic abnormalities. Moreover, the
karyotype differs from PPMF, where +1q is the main anomaly,
compared with PMF where +1q is rare and del(13q) or
del(20q) are far more common.[60,62] Almost 100% of PV cases
that develop dysplasia or progress to an acute phase have
cytogenetic abnormalities, including those associated with
therapy-related myelodysplasia or AML[4] and, interestingly,
the leukemic blasts may loose $JAK2$-^{V617F} expression.[63]

The bone marrow biopsy in PV

The BMTB is less often performed since the advent of detection of $JAK2^{V617F}$ and related mutations as a reliable diagnostic test.[6] However, the BMTB is very useful in the elucidation
of atypical or pre-polycythemic cases and in the assessment
of cytopenias due to the effects of therapy or the development of PPMF.

In classical cases,[53] the BM is hypercellular due to panmyelosis: proliferation of generally morphologically normal
erythropoiesis and granulopoiesis accompanied by abnormal megakaryopoiesis (Fig. 22.3A–F). Megakaryocytes are
increased in numbers, sometimes quite markedly in cases
with pronounced thrombocytosis, and have hyperlobated
nuclei. They are typically pleomorphic, with a mixture of
cell sizes, and loosely clustered. In the polycythemic phase

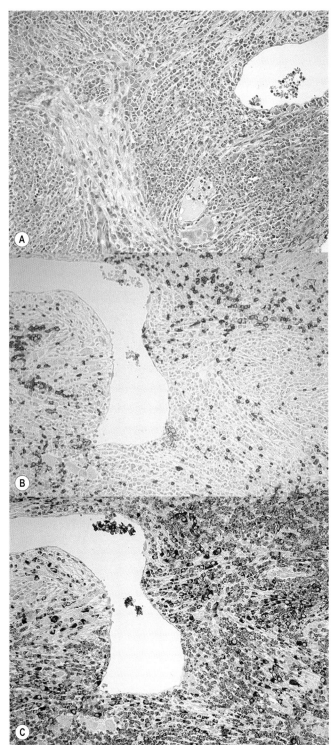

Fig. 22.5 (A–C) Post-polycythemic myelofibrosis, late stage. (A) Frank
collagen fibrosis is seen and sinusoidal dilation is apparent. (B) Erythropoiesis
is diminished in the spent phase and (C) granulopoiesis relatively increased.

megakaryocytes lack significant dysplastic features (Fig.
22.3) but become hyperchromatic and morphologically
atypical as PPMF develops (Fig. 22.4A–D). Proliferation of
left-shifted neutrophil granulopoiesis and reduced nucleated
erythroid precursors is also a feature of PPMF (Fig.
22.5A–B).

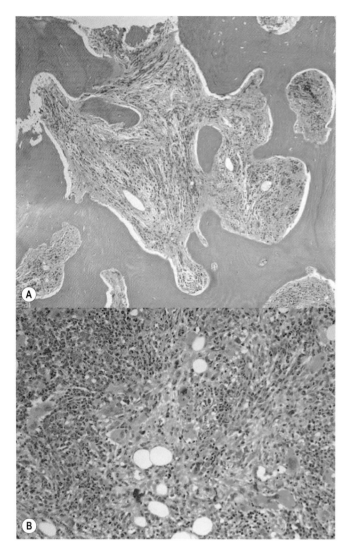

Fig. 22.6 (A, B) Post-polycythemic myelofibrosis, osteomyelofibrosis. (A) Bone changes are readily apparent. (B) More cellular areas may persist.

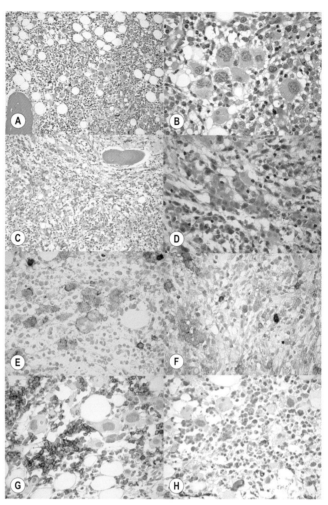

Fig. 22.7 (A–H) PV in accelerated phase. (A, B) Hemopoietic disorganization and increasing megakaryocytic dysplasia is present. (C, D) Dysplastic megakaryocytes proliferate within sinusoids. Immunocytochemistry is helpful in identifying mature cells and CD34[+] blasts. (E, F) Increasing megakaryocytic dysplasia is present. CD61 identifies micromegakaryocytes. (G) Glycophorin C identifies erythropoietic islands. (H) CD34 shows slight increase of blasts.

Reticulin is initially normal in 80% of cases, the rest showing varying degrees of increase.[4,53] There is a marked increase in the PPMF stage with increasing collagen fibrosis and finally osteomyelofibrosis (Fig. 22.6A, B). Sinusoidal dilatation and other feature of myelofibrosis are also seen (Fig. 22.7). Reticulin is typically not increased in cases of erythrocytosis.[53]

Iron deposits are absent (Perls staining) in approximately 95% of cases, in contrast to cases of erythrocytosis in which iron is readily identified.[53] Immunohistochemistry has no particular pattern but is useful in defining the components of hemopoiesis. CD34, CD117 and megakaryocyte markers such as CD61 and CD42 are useful in the diagnosis of the accelerated phase although CD117 positivity of immature erythroid precursors as well as early myeloid cells must be borne in mind[64] (Fig. 22.8A–C).

Frank dysplastic features develop in the accelerated phase[4] (Fig. 22.9A–D). The appearance of more than 20% blasts herald transformation to acute leukemia (Fig. 22.10A,B). Atypical morphology and reduced erythropoiesis may also be seen after cytoreductive therapy[4] (Fig. 22.11). This finding should not be mistaken for myelodysplasia. Thus, a complete clinical history is essential for the interpretation of a BMTB in PV.

Cases harboring the exon 12 *JAK2* mutation[65] have been reported to show predominant erythroid proliferation with normal megakaryocyte morphology and lack of clustering. However, others[66] and personal experience indicate that the megakaryocytes can be abnormal in some cases (Fig. 22.11A–C), with loose rather than tight clustering and variable nuclear morphology.

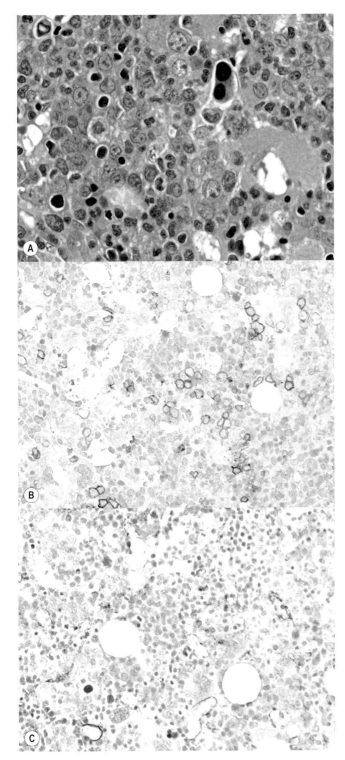

Fig. 22.8 (A–C) (A) An erythroid island showing dyserythropoiesis (B) and CD117 positivity (C) but no expression of CD34.

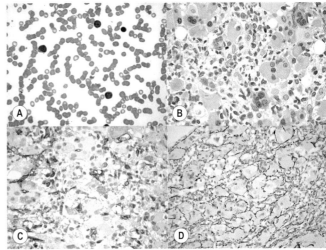

Fig. 22.9 (A–D) Transformation of PV to acute myeloid leukemia. (A) BM aspirate showing numerous blasts. (B) Severely dysplastic hemopoiesis is apparent and blasts exceed 20% of cells (C) CD34 immunostaining confirms increase of immature cells. (D) Reticulin is increased.

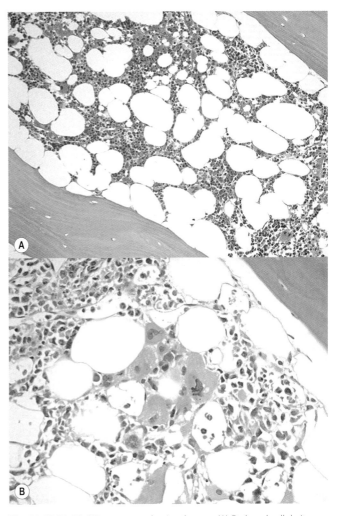

Fig. 22.10 (A, B) PV post-cytoreductive therapy. (A) Reduced cellularity and (B) dysplastic changes in megakaryocytes are apparent.

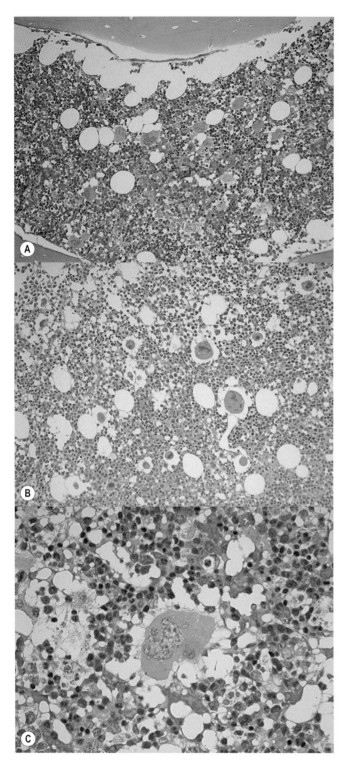

Fig. 22.11 (A–C) PV with exon 12 mutation. (A, B) Two cases showing varied morphology. Erythropoiesis dominates. Megakaryocytes do not show prominent clustering and display mild morphological abnormalities, partially resembling those seen in ET (C).

Familial PV

The familial nature of many primary erythrocytoses has already been described. Familial cases fulfilling the definition of the MPNs also occur but are rare. They differ from primary erythrocytoses because of clinical phenotype and multi-lineage proliferation in most instances.[67]

Only a small number of kindred have been described with four or more affected family members.[67,68] Affected family members have clonal hemopoiesis and form spontaneous erythroid colonies. Most but not all affected family members carry an acquired somatic mutation in the *JAK2* gene. This strongly suggests that only the predisposition to acquiring additional somatic mutations, such as *JAK2*[V617F], is inherited in these families, thus explaining the late onset and low penetrance of the MPN phenotype and the clonal hemopoiesis.[68]

Unclassifiable erythrocytosis

In the decades after the first analysis of the *Epo* gene, regulatory elements led to the discovery of HIF, which led in turn to the discovery of VHL and the PHDs.[20] Mutations in genes encoding all three of these essential components of the oxygen-sensing system have been identified in patients with familial erythrocytosis. Gain-of-function mutations in the *EpoR* gene also cause familial erythrocytosis.[3,6,20] It is highly likely that novel mutations in loci encoding other components of the O_2-sensing pathway remain to be identified.[20]

It is therefore essential that patients who have been fully investigated without a cause for the erythrocytosis having been found are identified and preferably referred to specialist centers. These patients should be placed in the 'unclassifiable erythrocytosis' category, which should not be used for incompletely investigated cases, as mentioned above.

In this group of patients with erythrocytosis in whom no cause has been identified after full investigation, one third has Epo levels below the normal range. A recent study[69] of so-called idiopathic erythrocytosis with low serum Epo levels showed that in fact 27% harbored the JAK2 exon 12 mutation. The other two thirds have normal or elevated Epo levels, and so have a secondary erythrocytosis of unknown cause.[70]

References

1. Messinezy M, van der Walt JD, Pearson TC. Polycythemia (the erythrocytoses). In: Wickramasinghe SN, McCullough J, editors. Blood and Bone Marrow Pathology. Edinburgh: Elsevier; 2002.

2. Hollowell JG, van Assendelft OW, Gunter EW, et al. Hematological and iron-related analytes – reference data for persons aged 1 year and over: United States, 1988–1994. Vital Health Stat 11; 2005;247: 1–156.

3. Patnaik MM, Tefferi A. The complete evaluation of erythrocytosis: congenital and acquired. Leukemia 2009;23:834–44.

4. Thiele J, Kvasnicka HM, Orazi A, et al. Polycythaemia vera. In: Swerlow SH, Campo E, Harris NL, et al, editors. WHO Classification of Tumours of Haematopoietic and Lymphoid Tissues. Lyon: IARC; 2008.

5. Spivak JL, Silver RT. The revised World Health Organization diagnostic criteria for polycythemia vera, essential thrombocythemia and primary myelofibrosis: an alternative proposal. Blood 2008;112:231–9.

6. McMullin MF. The classification and diagnosis of erythrocytosis. Int Jnl Lab Hem 2008;30:447–59.

7. Levine RL, Wadleigh M, Cools J, et al. Activating mutation in the tyrosine kinase JAK2 in polycythemia vera, essential thrombocythemia, and myeloid metaplasia with myelofibrosis. Cancer Cell 2005;7:387–97.

8. James C, Ugo V, Le Couedic JP, et al. A unique clonal JAK2 mutation leading to constitutive signalling causes polycythaemia vera. Nature 2005; 434:1144–8.

9. Kralovics R, Passamonti F, Buser AS, et al. A gain-of-function mutation of JAK2 in myeloproliferative disorders. N Engl J Med; 2005;352:1779–90.

10. Baxter EJ, Scott LM, Campbell PJ, et al. Acquired mutation of the tyrosine kinase JAK2 in human myeloproliferative disorders. Lancet 2005;365:1054–61.

11. Gonzalez Fernandez FA, Villegas A, Ropero P, et al. Haemoglobinopathies with high oxygen affinity. Experience of Erythropathology Cooperative Spanish Group. Ann Hematol 2009;88:235–8.

12. Rumi E, Passamonti F, Pagano L, et al. Blood p50 evaluation enhances diagnostic definition of isolated erythrocytosis. J Intern Med 2009;265:266–74.

13. Cartier P, Labie D, Leroux JP, et al. [Familial diphosphoglycerate mutase deficiency: hematological and biochemical study]. Nouv Rev Fr Hematol 1972;12: 269–87.

14. Rosa R, Prehu MO, Beuzard Y, Rosa J. The first case of a complete deficiency of diphosphoglycerate mutase in human erythrocytes. J Clin Invest 1978;62: 907–15.

15. Galacteros F, Rosa R, Prehu MO, et al. Diphosphoglyceromutase deficiency: new cases associated with erythrocytosis. Nouv Rev Fr Hematol 1984;26:69–74.

16. Hoyer JD, Steven LA, Beutler E, et al. Erythrocytosis due to bisphosphoglycerate mutase deficiency with concurrent glucose-6-phosphate dehydrogenase (G-6-PD) deficiency. Am J of Hematol 2004;75:205–8.

17. Yilmaz D, Cogulu O, Ozkinay F, et al. A novel mutation in the DIA1 gene in a patient with methemoglobinemia type II. Am J Med Genet A 2005;133A:101–2.

18. Fermo E, Bianchi P, Vercellati C, et al. Recessive hereditary methemoglobinemia: two novel mutations in the NADH-cytochrome b5 reductase gene. Blood Cells Mol Dis 2008;41:50–5.

19. Percy MJ, Lappin TR. Recessive congenital methaemoglobinaemia: cytochrome b5 reductase deficiency. B J of Haematol 2008;141:298–308.

20. Semenza GL. Involvement of oxygen-sensing pathways in physiologic and pathologic erythropoiesis. Blood 2009; 114:2015–19.

21. Liu E, Percy MJ, Amos CI, et al. The worldwide distribution of the VHL 598C>T mutation indicates a single founding event. Blood 2004;103:1937–40.

22. Percy MJ, McMullin MF, Jowitt SN, et al. Chuvash-type congenital polycythemia in 4 families of Asian and Western European ancestry. Blood 2003;102:1097–9.

23. Perrotta S, Nobili B, Ferraro M, et al. Von Hippel-Lindau-dependent polycythemia is endemic on the island of Ischia: identification of a novel cluster. Blood 2006;107:514–19.

24. Ang SO, Chen H, Gordeuk VR, et al. Endemic polycythemia in Russia: mutation in the VHL gene. Blood Cells Mol Dis 2002;28:57–62.

25. Ang SO, Chen H, Hirota K, et al. Disruption of oxygen homeostasis underlies congenital Chuvash polycythemia. Nat Genet 2002;32: 614–21.

26. Niu X, Miasnikova GY, Sergueeva AI, et al. Altered cytokine profiles in patients with Chuvash polycythemia. Am J Hematol 2009;84:74–8.

27. Ladroue C, Carcenac R, Leporrier M, et al. PHD2 mutation and congenital erythrocytosis with paraganglioma. N Engl J Med 2008;359:2685–92.

28. Furlow PW, Percy MJ, Sutherland S, et al. Erythrocytosis-associated HIF-2alpha mutations demonstrate a critical role for residues C-terminal to the hydroxylacceptor proline. J Biol Chem 2009;284:9050–8.

29. Percy ML. Genetically heterogeneous origins of idiopathic erythrocytosis. Hematology 2007;12:131–9.

30. Al-Sheikh M, Mazurier E, Gardie B, et al. A study of 36 unrelated cases with pure erythrocytosis revealed three new mutations in the erythropoietin receptor gene. Haematologica 2008;93:1072–5.

31. Percy MJ, Lee FS. Familial erythrocytosis: molecular links to red blood cell control. Haematologica 2008;93:963–7.

32. Hadland BK, Longmore GD. Erythroid-stimulating agents in cancer therapy: potential dangers and biologic mechanisms. J Clin Oncol 2009;27: 4217–26.

33. Jelkmann W. Erythropoiesis stimulating agents and techniques: a challenge for doping analysts. Curr Med Chem 2009;16:1236–47.

34. Stergiopoulos K, Brennan JJ, Mathews R, et al. Anabolic steroids, acute myocardial infarction and polycythemia: a case report and review of the literature. Vasc Health Risk Man 2008;4:1475–80.

35. Marinella MA. Hematologic abnormalities following renal transplantation. Int Urol Nephrol [Epub ahead of print]. 2009.

36. Garewal G, Ahluwalia J, Kumar V, et al. The utility of bone marrow examination in renal transplantation: nine years of experience from north India. Transplantation 2006;81:1354–6.

37. Vlasveld LT, de Wit CW, Verweij RA. Myomatous erythrocytosis syndrome: further proof for the pathogenic role of erythropoietin. Neth J Med 2008;66: 283–5.

38. Shiramizu M, Katsuoka Y, Grodberg J, et al. Constitutive secretion of erythropoietin by human renal adenocarcinoma cells in vivo and in vitro. Exp Cell Res 1994;215:249–56.

39. Burk JR, Lertora JJ, Martinez IR Jr, Fisher JW. Renal cell carcinoma with erythrocytosis and elevated erythropoietic stimulatory activity. South Med J 1977; 70:955–58.

40. Hama Y, Kaji T, Ito K, et al. Erythropoietin-producing renal cell carcinoma arising from autosomal dominant polycystic kidney disease. Br J Radiol 2005;78:269–71.

41. Blake-James B, Attar KH, Rabbani S, et al. Secondary polycythaemia associated with unilateral renal cystic disease. Int Urol Nephrol 2007;39:955–8.

42. Godeau P, Bletry O, Brochard C, Hussonois C. Polycythemia vera and primary hyperparathyroidism. Arch Intern Med 1981;141:951–3.

43. Drenou B, Le Tulzo Y, Caulet-Maugendre S, et al. Pheochromocytoma and secondary erythrocytosis: role of tumour erythropoietin secretion. Nouv Rev Fr Hematol 1995;37:197–9.

44. Vik A, Cui G, Isaksen V, Wik T, Hansen JB. Erythropoietin production by a hepatic adenoma in a patient with severe

erythrocytosis. Acta Haematol 2009; 121:52–5.

45. Matsuyama M, Yamazaki O, Horii K, et al. Erythrocytosis caused by an erythropoietin-producing hepatocellular carcinoma. J Surg Oncol 2000;75: 197–202.

46. Trimble M, Caro J, Talalla A, Brain M. Secondary erythrocytosis due to a cerebellar hemangioblastoma: demonstration of erythropoietin mRNA in the tumor. Blood 1991;78:599–601.

47. Bruneval P, Sassy C, Mayeux P, et al. Erythropoietin synthesis by tumor cells in a case of meningioma associated with erythrocytosis. Blood 1993;81:1593–7.

48. Thiele J. Is it justified to perform a bone marrow biopsy examination in sustained erythrocytosis? Cur Hematol Malig Rep 2006;1:87–92.

49. Thiele J, Kvasnicka HM, Diehl V. Bone marrow features of diagnostic impact in erythrocytosis. Ann Hematol 2005;84:362–7.

50. Tutaeva V, Misurin AV, Michiels JJ, et al. Application of PRV-1 mRNA expression level and JAK2-V617F mutation for the differentiating between polycythemia vera and secondary erythrocytosis and assessment of treatment by interferon or hydroxyurea. Hematol 2007;12:473–9.

51. Vannucchi AM, Guglielmelli P, Ayalew Tefferi A. Advances in understanding and management of myeloproliferative neoplasms. CA Cancer J Clin 2009; 59:171–91.

52. Campbell P, Scott LM, Buck G. Definition of subtypes of essential thrombocythaemia and relation to polycythaemia vera based on JAK2-V617F mutation status: a prospective study. Lancet 2005;366:1945–53.

53. Kvasnicka HM, Thiele J. Classification of Ph-negative chronic myeloproliferative disorders: morphology as the yardstick of classification. Pathobiology 2007;74: 63–71.

54. Gianelli U, Iurlo A, Vener C, et al. Early prepolycythemic phase of PV. The significance of bone marrow biopsy and JAK2-V617F Mutation in the differential diagnosis between the 'early' prepolycythemic phase of polycythemia vera and essential thrombocythemia. Am J Clin Pathol 2008;130:336–42.

55. Kvasnicka HM, Thiele J. Prodromal myeloproliferative neoplasms: The 2008 WHO classification. Am J Hematol 2010; 85:62–9.

56. Barosi G, Mesa RA, Thiele J, et al. Proposed criteria for the diagnosis of post-polycythemia vera and post-essential thrombocythemia myelofibrosis: a consensus statement from the International Working Group for Myelofibrosis Research and Treatment. Leukemia 2008;22:437–8.

57. Thiele J, Kvasnicka HM, Facchetti F, et al. European consensus on grading bone marrow fibrosis and assessment of cellularity. Haematologica 2005;90: 1128–32.

58. Manoharan A, Horsley R, Pitney WR. The reticulin content of bone marrow in acute leukaemia in adults. Br J Haematol 1979; 43:185–90.

59. Kralovics R. Genetic complexity of myeloproliferative neoplasms. Leukemia 2008;22:1841–8.

60. Andrieux J, Demory JL, Caulier MT, et al. Karyotypic abnormalities in myelofibrosis following polycythemia vera. Cancer Genet Cytogenet 2003; 140:118–23.

61. Andrieux JL, Demory JL. Karyotype and molecular cytogenetic studies in polycythemia vera. Curr Hematol Rep 2005;4:224–9.

62. Tefferi A, Skoda R, Vardiman JW. Myeloproliferative neoplasms: contemporary diagnosis using histology and genetics. Nat Rev Clin Oncol 2009; 6:627–37.

63. Theocharides A, Boissinot M, Girodon F, et al. Leukemic blasts in transformed JAK2-V617F-positive myeloproliferative disorders are frequently negative for the JAK2-V617F mutation. Blood 2007;1(110): 375–9.

64. Naresh KN, Lampert IA. CD117 Expression as an aid to identify immature myeloid cells and foci of ALIP in bone marrow trephines. Am J Hematol 2006; 81:79.

65. Scott LM, Tong W, Levine RL, et al. JAK2 exon 12 mutations in polycythemia vera and idiopathic erythrocytosis. N Engl J Med 2007;356(5)459–69.

66. Pardanani A, Lasho TL, Finke C, et al. Prevalence and clinicopathological correlates of JAK2 exon 12 mutations in JAK2V617F-negative polycythemia vera. Leukemia 2007;21:1960–3.

67. Rumi E. Familial chronic myeloproliferative disorders: the state of the art. Hematol Oncol 2008;26:131–8.

68. Skoda R. The genetic basis of myeloproliferative disorders. Hematology Am Soc Hematol Educ Program 2007: 1–10.

69. Percy MJ, Scott LM, Erber WN, et al. The frequency of JAK2 exon 12 mutations in idiopathic erythrocytosis patients with low serum erythropoietin levels. Haematologica 2007;92:1607–14.

70. McMullin MF. Idiopathic erythrocytosis: a disappearing entity. Hematology Am Soc Hematol Educ Program 2009:629–35.

CHAPTER 23

Essential thrombocythemia and primary myelofibrosis

HM Kvasnicka

Chapter contents

Introduction

Among the classical Philadelphia-chromosome-negative myeloproliferative neoplasms (MPN), essential thrombocythemia (ET) and primary myelofibrosis (PMF) represent two subtypes with considerable overlap in clinical and hematological presentation in particular at early stages of disease.[1] Differentiation between those two MPN subtypes is of clinical relevance, since PMF is characterized by a considerably higher risk of progression and leukemic transformation. In contrast, ET generally represents a stable disease with only minimal risk of myelofibrotic progression.[2] There is also a significant difference in long-term survival between both groups. The 15-year age-adjusted relative survival rate for ET is nearly 84%. In contrast, PMF is characterized by a significant loss in life expectancy. Even when diagnosed in very early stages of disease, PMF patients have a 15-year survival of only 55–67%.[2] Although the discovery of the JAK2^{V617F} mutation (see Chapter 21) led to important progress in the understanding of the molecular pathogenesis of ET and PMF,[3] the finding of this mutation in several MPN subtypes and the absence of the JAK2^{V617F} allele in many MPN patients preclude the use of JAK2^{V617F} testing alone to establish a diagnosis of ET or PMF. This is reflected in the revised WHO diagnostic criteria for ET and PMF (Box 23.1), which include mutation screening in the diagnostic work-up, but explicitly require a bone marrow (BM) morphological examination for making the diagnosis of both ET and PMF. Although a significantly lower JAK2^{V617F} allele burden has been found in ET when compared to early stages of PMF,[4] such variability in the allele burden does

not represent a sufficient criterion for distinguishing among different clinical entities. Furthermore, JAK2^{V617F}-negative cases reveal a similar clinical profile and outcome[5] and increase in JAK2^{V617F} allele frequencies is not linked to myelofibrotic transformation or progression to acute myeloid leukemia (AML).[6]

ET and PMF usually affect the elderly population, but they can occasionally be found in children, and in this instance, they raise age-related diagnostic and management issues.[7] Familial clustering of ET and also PMF is known, and this observation led to a suggestion of predisposition alleles even before the discovery of the JAK2^{V617F} mutation.[8] Relatives of patients with ET have a more than sevenfold increase in the relative risk of developing a similar MPN.[9] However, the coexistence of different clinical entities and of JAK2^{V617F}-positive and JAK2^{V617F}-negative diseases in the same family is noteworthy.[8,10]

When addressing the current WHO criteria (Box 23.1) for diagnosing the different MPN entities,[11,12] it is essential to emphasize that these guidelines do not claim that a single histological parameter defines a subgroup, but that the different subtypes of MPN are characterized by specific morphological BM patterns.[13] These patterns are composed of distinctive features and should always be reviewed in close relation to clinical, hematological and molecular-genetic findings to achieve a consensus-based working diagnosis.[1,3,14,15] In contrast to the determination of age-dependent cellularity and to the semiquantitative grading of myelofibrosis,[16,17] characterization of megakaryopoiesis may cause significant difficulties concerning definition and easy recognition of disease-related patterns among different observers.[18] Assessment of megakaryocytic histotopography, i.e.

Box 23.1 WHO criteria for the diagnosis of essential thrombocythemia (ET) and primary myelofibrosis (PMF)

Essential thrombocythemia (ET)

1. Sustained platelet count $\geq 450 \times 10^9/l$.
2. Bone marrow biopsy showing megakaryocyte proliferation with increased numbers of enlarged, mature megakaryocytes. No significant granulocyte or erythroid proliferation.
3. Not meeting WHO criteria for PV, PMF, BCR-ABL1-positive CML, or MDS or other MPN.
4. Demonstration of $JAK2^{V617F}$ or other clonal marker, or no evidence for reactive thrombocytosis.[a]

Diagnosis requires meeting all four criteria

Primary myelofibrosis (PMF)

Major criteria

1. Presence of megakaryocyte proliferation and atypia, usually accompanied by either reticulin and/or collagen fibrosis, or, in the absence of significant reticulin fibrosis, the megakaryocyte changes must be accompanied by an increased bone marrow cellularity characterized by granulocytic proliferation and often decreased erythropoiesis (i.e. prefibrotic/early phase disease).
2. Not meeting WHO criteria for PV, ET, BCR-ABL1-positive CML, MDS, or other MPN.
3. Demonstration of $JAK2^{V617F}$ or other clonal marker (e.g. MPLW515L/K), or no evidence for reactive bone marrow fibrosis.[b]

Minor criteria*

1. Leukoerythroblastosis.*
2. Increase in serum lactate dehydrogenase level (LDH).*
3. Anemia.*
4. Splenomegaly.*

Diagnosis requires meeting all three major criteria and two minor criteria*

---

*In prefibrotic/early stages these features are generally only borderline expressed.

[a]Causes of reactive thrombocytosis include iron deficiency, splenectomy, surgery, infection, inflammation, connective tissue disease, metastatic cancer, and lymphoproliferative disorders. The presence of a condition associated with reactive thrombocytosis does not exclude the possibility of ET if the first three criteria are met.

[b]Causes of bone marrow fibrosis include infection, autoimmune disorders or other chronic inflammatory conditions, hairy cell leukemia or other lymphoid neoplasm, metastatic malignancy, or toxic (chronic) myelopathies.

---

their arrangement within the BM space, and detection of certain nuclear abnormalities (besides maturation defects) are the keys to the diagnosis.[19] In contrast to the normal BM, in which megakaryocytes show a central distribution of single isolated cells, the overall increase of megakaryocytes in MPN is often associated with the uneven distribution such as group formation: from small clusters (at least three cells) to extensive groups (more than seven cells).[20] These megakaryocyte clusters may display either a loose (intermingled with other hematopoietic cells) or dense arrangement.[19] An abnormal dislocation of megakaryocytes towards the endosteal (paratrabecular) border is a highly conspicuous finding that is usually not seen in reactive disorders. Other features indicating a neoplastic process are peculiar nuclear aberrations and maturation defects that imply disturbances of the normal development of megakaryopoiesis.[1,21–23] These include:

- an atypical nuclear lobulation (extent and shape of nuclear foldings), i.e. hypolobulation, often described as cloud-like or bulbous (plumb, clumsy) nuclei
- hyperlobulation with marked segmentation mimicking a stag-horn-like formation
- anomalies of the chromatin pattern (mostly hyperchromasia).

Furthermore, maturation defects include a conspicuous deviation of the nuclear-cytoplasmic ratio or maturation with appearance of bizarre megakaryocytes. It is noteworthy that all these changes may be present in megakaryocytes of different sizes and ploidy status. Finally, so-called naked

(denuded, bare) nuclei with condensed chromatin pattern may frequently be found implicating a stimulated thrombocyte shedding and cell turnover.[20]

In other hematopoietic lineages, an increase and left-shifting of neutrophil granulopoiesis or erythropoiesis may be a prominent feature or a reduction in the amount of nucleated red cell precursors may be found, depending on disease entity and phase.[24]

Essential thrombocythemia (ET)

Essential thrombocythemia (ET) is a MPN that involves primarily the megakaryocytic lineage. It is characterized by sustained thrombocytosis $>450 \times 10^9/l$ in the peripheral blood (PB), increased numbers of large, mature megakaryocytes in the BM, and clinically by episodes of thrombosis and/or hemorrhage. Because there is no known genetic or biological marker specific for ET, other causes for thrombocytosis such as other MPN, inflammatory and infectious disorders, hemorrhage and other types of hematopoietic and non-hematopoietic neoplasms must be excluded.[12] The presence of the BCR-ABL1 fusion gene excludes the diagnosis of ET (Box 23.1). The reported annual incidence of ET ranges from 0.59 to 2.53/100 000 inhabitants and its prevalence is around 30/100 000, which is similar to that of polycythemia vera (PV).[25] The median age at diagnosis is 65–70 years,[26] but ET is occasionally found in children, and it is relatively common in female patients in their third or fourth decade of life.[27,28] In women of childbearing age, ET may be a risk factor for complications during pregnancy.[29] Venous thrombosis in unusual locations is typical in younger patients, and the thrombotic risk increases in patients over 60 years old.[26]

Clinical features

Many patients are asymptomatic when an excess in platelets is discovered by a routine blood count.[26,28,29] Most investigators have argued that the use of a threshold level $600 \times 10^9/l$ platelets compromises the detection of early-phase disease because the adjusted 95th percentile for normal platelet count is below $400 \times 10^9/l$.[30,31] Therefore, the platelet threshold count required for ET diagnosis has been lowered to $450 \times 10^9/l$ (Box 23.1). Initial presentation may include vascular occlusions, hemorrhage or microvascular complications that lead to transient ischemic attacks and digital ischemia with paresthesias.[32,33] Some patients may present with a thrombosis of major arteries and veins such as splenic or hepatic vein thrombosis as in the Budd–Chiari syndrome.[26,34,35] Increase in spleen size at time of diagnosis is seen only in a minority of patients.[2] Generally, there is no anemia, no circulating blasts, and serum levels of lactate dehydrogenase (LDH) are within the normal range.[23,36] In patients with borderline anemia, palpable spleen, slight elevation of LDH serum level or evidence of erythroid and/or granulopoietic precursors in the PB, a differential diagnosis of very early (prefibrotic) stages of PMF should be excluded by careful bone marrow trephine biopsy (BMTB) examination.[1,2,21,23,24,36,37] In contrast to PV cases, the utility of JAK2^{V617F} mutation screening for the diagnosis of ET is limited by suboptimal negative predictive value and lack of diagnostic specificity in the context of MPN.[14] Therefore, a BMTB is mandatory to differentiate ET from other MPN and to help with the differential diagnosis between JAK2^{V617F}-negative ET and reactive thrombocytosis.[1,14,21,24]

In most patients, ET is an indolent disorder characterized by long symptom-free intervals, interrupted by occasional life-threatening thromboembolic or hemorrhagic episodes.[26,28,38] Although after many years a few patients with ET may develop BM fibrosis such progression is very uncommon.[39–41] The exact incidence of myelofibrotic transformation in ET persists to be a controversial issue[42] and the reported results are certainly influenced by the risk status of the patients and the applied diagnostic criteria.[1,21,43,44] Careful morphological examination of BMTB is crucial in the diagnostic workup of post ET myelofibrosis (Post-ET MF), since appearance of BM fibrosis with a grade MF-2 or MF-3 is a prerequisite for the diagnosis (Box 23.2 and Fig. 23.1). Secondly, only cases with predefined and documented ET according to the WHO guidelines fall into this category.[45] Strict adherence to the WHO criteria (Box 23.1) is necessary to prevent diagnostic confusion associated with early PMF accompanied by thrombocytosis.[1,23,36] The frequency of true post-ET myelofibrosis is low; the transformation rate is 2.8% at a median follow-up of 9.1 years (or a 10-year risk of 3.9% and a 15-year risk of 6%).[46] Transformation of ET to acute myeloid leukemia or MDS occurs in fewer than 5% of patients, and in chemotherapy treated patients may be related to previous cytotoxic therapy.[26,28,47–49] The life expectancy in ET is near normal for most patients.[2,50,51]

Molecular data

A JAK2^{V617F} or a functionally similar mutation may be detected in approximately 40–50% of patients (see Chapter 21 for details).[5,52–55] However, these findings are not specific for ET and are also seen in other MPN subtypes. It has to be emphasized that significant differences in the JAK2^{V617F} allele burden were described between ET and early PMF.[4,6,56] As an independent marker this feature validates very nicely corresponding BMTB findings and thus supports the concept of differentiating ET from early PMF.[1,21,23,24,57] A gain-of-function mutation of MPL has been reported in approximately 1–3% of patients with ET.[58,59] None of these mutations are found in cases of reactive thrombocytosis. Although ET is usually characterized by a normal karyotype, an isolated del(5q) has been reported in few cases with ET. However, it is more likely that these cases represent MDS associated with this abnormality.[60,61]

Blood and bone marrow findings

Marked and sustained thrombocytosis is the hallmark of ET. The platelets often display anisocytosis, ranging from tiny forms to atypical large, giant platelets that may reveal bizarre shapes, pseudopods and agranularity. The white blood cell count (WBC) and leukocyte differential are usually normal, although a borderline elevation in the neutrophil lineage may occur.[28,62,63] In ET classified according to the histological guidelines of the WHO classification, neither a relevant increase in cellularity nor a significant left-shifted neutrophil granulopoiesis is observed.[1,3,57] Any case with a mild to moderate granulocytic and erythroid growth pattern (panmyelosis) and an EPO level below the reference range is suspicious for occult (pre-polycythemic) PV mimicking ET.[64,65] Regarding megakaryopoiesis, gross disturbances of the histological topography (significant abnormal localization and/or extensive dense clustering) are not seen (Figs 23.2 and 23.3). Megakaryocytes show a more or less random distribution, with scattered forms or a few loose clusters (Figs 23.4

Semiquantitative grading of bone marrow fibrosis (MF) in myeloproliferative neoplasms (MPN)

MF-0
Scattered linear reticulin with no intersections (cross-overs) corresponding to **normal bone marrow**

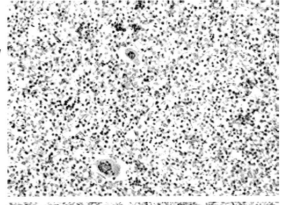

MF-1
Loose network of reticulin with many intersections, especially in perivascular areas

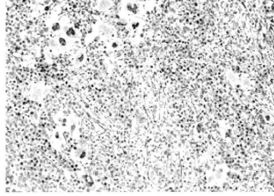

MF-2
Diffuse and dense increase in reticulin with extensive intersections, occasionally with only focal bundles of collagen and/or **focal osteosclerosis**

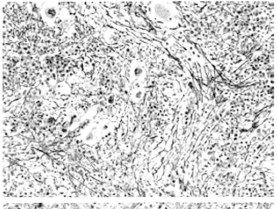

MF-3
Diffuse and dense increase in reticulin with extensive intersections with coarse bundles of collagen, often associated with **significant osteosclerosis**

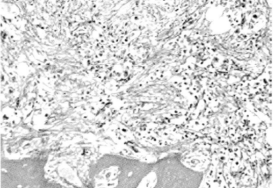

(fibre density should be assessed only in hematopoietic (cellular) areas)

Fig. 23.1 Semiquantitative grading of bone marrow fibrosis (MF) in myeloproliferative neoplasms (MPN).[17]

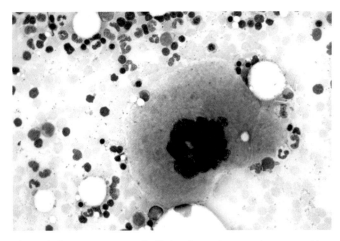

Fig. 23.2 Bone marrow smear in ET showing a giant megakaryocyte with hyperlobulated nucleus. MGG, ×63 objective.

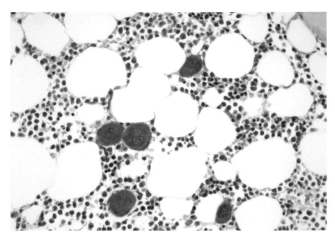

Fig. 23.5 Bone marrow biopsy section in ET showing loose clustering of large megakaryocytes. PAS, ×40 objective.

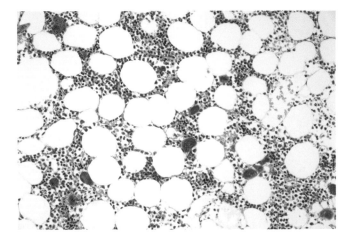

Fig. 23.3 Megakaryocytic proliferation in ET with random distribution within the bone marrow section. PAS, ×20 objective.

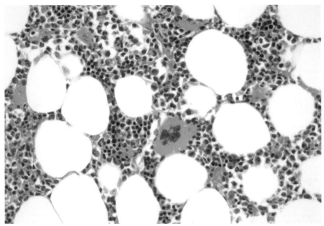

Fig. 23.6 Bone marrow biopsy section in ET showing a large, hyperlobulated (staghorn-like) megakaryocyte. H&E, ×40 objective.

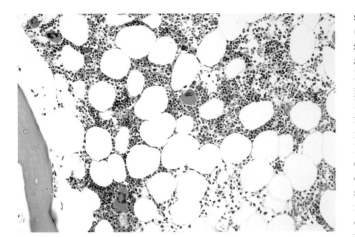

Fig. 23.4 Normocellular bone marrow biopsy section in ET with pronounced megakaryocytic proliferation. H&E, ×20 objective.

and 23.5). A predominance of large to giant mature megakaryocytes with extensively folded (staghorn-like) nuclei[19,20,22,24,66,67] surrounded by a correspondingly mature cytoplasm is found (Fig. 23.6). These features are clearly different from prefibrotic early PMF, where megakaryocytes show an extensive dense clustering and have hypolobulated (cloud-like or bulbous) and hyperchromatic nuclei with striking maturation defects (Fig. 23.7) leading to a marked anomaly of their nuclear-cytoplasmic ratio.[1,19–22,24,36,65,67] Finally, there is no substantial increase in reticulin fibers at presentation and collagen fibrosis is never observed in ET.[44] In a large series of ET patients, minimal to slight reticulin fibrosis was described in only 3% of cases.[19,40,41,68,69] Any marked increase in reticulin fibers is not compatible with ET,[1] in contrast to prefibrotic PMF, which is a differential diagnosis in patients with thrombocytosis.[2,21,22,57] In PMF cases, a relevant increase in age-matched cellularity and a significantly expressed left-shifted neutrophil granulopoiesis is regularly found. At times, the clinical and morphological distinction between ET and early phase PMF with associated thrombocytosis might not be clear cut. As the therapeutic relevance in these early stages is still unclear, a strict adherence to the WHO criteria for making a working diagnosis and close monitoring of the patient to capture any substantial changes that might warrant revision of diagnosis is recommended.[3,11,15]

Finally, when myelodysplastic and myeloproliferative BM features are simultaneously present and more than 15% ring sideroblasts are found in the aspirate, the case should be

Bone marrow morphology in early stage primary myelofibrosis and essential thrombocythemia

PMF (prefibrotic–early stage)
– Dense clustering of medium sized to giant megakaryocytes showing hyperchromatic, bulbous, or irregularly folded nuclei and an aberrant nuclear/cytoplasmic ratio
– Pronounced proliferation of granulopoiesis and reduction of erythroid/cytoplasmic ratio

ET
– Prominent large to giant megakaryocytes with deeply folded nuclei, dispersed or loosely clustered
– No significant increase in granulo- and erythropoiesis

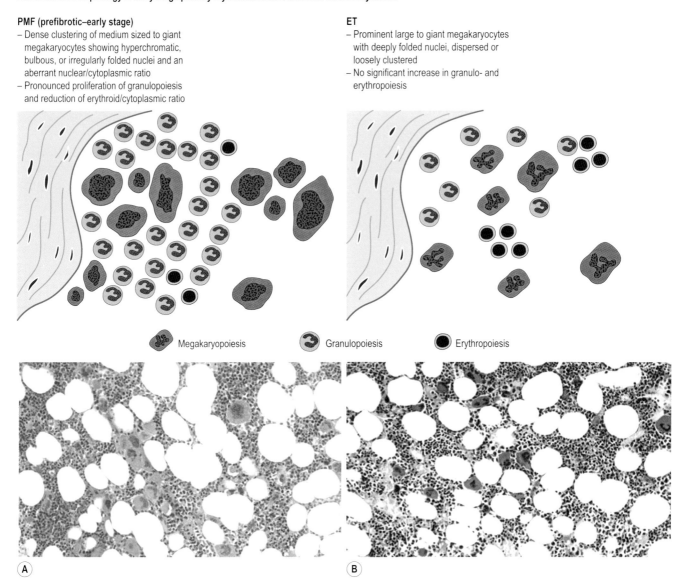

Megakaryopoiesis   Granulopoiesis   Erythropoiesis

(A)   (B)

Fig. 23.7 Bone marrow morphology in early stage primary myelofibrosis and essential thrombocythemia.

defined as refractory anemia with ring sideroblasts (RARS-T), an entity that is included in the MDS/MPN, unclassifiable category (see Chapter 27 for details).[11] It is important to note that the diagnostic criteria for RARS-T include not only the finding of an elevated platelet count in conjunction with anemia and presence of ring sideroblasts in the BM, but also morphologically abnormal megakaryocytes.[15]

Primary myelofibrosis (PMF)

PMF is a chronic hematologic malignancy characterized by a stepwise evolution from an initial prefibrotic phase revealing a hypercellular BM with absent or minimal reticulin fibrosis to an overt fibrotic phase with marked reticulin or collagen fibrosis that is often accompanied by osteosclerosis.[3,15,70,71] One of the hallmarks of PMF in the BM is a proliferation of predominantly megakaryocytes and

granulocytes[1,20,21,24,36] that in fully developed fibrotic disease stages is associated with hepatosplenomegaly, leukoerythroblastosis in the PB, cytopenias, teardrop-shaped red cells, extramedullary hematopoiesis, increased BM microvessel density[71–73] and constitutive mobilization of CD34+ hematopoietic progenitors and stem cells as well as endothelial progenitor cells into the peripheral blood.[74–76] However, endothelial progenitor cell mobilization predominates during the early phase of PMF, while hematopoietic stem and progenitor cell mobilization characteristically occurs in more clinically advanced phases of the disease.[74] This dysregulation of stem cell trafficking most likely leads to the seeding of extramedullary sites with primitive hematopoietic and endothelial cells, resulting in extramedullary hematopoiesis in the spleen, liver and in a variety of other organs. It has been documented that several proteolytic pathways play an important role in cytokine-mediated stem cell mobilization.[77] The interaction between stroma cells, endothelial cells and osteoblast-derived stroma cell derived factor-1 (SDF-1) and the CXC chemokine receptor-4 (CXCR-4) expressed by hematopoietic stem and progenitor cells is also believed to determine patterns of stem cell trafficking. Furthermore, proteases, including neutrophil elastase, soluble matrix metalloproteinase-9 (MMP-9) and cell bound MMP-9 have been shown to play a role in the constitutive mobilization of CD34[+] cells.[77]

In the overt stages, which were formerly termed agnogeneic myeloid metaplasia (AMM) or myelofibrosis with myeloid metaplasia (MMM),[45] profound BM fibrosis is a response to the clonal proliferation of hematopoietic stem cells.[78] Collagen type 3, also known as reticulin, and collagen type 1 are the predominant extracellular components of BM fibrosis in PMF.[79,80] These matrix components are produced by BM fibroblasts that do not belong to the malignant clone. This deposition of collagen is a result of the release of fibrogenic cytokines by abnormal megakaryocytes and monocytes derived from the malignant stem cell population.[73] However, BM fibrosis is not unique to PMF and may develop in the course of many other disorders.[79]

Prefibrotic, early stages of PMF presenting with only borderline or minimal clinical features indicating myelofibrosis with myeloid metaplasia have been more and more acknowledged.[1,3,20,21] The striking variability in the hematological findings of patients with PMF at the time of the first presentation is paralleled by corresponding BM features that may initially present only a hypercellular hematopoiesis without or with only slight increase of reticulin fibres.[1,21,24,36,39] Considering the dynamics of the disease process in PMF, the former gold standard for the diagnosis of AMM/MMM[72] should be avoided, because these criteria included only the advanced or overt stages of a wide spectrum of clinical and morphological disease manifestations. Therefore, overt myelofibrosis is not a necessary diagnostic feature of PMF, as outlined in Box 23.1. Furthermore, terminal stages of PV and ET presenting with findings of myeloid metaplasia[45,81] should not be included in this MPN category.[20,21,24,71]

The reported annual incidence of PMF is significantly biased by the change in diagnostic criteria.[82] When the manifest fibrotic stage is considered, the frequency is estimated at 0.5–1.5 per 100 000 individuals per year.[83,84] Disease onset is most common in the sixth to seventh decade of life,[71,73] but rarely even children may be affected.[85]

Clinical features

In the initial prefibrotic phase of PMF, the only relevant hematological finding may be sustained thrombocytosis mimicking ET and a borderline anemia and/or splenomegaly.[1,36,86] Depending on the grade of BM fibrosis, hepatosplenomegaly of varying degree is detected in many patients.[71,73,87] In the overt stages of the disease, extramedullary hematopoiesis in the spleen is a common finding, while liver, lymph nodes and other organs or soft tissue are other possible sites of involvement.[71] Early stages of PMF with only mild increase in reticulin (fibrosis grades MF-0 or MF-1; see Fig. 23.1) may not be recognized by clinical features alone. Many of these patients are asymptomatic at the time of diagnosis and only fortuitously discovered by the detection

of marginal splenomegaly during a routine physical examination and/or the presence of borderline anemia, leukocytosis and/or thrombocytosis in routine blood counts.[36] Only a minority of these cases are discovered due to unexplained leukoerythroblastosis or a significantly increased LDH serum level.[3,87]

Although younger patients may experience longer survival,[50,85] patients with symptomatic forms of PMF have a median survival of less than 5 years,[87,88] while appropriately treated ET is associated with nearly normal life expectancy. However, the overall prognosis significantly depends on the stage of PMF at diagnosis.[2,89] Adverse prognostic factors generally include higher age (>65 years), anemia (Hb <10 g/dl), WBC $>25 \times 10^9$/l, presence of circulating blast cells, thrombocytopenia (platelet count $<100 \times 10^9$/l), and an abnormal karyotype.[2,50,85,88,90,91] Major causes of death are related to the sequelae of portal hypertension or hepatic-splenoportal thrombosis, thromboses in various anatomic sites, heart failure due to splenic pooling, infections, pulmonary hypertension, bleeding caused by thrombocytopenia or hemostatic defects.[71–73] Terminal leukemic transformation is seen in about 5–30% of PMF patients as part of the natural history of this disease.[87,92]

Molecular data

Almost 50% of patients with PMF reveal a clonal hematopoiesis but lack JAK2[55] or MPL mutations (see Chapter 21 for details).[58,59] These patients, however, have a similar clinical history and prognosis to JAK2[V617F]-positive patients.[5] Thus, the presence of the mutations confirms the clonality of the proliferation, but it does not distinguish PMF from other MPN subtypes, in particular ET or PV.[3] A remarkable finding is that progression of prodromal PMF is not triggered by the JAK2[V617F] mutation status,[6] but by a number of relevant target genes that are involved in matrix modeling and regulation of fibrillogenesis.[93] Comparative genomic hybridization studies have shown that gains of cytogenetic material occur in more than 50% of patients with PMF and most commonly involve gains of 9p, 2q, 3p, chromosome 4, 12q and 13q.[94] Furthermore, an unbalanced translocation between chromosomes 1 and 6 with specific breakpoints t(1;6)(q21-23;p21.3) is strongly suggestive but not diagnostic of PMF.[95] Deletions affecting the long arms of chromosomes 7 and 5 have been reported as well, but may be associated with prior cytotoxic therapy used to control the myeloproliferation.[96]

Blood and bone marrow findings

It has been estimated that 30–40% of patients present with a prefibrotic or early fibrotic stage of PMF.[36,39,57,69] Clinical data in these prodromal stages of PMF are usually characterized by only minimal abnormalities such as borderline to slight anemia, minimal splenomegaly, a very low or missing peripheral blast count but often a pronounced thrombocytosis.[1,21,23] In the prodromal stages of PMF, the BMTB shows a marked hypercellularity with prominent granulocytic and megakaryocytic myeloproliferation (Figs 23.8, 23.9 and 23.10) and a concomitant reduction and/or maturation arrest of the nucleated erythroid precursors.[1,20,21,86] Reticulin fibrosis is minimal (Fig. 23.11) or even absent at this stage (corresponding to fibrosis grades MF-0 and MF-1; Box 23.2).

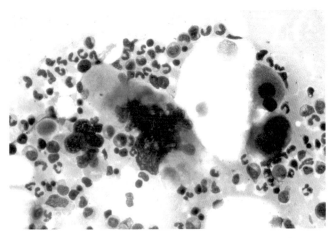

Fig. 23.8 Bone marrow smear in prefibrotic/early PMF with atypical clustering of medium sized to large megakaryocytes with abnormal bulbous and hyperchromatic nuclei. MGG, ×63 objective.

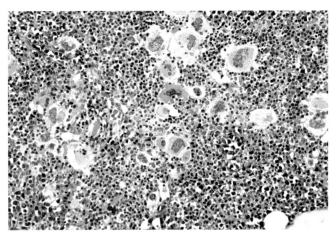

Fig. 23.10 Hypercellular bone marrow biopsy section in prefibrotic/early PMF with atypical dense clustering of abnormal megakaryocytes and granulocytic proliferation. Chloracetate esterase, ×20 objective.

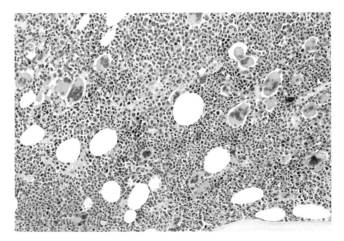

Fig. 23.9 Trephine biopsy section in prefibrotic/early PMF showing a clearly hypercellular bone marrow with pronounced megakaryocytic and granulocytic proliferation. H&E, ×20 objective.

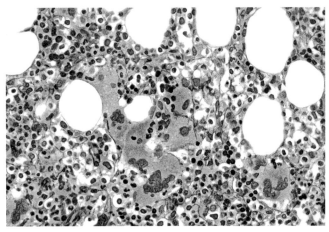

Fig. 23.11 Bone marrow biopsy section in prefibrotic/early PMF without increase in reticulin (fibrosis grade MF0). Gomori, ×40 objective.

If present, fibrosis is usually seen focally and tends to be concentrated around vessels.[17] There may be a mild left shift in granulopoiesis (see Fig. 23.10), with predominance of metamyelocytes, bands and segmented forms. Percentages of myeloblasts in BM aspirates are not increased and conspicuous clusters of blasts or CD34[+] progenitors are not observed.[1,36,86] Abnormal megakaryopoiesis is most conspicuous, and thus the histotopography and morphology of megakaryocytes is the key to the recognition of the prefibrotic stage of PMF.[1] Characteristically, an extensive clustering of megakaryocytes with loose to dense groupings with abnormal localization towards the endosteal borders is seen (Figs 23.12 and 23.13), but there are also striking abnormalities in megakaryocyte morphology and maturation.[1,19,21,24,36,86] Significant anomalies of megakaryocytes include a high degree of cellular pleomorphism with variations in size that range from small to giant forms. Abnormal nuclear folding and an aberration of the nuclear cytoplasmic ratio created by large, bulbous and hyperchromatic cloud-like nuclei are common. Apart from the disorganized nuclear lobulation of megakaryocytes, many so-called naked (bare) megakaryocytic nuclei are observed.[19,21,24,69,86] Increased

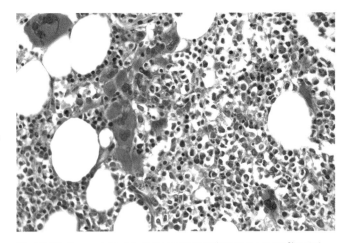

Fig. 23.12 Dense clustering of abnormal megakaryocytes in prefibrotic/early PMF. PAS, ×20 objective.

vascular proliferation is usual in the BM[97] and lymphoid nodules are found in about 20–30% of cases.[22,36]

Overall, the megakaryocytes in PMF are characterized by a higher degree of cytological atypia (megakaryocytic dysplasia) than any other subtype of MPN, in particular ET[1,19,21,24,66,67]

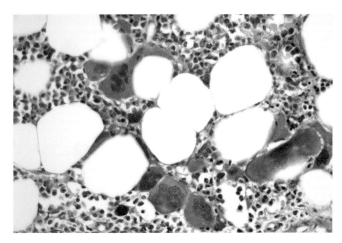

Fig. 23.13 Anomalies of megakaryocytes in prefibrotic/early PMF with variations in size, abnormal nuclear foldings with bulbous and hyperchromatic cloud-like shaped nuclei, and dense grouping. PAS, ×40 objective.

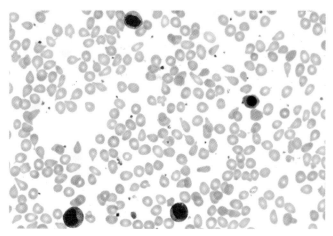

Fig. 23.14 Peripheral blood in advanced PMF showing marked teardrop poikilocytosis (dacrocytes) and nucleated erytrhoid precursor. MGG, ×63 objective.

Thus, megakaryocytic dysplasia is one of the most important features discriminating prefibrotic/early stage PMF from ET (Fig. 23.7). Careful morphological BMTB examination is crucial in distinguishing PMF cases with accompanying thrombocytosis from ET, because early stages of myelofibrosis with only borderline to mild increase in reticulin may not be recognized by clinical features alone.[2,3,14,21,22,24] The significant difference between these two MPN subtypes with regard to both survival and rate of myelofibrotic transformation has to be kept in mind.[2,21] An accurate distinction between both subtypes is not a matter of semantics, but ultimately does exert an influence on therapeutic strategies and, most importantly, is predictive of possible complications and outcome. The majority of patients with prefibrotic/early stages of PMF eventually transform into overt fibrotic/sclerotic myelofibrosis associated with extramedullary hematopoiesis.[36,39,41,69,98] It has been estimated that PMF patients have a more than 65% probability of progression to a full-blown myelofibrosis with a median time of 4.2 years.[2,44] However, usually this change in BM morphology is significantly preceding the clinical progression towards signs of myeloid metaplasia.[1]

The classical picture of advanced PMF includes a leukoerythroblastic PB smear with teardrop poikilocytosis (Fig. 23.14), splenomegaly and anemia of varying degree, associated with a marked reticulin and/or collagen BM fibrosis (fibrosis grades MF-2 and MF-3; see Fig. 23.1).[73,87] Progressive accumulation of fibrous tissue generally parallels disease progression; however, a striking variability in the hematological findings may be observed at the time of presentation.[21,87] Besides the significant amount of reticulin deposition and the appearance of coarse bundles of collagen fibers in the BM, additional features indicating an advanced to terminal PMF stage include plaque to bud-like osteosclerosis (endophytic bone formation) that is often associated with patchy hematopoiesis replaced by adipose tissue (Figs 23.15 and 23.16), i.e. progressive hypoplasia.[36,69] Foci of immature cells may be more prominent, although myeloblasts account for fewer than 10% of the BM cells.[36] As in prodromal stages, atypical megakaryopoiesis remains the most prominent feature, including the presence of large clusters or sheets of

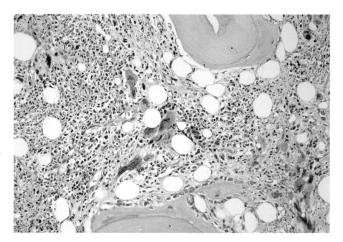

Fig. 23.15 Bone marrow biopsy section in advanced PMF with streaming of grossly atypical megakaryocytes and new bone formation. H&E, ×20 objective.

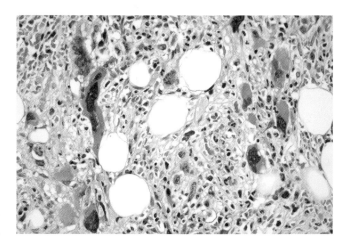

Fig. 23.16 Atypical megakaryocytes in advanced PMF with aberration of the nuclear cytoplasmic ration and hyperchromatic, dysplastic nuclei. H&E, ×40 objective.

megakaryocytes and numerous naked nuclei (Fig. 23.16). Dilated BM sinuses[97,99] with intraluminal hematopoiesis (Fig. 23.17), especially megakaryocytes, are prominent in most cases.[36,39] Rarely the BM is almost devoid of hematopoietic cells, showing mainly dense reticulin or collagen fibrosis with small islands of hematopoietic precursors situated mostly within the vascular sinuses.[36] In osteosclerotic

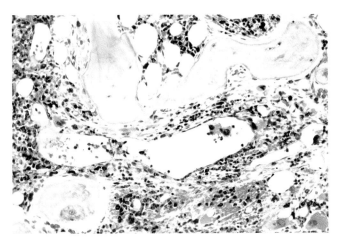

Fig. 23.17 Trephine biopsy section in advanced PMF showing dilated sinus with intrasinusoidal hematopoietic cells, in particular megakaryocytes. CAS, ×20 objective.

terminal phase of PMF, the marrow space is progressively replaced by broad, irregular trabeculae and appositional bud-like endophytic new bone formation.[69]

Increase in blood and/or BM blasts (<20%) as well as increased numbers of CD34+ cells with cluster formation and/or an abnormal endosteal location in the BM[36,100] indicate an accelerated phase of the disease, whereas 20% or more blasts in PB or BM are considered as blastic transformation, i.e. acute leukemia.

PMF usually displays an insidious onset and stepwise progression, which comprises the full spectrum of prodromal and terminal stages, the latter terminating in BM insufficiency, myelodysplastic changes and blast crisis (Fig. 23.18). Early stages may pose a diagnostic problem, because the classical clinical criteria for diagnosis may not be present at onset of the disease. Early PMF may be only recognized by careful BMTB examination in combination with clinical, hematological and molecular findings.[1] Therefore, demonstration of reticulin fibrosis, although characteristic, is not a required criterion for diagnosis of PMF. Instead, the cardinal and ultimately required features of PMF include an increase in megakaryocyte growth associated with conspicuous morphological abnormalities as well as granulocyte proliferation.[36] The speed of disease progression in the individual patient is unpredictable and development of myelofibrosis cannot be significantly influenced by treatment modalities with the exception of allogeneic stem cell transplantation.[37]

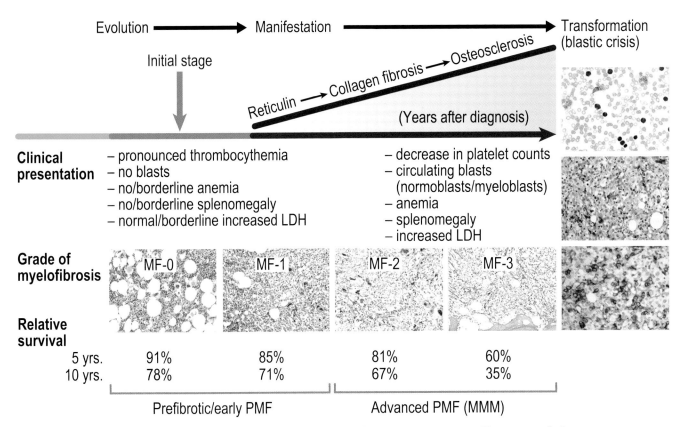

Fig. 23.18 Dynamics of the disease process in PMF with corresponding changes of the clinical presentation and bone marrow findings.

References

1. Kvasnicka HM, Thiele J. Prodromal myeloproliferative neoplasms: The 2008 WHO classification. Am J Hematol 2010 Jan;85(1):62–9.

2. Kvasnicka HM, Thiele J. The impact of clinicopathological studies on staging and survival in essential thrombocythemia, chronic idiopathic myelofibrosis, and polycythemia rubra vera. Semin Thromb Hemost 2006; 32:362–71.

3. Tefferi A, Thiele J, Orazi A, et al. Proposals and rationale for revision of the World Health Organization diagnostic criteria for polycythemia vera, essential thrombocythemia, and primary myelofibrosis: recommendations from an ad hoc international expert panel. Blood 2007;110:1092–7.

4. Malysz J, Crisan D. Correlation of JAK2 V617F mutant allele quantitation with clinical presentation and type of chronic myeloproliferative neoplasm. Ann Clin Lab Sci 2009;39:345–50.

5. Vannucchi AM, Guglielmelli P, Tefferi A. Advances in understanding and management of myeloproliferative neoplasms. CA Cancer J Clin 2009;59: 171–91.

6. Hussein K, Bock O, Theophile K, et al. JAK2(V617F) allele burden discriminates essential thrombocythemia from a subset of prefibrotic-stage primary myelofibrosis. Exp Hematol 2009; 37:1186–93.

7. Teofili L, Giona F, Martini M, et al. The revised WHO diagnostic criteria for Ph-negative myeloproliferative diseases are not appropriate for the diagnostic screening of childhood polycythemia vera and essential thrombocythemia. Blood 2007;110:3384–6.

8. Rumi E, Passamonti F, Della Porta MG, et al. Familial chronic myeloproliferative disorders: clinical phenotype and evidence of disease anticipation. J Clin Oncol 2007;25:5630–5.

9. Landgren O, Goldin LR, Kristinsson SY, et al. Increased risks of polycythemia vera, essential thrombocythemia, and myelofibrosis among 24,577 first-degree relatives of 11,039 patients with myeloproliferative neoplasms in Sweden. Blood 2008;112:2199–204.

10. Bellanne-Chantelot C, Chaumarel I, Labopin M, et al. Genetic and clinical implications of the Val617Phe JAK2 mutation in 72 families with myeloproliferative disorders. Blood 2006;108:346–52.

11. Vardiman JW, Thiele J, Arber DA, et al. The 2008 revision of the WHO classification of myeloid neoplasms and acute leukemia: rationale and important changes. Blood 2009;114:937–51.

12. Swerdlow SH, Campo E, Harris NL, et al. WHO Classification of Tumours of Haematopoietic and Lymphoid Tissues. 4th ed. Lyon: IARC Press; 2008.

13. Thiele J, Kvasnicka HM. A critical reappraisal of the WHO classification of the chronic myeloproliferative disorders. Leuk Lymphoma 2006;47:381–96.

14. Tefferi A, Vardiman JW. Classification and diagnosis of myeloproliferative neoplasms: the 2008 World Health Organization criteria and point-of-care diagnostic algorithms. Leukemia 2008;22:14–22.

15. Tefferi A, Thiele J, Vardiman JW. The 2008 World Health Organization classification system for myeloproliferative neoplasms: order out of chaos. Cancer 2009;115: 3842–7.

16. Vener C, Fracchiolla NS, Gianelli U, et al. Prognostic implications of the European consensus for grading of bone marrow fibrosis in chronic idiopathic myelofibrosis. Blood 2008;111: 1862–5.

17. Thiele J, Kvasnicka HM, Facchetti F, et al. European consensus on grading bone marrow fibrosis and assessment of cellularity. Haematologica 2005;90: 1128–32.

18. Wilkins BS, Erber WN, Bareford D, et al. Bone marrow pathology in essential thrombocythemia: interobserver reliability and utility for identifying disease subtypes. Blood 2008;111: 60–70.

19. Thiele J, Kvasnicka HM, Diehl V. Standardization of bone marrow features – does it work in hematopathology for histological discrimination of different disease patterns? Histol Histopathol 2005;20:633–44.

20. Thiele J, Kvasnicka HM, Orazi A. Bone marrow histopathology in myeloproliferative disorders – current diagnostic approach. Semin Hematol 2005;42:184–95.

21. Kvasnicka HM, Thiele J. Classification of Ph-negative chronic myeloproliferative disorders – morphology as the yardstick of classification. Pathobiology 2007; 74:63–71.

22. Thiele J, Kvasnicka HM. Diagnostic differentiation of essential thrombocythaemia from thrombocythaemias associated with chronic idiopathic myelofibrosis by discriminate analysis of bone marrow features – a clinicopathological study on 272 patients. Histol Histopathol 2003;18:93–102.

23. Thiele J, Kvasnicka HM. Clinicopathological criteria for differential diagnosis of thrombocythemias in various myeloproliferative disorders. Semin Thromb Hemost 2006;32: 219–30.

24. Thiele J, Kvasnicka HM, Vardiman J. Bone marrow histopathology in the diagnosis of chronic myeloproliferative disorders: a forgotten pearl. Best Pract Res Clin Haematol 2006;19: 413–37.

25. Johansson P. Epidemiology of the myeloproliferative disorders polycythemia vera and essential thrombocythemia. Semin Thromb Hemost 2006;32:171–3.

26. Fabris F, Randi ML. Essential thrombocythemia: past and present. Intern Emerg Med 2009.

27. Randi ML, Putti MC, Scapin M, et al. Pediatric patients with essential thrombocythemia are mostly polyclonal and V617FJAK2 negative. Blood 2006; 108:3600–2.

28. Finazzi G, Harrison C. Essential thrombocythemia. Semin Hematol 2005;42:230–8.

29. Tefferi A, Passamonti F. Essential thrombocythemia and pregnancy: observations from recent studies and management recommendations. Am J Hematol 2009;84:629–30.

30. Lengfelder E, Hochhaus A, Kronawitter U, et al. Should a platelet limit of 600 × 10(9)/l be used as a diagnostic criterion in essential thrombocythaemia? An analysis of the natural course including early stages. Br J Haematol 1998;100: 15–23.

31. Sacchi S, Vinci G, Gugliotta L, et al. Diagnosis of essential thrombocythemia at platelet counts between 400 and 600×10(9)/L. Gruppo Italiano Malattie Mieloproliferative Croniche(GIMMC). Haematologica 2000;85:492–5.

32. Besses C, Cervantes F, Pereira A, et al. Major vascular complications in essential thrombocythemia: a study of the predictive factors in a series of 148 patients. Leukemia 1999;13: 150–4.

33. Regev A, Stark P, Blickstein D, et al. Thrombotic complications in essential thrombocythemia with relatively low platelet counts. Am J Hematol 1997; 56:168–72.

34. Allegra A, Alonci A, Penna G, et al. JAK2 V617F-positive latent essential thrombocythemia and splanchnic vein thrombosis: the role of bone marrow biopsy for the diagnosis of myeloproliferative disease. Acta Haematol 2009;121:218–20.

35. Kiladjian JJ, Cervantes F, Leebeek FW, et al. The impact of JAK2 and MPL mutations on diagnosis and prognosis of splanchnic vein thrombosis: a report on 241 cases. Blood 2008;111:4922–9.

36. Thiele J, Kvasnicka HM. Hematopathologic findings in chronic idiopathic myelofibrosis. Semin Oncol 2005;32:380–94.

37. Thiele J, Kvasnicka HM. Grade of bone marrow fibrosis is associated with relevant hematological findings – a clinicopathological study on 865 patients with chronic idiopathic myelofibrosis. Ann Hematol 2006; 85:226–32.

38. Murphy S, Peterson P, Iland H, et al. Experience of the Polycythemia Vera Study Group with essential thrombocythemia: a final report on diagnostic criteria, survival, and leukemic transition by treatment. Semin Hematol 1997;34:29–39.

39. Buhr T, Busche G, Choritz H, et al. Evolution of myelofibrosis in chronic idiopathic myelofibrosis as evidenced in sequential bone marrow biopsy specimens. Am J Clin Pathol 2003; 119:152–8.

40. Thiele J, Kvasnicka HM, Schmitt-Graeff A, et al. Follow-up examinations including sequential bone marrow biopsies in essential thrombocythemia (ET): a retrospective clinicopathological study of 120 patients. Am J Hematol 2002;70:283–91.

41. Kreft A, Buche G, Ghalibafian M, et al. The incidence of myelofibrosis in essential thrombocythaemia, polycythaemia vera and chronic idiopathic myelofibrosis: a retrospective evaluation of sequential bone marrow biopsies. Acta Haematol 2005;113: 137–43.

42. Campbell PJ, Bareford D, Erber WN, et al. Reticulin accumulation in essential thrombocythemia: prognostic significance and relationship to therapy. J Clin Oncol 2009;27:2991–9.

43. Cervantes F, Alvarez-Larran A, Talarn C, et al. Myelofibrosis with myeloid metaplasia following essential thrombocythaemia: actuarial probability, presenting characteristics and evolution in a series of 195 patients. Br J Haematol 2002;118:786–90.

44. Thiele J, Kvasnicka HM, Vardiman JW, et al. Bone marrow fibrosis and diagnosis of essential thrombocythemia. J Clin Oncol 2009;27:e220–221; author reply e222–3.

45. Mesa RA, Verstovsek S, Cervantes F, et al. Primary myelofibrosis (PMF), post polycythemia vera myelofibrosis (post-PV MF), post essential thrombocythemia myelofibrosis (post-ET MF), blast phase PMF (PMF-BP): consensus on terminology by the international working group for myelofibrosis research and treatment (IWG-MRT). Leuk Res 2007; 31:737–40.

46. Passamonti F, Rumi E, Arcaini L, et al. Prognostic factors for thrombosis, myelofibrosis, and leukemia in essential thrombocythemia: a study of 605 patients. Haematologica 2008;93: 1645–51.

47. Passamonti F, Rumi E, Arcaini L, et al. Blast phase of essential

thrombocythemia: a single center study. Am J Hematol 2009;84:641–4.

48. Passamonti F, Rumi E, Arcaini L, et al. Leukemic transformation of polycythemia vera: a single center study of 23 patients. Cancer 2005;104:1032–6.

49. Radaelli F, Mazza R, Curioni E, et al. Acute megakaryocytic leukemia in essential thrombocythemia: an unusual evolution? Eur J Haematol 2002;69: 108–11.

50. Cervantes F, Passamonti F, Barosi G. Life expectancy and prognostic factors in the classic BCR/ABL-negative myeloproliferative disorders. Leukemia 2008;22:905–14.

51. Passamonti F, Rumi E, Pungolino E, et al. Life expectancy and prognostic factors for survival in patients with polycythemia vera and essential thrombocythemia. Am J Med 2004;117:755–61.

52. Kralovics R. Genetic complexity of myeloproliferative neoplasms. Leukemia 2008;22:1841–8.

53. Lippert E, Boissinot M, Kralovics R, et al. The JAK2-V617F mutation is frequently present at diagnosis in patients with essential thrombocythemia and polycythemia vera. Blood 2006; 108:1865–7.

54. Kralovics R, Passamonti F, Buser AS, et al. A gain-of-function mutation of JAK2 in myeloproliferative disorders. N Engl J Med 2005;352:1779–90.

55. Baxter EJ, Scott LM, Campbell PJ, et al. Acquired mutation of the tyrosine kinase JAK2 in human myeloproliferative disorders. Lancet 2005;365:1054–61.

56. Larsen TS, Pallisgaard N, Moller MB, et al. The JAK2 V617F allele burden in essential thrombocythemia, polycythemia vera and primary myelofibrosis – impact on disease phenotype. Eur J Haematol 2007;79: 508–15.

57. Thiele J, Kvasnicka HM. Chronic myeloproliferative disorders with thrombocythemia: a comparative study of two classification systems (PVSG, WHO) on 839 patients. Ann Hematol 2003;82:148–52.

58. Pardanani AD, Levine RL, Lasho T, et al. MPL515 mutations in myeloproliferative and other myeloid disorders: a study of 1182 patients. Blood 2006;108:3472–6.

59. Vannucchi AM, Antonioli E, Guglielmelli P, et al. Characteristics and clinical correlates of MPL 515W>L/K mutation in essential thrombocythemia. Blood 2008;112:844–7.

60. Panani AD. Cytogenetic findings in untreated patients with essential thrombocythemia. In Vivo 2006;20: 381–4.

61. Gangat N, Tefferi A, Thanarajasingam G, et al. Cytogenetic abnormalities in essential thrombocythemia: prevalence and prognostic significance. Eur J Haematol 2009;83:17–21.

62. Tefferi A, Murphy S. Current opinion in essential thrombocythemia: pathogenesis, diagnosis, and management. Blood Rev 2001;15:121–31.

63. Gisslinger H. Update on diagnosis and management of essential thrombocythemia. Semin Thromb Hemost 2006;32:430–6.

64. Thiele J, Kvasnicka HM, Diehl V. Initial (latent) polycythemia vera with thrombocytosis mimicking essential thrombocythemia. Acta Haematol 2005;113:213–19.

65. Gianelli U, Iurlo A, Vener C, et al. The significance of bone marrow biopsy and JAK2V617F mutation in the differential diagnosis between the 'early' prepolycythemic phase of polycythemia vera and essential thrombocythemia. Am J Clin Pathol 2008;130:336–42.

66. Gianelli U, Vener C, Raviele PR, et al. Essential thrombocythemia or chronic idiopathic myelofibrosis? A single-center study based on hematopoietic bone marrow histology. Leuk Lymphoma 2006;47:1774–81.

67. Florena AM, Tripodo C, Iannitto E, et al. Value of bone marrow biopsy in the diagnosis of essential thrombocythemia. Haematologica 2004;89:911–19.

68. Buhr T, Georgii A, Choritz H. Myelofibrosis in chronic myeloproliferative disorders. Incidence among subtypes according to the Hannover classification. Pathol Res Pract 1993;189:121–32.

69. Georgii A, Buesche G, Kreft A. The histopathology of chronic myeloproliferative diseases. Baillière's Clin Haematol 1998;11:721–49.

70. Tefferi A, Skoda R, Vardiman JW. Myeloproliferative neoplasms: contemporary diagnosis using histology and genetics. Nat Rev Clin Oncol 2009;6:627–37.

71. Tefferi A. Primary myelofibrosis. Cancer Treat Res 2008;142:29–49.

72. Barosi G. Myelofibrosis with myeloid metaplasia: diagnostic definition and prognostic classification for clinical studies and treatment guidelines. J Clin Oncol 1999;17:2954–70.

73. Barosi G, Hoffman R. Idiopathic myelofibrosis. Semin Hematol 2005; 42:248–58.

74. Massa M, Rosti V, Ramajoli I, et al. Circulating CD34+, CD133+, and vascular endothelial growth factor receptor 2-positive endothelial progenitor cells in myelofibrosis with myeloid metaplasia. J Clin Oncol 2005;23:5688–95.

75. Oppliger Leibundgut E, Horn MP, Brunold C, et al. Hematopoietic and endothelial progenitor cell trafficking in patients with myeloproliferative diseases. Haematologica 2006;91:1465–72.

76. Passamonti F, Rumi E, Pietra D, et al. Relation between JAK2 (V617F) mutation

status, granulocyte activation, and constitutive mobilization of CD34+ cells into peripheral blood in myeloproliferative disorders. Blood 2006;107:3676–82.

77. Xu M, Bruno E, Chao J, et al. Constitutive mobilization of CD34+ cells into the peripheral blood in idiopathic myelofibrosis may be due to the action of a number of proteases. Blood 2005;105:4508–15.

78. Le Bousse-Kerdiles MC, Martyre MC, Samson M. Cellular and molecular mechanisms underlying bone marrow and liver fibrosis: a review. Eur Cytokine Netw 2008;19:69–80.

79. Kuter DJ, Bain B, Mufti G, et al. Bone marrow fibrosis: pathophysiology and clinical significance of increased bone marrow stromal fibres. Br J Haematol 2007;139:351–62.

80. Bock O, Hoftmann J, Theophile K, et al. Bone morphogenetic proteins are overexpressed in the bone marrow of primary myelofibrosis and are apparently induced by fibrogenic cytokines. Am J Pathol 2008;172:951–60.

81. Alvarez-Larran A, Bellosillo B, Martinez-Aviles L, et al. Postpolycythaemic myelofibrosis: frequency and risk factors for this complication in 116 patients. Br J Haematol 2009;146:504–9.

82. Rollison DE, Howlader N, Smith MT, et al. Epidemiology of myelodysplastic syndromes and chronic myeloproliferative disorders in the United States, 2001–2004, using data from the NAACCR and SEER programs. Blood 2008;112:45–52.

83. Mesa RA, Silverstein MN, Jacobsen SJ, et al. Population-based incidence and survival figures in essential thrombocythemia and agnogenic myeloid metaplasia: an Olmsted County study, 1976–1995. Am J Hematol 1999;61:10–15.

84. Johansson P, Kutti J, Andreasson B, et al. Trends in the incidence of chronic Philadelphia chromosome negative (Ph−) myeloproliferative disorders in the city of Goteborg, Sweden, during 1983–99. J Intern Med 2004;256:161–5.

85. Cervantes F, Barosi G, Demory JL, et al. Myelofibrosis with myeloid metaplasia in young individuals: disease characteristics, prognostic factors and identification of risk groups. Br J Haematol 1998;102:684–90.

86. Thiele J, Kvasnicka HM. Prefibrotic chronic idiopathic myelofibrosis – a diagnostic enigma? Acta Haematol 2004;111:155–9.

87. Cervantes F, Barosi G. Myelofibrosis with myeloid metaplasia: diagnosis, prognostic factors, and staging. Semin Oncol 2005;32:395–402.

88. Cervantes F, Dupriez B, Pereira A, et al. New prognostic scoring system for primary myelofibrosis based on a study of the International Working Group for Myelofibrosis Research and Treatment. Blood 2009;113:2895–901.

89. Kvasnicka HM, Thiele J, Werden C, et al. Prognostic factors in idiopathic (primary) osteomyelofibrosis. Cancer 1997;80:708–19.

90. Hussein K, Huang J, Lasho T, et al. Karyotype complements the International Prognostic Scoring System for primary myelofibrosis. Eur J Haematol 2009;82:255–9.

91. Tam CS, Abruzzo LV, Lin KI, et al. The role of cytogenetic abnormalities as a prognostic marker in primary myelofibrosis: applicability at the time of diagnosis and later during disease course. Blood 2009;113:4171–8.

92. Huang J, Li CY, Mesa RA, et al. Risk factors for leukemic transformation in patients with primary myelofibrosis. Cancer 2008;112:2726–32.

93. Bock O, Neuse J, Hussein K, et al. Aberrant collagenase expression in chronic idiopathic myelofibrosis is related to the stage of disease but not to the JAK2 mutation status. Am J Pathol 2006;169:471–81.

94. Al-Assar O, Ul-Hassan A, Brown R, et al. Gains on 9p are common genomic aberrations in idiopathic myelofibrosis: a comparative genomic hybridization study. Br J Haematol 2005;129:66–71.

95. Dingli D, Grand FH, Mahaffey V, et al. Der(6)t(1;6)(q21-23;p21.3): a specific cytogenetic abnormality in myelofibrosis with myeloid metaplasia. Br J Haematol 2005;130:229–32.

96. Hussein K, Van Dyke DL, Tefferi A. Conventional cytogenetics in myelofibrosis: literature review and discussion. Eur J Haematol 2009;82:329–38.

97. Kvasnicka HM, Thiele J. Bone marrow angiogenesis: methods of quantification and changes evolving in chronic myeloproliferative disorders. Histol Histopathol 2004;19:1245–60.

98. Thiele J, Kvasnicka HM, Schmitt-Graeff A, et al. Dynamics of fibrosis in chronic idiopathic (primary) myelofibrosis during therapy: a follow-up study on 309 patients. Leuk Lymphoma 2003;44:949–53.

99. Mesa RA, Hanson CA, Rajkumar SV, et al. Evaluation and clinical correlations of bone marrow angiogenesis in myelofibrosis with myeloid metaplasia. Blood 2000;96:3374–80.

100. Thiele J, Kvasnicka HM. CD34+ stem cells in chronic myeloproliferative disorders. Histol Histopathol 2002;17:507–21.

CHAPTER 24

Chronic myelogenous leukemia

G Büsche, HH Kreipe

Chapter contents

Introduction

Chronic myelogenous leukemia (CML) is a myeloproliferative neoplasm consistently associated with the *BCR-ABL1* fusion gene (reviewed in[1]). CML is characterized by neutrophilic granulocytosis and pathologic left shift in the peripheral blood (PB) with less than 20% (WHO) or 30% (European LeukemiaNet) blasts in blood and bone marrow (BM).[2,3] CML is a disease most frequently occurring in the middle age with a peak in the 5th and 6th decades of life, affecting about 1–2 persons/100 000.[3] It may also occur in younger and older patients, but it is rarely seen in childhood.

Increased risk of CML had been observed in persons exposed to ionizing radiation.[5] However, history of radiation exposure is unusual in patients with CML so that the exact cause of disease remains unclear in the great majority of patients.[5] Inherited predisposition to CML has not been reported, but risk of CML appears to be reduced in persons with HLA-B3 and -B8 phenotype, indicating that some unknown predisposing factors may exist.[6]

Animal models[7] and the success of BCR-ABL tyrosine kinase (TK) inhibitors in inducing a remission of CML[8] have impressively demonstrated the relevance of the *BCR-ABL1* fusion to the pathogenesis of CML (described in detail in Chapter 21). Monotherapy with BCR-ABL TK inhibitors induces a complete cytogenetic (CCyR) and a major molecular (MMR) remission in the great majority of patients.[9,10]

Clinical features and course of disease

CML shows a characteristic bi- or triphasic course, starting with a rather indolent chronic phase (CP) and transforming to a usually lethal final acute phase, a dramatic clinical picture called 'blast crisis' (Table 24.1). In more than 95% of patients, CML is diagnosed in CP. Rarely, CML is diagnosed in acute phase with a clinical picture of a *BCR-ABL1*-positive acute myeloid (AML) or lymphatic leukemia (ALL).

In early CP, CML is usually asymptomatic and diagnosis may be incidental, due to the detection of leuko- or thrombocytosis, pathologic left shift or basophilia in the differential count. In late CP, the main symptoms causing contact with the physician are abdominal pain due to splenomegaly, fatigue or bleeding.

During the last 3 decades, the median duration of the CP could be markedly prolonged from less than 5[11] to more than

Table 24.1 Diagnostic criteria of various phases of CML

		Diagnosis of disease				CP		AP	BC
		Typical[1]	Often[2]	Unlikely[3]	General[6]	Early CP	Late CP		
PB	Neutrophils	+++	++	−−→−−−		+	+++	+++[7]	Variable
	Left shift	++	+			0→+	++	+++[8]	Variable
	Basophilia	++	+	0	<20%[4]	+	++	≥20%[4,9]	Variable
	Eosonophilia	++	+			0→+	++	++[8]	Variable
	Blast count	+	++		<10% (WHO), <15% (ELN)	<1%	≥5%	10–19%[9] (WHO), 15–29%[9] (ELN)	≥20%[10] (WHO), ≥30%[10] (ELN)
	Blasts + promyelocytes				<30 % (ELN)			≥30%[5,9] (ELN)	
	Platelets	+	++	−→−−−	10[11]–10[12] / l[4]	0→+	++	<10[11] or >10[12] / l[4,9]	Variable
	Erythrocytes	−	−	+→+++		0	−−−→−−−	−−−→−−−[8]	−−−→−−−[8]
BM	Granulopoiesis	+++	++	−−→−−−		+	+++	+++[8]	Variable
	Basophilia	+	++	0		0→+	++	+++[8]	Variable
	Eosinophilia	+	++	0		0→+	++	+++[8]	Variable
	Blast count	0	+		<10% (WHO), <15% (ELN)	<5%	≥5%	10–19%[9] (WHO), 15–29%[9] (ELN)	≥20%[10] (WHO), ≥30%[10] (ELN)
	Blasts + promyelocytes				<30% (ELN)			≥30%[5,9] (ELN)	
	Megakaryopoiesis	+	++	−−−→−−−		0→+	++→+++	+++[8]	Variable
	% Micromega-karyocytes	+++	++	0		++	+++	+++[8]	+++[8]
	Erythropoiesis	−	0	+→+++		0	−−−→−−−	−−−→−−−[8]	−−−[8]
	Pseudo-Gaucher cells	+	++			0→+	++	++[8]	Variable
	Marrow fibrosis	0	++			0	0→++	++→+++[8]	Variable
Other	Splenomegaly	++	+++			0	+++	+++[7]	+++[8]

A precise and widely accepted definition distinguishing early and late CP does not exist as yet. 0 = unchanged or no evidence, −−−, −−, − = significant, moderate, slight decrease; +++, ++, + = significant, moderate, slight increase.[1] >50%,[2] >10% of cases,[3] evidence of any of these criteria questions the diagnosis 'CML';[4] defined by WHO and ELN, all the other criteria not defined by WHO or ELN are not generally accepted;[5] but <30% blasts ;[6] all these criteria must be fulfilled, otherwise AP or BC should be diagnosed;[7] increasing leukocytosis or splenomegaly during therapy (WHO);[8] not defined by WHO and ELN;[9] occurrence of any of these criteria justifies the diagnosis AP or[10] BC.

10 years.[12] Before the use of TK inhibitors, the majority of patients developed blast crisis several years after diagnosis of CML.[11,12] After diagnosis of blast crisis, patients die within few months, usually from fatal infection or bleeding or organic failure due to blast infiltration.[13]

In the majority of patients, blast phase is preceded by an accelerated phase characterized by therapy resistance with increasing leuko- or thrombocytosis, increasing counts of immature myeloid precursors in PB, progressive basophilia, splenomegaly or hepatomegaly, and reduced quality of life. From the time of diagnosis of accelerated phase, the survival time is markedly reduced (median less than 2 years).[1]

With the application of BCR-ABL specific TK inhibitors for therapy of CML, prognosis and quality of life of patients have dramatically improved since the risk of progression to accelerated or acute phase has been significantly reduced when compared to earlier therapy concepts.[10,14]

Diagnostic procedures

Genetics

Evidence of the Philadelphia chromosome or the reciprocal translocation t(9;22)(q34;q11.2) confirms the CML diagnosis[3] in patients with characteristic morphologic changes in blood and BM (see below). Molecular evidence of the *BCR-ABL1* fusion is mandatory in patients without the Philadelphia chromosome. Cytogenetic and molecular studies are also used to control the efficacy of treatment (see Chapter

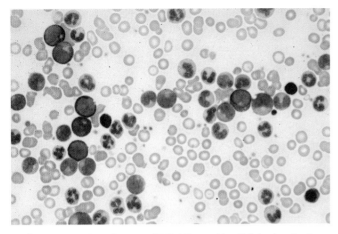

Fig. 24.1 Morphologic features of BCR-ABL1 positive CML in chronic phase: leukocytosis, pathologic left shift and increase of basophils in the peripheral blood. May–Grünwald–Giemsa, ×500.

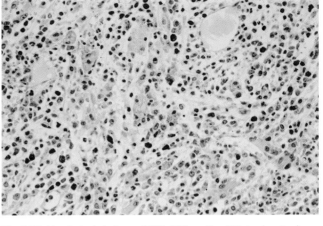

Fig. 24.2 Morphologic features of BCR-ABL1 positive CML in chronic phase: marked increase of granulopoiesis within bone marrow ('granulocyte-rich CML'), occurrence of pseudo-Gaucher cells. Giemsa, ×250.

21 for details). Nowadays, disease is considered therapy-resistant in patients who do not achieve cytogenetic remission[2] but patients who achieve a continuing CyCR have an excellent prognosis.[15]

Whereas additional chromosomal changes besides t(9;22)(q34;q11.2) do not appear to provide independent prognostic information when occurring prior to anti-neoplastic therapy,[16] clonal evolution may support diagnosis of therapy resistance or accelerated phase when occurring during the course of CML.[17,18]

BCR-ABL1 mutations are frequent in patients who become resistant to a therapy with a TK inhibitor.[17,19] Therefore, molecular analysis of BCR-ABL1 mutations has become a further standard procedure in patients losing their cytogenetic or molecular response to therapy.[2]

Morphology

Morphological diagnosis of CML is based on characteristic changes in blood and BM (Table 24.1). Organomegaly (splenomegaly, hepatomegaly) may also be present at diagnosis, indicating extramedullary expansion of disease.[16]

At diagnosis

Peripheral blood. The first diagnostic feature usually arousing suspicion of CML is a leukemic PB picture. Granulocytosis with a pathologic left shift without *hiatus leukaemicus* is the main characteristic (Fig. 24.1). Granulocytosis comprises neutrophils, eosinophils and basophils. Myelocytes usually predominate among immature precursors mobilized into PB, but promyelocytes and myeloblasts may also occur especially in the late chronic or the accelerated phase (Fig. 24.1). The WHO classification defines a blast count of less than 20%, otherwise the disease should be classified as an acute leukemia.[3] Some therapy trials use the previous FAB classification definition, where the count of blasts and promyelocytes should be less than 30%.[2] Thrombocytosis is a common finding and when excessive (>10[6]/l) may lead to the misdiagnosis of 'essential thrombocythemia' (ET).[20,21] However, CML with thrombocytosis differ from ET by a pathologic left shift and basophilia in the differential count, characteristic

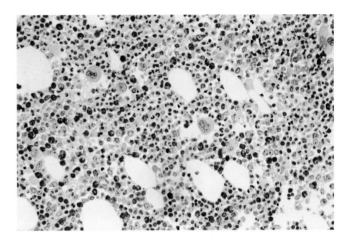

Fig. 24.3 Morphologic features of BCR-ABL1 positive CML in early chronic phase: increased number of basophils within bone marrow. May–Grünwald–Giemsa, ×500.

morphologic changes in BM (see below), evidence of the BCR-ABL1 fusion, and in most cases, lack of the JAK2[V617F] mutation (see Chapters 21 and 23 for details).

Although the BCR-ABL1 fusion affects a pluripotent hematopoietic stem cell involving all hematopoietic cell lines, mobilization of precursors of erythro- and megakaryopoiesis is less common than the mobilization of granulopoietic precursors. Erythrocytosis is not seen in CML. A significant proportion of patients develop anemia, thus indicating differences in the effects of the BCR-ABL1 fusion in various hematopoietic cell lines. Nevertheless, mobilization of normoblasts or megakaryoblasts to PB may occur, especially in late chronic, advanced or blastic phase of disease.

Bone marrow. BCR-ABL1 mediated inhibition of apoptosis leads to an excessive expansion of the neoplastic clone in BM replacing non-neoplastic hematopoietic and mesenchymal cells (adipocytes).

Changes in hematopoiesis. First obvious morphologic feature in microscopic evaluation at low magnification is a marked expansion of neutrophilic granulopoiesis (Fig. 24.2). In the majority of patients, eosinophilic granulopoiesis is also increased. Basophilic granulopoiesis is at least slightly increased in almost all patients (Fig. 24.3). In the majority

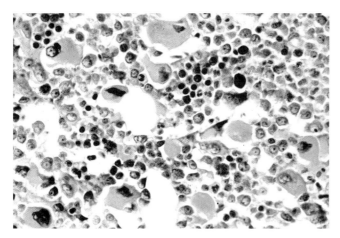

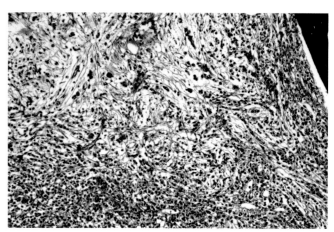

Fig. 24.4 Morphologic features of BCR-ABL1 positive CML in early chronic phase: increased number of micromegakaryocytes with hypolobulated nucleus ('megakaryocyte-rich CML'). Giemsa, ×250.

Fig. 24.6 Morphologic features of BCR-ABL1 positive CML: bone marrow fibrosis as shown by Gomori silver impregnation. ×125.

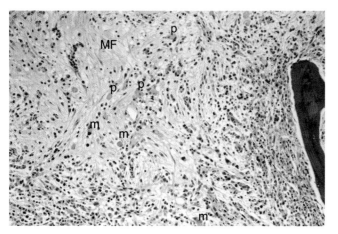

Fig. 24.5 Morphologic features of BCR-ABL1 positive CML in accelerated phase: focal marrow fibrosis (MF) with micromegakaryocytes (m) and pseudo-Gaucher cells (p). ×125.

of patients, granulopoiesis shows a complete maturation (Fig. 24.2), but it is often left shifted with a slight relative increase of myelocytes. In some patients, numbers of promyelocytes and myeloblasts are also increased. The myeloblast count is usually lower than 10%. The neoplastic granulocytes show a reduced leukocyte alkaline phosphatase (LAP) index, which distinguishes them from non-neoplastic granulocytes in leukemoid reactions.[22] However, this does not significantly influence their function so that infections due to granulocytic dysfunction are uncommon in CP of CML. In the past, determination of the LAP index of granulocytes was a standard method applied at diagnosis of CML. Molecular investigation for the presence of the *BCR-ABL1* fusion has replaced this procedure.

A further characteristic feature is an increase of micromegakaryocytes with a central hypolobulated nucleus, which is due to a reduction of mature hyperploid megakaryocytes[23,24] (Figs 24.4 and 24.5). The exact mechanism leading to the lack of hyperploid megakaryocytes is not clear as yet. This feature is pathognomonic for CML and lack of it should question the diagnosis of CML. Some authors have divided

CML according to the count of micromegakaryocytes into a megakaryocytic-rich and a granulocytic subtype.[23,25] The megakaryocytic-rich subtype differs from the granulocytic by an increased risk of BM fibrosis.

Although erythropoiesis in CML is also *BCR-ABL1* positive, it is usually not expanded. In the majority of patients, erythropoiesis is rather reduced, particularly in late chronic, accelerated or blastic phase, correlating with a varying degree of anemia.[25]

Except for micromegakaryocytes, dysplastic features of hematopoiesis are uncommon in CP of CML. Platelets may show dysfunction with increased risk of bleeding, but thromboembolic events are uncommon.[26]

A blast count exceeding 10% of marrow cells is not common at diagnosis, but a typical feature during the course of CML, especially in accelerated or blastic phase (Fig. 24.7). Blasts occur mainly within the proliferation zone of granulopoiesis (myeloblasts; Fig. 24.7), but they may also be observed outside of it, particularly lymphoblasts or megakaryoblasts (Fig. 24.8). By immunohistochemistry, myeloblasts are often but not always CD34 or CD117 positive with co-expression of CD33, myeloperoxidase or lysozyme. Megakaryoblasts are CD42b or CD61, and lymphoblasts have B-precursor related phenotype: TdT, CD34, CD10, CD20 and CD79a positive. Flow cytometry may be useful by demonstrating aberrant CD56 expression in granulopoiesis, which is, however, also observed in other myeloproliferative and myelodysplastic disorders.[27] This method can also help in early detection of incipient blast crisis and in differentiating between lymphatic and myeloid blastic transformation.[28]

Changes of non-hematopoietic tissue. First obvious morphologic feature in microscopic evaluation at low magnification is the replacement of the adipose BM tissue usually to less than 5% of marrow volume (Figs 24.2, 24.5–7). A further typical feature is the occurrence of storage histiocytes resembling Gaucher cells, the so-called pseudo-Gaucher cells[29] (Figs 24.2, 24.5). These histiocytes belong to the neoplastic clone,[30] and their Gaucher-like appearance is caused by a relative enzyme insufficiency as a result of an excessive phagocytosis of leukemic cells whereas the mesenchymal stem cells, which differentiate into adipocytes, fibroblasts

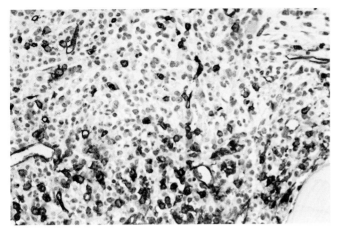

Fig. 24.7 Morphologic features of BCR-ABL1 positive CML in accelerated phase: increased vascularity and focal excess of blasts illustrated by CD34 immunohistochemistry (alkaline phosphatase-anti alkaline phosphatase method = red). ×250.

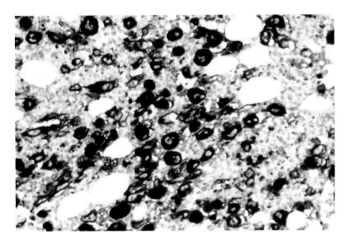

Fig. 24.8 Morphologic features of BCR-ABL1 positive CML in accelerated phase: large cluster of micromegakaryocytes and megakaryoblasts illustrated by CD42b immunohistochemistry (immunoperoxidase = brown). ×250.

and osteoblasts are not involved in the neoplastic proliferation.[31]

BM fibrosis is another typical feature of CML (Figs 24.5, 24.6).[32] It affects only a minority of patients at diagnosis, but a significant proportion of patients develop fibrosis during the course of disease, especially when therapy has lost its efficacy.[33,34] In patients not responding to therapy, the cumulative proportion of cases with BM fibrosis amounts to more than 90%.[33] Therefore, CML is the second myeloproliferative neoplasm besides primary myelofibrosis (PMF) characterized by a high risk of BM fibrosis.

Marrow fibrosis usually starts focally (patchily), followed by transformation to diffuse extensive fibrosis developing during course of disease.[34] As in PMF, the fiber-producing cells (fibroblasts) are not part of the neoplastic clone.[31] However, their fiber production is up-regulated by growth factors produced by the neoplastic hematopoiesis, particularly platelet-derived growth factor and transforming growth factor-β, resulting in increased collagen type I and III (reticulin) fiber deposits.[35]

Fibrosis becomes visible after silver impregnation (Fig. 24.6). Various methods were presented with respect to grading of marrow fibrosis (see Chapter 3), but a worldwide uniform approach to diagnosis and quantification of marrow fibrosis does not exist so far. In general, more than 5% of marrow volume per μm thickness of tissue section with fiber deposits $>10^4$ mm/mm^3 are uncommon in normal healthy subjects so that this limit can be applied to diagnose BM fibrosis.[36] In fibrotic BM regions in CML, the density of the fiber deposits usually exceeds 10^4 mm/mm^3.[36]

BM fibrosis correlates with an increased megakaryocyte count, splenomegaly and mobilization of normoblasts in PB.[25] It may also correlate with an excess of blasts. Extensive diffuse fibrosis may be accompanied with osteosclerosis.

Another characteristic feature that CML shares with other neoplastic disorders is an increased BM vascularity[37] (Fig. 24.7). It results from an increased production of pro-angiogenic growth factors by the neoplastic clone, especially the vascular endothelial growth factor A (VEGF). It has been found that BCR-ABL1 oncoprotein could *in vitro* induce *VEGF* promoter activity and increased VEGF protein levels in Ba/F3 cells as well as promote the expression of functionally active hypoxia-inducible factor-1 (HIF-1), a major transcriptional regulator of *VEGF* gene expression.[38] Furthermore, the pluripotent neoplastic stem cell appears to be able to differentiate into endothelial cells.[39] Thus, CML seems to be able to induce BM hypervascularity as a part of the neoplastic proliferation.

Extramedullary manifestations. Up to 70% of CML patients at diagnosis show a varying degree of hepato- and splenomegaly.[16] Spleen enlargement results from an infiltration of red pulp cords by neoplastic hematopoiesis, mainly granulopoiesis. Hepatomegaly is a result of intrasinusoidal and periportal infiltration by hematopoiesis.

Phases of disease

The phase of disease as defined by blood and BM morphology is still the most important prognostic factor of CML and its prognostic significance has not been abolished by current therapy, including allogenic stem cell transplantation and TK inhibitors. However, worldwide uniform approach to the definitions of these phases has not been achieved as yet. Two definitions are widely applied (Table 24.1), the criteria proposed by the WHO, and the definitions recommended by the European LeukemiaNet.[2,3]

Chronic phase (CP)

CML is usually diagnosed in chronic phase (CP). It is defined by less than 10% (WHO) or 15% (European LeukemiaNet) blasts within blood and BM, and less than 20% basophils in the PB. If these criteria are not fulfilled, the diagnosis of accelerated or acute phase is made. During therapy, persistent thrombocytopenia $<100 \times 10^9$/l unrelated to treatment should not occur. Furthermore, the WHO classification mentions additional following criteria for CP CML: absence of therapy-resistant progressive disease (increasing splenomegaly, increasing white blood cell count (WBC), thrombocytosis $>1000 \times 10^9$/l) and absence of cytogenetic evidence of clonal evolution.[3]

At diagnosis, BM fibrosis may occur in up to 30% of patients otherwise fulfilling criteria of CP (Figs 24.5, 24.6). Currently, BM fibrosis is not considered as a significant factor in the definition of the phase of disease. However, the prognosis of patients presenting with fibrosis appears to be rather poor, resembling accelerated phase.[34] Therefore, as long as a final consensus of opinions does not exist and as long as these patients do not show other signs of acceleration, we recommend omitting differentiation between chronic and accelerated phase in these patients and report the findings as 'CML with fibrosis'.

Early CP

A clear definition of 'early' and 'late' CP does not exist so far, although it is well accepted that less and more advanced stages of CP do exist.[40] The success of BCR-ABL TK inhibitors in inducing remission in CML has led to an increased awareness of CML and its symptoms, so that earlier stages of this disease are diagnosed more frequently. Patients with early chronic phase of CML (eCP) show relatively low WBC (e.g. $<20 \times 10^9$/l), less obvious left shift in the differential count, often with only few myelocytes, no or minimal thrombocytosis (platelets $<600 \times 10^9$/l), no organomegaly, no anemia and usually no general symptoms. In the PB, basophil count is often slightly increased, the eosinophil count is variable. Sometimes, thrombocytosis is the only conspicuous change in the PB. BM shows a varying increase of micromegakaryocytes with hypolobulated nucleus (Figs 24.3 and 24.4). There is often no or only a slight increase of granulopoiesis with slight left shift due to a relative increase of myelocytes and promyelocytes, as well as a slight relative increase of eosinophilic and/or basophilic granulopoiesis (Figs 24.3 and 24.4). Morphology of erythropoiesis and adipose marrow tissue do not appear altered (no significant reduction). BM fibrosis, blast excess and splenomegaly are uncommon. Among the morphologic changes, relative increase of basophils within the PB and the increase of micromegakaryocytes with hypolobulated nucleus in BM are most characteristic and should be followed by test for the *BCR-ABL1* fusion. CML in eCP is often detected by chance, due to the alterations of the blood cell counts.

Late chronic phase (lCP)

In the past, CML was diagnosed usually in the full-blown stage with marked leukocytosis and splenomegaly, which corresponded to a late CP. Nowadays late chronic phase (lCP) is less frequent at diagnosis but develops during the course of disease when therapy has lost its efficacy or the patient's compliance to therapy is low. Patients usually become symptomatic due to organomegaly (splenomegaly, hepatomegaly) and/or anemia.

In lCP, CML diagnosis on the basis of the morphologic alterations of blood and BM is rather straightforward. The WBC often exceeds 100×10^9/l, the blood basophil count may exceed 3%, and a pathologic left shift down to myeloblasts is common. The PB blast count may exceed 5% and normoblasts may occur. The thrombocyte count may exceed 1000×10^9/l.

In BM biopsy, replacement of erythropoiesis and adipose marrow due to excessive expansion of neutro-, eosino- and basophilic granulopoiesis is characteristic; adipose BM tissue is usually lower than 2% of BM volume (Fig. 24.2). The BM blast count often exceeds 5%. Micromegakaryocytes with hypolobulated nuclei may be excessively increased and they may show a larger variation of size than those seen in eCP.[23] Focal BM fibrosis may occur, and it is usually associated with a marked increase of megakaryopoiesis.

Accelerated phase (AP)

Accelerated phase (AP) is seen only in a minority of patients at CML diagnosis, but it is a common finding when therapy has lost its efficacy.[2,33] By definition, AP differs from lCP in four variables: (1) the percentages of blasts in PB and (2) the percentages of blasts in BM, (3) the thrombocyte counts, and (4) the basophil counts in PB. A basophil count $\geq 20\%$ of leukocytes or a persistent thrombocytopenia $<100 \times 10^9$/l unrelated to therapy are generally accepted criteria. Blast counts of 10–19% (WHO) or 15–29% (European LeukemiaNet) within blood or BM are further requirements.[2,3] The European LeukemiaNet has defined a BM or blood blast + promyelocyte count >30% with less than 30% blasts in blood and BM as a further fifth criterion for AP[2] whereas the WHO has proposed therapy-resistant progressive disease (increasing splenomegaly, increasing WBC, thrombocytosis $>1000 \times 10^9$/l) or cytogenetic evidence of clonal evolution as additional criteria.[3] Occurrence of any of these criteria justifies the diagnosis of AP. In most recent therapeutic trials, the criteria proposed by the European LeukemiaNet are used whereas the criteria proposed by the WHO classification are applied less commonly.

The BM alterations in AP resemble those observed in lCP. The BM blast or basophil counts are usually higher, and focal clusters of blasts may occur (Fig. 24.7). Focal accumulations of more than 30 blast cells should give a suspicion of evolving blast crisis and should therefore be mentioned in the pathology report. Megakaryopoiesis is usually significantly increased (Fig. 24.8), but megakaryocytes rarely exceed 50% of BM cells.[23] In a minority of patients, megakaryopoiesis may be reduced. BM fibrosis is a typical finding affecting up to 90% of patients (Figs 24.5 and 24.6).[33] In the majority of patients, fibrosis correlates with a markedly increased count of megakaryocytes. Osteosclerosis may also occur, especially in advanced stage of BM fibrosis.[23] AP may also show dysplastic features of hematopoiesis resembling those observed in myelodysplastic syndromes (MDS). After detection of AP, the overall survival time of patients is usually reduced to less than 2 years.[41] In the majority of patients, there is a continuous transition from lCP to AP of disease. The criteria for diagnosis of AP are based on the experience collected from patients treated with interferon-α or chemotherapy. Optimization of AP criteria for patients treated with TK inhibitors are pending so far.

Acute phase, blast crisis (BC)

Blast crisis (BC) is defined by the percentage of blasts in blood and BM. Whereas the WHO defines BC as $\geq 20\%$ blasts in blood or BM, the European Leukemia Net applies a blast count $\geq 30\%$, which is used in current European studies.[2] Furthermore, the WHO classification mentions

Table 24.2 Clinical risk scores for CML in chronic phase*

	Sokal index[45]	Hasford score[16]
Age (years)	+ 0.116 × (age − 43.3)	+ 0.666 if age ≥50 years
Spleen size (below costal margin)	+ 0.0345 × (spleen size [cm] − 7.51)	+ 0.042 × spleen size [cm]
Thrombocyte count	+ 0.188 × ((platelets × 10⁹/l: 700)² − 0.563	+ 1.0956 if platelets ≥1500 × 10⁹/l
% Blasts (differential blood count)	+ 0.0887 × (blast count [%] − 2.1)	+ 0.0584 × blast count [%]
% Basophils (differential count)	− not applied −	+ 0.20399 if >3% basophils
% Eosinophils (differential count)	− not applied −	+ 0.0413 × eosinophils [%]
Score value W	= e^{sum of score values}	= sum of score values × 1000
Risk groups: low	if W <0.8	if W ≤780
intermediate	if 0.8 ≤W ≤1.2	if 780 < W ≤1480
high	if W >1.2	if W >1480

*Based on observations of patients treated with interferon- or chemotherapy. A risk score based on results of treatment with BCR-ABL specific TK inhibitors is not available so far.

Box 24.1 Differential diagnosis of CML

1. Non-neoplastic changes, particularly leukemoid reaction
2. Other myeloproliferative neoplasms, especially primary myelofibrosis and essential thrombocythemia
3. Myelodysplastic/myeloproliferative neoplasms, particularly atypical CML and CMML
4. Myelodysplastic syndrome with del(5q) chromosome aberration
5. *De novo* acute leukemia.

extramedullary blast proliferation or large foci or clusters of blasts in the BM biopsy as indicators of BC.[3]

In the majority of patients BC evolves from AP, but occasionally it emerges suddenly from CP without obvious transient AP.[42] BC is rarely detected at diagnosis of CML. It usually occurs during the course of disease, especially after therapy failure. BC was more common during earlier applied treatment modalities, for example, treatment with chemotherapy.[11] Acquired loss of p53 appears to play a central role in a significant proportion of patients.[43]

In about 70% of patients BC is myeloid and in about 30% it is of lymphoid origin, fulfilling, respectively, the criteria of acute myeloid or B-lymphoblastic leukemia. Megakaryoblastic crisis may occur, particularly in patients with prior excess of megakaryopoiesis. Erythroblastic crisis is rare. In about 20–30% of patients, BC shows mixed phenotype involving both myeloblasts/megakaryoblasts and lymphoblasts.[44]

Prognostic factors in CML

TK inhibitors (imatinib mesylate and other drugs) have significantly improved the survival time of patients due to a reduction of the risk of transformation into AP or BC.[14] However, this has not substantially improved the survival time in AP or BC.[41] Thus, AP and BC are still the main disease-related causes of death in CML patients. To predict the outcome in CP, prognostic scores were presented in the literature, comprising clinical, morphological and genetic variables (Table 24.2). Age, spleen size, platelet count and percentage of blasts in blood have been established as prognostic factors at CML diagnosis.[16,45] Dynamics and degree of hematologic, cytogenetic and molecular remission are important prognostic factors during therapy. Other variables,

such as clonal evolution or BM fibrosis, may also be significant. However, these variables are not considered in the majority of recent therapy studies. The established scoring systems are based mainly on observation of patients treated with interferon-α or chemotherapy.[16,45] Due to excellent survival time of patients treated with BCR-ABL specific TK inhibitors, it appears to be too early to make definite recommendations concerning prognostic scoring and overall survival time during this new type of treatment.

Differential diagnoses

CML can be mimicked by numerous other neoplastic or non-neoplastic disorders with leuko-/thrombocytosis or left shift in the PB (Box 24.1). Molecular evaluation of hematopoiesis in such cases is mandatory, since evidence or lack of the *BCR-ABL1* fusion allows a clear distinction. Nevertheless, careful morphologic evaluation usually allows correct diagnosis in the most cases. Furthermore, the course of CML may be complicated by the evolution of *BCR-ABL1* negative myeloid neoplasms leading to a misdiagnosis or a misclassification of the phase of CML.

Non-neoplastic changes

Reactive changes may be excessive resulting in a marked leukocytosis and increase of BM granulopoiesis (leukemoid reaction). LAP score is usually high in leukemoid reaction. A pathologic left shift is uncommon in reactive leukocytosis. However, BM involvement by metastatic tumor or by processes replacing hematopoiesis may result in a mobilization of immature myeloid and/or erythroid precursors into the PB. Increase of blood or BM basophils, increase of micromegakaryocytes with central hypolobulated nucleus, excess of blasts, or BM fibrosis are uncommon in reactive changes of hematopoiesis, thus allowing a distinction from CML in the majority of cases. Evidence of inflammatory changes (i.e. pericapillary increase of plasma cells) or evidence of metastatic tumor is suggestive of leukemoid reaction. Nevertheless, advanced stages of CML may also be accompanied by inflammatory changes due to complicating infections so that none of the reactive changes typical for a leukemoid reaction are sufficient to exclude *BCR-ABL1* positive CML.

Neoplastic disorders

Atypical CML

In the past, it was assumed that a minority of cases morphologically and clinically corresponding to CML may lack the

BCR-ABL1 fusion. Therefore, it is has been accepted that a BCR-ABL1 negative leukemic disease similar to CML exists, but should be distinguished from it by applying the term 'atypical CML'.[46] It has been shown that BCR-ABL1 negative patients poorly respond to treatment and show an unfavorable prognosis.[47]

Although atypical CML shares many morphologic features with BCR-ABL1 positive CML, it differs in several characteristic features allowing discrimination. Firstly, increase of basophils in blood or BM and thrombocytosis are uncommon in atypical CML.[46] Although atypical CML may also show an increase of micromegakaryocytes, megakaryocytes show a wider variation in size and morphology, may contain hyperlobulated nuclei or may be multinucleated. Erythropoiesis may be slightly increased and it may show macrocytic changes or dysplastic features. Granulopoiesis in atypical CML frequently shows dysplastic features, such as an abnormal chromatin clumping, which is very uncommon in CP of CML.[48] Nevertheless, cases by morphology almost indistinguishable from BCR-ABL1 positive CML exist, thus requiring molecular exclusion of the BCR-ABL1 fusion.

Chronic neutrophilic leukemia

Chronic neutrophilic leukemia is a very rare disease. It shares with CML features of neutrophilic granulocytosis and splenomegaly, and (few) immature precursors of granulopoiesis may also occur in PB. Usually, it can be distinguished from CML by lack of basophilia and lack of micromegakaryocytes with hypolobulated nuclei. However, in patients with a BCR-ABL1 fusion at e19a2, which results in a p230 oncoprotein, neutrophilia is a characteristic feature[49] so that molecular exclusion of the BCR-ABL1 fusion is mandatory for discrimination from CML.

Chronic eosinophilic leukemia

CML may show a marked eosinophilia requiring distinction from chronic eosinophilic leukemia (CEL), another rare myeloproliferative neoplasm (see Chapter 25 for details). CML usually differs from CEL by a higher basophil count in blood and BM as well as by the presence of micromegakaryocytes with hypolobulated nucleus. However, some cases with CEL may also show a slight basophilia or micromegakaryocytes and differential diagnosis will rely on molecular studies.

Chronic myelomonocytic leukemia

Although the absolute monocyte count within the PB is usually slightly increased, relative monocytosis exceeding 10% in the differential count and significant increase of monocytes in BM are uncommon in CML. However, in cases with a BCR-ABL1 fusion at e1a2 with resulting P190 oncoprotein, monocytosis is frequent.[49]

Primary myelofibrosis

In early cellular phase of PMF, marked leukocytosis, pathologic left shift and thrombocytosis in blood, and marked increase of granulopoiesis may mimic CML. In its advanced stage, excessive BM fibrosis with marked increase of megakaryopoiesis or excess of blasts may cause problems in distinguishing from AP of CML. Most important morphologic differences to BCR-ABL1 positive CML are megakaryocytes and basophils. In PMF, megakaryocytes are usually larger than normal, containing an enlarged hypolobulated nucleus with low density of chromatin (see Chapter 23). Basophilia in blood or BM is uncommon even in advanced stage of PMF, but it is a typical feature of AP of CML. PMF frequently shows a JAK2^{V617F} mutation (see Chapter 21), which is uncommon in BCR-ABL1 positive CML and in atypical CML. However, in patients with a BCR-ABL1 fusion at e19a2 which results in a p230 oncoprotein, basophilia may be missing or insignificant[49] so that molecular exclusion of the BCR-ABL1 fusion is also recommended for PMF cases.

Polycythemia vera (PV)

Long-standing PV may transform into a disease resembling CML with marked leukocytosis and anemia. Eosinophilia, basophilia, left shift in the PB, BM fibrosis, and splenomegaly may also occur. CML-like PV differs from CML by giant megakaryocytes which do not occur in CML, and by the JAK2^{V617F} mutation (see Chapters 21 and 22). BCR-ABL1 positive CML occurring during the course of PV is extremely rare.[50] Nevertheless, if doubts remain, PB should be examined for the BCR-ABL1 fusion.

Essential thrombocythemia

In a minority of cases, BCR-ABL1 positive CML may show a marked thrombocytosis that may exceed $2000 \times 10^9/l$, whereas leukocytosis is mild or lacking. However, megakaryopoiesis significantly differs from that usually seen in ET; the megakaryocytes are not enlarged as it is characteristic in ET and their morphology resembles that of 'classic' CML. Therefore, it is nowadays accepted that BCR-ABL1 positive ET does not exist; BCR-ABL1 positive MPN presenting with thrombocythemia only is regarded as a variant of CML.[51]

Myelodysplastic syndromes

In AP, CML may develop some dysplastic features of hematopoiesis which may be suggestive of MDS. However, CML morphology usually significantly differs from an MDS phenotype. Erythropoiesis is reduced in the majority of CML patients whereas most MDS cases show an increase of erythropoiesis. In MDS, leukocytosis occurs rarely, whereas CML usually shows a marked leukocytosis. Furthermore, a continuous left shift in the differential count is unusual in MDS, but typical in CML.

Nevertheless, patients with MDS with a del(5q) (see Chapter 20 for details) often show a thrombocytosis; they may also show a slight leukocytosis. Atypical megakaryocytes with hypolobulated nucleus similar to those observed in CML occur in the BM, the granulopoiesis may be increased, and erythropoiesis is often reduced.[52] Most important differences between MDS with del(5q) and CML are a less prominent proliferation of granulopoiesis, lower counts of eosinophils and basophils, no continuous left shift in the blood, and macrocytosis of erythrocytes. A cytogenetic evaluation provides final diagnosis.

Acute leukemia

By definition, AML is distinguished from CML by the blast count within blood and bone marrow (see Chapter 18). BCR-ABL1 positive primary AML is rare.[53] If residual hematopoiesis shows morphologic features characteristic for CML and the BCR-ABL1 fusion is detected in a case presenting as AML, it is more likely a BC of CML rather than a primary AML. BCR-ABL1 positive acute lymphoblastic leukemia (ALL) occurs more frequently (see Chapter 19). Nevertheless, it cannot be excluded that some BCR-ABL1 positive B-precursor ALL in adults may be lymphatic BC of CML, particularly if p210 BCR-ABL1 is detected.

Coincidence of other myeloid neoplasms

In a minority of patients with CML, a BCR-ABL1 negative and sometimes JAK2^{V617F}-mutated clone exists or evolves besides the BCR-ABL1 positive clone (see Chapter 21).

Co-existence of another neoplastic BCR-ABL1 negative clone should be considered in cases with discordant morphologic findings – e.g. CML-like changes of granulopoiesis, but PMF-like changes of megakaryopoiesis or if cytogenetic and/or molecular analyses indicate remission of CML, but morphology gives evidence of myeloproliferative neoplasia.

References

1. Vardiman JW. Chronic myelogenous leukmia, BCR-ABL1+. Am J Clin Pathol 2009;132:250–60.

2. Baccarani M, Saglio G, Goldman J, et al. Evolving concepts in the management of chronic myeloid leukemia: recommendations from an expert panel on behalf of the European LeukemiaNet. Blood 2006;108:1809–20.

3. Swerdlow SH, Campo E, Harris NL, et al. WHO Classification of Tumours of Haematopoietic and Lymphatic Tissues. Lyon: IARC; 2008.

4. Rohrbacher M, Hasford J. Epidemiology of chronic myeloid leukaemia (CML). Best Pract Res Clin Haematol 2009;22: 295–302.

5. Corso A, Lazzarino M, Morra E, et al. Chronic myelogenous leukemia and exposure to ionizing radiation – a retrospective study of 443 patients. Ann Hematol 1995;70:79–82.

6. Posthuma EF, Falkenburg JH, Apperley JF, et al. HLA-B8 and HLA-A3 coexpressed with HLA-B8 are associated with a reduced risk of the development of chronic myeloid leukemia. Chronic Leukemia Working Party of the EBMT. Blood 1999;93:3863–5.

7. Zhang X, Ren R. Bcr-Abl efficiently induces a myeloproliferative disease and production of excess interleukin-3 and granulocyte-macrophage colony-stimulating factor in mice: a novel model for chronic myelogenous leukemia. Blood 1998;92:3829–40.

8. Jabbour E, Fava C, Kantarjian H. Advances in the biology and therapy of patients with chronic myeloid leukaemia. Best Pract Res Clin Haematol 2009;22: 395–407.

9. Hughes TP, Kaeda J, Branford S, et al. Frequency of major molecular responses to imatinib or interferon alfa plus cytarabine in newly diagnosed chronic myeloid leukemia. N Engl J Med 2003;349:1423–32.

10. O'Brien SG, Guilhot F, Larson RA, et al. Imatinib compared with interferon and low-dose cytarabine for newly diagnosed chronic-phase chronic myeloid leukemia. N Engl J Med 2003;348:994–1004.

11. Interferon alfa versus chemotherapy for chronic myeloid leukemia: a meta-analysis of seven randomized trials: Chronic Myeloid Leukemia Trialists' Collaborative Group. J Natl Cancer Inst 1997;89: 1616–20.

12. Hehlmann R, Berger U, Pfirrmann M, et al. Drug treatment is superior to allografting as first-line therapy in chronic myeloid leukemia. Blood 2007;109: 4686–92.

13. Silver RT. The blast phase of chronic myeloid leukaemia. Best Pract Res Clin Haematol 2009;22:387–94.

14. Druker BJ, Guilhot F, O'Brien SG, et al. Five-year follow-up of patients receiving imatinib for chronic myeloid leukemia. N Engl J Med 2006;355:2408–17.

15. Piazza RG, Magistroni V, Franceschino A, et al. The achievement of durable complete cytogenetic remission in late chronic and accelerated phase patients with CML treated with imatinib mesylate predicts for prolonged response at 6 years. Blood Cells Mol Dis 2006;37:111–15.

16. Hasford J, Pfirrmann M, Hehlmann R, et al. A new prognostic score for survival of patients with chronic myeloid leukemia treated with interferon alfa. Writing Committee for the Collaborative CML Prognostic Factors Project Group. J Natl Cancer Inst 1998;90:850–8.

17. Hochhaus A, Kreil S, Corbin AS, et al. Molecular and chromosomal mechanisms of resistance to imatinib (STI571) therapy. Leukemia 2002;16:2190–6.

18. Cortes JE, Talpaz M, Giles F, et al. Prognostic significance of cytogenetic clonal evolution in patients with chronic myelogenous leukemia on imatinib mesylate therapy. Blood 2003;101: 3794–800.

19. Jabbour E, Kantarjian H, Jones D, et al. Frequency and clinical significance of BCR-ABL mutations in patients with chronic myeloid leukemia treated with imatinib mesylate. Leukemia 2006; 20:1767–73.

20. Michiels JJ, Berneman Z, Schroyens W, et al. Philadelphia (Ph) chromosome-positive thrombocythemia without features of chronic myeloid leukemia in peripheral blood: natural history and diagnostic differentiation from Ph-negative essential thrombocythemia. Ann Hematol 2004;83:504–12.

21. Rice L, Popat U. Every case of essential thrombocythemia should be tested for the Philadelphia chromosome. Am J Hematol 2005;78:71–3.

22. Okun DB, Tanaka KR. Leukocyte alkaline phosphatase. Am J Hematol 1978;4: 293–9.

23. Georgii A, Buesche G, Kreft A. The histopathology of chronic myeloproliferative diseases. Baillière's Clin Haematol 1998;11:721–49.

24. Jacobsson S, Wadenvik H, Kutti J, Swolin B. Low megakaryocyte ploidy in Ph-positive chronic myelogenous leukemia measured by flow cytometry. Am J Clin Pathol 1999;111:185–90.

25. Thiele J, Kvasnicka HM, Fischer R. Bone marrow histopathology in chronic myelogenous leukemia (CML) – evaluation of distinctive features with clinical impact. Histol Histopathol 1999;14:1241–56.

26. Savage DG, Szydlo RM, Goldman JM. Clinical features at diagnosis in 430 patients with chronic myeloid leukaemia seen at a referral centre over a 16-year period. Br J Haematol 1997;96:111–16.

27. Lanza F, Bi S, Castoldi G, Goldman JM. Abnormal expression of N-CAM (CD56) adhesion molecule on myeloid and progenitor cells from chronic myeloid leukemia. Leukemia 1993;7:1570–5.

28. Urbano-Ispizua A, Cervantes F, Matutes E, et al. Immunophenotypic characteristics of blast crisis of chronic myeloid leukaemia: correlations with clinico-biological features and survival. Leukemia 1993;7:1349–54.

29. Busche G, Majewski H, Schlue J, et al. Frequency of pseudo-Gaucher cells in diagnostic bone marrow biopsies from patients with Ph-positive chronic myeloid leukaemia. Virchows Arch 1997;430: 139–48.

30. Anastasi J, Musvee T, Roulston D, et al. Pseudo-Gaucher histiocytes identified up to 1 year after transplantation for CML are BCR/ABL-positive. Leukemia 1998; 12:233–7.

31. Carrara RC, Orellana MD, Fontes AM, et al. Mesenchymal stem cells from patients with chronic myeloid leukemia do not express BCR-ABL and have absence of chimerism after allogeneic bone marrow transplant. Braz J Med Biol Res 2007;40:57–67.

32. Nowell PC, Kant JA, Finan JB, et al. Marrow fibrosis associated with a Philadelphia chromosome. Cancer Genet Cytogenet 1992;59:89–92.

33. Buesche G, Hehlmann R, Hecker H, et al. Marrow fibrosis, indicator of therapy failure in chronic myeloid leukemia – prospective long-term results from a randomized-controlled trial. Leukemia 2003;17:2444–53.

34. Buesche G, Ganser A, Schlegelberger B, et al. Marrow fibrosis and its relevance during imatinib treatment of chronic myeloid leukemia. Leukemia 2007; 21:2420–7.

35. Kimura A, Katoh O, Hyodo H, et al. Platelet derived growth factor expression, myelofibrosis and chronic myelogenous leukemia. Leuk Lymphoma 1995;18: 237–42.

36. Buesche G, Georgii A, Duensing A, et al. Evaluating the volume ratio of bone marrow affected by fibrosis: a parameter crucial for the prognostic significance of marrow fibrosis in chronic myeloid leukemia. Hum Pathol 2003;34:391–401.

37. Korkolopoulou P, Viniou N, Kavantzas N, et al. Clinicopathologic correlations of bone marrow angiogenesis in chronic myeloid leukemia: a morphometric study. Leukemia 2003;17:89–97.

38. Mayerhofer M, Valent P, Sperr WR, et al. BCR/ABL induces expression of vascular endothelial growth factor and its transcriptional activator, hypoxia inducible factor-1alpha, through a pathway involving phosphoinositide 3-kinase and the mammalian target of rapamycin. Blood 2002;100:3767–75.

39. Kvasnicka HM, Wickenhauser C, Thiele J, et al. Mixed chimerism of bone marrow vessels (endothelial cells, myofibroblasts) following allogeneic transplantation for chronic myelogenous leukemia. Leuk Lymphoma 2003;44:321–8.

40. Palandri F, Iacobucci I, Quarantelli F, et al. Long-term molecular responses to imatinib in patients with chronic myeloid leukemia: comparison between complete cytogenetic responders treated in early and in late chronic phase. Haematologica 2007;92:1579–80.

41. Kantarjian HM, O'Brien S, Cortes JE, et al. Treatment of Philadelphia chromosome-positive, accelerated-phase chronic myelogenous leukemia with imatinib mesylate. Clin Cancer Res 2002;8: 2167–76.

42. Alimena G, Breccia M, Latagliata R, et al. Sudden blast crisis in patients with Philadelphia chromosome-positive chronic myeloid leukemia who achieved complete cytogenetic remission after imatinib therapy. Cancer 2006;107: 1008–13.

43. Calabretta B, Perrotti D. The biology of CML blast crisis. Blood 2004;103: 4010–22.

44. Reid AG, De Melo VA, Elderfield K, et al. Phenotype of blasts in chronic myeloid leukemia in blastic phase – analysis of bone marrow trephine biopsies and correlation with cytogenetics. Leuk Res 2009;33:418–25.

45. Sokal JE, Cox EB, Baccarani M, et al. Prognostic discrimination in 'good-risk' chronic granulocytic leukemia. Blood 1984;63:789–99.

46. Bennett JM, Catovsky D, Daniel MT, et al. The chronic myeloid leukaemias: guidelines for distinguishing chronic granulocytic, atypical chronic myeloid, and chronic myelomonocytic leukaemia. Proposals by the French-American-British Cooperative Leukaemia Group. Br J Haematol 1994;87:746–54.

47. Onida F, Ball G, Kantarjian HM, et al. Characteristics and outcome of patients with Philadelphia chromosome negative, bcr/abl negative chronic myelogenous leukemia. Cancer 2002;95:1673–84.

48. Invernizzi R, Custodi P, de Fazio P, et al. The syndrome of abnormal chromatin clumping in leucocytes: clinical and biological study of a case. Haematologica 1990;75:532–6.

49. Pane F, Intrieri M, Quintarelli C, et al. BCR/ABL genes and leukemic phenotype: from molecular mechanisms to clinical correlations. Oncogene 2002;21:8652–67.

50. Mirza I, Frantz C, Clarke G, et al. Transformation of polycythemia vera to chronic myelogenous leukemia. Arch Pathol Lab Med 2007;131:1719–24.

51. Damaj G, Delabesse E, Le Bihan C, et al. Typical essential thrombocythaemia does not express bcr-abelson fusion transcript. Br J Haematol 2002;116:812–6.

52. Washington LT, Doherty D, Glassman A, et al. Myeloid disorders with deletion of 5q as the sole karyotypic abnormality: the clinical and pathologic spectrum. Leuk Lymphoma 2002;43:761–5.

53. Mrozek K, Heerema NA, Bloomfield CD. Cytogenetics in acute leukemia. Blood Rev 2004;18:115–36.

CHAPTER 25

Myeloproliferative neoplasms with eosinophilia

BJ Bain

In the 2008 World Health Organization (WHO) *Classification of Tumours of Haematopoietic and Lymphoid Tissues*[1] the term 'myeloproliferative neoplasm' (MPN) is preferrred to myeloproliferative disorder. Within the group of MPN is chronic eosinophilic leukemia, not otherwise specified.[2] Other neoplasms in which eosinophils constitute a dominant or major component are categorized according to the underlying molecular defect, a fusion gene incorporating part of *PDGFRA*, *PDGFRB* or *FGFR1*.[3] In the first and last of these groups of disorders there can also be a lymphoid component to the neoplasm, indicating that the responsible mutation occurred in a pluripotent lymphoid-myeloid stem cell. There are other MPN in which eosinophils are part of the neoplastic population but they are not usually a dominant feature. These include chronic myelogenous leukemia (*BCR-ABL1* positive) and systemic mastocytosis (SM). In addition, other well-defined MPN can undergo an eosinophilic transformation. The WHO categories of MPN with eosinophilia and a well defined genetic abnormality will be discussed first since a diagnosis of eosinophilic leukemia, not otherwise specified, can be made only when they have been excluded. Non-neoplastic disorders with eosinophilia are discussed in Chapter 16.

Myeloid and lymphoid neoplasms with *PDGFRA* rearrangement

Most neoplasms resulting from rearrangement of *PDGFRA* present as chronic eosophilic leukemia (CEL).[3,4] The natural history of this condition includes blastic transformation including myeloid sarcoma. A minority of patients present with acute leukemia, either myeloid or T-lymphoblastic with

Table 25.1 Possible clinicopathological features of chronic eosinophilic leukemias

Organ or system	Features
General	Fatigue, fever, weight loss, night sweats, headache
Hematological	Eosinophilia (by definition), variable increase in other leukocytes and their precursors, anemia, thrombocytopenia, increased bone marrow mast cells (in some subtypes), increased bone marrow reticulin, clonal cytogenetic or molecular abnormalities, increased serum vitamin B12, increased serum tryptase (in some subtypes)
Spleen	Splenomegaly, splenic infarction
Liver	Hepatomegaly
Lymph nodes	Lymphadenopathy (some subtypes)
Cardiovascular	Endocardial, myocardial and pericardial infiltration and damage, increased serum troponin, restrictive cardiomegaly, dilated cardiomyopathy, valvular incompetence, intracardiac thrombi and systemic embolization, cardiac failure, vasculitis, arterial thrombosis, Raynaud's phenomenon, digital necrosis, venous thromboembolism and pulmonary embolism
Respiratory	Cough, dyspnea as a result of infiltration, restrictive or obstructive pulmonary disease, pleural effusion
Skin	Pruritis, urticaria, angioedema, papules or nodules due to infiltration, vasculitis
Central and peripheral nervous system	Cranial nerve palsies, paraspinal masses, cerebral embolism, peripheral neuropathy
Gastrointestinal	Diarrhea as a result of infiltration, malabsorption, mucosal ulcers
Musculoskeletal	Myalgia, bone pain

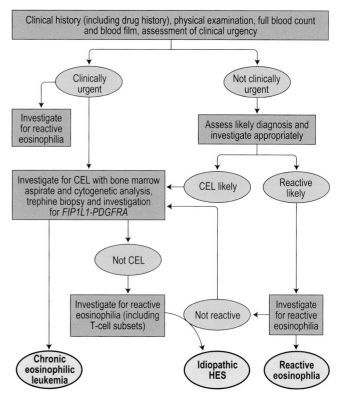

Fig. 25.1 An algorithm showing a diagnostic approach to eosinophilia and suspected eosinophilic leukemia

preceding eosinophilia being documented or being present at the time of diagnosis.[5]

The prototype of this group of neoplasms is CEL associated with a *FIP1L1-PDGFRA* fusion gene that has resulted from a cryptic interstitial deletion at 4q12. Until the discovery of this recurrent molecular abnormality[6] these patients were regarded as having the idiopathic hypereosinophilic syndrome (HES). The diagnosis of idiopathic HES can now not be made without exclusion of *FIP1L1-PDGFRA*.

Clinicopathological features result from tissue infiltration by eosinophils and organ damage by release of eosinophil granule contents (Table 25.1). Endocardial and myocardial damage is prominent, as is thrombosis.

Precise diagnosis of this condition is very important because of its sensitivity to treatment with imatinib and other tyrosine kinase inhibitors (TKI). Even patients who present in acute transformation can respond to imatinib. Because of the possibility of cardiac damage, rapid diagnosis can also be important. An algorithm showing a diagnostic approach to suspected eosinophilic leukemia is shown in Fig. 25.1.

Clinical features

This disease shows a remarkable male predominance (≥17:1), which is unexplained. It occurs at all ages but with the peak incidence in early adult life and middle age.

Presentation may be with systemic, respiratory, cardiac, gastrointestinal or cutaneous symptoms. Specifically there may be fatigue, cough, dyspnea, diarrhea, pruritis and syncope. The majority of patients have some degree of splenic enlargement. Other abnormalities on physical examination may include features of cardiac valve dysfunction and sometimes there is cardiac failure. Endocardial and valve disease can lead to embolization of brain, internal organs or limbs. Splinter hemorrhages may be present and represent the result of embolization. There may be a rash, cutaneous vasculitis or peripheral neuropathy. Urticaria pigmentosa has been observed but is quite uncommon. There may be mucosal ulcers affecting the mouth, the genitalia or the anus.

Pathologic features

Peripheral blood

There is eosinophilia and often neutrophilia. Some patients are anemic or thrombocytopenic. The eosinophils may be

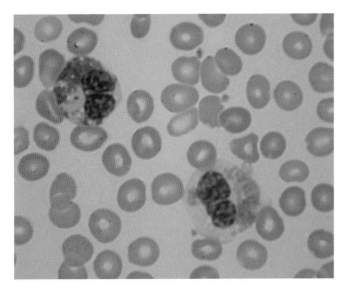

Fig. 25.2 Peripheral blood film from a patient with chronic eosinophilic leukemia (CEL) associated with a *FIP1L1-PDGFRA* fusion gene showing partially degranulated eosinophils. May–Grünwald–Giemsa (MGG) stain, ×100 objective.

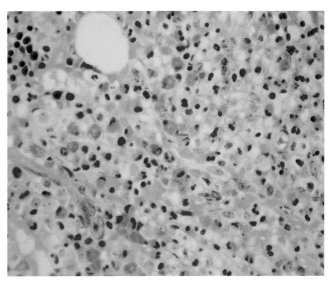

Fig. 25.4 Bone marrow trephine biopsy section from a patient with CEL associated with a *FIP1L1-PDGFRA* fusion gene showing hypercellularity and an increase of eosinophils and their precursors. Giemsa stain, ×100 objective.

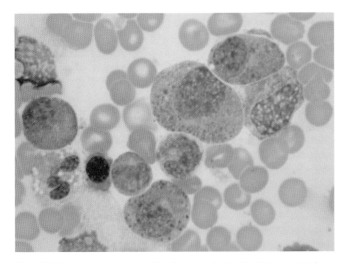

Fig. 25.3 Bone marrow aspirate film from a patient with CEL associated with a *FIP1L1-PDGFRA* fusion gene showing an increase of eosinophils and their precursors. May–Grünwald–Giemsa (MGG) stain, ×100 objective.

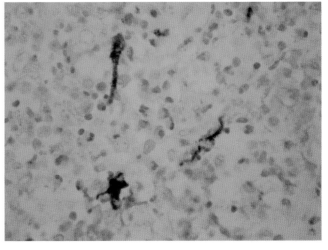

Fig. 25.5 Bone marrow trephine biopsy section from a patient with CEL associated with a *FIP1L1-PDGFRA* fusion gene showing an increase of spindle-shaped mast cells. Mast cell tryptase stain, ×50 objective.

cytologically normal but often there is degranulation, cytoplasmic vacuolation or nuclear abnormalities – either lack of segmentation or hypersegmentation (Fig. 25.2). Eosinophils may be sufficiently abnormal that they are not recognized by automated blood analyzers.

Bone marrow

The bone marrow (BM) aspirate is hypercellular as the result of an increase in eosinophils and their precursors. Eosinophil precursors may have purple-staining proeosinophilic granules (Fig. 25.3). There may also be an increase in neutrophils and precursors. Bone marrow trephine biopsy (BMTB) sections show dominance of granulopoiesis with prominent eosinophilia (Fig. 25.4). Reticulin is increased. The majority of patients also have increased mast cells (Fig.

25.5). These are often spindle-shaped and usually dispersed or in loose clusters but in occasional patients they form cohesive infiltrates similar to those of SM. The mast cells can express CD25, an abnormality that is also a feature of SM; they may or may not express CD2, which is usually expressed in SM.[3,7] CEL with increased BM mast cells has sometimes been misinterpreted as SM but it must be appreciated that SM with a *KIT* mutation and CEL with rearrangement of *PDGFRA* are distinct and different diseases.

Other tissues

Tissue infiltration by eosinophils is usual, and is notable in the respiratory and gastrointestinal tracts, endocardium and myocardium. The myocardium may show necrosis and both the endocardium and myocardium may show fibrosis.

Cardiac valve damage may be prominent. There may be arterial, venous or intracardiac thrombosis and peripheral or pulmonary embolism can occur.

Supplementary investigations

Serum tryptase is usually elevated. Serum vitamin B_{12} is markedly elevated as a result of increased transcobalamin I (haptocorrin). Serum troponin may be elevated in patients with active cardiac damage.

Cytogenetic analysis is usually normal but a minority of patients have a translocation with a 4q12 breakpoint or an unrelated abnormality such as trisomy 8. A secondary cytogenetic abnormality such as trisomy 8 may appear for the first time at evolution to AML.[8] Diagnosis is dependent on molecular analysis or fluorescence *in situ* hybridization (FISH) analysis. The reverse transcriptase polymerase chain reaction (RT-PCR) may demonstrate the *FIP1L1-PDGFRA* fusion gene but sometimes RT-PCR is negative and nested RT-PCR is required for demonstration of the fusion gene. Various FISH techniques are used. Mainly they rely on demonstration of deletion of the *CHIC2* gene, which is located between *FIP1L1* and *PDGFRA* and is thus included in the cryptic deletion (Fig. 25.6).[9] Probes flanking *FIP1L1* and *PDGFRA* can also be used with a dual-color break-apart technique.

A minority of patients have a different rearrangement of *PDGFRA*, usually as a result of a translocation. These include single patients with the hematological features of CEL associated with t(2;4)(p24;q12) and *STRN-PDGFRA*, t(4;12)(q12;p13) and *ETV6-PDGFRA* fusion, ins(9;4)(q33;q12q25) with *CDK5RAP2-PDGFRA* fusion and a complex rearrangement involving chromosomes 3, 4, 10 and probably 13 with *KIF5B-PDGFRA*. In addition a small number of patients have been described with hematological features intermediate between CEL and chronic myelogenous leukemia (CML) associated with t(4;22)(q12;q11) and *BCR-PDGFRA* fusion; T and B lymphoid transformations have occurred in this subgroup suggesting that the variant chromosomal rearrangements involving *PDGFRA* also occur in a pluripotent stem cell. Acquisition of a further mutation in the *FIP1L1-PDGFRA* fusion gene conveying imatinib resistance may be associated with refractoriness to imatinib and in some cases with evolution to AML.[8] The specific second mutation is of relevance since with T674I there is responsiveness to second line tyrosine kinase inhibitors whereas S801P is associated with resistance at least to imatinib and sorafenib[10] and D842V is associated with multiresistant disease.[11]

It should be noted that neither demonstration of a clonal rearrangement of a T-cell receptor gene[12] nor the occasional observation of an elevated serum immunoglobulin E^{7} excludes *FIP1L1-PDGFRA*-related CEL.

Myeloid neoplasms with *PDGFRB* rearrangement

The partner genes of myeloid neoplasms with a *PDGFRB* rearrangement are more numerous (Table 25.2) than is the case for myeloid neoplasms associated with rearrangement of *PDGFRA* and their clinicopathological features are more heterogeneous.[3] The most frequently observed causative

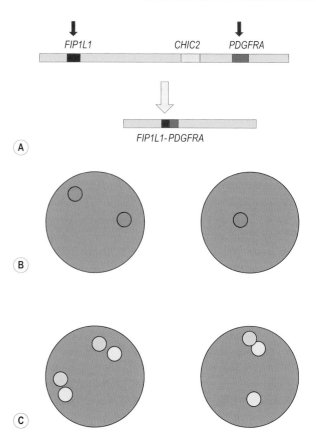

Fig. 25.6 (A–C) Diagram showing the principles of fluorescence *in situ* hybridization (FISH) analysis to demonstrate *CHIC2* loss, as a surrogate marker for *FIP1L1-PDGFRA* fusion: (A) illustration of the cryptic deletion that leads to loss of *CHIC2* and formation of a *FIP1L1-PDGFRA* fusion; the red arrows show the breakpoints and the yellow arrow the fusion gene; (B) single color probe for *CHIC2*; the normal cell (left) has two signals while the leukemic cell (right) has a single signal; (C) double color probes for *CHIC2* (orange) and the gene on the short arm of chromosome 4 (green); the normal cell (left) has two pairs of signals while the leukemic cell (right) has lost one of the *CHIC2* signals. *(Reproduced with permission from Bain BJ, Leukaemia Diagnosis, 4th Edn, Blackwell Publishing, Oxford, 2010.)*

cytogenetic/molecular abnormality is t(5;12)(q31-q33;p12) with *ETV6-PDGFRB* fusion. These neoplasms are responsive to TKI.

Clinical features

These neoplasms occur at all ages. There is a male predominance but this is much less striking than is the case for *PDGFRA*-related neoplasms, being about 2 : 1. Symptoms and signs are those related to the leukemic process (e.g. splenomegaly and less often hepatomegaly or skin infiltration) and those related specifically to the damaging effects of eosinophils on various tissues (e.g. cardiac damage). Acute transformation can occur.

Pathologic features

Peripheral blood

The hematological presentation may be as CEL but often there is more prominent involvement of other lineages so that the condition is better described as chronic myelo-

Table 25.2 Chronic eosinophilic leukemia and related conditions associated with rearrangement of *PDGFRB* (reproduced with minor modifications from[9])

Chromosomal rearrangement	Fusion gene	Hematological presentation
t(5;12)(q31-q33;p12) or variant	ETV6-PDGFRB	CEL or other MPN (CML, primary myelofibrosis transforming to AML) or MDS/MPN (CMML, aCML), usually with eosinophilia; bone marrow mast cells may be increased; AML
t(1;3;5)(p36;p21;q33)	WDR48-PDGFRB (WDR48 is at 3p22)	CEL
der(1)t(1;5)(p34;q33), der(5)t(1;5)(p34;q15), der(11)ins(11;5)(p12;q15q33)	GPIAP1-PDGRFB (GPIAP1 is at 11p13)	CEL
t(1;5)(q21;q33)	TPM3-PDGFRB	CEL
t(1;5)(q23;q33)	PDE4DIP-PDGFRB	MDS/MPN with eosinophilia
t(2;5)(p21;q33)	SPTBN1-PDGFRB	MPN with eosinophilia
t(3;5)(p21-25;q31-35)	GOLGA4-PDGFRB	CEL
t(4;5;5)(q23;q31;q33), t(4;5)(q21.2;q31.3) or t(4;5)(q21;q33)	PRKG2-PDGFRB	Two cases with chronic basophilic leukemia and abnormal bone marrow mast cells, one case with MPN with abnormal mast cells and an eosinophil count of 1.1×10^9/l
t(5;7)(q33;q11.2)	HIP1-PDGFRB	CMML with eosinophilia
t(5;10)(q33;q21)	CCDC6-PDGFRB	MPN with eosinophilia or aCML
t(5;12)(q31-33;q24)	GIT2-PDGFRB	CEL
t(5;12)(q33;p13.3)	ERC1-PDGFRB	AML (without eosinophilia)
t(5;14)(q33;q24)	NIN-PDGFRB	Ph-negative CML (13% eosinophils)
t(5;14)(q33;q32)	TRIP11-PDGFRB	Occurred at relapse of AML, associated with appearance of eosinophilia
t(5;14)(q33;q32)	CCDC88C-PDGFRB	CMML with eosinophilia
t(5;15)(q33;q22)	TP53BP1-PDGFRB	Ph-negative CML with prominent eosinophilia
t(5;16)(q33;p13)	NDE1-PDGFRB	CMML with eosinophilia
t(5;17)(q33;p11.2)	SPECC1-PDGFRB	JMML with eosinophilia
t(5;17)(q33;p13)	RABEP1-PDGFRB	CMML (without eosinophilia)
t(5;17)(q33-34;q11.2)	MYO18A-PDGFRB	MPN with eosinophilia

aCML, atypical chronic myeloid leukemia; CEL, chronic eosinophilic leukemia; CML, chronic myeloid leukemia; CMML, chronic myelomonocytic leukemia; JMML, juvenile myelomonocytic leukemia; MDS/MPN, myelodysplastic/myeloproliferative neoplasm; MPN, myeloproliferative neoplasm.

monocytic leukemia (CMML) with eosinophilia or, sometimes, atypical CML with eosinophilia. In a minority of patients eosinophilia has been absent. In the case of t(4;5) and related chromosomal rearrangements associated with *PRKG2-PDGFRB*, differentiation may be predominantly basophilic.[13,14] Otherwise there is a variable increase of neutrophils, monocytes, eosinophils and granulocyte precursors. There may be anemia or thrombocytopenia and trilineage dysplasia.

Bone marrow

The BM shows increased cellularity due to a variable increase of cells of neutrophil, eosinophil and monocyte lineages. The BMTB may show, in addition, an increase of mast cells, which may be spindle shaped, and reticulin may be increased. Mast cells resemble those of SM in expressing CD2 and CD25.

Other tissues

The spleen and other extramedullary sites may be infiltrated.

Supplementary investigations

Serum tryptase and serum vitamin B_{12} may be elevated. Cytogenetic analysis is essential for confirmation of the diagnosis. Unless there is a chromosomal rearrangement with a breakpoint it does not seem worthwhile to carry out molecular analysis to look for *PDGFRB* rearrangement, since cryptic rearrangements have rarely been described. It should be noted that FISH has occasionally been negative when Southern blot analysis was positive. The causative cytogenetic molecular lesions that have been described are summarized in Table 25.2.[9]

Myeloid and lymphoid neoplasms with *FGFR1* rearrangement

These rare neoplasms result from a number of translocations involving *FGFR1* occurring in a pluripotent lymphoid myeloid stem cell.[3,15,16] The most frequently observed translocations are t(8;13)(p11;q12), t(8;9)(p11;q33), t(6;8) (q27;p11-12) and t(8;22)(p11;q11). Common presentations are with CEL or other CML with eosinophilia, T lymphoblastic leukemia/lymphoma and myeloid sarcoma or acute myeloid leukemia (AML). However, B-lineage lymphoblastic leukemia/lymphoma also occurs. Mixed phenotype (B-myeloid) acute leukemia has been described. Often patients who present with AML or lymphoblastic leukemia/ lymphoma also have eosinophilia with the eosinophils being part of the leukemic clone. Patients who present in chronic phase as CEL may subsequently undergo lymphoid or myeloid transformation or even both.

Clinical features

The age range is wide with peak incidence being in young adults. There is a moderate male preponderance. The most frequently observed clinical features are lymphadenopathy and splenomegaly. Tonsillar involvement has been prominent among patients with t(8;9).[17] Systemic symptoms may be present. Prognosis is poor with those patients who present in chronic phase usually showing disease transformation within a year.

Pathologic features

Peripheral blood

Eosinophilia is almost always a feature. Other abnormalities depend on the specific form of leukemia or lymphoma present. There may be anemia, thrombocytopenia, neutrophilia, monocytosis, and circulating lymphoblasts or myeloblasts. Basophilia has been observed in association with *BCR-FGFR1* fusion and patients with this fusion gene have a disease that is phenotypically closer to chronic myelogenous leukemia.

Bone marrow

The BM may show only increased cellularity with an increase in eosinophils and precursors or there may be infiltration by lymphoblasts or myeloblasts (Fig. 25.7).

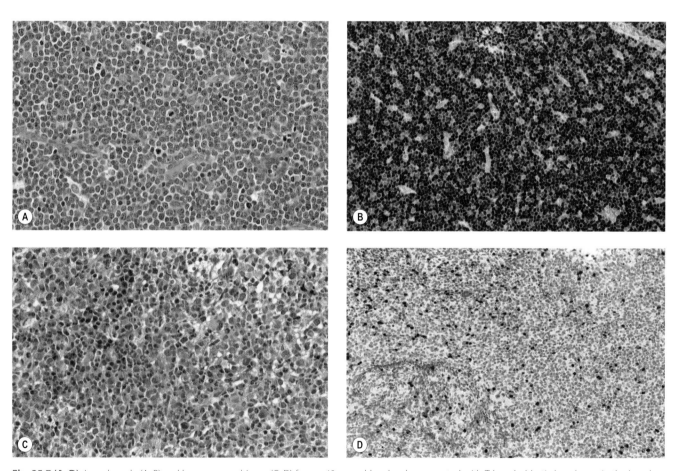

Fig. 25.7 (A–D) Lymph node (A, B) and bone marrow biopsy (C, D) from a 42-year-old male who presented with T-lymphoblastic lymphoma in the lymph node and chronic eosinophilic leukemia. In the lymph node there was a proliferation of blasts (A, ×40 objective) positive for terminal deoxynucleotidyl transferase (TdT) (B, ×20 objective) and cytoplasmic CD3 (not shown). The bone marrow showed a myeloproliferative neoplasm with a marked increase in eosinophils (C, ×40 objective) but only a few TdT-positive cells (D, ×20 objective). RT-PCR analysis showed *FIP1L1-PDGFRA* fusion transcripts in both lymph node and bone marrow samples. The patient responded well to combined chemotherapy and imatinib treatment. *(Photos courtesy of Dr Ugnius Mickys, National Centre of Pathology, Vilnius, Lithuania.)*

Table 25.3 Lymphoid and myeloid neoplasms associated with rearrangement of *FGFR1** (*modified from*[9])

Cytogenetics	Molecular genetics	Number	Hematological syndromes
t(8;13)(p11;q12)	ZNF198-FGFR1	21	CEL, T-ALL/T-LBL, AML, B-lineage ALL
t(8;9)(p11;q33)	CEP110-FGFR1	8	CEL, T-ALL/T-LBL; sometimes there is monocytosis or thrombocytosis
t(6;8)(q27;p11-12)	FGFR1OP1-FGFR1	6	CEL, T-ALL, AML, B-lineage ALL, polycythemia in four patients
t(8;22)(p11;q11)	BCR-FGFR1	5	CML; myeloid transformation may occur; one T + B lymphoid transformation
t(2;8)(q37;p11)[15]	LRRFIP1-FGFR1	1	RAEB; the translocation appeared 5 years later when eosinophilia developed; later evolved to AML
t(7;8)(q34;p11)	TRIM24-FGFR1	1	AML with eosinophilia
t(8;12)(p11;q15)[16]	CPSF6-FGFR1	1	T lymphoblastic lymphoma with mild eosinophilia
t(8;17)(p11;q23)	MYO18A-FGFR1	1	CML with severe thrombocytopenia
t(8;19)(p12;q13.3)	HERVK-FGFR1	1	AML with 45% bone marrow eosinophils
ins(12;8)(p11;p11p22)	FGFR1OP2-FGFR1	1	T-LBL and mild eosinophilia that progressed rapidly to AML

ALL, acute lymphoblastic leukemia; AML, acute myeloid leukemia; CEL, chronic eosinophilic leukemia; CML, chronic myeloid leukemia; RAEB, refractory anemia with excess of blasts; T-ALL, T-lineage acute lymphoblastic leukemia; T-LBL, T-lineage lymphoblastic lymphoma.

*In addition, *FGFR1* rearrangement has been found in association with t(8;12)(p11;q15) associated with T lymphoblastic lymphoma and MPN and with t(8;17)(p11;q25) associated with CML and systemic mastocytosis but the suspected involvement of *FGFR1* in t(8;11)(p11;p15) was not confirmed.

Other tissues

Lymph nodes may show lymphoblastic lymphoma with often eosinophilic infiltration. Myeloid sarcomas of soft tissues occur.

Supplementary investigations

Cytogenetic analysis is essential for the diagnosis. The reported cytogenetic abnormalities and equivalent molecular abnormalities are summarized in Table 25.3. Trisomy 21 is the most frequently observed secondary chromosomal abnormality.

Chronic eosinophilic leukemia, not otherwise specified

This diagnosis is made when there is eosinophilia (eosinophil count at least 1.5×10^9/l) with evidence that the disorder is leukemic in nature and there is no *BCR-ABL1* fusion or rearrangement of *PDGFRA. PDGFRB* or *FGFR1*. Cases with *RUNX1-RUNX1T1* and *CBFB-MYH11* fusion are also excluded. In the WHO classification[2] the evidence that the condition is leukemic may be either that blast cells are increased (more than 2% in the blood or more than 5% in the BM) or that there is a clonal cytogenetic or molecular genetic abnormality.

Clinical features

In some patients the diagnosis is an incidental one. In others there are symptoms such as fatigue, cough, diarrhea and pruritis. There may be enlargement of the liver and spleen. There may be cardiac damage and peripheral embolism, peripheral neuropathy and central nervous system dysfunction.

Pathologic features

Peripheral blood

There is eosinophilia as the dominant feature but there may be some increase of neutrophils or monocytes or the presence of granulocyte precursors including blast cells (Fig. 25.8). There may be anemia or thrombocytopenia.

Bone marrow

The BM shows an increase of eosinophils and precursors. Blast cells may be increased but are less than 20%. BMTB may show increased blast cells in addition to increased eosinophils and precursors (Fig. 25.9) as well as increased reticulin.

Other tissues

The spleen and liver are often infiltrated.

Supplementary investigations

Cytogenetic analysis may show a clonal cytogenetic abnormality such as trisomy 8, del(20q), i(17)(q10), trisomy 10, −Y (not necessarily a clonal abnormality), monosomy 11 plus monosomy 19[18] or del(16)(q22).[19] A few patients have t(8;9)(p23;p24) with *PCM1-JAK2* fusion.[20] Occasional patients have other translocations such as t(1;4)(q24;q35)[21] and a variety of translocations involving chromosome 9 producing an *ETV6-ABL1* fusion gene (at least four patients

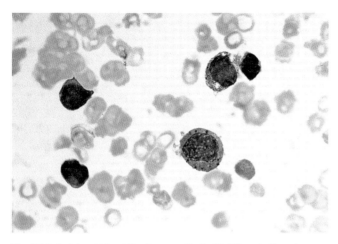

Fig. 25.8 Peripheral blood film from a patient with CEL, not otherwise specified, showing an abnormal non-lobulated eosinophil, an eosinophil myelocyte and three unidentifiable leukemic cells. MGG, ×100 objective.

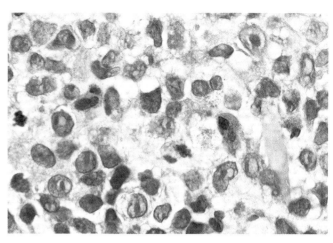

Fig. 25.9 Bone marrow trephine biopsy section from a patient with CEL, not otherwise specified, showing three mature eosinophils, eosinophil precursors (promyelocytes and myelocytes) and several blast cells. Hematoxylin and eosin, ×100 objective.

reported).[22] Other patients have a clonal molecular abnormality. $JAK2^{V617F}$ has been described in at least seven patients[18,23] but this is an uncommon finding in eosinophilic leukemia (2/36 of cases in one systematic study and 2/134 in another[18]).

Eosinophilia in other myeloproliferative neoplasms

Dominant eosinophilia is uncommon in MPN but well documented cases have been reported.

Chronic myelogenous leukemia

Philadelphia-positive, *BCR-ABL1*-positive CML usually has an absolute eosinophilia but it is very unusual for eosinophilia to be the predominant manifestation. Occasional such cases have been reported.[24,25] The poor prognosis that has been reported suggests that these cases may represent disease already in evolution. Interpretation of dominant eosinophilia as a manifestation of accelerated phase disease is suggested by a patient in whom only 60% of BM metaphases showed t(9;22).[25]

Primary myelofibrosis

Eosinophilic leukemia has been reported in myelofibrosis but without detailed documentation of the nature of the condition;[26,27] these two cases were not investigated for a *JAK2* or *MPL* mutation or for *FIP1L1-PDGRA* fusion although the first case did have typical clinicopathological features of primary myelofibrosis.

Systemic mastocytosis

Eosinophilia is recognized as a feature of SM. The mechanism is likely to be complex. Eosinophils could be part of the neoplastic clone, they could be non-clonal eosinophils

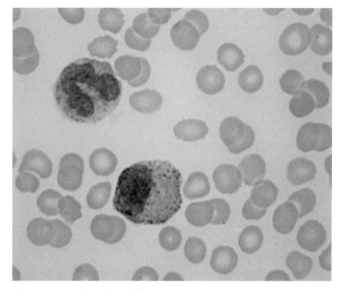

Fig. 25.10 Peripheral blood film showing eosinophilic transformation of primary myelofibrosis. Two highly dysplastic eosinophils have granules that stain unusual colors. MGG, ×100 objective.

present in increased numbers because of cytokines secreted by neoplastic mast cells or they could be clonal eosinophils with production further augmented by mast cell-derived cytokines. It is likely that all three possibilities actually occur.

Eosinophilic transformation of other myeloid neoplasms

CEL can occur as part of the disease evolution of MPN, e.g. in *BCR-ABL1*-positive CML, polycythemia vera[28] or primary myelofibrosis (Fig. 25.10). Eosinophilic transformation of myelodysplastic/myeloproliferative neoplasms (MDS/MPN) such as CMML can also occur.[29] Eosinophilic transformation can occur in MDS but is uncommon. In one survey of 322 patients defined as MDS by French-American-British (FAB) criteria (therefore including CMML and refractory anemia with excess of blasts in transformation) one patient with CMML developed an eosinophil/basophil transformation (both cell types at least 20%) and a further seven patients (2.1%) developed an eosinophil transformation (eosinophils at least 20%).[29]

Conclusions

Eosinophilia may be the sole or dominant manifestation of an MPN. In other patients eosinophilia is just one feature of the disease. The presence of eosinophilia is significant since there may be resultant tissue damage. Determining the underlying cytogenetic/molecular genetic abnormality may be crucial since some of these conditions show sensitivity to tyrosine kinase inhibitors.

References

1. Swerdlow SH, Campo E, Harris NL, et al. WHO Classification of Tumours of Haematopoietic and Lymphatic Tissues. Lyon: IARC; 2008.
2. Bain B, Gilliland DG, Vardiman J, Horny HP. Chronic eosinophilic leukaemia, not otherwise specified. World Health Organization Classification of Tumours of Haematopoietic and Lymphoid Tissue. Lyon: IARC Press; 2008. p. 51–3.
3. Bain B, Gilliland DG, Horny HP, Vardiman J. Myeloid and lymphoid neoplasms with eosinophilia and abnormalities of PDGFRA, PDGFRB and FGFR1. World Health Organization Classification of Tumours of Haematopoietic and Lymphoid Tissue. Lyon: IARC Press; 2008.
4. Gleich GJ, Leiferman KM. The hypereosinophilic syndromes: current concepts and treatments. Br J Haematol 2009;145:271–85.
5. Metzgeroth G, Walz C, Score J, et al. Recurrent finding of the FIP1L1-PDGFRA fusion gene in eosinophilia-associated acute myeloid leukemia and lymphoblastic T-cell lymphoma. Leukemia 2007;21:1183–8.
6. Cools J, DeAngelo DJ, Gotlib J, et al. A tyrosine kinase created by fusion of the PDGFRA and FIP1L1 genes as a therapeutic target of imatinib in idiopathic hypereosinophilic syndrome. N Engl J Med 2003;348:1201–14.
7. Metzgeroth G, Walz C, Erben P, et al. Safety and efficacy of imatinib in chronic eosinophilic leukaemia and hypereosinophilic syndrome: a phase-II study. Br J Haematol 2008;143:707–15.
8. von Bubnoff N, Sandherr M, Schlimok G, et al. Myeloid blast crisis evolving during imatinib treatment of an FIP1L1-PDGFR alpha-positive chronic myeloproliferative disease with prominent eosinophilia. Leukemia 2005;19:286–7.
9. Bain B. Leukemia Diagnosis. Oxford: Blackwell Publishing; 2010.
10. Salemi S, Yousefi S, Simon D, et al. A novel FIP1L1-PDGFRA mutant destabilizing the inactive conformation of the kinase domain in chronic eosinophilic leukemia/hypereosinophilic syndrome. Allergy 2009;64:913–8.
11. Lierman E, Michaux L, Beullens E, et al. FIP1L1-PDGFRalpha D842V, a novel panresistant mutant, emerging after treatment of FIP1L1-PDGFRalpha T674I eosinophilic leukemia with single agent sorafenib. Leukemia 2009;23:845–51.
12. Helbig G, Moskwa A, Swiderska A, et al. Weekly imatinib dosage for chronic eosinophilic leukaemia expressing FIP1L1-PDGFRA fusion transcript: extended follow-up. Br J Haematol 2009;145:132–4.
13. Walz C, Metzgeroth G, Haferlach C, et al. Characterization of three new imatinib-responsive fusion genes in chronic myeloproliferative disorders generated by disruption of the platelet-derived growth factor receptor beta gene. Haematologica 2007;92:163–9.
14. Lahortiga I, Akin C, Cools J, et al. Activity of imatinib in systemic mastocytosis with chronic basophilic leukemia and a PRKG2-PDGFRB fusion. Haematologica 2008;93:49–56.
15. Soler G, Nusbaum S, Varet B, et al. LRRFIP1, a new FGFR1 partner gene associated with 8p11 myeloproliferative syndrome. Leukemia 2009;23:1359–61.
16. Hidalgo-Curtis C, Chase A, Drachenberg M, et al. The t(1;9)(p34;q34) and t(8;12) (p11;q15) fuse pre-mRNA processing proteins SFPQ (PSF) and CPSF6 to ABL and FGFR1. Genes Chromosomes Cancer 2008;47:379–85.
17. Park TS, Song J, Kim JS, et al. 8p11 myeloproliferative syndrome preceded by t(8;9)(p11;q33), CEP110/FGFR1 fusion transcript: morphologic, molecular, and cytogenetic characterization of myeloid neoplasms associated with eosinophilia and FGFR1 abnormality. Cancer Genet Cytogenet 2008;181:93–9.
18. Helbig G, Majewski M, Wieczorkiewicz A, et al. Screening for JAK2 V617F point mutation in patients with hypereosinophilic syndrome – in response to 'Hypereosinophilic syndrome: another face of Janus?' by Dahabreh et al. published in Leukemia Research, in press. Leuk.Res 2009;33:e1–2.
19. Kamineni P, Baptiste A, Hassan M, et al. Case of chronic eosinophilic leukemia with deletion of chromosome 16 and hepatitis C. J Natl Med Assoc 2006;98:1356–60.
20. Cornfield DB, Gheith SM, Friedman EL. A third case of chronic eosinophilic leukemia with the (8;9)(p23;p24) translocation. Cancer Genet Cytogenet 2008;185:60–1.
21. Arora RS. Chronic eosinophilic leukemia with a unique translocation. Indian Pediatr 2009;46:525–7.
22. Keung YK, Beaty M, Steward W, et al. Chronic myelocytic leukemia with eosinophilia, t(9;12)(q34;p13), and ETV6-ABL gene rearrangement: case report and review of the literature. Cancer Genet Cytogenet 2002;138:139–42.
23. Dahabreh IJ, Giannouli S, Zoi C, et al. Hypereosinophilic syndrome: another face of Janus? Leuk Res 2008;32:1483–5.
24. Gotlib V, Darji J, Bloomfield K, et al. Eosinophilic variant of chronic myeloid leukemia with vascular complications. Leuk Lymphoma 2003;44:1609–13.
25. Aggrawal DK, Bhargava R, Dolai TK, et al. An unusual presentation of eosinophilic variant of chronic myeloid leukemia (eoCML). Ann Hematol 2009;88:89–90.
26. Cox MC, Panetta P, Venditti A, et al. New reciprocal translocation t(6;10) (q27;q11) associated with idiopathic myelofibrosis and eosinophilia. Leuk Res 2001;25:349–51.
27. Ishii Y, Ito Y, Kuriyama Y, et al. Successful treatment with imatinib mesylate of hypereosinophilic syndrome (chronic eosinophilic leukemia) with myelofibrosis. Leuk Res 2004;28(Suppl 1):S79–80.
28. Chim CS, Ma SK. Eosinophilic leukemic transformation in polycythemia rubra vera (PRV). Leuk Lymphoma 2005;46:447–50.
29. Wimazal F, Baumgartner C, Sonneck K, et al. Mixed-lineage eosinophil/basophil crisis in MDS: a rare form of progression. Eur J Clin Invest 2008;38:447–55.

Systemic mastocytosis

H-P Horny

Definition

Systemic mastocytosis (SM) is a clonal disease derived from transformed bone marrow (BM) progenitor cells, histologically characterized by accumulations of atypical mast cells in various tissue sites. SM presents an unusually broad spectrum of morphological and clinical features. In approximately 30% of SM patients, a systemic mastocytosis-associated hematologic non-mast cell disorder (SM-AHNMD) is diagnosed simultaneously, before or after SM diagnosis.

Introduction

SM diagnosis is based on morphology and cannot be established on the basis of clinical findings alone. Therefore, the pathologist should be familiar with the diagnostic criteria defined for mastocytosis and also to recognize its mimickers.[1,2] Important mimickers of mastocytosis are reactive states of mast cell hyperplasia and a few rare neoplastic hematological disorders such as tryptase-positive acute myeloid leukemia (AML) or myelomastocytic leukemia. Diagnostic criteria of SM are given in Box 26.1.

The major and two of four minor diagnostic criteria are morphology-based. Diagnosis of SM can be established if the major and one minor criterion are fulfilled. In cases lacking the major criterion, SM diagnosis can be established if at least three minor criteria are found.[1,2] Most cases of SM can be easily diagnosed when focal compact infiltrates with a significant proportion of spindle-shaped mast cells are present. SM exhibiting exclusively round mast cells can be diagnosed after demonstration of an atypical immunophenotype with expression of CD25, which is not present in normal mast cells.[3] If compact mast cell infiltrates are missing, diffusely scattered spindle-shaped mast cells with CD25 expression alone are not enough to establish a diagnosis of mastocytosis. In these patients, demonstration of the KIT^{D816V} mutation and/or chronically elevated serum tryptase enables diagnosis of mastocytosis since three of four minor criteria are fulfilled.[4,5,6]

BM is the main tissue where diagnosis of SM can be established. However, demonstration of compact mast cell infiltrates in extramedullary tissues like lymph node, spleen, liver and/or mucosa should also be regarded as strong indication for SM.[7,8,9] Rarely, the diagnosis of mastocytosis is first established in the mucosa of the gastrointestinal (GI) tract and BM involvement is confirmed later. It is rather unlikely that pure GI form exists. In all patients with GI involvement, the meticulous investigation of the BM should be performed using immunohistochemistry and molecular biology. In a considerable proportion of SM patients, the degree of tissue infiltration is very low. The WHO 2008 classification of mastocytosis is given in Box 26.2.[2] The approach to the diagnosis of mastocytosis is complex and considering its relatively low incidence, the diagnosis is usually more difficult than in most other hematological malignancies. The different forms of SM can only be recognized when the pathologist is aware of important clinical findings, especially the so-called 'B-findings', including organomegaly, and

Major diagnostic criterion

Focal compact tissue infiltrate predominantly or *exclusively* composed of mast cells.

Minor diagnostic criteria

1. Prominent spindling of mast cells (>25%).
2. Atypical immunophenotype of mast cells with expression of CD25 and/or CD2.
3. Activating point mutation of c-kit in codon 816 (usually: KITD816V).
4. Chronically elevated serum tryptase (>20 ng/ml).

Box 26.2 Classification of mastocytosis (WHO 2008)[2]

1. Cutaneous mastocytosis (CM) includes urticaria pigmentosa/maculopapular cutaneous mastocytosis, diffuse cutaneous mastocytosis and solitary mastocytoma of the skin.
2. Systemic mastocytosis (SM) (meets criteria in Box 26.1)
   i. Indolent systemic mastocytosis (ISM) has no 'C' findings (see below). Includes BM mastocytosis (with no skin involvement) and smoldering SM (two or more B findings)
   ii. SM-associated hematologic non-mast cell disorder (SM-AHNMD)
   iii. Aggressive systemic mastocytosis (ASM) has one or more C findings but no evidence of mast cell leukemia.
   iv. Mast cell leukemia (MCL) must show 20% or more mast cells in BM smears
3. Mast cell sarcoma (MCS) is a unifocal mast cell tumor with high-grade cytology and destructive growth pattern.
4. Extracutaneous mastocytoma (ECM) is a unifocal mast cell tumor with low-grade cytology and no destructive growth pattern.

'B' findings

1. BM biopsy showing >30% infiltration of mast cells and/or serum tryptase level >200 ng/ml.
2. Signs of dysplasia or myeloproliferation in non-mast cell lineages but criteria for definitive diagnosis of AHNMD are not fulfilled.
3. Hepatomegaly without impairment of liver function and/or palpable splenomegaly without hypersplenisn and/or lymphadenopathy.

'C' findings

1. One or more cytopenia (ANC <1 × 10^9/l, Hb<10 g/l, or platelets <100 × 10^9/l) but no criteria for AHNMD.
2. Hepatomegaly with impairment of liver function, ascites and/or portal hypertension.
3. Skeletal involvement with osteolytic lesions and/or pathological fractures.
4. Splenomegaly with hypersplenism.
5. Malabsorption of weight loss due to GI mast cell infiltrates.

'C-findings', indicating organ dysfunction due to widespread mast cell infiltration (Box 26.2).

Molecular genetics aspects

Mast cells of most patients with SM carry the activating point mutation KIT^{D816V} of the *c-kit* gene.[10] However, the frequency of KIT^{D816V} varies between subtypes of the disease. It has been found in almost 100% of patients with SM-AHNMD but only in about 50–60% of patients with aggressive SM and mast cell leukemia (MCL). Indolent SM assumes an intermediate position. Other than D816V point mutations of *c-kit* (e.g. D816Y or D816H) do occur but are rarely detected in SM.[11] A considerable number of patients with SM-AHNMD were found to carry KIT^{D816V} not only in the SM but also in the AHNMD compartment of the disease. The frequency of KIT^{D816V} depends on the subtype of hematological disorder. SM-associated chronic myelomonocytic leukemia (CMML) exhibits KIT^{D816V} in almost all cases. The mutation is found both in the SM and the AHNMD compartment of the disease, which underlines a close clonal relationship between SM and CMML in the setting of SM-AHNMD. In SM associated with a myeloproliferative neoplasm with eosinophilia (MPNEo), KIT^{D816V} is usually not found in the MPNEo. Very surprisingly, it is also lacking in the SM compartment, although compact infiltrates of CD25$^+$ mast cells are present in a few cases thus enabling the morphological diagnosis of SM.[12] In other types of SM-AHNMD (SM with myelodysplastic syndrome (SM-MDS), SM-AML, and SM with myeloproliferative neoplasms (SM-MPN)), the incidence of KIT^{D816V} in the associated disorder varies between 20% and 60% of patients. Interestingly, it has been shown that in cases of SM-MPN (e.g. primary myelofibrosis), both mast cells and cells of neutrophilic lineage could carry *both* activating point mutations KIT^{D816V} *and* JAK-2^{V617F}, further indicating the close relationship between SM and 'AHNMD'.[13]

Important messages

1. Indolent SM (ISM) is the most frequent subtype of the disease. In more than 90% of patients with long-standing adult-type cutaneous mastocytosis (CM), mostly urticaria pigmentosa, bone marrow trephine biopsies (BMTB) exhibit features of ISM when the sample is investigated with appropriate immunological and molecular methods.[14]
2. SM-AHNMD is the most frequent diagnosis in patients without cutaneous disease.[15,16,17] In up to 10% of BMTB from patients with all myeloid neoplasms irrespective of the subtype (MDS, myelodysplastic/myeloproliferative neoplasms (MDS/MPN such as CMML), MPN, and AML) investigated with antibodies against tryptase, CD25 and CD117, atypical spindle-shaped CD25-expressing mast cells are found. Overt SM is present in about 5% of these patients. Almost all of SM-AHNMD patients carry the KIT^{D816V} mutation. In many of these patients, KIT^{D816V} mutation is not limited to the SM compartment but can be detected in a significant proportion of malignant cells of hematological disorder, especially when analyses are performed using microdissection technique.[13]
3. CMML is the hematological disorder most frequently associated with SM. Myeloid neoplasms, in particular AML and MPN, may even obscure SM, which is detected only after chemotherapy and remission of the basic disease (= 'occult mastocytosis').[18]
4. Juvenile patients almost exclusively present with CM without clinical signs of systemic involvement and a good chance of spontaneous regression at puberty.[19] Adults with CM should be monitored for systemic

spread of the disease (ISM), when the serum tryptase is chronically elevated and/or the cutaneous mast cells exhibit an atypical immunophenotype with expression of CD25. Detection of the KIT[D816V] mutation in the skin should prompt suspicion of SM and investigation of a BMTB is strongly recommended in such patients.

Routine work-up of cases with suspected systemic mastocytosis

To be able to establish a proper diagnosis including classification of SM, the hematopathologist must be provided with clinical data concerning presence of urticaria pigmentosa or another mastocytosis-related rash, hepatosplenomegaly and/or lymphadenopathy, cytopenia or increase in blood cells such as thrombocytosis, allergy, and elevated serum tryptase.

Bone marrow trephine biopsy

The adequate BMTB specimen should be above 2 cm in length. Antibodies against CD25, CD117 and tryptase should be applied.[20,21,22,23] In cases of suspected SM-AHNMD further immunohistochemical stainings with appropriate antibodies depending on the subtype of the hematological disorder should also be performed. The tissue can also be used for demonstration of the KIT[D816V] mutation, which is best detected if the biopsy is fixed in 5% buffered neutral formalin and mildly decalcified in ethylenediaminetetraacetic acid (EDTA) overnight. Peripheral blood (PB) and BM smears are crucial for differential diagnosis between aggressive SM (ASM) and aleukemic MCL or aleukemic from leukemic MCL, respectively.

General morphological aspects of SM

Diagnosis of SM is usually established on the basis of BM findings. Investigation of a BMTB specimen is necessary in all cases with the exception of the very rare cases of MCL where evaluation of BM and blood smears is sufficient for diagnosis. There are various infiltration patterns that can be associated with the different subtypes of SM:

1. *Multifocal infiltration.* If the degree of involvement is low (5% or less of the section area), the most probable diagnoses are indolent SM or isolated SM of the bone marrow. However, mild multifocal involvement is also found in most cases of SM-AHNMD. In cases with more pronounced infiltration, smouldering SM or even ASM are the most probable diagnoses.
2. *Diffuse compact infiltration* is associated with aggressive or even leukemic SM.
3. *Diffuse interstitial infiltration* is usually associated with indolent or occult SM. However, the diagnosis of SM cannot be established here by morphology alone. The important major criterion is usually missing and only two of three required minor criteria are present, namely prominent spindling and aberrant immunophenotype of mast cells (expression of CD25). In these patients, it is crucial to detect at least one non-morphological minor criterion such as chronically elevated serum tryptase and/or the KIT[D816V] point mutation to establish SM diagnosis.

Size and cytological composition of compact (diagnostic) mast cell infiltrates varies greatly. Mast cells are not always dominant and may be obscured by follicle-like aggregates of lymphocytes. The lymphocyte-dominated infiltrates may mimic lymphocytic lymphoma, which is almost always accompanied by an increase in reactive (round, strongly metachromatic) mast cells posing considerable differential diagnostic problems in some cases (Fig. 26.1A).[24] In contrast

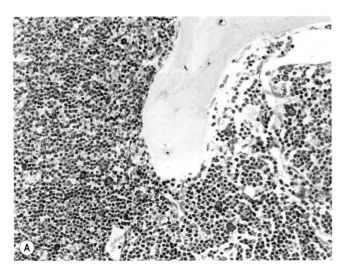
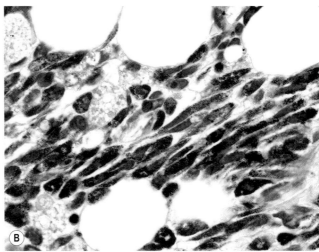

Fig. 26.1 (A,B) (A) Mast cell hyperplasia. Giemsa stained bone marrow trephine biopsy shows extremely hypercellular bone marrow with diffuse compact infiltration by a non-Hodgkin's lymphoma of lymphocytic subtype. A significant increase in loosely scattered, round, strongly metachromatic mast cells is almost always seen in this particular subtype of malignant lymphoma. This is the typical finding of a reactive increase in mast cells termed mast cell hyperplasia. (B) Systemic mastocytosis (focal infiltration of bone marrow). Giemsa stained bone marrow trephine biopsy with a focal compact infiltrate consisting of atypical spindle-shaped hypogranulated mast cells exhibiting elongated nuclei without inconspicuous nucleoli. The diagnosis of systemic mastocytosis is possible on the basis of this finding alone since the major criterion (compact mast infiltrate) and one minor criterion (predominance of spindle-shaped mast cells) are fulfilled, ×10, ×40 objective.

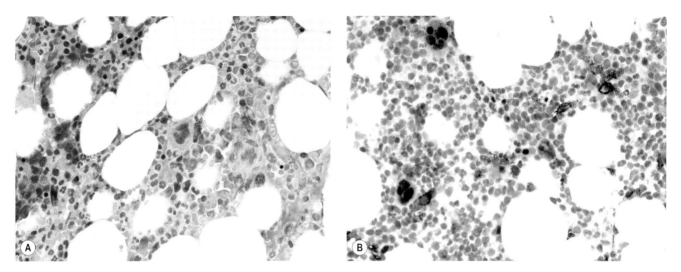

Fig. 26.2 (A, B) (A) Systemic mastocytosis with diffuse interstitial infiltration of bone marrow. Giemsa stained bone marrow trephine biopsy with an increase in loosely scattered atypical spindle-shaped hypogranulated mast cells before the background of a normal hemopoiesis. (B) Systemic mastocytosis with diffuse interstitial infiltration of bone marrow. Immunohistochemistry anti-CD25 (ABC method) reveals an aberrant phenotype of mast cells expressing CD25 (an antigen, which is not detected on normal/reactive mast cells). Note that CD25-positivity of megakaryocytes can be used as an internal control since CD25-expressing lymphoid cells are rarely found in the bone marrow. Such findings are seen in a considerable number of adults with long-standing urticaria pigmentosa (cutaneous mastocytosis). Since compact mast cell infiltrates are missing and only two of at least three minor criteria (prominent spindling, CD25-expression) are fulfilled, diagnosis of systemic mastocytosis cannot be established on the basis of morphology alone. An additional finding (activating point mutation KITD816V and/or chronically elevated serum tryptase), however, is sufficient for diagnosis of systemic mastocytosis, ×25, ×25 objective.

to mast cell hyperplasia, most SM cases exhibit at least one compact infiltrate consisting of slightly atypical often spindle-shaped and hypogranulated mast cells (Fig. 26.1B). Increased numbers of eosinophils are also usually found, admixed to lymphocytes and mast cells. Eosinophilic micro-abscesses are rarely detected. Focal increase in eosinophils within these compact infiltrates is only rarely accompanied by a significant eosinophilia in the hematopoietic islands. Stromal reaction shows almost always a dense network of reticulin fibers with the possibility to transform into collagen fibrosis. In some cases, the infiltrates may show striking variation in morphological appearance within the same biopsy specimen, ranging from large foci of collagen fibrosis with loosely scattered spindle-shaped mast cells to smaller lymphoid follicle-like structures with adjacent compact micronodules of round hypogranulated mast cells containing only slightly increased amounts of reticulin fibers. In larger infiltrates, there is also a significant angio-neogenesis with increase in small blood vessels. In most cases, mast cell infiltrates show a predominant peritrabecular localization leading to focal sclerosis of the adjacent bone. Cytomorphology of mast cells also varies greatly, ranging from cases with a predominance of spindle-shaped, markedly hypogranulated cells to cases containing exclusively round hypergranulated, mature-appearing mast cells, posing here the differential diagnosis of well-differentiated SM. The numbers of loosely scattered atypical mast cells are usually hard to estimate in Giemsa-stained sections (Fig. 26.2A), but they can be easily seen in CD25 immunostaining (Fig. 26.2B). It is crucial to apply all three antibodies: CD25, CD117 (KIT) and tryptase in all cases of suspected SM, in order to identify spindle-shaped, hypogranulated, fibroblast-like cells as mast cells, to recognize an aberrant immunophenotype with CD25-expression, and to be able to estimate the degree of

the diffuse involvement of the BM aside from the compact mast cell infiltrates However, co-expression of tryptase and CD117 defines both normal/reactive and clonal-neoplastic mast cells of all stages of maturation and all degrees of atypia. Tryptase-expressing cells without CD117 are not mast cells but can be regarded as (neoplastic) basophils or myeloblasts. Such tryptase-positive CD117-negative cells are small to medium-sized and exclusively round. CD117-positive tryptase-negative cells are not mast cells but most likely BM progenitor cells of granulopoietic and/or erythropoietic lineage. Mast cells of high-grade subtypes like aggressive or leukemic SM may express some other aberrant markers like CD30 and/or CD33 that easily may lead to an erroneous diagnosis when the relevant mast cell-associated antibodies are not applied. In most patients with ISM or isolated SM of the bone marrow, the hematopoiesis is completely normal. Some signs of so-called inflammatory reaction like plasmacytosis, ceroid histiocytosis and eosinophilia are often present. In cases with aggressive SM or MCL, the hematopoiesis is often markedly reduced or almost completely effaced. It may be very difficult to assess or exclude the diagnosis of an 'AHNMD' (i.e., ASM-AHNMD or MCL-AHMD) in such cases. It is therefore strongly recommended to analyse BM and PB smears carefully in order not to miss an associated hematological malignancy. There are cases of ASM with subtotal involvement of the BM, where PB investigation revealed a diagnosis of CMML thus leading to the ultimate diagnosis of ASM-CMML. It is likely that 'pure' aggressive SM is a very uncommon disorder and ASM-AHNMD is the common setting (own unpublished observations).

In cases of SM-AHNMD, each disease component has to be properly classified. Accordingly, the histological BM picture shows an extremely broad variation ranging from occult SM

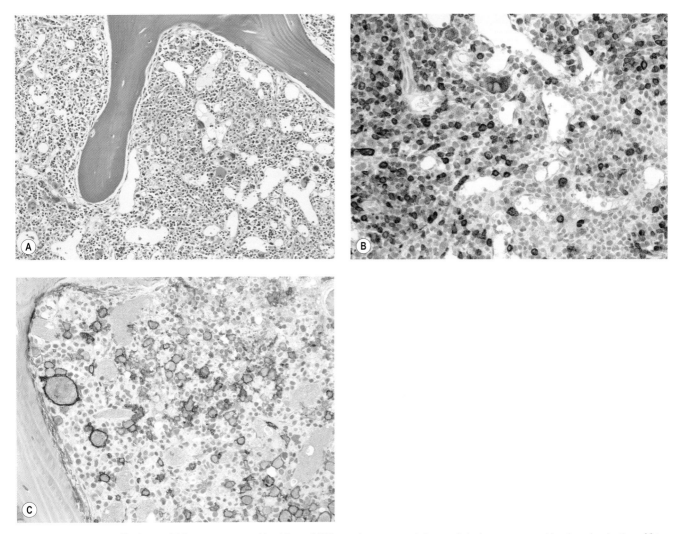

Fig. 26.3 (A–C) Mast cell leukemia. (A) Bone marrow trephine biopsy (H&E) reveals an extremely hypercellular bone marrow with subtotal reduction of fat cells and normal blood cell precursors. Note the prominent sinus-like structures. The picture is dominated by medium-sized to large sometimes bizarre and multinucleated blast-like cells forming dense infiltrates. A few groups of atypical grouped megakaryocytes can also be seen. Tryptase immunohistochemistry (B) reveals that blast cells are in fact atypical mast cells. A minor portion of mast cells co-express the activation antigen CD30, which is not found on normal/reactive mast cells and on mast cells of 'low-grade' systemic mastocytosis (C; author's unpublished observation), ×10, ×25, ×25 objective.

only detectable by a meticulous immunohistochemical investigation and additional molecular analysis, to aggressive or leukemic SM obscuring the associated neoplasm (AHNMD). The morphological aspects vary dependent on the subtype of the AHNMD, among which myeloid neoplasms are much more common than lymphatic tumors. Among myeloid neoplasms, CMML is most frequent, while among the lymphatic tumors plasma cell myeloma predominates.

TROCI-bm (= tryptase positive round cell infiltrate of the bone marrow)[25] is a recently described immunohistochemical phenomenon, defined as focal or diffuse but always compact tissue infiltrates consisting exclusively of tryptase-expressing *round* cells in the BM. TROCI-bm is only seen in some rare hematological neoplasms. Diffuse TROCI-bm is encountered in myelomastocytic leukemia, MCL or chronic basophilic leukemia. Focal TROCI-bm is seen in common type systemic mastocytosis, well-differentiated mastocytosis or chronic basophilic leukemia, as well as in accelerated phase of chronic myeloid leukemia (CML).

Bone marrow smears

In most cases, evaluation of BM smears is not sufficient for diagnosis of SM. However, cytomorphologic evaluation and differential count of BM smears is inevitable for differentiation of ASM from MCL.[26] If numbers of mast cells exceed 20% of nucleated BM cells, diagnosis of MCL is confirmed (Fig. 26.3A–C). Conversely, mast cell numbers are lower than 0.1% of nucleated cells in BM smears from patients with indolent SM and therefore it is challenging to search for mast cells and estimate their frequency. In patients with ISM, cytomorphological evaluation usually confirms mild atypia of mast cells. The mast cells here are often spindle-shaped and contain plump cigar-like nuclei together with a hypogranulated cytoplasm. The presence of such mast cells in patients with cutaneous mastocytosis (usually urticaria pigmentosa) must prompt suspicion of ISM and can be regarded as an indication for histological investigation of a BMTB specimen.

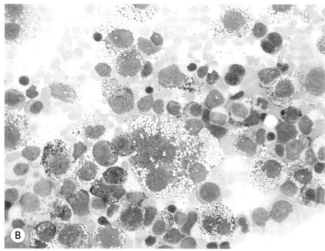

Fig. 26.4 (A, B) Mast cell leukemia. Cytomorphology of smears (Pappenheim/Wright–Giemsa stain) reveals cellular bone marrow smears with marked increase in medium sized to large atypical mast cells often with vacuolated cytoplasm and scarce metachromatic granules. Some atypical neutrophils and megakaryocytes are intermingled leading to an ultimate diagnosis of SM-AHNMD in form of an aleukemic mast cell leukemia (aMCL) associated with a myeloid neoplasm which is nearly obscured by the MCL but can be diagnosed as myelodysplastic syndrome (aMCL-MDS), ×25, ×40 objective.

Blood smears

Apart from rare patients with MCL, blood findings are not indicative of SM.[15] MCL shows a significant increase in circulating mast cells, which exhibit varying degrees of atypia. Some cases show mature round mast cells with abundant metachromatic granules leading to a correct diagnosis at first glance. Other MCL contain highly atypical hypogranulated circulating mast cells with pale large cytoplasm mimicking monocytoid or hairy cells. In most patients with indolent SM, PB exhibits no significant changes but some patients may show mild eosinophilia. Major alterations of blood cells are detected in most cases of SM-AHNMD, in particular those with associated myeloid leukemia. It has to be emphasized that sometimes a diagnosis of SM-AHNMD can only be established when a BMTB specimen and blood smears are investigated together because SM shows diffuse-compact BM infiltration thus obscuring the AHNMD. In every patient with aggressive SM or MCL, blood smears have to be analyzed in order not to overlook the AHNMD.

Morphology of the various defined subtypes of SM in the bone marrow

Main subtypes of SM

1. *Indolent SM.* Multifocal BM involvement, usually comprising 5% or less of the section area enables diagnosis of SM at first glance especially when there is prominent spindling and CD25-expression of mast cells. The hematopoiesis is intact with no signs of MDS or MPN. In cases with a slight diffuse increase of spindle-shaped CD25-expressing mast cells without any compact infiltrate, another minor criterion (KIT^{D816V} or elevated serum tryptase) is necessary to definitively establish the diagnosis.
2. *SM-AHNMD.* Here the morphological picture may be very difficult to interpret because in most cases the associated disorder dominates and even may obscure the SM (occult SM). Usually there is also multifocal BM involvement, comprising from <1% to 30% of the section area. In up to 10% of cases, SM is revealed only by using anti-tryptase and anti-CD25 immunostaining, thus enabling detection of even small compact infiltrates or a mere diffuse increase in atypical mast cells. Both compartments of the disease should be subcategorized. AHNMD in about 30–40% of the patients presents as CMML, while other disorders of the MDS/MPN group are rarely found. SM should also be further classified and usually presents as isolated BM mastocytosis, which is a subtype of indolent SM. SM-AHNMD is very heterogeneous not only morphologically but also on a molecular level (see above).
3. *Aggressive SM.*[27] In these patients, the BMTB is strongly infiltrated by large multifocal sometimes confluent sheets of mast cells (>30% of section area). In cases of ASM with diffuse-compact BM infiltration mast cell leukemia (MCL) can only be decided by investigation of BM and PB smears. In ASM, the BM smear contains <20% mast cells and the blood smear is without circulating mast cells. To establish a diagnosis of ASM, signs of organ dysfunction ('C-findings') should be present. ASM is almost always accompanied by significant cytopenia. Accordingly, the hematopoiesis is often markedly reduced and/or exhibits signs of dysplasia, which is indicative of an AHNMD (ASM-AHNMD).
4. *Mast cell leukemia/MCL.*[28] BM is usually diffusely infiltrated by sheets of mast cells (70% of section area or more). Numbers of fat cells and blood cell precursors are markedly reduced. Diagnosis of MCL, however, can only be established when more than 20% atypical mast cells are found in BM smears. Further classification (aleukemic versus leukemic MCL) depends on the presence of circulating mast cells

(usually >10% of leukocytes). In aleukemic MCL, the BM smear shows >20% mast cells and PB is without evidence of circulating mast cells. In MCL, the BM smear shows >20% mast cells and blood smear shows circulating mast cells.

5. *Mast cell sarcoma/MCS.*[29,30,31] MCS is extremely rare and almost always primarily involves extramedullary tissues. The terminal phase of the disease usually is a MCL.

Provisional entities

1. *Smoldering systemic mastocytosis/SSM.*[32,33] SSM assumes an intermediate position between indolent and aggressive SM showing a more pronounced BM involvement (20% and more of the BMTB section area) and organomegaly ('B findings') while 'C findings' are missing. SSM usually exhibits expansion of the KIT[D816V] mutation to non-mast cell lineages, usually neutrophils, but may also show minor degrees of dysplasia making the differential diagnosis to overt MDS (SM-MDS) very difficult in some of the cases.

2. *Isolated BM mastocytosis* morphologically presents like indolent SM but cutaneous (urticaria pigmentosa) involvement is missing. Isolated BM mastocytosis is usually found in patients with hymenoptera allergy and in some cases of SM-AHNMD.

3. *Well-differentiated systemic mastocytosis*[34] presents as exclusively round-cell type of the disease with compact multifocal infiltrates lacking expression of CD25. Since the demonstration of a point mutation outside codon 816 of c-kit (KIT[F522P]) does not meet the defined minor criterion it is necessary to investigate the serum tryptase level of the patient. If serum tryptase is persistently elevated, a diagnosis of SM can be established.

4. *'Occult' mastocytosis* can be used as a preliminary term for rare cases of SM that were initially obscured by a malignant hematological disorder in the setting of SM-AHNMD. After chemotherapy and disappearance of the associated neoplasm, typical compact mast cell infiltrates are disclosed.[18,11] As a rule, appropriate investigation of the primary BMTB specimen enables to diagnose occult mastocytosis retrospectively, usually based on three minor criteria (spindling, CD25 expression and KIT[D816V]). The term occult mastocytosis can also be used in rare patients, in whom previously examined tissue is available for re-evaluation. For example: in a patient with KIT[D816V]-positive SM with multifocal BM infiltration, lymph nodes previously removed on the occasion of removal of cystadenolymphoma of the parotid gland lacked morphological signs of mastocytosis but demonstrated the molecular evidence of KIT[D816V] mutation.[11]

Differential diagnosis

Mastocytosis has to be strictly separated both from reactive states of mast cell hyperplasia and from neoplastic diseases exhibiting signs of mast cell differentiation. The so-called 'monoclonal mast cell activation syndrome' (MMAS) is only roughly defined until now with respect to morphology. MMAS can be applied to cases showing disseminated scattered mast cells carrying the KIT[D816V] mutation but not fulfilling other criteria for mastocytosis, in particular missing compact infiltrates. MMAS is somewhat analogous to a monoclonal gammopathy of undetermined significance (MGUS, see Chapter 30) and at present is a preliminary description of a still ill-defined status.

The following neoplastic hematological disorders have to be included in the morphological differential diagnosis of mastocytosis:

1. *Myelomastocytic leukemia*[35,36] represents an extremely rare type of AML with prominent signs of mast cell differentiation but not fulfilling criteria for SM, especially when compact mast cell infiltrates and the KIT[D816V] mutation are missing. The histological picture is dominated by blast cells expressing myeloid and mast cell-associated antigens such as tryptase and/or chymase. A few cases exhibiting marked dysplastic features (similar to MDS of RAEB-2 type) have been encountered (author's unpublished observation).

2. *Tryptase positive acute myeloid leukemia*[37] is also a rare subtype of AML, usually within the WHO categories of AML with minimal differentiation or AML without maturation, showing strong expression of tryptase but lacking other features of mastocytosis or myelomastocytic leukemia. Since serum tryptase is usually markedly elevated, it is possible to monitor the disease serologically. Similar to myelomastocytic leukemia, tryptase positive AML is only recognized when tryptase immunohistochemistry is applied.

3. *Chronic basophilic leukemia* (Fig. 26.5A–D) is a very rare myeloid leukemia usually presenting as secondary 'basophilic crisis' in preexisting BCR-ABL1+ CML. De novo/primary chronic basophilic leukemia is exceedingly rare but does exist. Since only neoplastic basophils express tryptase in immunohistochemically detectable amounts, it is important differentiate basophils from mast cells. Cytomorphologically basophils are small to medium-sized round cells while mast cells in SM are usually large and often spindle-shaped. Immunostaining with CD117 is crucial to confirm the mast cell nature of a tryptase+ round cell, since basophils in contrast to mast cells are always CD117 negative. Antibodies against basophil-associated antigens like CD123, 2D7 or BB1 can also be used in such cases.

4. *Myeloproliferative neoplasm with eosinophilia (MPNEo)*[38,12] was formerly termed chronic eosinophilic leukemia/hypereosinophilic syndrome and is now regarded as a distinct group of disorders within myeloid neoplasms (see Chapter 25 for details). Morphologically more than 50% of cases with MPNEo exhibit a significant increase in spindle-shaped mast cells with an atypical immunophenotype and expression of CD25. However, criteria for diagnosis of SM, in particular SM-AHNMD, are not fulfilled in almost all cases since compact mast cell infiltrates are not present and the KIT[D816V] mutation is not detectable.

It is important to be aware that even the different forms of mastocytosis include a considerable spectrum of differential diagnoses. These are summarized in Box 26.3.

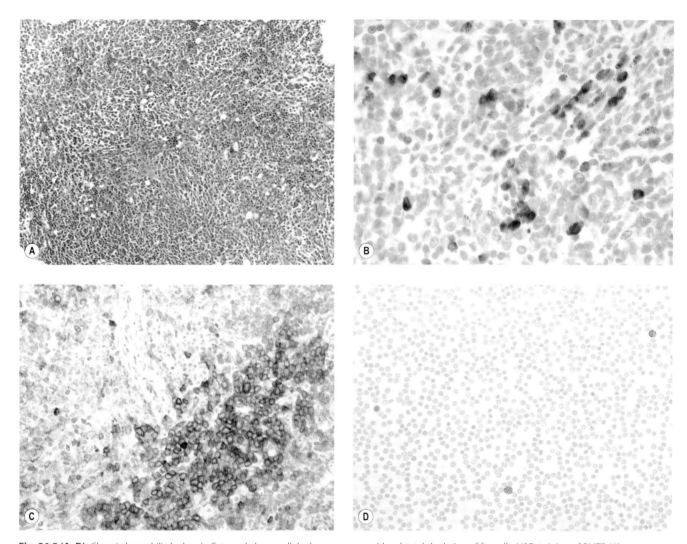

Fig. 26.5 (A–D) Chronic basophilic leukemia. Extremely hypercellular bone marrow with subtotal depletion of fat cells; H&E staining of BMTB (A) suggests a myeloid neoplasm but does not allow definitive classification of the disease. Immunostaining with anti-tryptase antibody (B; ABC method) reveals a significant increase in small to medium sized round cells. Since the tryptase-positive cells do not coexpress CD117 (C; ABC method), they cannot be classified as mast cells and thus obviously represent basophilic granulocytes, which in a neoplastic state may express detectable amounts of tryptase using light microscopy. Blood smear (D; Pappenheim/Wright–Giemsa) reveals a striking predominance of atypical circulating basophils but not the findings of chronic myeloid leukemia. The atypical fusion gene *BCR-ABL1* was found to be present enabling a diagnosis of *BCR-ABL1*-positive chronic basophilic leukemia to be established (possibly presenting as 'basophilic crisis' of previously undetected CML), ×10, ×25, ×25, ×25 objective.

Box 26.3 Differential diagnoses of various forms of mastocytosis

1. Differential diagnoses of *cutaneous mastocytosis*:
   i. mast cell hyperplasia
   ii. indolent SM.
2. Differential diagnoses of *indolent SM*:
   i. well-differentiated SM
   ii. isolated bone marrow mastocytosis
   iii. smoldering SM
   iv. mast cell hyperplasia
   v. monoclonal mast cell activation syndrome
   vi. lymphoplasmacytic lymphoma (cases with pronounced bone marrow lymphocytosis)
   vii. fibromastocytic lesion (ill-defined lesion with localized bone marrow fibrosis and increased numbers of spindle-shaped mast cells *lacking* CD25 and KITD816V).
3. Differential diagnoses of *SM-AHNMD*:
   i. 'occult' mastocytosis
   ii. tryptase positive AML
   iii. myelomastocytic leukemia
   iv. myeloproliferative neoplasm with eosinophilia (MPNEo).

4. Differential diagnoses of *aggressive SM*:
   i. smoldering SM, SM-AHNMD
   ii. aleukemic mast cell leukemia
   iii. myelomastocytic leukemia
   iv. tryptase positive AML
   v. Hodgkin's lymphoma and anaplastic large cell lymphoma in cases with prominent expression of CD30 by the neoplastic mast cells.
5. Differential diagnoses of *mast cell leukemia*:
   i. myelomastocytic leukemia
   ii. tryptase positive AML
   iii. basophilic leukemia
   iv. monocytic leukemia
   v. malignant histiocytosis
   vi. SM-AHNMD
   vii. hairy cell leukemia
   viii. aggressive SM (in cases of aleukemic mast cell leukemia).

References

1. Valent P, Horny HP, Escribano L, et al. Diagnostic criteria and classification of mastocytosis: a consensus proposal. Leuk Res 2001a;25:603–25.
2. Horny HP, Metcalfe DD, Bennett J, et al. Mastocytosis. World Health Organization Classification of Tumours of Haematopoietic and Lymphoid Tissue. Lyon: IARC Press; 2008. p. 54–63.
3. Sotlar K, Horny HP, Simonitsch I, et al. CD25 indicates the neoplastic phenotype of mast cells: a novel immunohistochemical marker for the diagnosis of systemic mastocytosis (SM) in routinely processed bone marrow biopsy specimens. Am J Surg Pathol 2004;28:1319–25.
4. Sotlar K, Marafioti T, Griesser H, et al. Detection of c-kit mutation Asp 816 to Val in microdissected bone marrow infiltrates in a case of systemic mastocytosis associated with chronic myelomonocytic leukaemia. Mol Pathol 2000;53:188–93.
5. Feger F, Ribadeau DA, Leriche L, et al. Kit and c-kit mutations in mastocytosis: a short overview with special reference to novel molecular and diagnostic concepts. Int Arch Allergy Immunol 2002;127: 110–4.
6. Sperr WR, Jordan JH, Fiegl M, et al. Serum tryptase levels in patients with mastocytosis: correlation with mast cell burden and implication for defining the category of disease. Int Arch Allergy Immunol 2002;128:136–41.
7. Horny HP, Valent P. Diagnosis of mastocytosis: general histopathological aspects, morphological criteria, and immunohistochemical findings. Leuk Res 2001;25:543–51.
8. Horny HP, Valent P. Histopathological and immunohistochemical aspects of mastocytosis. Int Arch Allergy Immunol 2002;127:115–17.
9. Horny HP, Ruck MT, Kaiserling E. Spleen findings in generalized mastocytosis. A clinicopathologic study. Cancer 1992;70:459–68.
10. Furitsu T, Tsujimura T, Tono T, et al. Identification of mutations in the coding sequence of the proto-oncogene c-kit in a human mast cell leukemia cell line causing ligand-independent activation of c-kit product. J Clin Invest 1993;92: 1736–44.
11. Sotlar K, Saeger W, Stellmacher F, et al. 'Occult' mastocytosis with activating c-kit point mutation evolving into systemic mastocytosis associated with plasma cell myeloma and secondary amyloidosis. J Clin Pathol 2006;59:875–8.
12. Maric I, Robyn J, Metcalfe DD, et al. KIT D816V-associated systemic mastocytosis with eosinophilia and FIP1L1/PDGFRA-associated chronic eosinophilic leukemia are distinct entities. J Allergy Clin Immunol 2007;120:680–7.
13. Sotlar K, Bache A, Stellmacher F, et al. Systemic mastocytosis associated with chronic idiopathic myelofibrosis: a distinct subtype of systemic mastocytosis associated with a [corrected] clonal hematological non-mast [corrected] cell lineage disorder carrying the activating point mutations KITD816V and JAK2V617F. J Mol Diagn 2008;10:58–66.
14. Escribano L, Orfao A, Diaz-Agustin B, et al. Indolent systemic mast cell disease in adults: immunophenotypic characterization of bone marrow mast cells and its diagnostic implications. Blood 1998;91:2731–6.
15. Horny HP, Ruck M, Wehrmann M, Kaiserling E. Blood findings in generalized mastocytosis: evidence of frequent simultaneous occurrence of myeloproliferative disorders. Br J Haematol 1990;76:186–93.
16. Sperr WR, Horny HP, Lechner K, Valent P. Clinical and biologic diversity of leukemias occurring in patients with mastocytosis. Leuk Lymphoma 2000; 37:473–86.
17. Horny HP, Sotlar K, Sperr WR, Valent P. Systemic mastocytosis with associated clonal haematological non-mast cell lineage diseases: a histopathological challenge. J Clin Pathol 2004;57: 604–8.
18. Bernd HW, Sotlar K, Lorenzen J, et al. Acute myeloid leukaemia with t(8;21) associated with 'occult' mastocytosis. Report of an unusual case and review of the literature. J Clin Pathol 2004;57: 324–8.
19. Caplan RM. The natural course of urticaria pigmentosa. Analysis and follow-up of 112 cases. Arch Dermatol 1963;87: 146–57.
20. Li CY. Diagnosis of mastocytosis: value of cytochemistry and immunohistochemistry. Leuk Res 2001;25:537–41.
21. Horny H.P, Sillaber C, Menke D, et al. Diagnostic value of immunostaining for

tryptase in patients with mastocytosis. Am J Surg Pathol 1998;22:1132–40.

22. Li WV, Kapadia SB, Sonmez-Alpan E, Swerdlow SH. Immunohistochemical characterization of mast cell disease in paraffin sections using tryptase, CD68, myeloperoxidase, lysozyme, and CD20 antibodies. Mod Pathol 1996;9:982–8.

23. Jordan JH, Walchshofer S, Jurecka W, et al. Immunohistochemical properties of bone marrow mast cells in systemic mastocytosis: evidence for expression of CD2, CD117/Kit, and bcl-x(L). Hum Pathol 2001b;32:545–52.

24. Horny HP, Sotlar K, Stellmacher F, et al. An unusual case of systemic mastocytosis associated with chronic lymphocytic leukaemia (SM-CLL). J Clin Pathol 2006b;59:264–8.

25. Horny HP, Sotlar K, Stellmacher F, et al. The tryptase positive compact round cell infiltrate of the bone marrow (TROCI-BM): a novel histopathological finding requiring the application of lineage specific markers. J Clin Pathol 2006a; 59:298–302.

26. Sperr WR, Escribano L, Jordan JH, et al. Morphologic properties of neoplastic mast cells: delineation of stages of maturation and implication for cytological grading of mastocytosis. Leuk Res 2001a;25:529–36.

27. Valent P, Akin C, Sperr WR, et al. Aggressive systemic mastocytosis and related mast cell disorders: current treatment options and proposed response criteria. Leuk Res 2003;27:635–41.

28. Travis WD, Li CY, Hoagland HC, et al. Mast cell leukemia: report of a case and review of the literature. Mayo Clin Proc 1986;61:957–66.

29. Horny HP, Parwaresch MR, Kaiserling E, et al. Mast cell sarcoma of the larynx. J Clin Pathol 1986;39:596–602.

30. Kojima M, Nakamura S, Itoh H, et al. Mast cell sarcoma with tissue eosinophilia arising in the ascending colon. Mod Pathol 1999;12:739–43.

31. Guenther PP, Huebner A, Sobottka SB, et al. Temporary response of localized intracranial mast cell sarcoma to combination chemotherapy. J Pediatr Hematol Oncol 2001;23:134–8.

32. Hauswirth AW, Sperr WR, Ghannadan M, et al. A case of smouldering mastocytosis with peripheral blood eosinophilia and lymphadenopathy. Leuk Res 2002;26: 601–6.

33. Jordan JH, Fritsche-Polanz R, Sperr WR, et al. A case of 'smouldering' mastocytosis with high mast cell burden, monoclonal myeloid cells, and C-KIT mutation

Asp-816-Val. Leuk Res 2001a;25: 627–34.

34. Akin C, Fumo G, Yavuz AS, et al. A novel form of mastocytosis associated with a transmembrane c-kit mutation and response to imatinib. Blood 2004; 103:3222–5.

35. Valent P, Samorapoompichit P, Sperr WR, et al. Myelomastocytic leukemia: myeloid neoplasm characterized by partial differentiation of mast cell-lineage cells. Hematol J 2002;3:90–4.

36. Valent P, Sperr WR, Samorapoompichit P, et al. Myelomastocytic overlap syndromes: biology, criteria, and relationship to mastocytosis. Leuk Res 2001b;25:595–602.

37. Sperr WR, Jordan JH, Baghestanian M, et al. Expression of mast cell tryptase by myeloblasts in a group of patients with acute myeloid leukemia. Blood 2001b; 98:2200–9.

38. Pardanani A, Ketterling RP, Brockman SR, et al. CHIC2 deletion, a surrogate for FIP1L1-PDGFRA fusion, occurs in systemic mastocytosis associated with eosinophilia and predicts response to imatinib mesylate therapy. Blood 2003;102:3093–6.

Myelodysplastic/myeloproliferative neoplasms

M Czader, A Orazi

Chapter contents

Introduction

Myelodysplastic/myeloproliferative neoplasms (MDS/MPN) are clonal hematopoietic malignancies with hybrid myelodysplastic and myeloproliferative features. In these disorders, cytopenias and dysplasia may coexist with elevated white blood cell counts, thrombocytosis and/or organomegaly making it difficult to assign individual cases into a myelodysplastic or myeloproliferative category. Even though disorders with mixed myelodysplastic and myeloproliferative features have been recognized for many years, the precise diagnosis and assignment to a biologically defined category has been challenging. Acknowledging the unique characteristics of these diseases, in 2001 the World Health Organization classification of hematopoietic and lymphoid malignancies created a separate group of MDS/MPN.[1] Chronic myelomonocytic leukemia (CMML) is perhaps the most well known example of a MDS/MPN. Depending on WBC count, CMML may resemble more closely a myelodysplastic syndrome (MDS) or a myeloproliferative neoplasm (MPN). The disease is clinically heterogeneous and lacks a precise biological connotation. Similar to CMML, other categories of MDS/MPNs are also a genetically heterogeneous group of diseases with variable patient outcomes. They are frequently positioned on a continuum between MDS and MPN, and thus are challenging to diagnose using traditional morphology-based approaches. Integration of morphologic features with laboratory data, clinical presentation, immunophenotype and cytogenetic/molecular tests is required to categorize MDS/MPNs according to current WHO 2008 classification.[2] It is critical to diagnose patients at the time of original presentation, i.e. before bone marrow (BM) and peripheral blood (PB) features are modified by therapy or progression of the disease. If a patient has been previously diagnosed elsewhere, a complete review of the original diagnostic material is mandatory. 'Re-classification' based on the review of post-treatment and/or follow-up BM sample is strongly discouraged.

Three discrete MDS/MPN entities can be reliably classified using the above described integrated multiparametric approach: chronic myelomonocytic leukemia (CMML), atypical chronic myeloid leukemia (aCML), BCR-ABL1 negative and juvenile myelomonocytic leukemia (JMML). Occasionally, a myeloid neoplasm with myelodysplastic and myeloproliferative features cannot be assigned to any of these 'classical' categories. Such cases should be diagnosed as MDS/MPN, unclassifiable.[2] This group includes also the provisional entity known as refractory anemia with ring sideroblasts associated with marked thrombocytosis (RARS-T). Additionally, there are rare disorders, which may qualify for inclusion in the MDS/MPN group in the future. One such disease is known as myeloid neoplasm with an isolated isochromosome 17q. This is a rare entity with a rapidly progressive clinical course that may occasionally morphologically resemble CMML.

A detailed discussion of the MDS/MPNs is presented below. The main diagnostic features of these neoplasms are summarized in Table 27.1. Some cytogenetic and genetic features are also addressed in Chapter 21.

Chronic myelomonocytic leukemia

Definition and diagnostic criteria

CMML is a hematopoietic malignancy with hybrid myeloproliferative and myelodysplastic features. The diagnostic criteria include: 1) persistent unexplained monocytosis (>1 × 10^9/l with >10% monocytes on the differential count); 2) absence of defining genetic features such as BCR-ABL1 fusion or rearrangements of PDGFRA and PDGFRB; 3) less than 20% blasts; and 4) dysplasia in one or more myeloid lineages. In the absence of definitive dysplastic features, the diagnosis of CMML can be rendered if unexplained monocytosis persists longer than 3 months or if cytogenetic/molecular studies demonstrate the presence of acquired clonal cytogenetic or molecular genetic abnormality.[2]

Epidemiology, clinical and laboratory features

CMML is a rare disease with estimated incidence of 3 cases per 100 000 people.[3] The disease is more prevalent in men with a predominance of 1.5–3 : 1 and has a median age of presentation between 65 and 75 years.[4,5] The disease is more common in Western countries as compared to Asian population.[6] Patients can present with elevated WBC or with leukopenia. Signs and symptoms of BM failure are common and include fatigue, susceptibility to infections and bleeding. Weight loss, night sweats, fever, organomegaly, tissue infiltration (e.g. skin lesions) and serous effusions are also seen. Depending on the WBC (threshold 13 × 10^9/l), CMML has been previously divided into myeloproliferative or myelodysplastic categories.[7] Splenomegaly and increased LDH are more common in the myeloproliferative subtype of CMML.[8,9] Other clinical and laboratory features, and prognosis, including overall survival and incidence of transformation into acute leukemia, are similar for both groups.[8–10] Whether the myelodysplastic and myeloproliferative CMML should be considered different phases of the disease or represent distinct entities is at present unclear. The separation is not required by the WHO 2008 classification.

Morphology and immunophenotypic features

PB shows significant monocytosis (>1 × 10^9/l with >10% monocytes on the differential count), variable WBC (neutrophilia is seen in about 50% of the cases), anemia and thrombocytopenia. The majority of monocytes are mature, and they frequently display abnormal nuclear and cytoplasmic features. These include abnormal nuclear lobulation or chromatin pattern, prominent granulation or increased basophilia of cytoplasm (Fig. 27.1). Morphological definition of 'abnormal monocytes' and promonocytes has been a matter of debate and is thoroughly described in the WHO 2008 classification.[2] In most cases, peripheral blood blasts, including monoblasts and promonocytes constitute less than 5% of the differential count. Neutrophilia may be present with dysgranulopoiesis including pseudo-Pelger–Huët cells and hypogranulation. Circulating neutrophilic precursors (promyelocytes and myelocytes) usually constitute less than 10% of white blood cells. In cases with significant eosinophilia (≥1.5 × 10^9/l), molecular studies excluding the rearrangements in PDGFRA and PDGFRB genes are necessary to further consider the diagnosis of CMML. Basophilia is uncommon. Giant platelets can be seen. Red blood cells are more often normochromic and normocytic but macrocytosis can also be seen.

Even though peripheral blood monocytosis is the single most important diagnostic finding, the final diagnosis of CMML should never be rendered without BM evaluation. The population of promonocytes, which are morphologically more differentiated than blasts in the bone marrow is not infrequently present in PB of patients with acute myelomonocytic and monocytic leukemia. Also, increase in monocytes largely confined to the BM without absolute monocytosis in PB can be seen in rare cases of 'marrow predominant' CMML. These diagnoses can be missed if a BM

Table 27.1 Main diagnostic features of MDS/MPNs and related neoplasms

CMML	aCML	JMML	MDS/MPN, U	RARS-T (provisional entity)	MDS with isolated del(5q) and $JAK2^{V617F}$ mutation	MDS/MPN with an isolated isochromosome 17q
Persistent unexplained monocytosis (>1 × 10^9/l) with >10% monocytes); absence of defining genetic features such as *BCR-ABL1* fusion or rearrangements of *PDGFRA* and *PDGFRB*; less than 20% blasts; dysplasia in ≥1 myeloid lineages	Neutrophilia with significant dysplasia and left shift; absence of *BCR-ABL1* rearrangement	Monocytosis (>1 × 10^9/l); blast and promonocyte count <20%; absence of *BCR-ABL1* rearrangement. Additional diagnostic criteria (≥2 required): increase in hemoglobin F for age; granulocytic precursors in peripheral blood, WBC above 10 × 10^9/l; clonal chromosomal abnormality and/or GM-CSF hypersensitivity of myeloid progenitors in vitro	Diagnosis of exclusion-neoplasm with myelodysplastic and myeloproliferative features that does not fulfill diagnostic criteria for CMML, aCML, JMML	Thrombocytosis ≥450 × 10^9/l; dysplasia of erythroid lineage; ≥15% ring sideroblasts; bone marrow shows large atypical megakaryocytes and dyserythropoiesis	Coexistence of isolated 5q deletion and $JAK2^{V617F}$ mutation; hypolobated/monolobated megakaryocytes and frequent prominent granulocytic hyperplasia with higher WBC and a trend for higher platelet counts	Neutrophilia with frequent non-segmented forms, hyposegmented neutrophils, ring nuclei, hypogranularity and chromatin clumping; monocytosis is reported and a proportion of cases fulfill the criteria for CMML; hypercellular bone marrow with significant granulocytic proliferation, dysgranulopoiesis and <5% blasts; dysplastic changes in erythroid progenitors and megakaryocytes; significant fibrosis
In the absence of definitive dysplastic features, the unexplained monocytosis has to persist >3 months or cytogenetic/molecular studies have to demonstrate the presence of acquired clonal cytogenetic or molecular genetic abnormality	No basophilia or monocytosis (<10% monocytes in peripheral blood); neutrophils with chromatin clumping may be present; bone marrow findings similar to CML	Demonstration of mutations in genes regulating *RAS* pathway or HUMARA assay may be helpful to solidify diagnosis in challenging cases	Diagnosis requires extensive work-up to exclude e.g. preexisting myeloid neoplasm, effects of previous treatment with growth factors or cytotoxic drugs	Absence of isolated deletion of chromosome 5, abnormalities of chromosome 3 and *BCR-ABL1* rearrangement. Clinical correlation to rule out conditions and medications associated with increase in ring sideroblasts is required		Cases which do not fulfill criteria for CMML diagnosis often show pleomorphic megakaryocyte morphology and should be classified as MDS/MPN, U with isolated isochromosome 17q

aCML, atypical chronic myeloid leukemia; CMML, chronic myelomonocytic leukemia; JMML, juvenile myelomonocytic leukemia; MDS/MPN, U, myelodysplastic/myeloproliferative neoplasm, unclassifiable; MDS, myelodysplastic syndrome; MDS/MPN, myelodysplastic/myeloproliferative neoplasm.

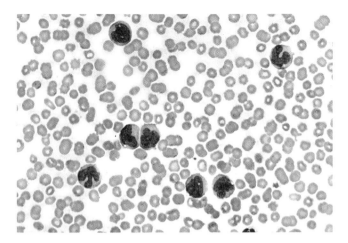

Fig. 27.1 CMML. Abnormal monocytes.

examination is not performed. Conversely, significant mono-cytosis can also be seen in some cases of *BCR-ABL1*+ chronic myelogenous leukemia (CML), which should always be excluded (see Chapter 24).

BM is significantly hypercellular in a majority of CMML cases, a finding easily appreciated in a predominantly elderly population, in which this disease occurs (Fig. 27.2A). Rarely, BM may be normo- or hypocellular.[11] A prominent myeloid proliferation is usually seen (Fig. 27.2B). This includes both an increased number of neutrophilic forms as well as mono-cytes, which can be difficult to appreciate in the absence of non-specific esterase cytochemistry. In a significant number of cases, the granulopoiesis may be left shifted and show significant dysplasia including hypogranulation and nuclear abnormalities.[7] Due to difficulties in differentiating mono-cytes from immature granulocytic cells (e.g. myelocytes and metamyelocytes), the quantification of the monocytic com-ponent may be challenging, which causes a significant vari-ability between observers. The most significant practical issue is the differentiation of abnormal monocytes from monoblasts and promonocytes. The early stages of mono-cytic differentiation in the bone marrow of CMML patient are shown in Fig. 27.2C.

The application of nonspecific esterase and immunophe-notyping by flow cytometry or immunohistochemistry are helpful in quantifying the monocytic component. Nonspecific esterase staining (alpha-naphthyl butyrate or alpha-naphthyl acetate esterase) is an effective method of demonstrating monocytic differentiation. The stain is useful to confirm the increased number of esterase positive cells in cases of CMML. Median values of 10–20% esterase positive cells are found in the majority of CMML patients[12,13] (Fig. 27.2D). Multiparametric flow cytometry has the added ben-efits of separating various stages of monocytic differentiation and demonstrating an aberrant antigen expression. The former can be accomplished by profiling the expression of the different epitopes of CD14 antigen in combination with CD64 and CD33, which reveals the presence of promono-cytes and more mature monocytic forms.[14] Aberrant expres-sion of myeloid antigens, both loss and altered antigen density, and expression of non-myeloid markers, are fre-quently seen in monocytes and in the granulocytic popula-tion. Monocytes show altered density of HLA-DR, CD13 and

CD64, and may show co-expression of CD2 and CD56 (Fig. 27.3A). In comparison to reactive monocytes, the aberrant expression of CD56 on CMML monocytes was much higher.[15,16] The decrease in right-angle light scatter is not infrequent and reflects the hypogranulation of granulocytic series (Fig. 27.3B). Increase in the number of CD34 and/or CD117 positive blasts may indicate progression of the disease and alert to the impending transformation.

With the exception of demonstrating an increased number of blasts and blast clusters using immunohistochemical stain for CD34, the value of immunohistochemistry in CMML has been limited. Common myeloid/monocyte/macrophage immunohistochemical markers such as lysozyme and CD68 (KP1) applied to BM trephine biopsies (BMTB), are generally not reliable in quantifying monocytic component.[12] CD68R and CD163 have been shown to be more restricted to mono-cytes and macrophages. However, these markers usually stain significantly lower numbers of monocytic cells as com-pared to naphthyl butyrate esterase[12,17] (Fig. 27.2E). Some investigators reported that staining pattern of CD68R (fine vs coarse granules) in conjunction with cell morphology can discriminate between monocyte precursors and mature monocytes.[18] The success of this approach may, however, be dependent on the processing of BMTB and staining methodology used, and needs further validation and stand-ardization in a multi-institutional setting. New antibodies applicable to paraffin embedded material have recently been reported to aid in enumeration of the monocytic component in BMTB. A combined use of CD14 and CD16 allowed dis-criminating between monocyte population and dysplastic granulocytes in this setting.[17]

Numerous studies confirmed that the number of blasts and promonocytes is the most reliable predictor of patient prognosis and of the risk of transformation to acute leuke-mia. Recognizing the importance of the increase in blasts, CMML is divided into two groups: CMML-1 with less than 5% blasts in PB and less than 10% in BM; and CMML-2 with 5–19% of blasts in PB and 10–19% in BM. The prognostic value of this classification has been previously confirmed.[19]

Erythropoiesis is usually normal to decreased and may show dysplastic changes.[20] These include megaloblastoid change with asynchrony in maturation of nucleus and cyto-plasm, and nuclear abnormalities such as nuclear fragmenta-tion, irregularity of nuclear outline and multinucleation. Increased megakaryopoiesis is not uncommon; however, it is usually less pronounced than that seen in cases of *BCR-ABL1*+ CML.[12] Dysmegakaryopoiesis is seen in the majority of CMML cases.[21] Dysplastic megakaryocytes display abnormal nuclear lobation including mononuclear or hypolobated forms, or separated nuclear lobes. Micromeg-akaryocytes can also be seen. Approximately 20% of cases show significant reticulin fibrosis.[13]

Approximately 20% of CMML cases show nodular prolif-erations of plasmacytoid dendritic cells[12] (Fig. 27.4). The lineage and origin of these cells have long been debated and is reflected by changing nomenclature starting from the designation of 'T-associated plasma cells' and 'plasmacy-toid T-cells' to 'plasmacytoid monocytes'. Currently, plasma-cytoid dendritic cells are believed to be derived from myeloid progenitors. Thus, it is perhaps not surprising that focal proliferations of these cells are seen in association with myeloid neoplasms with monocytic differentiation, most

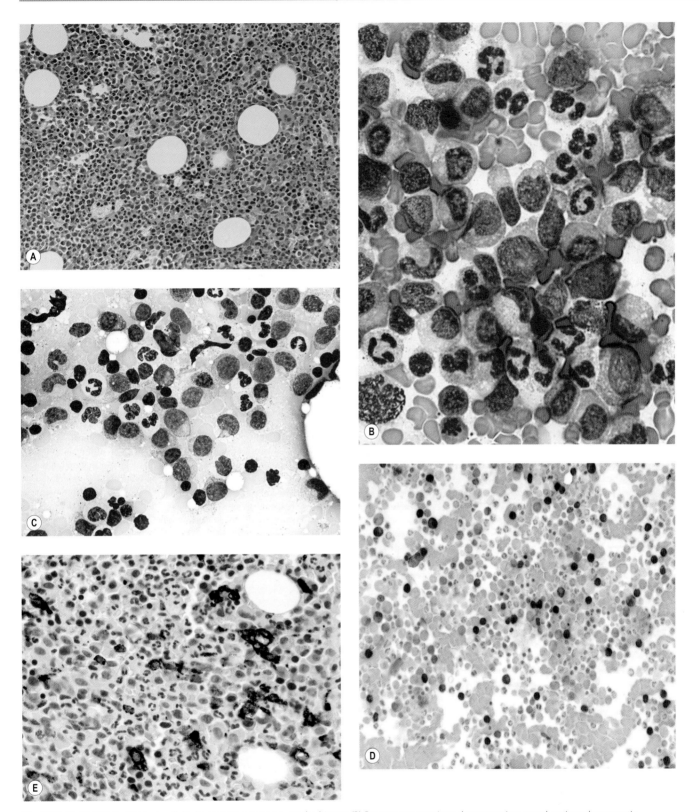

Fig. 27.2 (A–E) CMML. (A) Hypercellular bone marrow as seen on the biopsy. (B) Bone marrow aspirate demonstrating granulocytic and monocytic hyperplasia. The monocytes are difficult to discern in the absence of cytochemistry. (C) Monoblasts and promonocytes. (D) Butyrate esterase facilitates identification of monocytic series. (E) Immunohistology with CD68R can be used to identify the monocytic cells, however it frequently shows relatively low number of monocytes and scattered macrophages.

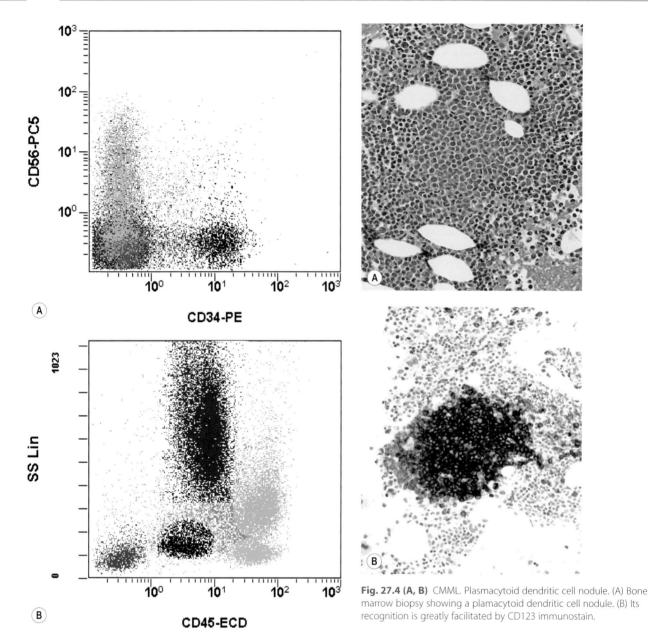

Fig. 27.3 (A, B) Flow cytometric evaluation of bone marrow with CMML. (A) Coexpression of CD56 antigen on monocytes is frequently seen in CMML (monocytes presented in green). (B) Decreased side-scatter demonstrates hypogranular neutrophils.

Fig. 27.4 (A, B) CMML. Plasmacytoid dendritic cell nodule. (A) Bone marrow biopsy showing a plamacytoid dendritic cell nodule. (B) Its recognition is greatly facilitated by CD123 immunostain.

commonly in CMML. These nodules are considered clonal and in select cases have been shown to be clonally related to the underlying myeloid neoplasm.[22,23] Plasmacytoid dendritic cells are intermediate in size with round to oval nucleus, with or without indentation, finely dispersed chromatin and moderately abundant cytoplasm with distinct cytoplasmic border. Their identification is facilitated by immunohistochemical stains including CD123, CD68, CD68R, CD4 and CD14. Plasmacytoid dendritic cells are also positive for granzyme B and occasionally for CD56, CD2 and CD5. They are negative for other lymphoid markers, and for CD13, CD11c, myeloperoxidase and CD34.

Prognosis

The survival of patients with CMML is extremely variable, ranging from 1 to 100 months.[2,4,12,24] Considerable efforts have been made in the past to design a predictor of clinical outcome. All scoring systems shown to be useful in predicting the clinical outcome (such as modified Bournemouth score, Dusseldorf score, MD Anderson prognostic score and Spanish CMML score) used a combination of BM blast count with PB counts to predict survival.[5,24] In multivariate analysis, PB and BM blast percentage proved to be the strongest predictor of survival and of transformation into acute myeloid leukemia (AML).[4,13,19,25,26] PB and BM blast counts are the keystones to distinguish between CMML-1 and CMML-2. These two subcategories were shown to be highly predictive of overall survival and correlated well with transformation into AML. Specifically, at 5-year follow-up, 63% of patients with a BM blast count of 10% or greater developed AML as compared to 18% of patients with blast count below 10%.[19] Previously discussed myelodysplastic and myeloproliferative subtypes of CMML were not significant for predicting patient outcome.[19]

As our knowledge on the pathogenesis of myeloid neoplasms expands, new prognostic factors emerge. *TET2* gene mutations have been recently reported to occur in 50% of CMML patients (see Chapter 21) and have been associated with poor survival in the CMML-1 subgroup.[27] *RUNX1* mutations occur in up to 40% of CMML cases and abnormalities of C-terminal portion of this gene are associated with progression to AML.[28]

Special considerations

Chronic myelomonocytic leukemia developing in a course of myelodysplastic syndrome

The evolution of previously diagnosed MDS to CMML is well documented.[29-32] The pathogenesis of this phenomenon is not well understood with only rare studies testing select genes implicated in myeloid neoplasms.[32] The interval between the initial MDS diagnosis and the evolution to CMML ranged between 2 and 59 months.

Approximately 20% of MDS patients show relative peripheral blood monocytosis (more than 10% monocytes but with absolute monocyte count less than $1 \times 10^9/l$) at the time of their initial diagnosis. Over time, a significant proportion of these patients may develop CMML. Conversely, up to 24% of patients with CMML have a documented preceding MDS phase.[13,32] Both groups, whether originally presenting with or without relative monocytosis, initially show less than $1 \times 10^9/l$ monocytes in PB. Rigolin et al. reported the distinct clinicopathological features of MDS cases with relative monocytosis (>10% monocytes).[29] In comparison to MDS without monocytosis, these patients showed higher marrow cellularity, higher incidence of chromosomal abnormalities, and a more aggressive disease with high incidence of progression to CMML and transformation into acute myelomonocytic or monocytic leukemia.[29] When CMML evolving from the MDS phase was compared to myelodysplastic type of *de novo* CMML, the former showed a superior survival.[31,32]

Therapy-related CMML

The majority of CMML cases represent *de novo* disease arising in patients without a pre-existing hematologic or non-hematopoietic neoplasm. Occasionally, CMML may develop after treatment with chemotherapeutic agents and/or radiotherapy for malignancies or non-neoplastic diseases.[33-35] Even though the numbers of reported cases are low, therapy-related CMML seems to show morphologic and immunophenotypic features similar to those of *de novo* CMML. However, a proportion of these cases show the rearrangement of *MLL* gene, a finding which is usually seen only in acute leukemia. Regardless of morphologic features, current WHO classification recommends to classify all therapy-related cases under the umbrella of therapy-related myeloid neoplasms. Therefore, all therapy-related CMML cases should be included in this category. Thus, the detailed knowledge of patient's previous medical history is critical while diagnosing CMML.

Atypical chronic myeloid leukemia, *BCR-ABL1* negative

Definition and diagnostic criteria

Atypical chronic myeloid leukemia (aCML) is a MDS/MPN with a predominant involvement of the granulocytic series, which in addition to a marked granulocytic proliferation shows significant dysplasia. Some of the clinical and morphologic features of aCML are similar to those seen in *BCR-ABL1*+ CML; however, the *BCR-ABL1* rearrangement is absent. The presence of a granulocytic proliferation associated with marked dysgranulopoiesis and the absence of *BCR-ABL1* translocation are the defining features of aCML.

Epidemiology, clinical and laboratory features

The aCML is a rare myeloid neoplasm with an incidence of 1–2 cases for every 100 cases of Philadelphia-positive CML.[36] Patients present in the 7th or 8th decade of life with leukocytosis, splenomegaly, frequent anemia and variable platelet counts. Both genders are equally affected. The $JAK2^{V617F}$ mutation is absent.[37]

Morphology and immunophenotypic features

By definition, the WBC is elevated in the range of $18-300 \times 10^9/l$ (median $24-36 \times 10^9/l$)[36-39] and is frequently accompanied by anemia and thrombocytopenia. The majority of cases show more than 10% of circulating immature granulocytic cells, which is roughly similar to what is seen in CML. Blast count is low, usually less than 5%. Prominent dysgranulopoiesis differentiates aCML from CML (Fig. 27.5A). CML usually does not show dysgranulopoieis at the time of the initial diagnosis but may develop severe dysplastic changes upon progression of the disease.

Dysgranulopoiesis seen in aCML includes the presence of neutrophils with abnormally lobated nuclei such as pseudo-Pelger–Huët cells, abnormally condensed chromatin and hypogranulation. In a proportion of cases, the dysplastic neutrophils have abnormally hyperlobulated nuclei and abnormal chromatin clumping (syndrome of abnormal chromatin clumping). Due to leukocytosis, the absolute monocyte count can be higher than $1 \times 10^9/l$. However, monocytes never exceed 10% of the differential count. Significant basophilia, as seen in CML cases, is not present and basophils rarely exceed 2% of the differential count. Anemia may be macrocytic with macroovalocytes as evidence of dysplastic erythroid maturation. Platelets are frequently decreased. However, cases with thrombocytosis have been reported (range $9-2675 \times 10^9/l$). In the original study by the French-American-British (FAB) Cooperative Leukemia Group, the parameters most strongly associated with the diagnosis of aCML were: peripheral blood leukocytosis with immature myeloid forms, dysgranulopoiesis, and the absence of basophilia and monocytosis.[40]

In the majority of cases, BM is hypercellular with a significantly increased granulopoiesis (Fig. 27.5B). Dysgranulopoiesis is seen in all cases. By definition, blast count is below 20% and, in most instances, blasts represent less than 5% of marrow elements. The M:E ratio is commonly increased

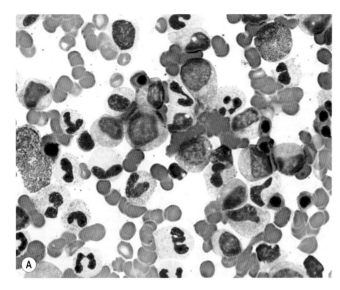

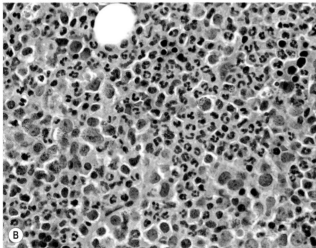

Fig. 27.5 (A, B) aCML. (A) Bone marrow aspirate smear of aCML showing dysplastic granulocytes. (B) Bone marrow biopsy of aCML showing a hypercellular marrow.

with erythroid series frequently accounting for less than 10% of BM elements.[40] Dyserythropoiesis is common. The number of megakaryocytes is variable and not uncommonly decreased. Dysmegakaryopoiesis is usually seen. Hypolobated and/or monolobated forms and micromegakaryocytes are most common. As in other subtypes of MDS/MPN, reticulin fibers may be increased.

Prognosis

aCML is an aggressive disease with a median survival of 14–37 months depending on the therapy received.[36,38,39,41] The majority of patients succumb to BM failure and approximately 20–40% of cases transform to AML. The rate and time to transformation is variable, dependent on the initial treatment (conservative vs intensive induction-like therapy). In younger patients, the outcome is improved by hematopoietic stem cell transplantation.[42]

Variables associated with shorter survival times include older age, female gender, leukocyte count of more than 50 × 10⁹/l, and circulating immature precursors. The percentage

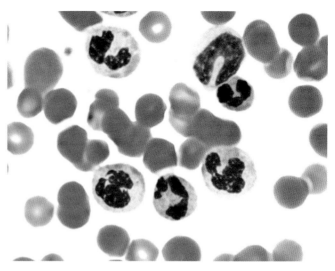

Fig. 27.6 PB with abnormal chromatin clumping.

of BM blasts (>5%) and marked dyserythropoiesis were the most significant factors associated with leukemic transformation.[36]

Special considerations

Syndrome of abnormal chromatin clumping

The syndrome of abnormal chromatin clumping, which has long been recognized as representing a hematologic neoplasm with both myelodysplastic and myeloproliferative features is, in most cases, simply a morphologic variant of aCML.[43-47] The majority of patients from the original series with abnormal chromatin clumping developed leukocytosis, anemia and thrombocytopenia. Rare patients showed neutropenia at the onset of the disease. The defining feature of this disease is a characteristic neutrophil morphology – excessive 'clumping' of chromatin into large well separated blocks of heterochromatin and euchromatin. This feature is commonly accompanied by a loss of segmentation and is best appreciated in mature neutrophils (Fig. 27.6).

BM features are similar to those seen in other cases of aCML and include granulocytic hyperplasia, megaloblastoid erythropoiesis, the presence of micromegakaryocytes and other dysplastic megakaryocyte forms. The risk of leukemic transformation is approximately 30%. The majority of patients die of BM failure.

Abnormal chromatin clumping is not limited to the syndrome described above. Rare cases of *BCR-ABL1*+ CML have been reported to show an identical morphology.[48] In addition, reversible chromatin clumping is seen in neutrophils of patients treated with mycophenolate mofetil, in HIV infection, and in select patients treated for lymphoproliferative disorders.[49,50] Thus, as in all hematologic malignancies, the final diagnosis has to be made in correlation with laboratory data and in the context of clinical presentation.

Atypical chronic myeloid leukemia with t(8;9)(p22;p24)/*PCM1-JAK2*

A number of cases classified as aCML and carrying fusion of *PCM1-JAK2* genes have been described.[51,52] Detailed description of the morphologic features of PB and BM is not available in all cases. However, in many instances, significant eosinophilia of a degree comparable to that seen in chronic eosinophilic leukemia has been reported. Other cases showed more complex morphologic characteristics and multilineage involvement. *PCM1-JAK2* abnormality can also present as de novo AML or acute lymphoblastic leukemia. Thus, in cases with t(8;9)(p22;p24), a detailed review of cellular morphology and correlation with laboratory values is necessary for a definitive classification.

Juvenile myelomonocytic leukemia (JMML)

Definition and diagnostic criteria

JMML is a myelodysplastic/myeloproliferative neoplasm with predominant granulocytic and monocytic proliferation. PB monocytosis ($>1 \times 10^9/l$), blast and promonocyte count of less than 20% and the absence of *BCR-ABL1* rearrangement are required for the diagnosis. Additional diagnostic criteria (two or more required at the time of presentation) include: increase in fetal hemoglobin (HbF) for age, granulocytic precursors in peripheral blood, WBC above $10 \times 10^9/l$, clonal chromosomal abnormality and/or granulocyte-macrophage colony stimulating factor (GM-CSF) hypersensitivity of myeloid progenitors *in vitro*.

Epidemiology, clinical and laboratory features

In the past, JMML has been referred to as juvenile chronic myeloid leukemia, chronic myelomonocytic leukemia and infantile monosomy 7 syndrome. The incidence of this disease is approximately 1 case per million children younger than 14 years.[53-55] It is most common in children below 3 years of age; however, early adolescent patients have also been reported. Males are affected more frequently than females. There is an association with neurofibromatosis type 1 and to lesser extent with Noonan syndrome, related to the activation of *RAS* pathway through mutations in tumor suppressor gene *NF1*, and *PTPN11*, *KRAS* or *SOS1* genes. Presenting features include leukocytosis with monocytosis, anemia and thrombocytopenia leading to pallor, malaise, infections and bleeding. Similar to adult CMML, a maculopapular rash also occurs. Organ infiltration by leukemic cells leads to hepatosplenomegaly and lymphadenopathy. Leukemic infiltrates in the lungs and gastrointestinal tract clinically manifest as respiratory failure and diarrhea. In cases of neurofibromatosis type 1 or Noonan syndrome, additional features related to primary disorder, such as café au lait spots, may also be present.

Two additional laboratory features are keystones of JMML diagnosis. At least half of the patients show elevation of the HbF level corrected for age. This feature is seen predominantly in patients without monosomy 7.[56] In vitro hypersensitivity of myeloid progenitors to GM-CSF is another important diagnostic parameter.[57] In contrast to other neoplasms with myeloproliferative features, this hypersensitivity is limited to GM-CSF. The response of JMML cells to interleukin(IL)-3 or G-CSF is normal. *In vitro* hypersensitivity to GM-CSF is a labor intensive and challenging assay and

may, in the future, be replaced by flow cytometry testing hyperphosphorylation of signal transducer and activator of transcription (STAT)-5 . In this assay, BM cells are stimulated by a low-dose of GM-CSF with subsequent measurement of STAT3 phosphorylation. JMML marrows show a significantly higher percentage of phospho-STAT5 positive cells upon stimulation than that observed in normal BM and in select other pediatric myeloid disorders. This test can be easily performed in clinical flow cytometry laboratory.[58]

Many JMML patients show polyclonal hyperglobulinemia; however, this finding does not play a role in the diagnosis.

Morphology and immunophenotypic features

PB shows leukocytosis with reported medians in the range of $30 \times 10^9/l$. Approximately 10% of patients have WBC exceeding $100 \times 10^9/l$. Absolute monocytosis is the defining feature of this disease and is even evident in rare patients who present with WBC within normal limits (Fig. 27.7A). The degree of monocytosis is variable with the majority of patients showing more than $5 \times 10^9/l$ monocytes. The reported range for an absolute monocyte count is between 1.1 and $60.8 \times 10^9/l$.[56] Both mature monocytes and their precursors can be seen in the PB. However, the combined blast and promonocyte count is below 5% in the majority of patients. Immature granulocytes and erythroid precursors

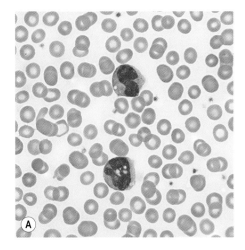

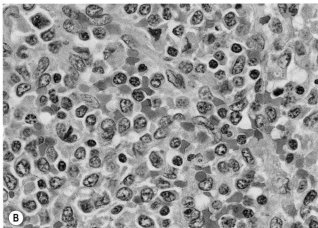

Fig. 27.7 (A, B) JMML. (A) Monocytes in peripheral blood. (B) Extramedullary manifestation (spleen) in JMML.

can also be seen in PB. A proportion of cases show macrocytic red blood cells; however, normocytic or microcytic anemia are not infrequent. Thrombocytopenia is common with close to 20% of patients showing platelet count below $20 \times 10^9/l$.[56]

BM findings are not specific for this disease and the diagnosis of JMML based on BM morphology alone is challenging. Common findings are granulocytic hyperplasia and a left shift. Similar to CMML, the monocytic component is not always prominent but usually at least a mild monocytosis is apparent. Cytochemical stains for nonspecific esterases may help in quantification of monocytic component. Blasts and promonocytes always account for less than 20% of BM elements. Marked dysplasia is not seen; however, rare cases may show mild dysgranulopoiesis, megaloblastoid erythroid series or hypolobated megakaryocytes. The number of megakaryocytes may be decreased. Reticulin fibrosis may be seen.

Flow cytometric immunophenotyping may show abnormalities in the monocyte population and in blasts. However, these changes are not specific for the diagnosis of JMML.

The leukemic infiltrates of extramedullary organs such as lymph nodes, spleen, liver, lungs and skin are composed of a myelomonocytic population similar to that seen in the BM (Fig. 27.7B).

Prognosis

JMML is an aggressive disease with a 5-year survival of 40%.[53] Prognostic factors associated with shorter survival include platelet count below $40 \times 10^9/l$, an increased HbF level, and age above 2 years. Combined HbF, platelet count and cytogenetics (FPC) score has previously been shown to be highly predictive of survival in JMML.[53,59]

Without intensive treatment, the majority of patients succumb to rapidly progressive BM and organ failure. Rare cases transform into an acute phase. Hematopoietic stem cell transplant is curative in approximately 50% of children with JMML.

Rare cases of spontaneous improvement of the disease were reported in the association with Noonan syndrome and in *de novo* JMML with glycine to serine substitution of codon 12 of *RAS* genes.[60–62] The latter observation has been subsequently disputed.[63] Thus, further large-scale studies are required to determine the association of genotype with clinical features and to warrant the withholding of currently available and potentially curative treatment regimens.

Special considerations

Differential diagnosis between JMML and viral infection

The most significant differential diagnosis, especially in young children, is viral infection. Similar to JMML, infections can be accompanied by a leukemoid reaction and monocytosis. Infections with EBV, CMV and HHV6, and other microorganisms such as *Histoplasma, Toxoplasma* and mycobacteria can mimic BM findings and clinical presentation of JMML.[64–67] BM morphology is not useful in distinguishing between JMML and an infectious process. The demonstration of clonality, either with cytogenetic or molecular analysis, is most helpful to resolve this differential

diagnosis. Even though cytogenetic abnormalities are seen only in a third of patients with JMML, 75% of children harbor mutations in genes regulating *RAS* pathway (*NRAS, KRAS, PTPN11* and *NF1*). Recently described mutations in *CBL* gene bring the number of JMML cases with identifiable genetic lesion to over 90%. In female patients with normal cytogenetics and no mutations of genes involved in the regulation of *RAS* activation, human androgen receptor gene analysis (HUMARA assay) may be helpful in establishing a definitive diagnosis.[61]

JMML and transient polyclonal myeloproliferation of Noonan syndrome

Patients with Noonan syndrome are at increased risk of developing JMML due to mutations in genes regulating the *RAS* pathway. They can also exhibit a constitutional nonclonal myelomonocytic proliferation, which can fulfill current diagnostic criteria for JMML and present with similar clinical features.[60,61] These patients can develop a clonal monocyte population and/or cytogenetic abnormality leading to progression of the disease or they can undergo spontaneous remission despite persistent hypersensitivity to GM-CSF.[61] It is critical to distinguish between the transient polyclonal myeloproliferation of Noonan syndrome and true JMML to avoid unnecessary therapy.

Myelodysplastic/myeloproliferative neoplasm, unclassifiable

Definition and diagnostic criteria

Myelodysplastic/myeloproliferative neoplasm, unclassifiable (MDS/MPN,U) includes hematologic malignancies with hybrid myelodysplastic and myeloproliferative features, which at the time of the original diagnosis do not fulfill the diagnostic criteria for CMML, aCML, JMML and for any other form of MPN and/or MDS. It is a diagnosis of exclusion, which requires an extensive work-up. This includes cytogenetic and molecular analysis, and correlation with clinical history to exclude a pre-existing myeloid neoplasm and/or the effects of previous treatment with growth factors or cytotoxic drugs. As previously discussed, the 're-classification' of myeloid neoplasm as MDS/MPN,U based on post-treatment samples obtained at follow-up or upon progression of the disease, even if hybrid myelodysplastic and myeloproliferative features are documented, is not appropriate, at least in most cases.

Epidemiology, clinical and laboratory features

This is a rare entity and demographic data are not readily available. Clinical features reflect a mixed myelodysplastic and myeloproliferative nature of this disease. Manifestations of ineffective hematopoiesis such as cytopenias and excessive proliferation of other lineages, including leukocytosis of more than $13 \times 10^9/l$ and platelet counts higher than $450 \times 10^9/l$, can be seen. Splenomegaly, hepatomegaly and infiltration of other extramedullary organs can also be present.

Morphology and immunophenotypic features

PB can show leukocytosis and/or thrombocytosis with variable degrees of dysplastic features such as pelgeroid and hypogranular forms, and giant and hypogranular platelets. Macrocytic anemia or dimorphic red blood cells may be seen. Increase in blasts cells above 10% may indicate the progression of the disease.[2]

BM is hypercellular with myeloid hyperplasia and dysplasia in at least one of the hematopoietic lineages.

There are no specific cytochemical features. Immunophenotype has not been well studied.

Provisional entity in myelodysplastic/myeloproliferative neoplasm, unclassifiable: refractory anemia with ring sideroblasts associated with marked thrombocytosis

Definition and diagnostic criteria

Refractory anemia with ring sideroblasts associated with marked thrombocytosis (RARS-T) is a provisional entity characterized by anemia, dysplasia of the erythroid lineage, at least 15% ring sideroblasts, thrombocytosis (platelet counts higher than $450 \times 10^9/l$) and large atypical megakaryocytes. The exclusion of cases of MDS with an isolated deletion of chromosome 5, myeloid neoplasms with abnormalities of chromosome 3, as well as cases positive for BCR-ABL1 rearrangement is critical, since all of these entities can present with thrombocytosis and/or dyserythropoiesis. Correlation with clinical data is critical to rule out conditions and medications associated with increase in ring sideroblasts. Finally, the diagnosis of RARS-T is reserved for de novo disease arising in a patient with no previous myeloid neoplasm.

Epidemiology, clinical and laboratory features

RARS-T is rare and accounted for only 0.7% of FAB-defined MDS cases (data from the MDS registry, Dusseldorf, Germany).[68,69] It predominantly affects older adults with a reported median age of presentation ranging from 59 to 73 years. Men and women are equally affected. Anemia and thrombocytosis can be significant; however, the majority of patients present with a median hemoglobin level of 10.1 g/dl and moderate thrombocytosis below $1000 \times 10^9/l$.[70] In a recent study, Raya et al. compared RARS-T cases with marked thrombocytosis to those with only borderline platelet elevation.[71] The former group showed more prominent myeloproliferative features including a higher WBC, higher incidence of splenomegaly and more frequent $JAK2^{V617F}$ mutations. However, rare cases of RARS-T with the $JAK2^{V617F}$ mutation and platelet counts within the normal range have also been reported.

Morphology and immunophenotypic features

Peripheral blood shows thrombocytosis. Although giant platelets can be seen, abnormalities of platelet granulation are not common. Anisopoikilocytosis with dimorphic red blood cells and basophilic stippling are reported. WBC count is usually within normal limits and dysgranulopoiesis is uncommon. Blasts are not seen.

Most cases show hypercellular BM (Fig. 27.8A). The most significant BM findings differentiating RARS-T from other myeloid neoplasms presenting with thrombocytosis and increased numbers of ring sideroblasts, are megakaryocyte morphology accompanied by dyserythropoiesis (Fig. 27.8B). Large pleomorphic megakaryocytes similar to those seen in BCR-ABL1 negative MPN are frequently seen. Although small hypolobated and monolobated forms can also be present, true micromegakaryocytes (diameter of less than 15 microns) are not common. Dyserythropoiesis is a constant finding and includes maturation asynchrony, nuclear budding and megaloblastoid chromatin. Ring sideroblasts are defined as erythroid cells with at least five siderotic granules surrounding at least one third of the nuclear circumference[72] (Fig. 27.8C). In RARS-T, by definition, ring sideroblasts constitute at least 15% of erythroid precursors. It is important to remember that ring sideroblasts per se are not a feature of dysplasia. They can also be seen in a variety of reactive states and appear transiently in association with exposure to medications and toxins. The review of clinical history to exclude reactive causes of ring sideroblasts is an integral part of BM evaluation. BM blasts constitute less than 5% of the differential count. Abnormal localization of immature precursors has not been reported in this entity. Mast cell hyperplasia can be seen in some cases. The majority of cases show at least a mild increase in reticulin fibers. Significant reticulin fibrosis can also be observed.

Prognosis

Prognosis of patients with RARS-T is better than that of other subtypes of MDS/MPNs. Reported median survivals are variable (range between 71 and 101 months).[73,74] However, most reports agree that survival in RARS-T is inferior to that seen in essential thrombocythemia (ET) and comparable to that of RA-RS category of MDS. The initial report on the $JAK2^{V617F}$ mutation suggested that cases with mutated JAK2 have a survival advantage.[75] This finding has not been confirmed in more recent reports and requires further study.[71] Transformation to acute leukemia has been reported.[76]

Special considerations

Differentiation of RARS-T from myeloproliferative neoplasms with thrombocytosis and ring sideroblasts

The presence of ring sideroblasts in MPN has been linked to mutations in genes associated with hemochromatosis.[77] Ring sideroblasts can be seen in approximately 5% of BCR-ABL1 negative MPN including ET and primary myelofibrosis (PMF). These disorders can overlap with RARS-T in regards to the presence of thrombocytosis, degree of megakaryocytic proliferation seen in the bone marrow, and the presence of the $JAK2^{V617F}$ mutation. ET presents with normocellular or slightly hypercellular BM and, in most cases, lacks erythroid or granulocytic hyperplasia. Rare cases can show a borderline increase in the erythroid series; however, dyserythropoiesis

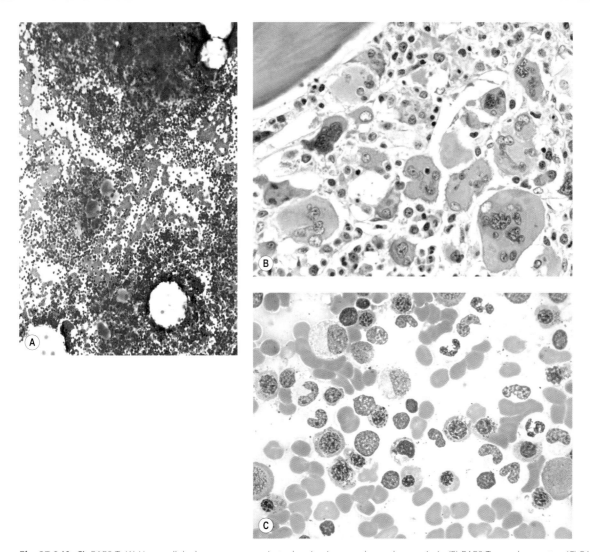

Fig. 27.8 (A–C) RARS-T. (A) Hypercellular bone marrow aspirate showing increased megakaryopoiesis. (B) RARS-T megakaryocytes. (C) RARS-T ring sideroblasts.

is not present. On the contrary, the diagnosis of RARS-T requires the presence of dyserythropoiesis. Similarly, in early prefibrotic stage, PMF presents with thrombocytosis and hypercellular marrow with megakaryocytic hyperplasia. In the majority of these cases, the reduction in the erythroid series, more pronounced dysmegakaryopoiesis and megakaryocyte clustering are helpful in establishing the diagnosis of PMF.

RARS and RARS-T, distinct entities or clinical continuum

Considering overlapping clinicopathological features of this disease, the designation of RARS-T as a distinct entity has been previously disputed. The overlap with myeloproliferative neoplasms has been discussed above. Cases overlapping with MDS of RA-RS category have also been reported. Perhaps the most compelling evidence for the existence of the biological and clinical continuum between these two entities is the development of elevated platelet counts in classical cases of RARS.[70] In a few reported cases of RARS, the onset of thrombocytosis coincided with the appearance of the $JAK2^{V617F}$ mutation in a subset of granulocytes. Of note,

$JAK2$ mutation has been reported in 60% to over 90% of RARS-T cases, and is more frequent in cases with marked thrombocytosis.[71] The latter cases show also higher WBC and more frequent splenomegaly. Thus, the acquisition of the $JAK2^{V617F}$ mutation may indeed confer a myeloproliferative phenotype to what would be otherwise a case of RARS. The more definitive studies to elucidate pathogenesis of RARS-T are needed to clarify its position in the taxonomy of MPN. Until these data are available, the set of features most useful in separating RARS-T from RARS is megakaryocyte morphology and the presence of the $JAK2^{V617F}$ mutation.

Miscellaneous myeloid neoplasms with myelodysplastic and myeloproliferative features

Myelodysplastic syndrome with isolated del(5q) and $JAK2^{V617F}$ mutation

A small subset of MDS with isolated 5q deletion has been recently shown to harbor $JAK2^{V617F}$ mutations.[78] In addition to typical features of MDS with isolated del(5q) such as

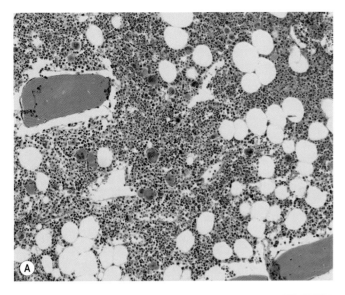

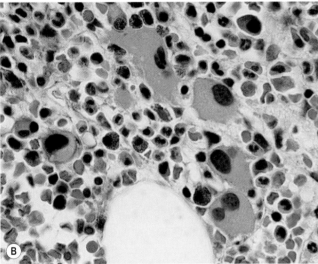

Fig. 27.9 (A, B) Myelodysplastic syndrome with isolated del(5q) and *JAK2*[V617F] mutation. (A) Hypercellular bone marrow with granulocytic hyperplasia and dysmegakaryopoiesis. (B) Higher magnification showing the typical '5q- megakaryocytes'.

hypolobated/monolobated megakaryocytes, these cases more frequently demonstrated a prominent granulocytic hyperplasia with a higher WBC (5.21 vs. 4.45 × 10⁹/l in cases with wild type *JAK2* gene) and a trend for higher platelet counts (Fig. 27.9). A proportion of these cases are responsive to lenalidomide treatment.[79] Until further clinicopathological data are available, the WHO classification recommends that these cases be classified as MDS with isolated del(5q) and the *JAK2*[V617F] mutation.

Myelodysplastic/myeloproliferative neoplasm with isolated isochromosome 17q

MDS/MPN with isochromosome 17q is not uncommon in myeloid neoplasms both within a complex karyotype and as secondary abnormality in patients with CML in accelerated

or blast phase.[80] It can also present as a sole abnormality in cases with mixed myelodysplastic and myeloproliferative features.[81–83] The patient age varies with a median of 60 years. There is a male predominance. The majority of patients present with anemia, leukocytosis due to neutrophilia and organomegaly. Monocytosis is commonly reported and a proportion of cases fulfill the criteria for CMML-1.[83] Dysgranulopoiesis including frequent non-segmented forms, hyposegmented neutrophils (pseudo-Pelger–Huët cells), ring nuclei, hypogranularity and chromatin clumping is prominent (Fig. 27.10A). Blasts represent less than 5% of the differential count in the majority of cases. Platelet counts are variable and abnormal hypogranular and/or giant platelets are often seen. The BM is markedly hypercellular with significant granulocytic proliferation and dysgranulopoiesis (Fig. 27.10B). Blasts constitute less than 5% of the cellularity. Dysplastic changes are also seen in erythroid progenitors and megakaryocytes (Fig. 27.10B). Dysplastic small megakaryocytes and large multinucleated ones have both been reported. Significant fibrosis is frequent (Fig. 27.10C). The median survival was 2.5 years and 64% of patients progressed to AML.[83]

The cases which do not fulfill the criteria for CMML, often show a more pleomorphic megakaryocyte morphology, including large abnormal forms associated with marked fibrosis and organomegaly. These features are more reminiscent of a MPN. Such cases are best left in the category of MDS/MPN, unclassifiable. Cases, which fulfill the diagnostic criteria of CMML can be placed in this category. However, if we consider that the goal of nosology is to define biologically and clinically relevant disease categories, assigning patients with isolated isochromosome 17q to the CMML group does not reflect the dismal prognosis associated with this cytogenetic abnormality. The majority of these patients can be placed in the CMML-1 category, which carries a far better prognosis and lower rate of transformation to AML than cases with the isolated isochromosome 17q. Comprehensive studies of larger case series may allow the more appropriate categorization of these cases in the future.

Concluding remarks

Despite significant advances in our understanding of myelodysplastic/myeloproliferative neoplasms, the diagnosis of these diseases still relies heavily on a careful clinicopathological correlation. In addition to the presence of overlapping features between various entities, the possibility of evolution from another pre-existing myeloid disease should also be considered. This possibility is particularly important in CMML and in cases of RARS-T. Thus, one should remain vigilant to changes in phenotype related to acquisition of secondary genetic lesions. The latter is not uncommon considering the inherent genomic instability of neoplastic cells and can significantly alter the designation of the disease. Unraveling of the specific associations between genotype and phenotype and the discovery of initiating pathogenetic abnormalities will allow us to improve the existing classification so it is more biologically and clinically relevant. This should facilitate patient selection for modern target therapy trials.

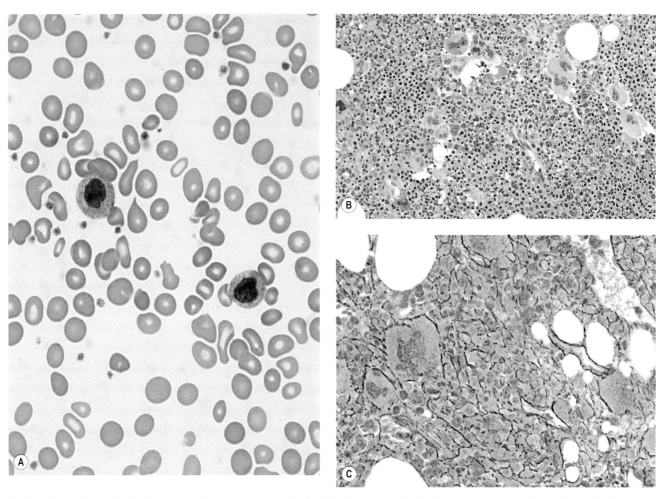

Fig. 27.10 (A–C) Myelodysplastic/myeloproliferative neoplasm with isolated isochromosome 17q. (A) Dysplastic granulocytes in peripheral blood. (B) Hypercellular bone marrow biopsy with granulocytic hyperplasia and dysmegakaryopoiesis. (C) Frequent bone marrow fibrosis (reticulin stain).

References

1. Jaffe E, Harris N, Stein H, editors. WHO Classification of Tumours Pathology and Genetics of Tumours of Hematopoietic and Lymphoid Tissues. Lyon: IARC Press; 2001.

2. Swerdlow S, Campo E, Harris N, editors. WHO Classification of Tumours of Haematopoietic and Lymphoid Tissues. Lyon: IARC Press; 2008.

3. Bennett JM, Catovsky D, Daniel MT, et al. Proposals for the classification of the myelodysplastic syndromes. Br J Haematol 1982;51:189–99.

4. Fenaux P, Beuscart R, Lai JL, et al. Prognostic factors in adult chronic myelomonocytic leukemia: an analysis of 107 cases. J Clin Oncol 1988;6:1417–24.

5. Onida F, Kantarjian HM, Smith TL, et al. Prognostic factors and scoring systems in chronic myelomonocytic leukemia: a retrospective analysis of 213 patients. Blood 2002;99:840–9.

6. Bowen DT. Chronic myelomonocytic leukemia: lost in classification? Hematol Oncol 2005;23:26–33.

7. Bennett JM, Catovsky D, Daniel MT, et al. Proposals for the classification of the acute leukaemias. French-American-British (FAB) co-operative group. Br J Haematol 1976;33:451–8.

8. Germing U, Gattermann N, Minning H, et al. Problems in the classification of CMML – dysplastic versus proliferative type. Leuk Res 1998;22:871–8.

9. Voglová J, Chrobák L, Neuwirtová R, et al. Myelodysplastic and myeloproliferative type of chronic myelomonocytic leukemia – distinct subgroups or two stages of the same disease? Leuk Res 2001 2001;25:493–9.

10. Nösslinger T, Reisner R, Grüner H, et al. Dysplastic versus proliferative CMML – a retrospective analysis of 91 patients from a single institution. Leuk Res 2001;25:741–7.

11. Storniolo AM, Moloney WC, Rosenthal DS, et al. Chronic myelomonocytic leukemia. Leukemia 2002;4:766–70.

12. Orazi A, Chiu R, O'Malley DP, et al. Chronic myelomonocytic leukemia:

the role of bone marrow biopsy immunohistology. Mod Pathol 2006;19:1536–45.

13. Tefferi A, Hoagland HC, Therneau TM, et al. Chronic myelomonocytic leukemia: natural history and prognostic determinants. Mayo Clin Proc 1989;64:1246–54.

14. Yang DT, Greenwood JH, Hartung L, et al. Flow cytometric analysis of different CD14 epitopes can help identify immature monocytic populations. Am J Clin Pathol 2005;124:930–6.

15. Xu Y, McKenna R, Karandikar N, et al. Flow cytometric analysis of monocytes as a tool for distinguishing chronic myelomonocytic leukemia from reactive monocytosis. Am J Clin Pathol 2005;124:799–806.

16. Lacronique-Gazaille C, Chaury, M, Le Guyader, A, et al. A simple method for detection of major phenotypic abnormalities in myelodysplastic syndromes: expression of CD56 in CMML. Haematologica 2007;92:859–60.

17. Qubaja M, Marmey B, Le Tourneau A, et al. The detection of CD14 and CD16 in paraffin-embedded bone marrow biopsies is useful for the diagnosis of chronic myelomonocytic leukemia. Virchows Arch 2009;454:411–19.

18. Ngo N, Lampert I, Naresh, K. Bone marrow trephine morphology and immunohistochemical findings in chronic myelomonocytic leukaemia. Br J Haematol 2008;141:771–81.

19. Germing U, Strupp C, Knipp S, et al. Chronic myelomonocytic leukemia in the light of the WHO proposals. Haematologica 2007;92:974–7.

20. Van der Weide M, Sizoo W, Nauta JJ, et al. Myelodysplastic syndromes: analysis of clinical and prognostic features in 96 patients. Eur J Haematol 1988;41:115–22.

21. Martiat P, Michaux JL, Rodhain J. Philadelphia-negative (Ph−) chronic myeloid leukemia (CML): comparison with Ph+ CML and chronic myelomonocytic leukemia. Groupe Français de Cytogénétique Hématologique. Blood 1991;1:205–111.

22. Chen YC, Chou JM, Ketterling RP, et al. Histologic and immunohistochemical study of bone marrow monocytic nodules in 21 cases with myelodysplasia. Am J Clin Pathol 2003;120:874–81.

23. Vermi W, Facchetti F, Rosati S, et al. Nodal and extranodal tumor-forming accumulation of plasmacytoid monocytes/ interferon-producing cells associated with myeloid disorders. Am J Surg Pathol 2004;28:585–95.

24. Germing U, Kündgen A, Gattermann N. Risk assessment in chronic myelomonocytic leukemia (CMML). Leuk Lymphoma 2004;45:1311–18.

25. Storniolo AM, Moloney WC, Rosenthal DS, et al. Chronic myelomonocytic leukemia. Leukemia 1990;4:766–70.

26. Germing U, Strupp C, Aivado M, et al. New prognostic parameters for chronic myelomonocytic leukemia. Blood 2002; 100:731–2.

27. Kosmider O, Gelsi-Boyer V, Ciudad M, et al. TET2 gene mutation is a frequent and adverse event in chronic myelomonocytic leukemia. Haematologica 2009;94:1676–81.

28. Kuo MC, Liang DC, Huang CF, et al. RUNX1 mutations are frequent in chronic myelomonocytic leukemia and mutations at the C-terminal region might predict acute myeloid leukemia transformation. Leukemia 2009;23:1426–31.

29. Rigolin GM, Cuneo A, Roberti MG, et al. Myelodysplastic syndromes with monocytic component: hematologic and cytogenetic characterization. Haematologica 1997;82:25–30.

30. Rosati S, Mick R, Xu F, et al. Refractory cytopenia with multilineage dysplasia: further characterization of an 'unclassifiable' myelodysplastic syndrome. Leukemia 1996;10:20–6.

31. Breccia M, Cannella L, Frustaci A, et al. Chronic myelomonocytic leukemia with antecedent refractory anemia with excess blasts: further evidence for the arbitrary nature of current classification systems. Leuk Lymphoma 2008 2008;49: 1292–1296.

32. Wang SA, Galili N, Cerny J, et al. Chronic myelomonocytic leukemia evolving from preexisting myelodysplasia shares many features with de novo disease. Am J Clin Pathol 2006;126:789–97.

33. George R, Pearson AD, Evans J, et al. Secondary chronic myelomonocytic leukemia with t(9;11) in a child. Cancer Gen Cytogenet 1994;75:64–6.

34. Noriko S, Yasushi I, Yoshiko O, et al. Novel MLL-CBP fusion transcript in therapy-related chronic myelomonocytic leukemia with a t(11;16) (q23;p13) chromosome translocation. Genes Chromosome and Cancer 1997;20: 60–3.

35. Czader M, Orazi A. Therapy-related myeloid neoplasms. Am J Clin Pathol 2009;132:410–25.

36. Breccia M, Biondo F, Latagliata R, et al. Identification of risk factors in atypical chronic myeloid leukemia. Haematologica 2006;91:1566–8.

37. Fend F, Horn T, Koch I, et al. Atypical chronic myeloid leukemia as defined in the WHO classification is a JAK2 V617F negative neoplasm. Leukemia Res 2008; 32:1931–5.

38. Hernández JM, del Cañizo MC, Cuneo A, et al. Clinical, hematological and cytogenetic characteristics of atypical chronic myeloid leukemia. Ann Oncol 2000;11:441–4.

39. Kurzrock R, Bueso-Ramos CE, Kantarjian H, et al. BCR rearrangement-negative chronic myelogenous leukemia revisited. J Clin Oncol 2001;19:2915–26.

40. Bennett JM, Catovsky D, Daniel MT, et al. The chronic myeloid leukaemias: guidelines for distinguishing chronic granulocytic, atypical chronic myeloid, and chronic myelomonocytic leukaemia. Proposals by the French-American-British Cooperative Leukaemia Group. Br J Haematol 1994;87:746–54.

41. Costello R, Sainty D, Lafage-Pochitaloff M, et al. Clinical and biological aspects of Philadelphia-negative/BCR-negative chronic myeloid leukemia. Leuk Lymphoma 1997;25:225–32.

42. Koldehoff M, Beelen DW, Trenschel R, et al. Outcome of hematopoietic stem cell transplantation in patients with atypical chronic myeloid leukemia. Bone Marrow Transplant 2004;34:1047–50.

43. Morel P, Bryon, P, Guyon J, et al. Hémopathie maligne de type aplastique avec anomalies nucléaires majeures des granulocytes. Semaine des Hôpitaux 1968;49:3026–8.

44. Gustke SS, Becker GA, Garancis JC, et al. Chromatin clumping in mature leukocytes: a hitherto unrecognized abnormality. Blood 1970;35:637–58.

45. Felman P, Bryon PA, Gentilhomme O, et al. The syndrome of abnormal chromatin clumping in leucocytes: a myelodysplastic disorder with proliferative features? Br J Haematol 1988;70:49–54.

46. Brizard A, Huret JL, Lamotte F, et al. Three cases of myelodysplastic-myeloproliferative disorder with abnormal chromatin clumping in granulocytes. Br J Haematol 1989;72:294–5.

47. Jaen A, Irriguible D, Milla F, et al. Abnormal chromatin clumping in leucocytes: a clue to a new subtype of myelodysplastic syndrome. Eur J Haematol 1990;45:209–14.

48. Adhya, A, Ahluwalia J, Varma N, et al. Abnormal chromatin clumping in leucocytes of Ph positive chronic myeloid leukemia cases – extending the morphological spectrum. Indian J Pathol Microbiol 2008;51:548–50.

49. Banerjee R, Halil O, Bain BJ, et al. Neutrophil dysplasia caused by mycophenolate mofetil. Transplantation 2000;70:1608–10.

50. Daliphard, S, Accard F, Delattre C, et al. Reversible abnormal chromatin clumping in granulocytes from six transplant patients treated with mycophenolate mofetil: a rare adverse effect mimicking abnormal chromatin clumping syndrome. Br J Haematol 2002;116:725–8.

51. Reiter A, Walz C, Watmore A, et al. The t(8;9)(p22;p24) is a recurrent abnormality in chronic and acute leukemia that fuses PCM1 to JAK2. Cancer Res 2005;65: 2662–7.

52. Bousquet M, Quelen C, De Mas V, et al. The t(8;9)(p22;p24) translocation in atypical chronic myeloid leukaemia yields a new PCM1-JAK2 fusion gene. Oncogene 2005;24:7248–52.

53. Passmore SJ, Chessells JM, Kempski H, et al. Paediatric myelodysplastic syndromes and juvenile myelomonocytic leukaemia in the UK: a population-based study of incidence and survival. Br J Haematol 2003;121:758–67.

54. Hasle H, Niemeyer CM, Chessells JM, et al. A pediatric approach to the WHO classification of myelodysplastic and myeloproliferative diseases. Leukemia 2003;17:277–82.

55. Chan RJ, Cooper T, Kratz CP, et al. Juvenile myelomonocytic leukemia: a report from the 2nd International JMML Symposium. Leuk Res 2009;33:355–62.

56. Niemeyer CM, Arico M, Basso G, et al. Chronic myelomonocytic leukemia in childhood: a retrospective analysis of 110 cases. European Working Group on Myelodysplastic Syndromes in Childhood (EWOG-MDS). Blood 1997;89:3534–343.

57. Emanuel PD, Bates LJ, Castleberry RP, et al. Selective hypersensitivity to granulocyte-macrophage colony-stimulating factor by juvenile chronic

myeloid leukemia hematopoietic progenitors. Blood 1991;77:925–9.

58. Kotecha N, Flores N, Irish J, et al. Single cell profiling identifies aberrant STAT5 activation in myeloid malignancies with specific clinical and biologic correlates. Cancer Cell 2008;14:335–43.

59. Passmore SJ, Hann IM, Stiller CA, et al. Pediatric myelodysplasia: a study of 68 children and a new prognostic scoring system. Blood 1995;1:1742–50.

60. Bader-Meunier B, Tchernia G, Miélot F, et al. Occurrence of myeloproliferative disorder in patients with Noonan syndrome. J Pediatr 1997;130:885–9.

61. Lavin VA, Hamid R, Patterson J, et al. Use of human androgen receptor gene analysis to aid the diagnosis of JMML in female Noonan syndrome patients. Pediatr Blood Cancer 2008;51:298–302.

62. Matsuda K, Shimada A, Yoshida N, et al. Spontaneous improvement of hematologic abnormalities in patients having juvenile myelomonocytic leukemia with specific RAS mutations. Blood 2007;109:5477–80.

63. Flotho C, Kratz C, Bergstrasser E, et al. Genotype-phenotype correlation in cases of juvenile myelomonocytic leukemia with clonal RAS mutations. Blood 2008;111:966–7.

64. Herrod H, Dow L, Sullivan J. Persistent Epstein–Barr virus infection mimicking juvenile chronic myelogenous leukemia: immunologic and hematologic studies. Blood 1983;61:1098–104.

65. Kirby M, Weitzman S, Freedman MH. Juvenile chronic myelogenous leukemia: differentiation from infantile cytomegalovirus infection. Am J Pediatr Hematal Oncol 1990;12:292–6.

66. Pinkel D. Differentiating juvenile myelomonocytic leukemia from infectious disease. Blood 1998;91:365–7.

67. Lorenzana A, Lyons H, Sawaf H, et al. Human herpesvirus 6 infection mimicking juvenile myelomonocytic leukemia in an infant. J Pediatr Hematol 2002;24:136–41.

68. Gattermann N, Billiet J, Kronenwett R, et al. High frequency of the JAK2 V617F mutation in patients with thrombocytosis (platelet count>600 × 10⁹/L) and ringed sideroblasts more than 15% considered as MDS/MPD, unclassifiable. Blood 2007;1:1334–5.

69. Orazi A, Germing U. The myelodysplastic/myeloproliferative neoplasms: myeloproliferative diseases with dysplastic features. Leukemia 2008;22:1308–19.

70. Malcovati L, Della Porta MG, Pietra D, et al. Molecular and clinical features of refractory anemia with ringed sideroblasts associated with marked thrombocytosis. Blood 2009;22:3538–45.

71. Raya JM, Arenillas L, Domingo A, et al. Refractory anemia with ringed sideroblasts associated with thrombocytosis: comparative analysis of marked with non-marked thrombocytosis, and relationship with JAK2 V617F mutational status. Int J Hematol 2008;88:387–95.

72. Mufti GJ, Bennett JM, Goasguen J, et al. Diagnosis and classification of myelodysplastic syndrome: International Working Group on Morphology of Myelodysplastic Syndrome (IWGM-MDS) consensus proposals for the definition and enumeration of myeloblasts and ring sideroblasts. Haematologica 2008;93:1712–7.

73. Shaw GR. Ringed sideroblasts with thrombocytosis: an uncommon mixed myelodysplastic/myeloproliferative disease of older adults. Br J Haematol 2005;131:180–4.

74. Wang SA, Hasserjian RP, Loew JM, et al. Refractory anemia with ringed sideroblasts associated with marked thrombocytosis harbors JAK2 mutation and shows overlapping myeloproliferative and myelodysplastic features. Leukemia 2006;20:1641–4.

75. Schmitt-Graeff A, Thiele J, Zuk I, et al. Essential thrombocythemia with ringed sideroblasts: a heterogeneous spectrum of diseases, but not a distinct entity. Haematologica 2002;87:392–9.

76. Pich A, Riera L, Sismondi F, et al. JAK2V617F activating mutation is associated with the myeloproliferative type of chronic myelomonocytic leukaemia. J Clin Pathol 2009;62:798–801.

77. Szpurka H, Tiu R, Murugesan G, et al. Refractory anemia with ringed sideroblasts associated with marked thrombocytosis (RARS-T), another myeloproliferative condition characterized by JAK2 V617F mutation. Blood 2006;1:2173–81.

78. Ingram W, Lea NC, Cervera J, et al. The JAK2 V617F mutation identifies a subgroup of MDS patients with isolated deletion 5q and a proliferative bone marrow. Leukemia 2006;20:1319–21.

79. Melchert M, Kale V, List A. The role of lenalidomide in the treatment of patients with chromosome5q deletion and other myelodysplastic syndromes. Curr Opin Hematol 2007;14:123–9.

80. Hernandez-Boluda JC, Cervantes F, Costa D, et al. Blast crisis of Philadelphia-positive chronic myeloid leukemia with isochromosome 17q: report of 12 cases and review of the literature. Leuk Lymphoma 2000;38:83–90.

81. Weh HJ, Kuse R, Hossfeld DK. Acute nonlymphocytic leukemia (ANLL) with isochromosome i(17q) as the sole chromosomal anomaly: a distinct entity? Eur J Haematol 1990;44:312–14.

82. Sole F, Torrabadella M, Granada I, et al. Isochromosome 17q as a sole anomaly: a distinct myelodysplastic syndrome entity? Leuk Res 1993;17:717–20.

83. McClure RF, Dewald GW, Hoyer JD, et al. Isolated isochromosome 17q: a distinct type of mixed myeloproliferative disorder/myelodysplastic syndrome with aggressive clinical course. Br J Haematol 1999;106:445–54.

CHAPTER 28

The chronic lymphoid leukemias

R Rosenquist, A Porwit

Chapter contents

In this chapter we deal with the chronic lymphoproliferative disorders that usually present with lymphocytosis (i.e. as leukemia). We discuss these conditions using the newest edition of the World Health Organization (WHO 2008) classification as a framework;[1] bone marrow (BM) involvement by lymphoid neoplasms more often presenting as lymphoma is described in Chapter 29.

Chronic lymphocytic leukemia

B-cell chronic lymphocytic leukemia (CLL) is a chronic leukemia resulting from the proliferation of a neoplastic clone of monoclonal B-lymphocytes with a very characteristic immunophenotype (CD19$^+$/CD5$^+$/CD23$^+$).The CLL diagnosis can be readily established if these cells are more than or equal to 5×10^9/l in peripheral blood (PB).[1]

In the WHO 2008 classification, CLL falls into the category designated CLL/small lymphocytic lymphoma (SLL). Cases of SLL differ from CLL only in that there is no PB lymphocytosis at presentation. However, lymphocytosis may or may not develop during the course of the disease.

CLL patients often have an indolent disease course and will survive for many years, even decades, and may die from unrelated causes rather than from the leukemia. However, patients with advanced-stage disease may succumb rapidly from disease progression or, in a minority, following transformation (i.e. Richter's syndrome).

Clinical features

CLL is the most common leukemia in the Western world with an incidence of the order of 6/100 000/year, whereas

DOI: 10.1016/B978-0-7020-3147-2.00028-6

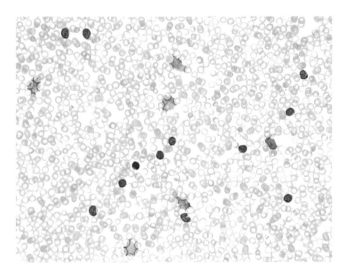

Fig. 28.1 Peripheral blood smear in chronic lymphocytic leukemia showing lymphocytosis and frequent smear cells. MGG, ×60 objective.

the disease is much less prevalent in Asian countries.[2] It is mainly a disease of the middle-aged and elderly, and with a male:female ratio of approximately 2:1 (http://www.hmrn.org/Statistics/Incidence.aspx).

In most patients, the diagnosis of CLL is an incidental one, made when a blood count is performed without any clinical suspicion of leukemia. These patients have no abnormal physical findings nor any symptoms resulting from the leukemia. In other patients with more advanced disease, the typical clinical findings are lymphadenopathy, splenomegaly and, less often, hepatomegaly. In some patients, the initial presentation is with herpes zoster or with symptoms and signs of anemia resulting from autoimmune hemolytic anemia with a positive direct antiglobulin test. Usually, there is a reduction of normal serum immunoglobulins, particularly in patients with advanced disease. A minority of patients may have a paraproteinemia.

Pathologic features

Peripheral blood

In early-stage disease, the only PB abnormality is lymphocytosis with an increase of mature small lymphocytes, which are relatively uniform in their cytologic features (Fig. 28.1). The lymphocytes typically have a high nucleocytoplasmic ratio, condensed chromatin and an inapparent or barely apparent nucleolus. Sometimes the chromatin is condensed into a mosaic pattern. Smear cells are typically seen in blood films, but are not pathognomonic (Fig. 28.1). The presence of some plasmacytoid lymphocytes and small numbers of cells with cleft or irregular nuclei is compatible with a diagnosis of CLL. There may be up to 10% prolymphocytes (atypical cells with larger, more prominent nucleoli). The presence of more than 10% prolymphocytes or of a spectrum of cells from small to large, with cytoplasmic basophilia, may be associated with increased proliferation and disease progression. If the number of prolymphocytes exceeds 55% a diagnosis of prolymphocytic leukemia should be considered.

In patients with more advanced disease, there is anemia and thrombocytopenia. The anemia is usually normocytic

and normochromic with no specific morphologic features. In patients with complicating autoimmune hemolytic anemia, there are spherocytes and polychromasia. In untreated patients, neutropenia is uncommon.

Bone marrow

The BM aspirate is hypercellular as the result of an increase in small mature lymphocytes with the same cytologic features as those in blood. A threshold of 30% lymphocytes has been previously applied as a diagnostic criterion of CLL involvement in BM aspirate; nowadays it is usually replaced by detection of monoclonal B-cell population >5 × 10⁹/l with CLL phenotype by flow cytometry (FCM) (Fig. 28.2).

The BM trephine biopsy (BMTB) shows variable degree of infiltration. The neoplastic infiltrate is composed predominantly of small lymphocytes with low numbers of prolymphocytes and para-immunoblasts (Fig. 28.3). The small lymphocytes have coarsely clumped chromatin and scanty cytoplasm. Prolymphocytes are slightly larger than small lymphocytes with a dispersed chromatin pattern and a small central nucleolus. Para-immunoblasts are medium-sized cells with an open chromatin pattern, prominent central nucleolus and moderate amounts of basophilic cytoplasm. Prolymphocytes and para-immunoblasts may be present in greater numbers in some areas of the infiltrate. Those areas usually show higher proliferation and are called proliferation centers (Fig. 28.4A). Four patterns of infiltration are seen – interstitial, nodular, nodular-interstitial and diffuse. The interstitial pattern is characterized by neoplastic cells infiltrating individually between normal hemopoietic precursors and fat cells. Nodular infiltrates focally replace fat and hemopoietic cells. Nodular-interstitial infiltration is a combination of the nodular and interstitial patterns (Fig. 28.4B). In cases with diffuse infiltration there is complete replacement of hemopoietic precursors and fat cells. Unlike many other BM lymphoid infiltrates, there is usually little or no increase in reticulin associated with infiltration by CLL.

Other tissues

Lymph node involvement in CLL is characterized by effacement of nodal architecture by a diffuse infiltrate of small lymphocytes with the formation of proliferation centers in which there are increased numbers of prolymphocytes and para-immunoblasts. At low power proliferation centers appear paler than the surrounding areas, and if numerous can give the infiltrate an appearance of nodularity (Fig. 28.5).

In the spleen, infiltration leads to expansion of the white pulp, with some cases also having involvement of the red pulp.[3] Infiltration of the liver involves both portal tracts and sinusoids. Rarely there may be symptomatic infiltration of the skin,[4] CNS[5] or prostate.[6] In all these tissues the infiltrate is made up predominantly of small lymphocytes.

Rapid development of an extramedullary tumor is the typical presentation of Richter's syndrome, which represents the clinico-pathologic transformation of CLL to an aggressive lymphoma, most commonly diffuse large B-cell lymphoma (DLBCL).[7] In most cases, CLL transform to a clonally related DLBCL, but development of a DLBCL unrelated to the CLL clone has also been described.[7] In some patients

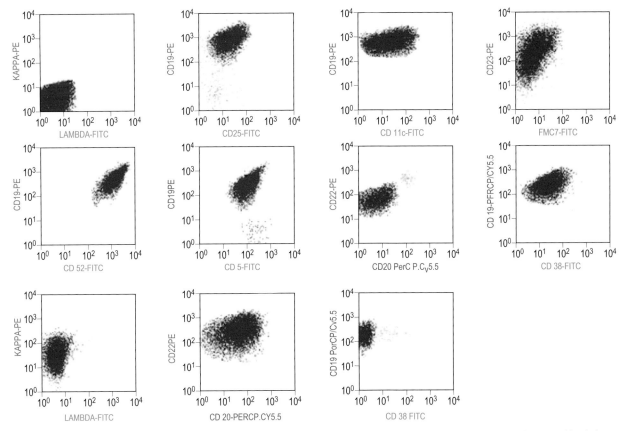

Fig. 28.2 Flow cytometry of CLL. The upper and middle rows show a CLL case (red dots) with typical immunophenotype: kappa and lambda negative, CD20 negative, FMC7 negative, CD5 dim, CD23 positive, CD22 dim, CD52 bright. Normal B-cells can be seen in green on CD20/CD22 plot and normal T-cells in blue on the CD19/CD5 plot. The lower row shows another CLL case positive for CD20 and with membrane kappa.

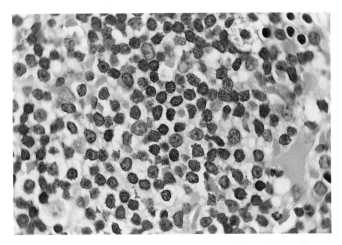

Fig. 28.3 Trephine biopsy section of CLL showing infiltration by small lymphocytes with low numbers of prolymphocytes. H&E, ×100 objective.

the infiltration by CLL and DLBCL can be seen in the same biopsy material. In rare patients, a transformation towards Hodgkin lymphoma has been described and Epstein–Barr virus has been implicated in pathogenesis of this transformation.[8]

Immunophenotype

Besides characteristic CD19/CD5/CD23 phenotype, FCM studies show a weak surface membrane expression of monotypic (kappa or lambda) immunoglobulin, usually IgM with or without IgD and a weak expression of certain B-cell markers, specifically CD20, CD22 and CD79b[9] (Fig. 28.2). FMC7, which is expressed by most other mature B-cell neoplasms, is usually weak or negative, while CD43 and CD200 are positive. CD11c and CD25 are variably expressed.

Modern FCM technology can now detect low levels of cells with CLL phenotype in 0.6–12%[10] of healthy population with a male:female ratio of approximately 2:1. The prevalence increases with age and in individuals with first-degree relatives with CLL. The absolute numbers of cells with CLL phenotype are low (median 13, range 3–1458 per mm^3) and represent a minor proportion of total B-lymphocytes in most cases (5–10%).[10] It has been demonstrated that virtually all cases of CLL have been preceded by CLL-type MBL several years prior to diagnosis.[11] However, the risk for an individual with CLL-type MBL to develop CLL is likely to be low and currently estimated as approximately 1% per year.

Cytogenetics and molecular genetics

In recent years, molecular genetic studies have revealed new prognostic markers which have significantly improved the subdivision of CLL. One of the most stable molecular markers, the somatic hypermutation status of the immunoglobulin heavy variable (IGHV) genes, divides CLL into two clinical subgroups, where patients with unmutated IGHV genes (≥98% identity to the corresponding germline gene; ~30–40% of patients) show a considerably worse prognosis than patients with mutated IGHV genes (<98%

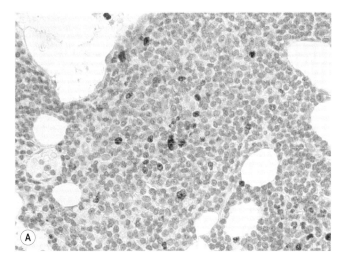

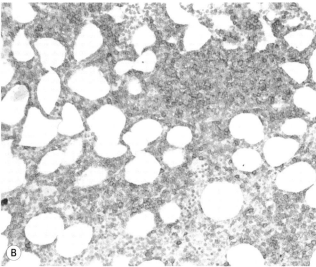

Fig. 28.4 (A, B) (A) Nodular infiltrate of CLL in trephine biopsy showing a proliferation center visualized by immunostaining for proliferation marker Ki67 (MIB-1 antibody). (B) Trephine biopsy section with CLL involvement with nodular and interstitial infiltration visualized by staining for B-cell marker CD20.

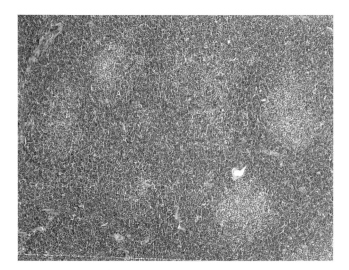

Fig. 28.5 Lymph node biopsy section in chronic lymphocytic leukemia showing a pseudonodular pattern of involvement.

identity to the corresponding germline gene; 60–70% of patients).[12,13] IGHV unmutated CLL patients also display a more progressive disease, more frequently carry high-risk genomic aberrations and require chemotherapy at an earlier stage than IGHV mutated CLL patients. IGHV mutational analysis can be performed at any time point during the disease course, since the mutational status will remain unchanged in CLL.

Immunogenetic studies have suggested that antigen stimulation may be involved in disease development.[14] This is supported by the finding of non-random combinations of specific IGHV-D-J genes and homologous complementarity determining region 3 (CDR3) leading to structural similarity of the B-cell receptor (BCR) in a significant proportion of CLL patients.[15,16] The similarity of the BCR among patients belonging to a 'stereotyped' subset suggests that the antigens these receptors bind to are similar and potentially relevant to disease pathogenesis. Interestingly, it was recently indicated that stereotyped subsets may not only share biological but also clinical features.[16] For instance, the IGHV3-21/IGLV3-21 subset has been associated with a poor outcome irrespective of IGHV gene mutational status.

Potential surrogate markers for the IGHV mutational status have been suggested, e.g. the expression levels of CD38 and ZAP70 as determined by flow cytometry.[13,17] Although studies have shown an insufficient correlation between the CD38 level and IGHV mutational status, CD38 may still serve as an independent prognostic factor.[18] More promising is the expression level of the tyrosine kinase ZAP70, which predict the IGHV gene mutation status with high accuracy,[17,19] although discordant results have been reported.[18]

In contrast to many other B-cell lymphoma entities, there are no genetic aberrations that are common to all CLL patients. Several recurrent aberrations have been characterized, where the most frequent are deletion of 13q14 (50–55%), deletion of 11q22-23 (12–18%), trisomy 12 (11–16%) and deletion of 17p13 (5–10%).[20] These recurrent aberrations are often present only in a proportion of cells of the leukemic clone, indicating that they do not reflect the initial leukemogenic event. The 11q22-23 deletion encompasses the *ATM* gene and the 17p13 deletion covers the *TP53* gene, where both of these genes are crucial in maintaining cell cycle control. Interestingly, two micro-RNAs, *miR-15* and *miR-16*, have recently been shown to be encoded in the deleted region of 13q, and have been proposed to be of pathogenetic importance in CLL.[21]

Patients with 13q deletion, if present as a single aberration, are known to have a better outcome compared to patients with 11q and especially 17p deletions, whereas trisomy 12 patients show a more intermediate risk-profile.[20] Patients with poor-risk aberrations also respond poorly to current treatment protocols, in particular the 17p-deleted subgroup. Since conventional cytogenetics give a low success rate (will only detect ~40–50% aberrations), fluorescence *in situ* hybridization (FISH) analysis has became the gold standard in CLL using a commercially available panel of FISH probes to screen for 11q-, 13q-, +12 and 17p-. This FISH analysis is usually performed on interphase cells from a peripheral blood smear where the proportion of aberrant cells is counted (Fig. 28.6). Since clonal evolution can occur in CLL and high-risk aberrations can emerge over time, it is

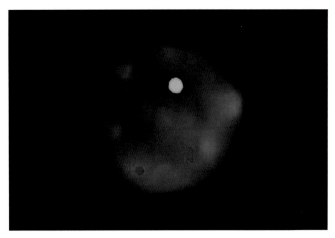

Fig. 28.6 FISH analysis of 11q/17p in CLL. A CLL cell is analyzed using FISH probes directed to the *ATM* gene on 11q (green color) and the *TP53* gene on 17p (red color). Both copies of *TP53* are present while one copy of the *ATM* gene is deleted.

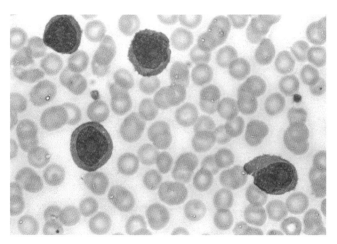

Fig. 28.7 Peripheral blood film in B-lineage prolymphocytic leukemia showing large lymphoid cells with a regular outline and a round nucleus; each cell has a single large vesicular nucleolus. MGG, ×100 objective.

important to perform FISH analysis if there is a change in clinical course or if the patient does not respond to therapy as expected.

Leukemic presentations of other B-cell lymphomas

Blood and BM presentatations of other B-cell lymphomas are described in detail in Chapter 29. Frequency of leukemic presentation and immunophenotypes of cells that can be found in blood and bone marrow are summarized in Table 29.1.

Prolymphocytic leukemias

B-lineage prolymphocytic leukemia

B-cell prolymphocytic leukemia (B-PLL) is an uncommon chronic leukemia (1% of lymphocytic leukemias) resulting from the proliferation of a neoplastic clone of mature B-lymphocytes with specific cytologic features of prolymphocytes. Cases of transformed CLL and cases carrying translocation t(11;14)(q13;q32) are excluded.

Clinical features

B-PLL is usually a disease of the elderly (median age 70 years) with a slight male preponderance. Typically, there is splenomegaly with only minor lymphadenopathy. In most patients the rate of disease progression is much more rapid than that of CLL. A paraprotein is present more often than in CLL. Prognosis is considerably worse than that of CLL with the median survival being about 3 years.[22]

Pathologic features

Peripheral blood

The white cell count is usually markedly elevated as the result of the presence of considerable numbers of abnormal lymphoid cells. Prolymphocytes are medium-sized to large

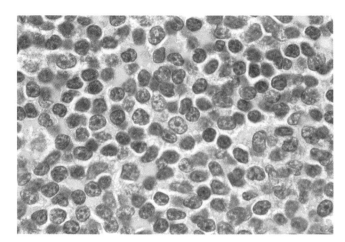

Fig. 28.8 Trephine biopsy section in B-prolymphocytic leukemia. H&E, ×100 objective.

cells, characterized by a prominent nucleolus which appears vesicular because of perinucleolar chromatin condensation (Fig. 28.7). In some patients, the majority of neoplastic cells are typical large prolymphocytes with large prominent nucleoli. In others, there is a spectrum of cells with the medium-sized and smaller cells having less prominent nucleoli. Prolymphocytes must exceed 55% of blood cells. Smear cells are not a typical feature. Anemia and thrombocytopenia are common.

Bone marrow

The bone marrow is infiltrated by cells with similar cytologic features to those in the peripheral blood.

The bone marrow trephine biopsy usually shows an interstitial pattern of infiltration, but nodular–interstitial and diffuse patterns are also seen. The neoplastic cells are slightly larger than the small lymphocytes seen in CLL and have coarsely clumped chromatin and a prominent nucleolus (Fig. 28.8). There is usually an increase in reticulin fibers in the areas of infiltration.

Other tissues

The spleen shows expansion of the white-pulp marginal zone by cells similar to those seen in the bone marrow; there is often also infiltration of the red pulp. Clinically significant involvement of other tissues, including lymph nodes, is uncommon.

Immunophenotype

The neoplastic cells in the majority of patients show strong expression of surface membrane immunoglobulin. This is usually IgM, with or without IgD. CD5 and CD23 are not expressed whereas there is strong expression of CD19, CD20, CD22, CD79a, CD79b, FMC7 and often CD11c.[22] Previously described cases with CD5 expression represent probably leukemic presentations of mantle cell lymphoma.

Cytogenetics and molecular genetics

Roughly half of B-PLL cases display unmutated IGHV genes, but in contrast to CLL this has no prognostic impact.[23] There is no specific cytogenetic aberration characteristic for B-PLL. These patients often show complex karyotypes which may include deletion of 6q and structural aberration of chromosome 1. Initially, t(11;14) was demontrated in up to 20% of B-PLL but these cases are now instead considered as leukemic variants of MCL and excluded from B-PLL category. *TP53* abnormalities (e.g. deletions and/or mutations) are very common in B-PLL, which may be related to the observed poor outcome.[24] Deletion of 11q22-23 and 13q14 are also frequent,[25] whereas trisomy 12 is present at a lower frequency than in CLL. Gene expression analysis showed that B-PLL has a specific signature, which differs from that of CLL.[26] The overexpression of *C-MYC* and *AKT* combined with *TP53* impairment may have a central role in the pathogenesis of B-PLL, promoting apoptosis inhibition and cell proliferation.[26]

T-lineage prolymphocytic leukemia

T-lineage prolymphocytic leukemia (T-PLL) is a rare lymphoproliferative disorder (3% of all T-cell lymphoproliferative disorders, 1% of chronic leukemias).[27] It results from proliferation of small-medium sized T-cells with a mature post-thymic TCL1 phenotype and characteristic overexpression of the TCL1 protein. It has no relationship to the B-lineage prolymphocytic leukemia.

Clinical features

The disease occurs in late middle and old age and is somewhat more common in men than in women (M:F 1.4). Patients usually present with general symptoms, splenomegaly and in about a half of patients there is also lymphadenopathy and/or hepatomegaly. Skin infiltration occurs in about a third of patients and typically leads to either a papular, non-itchy rash on the trunk, face and arms or to a generalized erythroderma.[22,28] Prognosis is very poor with survival usually being less than a year.[28] However, in one third of patients treatment with humanized anti-CD52 monoclonal antibody resulted in complete remission and prolonged survival was achieved in patients who received consolidation with stem cells transplant.[29,30]

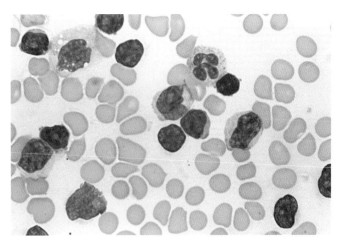

Fig. 28.9 Peripheral blood film in T-lineage prolymphocytic leukemia showing medium sized lymphoid cells with irregular nuclei; some cells have prominent medium-sized nucleoli. MGG, ×100.

Pathologic features

Peripheral blood

There is anemia in 25% of patients and moderate to marked lymphocytosis with WBC >100 × 10^9/l in above 70% of patients.[31] The prolymphocytes of T-PLL are usually readily differentiated from those of B-PLL. T-PLL cells are more irregular in shape and may show cytoplasmic basophilia (Fig. 28.9). The nucleolus may be less prominent. Often they are smaller than B-PLL cells and in 20% of cases are no larger than the cells of CLL. They can, however, be distinguished from CLL cells by their cytoplasmic basophilia, cytoplasmic blebs and irregular, hyperchromatic nucleus with a nucleolus. The term 'small cell variant' of T-PLL is often used for the latter cases, although they do not differ in any important respect from cases with larger cells. In 5% of cases, irregular, so-called cerebriform nuclei are observed.[31]

Bone marrow

The BM is infiltrated by cells with similar cytologic features to those in the blood. Trephine-biopsy histology usually shows a mixed interstitial–diffuse pattern of infiltration. The infiltrating cells resemble those of B-PLL although in many cases the cells of T-PLL have more irregular nuclear outlines (Fig. 28.10). Immunophenotyping is required to make the distinction on histologic sections. A minority of patients have either very little infiltration or a heavy diffuse infiltrate.

Other tissues

The spleen shows expansion of the white pulp and infiltration of the red pulp.[32] Lymph node architecture is effaced by a diffuse infiltrate that initially replaces the paracortex. An important feature in making a distinction from CLL is the absence of proliferation centers. Skin infiltration is dermal, sometimes with extension into the subcutaneous fat; infiltration is preferentially around skin appendages and blood vessels.[33]

Immunophenotype

Leukemic cells are usually positive for CD7 and CD3 although about 20% express cytoplasmic but not surface

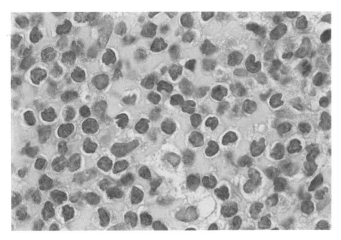

Fig. 28.10 Trephine biopsy in T-lineage prolymphocytic leukemia. H&E, ×100 objective.

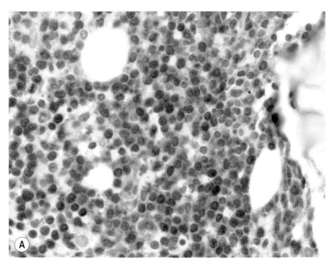

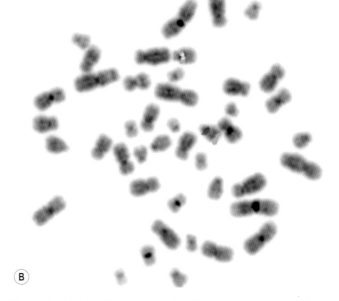

CD3. They are usually CD4 positive and CD8 negative (60%) but in a minority of cases cells either express both CD4 and CD8 or are CD4 negative and CD8 positive. TCL1 protein is present in most cases (Fig. 28.11A). T-PLL cells usually do not express CD25 or express it only weakly, a useful feature in making a distinction from adult T-cell leukemia lymphoma. NK-cell markers (CD56, CD57, CD16), as well as T-precursor related markers CD1a and Tdt, are negative.[31,34]

Cytogenetics and molecular genetics

T-cell receptor (TCR) β and/or γ are rearranged in all cases of T-PLL.[29] The most characteristic cytogenetic aberrations in T-PLL, observed in about 80% of patients, is inversion of chromosome 14, inv(14)(q11q32), where the *TCL1* gene at 14q32 is rearranged to the T-cell receptor αδ locus at 14q11.[35] In a minor proportion of cases a translocation between two chromosome 14, t(14;14)(q11;q32), may instead occur. Both these rearrangements lead to constitutive activation of *TCL1* which has oncogenetic properites and hence prevent apoptosis. inv(14) or t(14;14) can be indicated by FISH analysis using a probe directed to the TCR αδ locus (Fig. 28.11B).

Conventional cytogenetics usually reveals complex karyotypes in T-PLL. Structural abnormalities of chromosome 8 are observed in 70–80% of cases.[36] Furthermore, deletion of 11q22-23 and *ATM* mutations are frequent in T-PLL[37] as well as aberrations of chromosome 6 and 17.

T-cell large granular lymphocyte leukemia and lymphoproliferative disorders of NK cells

Chronic leukemias of large granular lymphocytes (LGL) may be of either T-lineage or natural killer (NK) lineage. The WHO classification recognizes these as separate entities, using the names T-cell large granular lymphocytic leukemia and chronic lymphoproliferative disorders of NK cells.[1] Both are rare disorders, representing together 2–3% of mature lymphocytic leukemias and have indolent character with most patients surviving >10 years. The majority of patients

Fig. 28.11 (A, B) (A) TCL-1 expression in T-PLL *(courtesy of Dr Elizabeth Hyjek, Department of Pathology, University of Chicago, USA)*. (B) FISH analysis of T-PLL. The TCR alfa/delta break-apart FISH probe (yellow color) is directed to the *TCR* alfa/delta locus on chromosome 14q. In a normal cell two yellow signals will appear, while in the presence of inv(14) the FISH probe will be split into one red and one green signal.

are older than 45 years of age.[1] In contrast, most patients with a very rare aggressive NK-cell leukemia that is in most cases Epstein–Barr virus related survive only a few months. This type of leukemia occurs mostly in young adults and it is much commoner in Asia, among Japanese and Chinese people, than among Europeans.[38]

Clinical features

T-cell LGL leukemia may be an incidental diagnosis or patients may present with recurrent infections, resulting from neutropenia. Splenomegaly is common (60% of patients), hepatomegaly is seen in 20% of patients but lymphadenopathy is not a constant feature. There is an association with rheumatoid arthritis, including Felty's syndrome.

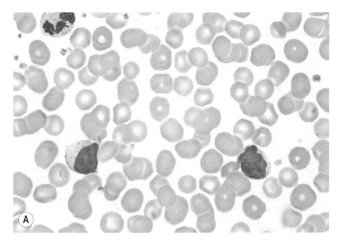

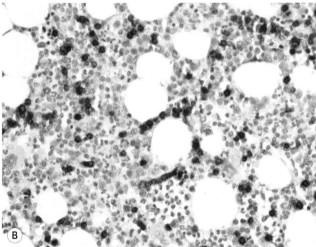

Fig. 28.12 (A, B) (A) Peripheral blood film in large granular lymphocyte leukemia. MGG, ×100 objective. (B) BM biopsy in T-LGL leukemia. CD57 immunostaining reveals sinusoid infiltrates of T-LGL cells. ×40 objective.

It has been estimated that as many as 40% of patients with Felty's syndrome have T-cell LGL leukemia. Rheumatoid factor antibodies are present in about 60% of patients and antinuclear antibodies in about 40%. A polyclonal hypergammaglobulinemia is usual.[39]

The majority of patients with NK-cell leukemia are asymptomatic, but patients with an aggressive variant usually have hepatomegaly and splenomegaly and often have B symptoms. About a third have lymphadenopathy and extranodal involvement may also occur. On average, patients are younger than those with T-cell LGL leukemia. There is a strong association with EBV infection with the leukemic cells carrying the clonal episomal form of the virus.[38]

Pathologic features

Peripheral blood

Lymphocytosis is seen in about 50% of patients with T-cell LGL leukemia. An increase in large granular lymphocytes is present in virtually all patients (Fig. 28.12A). The neoplastic cells are cytologically very similar to normal large granular lymphocytes. They are medium-sized cells with abundant weakly basophilic granular cytoplasm and prominent azurophilic granules. In occasional patients the neoplastic cells lack granules. Neutropenia is seen in up to 85% of patients, around 50% of patients are anemic and about a fifth are thrombocytopenic. The white cell count is not usually greatly elevated but large granular lymphocytes constitute more than 25% of WBC and reach $2-20 \times 10^9/l$.[39]

In aggressive NK-cell leukemia the leukemic cells also resemble normal large granular lymphocytes but they may be cytologically atypical, being larger with a higher nucleocytoplasmic ratio, basophilic cytoplasm of a visible nucleolus. Anemia and thrombocytopenia are common but neutropenia is less common than in T-cell LGL leukemia.[40]

Bone marrow

In T-cell LGL, the BM may be infiltrated with cells that are cytologically similar to those in the PB. Associated abnormalities that may be present in T-cell LGL leukemia include pure red cell aplasia and an apparent maturation arrest in the granulocytic series. In aggressive NK-cell leukemia there may be increased hemophagocytic macrophages.

On BMTB the infiltration in T-cell LGL leukemia may be subtle and more readily detected by immunohistochemical staining for CD3, CD8 and CD57 than by examination of H&E-stained sections (Fig. 28.12B). Infiltration may be interstitial or there may be small focal infiltrates. The neoplastic cells are small to medium sized with irregular nuclear contours and condensed chromatin; cytoplasmic granules are not visible in histologic sections. Aggressive NK-cell leukemia may have variable level of infiltration and variable morphological features. Usually, there are foci of monotonous infiltrates of destructive character. Necrosis, apoptosis, angioinvasion, angiodestruction and hemophagocytosis may be present.[40]

Other tissues

Splenic histology in T-cell LGL leukemia shows marked expansion of the red pulp as a result of infiltration predominantly within the sinuses. The splenic white pulp is preserved and some patients have prominent reactive germinal centers.[32,39] In the liver infiltration is predominantly sinusoidal, but portal tracts may also be infiltrated. Lymph nodes are rarely biopsied but have been reported to show paracortical and interfollicular infiltration. In cases with skin involvement, there is dermal infiltration, preferentially around skin appendages.

Immunophenotype

T-cell LGL leukemia is characterized by an expansion of CD3+ CD8+ TCR-αβ T-cells, though rarely CD3+CD4+ CD8+ TCR-αβ or CD4− CD8− TCR-γδ T cells are also involved. It was recently shown that leukemic T-LGLs have CD3+CD8+ CD45RA+ CD62L− phenotype consistent with effector/memory RA T cells (TEMRA). Leukemic T-LGLs often express CD57.[41] Chronic NK-cell proliferations are characterized by CD3− CD56+ and/or CD16+ cells.[41] Further information can be obtained by investigation of expression pattern of killer cell Ig-like receptors (KIRa, CD158) on these cells. These receptors are encoded by at least two distinct families of genes and gene products, which are members of the immunoglobulin gene superfamily.[42] In NK-LGL, approximately one third of cases exhibit restricted expression of a single (or multiple) KIR isoform. The remaining NK-LGL cases lack detectable expression of the three ubiquitously expressed KIRs, CD158a, CD158b, and CD158e. The uniform absence of these KIRs on NK cells is aberrant because in normal NK-cell populations, there are subsets positive for each.[43] In contrast to normal NK cells that show variable staining intensity, NK lymphoproliferations often show uniform bright expression of CD94 exclusively paired with NKG2A to form an inhibitory receptor complex. Abnormal loss of CD161 expression is also frequent in NK-LGL.[43]

In aggressive NK-cell leukemia the typical immunophenotype is positivity for CD2, CD16 and CD56 with loss of CD7 and variable expression of CD8 and CD57.[40,44]

Cytogenetics and molecular genetics

Deletion of 6q have been detected in T-cell LGL leukemia but besides that there is no specific rearrangements that have yet been associated with the disease.[39] TCRG genes are always rearranged in T-LGL leukemia but not in chronic lymphoproliferative disorders of NK cells, which usually present with normal karyotype and germline TCR. In aggressive NK-cell leukemia, various clonal cytogenetic abnormalities have been described, where the most common is del(6q) and del(11q).[1,44]

Sézary syndrome

Sézary syndrome (SS) and mycosis fungoides (MF) are closely related cutaneous lymphomas. Sézary syndrome is characterized by circulating neoplastic cells and an erythrodermic rash whereas MF is initially confined to the skin. MF is the most common cutaneous T-cell lymphoma (72%), while SS is a rare disease (2.5% of cutaneous T-cell lymphomas).[45] Large cell transformation may occur in both conditions, including transformation to large cell anaplastic lymphoma. WHO 2008 criteria for SS include at least one of the following: an absolute count of Sézary cells $\geq 1 \times 10^9$/l, an expanded CD4$^+$ T-cell population resulting in CD4/CD8 ratio >10 and/or loss of one or more T-cell antigens.[1]

Clinical features

Both SS and MF are mainly diseases of the elderly. In SS there is widespread skin infiltration leading to generalized erythroderma with or without plaque-like skin lesions and cutaneous tumors. Lymphadenopathy is a common feature. MF is characterized initially by pruritic eczematous skin lesions, and later by thickened plaques and tumor formation. In the early stages, lymphadenopathy is usually a result of a type of reactive lymphadenitis that is also seen in association with other non-neoplastic skin conditions (dermatopathic lymphadenopathy). However, later in the disease course there is infiltration of lymph nodes and also hepatomegaly and/or splenomegaly. Peripheral blood and bone marrow involvement occur late in the course of MF and presence of $\geq 1 \times 10^9$/l tumor cells in blood defines high tumor burden (Table 28.1).[45]

Table 28.1 Blood (B) rating in ISCL/EORTC staging of mycosis fungoides and Sézary syndrome[45]

B0	Absence of significant blood involvement (≤5% of blood lymphocytes are atypical (Sézary[†]) cells)
B0a*	Clone negative
B0b*	Clone positive
B1	Low tumor burden, does not meet criteria for B0 or B2
B1a*	Clone negative
B1b*	Clone positive
B2	High blood tumor burden: $\geq 1 \times 10^9$/l Sézary cells with positive clone*

*A T-cell clone is defined by PCR or Southern blot analysis of the T-cell receptor gene.

†Sézary cells are defined by morphology or characteristic abnormal immunophenotype.

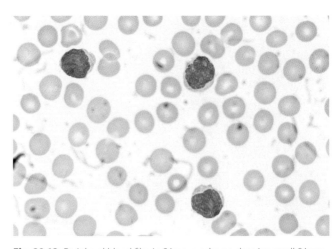

Fig. 28.13 Peripheral blood film in Sézary syndrome showing small Sézary cells with grooved nuclear surfaces. MGG, ×100 objective.

Pathologic features

Peripheral blood

Circulating neoplastic cells are cytologically very variable between patients. Morphology is similar in MF and SS patients. Small Sézary cells have a high nucleocytoplasmic ratio and a 'cerebriform' nucleus with intertwined lobes and hyperchromatic chromatin; the surface of the nucleus often appears grooved (Fig. 28.13). Large Sézary cells have more plentiful cytoplasm and lobulated or cerebriform nuclei. Individual patients may have only small cells, a mixture of large and small cells or mainly large cells. There may be a minority of cells with a flower-shaped nucleus, resembling the cells seen in adult T-cell leukemia/lymphoma. Sometimes Sézary cells have a ring of vacuoles; this appearance, which reflects glycogen in the cytoplasm, has been likened to a string of rosary beads. Reactive eosinophilia is sometimes present.

Bone marrow

Early in the course of the disease bone marrow infiltration is absent or minimal and difficult to detect. The BM involvement had no impact on prognosis in multivariate analysis and therefore is recommended only in patients with B2 level of blood involvement[45] (Table 28.1). Even in patients with Sézary syndrome with significant numbers of circulating neoplastic cells it may be difficult to detect lymphoma cells in BM without immunohistochemistry. Heavier infiltration is seen late in the disease course. In BMTB, the neoplastic cells are small with irregular, often convoluted nuclear outlines and condensed chromatin. Some cases also have a population of larger cells with prominent nucleoli.

Other tissues

In the early stages of the disease the histologic changes within the skin are often nonspecific, and repeated biopsies may be required to establish the diagnosis. There is a diffuse infiltrate of medium-sized lymphoid cells with irregular convoluted (cerebriform) nuclei in the upper dermis which can obscure the dermo-epidermal junction. Smaller numbers of larger cells with prominent nucleoli are often present. A diagnostically useful feature is infiltration of the epidermis by small groups of neoplastic cells forming Pautrier microabscesses. As the disease progresses with the formation of tumor nodules the number of larger cells within the infiltrate increases.[46]

Dermatopathic lymphadenopathy is characterized by expansion of the lymph node paracortex with numerous Langerhans cells and macrophages containing phagocytosed melanin. In infiltrated lymph nodes, aggregates of small to medium-sized lymphoid cells with cerebriform nuclei are seen in the paracortex. Early involvement is often difficult to recognize, particularly if there are also changes of dermatopathic lymphadenopathy. In the late stages of the disease, other tissues, including liver, spleen and lung, may be infiltrated by neoplastic cells with typical convoluted nuclei.

Immunophenotype

The typical immunophenotype is positivity for CD2, CD3, CD4, CD5, but CD7 is expressed only in 50% of patients. CD8 and CD25 are usually negative; if expressed, CD25 is weak. Recent studies have shown that Sézary cells have an immunophenotype similar to T-central memory cells (CD4$^+$CD27$^+$CD26$^-$CD45RA$^-$), while CD4$^+$ cells in patients with inflammatory erythroderma were CD27 negative.[47]

Cytogenetics and molecular genetics

PCR analysis shows TCR rearrangements in great majority of MF and SS patients.[45] Conventional cytogenetic analysis and comparative genomic hybridization (CGH) has shown aberrations in approximately 60% of patients with Sézary syndrome. Common aberrations include losses on chromosome 10 and 17, and gain on chromosome 8, often harboring the *MYC* oncogene.[48–50] Patterns of genomic alterations in MF differ from those in SS and often include gain of 7q, and loss of 5q and 9p.[50]

Adult T-cell leukemia/lymphoma

Adult T-cell leukemia/lymphoma (ATLL) occurs only in individuals who are carriers of the human T-cell leukemia virus type I (HTLV-I). This disease is most common in areas where this virus is endemic, particularly Japan and the West Indies, but sporadic cases occur in many other parts of the world where the virus is found, albeit less frequently. The disease may thus occur in the Middle East, Central and West Africa and South America. Most HTLV-1 carriers remain infected lifelong without developing leukemia but a small proportion (2.1% for females and 6.6% for males) will progress to ATLL. HTLV-1 regulatory factors such as TAX and HBZ allow favored proliferation of infected cells. Permanent TAX-induced proliferation and abnormal expansion of infected cells generate DNA lesions characteristic of ATLL. Inhibition of host checkpoint machinery allows further proliferation of infected cells harboring DNA damage. Progressive stabilization of these abnormalities provides an increased proliferative capacity to the infected cells and ultimately leads to ATLL.[51]

Clinical features

About 90% of patients present with leukemia and about 10% with lymphoma. Common clinical features are skin rash (reflecting cutaneous infiltration), lymphadenopathy, hepatomegaly, splenomegaly and hypercalcemia. The latter manifestation is caused by activation of osteoclasts by cytokines secreted by the neoplastic cells. Opportunistic infections are quite common. They include cryptococcosis, infection with *Pneumocystis carinii* and hyperinfection with *Stronglyoides stercoralis*. Some patients have not only ATLL but also other HTLV-I-related conditions such as tropical spastic paraparesis or uveitis. Three clinical subtypes have been defined:

- smoldering (with dominance of skin changes, normal lactate dehydrogenase (LDH), low numbers of pathological cells in blood)
- chronic (with lymphocytosis, slightly increased LDH and variable skin manifestations)
- acute (with high lymphocytosis, high LDH, variable extent of other organ involvement).[52]

Pathologic features

Peripheral blood

In the 90% of patients who present with leukemia rather than lymphoma there are varying numbers of abnormal lymphoid cells in the blood. These cells are very pleomorphic with a moderate amount of cytoplasm and irregularly shaped nuclei that are often nucleolated. A proportion of the cells are lobulated in such a manner that the nuclear shape resembles a flower (Fig. 28.14A). A smaller number of cells have a high nucleocytoplasmic ratio and less obvious lobulation so that they resemble Sézary cells. Some cells may have a more diffuse chromatin pattern and some resemble immunoblasts; these are large cells with a prominent nucleolus and plentiful basophilic cytoplasm. There may be reactive eosinophilia and neutrophilia.

Bone marrow

The BM infiltration is often subtle, even in patients who have quite numerous circulating neoplastic cells. In trephine

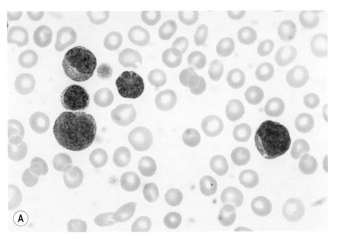
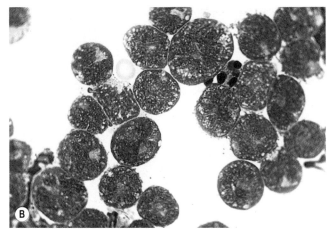

Fig. 28 14 (A, B) (A) Peripheral blood film in adult T-cell leukemia/lymphoma showing pleomorphic lymphoid cells, one of which has a flower-shaped nucleus. MGG, ×100. (B) Film of ascitic fluid from a patient with ascites caused by adult leukemia/lymphoma showing highly pleomorphic medium sized and large lymphoid cell. MGG, ×100 objective.

biopsy sections the pattern of infiltration may be interstitial, focal or diffuse. There is marked variation in the morphology of the neoplastic cells. In most cases the cells have medium-sized or large hyperchromatic nuclei showing marked pleomorphism with irregular, convoluted or lobated outlines and prominent nucleoli. Increased numbers of plasma cells and eosinophils are often present within areas of infiltration. Some cases have increased bone resorption with prominent Howship's lacunae containing osteoclasts.

Other tissues

Lymph node infiltration is initially paracortical, but later there is diffuse effacement of the nodal architecture. The infiltrate is often polymorphous with a mixture of medium-sized and large cells showing marked nuclear pleomorphism. Some cases have multinucleate tumor cells resembling Reed–Sternberg cells.

Skin infiltration is common. There is a dense lymphoid infiltrate within the dermis often extending into the subcutis. There may be epidermal invasion resembling that seen in mycosis fungoides. The neoplastic cells resemble those seen in the lymph nodes and bone marrow.

Pleural and peritoneal effusions sometimes occur and highly atypical cells are then present in the exudate (Fig. 28.14B).

Immunophenotype

In most patients, ATLL cells exhibit the phenotype of activated CD4+ memory T cells and express CD2, CD5, CD25, CD45RO, CD29, TCR αβ, and HLA-DR. ATLL cells usually lack CD7 and CD26 and exhibit lower CD3 expression than normal T-cells.[53]

Cytogenetics and molecular genetics

Most patients with ATLL show complex and variable karyotypes, where an increasing number of genomic aberrations has been associated with more aggressive forms.[54] Array-CGH recently showed that the lymphoma subtype more frequently displays gains at 1q, 2p, 4q, 7p, and 7q and losses of 10p, 13q, 16q, and 18p, whereas the acute subtype demonstrates gain of 3/3p.[53] Mutation or deletion of tumor suppressor genes, such as *TP53* or *p15INK4B/p16INK4A*, is observed in approximately half of the patients.[53]

References

1. Swerdlow SH, Campo E, Harris NL, et al. WHO Classification of Tumours of Haematopoietic and Lymphatic Tissues. Lyon: IARC; 2008.

2. Tamura K, Sawada H, Izumi Y, et al. Chronic lymphocytic leukemia (CLL) is rare, but the proportion of T-CLL is high in Japan. Eur J Haematol 2001;67:152–7.

3. Wilkins B, Wright DH. Illustrated pathology of the spleen. Cambridge, UK: Cambridge University Press; 2000.

4. Greenwood R, Barker DJ, Tring FC, et al. Clinical and immunohistological characterization of cutaneous lesions in chronic lymphocytic leukaemia. Br J Dermatol 1985;113:447–53.

5. Brick WG, Majmundar M, Hendricks LK, et al. Leukemic leptomeningeal involvement in stage 0 and stage 1 chronic lymphocytic leukemia. Leuk Lymphoma 2002;43:199–201.

6. Chu PG, Huang Q, Weiss LM. Incidental and concurrent malignant lymphomas discovered at the time of prostatectomy and prostate biopsy: a study of 29 cases. Am J Surg Pathol 2005;29:693–9.

7. Rossi D, Gaidano G. Richter syndrome: molecular insights and clinical perspectives. Hematol Oncol 2009;27: 1–10.

8. Tzankov A, Fong D. Hodgkin's disease variant of Richter's syndrome clonally

related to chronic lymphocytic leukemia arises in ZAP-70 negative mutated CLL. Med Hypotheses 2006;66:577–9.

9. Matutes E, Wotherspoon A, Catovsky D. Differential diagnosis in chronic lymphocytic leukaemia. Best Pract Res Clin Haematol 2007;20:367–84.

10. Rawstron AC. Monoclonal B-cell lymphocytosis. Hematology Am Soc Hematol Educ Program 2009;430–9.

11. Landgren O, Albitar M, Ma W, et al. B-cell clones as early markers for chronic lymphocytic leukemia. N Engl J Med 2009;360:659–67.

12. Hamblin TJ, Davis Z, Gardiner A, et al. Unmutated Ig V(H) genes are associated

with a more aggressive form of chronic lymphocytic leukemia. Blood 1999; 94:1848–54.

13. Damle RN, Wasil T, Fais F, et al. Ig V gene mutation status and CD38 expression as novel prognostic indicators in chronic lymphocytic leukemia. Blood 1999; 94:1840–7.

14. Caligaris-Cappio F, Ghia P. Novel insights in chronic lymphocytic leukemia: are we getting closer to understanding the pathogenesis of the disease? J Clin Oncol 2008;26:4497–503.

15. Tobin G, Thunberg U, Karlsson K, et al. Subsets with restricted immunoglobulin gene rearrangement features indicate a role for antigen selection in the development of chronic lymphocytic leukemia. Blood 2004;104:2879–85.

16. Stamatopoulos K, Belessi C, Moreno C, et al. Over 20% of patients with chronic lymphocytic leukemia carry stereotyped receptors: pathogenetic implications and clinical correlations. Blood 2007;109:259–70.

17. Crespo M, Bosch F, Villamor N, et al. ZAP-70 expression as a surrogate for immunoglobulin-variable-region mutations in chronic lymphocytic leukemia. N Engl J Med 2003;348:1764–75.

18. Rassenti LZ, Kipps TJ. Clinical utility of assessing ZAP-70 and CD38 in chronic lymphocytic leukemia. Cytometry B Clin Cytom 2006;70:209–13.

19. Orchard JA, Ibbotson RE, Davis Z, et al. ZAP-70 expression and prognosis in chronic lymphocytic leukaemia. Lancet 2004;363:105–11.

20. Dohner H, Stilgenbauer S, Benner A, et al. Genomic aberrations and survival in chronic lymphocytic leukemia. N Engl J Med 2000;343:1910–16.

21. Calin GA, Ferracin M, Cimmino A, et al. A MicroRNA signature associated with prognosis and progression in chronic lymphocytic leukemia. N Engl J Med 2005;353:1793–801.

22. Dungarwalla M, Matutes E, Dearden CE. Prolymphocytic leukaemia of B- and T-cell subtype: a state-of-the-art paper. Eur J Haematol 2008;80:469–76.

23. Del Giudice I, Davis Z, Matutes E, et al. IgVH genes mutation and usage, ZAP-70 and CD38 expression provide new insights on B-cell prolymphocytic leukemia (B-PLL). Leukemia 2006;20:1231–7.

24. Lens D, Coignet LJ, Brito-Babapulle V, et al. B cell prolymphocytic leukaemia (B-PLL) with complex karyotype and concurrent abnormalities of the p53 and c-MYC gene. Leukemia 1999;13:873–6.

25. Lens D, Matutes E, Catovsky D, Coignet LJ. Frequent deletions at 11q23 and 13q14 in B cell prolymphocytic leukemia (B-PLL). Leukemia 2000;14:427–30.

26. Del Giudice I, Osuji N, Dexter T, et al. B-cell prolymphocytic leukemia and chronic lymphocytic leukemia have distinctive gene expression signatures. Leukemia 2009;23:2160–7.

27. Bartlett NL, Longo DL. T-small lymphocyte disorders. Semin Hematol 1999;36:164–70.

28. Matutes E, Brito-Babapulle V, Swansbury J, et al. Clinical and laboratory features of 78 cases of T-prolymphocytic leukemia. Blood 1991;78:3269–74.

29. Dearden CE. T-cell prolymphocytic leukemia. Clin Lymphoma Myeloma 2009;9(Suppl. 3):S239–43.

30. Krishnan B, Else M, Tjonnfjord GE, et al. Stem cell transplantation after alemtuzumab in T-cell prolymphocytic leukaemia results in longer survival than after alemtuzumab alone: a multicentre retrospective study. Br J Haematol 2010 Jun;149(6):907–10.

31. Matutes E. T-cell prolymphocytic leukemia. Cancer Control 1998;5:19–24.

32. Osuji N, Matutes E, Catovsky D, et al. Histopathology of the spleen in T-cell large granular lymphocyte leukemia and T-cell prolymphocytic leukemia: a comparative review. Am J Surg Pathol 2005;29:935–41.

33. Mallett RB, Matutes E, Catovsky D, et al. Cutaneous infiltration in T-cell prolymphocytic leukaemia. Br J Dermatol 1995;132:263–6.

34. Herling M, Khoury JD, Washington LT, et al. A systematic approach to diagnosis of mature T-cell leukemias reveals heterogeneity among WHO categories. Blood 2004;104:328–35.

35. Brito-Babapulle V, Pomfret M, Matutes E, Catovsky D. Cytogenetic studies on prolymphocytic leukemia. II. T cell prolymphocytic leukemia. Blood 1987; 70:926–31.

36. Sorour A, Brito-Babapulle V, Smedley D, et al. Unusual breakpoint distribution of 8p abnormalities in T-prolymphocytic leukemia: a study with YACS mapping to 8p11-p12. Cancer Genet Cytogenet 2000;121:128–32.

37. Yuille MA, Coignet LJ, Abraham SM, et al. ATM is usually rearranged in T-cell prolymphocytic leukaemia. Oncogene 1998;16:789–96.

38. Kwong YL. Natural killer-cell malignancies: diagnosis and treatment. Leukemia 2005;19:2186–94.

39. O'Malley DP. T-cell large granular leukemia and related proliferations. Am J Clin Pathol 2007;127:850–9.

40. Liang X, Graham DK. Natural killer cell neoplasms. Cancer 2008;112:1425–36.

41. Shah MV, Zhang R, Loughran TP Jr. Never say die: survival signaling in large granular lymphocyte leukemia. Clin Lymphoma Myeloma 2009;9(Suppl. 3):S244–53.

42. Purdy AK, Campbell KS. Natural killer cells and cancer: regulation by the killer cell Ig-like receptors (KIR). Cancer Biol Ther 2009;8:2211–20.

43. Morice WG. The immunophenotypic attributes of NK cells and NK–cell lineage lymphoproliferative disorders. Am J Clin Pathol 2007;127:881–6.

44. Yoo EH, Kim HJ, Lee ST, et al. Frequent CD7 Antigen loss in aggressive natural killer-cell leukemia: a useful diagnostic marker. Korean J Lab Med 2009;29:491–6.

45. Olsen E, Vonderheid E, Pimpinelli N, et al. Revisions to the staging and classification of mycosis fungoides and Sézary syndrome: a proposal of the International Society for Cutaneous Lymphomas (ISCL) and the cutaneous lymphoma task force of the European Organization of Research and Treatment of Cancer (EORTC). Blood 2007;110:1713–22.

46. Kempf W, Sander CA. Classification of cutaneous lymphomas – an update. Histopathology 2010;56:57–70.

47. Fierro MT, Novelli M, Quaglino P, et al. Heterogeneity of circulating CD4+ memory T-cell subsets in erythrodermic patients: CD27 analysis can help to distinguish cutaneous T-cell lymphomas from inflammatory erythroderma. Dermatology 2008;216:213–21.

48. Mao X, Lillington DM, Czepulkowski B, et al. Molecular cytogenetic characterization of Sézary syndrome. Genes Chromosomes Cancer 2003;36:250–60.

49. Barba G, Matteucci C, Girolomoni G, et al. Comparative genomic hybridization identifies 17q11.2 approximately q12 duplication as an early event in cutaneous T-cell lymphomas. Cancer Genet Cytogenet 2008;184:48–51.

50. van Doorn R, van Kester MS, Dijkman R, et al. Oncogenomic analysis of mycosis fungoides reveals major differences with Sézary syndrome. Blood 2009;113:127–36.

51. Boxus M, Willems L. Mechanisms of HTLV-1 persistence and transformation. Br J Cancer 2009;101:1497–501.

52. Shimoyama M. Diagnostic criteria and classification of clinical subtypes of adult T-cell leukaemia-lymphoma. A report from the Lymphoma Study Group (1984–87). Br J Haematol 1991;79:428–37.

53. Tsukasaki K, Hermine O, Bazarbachi A, et al. Definition, prognostic factors, treatment, and response criteria of adult T-cell leukemia-lymphoma: a proposal from an international consensus meeting. J Clin Oncol 2009;27:453–9.

54. Tsukasaki K, Krebs J, Nagai K, et al. Comparative genomic hybridization analysis in adult T-cell leukemia/lymphoma: correlation with clinical course. Blood 2001;97:3875–81.

Lymphoma

BS Wilkins

Introduction

Peripheral blood (PB) and bone marrow (BM) are relatively frequently involved by lymphomas, particularly those with low-grade clinical behavior.[1] BM aspiration and bone marrow trephine biopsy (BMTB) are currently performed at diagnosis as part of the staging of most patients with non-Hodgkin lymphomas (NHL) and in selected patients with Hodgkin lymphoma (HL). Criteria for patient selection for these procedures vary between treatment centers and are undergoing revision as techniques such as magnetic resonance imaging and positron emission tomography are refined to permit non-invasive assessment of disease spread. Evidence that BM involvement influences clinical outcome varies for different disease entities within the spectrum of lymphoproliferative disorders.[2-9] BM involvement, and its extent, can be important factors in making clinical decisions concerning choice of treatment.

Lymphoproliferative diseases that present as leukemias have been considered elsewhere (see Chapter 28), as has plasma cell neoplasia (see Chapter 30). In this chapter, blood and BM involvement by lymphomas presenting primarily with lymph node or other solid organ involvement is discussed.

©2011 Elsevier Ltd
DOI: 10.1016/B978-0-7020-3147-2.00029-8

General comments on bone marrow (BM) examination in lymphoproliferative diseases

Patients with lymphoma do not always present with lymph node enlargement or obvious tumor formation at other sites. Instead, they may have unexplained cytopenias, a leuko-erythroblastic blood picture, paraprotein, immune paresis or fever requiring BM examination for diagnostic purposes. Diagnostic lymph node biopsy may not be feasible in frail or elderly patients with disease involvement only at deep sites.

The full blood count, blood film, BM aspirate and BMTB have complementary roles in the investigation of BM involvement by lymphoma. In different lymphoproliferative diseases, each of these types of specimen may be of greater or lesser value.[10-14] In lymphomas that do not readily display leukemic behavior, BMTB sections are frequently found to contain lymphoma when none is evident in the blood or BM aspirate.

Where circulating lymphoma cells are available in sufficient number in the peripheral blood (PB), these give the most consistent morphology and phenotyping by flow cytometry (FCM). BM aspiration without accompanying BMTB may be valuable if representation of disease in the PB is inadequate for diagnosis, permitting cytologic and immunocytochemical assessment of larger numbers of neoplastic cells. However, aspiration for the evaluation of BM involvement by lymphoma has a high false negative rate.[13] Deposits of disease frequently occupy sites within the BM microenvironment that are suboptimally sampled by aspiration (e.g. paratrabecular zones). They may also be adherent to stromal components inducing focal fibrosis and less readily aspirated than BM hemopoietic elements. For these reasons BMTB in addition to aspiration is always recommended for the evaluation of BM involvement by lymphoma. Exceptionally, if BM aspiration alone is possible in some patients for whom BMTB cannot be performed, the aspirate films can still provide valuable information about hemopoietic reserve and iron stores. If aspiration proves technically difficult or a poor sample is obtained, BMTB should definitely be performed and an imprint or roll preparation made for cytologic assessment.

BM aspiration provides a potential source of cells for morphologic assessment, FCM immunophenotyping, cytogenetic analysis and molecular genetic studies. The latter investigations include clonality analysis, assessment of immunoglobulin (Ig) variable gene mutation status, reverse transcription-polymerase chain reaction (RT-PCR), fluorescent in situ DNA hybridization (FISH) and studies of loss of heterozygosity. Aspirated cells may also be a source of material for DNA vaccine development for the treatment of lymphomas.

BMTB sections are used primarily for morphologic assessment, including analysis of the spatial distribution and extent of lymphomatous deposits.[4,8-10,12,14-25] Spatial and cytologic assessment often provide clues to lymphoma subtype (e.g. the pattern of paratrabecular infiltration typical of follicular lymphoma) and can, as a minimum, be used to assess whether disease involvement represents indolent or aggressive lymphoma. Histologic sections can also be used for immunohistochemistry (IHC), FISH and PCR; these additional investigations are particularly useful if PB or aspirated BM cells do not provide adequate representation of lymphoma. Where decalcification is employed in association with paraffin wax embedding of trephine cores, use of ethylene diamine tetra-acetic acid (EDTA) to decalcify by chelation, rather than acid exposure, offers excellent antigen and nucleic acid preservation.[26-28] For immunophenotyping of lymphoid cell infiltrates in BMTB sections a similar, marginally more restricted, range of antibodies is employed to that used for FCM. Antibodies reactive with additional antigens such as CD79a, cyclin D1, IRF4/MUM1, PAX5 and Ki67 are also available which have been developed specifically for IHC use; these are referred to individually in the text that follows, where appropriate.

Differential diagnosis of reactive lymphoid aggregates vs lymphoma

Nodular aggregates of small lymphoid cells may be found in BMTB sections as a reactive phenomenon, unrelated to any neoplastic lymphoid proliferation. Criteria for distinguishing such aggregates from neoplastic lymphoid infiltrates remain imperfect and controversial.[29-31] Immunostaining is helpful in only a minority of examples. Morphologic features remain the best guide, supported by application of molecular genetic techniques, such as PCR amplification and IGH/TCR rearrangement studies, in appropriately processed specimens. However, the sensitivity and specificity of the PCR methods employed may vary and the finding of a monoclonal IGH/TCR rearrangement cannot be assumed to equate with a diagnosis of lymphoma without other supportive evidence.[32] In limited circumstances FISH performed using intact sections may be informative (consideration of t(11;14) and t(14;18), for example). For any techniques performed in addition to histological assessment of the original sections, there is a significant likelihood that small or few lymphoid aggregates will not be represented in the material available for testing.

The position of a lymphoid aggregate within BM is important in assessing whether it is reactive or neoplastic. It is never normal for lymphoid cells to aggregate at trabecular margins or the edges of sinusoids. As discussed earlier, paratrabecular lymphoid infiltrates are most likely to represent lymphoma. Perisinusoidal infiltrates may be subtle but declare themselves on low-power histologic examination because they distort and pull open the lumen of the adjacent sinusoid, as a result of an accompanying increase in stromal reticulin.

To be accepted as reactive, lymphoid nodules should be few in number, centrally placed within intertrabecular spaces, small and round in profile with well-demarcated margins. A small capillary may be present, running from the periphery into the center of the nodule (Fig. 29.1) and there may be reactive changes such as aggregation of eosinophils in the adjacent hemopoietic tissue. An underlying meshwork of reticulin or CD23+ follicular dendritic cells may be present or absent, probably more dependent on the size of a particular nodule than on its reactive or neoplastic nature. The subjective nature of these criteria will be obvious to the reader but, to date, an objective gold standard for assessment of BM lymphoid nodules remains elusive.

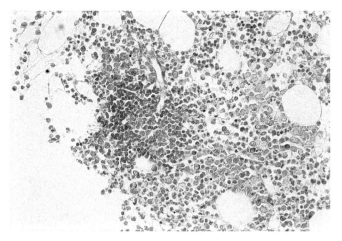

Fig. 29.1 Lymphoid nodule in a bone marrow trephine biopsy section demonstrated with a Giemsa stain. Closely packed lymphoid cell nuclei result in intense blue staining of the nodule relative to the background hemopoietic tissue, which has a mauve/pink tone overall. Note also the reactive eosinophils around the margin of the nodule, which stain orange/red with Giemsa. Eosinophil aggregation at the periphery of lymphoid nodules is more commonly seen accompanying reactive nodules than neoplastic lymphoid infiltrates but may also occur with the latter, especially following chemotherapy. Decalcified, wax-embedded bone marrow trephine biopsy section; Giemsa stain, original magnification ×20.

The cytologic composition of lymphoid infiltrates is also critical to their interpretation. Most non-neoplastic aggregates consist of small lymphocytes with only occasional large blast cells; they show little evidence of plasma cell differentiation. Reactive germinal center formation is distinctly uncommon but, when it occurs, the composition of the lymphoid follicle recapitulates that found in lymph nodes and other organized lymphoid tissues. Formation of reactive germinal centers within BM lymphoid aggregates is said to be increased in patients with rheumatoid arthritis and other systemic chronic inflammatory disorders.[32] Reactive lymphocytes, predominantly T-cells, also form a significant component of many granulomas in the BM, and the compact infiltrates of systemic mastocytosis; these lesions can be confirmed by IHC, if suspected, and should not be mistaken either for lymphoma or incidental reactive lymphoid nodules.

Interpreting necrotic deposits of possible lymphoma

The situation may be encountered, usually in patients with large cell or other high-grade lymphomas, in which extensive BM infiltration is present but represented only by necrotic tissue. Loss of the outlines of fat spaces in areas of necrosis indicates that the BM is infiltrated and the picture is not one of infarction of normal hemopoietic tissue. Reticulin staining generally confirms an underlying disturbance of stromal architecture. Stains such as hematoxylin and eosin (H&E), Giemsa and periodic acid–Schiff (PAS) offer little further insight into the nature of necrotic tissue in the BM but immunostaining, applied with care, can be very helpful. In particular, CD20 is well preserved in necrotic lymphoid cells and can demonstrate the B-cell nature of a lymphomatous infiltrate, often highlighting the size and outline of

individual cells so that at least a partial impression of cell morphology can be gained. Since most cases of necrotic lymphoma in the BM are examples of DLBCL, this is of considerable practical value.

Demonstration of most T-cell-associated antigens in this context is unreliable, since these are not well preserved on necrotic lymphoid cells and the antibodies used for their detection will cross-react with myelomonocytic cells, including macrophages attracted to the site in response to the presence of necrosis. Alone of the T-cell markers, CD3 may be adequately preserved and false positive results are not generally found. For the differential diagnosis of classical HL, use of CD30 and CD15 immunostaining is unreliable. In rare cases of metastatic carcinoma mimicking necrotic lymphoma, high- and low-molecular weight cytokeratins may be stained successfully without nonspecific positive results. Immunostaining for melanoma markers is unreliable in necrotic tissue due to poor antigen preservation and, in the case of S100 protein, cross-reactivity with macrophages.

The laboratory investigation of blood and BM specimens suspected or known to have involvement by lymphoma

The general principles of investigations that should be performed using blood and BM specimens in all cases of suspected involvement by lymphoma are outlined below.

Blood

A full blood count and differential white cell count should always be performed. The blood film should be stained using May–Grünwald–Giemsa (MGG) or Wright's method to assess cytologic features. When circulating abnormal cells are known or suspected to be present immunophenotyping by FCM should be performed; a useful basic antibody panel is shown in Table 29.1. PB cells should also be analyzed by classical cytogenetic and/or molecular genetic methods when the differential diagnosis includes lymphomas known to be associated consistently with abnormal genetic features.

Bone marrow aspirate

A minimum of three films should be prepared and air-dried, using MGG stain for cytologic assessment and differential cell count.[33] A Perls stain is also desirable as a routine, for assessment of iron stores. Aspirated BM cells should also be sent in suspension for FCM immunophenotyping and genetic analysis.

Bone marrow trephine biopsy (BMTB)

Cores of tissue should be collected that will contain at least 1 cm of interpretable, uncrushed BM after histologic processing. In practice, because of likely inclusion of cortex at the outer end and crushed tissue at the inner end, plus shrinkage that occurs during processing, unfixed cores at the time of collection should be at least 1.5 cm long[10,34–36] If aspiration has been unsuccessful, touch preparations should be made

Table 29.1 Typical antigen expression patterns found in subtypes of mature B-cell non-Hodgkin lymphoma

WHO category	Frequency of leukemic presentation	SIg	CD20	CD79b	CD5	CD10	CD23	FMC7	CD25	CD11c	CD103	Other markers	%Ki67
CLL/SLL	90%	d	-/d	-/d	+	-	+	-(+)	-/+	-(+)	-	CD38+/-, CD200+, Zap70-/+, MUM1-/+	<20%
PLL	100%	b	+	+	-	-	-/+	+	-	-	-		20-40%
LPL	10%	+/d	+/d	+	-	-	-	+	-	-	-	MUM1 +	<20%
HCL	<10%	b	+	+	-	-/+	-	+	+	+	+	CD123+, CD72+, Annexin1+, TRAP+, cyclin D1+	<20%
HCLv	100%	b	+	+	-	-	-	+	-	+	+	CD72+/-	<20%
MZL (MALT)	0%	b	+	+	-	-	-	+	-	-	-	CD21+ CD35+	<20%
MZL (nodal)	<10%	b	+	+	-	-	-/+	+	-	+/-	-	CD21+ CD35+	10-30%
SMZL	75%	b	+	+	-	-	-/+	+	-/+	+	-	TRAP+	<20%
FL	<10%	b/d	+	+	-	+	-(+)	+	-	-	-	Bcl6+	10-60%
MCL	30%	b	+	+	+	-	-	+	-	-	-	cyclinD1+	10-60%
DLBCL	<10%	b/d	+(-)	+	-/+	+/-	-/+	-/+	-/+	-/+	-	Bcl6, MUM1	30-90%
BL	30%	b	+	+	-	+	-	-	-	-	-	Bcl2-	100%

Abbreviations: diagnostic categories abbreviated as in main text. SIg, surface immunoglobulin; d, dim (weak) positive staining; b (bright) strong, (+) some cases positive.

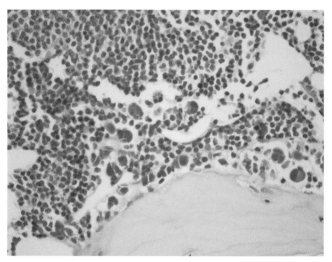

Fig. 29.3 Intracellular immunoglobulin in a case of lymphoplasmacytic lymphoma. Decalcified, wax-embedded bone marrow trephine biopsy section; PAS stain, original magnification ×40.

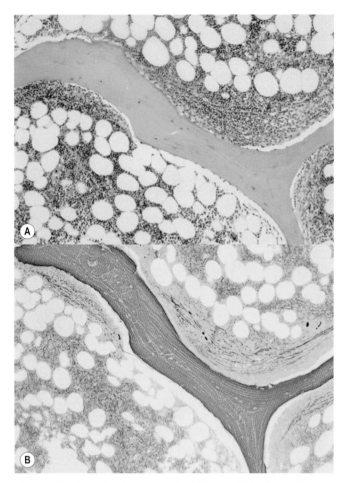

Fig. 29.2 (A, B) Localized paratrabecular infiltrates of follicular lymphoma as seen in standard decalcified, wax-embedded bone marrow trephine biopsy sections. (A) H&E and (B) Gordon and Sweet's silver stain for reticulin fibers. Original magnification ×10.

using the trephine biopsy core by rolling it gently between two slides and then staining both air-dried slides with MGG. A detailed discussion of technical matters is beyond the scope of this chapter and only brief comments are made here. Further guidance can be found in references.[26,37] Plastic-embedded specimens (usually in methyl or glycol methacrylate resin) require modifications to be made to standard tinctorial and IHC methods that may be difficult to incorporate into automated staining schedules but a wide range of immunostains can none the less be performed in laboratories specialized to handle these specimens. After processing the core for histology, thin sections (1–2 µm for plastic-embedded specimens; 3–4 µm for decalcified, paraffin wax-embedded ones) should be cut and stained with H&E from a minimum of three levels through the core. Levels are usually cut 25–50 µm apart, depending on local practice and the diameter of the specimen. On sections from the middle or deepest level, reticulin, PAS and Giemsa stains should be performed routinely. H&E provides a basic and familiar stain with which to assess cell morphology (Fig. 29.2A). Lymphoid infiltrates are often associated with increased reticulin deposition and a disturbance of the normal pattern of reticulin fiber distribution (Fig. 29.2B). PAS stain highlights carbohydrate-rich molecules and consequently stains immunoglobulin if it is of the IgM class and sufficiently abundant.

IgM is richly glycosylated; consequently, intracellular and, occasionally, extracellular accumulation of this Ig can be detected in some cases of lymphoplasmacytic lymphoma (Fig. 29.3). The key importance of high-quality Giemsa staining in trephine biopsy sections cannot be over-emphasized (see Chapter 3). Any collection of lymphoid cells will stand out as being turquoise/blue in color, against a generally mauve/pink background (Fig. 29.1). IHC can be useful in confirming the precise diagnosis of lymphoma and in assessing its grade but is of limited value in differentiating reactive lymphoid aggregates in the BM from small deposits of low-grade lymphoma. For the latter task, molecular genetic analysis is gaining importance.[30,32]

The World Health Organization (WHO) classification of lymphomas

At the end of 1999, an outline version of a new lymphoma classification was published as a result of the WHO lymphoma classification project.[38] This embodied the principles of the revised European–American lymphoma (REAL) classification,[39] which was published in 1994 and has since become widely accepted in lymphoma diagnostic practice. A revision of the WHO classification was published in 2008 (Box 29.1).[40]

A novel and fundamental principle of the REAL classification was the definition of lymphomas according to their distinctive clinical, as well as pathologic, features. Much of the REAL classification remains little changed by the WHO, except for alterations in terminology, but considerable advances in the immunophenotypic and genetic contributions to defining lymphoma types have been incorporated. Some lymphomas considered as provisional entities in the REAL system became accepted as definite entities within the initial WHO classification, and this process, including the addition of new provisional entities, has continued with the 2008 revision. Box 29.1 summarizes the lymphoma categories recognized by the WHO 2008 scheme. Areas of uncertainty in lymphoma classification remain, however, and an important feature of the WHO classification is that it has

Box 29.1 Summary of the revised World Health Organization classification of lymphomas (2008)[40]

B-cell neoplasms
Precursor B-cell origin:
B-lymphoblastic leukemia/lymphoma, NOS

B-lymphoblastic leukemia/lymphoma with recurrent genetic abnormalities:

t(9;22)(q34;q11.2); *BCR-ABL1*

t(v;11q23); *MLL* rearranged

t(12;21)(p13;q22); *TEL-AML* (*ETV6-RUNX1*)

hyperdiploidy

hypodiploidy

t(5;14)(q31;q32); *IL3-IGH*

t(1;19)(q23;p13.3); *E2A-PBX1* (*TCF3-PBX1*)

Mature B-cell origin:
Chronic lymphocytic leukemia/small lymphocytic lymphoma

B-cell prolymphocytic leukemia

Splenic B-cell marginal zone lymphoma

Hairy cell leukemia

Splenic B-cell lymphoma/leukemia, unclassifiable

    Splenic diffuse red pulp B cell lymphoma

    Hairy cell leukemia variant

Lymphoplasmacytic lymphoma

Heavy chain diseases (alpha, gamma, mu)

Plasma cell myeloma

Solitary plasmacytoma of bone

Extraosseous plasmacytoma

Extranodal marginal zone lymphoma of mucosa-associated lymphoid tissue

Nodal marginal zone lymphoma

    Pediatric nodal marginal zone lymphoma

Follicular lymphoma

    Pediatric follicular lymphoma

Primary cutaneous follicle centre lymphoma

Mantle cell lymphoma

Diffuse large B-cell lymphoma (DLBCL), NOS

    T-cell/histiocyte-rich large B-cell lymphoma

    Primary DLBCL of the CNS

    Primary cutaneous DLBCL, leg type

    EBV-positive DLBCL of the elderly

    DLBCL associated with chronic inflammation

Lymphomatoid granulomatosis

Primary mediastinal (thymic) large B-cell lymphoma

Intravascular large B-cell lymphoma

ALK-positive large B-cell lymphoma

Plasmablastic lymphoma

Large B-cell lymphoma arising in HHV8-associated multicentric Castleman disease

Primary effusion lymphoma

Burkitt lymphoma

B-cell lymphoma, unclassifiable, with features intermediate between DLBCL and Burkitt lymphoma

B-cell lymphoma, unclassifiable, with features intermediate between DLBCL and classical Hodgkin lymphoma

T- and NK-cell neoplasms
Precursor T-cell origin:
T-lymphoblastic leukemia/lymphoma

Mature T-cell and NK-cell origin:
T-cell prolymphocytic leukemia

T-cell large granular lymphocytic leukemia

Chronic lymphoproliferative disorder of NK-cells

Aggressive NK-cell leukemia

Systemic EBV-positive T-cell lymphoproliferative disease of childhood

Hydroa vacciniforme-like lymphoma

Adult T-cell leukemia/lymphoma

Extranodal NK/T-cell lymphoma, nasal type

Enteropathy-associated T-cell lymphoma

Hepatosplenic T-cell lymphoma

Subcutaneous panniculitis-like T-cell lymphoma

Mycosis fungoides

Sézary syndrome

Primary cutaneous CD30-positive T-cell lymphoproliferative disorders:

    Lymphomatoid papulosis

    Primary cutaneous anaplastic large cell lymphoma

Primary cutaneous gamma-delta T-cell lymphoma

Primary cutaneous CD8-positive aggressive epidermotropic cytotoxic T-cell lymphoma

Primary cutaneous CD4-positive small/medium T-cell lymphoma

Peripheral T-cell lymphoma, NOS

Angioimmunoblastic T-cell lymphoma

Anaplastic large cell lymphoma, ALK positive

Anaplastic large cell lymphoma, ALK negative

Hodgkin lymphoma
Nodular lymphocyte predominant Hodgkin lymphoma

Classical Hodgkin lymphoma:

    Nodular sclerosis classical Hodgkin lymphoma

    Lymphocyte-rich classical Hodgkin lymphoma

    Mixed cellularity classical Hodgkin lymphoma

    Lymphocyte-depleted classical Hodgkin lymphoma

Immunodeficiency-associated lymphoproliferative disorders
Post-transplant lymphoproliferative disorders (PTLD)

    Early lesions:

        Plasmacytic hyperplasia

        Infectious mononucleosis-like PTLD

    Polymorphic PTLD

    Monomorphic PTLD (B- and T/NK-cell types; classified according to the lymphoma/leukemia to which they correspond)

    Classical Hodgkin lymphoma-like PTLD

Lymphoproliferative diseases associated with primary immune disorders

Lymphomas associated with HIV infection

Other iatrogenic immunodeficiency-associated lymphoproliferative disorders

(Italic text denotes entities regarded as provisional in the WHO 2008 Classification)

flexibility to allow for further evolution in the understanding of hematological malignancies. An important advance in the WHO system over previous classifications is the recognition of subtypes of lymphoma that tend to exhibit leukemic behavior (see Chapter 28). Emerging information about the mutational status of immunoglobulin variable region genes in B-cell lymphomas[41–46] and gene expresssion micro-array patterns across a wider spectrum of lymphomas,[47–59] are likely to permit refinement of the classification as the biological significance of such data becomes clearer. However, while immunophenotypic, cytogenetic and molecular genetic features are central to the WHO classification, with expanded importance in the 2008 revision, little reference is made to the interpretation of patterns of BM involvement as a contribution to the definition of lymphoma entities.

Blood and BM involvement of lymphoma entities according to WHO classification

Description of entities primarily presenting as leukemias is provided in Chapter 28. Features of blood and BM involvement of lymphomas primarily presenting in lymph nodes or as extranodal infiltrates are described below.

Mature B-cell neoplasms

Lymphoplasmacytic lymphoma (LPL)

Clinical features, blood and bone marrow aspiration

Lymphoplasmacytic lymphoma is an indolent lymphoid neoplasm comprising 1–2% of all NHL.[40,60–62] Studies in southern Europe have suggested an association between hepatitis C (HCV) infection and LPL,[63–65] with treatment of the former being effective in controlling the lymphoma, but no similar association with HCV has been found elsewhere.

BM involvement is common at presentation and 30% of patients have splenomegaly and/or lymphadenopathy. The clinical presentation usually reflects the presence of a circulating paraprotein (IgM in almost all cases) with or without hyperviscosity symptoms. BM involvement by LPL with an IgM paraprotein underlies the clinical syndrome of Waldenström macrogobulinemia (see Chapter 30). There may be an associated peripheral neuropathy that is believed to be a paraneoplastic phenomenon.[62] Pancytopenia may be present as a consequence of tumor burden such as BM failure or fibrosis. Blood involvement is rare, except in advanced disease; it is characterized by the presence in the circulation of plasmacytoid cells with an eccentric nucleus and basophilic cytoplasm. BM aspirate films show a mixture of small lymphocytes, lymphoplasmacytoid cells and mature plasma cells (Fig. 29.4). There is frequently an accompanying increase in mast cells. Typical immunophenotype findings are summarized in Table 29.1.

Bone marrow trephine biopsy

Bone marrow is frequently the predominant site of disease involvement in LPL. BMTB sections show infiltrates in most patients, often with more extensive involvement than suggested by aspirate films.[10] The cells are predominantly small lymphocytes with varying numbers of plasma cells and cells

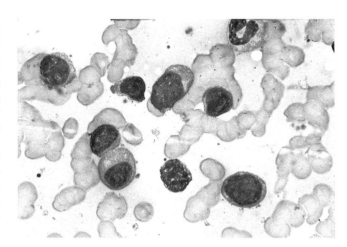

Fig. 29.4 Aspirated bone marrow showing cell mixture typical of LPL, with small lymphocytes, lymphoplasmacytoid cells and mature plasma cells represented. Bone marrow aspirate film; MGG stain, original magnification ×100.

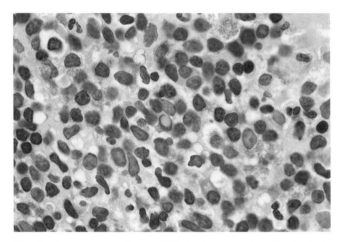

Fig. 29.5 Bone marrow infiltrate of LPL showing a prominent Dutcher body within a nucleus in the center of the field. Decalcified, wax-embedded bone marrow trephine biopsy section; H&E stain, original magnification ×100.

having intermediate (plasmacytoid) features. The plasma cells may contain Dutcher bodies, which are inclusions of immunoglobulin that invaginate the nuclear membrane and appear intranuclear in histologic sections (Fig. 29.5). Less commonly, single or multiple intracytoplasmic immunoglobulin inclusions (Russell bodies) are found. Scattered lymphoid blast cells may be seen but true para-immunoblasts are absent and no proliferation centers are formed; finding the latter would indicate a diagnosis of B-cell chronic lymphocytic leukemia (B-CLL) with plasmacytic differentiation, rather than LPL. The presence of increased numbers of reactive mast cells in the marrow interstitium, sometimes located preferentially in the periphery of lymphoid infiltrates, may be helpful in supporting a diagnosis of LPL (Fig. 29.6). This phenomenon, however, is also seen in a minority of cases of CLL and is possibly related to IgM expression rather than to other properties of either disease.[62,66] It has been suggested that mast cells contribute to B cell proliferation in LPL.[67,68] The pattern of infiltration is usually irregular, paratrabecular or diffuse throughout the interstitium; mixtures of these patterns are common in individual cases. Well-defined nodular infiltrates are unusual and when nodules occur in

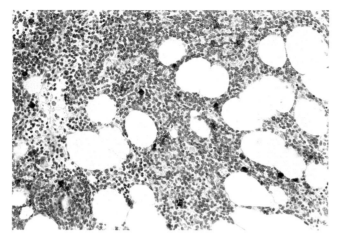

Fig. 29.6 Infiltrate of LPL in bone marrow accompanied by numerous mast cells, which have purple granular cytoplasm in this section stained with buffered thionin (a metachromatic stain similar to toluidine blue). Decalcified, wax-embedded bone marrow trephine biopsy section; original magnification ×20.

LPL they are usually small and more elliptical or irregular than those seen in other small B-cell lymphomas. The paratrabecular infiltrates of LPL are not usually as extensive or regular as those found in follicular lymphoma. In some patients who have an IgM paraprotein, sinusoids contain PAS-positive proteinaceous material that represents plasma rich in IgM; there may also be interstitial and, rarely, intracytoplasmic deposition of crystalline PAS-positive IgM (Fig. 29.3). IHC shows that the small B-lymphocytes of LPL express CD19, CD20 (which may be weak or absent in cases with prominent plasma cell differentiation), CD79a and PAX5 but lack expression of CD5, CD10, BCL6 and cyclin D1. In occasional cases, a proportion of the neoplastic cells expresses CD23. Plasma cell differentiation is often evident with staining for CD79a and can be demonstrated more clearly using antibodies reactive with CD138 or IRF4/MUM1, or antibody VS38c that reacts with rough endoplasmic reticulum-associated p63 protein.[69] Expression of monotypic immunoglobulin in the cytoplasm of cells showing plasmacytic differentiation is usually easily demonstrated, most commonly IgM kappa,[40,70] and light chain mRNA production by such cells can also be shown by *in situ* hybridization (Fig. 29.7). Transformation to large cell lymphoma may occur but is not very common.

Genetic studies

Initial studies reporting a t(9;14)(p13;q32) IGH/PAX5 translocation in association with LPL[70,70] have not been confirmed and no other consistent genetic associations have been identified. A variety of trisomies has been found, of unknown significance, and del(6q) may be associated with an adverse prognosis.[71] Immunoglobulin heavy chain genes typically show hypermutation without evidence of ongoing acquisition of further mutations.[72]

Hairy cell leukemia (HCL)

Clinical features and pathology in the spleen

Hairy cell leukemia is a rare disease accounting for 2% of leukemias and predominantly affecting middle-aged men.

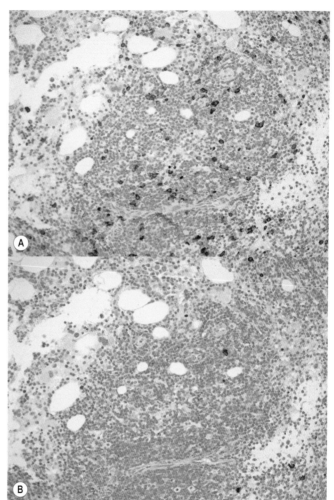

Fig. 29.7 (A, B) Lambda light chain restriction demonstrated within the plasma cell component of lymphoplasmacytic lymphoma using mRNA in situ hybridization for (A) lambda and (B) kappa. Decalcified, wax-embedded bone marrow trephine biopsy section; original magnification ×20.

The clinical presentation is with anemia, bleeding or infection (often with opportunistic organisms), reflecting PB cytopenias caused by hypersplenism and/or BM failure due to fibrosis associating tumor infiltrates.[40] At presentation 60% of patients have splenomegaly and 40% hepatomegaly. In the spleen, HCL is recognized by the presence of a diffuse infiltrate of typical hairy cells (see below), causing effacement of normal red and white pulp architecture. As in the BM, splenic infiltration is accompanied by reticulin deposition, interstitial hemorrhage, sinusoidal vascular ectasia and peliosis-like disruption.[73]

Blood and bone marrow aspiration

Most patients with HCL have circulating hairy cells although numbers are typically low. These are medium-sized to large lymphoid cells which have abundant, weakly basophilic cytoplasm and hair-like projections from the cell surface.[74] The nucleus is frequently indented and has a smooth chromatin pattern with indistinct nucleoli. Typical immunophenotyping results are summarized in Table 29.1. Peripheral cytopenias are common in HCL, particularly neutropenia and monocytopenia. BM aspiration is often unsuccessful

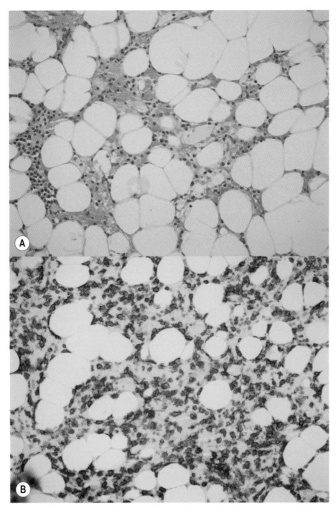

Fig. 29.8 (A, B) Hairy cell leukemia mimicking aplastic anemia, Decalcified, wax-embedded bone marrow trephine biopsy sections; (A) H&E and (B) CD20 immunohistochemistry. Original magnification ×40.

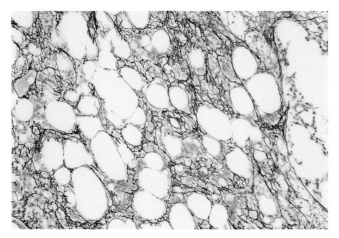

Fig. 29.9 Markedly increased stromal reticulin in bone marrow accompanying relatively subtle interstitial infiltration by HCL. Decalcified, wax-embedded bone marrow trephine biopsy section; Gordon and Sweet's stain for reticulin, original magnification ×20.

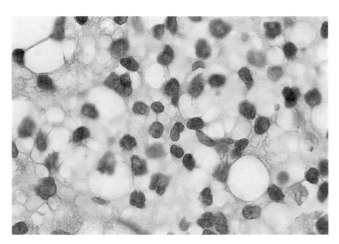

Fig. 29.10 High-power view of cells in HCL. They are widely spaced with abundant pale cytoplasm and irregular nuclei. One cell with a bilobed nucleus is present in the center of the field. Decalcified, wax-embedded bone marrow trephine biopsy section; H&E stain, original magnification ×100.

Bone marrow trephine biopsy

due to increased marrow reticulin associated with HCL infiltration; when neoplastic cells are obtained, they are essentially identical in morphology to those found in PB. They may be accompanied by reactive mast cells and plasma cells. In touch preparations from BMTB, HCL cells may lack typical 'hairy cell' cytology but present as lymphatic cells with abundant cytoplasm.

Bone marrow trephine biopsy

The degree of BM involvement is usually extensive at presentation, with large areas showing almost complete replacement of normal hemopoiesis by infiltrating hairy cells and partial or complete loss of fat spaces. Occasionally, the BM appears hypoplastic, with a subtle pattern of diffuse interstitial infiltration and partial preservation of hemopoiesis; granulopoiesis is often disproportionately reduced and this picture should not be confused with hypoplastic/aplastic anemia or a hypoplastic myelodysplastic syndrome (Fig. 29.8A). Subtle intrasinusoidal infiltration may also occur.[25] CD20 staining is essential to determine the extent of infiltrates (Fig. 29.8B). In almost all cases of HCL, interstitial reticulin is greatly increased (Fig. 29.9), which is rarely the case in other hypoplastic states. The infiltrating cells are of medium size with round, oval or bilobed nuclei and abundant, empty-looking cytoplasm (Fig. 29.10). Occasionally, they appear spindle-shaped. The abundant cytoplasm gives an appearance of the cells being widely spaced from one another. Extravasation of red cells into the interstitium is common and sinusoids appear prominent, with gaping lumens, as a result of the background of increased reticulin fibers (Fig. 29.11). Collagen fibrosis is rare. Osteosclerosis may also occur rarely in association with HCL and may regress with treatment.[75,76] Reactive mast cells are typically abundant throughout BM infiltrates and polytypic plasma cells may also be increased. Transformation of HCL to a more aggressive, large B-cell lymphoma occurs infrequently.[77]

In BMTB sections, hairy cells can be shown by IHC to express CD20, CD79a and CD45RA but not CD5 or CD23. Expression of tartrate-resistant acid phosphatase (TRAP) can usually be demonstrated in extensive infiltrates[78,79] although technical performance of anti-TRAP monoclonal antibodies varies and subtle HCL involvement may not be visible

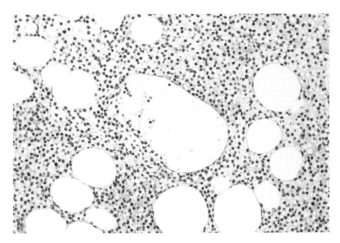

Fig. 29.11 Infiltrate of HCL causing a sinusoid to gape because of increased stromal reticulin deposition. The sinusoid can be distinguished from fat spaces elsewhere in the section by virtue of its larger size and its more irregular outline. Higher power examination would also allow its lining of flattened endothelium to be seen and blood cells within its lumen to be identified. Decalcified, wax-embedded bone marrow trephine biopsy section; H&E stain, original magnification ×20.

against background weak staining of hemopoietic cells. In many cases, hairy cells show heterogeneous, usually weaker than in mantle cell lymphoma, nuclear expression of cyclin D1 and, in a minority of cases, they are positive for CD10.[80] Dot-like cytoplasmic expression of CD68 may also be seen. Hairy cells are strongly positive for CD25 and CD123. Hairy cells react well with the monoclonal antibody DBA44,[79,81] which recognizes CD72[82] a B-cell surface antigen strongly associated with hairy cells but not entirely specific. Annexin A1 and T-cell associated transcription factor T-bet offer further and, to date, highly specific additional markers for HCL.[83,84]

After treatment, HCL infiltration usually appears dramatically reduced and the increased reticulin resolves rapidly in most patients.[75] Assessment of residual disease during and after therapy can be difficult in HCL, in which small interstitial clusters of scattered neoplastic cells may be all that remain; IHC usually reveals more disease than is readily apparent from standard tinctorial stains.

Genetic studies

Knowledge of genetic abnormalities associated with HCL is extremely limited and no consistent genetic associations have been found that appear causative. Immunoglobulin heavy chain genes are hypermutated but stable, without evidence of ongoing mutation. Partial understanding has been gained of genetic abnormalities underpinning the unusual properties of hairy cells;[85] over-expression of the activator protein-1 (AP-1) transcription factor drives the expression of CD11c, resulting in some of the unusual stromal interactions and adhesive properties of HCL cells. Up-regulation of AP-1 is secondary to *RAS* activation in HCL which, in turn, may be due to reduced expression of RhoH that normally competes with Ras proteins at GTP binding sites. Reconstitution of RhoH expression in a mouse xenograft model of HCL reduced proliferation of neoplastic cells and prolonged survival.[86]

HCL variant (HCLv)

Clinical features and pathology in the spleen

HCLv is a rare disease with incidence of 3 cases per 1 000 000. It may be more common in Asian countries. It has been recognized as a provisional entity in the WHO 2008 classification;[40] despite its name, it is clinically, immunophenotypically and genetically distinct from HCL.[87,88] Patients typically present with splenomegaly; anemia is common but neutropenia and monocytopenia are rare. HCLv shows overlap between HCL and B-cell prolymphocytic leukemia (B-PLL) in their pattern of splenic involvement, with predominant diffuse red pulp involvement.[40]

Blood and bone marrow aspiration

There are usually abundant circulating neoplastic cells in HCLv with WBC usually in the range of 20–40×10^9/l. Although HCLv cells have cytoplasmic projections as in HCL, they are larger and have nucleoli more akin to those seen in B-PLL. BM aspiration is usually successful because HCLv is not associated with significantly increased reticulin fiber production in the marrow stroma. The immunophenotype of cells in HCLv is distinct from that found in HCL (see Table 29.1); they are generally negative for CD25, CD123 and annexin A1, with weak or absent TRAP expression. They show CD11c, CD103, FMC7 and strong sIg reactivity as in HCL.

Bone marrow trephine biopsy

The histologic features of HCLv are different from those described above for HCL. They resemble those seen in CLL or B-PLL, with focal nodular and interstitial infiltration by small lymphoid cells, some having nucleoli. Infiltration is sometimes subtle and interstitial or intrasinusoidal. Cells in HCLv lack the distinctive nuclear and cytoplasmic characteristics of classical hairy cells and any increase in stromal reticulin is much less marked than in HCL. The immunophenotype in paraffin sections mirrors that described above; reactivity with DBA.44 (CD72) is similar to that found in HCL. It may in some cases be impossible to distinguish HCLv from splenic diffuse red pulp small B-cell lymphoma (see below).

Genetic studies

No specific genetic associations are known for HCLv; some patients have had translocations involving immunoglobulin gene regions and some have shown complex cytogenetic abnormalities.[89]

Splenic marginal zone B-cell lymphoma (SMZL)

Clinical features and pathology in the spleen

This disease accounts for fewer than 2% of lymphoid neoplasms and occurs mainly in older individuals, affecting men and women equally.[40] An association with hepatitis C has been noted in southern Europe.[63]

Patients typically present with splenomegaly, with or without hilar lymphadenopathy. Lymph node involvement elsewhere is distinctly uncommon. There may be a small paraprotein, usually IgM, but not as substantial as that found in many cases of lymphoplasmacytic lymphoma, and without secondary consequences of hyperviscosity. Autoimmune thrombocytopenia or anemia may accompany the lymphoma, and patients with substantial splenic enlargement may have hypersplenism. A proportion of patients are detected as a result of PB lymphocytosis, the cells typically appearing villous (see below); even in the absence of lymphocytosis, the BM is usually involved.

Within the spleen, there is widespread, generally uniform, involvement of the white pulp, giving a miliary appearance to the cut surfaces of splenectomy specimens.[90] The germinal centers and mantles of white pulp nodules are atrophic and replaced by densely clustered small lymphoid cells surrounded by expanded marginal zones of more mixed composition. Cells in the marginal zones are predominantly slightly larger, lymphoplasmacytoid or monocytoid cells with more cytoplasm than the lymphocytes present centrally within involved nodules. Within the marginal zones there are also scattered immunoblast-like cells in varying proportions. Small satellite collections of marginal zone-type cells are frequently also present surrounding red pulp capillaries, and are often accompanied by small collections of epithelioid macrophages.[73] There may be diffuse infiltration of red pulp cords and sinusoids by the small lymphoid cells. Appearances in splenunculi, when present, are identical to those in the main spleen; hilar lymph nodes show vaguely nodular replacement of follicles by small lymphocytes, usually without morphological evidence of marginal zone differentiation.

Blood and bone marrow aspiration

In PB, neoplastic cells in SMZL are slightly larger than normal lymphocytes, with a round nucleus and mature chromatin pattern. They have a relatively large volume of weakly basophilic cytoplasm and typically exhibit polar villi. BM involvement is almost always present and similar cells are usually readily apparent in aspirate. The immunophenotype (Table 29.1) shows usually positivity for CD19, CD20, surface IgM and in most cases IgD, no CD5 or CD10. CD23 and CD11c are positive in a fraction of cases. Cyclin D1 and Annexin A1 are negative.

Bone marrow trephine biopsy

There is usually nodular, interstitial and, less regularly, paratrabecular infiltration by neoplastic cells.[10,91] Intrasinusoidal infiltration is often an additional finding, demonstration of which may require IHC (Fig. 29.12). In occasional patients, a subtle and purely intrasinudoidal infiltrate may be present, requiring careful distinction from persistent polyclonal B-cell lymphocytosis (see below). A diffusely infiltrated, packed marrow is found only in rare patients.

Genetic studies

These neoplasms have clonally rearranged *IgH* and approximately 50% show hypermutation but evidence of ongoing acquisition of mutations is rare.[92] Trisomy 3q has been found in a high proportion of cases, regarded as a late or secondary event in the neoplasm development and of uncertain biological relevance. The occurrence of translocations or allelic losses involving 7q31-32 and 7q21 is believed to be

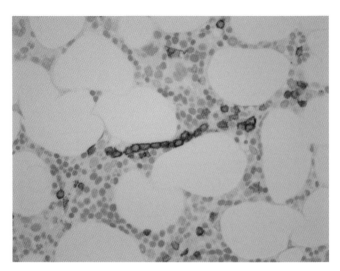

Fig. 29.12 Intrasinusoidal bone marrow infiltration by splenic marginal zone B-cell lymphoma. Decalcified, wax-embedded bone marrow trephine biopsy section; CD20 immunhistochemistry. Original magnification ×40.

more significant. The latter result in dysregulation of CDK6.[93] Microarray and CGH analysis suggests a distinctive profile involving up-regulation of gene expression within the AKT1 and B-cell receptor signaling pathways.[94,95] Of note, t(11;18), found in a high proportion of MALT-type marginal zone lymphomas, is absent from SMZL.

Splenic diffuse red pulp small B-cell lymphoma

Clinical features and pathology in the spleen

This lymphoma has been introduced as a provisional entity in the 2008 revision of the WHO classification[40] and has been described in patients predominantly of middle age and older, with men and women equally affected. Its clinical behavior is indolent.

Presentation is typically with splenomegaly accompanied by peripheral blood B-cell lymphocytosis. Cytopenias may be present, particularly neutropenia or thrombocytopenia. Skin involvement in the form of a pruritic papular rash has been described in some patients. Unlike typical SMZL, infiltration in the spleen is diffuse throughout the red pulp, involving cords and sinusoidal lumens and obscuring the distinction between red and white pulp structures. The destruction of underlying architecture and 'spaced out' appearance of HCL are absent and the immunophenotype is distinct from that of CLL or B-PLL.

Blood and bone marrow aspiration

Circulating lymphocytes often have villous processes and unusually basophilic cytoplasm.[96] They may be present only in low numbers. Similar cells are present in BM aspirate. Their imunophenotype resembles that of SMZL but sometimes overlaps with HCLv and increasing experience of these two provisional entities may in future reveal genuine biological overlap between them.

Bone marrow trephine biopsy

BM infiltration is present in all cases but may not be apparent in standard histological sections because it is almost exclusively intrasinusoidal. Absence of additional nodular, paratrabecular or diffuse infiltrates is in marked contrast with the findings in other spleen-predominant small B-cell lymphomas although this finding may be shared by some cases of HCLv. Differential diagnosis from persistent polyclonal B lymphocytosis is important but the clinical context and the cytology of circulating lymphocytes differ; cells in splenic diffuse red pulp small B-cell lymphoma express monotypic immunoglobulin light chains.

Genetic studies

Hypermutation patterns of *IGH* and the spectrum of variable region gene usage differ from those found in SMZL and resemble HCL in some cases. A translocation, t(9;14), involving *PAX5* and *IGH* has been found in some patients and genetic alterations associated with splenic, nodal and extranodal marginal zone lymphomas are absent.[40,97]

Extranodal marginal zone lymphoma of mucosa-associated lymphoid tissue (MALT)-type

Clinical features and pathology at presenting sites

Extranodal marginal zone lymphomas of MALT-type are indolent lymphoproliferative disorders with a 10-year survival of more than 80%.[60,61] The most common primary sites of MALT-type extranodal marginal zone lymphoma are within the gastrointestinal tract. Salivary glands, skin, orbit, lung and urogenital organs are the sites of origin in smaller numbers of patients. At presentation, 30% of patients have involvement of more than one mucosal site but lymph node spread is usually absent or localized to nodes close to the mucosal site(s) of involvement. As defined in the WHO classification, these lymphomas are low grade and arise in the context of normal or induced lymphoid tissue in the organs involved (e.g. that caused by infection with *Helicobacter pylori* in the stomach or *Chlamydia psittaci* in the orbit).[40] The neoplastic cells are typically centrocyte-like, with a tendency to infiltrate epithelial structures and form lympho-epithelial lesions; they show monocytoid or plasmacytic differentiation to varying extents in different individuals.

In some cases, progression to large B-cell lymphoma can be seen in MALT-type marginal zone lymphoma, indicating requirement for more aggressive management. In order to avoid confusion for patient management, the large cell component is classified separately (as diffuse large B-cell lymphoma, not otherwise specified, in most cases), so that the need for consideration of more intensive treatment is made clear.

Blood and bone marrow aspiration

Bone marrow involvement has been reported in 15–40% of cases.[98] Fifteen per cent of patients are anemic at presentation but circulating lymphoma cells are not seen. Bone marrow aspiration rarely reveals the presence of lymphoma cells, even when BMTB shows histologic evidence of involvement. Immunophenotype is similar to other marginal zone lymphomas, as summarized in Table 29.1.

Bone marrow trephine biopsy

When present, infiltrates of extranodal marginal zone lymphomas of MALT-type are usually nodular but paratrabecular and interstitial involvement has been described.[99]

The infiltrating cells are small but their centrocyte-like morphology can be difficult to appreciate due to admixture of reactive lymphocytes. For the same reason, IHC is often difficult to interpret but the neoplastic cells express CD20 and CD79a while lacking expression of CD5, CD10, CD23, CD43, BCL6 and cyclin D1.

Genetic studies

The translocation t(11;18)(q21;q21) has been found in some cases, particularly of gastric or pulmonary origin, associated with the formation of an *API2-MALT1* fusion gene.[100] This fusion gene is of uncertain functional significance at present but is absent from node-based and splenic forms of MZL. A t(14;18) translocation, distinct from that associated with FL, has been described mainly in orbital and salivary MALT lymphomas and t(3;14) in thyroid, orbital and skin lymphomas. These are associated with an abnormal API2-MALT1 fusion protein, in the case of t(11;18), or transcriptional deregulation of *BCL10, FOXP1* and *MALT1*. Trisomy 3 has been detected in more than 60% of cases using FISH and comparative genomic hybridization;[101,102] this (and other reported associated trisomies, of chromosome 8 and other chromosomes) is not specific for MALT lymphomas. Immunoglobulin genes show a hypermutated pattern indicative of a post-germinal center B cell[103,104] with ongoing mutations.

Nodal marginal zone lymphoma (+/– monocytoid B-cells)

Clinical features and lymph node pathology

Nodal marginal zone lymphoma (MZL) is rare, comprising less than 2% of all NHL. Presentation is usually with advanced disease characterized by peripheral and para-aortic lymphadenopathy; 5-year survival is 50–60%.[40]

The histologic appearances in lymph nodes can be similar to those of nodal involvement secondary to extranodal lymphoma of MALT-type and may also require distinction from reactive monocytoid B-cell hyperplasia. Monocytoid B-cells are medium-sized cells that are quite similar to hairy cells in histologic sections, having oval or bilobed nuclei and abundant, clear cytoplasm. However, infiltrates in nodal MZL are usually heterogeneous, including centrocyte-like cells and others showing marginal zone cell or plasmacytoid differentiation. Distinction from variants of FL with down-regulation of CD10 and, less consistently, of BCL6 can be difficult in some patients in whom nodular architecture is prominent within the lymphoma.[105,106]

Blood and bone marrow aspiration

The blood is involved in 10% of patients but up to 30% have BM involvement. The appearance of circulating cells varies between patients; they may resemble small lymphocytes or be larger, with monocytoid appearances. The immunophenotype is indistinguishable from extranodal, MALT-type marginal zone lymphoma in many cases (see Table 29.1) although with CD43 and/or weak CD23 expression in some.

Bone marrow trephine biopsy

Few descriptions have been published recording histologic features of BM involvement in nodal MZL. Nodular and paratrabecular patterns of infiltration have been described.[107]

The infiltrating cells are a mixture of lymphocytes, centrocyte-like cells, monocytoid cells and plasma cells. Clinical features, knowledge of the lymph node or splenic histology and immunophenotype usually exclude the other lymphoma categories. In histologic sections, the neoplastic cells can be shown to express CD20, CD79a but not CD5, CD10, CD23 or cyclin D1.

Genetic studies

Little is known about underlying genetic abnormalities in nodal MZL; trisomies 3, 7 and 18 have been found in a high proportion of cases[108] but, like most numerical chromosomal abnormalities in lymphomas, they are probably a secondary phenomenon. The t(11;18) and t(14;18) translocations associated with MALT-type extranodal MZL are not found.

Follicular lymphoma (FL)

Clinical features and lymph node pathology

Follicular lymphoma comprises approximately 35% of NHL. Disease is frequently widespread at diagnosis involving lymph nodes, spleen, and BM. Blood is involved in 10% of cases. The median survival is around 7–9 years and there is approximately 20% risk of transformation to diffuse large B-cell lymphoma within 10 years from diagnosis[108] although it is anticipated that intervention with anti-CD20 treatment will improve these outcomes.

In lymph nodes, FL typically replaces normal structures with well defined, uniformly sized germinal centers containing neoplastic centrocytes and centroblasts. The WHO classification divides FL into three grades, depending on the relative proportions of centrocytes and centroblasts present; precise details of how this grading is achieved are available elsewhere.[40] Grade 3 disease is further subdivided into grades 3A and 3B. Assessment of grade in FL is of prognostic value; grades 1 and 2 behave as low-grade lymphomas with a chronic course but long survival, while grade 3B disease is more aggressive and has an outcome equivalent to diffuse large B-cell lymphoma. The precise status of grade 3A disease remains controversial but it is generally regarded as more aggressive than grades 1 and 2.[109]

Blood and bone marrow aspiration

Follicular lymphoma cells, when present in the circulation, are usually centrocytes that appear smaller than those seen in BM or lymph nodes and have little or no cytoplasm. Nuclear chromatin is condensed and uniformly distributed; in typical cases a deep nuclear cleft can be seen (Fig. 29.13). Circulating centroblasts, which are larger cells with prominent nucleoli, are usually only seen in advanced disease. BM aspirate contains detectable centrocytes and/or centroblasts only infrequently, even when BMTB shows clear evidence of histological involvement. Typical immunophenotype findings in FL are summarized in Table 29.1.

Bone marrow trephine biopsy

BMTB sections from patients with FL show involvement in the majority of cases but deposits of disease may be small and focal. If no lymphomatous infiltration is detected in initial sections, immunostaining and examination of further sections representing deeper parts of the tissue core are

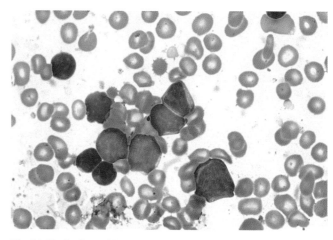

Fig. 29.13 Cytology of FL in a bone marrow aspirate film. A mixed population of atypical lymphoid cells is present, including large and small cells with irregular nuclear indentations. MGG stain, original magnification ×100.

mandatory to avoid missing focal deposits.[110] Small or crushed specimens, in which only limited histological assessment is possible, should be regarded as inadequate if no lymphoma is evident, and the biopsy repeated, since there is a high chance of false negative results from such specimens. At least three intact intertrabecular spaces, free from traumatic and other artifacts, are needed for adequate assessment.

The classical pattern of BM infiltration by FL is paratrabecular. Well-developed paratrabecular infiltrates form bands or 'crescent moon' shapes with the longest axis abutting and lying parallel to the trabecular surface (Figs 29.14 and 29.15). Nodular infiltrates are found less often and diffuse interstitial involvement is distinctly uncommon; in either case, typical areas of paratrabecular infiltration are usually also seen. In contrast with the lymph node features, neoplastic germinal centers are rarely formed in BM deposits of FL. If they are present (Fig. 29.16), care must be taken not to mistake them for focal transformation to large cell lymphoma, since they may contain prominent centroblasts. In paratrabecular infiltrates, the cells present are predominantly non-neoplastic small T-lymphocytes, with only small numbers of centrocytes and even fewer centroblasts usually being present. Consequently, immunostaining may be misleading and greater reliance should be placed on recognition of the distinctive paratrabecular distribution of FL infiltrates. It may be very difficult to distinguish minimal non-paratrabecular infiltrates of FL from non-neoplastic lymphoid infiltrates.

By IHC, neoplastic cells in BM infiltrates of FL are seen to express CD20 and CD79a but not CD5 or cyclin D1. They also usually lack CD23 and IRF4/MUM1 expression. In contrast with nodal disease, the cells may show partial or complete down-regulation of both CD10 and BCL6. Use of immunostaining to demonstrate BCL2 is not helpful in BMTB sections, since this antigen is expressed strongly by reactive T-cells; the latter, as described above, often outnumber and obscure the neoplastic cells.

Genetic studies

Immunoglobulin genes are rearranged and hypermutated with evidence of ongoing somatic mutation.[45,103] Most cases

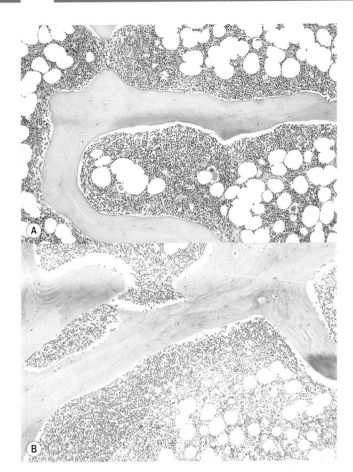

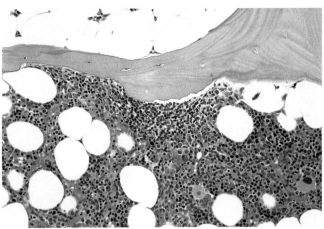

Fig. 29.15 Subtle involvement of bone marrow by FL. In contrast to the extensive linear paratrabecular infiltrates shown in Fig. 29.14, lymphoma in this example is represented by a small 'crescent moon' deposit of lymphoma. Although tiny, this deposit can still be seen clearly to be associated with the surface of the adjacent bony trabecula, having its longest axis along the trabecular margin. Decalcified, wax-embedded bone marrow trephine biopsy section; H&E stain, original magnification ×20.

Fig. 29.14 (A, B) Classical band-like paratrabecular infiltration of bone marrow by FL. (A) H&E stain; (B) Giemsa stain. At low magnification, loss of fat spaces and condensation of cellular tissue around the trabecular margin is a clue to the presence of lymphoma at this site and Giemsa staining highlights the presence of closely packed small lymphoid cells forming the paratrabecular infiltrates. Decalcified, wax-embedded bone marrow trephine biopsy section, original magnification ×10.

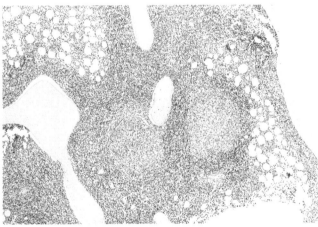

Fig. 29.16 Formation of neoplastic germinal centers within an infiltrate of FL in bone marrow. Note the additional component of paratrabecular infiltration in the background. Paler staining of the germinal centers relative to paratrabecular infiltrates in this example reflects the lesser admixture of small, non-neoplastic lymphocytes (predominantly T cells) in the former. Paratrabecular infiltrates are almost always accompanied by numerous reactive T-lymphocytes. Decalcified, wax-embedded bone marrow trephine biopsy section; H&E stain, original magnification ×5.

of FL have a t(14;18)(q32;q21) translocation which dysregulates the *BCL2* oncogene by placing it under the influence of the immunoglobulin heavy chain gene promoter. Variant translocations involving kappa and lambda light chain genes occur in a few patients; t(2;18)(p12;q21) and t(18;22)(q21;q11), respectively. High grade examples of FL may have additional *BCL6* rearrangements, as found in diffuse large B-cell lymphoma, and very aggressive variants have additional abnormalities of *TP53*, *p16*-INK4a and/or *MYC*.

Mantle cell lymphoma (MCL)

Clinical features and lymph node pathology

MCL comprises approximately 6% of NHL. The median age at diagnosis is 60 years and most patients present with widespread disease involving lymph nodes, spleen and, sometimes, the gastrointestinal (GI) tract ('lymphomatous polyposis'). Median survival is only 3–5 years.[40,111]

In lymph nodes, MCL grows in a diffuse or vaguely nodular fashion, sometimes showing a tendency to expand mantle zones around residual, non-neoplastic germinal centers. The cytology of classic MCL varies from lymphocytic to centrocytic but is usually uniform in any individual

patient; occasional patients have a so-called 'blastoid' variants of MCL, in which cells resemble either lymphoblasts or pleomorphic large blast cells. Growth in the spleen or at mucosal sites within the GI tract has essentially similar characteristics.

Blood and bone marrow aspiration

Sixty per cent of patients have BM involvement at diagnosis and circulating lymphoma cells are present in the blood in 30%, particularly those with advanced disease.[98] However, there is a subgroup of patients who present with lymphocytosis ± splenomegaly but with no lymphadenopathy and in whom the disease pursues a more indolent course.

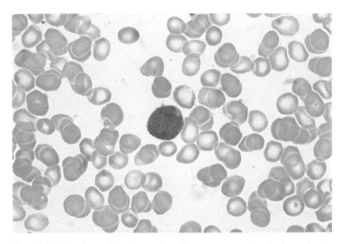

Fig. 29.17 Cytology of MCL in aspirated bone marrow. A typical neoplastic mantle cell is shown; medium-sized with scanty cytoplasm and an irregular nuclear outline. Bone marrow aspirate film; MGG stain, original magnification ×100.

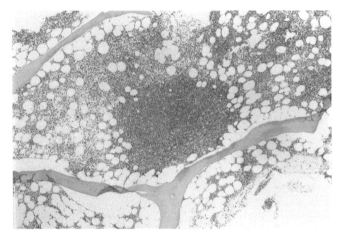

Fig. 29.18 Nodular infiltration of bone marrow by MCL. At this magnification, a minor degree of interstitial infiltration cannot be confirmed or excluded but predominance of the nodular pattern is clear. Decalcified, wax-embedded bone marrow trephine biopsy section; H&E stain, original magnification ×5.

Circulating cells, when present, are pleomorphic; the predominant cell type is medium-sized with moderately abundant chromatin, an irregular nuclear outline and dispersed chromatin. In the blastoid form of MCL, nucleoli are seen within tumor cell nuclei. Similar features characterize the cells in BM aspirate films (Fig. 29.17). By FCM, they have a distinctive immunophenotype (see Table 29.1).

Bone marrow trephine biopsy

Histologic evidence of BM involvement is found in more than 70% of patients with MCL. The pattern of infiltration varies widely: nodular, interstitial, diffuse and paratrabecular patterns have been described. Nodular infiltration (Fig. 29.18), with or without an additional interstitial component is probably the most commonly seen pattern. Paratrabecular infiltration occurs fairly frequently but, in contrast with FL, is less extensive and is often overshadowed by other patterns of involvement.[10,107] The cells are small and, as in lymph nodes, may be lymphocyte-like, may resemble centrocytes

or, in a minority of cases, have lymphoblast-like or pleomorphic features. The blastoid variant requires distinction from Burkitt lymphoma and acute lymphoblastic leukemia.

IHC enables demonstration of cyclin D1 expression in the nuclei of neoplastic cells in a great majority of cases of MCL.[112] This cell cycle regulatory protein is not detectable in normal lymphoid cells but endothelial cells are positive and may serve as internal positive control for cyclin D1 IHC. The neoplastic cells of CLL, SMZL and FL do not express this molecule. Rare cases of B-PLL have been reported as positive but these may in fact represent examples of leukemic presentation of MCL.[113] The cells of MCL also express CD20, CD79a and CD5 but not CD10, CD23 or terminal deoxynucleotidyl transferase (TdT). Expression of Ki67, as a marker of proliferative activity, is of prognostic importance, with high levels (40% or more of cells positive) indicating more aggressive clinical behavior. Accompanying CD23-positive follicular dendritic cell meshworks are less commonly found in bone marrow infiltrates than in involved lymph nodes and other tissue deposits. Occasional cases that appear cyclin D1 negative by IHC can usually be shown by FISH to have t(11;14), using aspirated marrow cells or BMTB sections.

Genetic studies

The translocation t(11;14)(q13;q32) is strongly associated with MCL and places the *BCL1* oncogene, which encodes cyclin D1, under regulation of the immunoglobulin heavy chain gene promoter. This leads to inappropriate expression of cyclin D1, as described above. A variant translocation, t(11;22)(q11;q13), juxtaposes *BCL1* with the lambda light chain gene in a minority of patients with MCL. Cells of MCL uncommonly show evidence of immunoglobulin variable region gene hypermutation; when present, only low levels of somatic mutation are evident[41] and, unlike CLL, the level in an individual patient does not appear to be of prognostic importance with current treatment regimes.

Diffuse large B-cell lymphoma not otherwise specified (DLBCL, NOS)

Clinical features and pathology at presenting sites

Diffuse large B cell lymphoma, not otherwise specified (DLBCL, NOS) comprises approximately 30% of NHL. Presentation may be with node-based or extranodal disease.[40] Thirty per cent of patients have B symptoms (fever, weight loss, night sweats) at the time of diagnosis. Assessment of prognostic factors is important for therapy; such factors include age, stage of disease, performance status and serum lactate dehydrogenase (LDH) concentration. Patients with low-risk factors have an 83% 5-year survival while 5-year survival is only 32% in those with high-risk disease.[40] A majority of cases of DLBCL, NOS arise *de novo* but a significant proportion occur following or accompanied by variants of small B-cell lymphoma (particularly B-cell CLL and FL).

Infiltration by DLBCL, NOS usually causes total or near-total loss of normal lymph node architecture and replacement by large blast cells. Most commonly these are centroblasts but a variable proportion of immunoblasts and plasmablasts may be present. The infiltrating cells may be monotonous or exhibit marked pleomorphism; in occasional cases, anaplastic cells resembling Reed–Sternberg

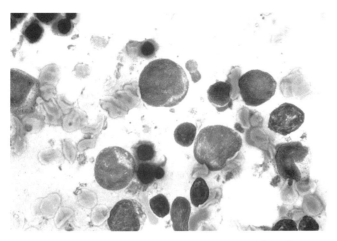

Fig. 29.19 Cytology of DLBCL in aspirated bone marrow. Cells are large with varying amounts of cytoplasm, irregular nuclear outlines and prominent nucleoli. Bone marrow aspirate film; MGG stain, original magnification ×100.

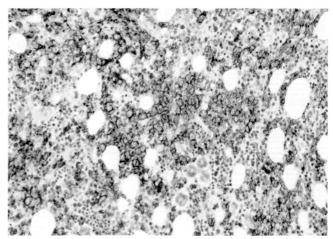

Fig. 29.20 CD20 immunostaining highlights patchy infiltrates of DLBCL in bone marrow trephine biosy. Original magnification ×40.

cells may be found. Cases of DLBCL, NOS also arise *de novo* at extranodal sites, particularly involving the GI system, testis and bone. At present, it is unclear whether variants of DLCBL with primary extranodal presentation are related pathogenetically to low-grade node-based or extranodal lymphomas. Large B-cell lymphomas arising in the CNS and mediastinum are recognized separately in the 2008 revision of the WHO classification, reflecting evidence that these are distinctive clinicopathological entities.

Blood and bone marrow aspiration

Blood involvement in DLBCL, NOS is rare and, when present, circulating lymphoma cells are usually large, with a large nucleus, prominent multiple nucleoli and abundant cytoplasm. BM aspirate involvement can be recognized by the presence of cells with these features (Fig. 29.19); immunophenotypic findings do not permit their distinction from some other NHL subtypes but remain important in supporting a putative diagnosis of DLCBL, NOS and excluding non-lymphoid blast cell proliferations, as well as contributing to assessment of prognosis.

Bone marrow trephine biopsy

Primary involvement of the BM by DLBCL, NOS is uncommon. When present, it shows no characteristic pattern of distribution within intertrabecular spaces; infiltrates usually form random, solid patches or are dispersed in the interstitium[10] (Fig. 29.20). The cellular morphology of large blast cells in BM infiltrates of DLBCL, NOS generally matches that seen at the primary site. In some cases, BM infiltration may be discordant and show low-grade histologic features, even when no accompanying low-grade lymphoma has been found in sections from a lymph node or other diagnostic specimen.[114-116] This is occasionally helpful in providing evidence to support origin of an apparently *de novo* DLBCL, NOS from FL, if typical paratrabecular infiltrates of FL are found in the BMTB sections. The presence of discordant low-grade lymphoma in the BM of patients with DLBCL, NOS does not appear to influence prognosis significantly, whereas the concordant presence of DLBCL, NOS in the BM is an adverse factor.[114] It is not always appropriate to assume that

the discordant elements represent a single lymphoma; some studies have shown a clonal relationship between *IGH* rearrangements in only approximately 50% of examples.[116] Examples of discordance involving low-grade lymphoma elsewhere and DLBCL, NOS in the BM are very rare. Primary DLCB of bone without any signs of other organ involvement is rare but has been reported to have rather good prognosis.[117]

The differential diagnosis of DLBCL, NOS in BM includes other subtypes of DLCBL, other large B-cell lymphomas, Burkitt lymphoma, myeloma, acute lymphoblastic leukemia and acute myeloid leukemia. Attention to clinical features, cytologic detail of the infiltrating cells and the appearances of hemopoietic tissue in the background usually permits discrimination between these alternatives. IHC can be used to confirm the B-cell phenotype of neoplastic cells, which express CD79a and in most cases CD20. Less consistently, there may be expression of PAX5, CD5, CD10, BCL2, BLC6, and/or IRF4/MUM1 but staining for myeloid markers and TdT will be negative. Occasionally, the neoplastic cells will be found to express CD30; in the context of a B-cell immunophenotype. Germinal center (GC)-like and non-GC-like immunophenotypes can be deduced from combinations of CD10, BCL6 and IRF4/MUM1 expression,[52] providing prognostic information similar to that available from microarray studies (see below). However, genetic and immunophenotypic results do not correlate completely and expression of combinations of different antigens has also been found to be of prognostic value.[48] Proliferative activity, conveniently demonstrated by Ki67 immunostaining, is variable but should always be investigated to ensure the differential diagnosis of BL is not missed. Immunocompromised patients, in whom primary presentation of their lymphoma may be in the BM rather than at a nodal or extranodal soft tissue site, are likely to have neoplastic cells harboring latent Epstein–Barr virus (EBV) infection, demonstrable by EBV-EBER *in situ* hybridization.

Genetic studies

Genetic findings in DLCBL are complex; aneuploidy is common and complex aberrant clones are often found. Cells may show t(14;18)(q32;q21), with *BCL2* dysregulation, as in FL. The translocation t(3;14)(q27;q32), and others involving 3q27 breakpoints, dysregulating *BCL6* are also relatively common in DLBCL of all morphologic varieties.[40] Immunoglobulin variable region genes show evidence of hypermutation with ongoing changes, implying continued exposure to somatic mutator mechanisms.[45] Microarray studies have defined germinal center (GC)-like and activated B-cell (ABC)-like molecular expression profiles[56,58,118] that are of prognostic significance for patients, even when treated with chemotherapy combinations incorporating anti-CD20. Alternative separation of patients into prognostic groups according to gene expression patterns reflecting immune/stromal response, proliferation characteristics and oxidative phosphorylation is under investigation.[54,55]

Other diffuse large B-cell lymphoma subtypes

As recognized in the WHO 2008 classification, these are T-cell/histiocyte-rich large B-cell lymphoma, primary DLBCL of the CNS, primary cutaneous DLBCL, leg type, and EBV-positive DLBCL of the elderly. Of these, only T-cell/histiocyte-rich large B cell lymphoma[40,119] involves BM with any frequency. Neoplastic cells are rarely represented in blood or aspirated marrow. The histological picture is one of random patchy or diffuse BM replacement by infiltrates that are, as the name implies, rich in reactive small T lymphocytes and macrophages. Large neoplastic blast cells variously resemble large centroblasts, mononuclear Hodgkin and Reed–Sternberg (HRS) cells and the so-called 'LH' cells of nodular lymphocyte-predominant Hodgkin lymphoma (NLPHL). Extensive immunophenotyping is often needed to highlight neoplastic cells, demonstrate their B cell phenotype and confirm absence of HRS features. Excluding an alternative diagnosis of NLPHL can be difficult and is controversial; NLPHL may have a growth pattern closely resembling T-cell/histiocyte-rich large B cell lymphoma and this may develop as a progression from a more typical pattern with repeated relapse over time.[120] The genetic basis of T-cell/histiocyte-rich large B cell lymphoma is poorly understood.

Other lymphomas of large B cells

These lymphomas, as recognized in the 2008 WHO classification, are primary mediastinal large B-cell lymphoma, intravascular large B cell lymphoma, DLBCL associated with chronic inflammation, lymphomatoid granulomatosis, ALK-positive large B-cell lymphoma, plasmablastic lymphoma, large B-cell lymphoma arising in HHV8-associated multicentric Castleman disease, and primary effusion lymphoma. BM is infrequently involved in most of these and, when it is, the features are similar to those found in DLBCL, NOS.

An exception is intravascular large B cell lymphoma, which is a rare and highly aggressive neoplasm that usually presents as a result of CNS or subcutaneous vascular infiltration but may have a primary presentation in BM.[6,22,40] Neoplastic cells are rarely recognized in blood or BM aspirate. They are large and anaplastic, resembling cells of Hodgkin or anaplastic large cell lymphoma. They show varying combinations of CD5, CD10 and IRF4/MUM1 expression in addition to expressing CD20 and other pan-B cell markers. Their pattern of BM infiltration is predominantly intrasinusoidal (Fig. 29.21); the marrow interstitium and lumens of

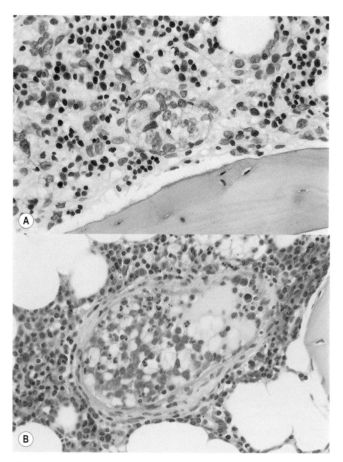

Fig. 29.21 (A, B) Intravascular large B-cell lymphoma in bone marrow. (A) Large malignant lymphoid cells apparently forming a cluster because of their confinement within a sinusoidal lumen. (B) Larger blood vessels within bone marrow, in this case probably a venule, can also contain malignant lymphoid cells in this variant of large B-cell lymphoma. Decalcified, wax-embedded bone marrow trephine biopsy sections; H&E stain, original magnification ×40.

larger blood vessels are involved less conspicuously and solid infiltrates are rare. The genetic basis of this rare lymphoma is unknown.

Burkitt lymphoma (BL)

Clinical features and pathology at presenting sites

Burkitt lymphoma (BL) is a rare and aggressive disease, accounting for fewer than 1% of all cases of NHL. Cure is possible with highly intensive chemotherapy regimens and hemopoietic stem cell transplantation.

The WHO classification recognizes three clinical subtypes of BL (endemic, sporadic and immunodeficiency-associated).[40] Aggressive lymphomas previously regarded as 'Burkitt-like' or 'atypical Burkitt's lymphoma' are now classified within the WHO 2008 revision as 'B-cell lymphoma, unclassifiable, with features intermediate between diffuse large B-cell lymphoma and Burkitt lymphoma'.[121] Endemic BL is a disease of childhood in sub-Saharan Africa and is frequently extranodal at presentation, with a high incidence of jaw tumors. Sporadic BL occurs in all parts of the world and has a wide age distribution; ileocecal tumor formation in young males is a common presentation. Burkitt lymphoma in the context of immunodeficiency is most commonly seen in association with human immunodeficiency virus (HIV) infection but may also occur as a form of post-transplant lymphoproliferative disease and in other immunodeficiency states; its histologic features resemble those of the sporadic disease. All subtypes of BL are characterized histologically by diffuse proliferation of medium-sized cells that typically have a round nucleus, small or inconspicuous nucleoli and a rim of basophilic cytoplasm that may contain lipid vacuoles. Cells in BL associated with immunosuppression may show more evidence of plasmablastic differentiation than those in the other subtypes. Much variation in cellular features occurs between patients, however, and BL cannot be diagnosed reliably on the basis of cell morphology. High cell turnover in all subtypes is reflected by the presence of abundant tingible body macrophages, responding to the high rate of apoptotic cell death and providing the well-known 'starry sky' appearance. It should be noted that this feature is not specific to BL but may also be found in other aggressive lymphomas with high rates of apoptotic cell death.

Blood and bone marrow aspiration

Circulating tumor cells are present in a minority of patients with BL; in effect, these patients have a mature B-cell acute leukemia, of ALL-L3 subtype as defined historically by the French-American-British (FAB) group.[122] The cells are fairly large, with cytoplasmic basophilia and vacuolation. Nuclear chromatin is dispersed and nucleoli are indistinct. The same morphology is represented in BM aspirate films, when involved, and the immunophenotype is distinguished from B-ALL by absence of nuclear TdT expression. Within the WHO classification, this presentation is categorized as Burkitt leukemia.[40]

Bone marrow trephine biopsy

The BM is not commonly involved by BL at presentation, except those patients who present with Burkitt leukemia. When present, BL cells in BMTB sections resemble those seen at other sites of disease involvement, being medium-sized with round nuclei, inconspicuous nucleoli and basophilic cytoplasm. Vacuolation of the cytoplasm is difficult to appreciate in histologic sections, even when prominent in cytology preparations. Mitotic figures are usually numerous. Infiltration may be interstitial, nodular or diffuse[10] and may be accompanied by tingible body macrophages, giving a similar 'starry sky' appearance to that seen at other sites of involvement. The differential diagnosis includes ALL, blastoid variants of MCL and aggressive morphologic variants of DLCBL; clinical context and immunophenotype are usually discriminatory. The cells of BL express CD20 (sometimes only weakly), CD79a and CD10 but not CD5, cyclin D1, TdT or IRF4/MUM1. BCL2 is absent in most cases. Demonstration of Ki67 expression provides indirect evidence that cell cycle control has been dysregulated to leave all BL cells active in the cell cycle. Essentially 100% of tumor cells in BL express Ki67, with uniformly strong intensity, a picture that is very uncommon in all other lymphomas. The presence of EBV in tumor cells can be demonstrated in BMTB sections by IHC for latent membrane protein-1 (LMP-1) or EBV nuclear antigen-2 (EBNA-2), or by *in situ* hybridization to demonstrate EBV early RNA species (EBER). As mentioned above,

however, EBV is less commonly associated with sporadic BL than with endemic and HIV-associated cases.

Genetic studies

At a genetic level, BL cells characteristically have translocations involving the *MYC* oncogene and immunoglobulin heavy or light chain genes: t(8;14)(q24;q32), t(2;8) (p12;q24), t(8;22)(q24;q11). The precise breakpoints vary between endemic, sporadic and immunodeficiency-associated subtypes and, in a substantial proportion of patients, the partner genes involved in *MYC* translocations are unknown. The subtypes also vary in their association with clonal latent infection by EBV; endemic BL is highly associated with EBV latency in tumor cells, sporadic BL less so and, of the immunodeficiency-associated cases, EBV latency is most frequently encountered in those arising in HIV-positive patients. Immunoglobulin variable region genes are hypermutated in BL. Gene profiling with microarray techniques shows an expression signature clearly distinct from that of DLCBL, although intermediate patterns are also found.[50]

B-cell lymphoma, unclassifiable, with features intermediate between DLBCL and BL

This category within the WHO 2008 classification includes aggressive lymphomas showing different combinations of the morphological, immunophenotypic and genetic features of both BL and DLCBL but not fully meeting all clinical and pathological criteria for either.[40,121] The lymphomas encompassed are heterogeneous. Most have cytomorphology that is intermediate between the two; others have typical BL morphology but an atypical immunophenotype. The presence of *MYC* rearrangement may be found in association with a complex karyotype or an additional t(14;18), the latter suggesting origin by transformation from FL and being associated with particularly aggressive clinical behavior. Additional *BCL6* rearrangement is also commonly found. Features in blood and BM have not been described specifically although patients may present with leukemia. When BM is involved, the infiltrates share the characteristics shown at other sites of involvement. This category should be used with caution in patients presenting with BM as the only diagnostic tissue unless extensive immunophenotyping and cytogenetic or FISH analysis is employed to provide the wide range of information needed.

B-cell lymphoma, unclassifiable, with features intermediate between DLBCL and classical Hodgkin lymphoma

This category has been created within the 2008 revision of the WHO classification of lymphomas to recognize rare large cell lymphomas which, as the name indicates, share characteristics of large B cell lymphoma (particularly primary mediastinal B cell lymphoma) and classical Hodgkin lymphoma (HL) without clearly meeting diagnostic criteria for either.[40,121] Typical presentation is in young men, with a large anterior mediastinal mass; unlike classical HL, EBV is present only in a relatively small minority of patients. Blood and BM features have not been described specifically although spread to BM is noted. Marrow infiltration, when present, would be expected to have similar features to those found at other sites. A high content of very pleomorphic large blast cells is usual, accompanied by fibrosis but relatively low numbers of inflammatory cells such as macrophages and eosinophils. There is more evidence of B cell-associated antigen expression than in classical HL, with both CD20 and CD79a being strongly expressed. There is retention of CD45 positivity by neoplastic cells, expression of CD30 and, in most cases, also of CD15. This category should be used with caution in patients for whom BM is the sole diagnostic tissue unless clinical features are strongly indicative and extensive immunophenotyping is employed to characterize infiltrates.

Mature T-cell and NK-cell neoplasms

Extranodal NK/T lymphoma, nasal type; enteropathy-associated T-cell lymphoma, subcutaneous panniculitis-like T-cell lymphoma

Clinical features and pathology at presenting sites

These are rare subtypes of T-cell and natural killer (NK)-cell lymphomas presenting in adults with distinctive, generally aggressive, clinical features but rarely involving BM; for this reason they are considered only briefly here.

Lymphomas of NK/T-cell, nasal type are much more common in Asia than anywhere else and are associated with latent EBV infection in most cases. It is important to note that, although the classical presentation is with a necrotizing mid-facial neoplasm, these lymphomas also occur at other body sites.[24,40] Inflammatory features frequently mask the presence of neoplastic cells and the diagnosis may be difficult to establish.

Enteropathy-associated T-cell lymphoma (EATL)[40] usually presents in adults with small bowel obstruction due to constricting tumor or with perforation due to tumor ulceration; multiple sites of small bowel tumor formation may be found at laparotomy. The neoplastic cells are medium-sized or large, with a cytotoxic T-cell phenotype, often associated with extensive tissue necrosis underlying the formation of ulcers. Most cases show background histologic features of gluten-sensitive enteropathy in non-neoplastic small bowel tissue and a proportion of patients have clinically overt celiac disease, usually of adult onset.

As its name implies, subcutaneous panniculitis-like T-cell lymphoma presents with clinical features of panniculitis and also has striking inflammatory histologic features accompanying dispersed malignant cells in subcutaneous tissue.[40] The neoplastic T/NK-cells in these lymphoma subtypes are large and frequently pleomorphic. They typically have cytotoxic features, with granules containing perforin, granzymes and TIA-1 contributing to their necrotizing/inflammatory behavior.

Blood and bone marrow aspirate findings

Rare patients with disseminated NK/T-cell nasal type lymphomas may have pancytopenia; circulating or aspirated neoplastic cells have large polymorphic nuclei and scanty basophilic cytoplasm. Blood and BM aspirate samples virtually never contain neoplastic cells in enteropathy-type or subcutaneous panniculitis-like T-cell lymphomas but PB cytopenias, accompanied by prominent BM aspirate features of hemophagocytosis, may be seen in the latter disease.

Bone marrow trephine biopsy

BMTB histology rarely shows evidence of direct involvement by these subtypes of T- and NK-cell lymphoma. In those few cases with involvement, appearances are indistinguishable from peripheral T-cell lymphoma, not otherwise specified. Random or diffuse patterns of infiltration may be present, with cells of medium to large size, often with high nucleocytoplasmic ratios and irregular nuclear outlines. IHC is needed to demonstrate expression of T-cell associated antigens such as CD2, CD3, CD4, CD5, CD7, CD8 and CD45RO, cytotoxic granule proteins and/or NK-associated antigens including CD16, CD56, CD57. There may be admixed inflammatory cells, including macrophages, and increased stromal reticulin may accompany the infiltrates. Subcutaneous panniculitis-like T-cell lymphoma may be accompanied by a severe hemophagocytic syndrome. The latter is represented in BMTB sections by prominence of large, round stromal macrophages containing abundant phagocytosed hemopoietic cells and other debris.

Genetic studies

TCR-beta and -gamma genes are in germline configuration in most examples of nasal type NK/T-cell lymphoma but are often clonally rearranged in rare cases presenting in the lymph nodes as well as in subcutaneous panniculitis-like T-cell lymphoma and EATL. Patients with EATL have a high frequency of an underlying constitutional HLA-DQA1*0501,DQB1*0201 genotype, which is present in a very high proportion of patients with celiac disease.[123] In contrast with other T cell lymphomas, complex abnormalities of 9q or deletions involving 16q are present in most cases of EATL.[124]

Hepatosplenic T-cell lymphoma

Clinical features, pathology, blood and bone marrow aspirate findings

This is a rare lymphoma with a median age at presentation of approximately 30 years. Most patients present with hepatosplenomegaly and have systemic symptoms.[40] Most are pancytopenic at presentation and approximately half have circulating lymphoma cells. The presence of the latter heralds aggressive, end-stage disease in some patients, although prognosis in all cases is poor.[11,17,125]

Liver and spleen are diffusely enlarged by intrasinusoidal lymphoid cell infiltration with little tendency for solid accumulation of neoplastic cells. The cells vary somewhat in morphology from patient to patient; they may be small, medium-sized or large with regular or folded nuclei, a condensed chromatin pattern and inconspicuous nucleoli. They have moderately abundant, pale cytoplasm. In the terminal stages of disease, transformation to blast cells with prominent nucleoli may occur. Identical cells are present in the BM and, when involved, in PB.

Bone marrow trephine biopsy

Histologic sections show erythroid and megakaryocytic hyperplasia, with interstitial and intrasinusoidal infiltration by neoplastic cells,[21,40] which may be subtle and almost invisible without IHC. The cells are of variable size, as described above, and are often pleomorphic; IHC stains reveal that they express CD2, CD3 and CD56 but usually neither CD4 nor CD8. They lack CD5 expression and show selective expression of the cytotoxic granule proteins TIA-1 and granzyme M without perforin or granzyme B. If involvement is slight, IHC staining of sinusoidal endothelium for von Willebrand factor, CD31 or CD34 may be useful to highlight the location of infiltrating cells. The presence of prominent intrasinusoidal infiltration by relatively large neoplastic cells permits distinction of this disease from other T-cell lymphomas. The marrow reaction and T-cell phenotype of the neoplastic cells distinguish it from intravascular large B-cell lymphoma. T-cell phenotype, cellular pleomorphism and absence of nodular infiltrates also distinguish hepatosplenic T-cell lymphoma from SMZL, which may show similar predominance of intrasinusoidal infiltration.

Genetic studies

Molecular genetic studies have shown monoclonal rearrangements of either gamma or beta or both sets of *TCR* genes in individual patients. *TCR*-beta rearrangement is generally unproductive but, while most cases express only alpha-beta T-cell receptor proteins, neoplastic cells in a minority of patients do express the alpha-beta T-cell receptor.[126-128] This does not alter clinical behavior compared with cases showing gamma-delta T-cell receptor expression. Most cases have an isochromosome 7q in the neoplastic cell clone and progression is associated with increased copies of this or with abnormalities involving the second chromosome 7.[129] EBV latent genes are not expressed in this lymphoma.

Anaplastic large cell lymphoma (ALCL), ALK-positive, and ALCL, ALK-negative

Clinical and pathologic features

Anaplastic large cell lymphoma (ALCL) accounts for 2% of adult and 13% of pediatric non-Hodgkin lymphoma.[61,130] Approximately 50% express the anaplastic lymphoma-associated kinase (ALK; CD246 – see below). Patients with ALK-positive disease have different clinical features from those with ALK-negative lymphoma. This has been recognized by creation of a new entity of ALK-negative ALCL in the 2008 revised WHO classification, distinct from ALK-positive ALCL.[40] ALK expression is associated with younger age, male sex, combinations of nodal and extranodal involvement and the occurrence of 'B' symptoms. Patients with ALK-positive disease have significantly better survival following intensive chemotherapy than do patients with ALK-negative disease.[131-133]

In ALCL, whether ALK positive or ALK negative, involved lymph nodes are infiltrated, sometimes only to a minor extent, by clusters and sheets of pleomorphic large cells. Reactive changes may be prominent, dominating the histologic picture. Skin infiltrates are frequently present in both ALK-positive and ALK-negative ALCL and may be indistinguishable histologically from those found in primary cutaneous CD30-positive T-cell lymphoproliferative disorders. The neoplastic cells usually resemble Reed–Sternberg cells of Hodgkin lymphoma but variants of ALCL occur that are characterized by smaller, mononuclear neoplastic cells (small cell variant) or by admixture of abundant non-neoplastic lymphocytes and macrophages (lymphohistiocytic variant). The neoplastic cells of ALK-positive and ALK-negative ALCL

typically express CD30 in association with epithelial membrane antigen (EMA). Very variable expression of antigens associated with either T- or NK-cell differentiation is found; usually there is positivity for CD4 and cytotoxic markers such as perforin, TIA-1 and/or granzyme B. Cells in a minority of cases appear null, lacking expression of T- and NK-cell markers. By contrast with Hodgkin lymphoma, IHC staining for CD45 is usually positive and for CD15 is usually negative.

In ALK-positive ALCL, variation in the precise nature of the underlying chromosomal translocation pairs *ALK* with one of several alternative partner genes. The nature of the fusion partner influences subcellular localization of the expressed ALK enzyme but this is not known to influence clinical behavior of the disease.[134] IHC can reveal the distribution of ALK within neoplastic cells, correlating well in most patients with the cytogenetic and molecular genetic findings.[135]

Blood and bone marrow aspiration

PB cytopenias occur and correlate with the presence of BM involvement but circulating tumor cells have been reported in only rare cases of ALCL with small cell cytology. Neoplastic cells are occasionally represented in aspirated BM; they can be recognized by their large size, abundant moderately basophilic cytoplasm and large irregular, sometimes multiple, nuclei with prominent nucleoli. Reactive hemophagocytosis may be found.[23]

Bone marrow trephine biopsy

BMTB sections reveal evidence of BM infiltration in 10–30% of patients, with the higher end of this range reflecting use of immunostains in addition to standard H&E staining. Few studies have attempted to assess ALK-positive and ALK-negative ALCL as distinct entities.[14] BM involvement is possibly more common in the elderly, who are more likely to have ALK-negative disease. Infiltration is usually interstitial or focal and may be subtle, with only small clusters or single cells present.[7,14] Morphology of the neoplastic cells resembles that at the primary site, with Reed–Sternberg cell-like features in most cases but small cell variants and admixed inflammatory cells may confuse the picture. IHC staining for T-cell associated antigens plus CD30 and ALK (CD246) is helpful, although expression of several T-cell associated antigens may be down-regulated. The major differential diagnosis is with Hodgkin lymphoma, but the characteristic background inflammatory infiltrate is missing. Alternative diagnoses of metastatic carcinoma, melanoma, Langerhans cell histiocytosis and large B cell lymphomas require consideration in some cases. Further IHC studies to demonstrate cytokeratins and other epithelial markers, melanoma markers (HMB45, MelanA, S100 protein) and antigens expressed by Langerhans cells (S100 protein, CD1a and CD2) and B-cells may be needed to establish the correct diagnosis.

Genetic studies

Most cases have clonally arranged *TCR* genes. The variation in *ALK* translocation fusion partners, the resultant subcellular localization of ALK protein expression and, where known, the molecular basis of this variation is summarized in the WHO 2008 classification.[40] Secondary structural and numerical chromosomal changes occur frequently, involving numerous targets that differ between ALK-positive and ALK-negative ALCL. Gene expression profiling by microarray techniques has also shown patterns which differ between the two,[53] further justifying their consideration as distinct entities.

Angioimmunoblastic T-cell lymphoma (AIL-T NHL)

Clinical features and lymph node pathology

Patients are usually adults and present with lymphadenopathy, often disseminated although not bulky. Additional features of fever, autoimmune phenomena, drug hypersensitivities and hypergammaglobulinemia (usually polyclonal) are common.[136]

Lymph nodes involved by AIL-T NHL usually show T-zone expansion with inactive B-cell follicles although greater histological variation has been recognized in recent years, including examples accompanied by marked follicular hyperplasia.[137,138] The expanded paracortex may contain vaguely nodular areas of infiltration. High endothelial venules and other arborizing small blood vessels are usually prominent and are seen well with PAS staining. The latter may also show deposits of extravascular PAS-positive material, of uncertain origin. Cells within infiltrated areas are mixed, with scattered blast cells, macrophages, plasma cells and single or clustered medium-sized lymphoid cells that have abundant clear cytoplasm. The clear cells may appear to be clustered around small blood vessels; immunostaining reveals these cells to be of T-cell phenotype, usually of CD4 subtype and expressing PD-1 (programmed death-1), indicative of a follicular helper T-cell phenotype.[139,140] The scattered blasts are a mixture of T- and B-cells. In most cases an irregular meshwork of dendritic cells expressing CD21 and CD23 is present underlying expanded areas of paracortex. Evidence of latent EBV infection can be demonstrated in most cases, with EBV-EBER expression in varying proportions of the B-cell blasts. Transformation to diffuse large B-cell lymphoma occurs occasionally via overgrowth of a monoclonal large B-cell population.[136]

Blood and bone marrow aspiration

Direct involvement of PB is very rare in AIL-T NHL but there may be cytopenias involving erythroid cells, platelets, granulocytes and lymphocytes in various combinations. Reactive increases in plasma cells, plasmacytoid cells and atypical lymphocytes may be seen[141] and there may be a polyclonal increase in plasma immunoglobulins. The presence of a leukoerythroblastic blood picture may reflect BM infiltration. BM aspirate films usually reflect similar nonspecific findings but neoplastic T-cells can occasionally be found; FACS and/or molecular genetic analysis are required for confirmation if cells are seen that raise suspicion of neoplasia.

Bone marrow trephine biopsy

BMTB sections show evidence of infiltration relatively frequently in AIL-T NHL, although the reported incidence varies widely between different studies.[17,19,20] Involvement is usually focal, with infiltrates distributed randomly within marrow spaces (Fig. 29.22).[20] Infiltrates have a similar mixed composition to those found in affected lymph nodes and the underlying stroma usually has increased reticulin fibers, sometimes

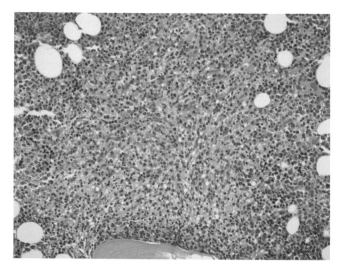

Fig. 29.22 Bone marrow infiltrated by AILTL. The marrow is hypercellular and disorderly with an irregular area of infiltration by a mixture of medium-sized and large pale cells. A hint of cell 'streaming' is present due to accompanying increased stromal reticulin and vascularity (reticulin staining would be needed for confirmation of these secondary features). Decalcified, wax-embedded bone marrow trephine biopsy section; H&E stain, original magnification ×20.

with a locally increased number of capillaries. Extracellular PAS-positive material is rarely seen. The background hemopoietic tissue frequently shows dysplastic features, with abnormalities of cell distribution within marrow spaces. Megakaryocytes and erythroid cells may show cytological atypia and granulopoiesis may be left-shifted, with relatively increased numbers of promyelocytes and myelocytes.

IHC may be helpful to confirm the presence of atypical T-cells and to exclude alternative diagnoses such as Hodgkin lymphoma and T-cell/histiocyte-rich large B-cell lymphoma. The histologic and IHC features of AIL-T NHL in BM show considerable overlap with those found in other peripheral T-cell lymphomas, particularly those of no specified subtype, and a conclusive diagnosis can usually only be made by lymph node biopsy. Demonstration of PD-1 expression, which is not generally found in peripheral T-cell lymphoma, NOS, may be helpful, as may in situ hybridization for EBV-EBER although B-cell blasts are less regularly demonstrable in BM infiltrates of AIL-T NHL than in involved lymph nodes.

Genetic studies

Clonal rearrangements of TCR genes are present in almost all cases and additional clonal or oligoclonal IGH rearrangements are also found in a substantial minority.[142] The latter correlate with the presence of EBV-positive B-cell blasts. Trisomies of chromosomes 3 and 5 are relatively frequent, as is an additional X chromosome. Gains of chromosomes 19, 22q and 11q plus losses of 13q have been found by comparative genomic hybridization studies.[143] Gene expression profiling confirms a molecular signature of follicular helper T-cells.[51]

Peripheral T-cell lymphoma, not otherwise specified (PTCL, NOS)

Clinical features and lymph node pathology

These lymphomas account for approximately 6% of NHL and occur in a wide age range of patients (median 61 years;

range 17–90 years).[61] There is usually extensive nodal involvement at presentation, with 65% of patients having stage IV disease.[98] Extranodal involvement occurs more frequently than in B-cell NHL and systemic features, such as fever, are also common. Peripheral T-cell lymphomas in this category are probably a mixture of different entities that cannot currently be separated into defined prognostic groups;[40] overall, they are aggressive neoplasms with worse prognoses than DLBCL.

Lymph node histology in PTCL, NOS varies considerably between cases. Underlying lymph node architecture is usually preserved and a mixed infiltrate replaces normal components to a variable extent. Frequently, but not always, the paracortex is preferentially involved. Reactive cells, including macrophages, eosinophils, lymphocytes and plasma cells are usually present and may be sufficiently numerous to obscure the neoplastic T-cells. The latter may be small, medium or large in size, often mixed in differing proportions, and may have aberrant T-cell phenotypes including loss of pan-T cell antigens, such as CD5 and CD7, and absent expression of both CD4 and CD8. IHC and molecular genetic demonstration of a monoclonal *TCR* gene rearrangement are usually needed to confirm the diagnosis.

Blood and bone marrow aspiration

PB involvement by PTCL, NOS occurs only rarely and, in keeping with lymph node cytologic features, the cells may vary in size from small to large or be highly pleomorphic. Bone marrow involvement is also recognized only infrequently in aspirate films or by FACS analysis of aspirated cells, despite the fact that trephine biopsy is positive relatively frequently.

Bone marrow trephine biopsy

While PTCL, NOS accounts for only a minority of non-Hodgkin lymphomas, BM involvement in this category of lymphoma is frequent, with the majority of reported cases in several series having positive BM staging biopsies.[17,19] Some patients with PTCL, NOS present with BM as the sole or predominant site of disease. Infiltration is usually focal and patchy or diffuse throughout the interstitium. Reactive cells are frequently admixed with the infiltrates, as in AIL-T NHL, but the neoplastic cells in PTCL, NOS are usually larger and more obviously atypical, with marked pleomorphism. There is usually a patchy or diffuse increase in reticulin, sometimes with increased capillaries in areas of focal infiltration. Dysplastic hemopoietic features may be seen in non-infiltrated areas of marrow,[16] as in AIL-T NHL. Lymph node histology is required to distinguish PTCL, NOS from AIL-T NHL. IHC may be necessary to exclude possible alternative diagnoses of BM involvement by Hodgkin lymphoma, DLBCL or ALCL. The BM histology may also mimic a post-transplant lymphoproliferative disorder or the polymorphous lymphoid aggregates found in some patients with HIV infection; clinical context usually suggests the likelihood of one or other of these latter types of infiltration.

Genetic studies

This is a heterogeneous group of T-cell lymphomas with complex karyotypes. A wide variety of recurring chromosomal gains and losses have been described that differ from those seen in AIL-T NHL and ALCL.[143] Gene expression

profiles also differ from other peripheral T cell lymphomas.[59] Accompanying EBV latent infection is relatively infrequent.

Hodgkin lymphoma (HL)

Nodular lymphocyte predominant Hodgkin lymphoma (NLPHL)

Clinical features and lymph node pathology

Nodular lymphocyte predominant Hodgkin lymphoma (NLPHL) comprises approximately 5% of all HL. The median age at presentation is mid-30s and males are affected significantly more often than females. The disease usually involves peripheral lymph nodes (neck, axillary or inguinal groups) and approximately 80% of patients have stage I or II disease at diagnosis. The prognosis is good; 90% of patients remain alive at 10 years from diagnosis, mostly having had removal of involved lymph nodes with or without adjunctive local radiotherapy as their sole treatment.[120] There is, however, a higher risk of late disease relapse than in classical Hodgkin lymphoma and relapse may involve disease transformation into large B cell lymphoma.

In lymph nodes, NLPHL is characterized histologically by replacement of normal structures with expanded, B-cell-rich nodules enclosing scattered CD30-negative large blast cells.[40] These large cells have distinctive 'popcorn cell' appearances, express CD45 and are positive for B-cell markers such as CD20 and CD79a; they are typically accompanied by scattered or loosely clustered macrophages and rosettes of T-lymphocytes. T-cells within rosettes show up-regulation of IRF4/MUM1 and express PD-1, indicating a follicular helper T-cell phenotype. Scattered as well as rosetted T-cells include a high proportion of CD57-positive cells, unlike the reactive T-cells accompanying classical Hodgkin lymphoma. True Reed–Sternberg cells are not present and the features of NLPHL may be accompanied by progressive transformation of germinal centers, a histologically distinctive reactive process; differential diagnosis between NLPHL and this reactive process is sometimes difficult when only few large cells are present. In other cases, diffuse architecture may lead to overlapping features with T-cell/histiocyte-rich large B cell lymphoma and the distinction of NLPHL from, or its possible relationship to, this variant of large B cell lymphoma is controversial.

Blood and bone marrow aspiration

PB involvement by NLPHL essentially does not occur. Bone marrow examination for staging is not usually performed in NLPHL and, consequently, involvement has rarely been reported in marrow aspirate films.

Bone marrow trephine biopsy

Involvement of the BM is distinctly uncommon in NLPHL and, like aspiration, BMTB for staging is performed relatively infrequently. The finding of lymphoid or lymphohistiocytic infiltrates in BMTB sections from a patient diagnosed as having NLPHL should prompt review of the original diagnosis, since stage IV disease occurs rarely. Most such cases, upon review, are found to represent lymphocyte-rich classical Hodgkin lymphoma or occur in patients with a history of multiply-relapsed NLPHL in whom a high stage, T cell/histiocyte-rich pattern of disease, overlapping with T-cell/

histiocyte-rich large B cell lymphoma may emerge over time.[9] Histological features in the BM in such patients resemble those at other sites. In typical NLPHL at first presentation, BM histology is usually entirely normal.

Genetic studies

The relative paucity of neoplastic cells in NLPHL renders clonal *IGH* rearrangement undetectable in most cases unless specialized techniques such as single-cell PCR are employed. Isolated neoplastic cells, however, have been shown to have clonally rearranged *IGH* with a high degree of somatic hypermutation. They demonstrate ongoing acquisition of further mutations[144] and have functional immunoglobulin production. Translocations and other abnormalities of BCL6 are relatively common.[145] Latent EBV infection is absent.

Classical Hodgkin lymphoma

Nodular sclerosis subtype (NSCHL)
Mixed cellularity subtype (MCCHL)
Lymphocyte-rich classical subtype (LRCHL)
Lymphocyte-depleted (LDCHL).

Clinical features and lymph node pathology

Classical Hodgkin lymphoma represents approximately 11% of all lymphoma diagnosis. Typical presentation is with supradiaphragmatic lymphadenopathy and approximately 30% of patients have 'B' symptoms. The disease has a bimodal age incidence, with peaks in childhood and after the age of 55 years.

All variants of classical Hodgkin lymphoma are characterized histologically by the presence of Reed–Sternberg (RS) cells.[40] These cells frequently have distinctive lacunar morphology in nodular sclerosing classical Hodgkin lymphoma (NSCHL) but, in the other subtypes, classical binucleate and multinucleate RS cells are found. They express CD30 and, in a majority of cases, CD15; they generally lack expression of CD45 and EMA. PAX5 and IRF4/MUM1 are consistently expressed but there is usually no demonstrable production of immunoglobulin or J-chain. CD20 and CD79a are only rarely positive (usually one or the other, but not both). The transcription factor OCT2 and its coactivator BOB1 are negative in a great majority of cases. Latent EBV infection in RS cells, and in occasional bystander small B cells, can be demonstrated in approximately 50% of cases; this is most frequent in MCCHL and occurs to a lesser extent in NSCHL. The pattern of latency is such that there is consistent expression of LMP1, which can be shown conveniently by IHC. Alternatively, *in situ* hybridization can be employed to demonstrate EBV-EBER. Mononuclear Hodgkin cells sharing these phenotypic properties are present in most cases and predominate in some. In all subtypes of classical Hodgkin lymphoma, RS cells are accompanied by reactive lymphoid cells, macrophages and eosinophils. Bands of fibrosis separating nodular areas of mixed, cellular infiltration are present in NSCHL. Lymphocyte-depleted Hodgkin lymphoma (LDCHL) is much less frequently diagnosed now than in pre-immunohistochemistry days, since many cases that would previously have been categorized as LDCHL can now be shown to be variants of anaplastic large cell lymphoma. Lymphocyte-rich classical Hodgkin lymphoma (LRCHL) is characterized by appearances superficially resembling NLPHL but with true RS cells and clinical behavior more in keeping with mixed cellularity Hodgkin lymphoma (MCCHL).[40]

Blood and bone marrow aspiration

A full blood count frequently shows normocytic, normochromic anemia and the erythrocyte sedimentation rate is often raised. In 10% of patients there is PB eosinophilia and there may be leukopenia due to a reduction in circulating $CD4^+$ T-lymphocytes. Bone marrow is involved in 10–14% of patients, usually those with advanced disease. Reed–Sternberg cells are exceptionally uncommon in aspirate films, since infiltrates of disease contain few neoplastic cells and are typically densely fibrotic; representative cells are only rarely yielded upon aspiration. Non-involved BM usually has reactive appearances with granulocytic and megakaryocytic hyperplasia, with or without increased cells of the eosinophil lineage, and shows reduced erythropoiesis in anemic patients.

Bone marrow trephine biopsy

BMTB is much more sensitive than aspiration for detection of BM involvement by classical HL, at least in part because the infiltrates cause stromal fibrosis and are difficult to aspirate. Depending on patient selection criteria, different studies have reported up to 15% of BMTB performed for staging in classical HL to be positive.[3] This figure is undoubtedly an over-estimate, since many patients with clinical stage IA or IIA disease do not undergo BM examination. Bilateral biopsies or single long-core biopsy increase the positive detection rate in classical HL and in non-Hodgkin lymphomas. However, the clinical value of BM staging in classical HL has been questioned,[1] since patient management is rarely influenced directly by the outcome. Occasionally, BM is the primary or sole site of involvement by classical HL; this is particularly the case in patients with HIV-associated disease.

Involvement of BM by classical HL is rarely subtle; the infiltrates usually form sizeable, irregular patches with dense underlying fibrosis. Occasionally, all or most of the biopsy core is replaced. Extensively involved BM may contain areas of necrosis, even in previously untreated patients. Classical RS cells may or may not be found and mononuclear Hodgkin cells are usually few, scattered widely within irregular areas of macrophage and lymphocyte infiltration (Fig. 29.23). Plasma cells and eosinophils are usually also present in these infiltrates but the number of these cells varies considerably between patients. Sometimes, the infiltrates appear densely fibrotic, or loose and edematous, with few cells of any type other than fibroblasts evident, and remodeling of trabecular bone may be seen; this pattern is relatively common in specimens taken for re-staging after treatment.

Criteria for interpretation of these features differ depending upon whether or not BMTB has been performed in a patient with a known diagnosis of classical HL, confirmed histologically at another site. If the diagnosis has already been established, it is generally regarded as adequate to see atypical large cells in an appropriate lymphohistiocytic background in order to confirm BM involvement. If the diagnosis has not been made by histologic study of tissue from a lymph node or other site, a diagnosis of classical HL in the BM can only be made with certainty if true RS cells are identified. This may require examination of multiple sections, cut

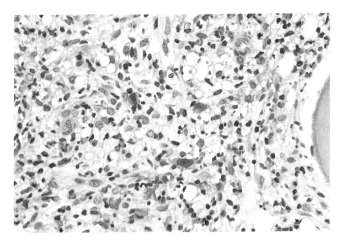

Fig. 29.23 Extensive infiltration by a mixed population of cells in bone marrow involved by classical HL. Occasional large cells representing mononuclear Hodgkin cells are present although true Reed–Sternberg cells are uncommon. Decalcified, wax-embedded bone marrow trephine biopsy section; H&E stain, original magnification ×40.

at different levels from the tissue core. Identification of RS cells and mononuclear Hodgkin cells is greatly assisted by IHC for CD30, CD15, B- and T-cell-associated antigens and markers of ALK-positive and ALK-negative ALCL. Immunostaining for EBV-LMP1 or *in situ* hybridization for EBV-EBER are also extremely helpful in difficult cases since EBV is not associated with most lymphomas that are in the differential diagnosis.

Appearances of NSCHL and MCCHL in biopsy sections are similar and it is not possible to subtype classical HL variants on the basis of BM histology. The lymphocyte-rich subtype spreads to BM relatively rarely and may mimic NLPHL or small cell types of NHL when it does so, with few neoplastic cells admixed with abundant small lymphoid cells. However, the RS cells retain a typical classical HL immunophenotype. The differential diagnosis includes ALCL, other T-cell lymphomas, T-cell/histiocyte-rich large B-cell lymphoma and the polymorphous reactive lymphohistiocytic infiltrates which occur in some HIV-positive patients. If fibrosis is severe, idiopathic myelofibrosis and metastatic carcinoma also require consideration.

It is important to realize that, in focally involved and uninvolved BM from patients with classical HL there is frequently marked granulocytic and megakaryocytic hyperplasia, often with increased eosinophil production. Erythropoiesis is usually normal or somewhat reduced. Prominent megakaryocytes should not be mistaken for RS cells. These reactive changes, which are believed to be cytokine-mediated, are most marked in younger patients but should not be overlooked in older individuals, in whom overall hemopoietic cellularity may not appear to be greatly increased. Common findings in association with these hyperplastic appearances are scattered sarcoid-like granulomas and aggregates of apoptotic neutrophil nuclei within the cytoplasm of stromal macrophages. Rarely, generalized marrow hypoplasia is found, without evidence of infiltration by disease.

Genetic studies

Reed–Sternberg cells in cases of classical HL studied by single-cell PCR techniques have been shown to have clonally rearranged and hypermutated *IGH* without intraclonal heterogeneity (i.e., with no evidence of ongoing somatic mutation).[146] However, immunoglobulins are not transcribed, due either to crippling mutations or defective regulatory elements such as OCT2 and BOB1. Integrated, clonal, EBV is present in RS and bystander B-cells in a high proportion of cases of classical HL, particularly in MCCHL and in classical HL arising in immunocompromised patients, with a distinctive pattern of latent gene expression including LMP1 and EBNA2 expression.[147] Intracellular signaling pathways involving NFkappaB are constitutively activated, and regulation of the JAK/STAT pathway is disrupted, promoting proliferation and inhibiting apoptosis.[148] Gene expression studies using microarray techniques show a molecular signal reflecting these disturbances and closely resembling that found in primary mediastinal large B cell lymphoma;[149] the WHO 2008 classification recognizes overlap between large B cell lymphoma, predominantly of mediastinal type, and classical HL.[40]

Post-transplant lymphoproliferative disorders (PTLD) and other lymphoid proliferations associated with impaired immunity

Clinical and pathologic features

The clinical presentation of PTLD is very variable. Patients presenting in the early post-transplant period often have an infectious mononucleosis-like disease characterized by constitutional symptoms and rapid enlargement of tonsils and cervical lymph nodes. Patients with PTLD of late onset, usually a year or more after transplantation, have less severe constitutional symptoms and frequently have extranodal disease similar to HIV-related lymphomas. The cumulative incidence of PTLD at 10 years is in the order of 5% following heart transplantation and 1% following renal or BM transplantation.[150,151] The incidence of PTLD is higher in patients who are seronegative for EBV at the time of transplantation, compared with those who are seropositive. In solid organ recipients, PTLD is almost always of host origin while, in recipients of allogeneic BM grafts, not surprisingly it arises from donor cells.

Lymphoproliferative disorders arising after solid organ or BM transplantation also vary greatly in histologic appearance and immunophenotype between individuals.[40,152] Although they may appear to arise from either T- or B-cells, EBV infection is associated with the majority of cases, through reactivation of latent infection in the graft recipient or as a result of primary infection acquired from graft tissue. Similar EBV-associated lymphoid proliferations occur in other acquired and inherited immune deficiency states and in association with age-related decline in immunity in some elderly patients.[153] Morphologically, examples of PTLD have been reported that are equivalent to most subtypes of large B-cell, Burkitt, peripheral T-cell and Hodgkin lymphomas, plus polyclonal and monoclonal plasmacytic proliferations. Also well described in the spectrum of PTLD are polymorphous lymphoid infiltrates composed of complex mixtures of inflammatory cells and atypical lymphoid cells, including B-cells at all stages of maturation.

Cases of PTLD may be polyclonal or monoclonal, and their clonal status does not necessarily indicate their likely

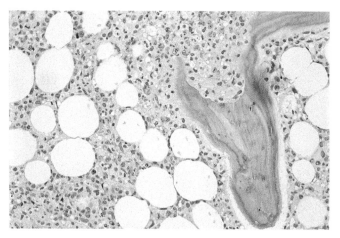

Fig. 29.24 Poorly-defined interstitial and nodular replacement of bone marrow by a polymorphous infiltrate of PTLD, in this example showing erosion of trabecular bone. Decalcified, wax-embedded bone marrow trephine biopsy section; H&E stain, original magnification ×20.

aggressiveness. Factors predicting responsiveness to modulation of immunosuppressive therapy versus requirement for cytotoxic chemotherapy remain uncertain. In an appropriate context, EBV-negative examples are still regarded as PTLD and may respond to immune modulation; some of these may harbor undetectable EBV while others may be due to alternative viruses or other factors that can be influenced by host immune regulation.

Blood and BM aspiration

PB rarely contains detectable disease and BM aspiration is also usually negative. In examples equivalent to subtypes of NHL arising unrelated to transplantation or immunodeficiency, there may occasionally be involvement with the same cytologic features as those described in individual sections above. Blood or BM plasmacytosis (polyclonal or monoclonal) may be encountered in cases with plasma cell-predominant lymphoid proliferations.

Bone marrow trephine biopsy

Approximately 50% of patients with polymorphous PTLD have BM involvement, seen in trephine biopsy sections as poorly defined irregular or nodular infiltrates of mixed cells (Fig. 29.24). BM involvement by PTLD in patients who have variants equivalent to B-cell, T-cell or Hodgkin lymphomas shares the morphology of the primary tumor and has features as described above for the equivalent lymphomas seen in immunocompetent individuals. The presence of EBV can be demonstrated in a majority of patients by *in situ* hybridization for EBER but LMP1 is often not expressed and immunostaining for the latter should not be relied upon in this context. BM involvement has been associated with poor prognosis.[154]

Appearances of lymphoma infiltrates following therapy

In patients with known lymphoma, BM examination may be required to assess efficacy of treatment or to investigate cytopenias which may result from complications of treatment, intercurrent illness, relapse or progression of disease. BM examination may also be performed to assess the extent of any residual disease, particularly before stem cell harvesting for autograft transplantation.

Apart from quantitative changes in the degree of BM infiltration by lymphoma following chemotherapy, there may also be changes in the morphology of cell infiltrates. At present, it remains controversial whether nodular lymphoid infiltrates (a common finding in this context), not occupying paratrabecular or perisinusoidal locations, are reactive phenomena or residual deposits of low-grade lymphoma. A prominent, hypercellular rim of granulocytes, particularly eosinophils, often surrounds such nodules and they are usually composed predominantly of small T-lymphocytes, with few B-cells, regardless of the original lymphoma diagnosis (Fig. 29.25).[155] It is relatively common to see such nodules following anti-CD20 immunotherapy of low-grade lymphoma. This treatment leads to down-regulation of CD20 expression by B-cells, an effect which may persist for long periods, so that use of CD20 as a B-cell marker for IHC in this context is unreliable. Typical findings are normal expression of antigens such as CD19 and CD79a in the almost complete absence of CD20. Absence of demonstrable clonal *IGH* rearrangement in microdissected nodules of this type has led some authors to conclude that they are not neoplastic,[156,157] but they may represent 'tombstone' lesions rather than newly formed reactive lymphoid nodules; whether or not they are truly inert in terms of potential for re-growth of lymphoma is unproven.

BM hyperplastic, dysplastic and stromal reactions to lymphoma

Hemopoiesis often appears remarkably unaffected by significant levels of BM infiltration by lymphoma. However, certain types of lymphoma are regularly associated with spatial and cytologic abnormalities of hemopoiesis, often with increased stromal reticulin. Such effects are presumably secondary to cytokine production by the neoplastic cells themselves or by inflammatory cells stimulated in consequence of their presence. Infiltration of the BM by angioimmunoblastic T-cell lymphoma or peripheral T-cell lymphoma, not otherwise specified, has particularly been reported in association with such phenomena.[4,16,19,158] However, in occasional patients, B-cell lymphomas of various subtypes are also accompanied by marked hemopoietic cell hyperplasia and/or by stromal edema and fibrosis. In these cases, the presence of lymphomatous infiltrates is usually obvious; attention to megakaryocyte morphology usually excludes a myeloproliferative neoplasm but it can be difficult to determine whether or not a myelodysplastic syndrome is represented. Immunostaining for CD42b or CD61 can assist by revealing the full spectrum of megakaryocytes, including any true micromegakaryocytes. The latter would not be expected in a reactive myelopathy. Lack of an increase in CD34-positive early hemopoietic cells may be additionally reassuring. Hematological follow-up, with BM aspiration and cytogenetic studies ± repeat trephine biopsy may be helpful.

Epithelioid granulomas are occasionally encountered accompanying BM infiltration with lymphomas, particularly low-grade B-cell NHL. They may be epiphenomena for which no cause can be established but it is important to exclude mycobacterial infection, particularly tuberculosis, in

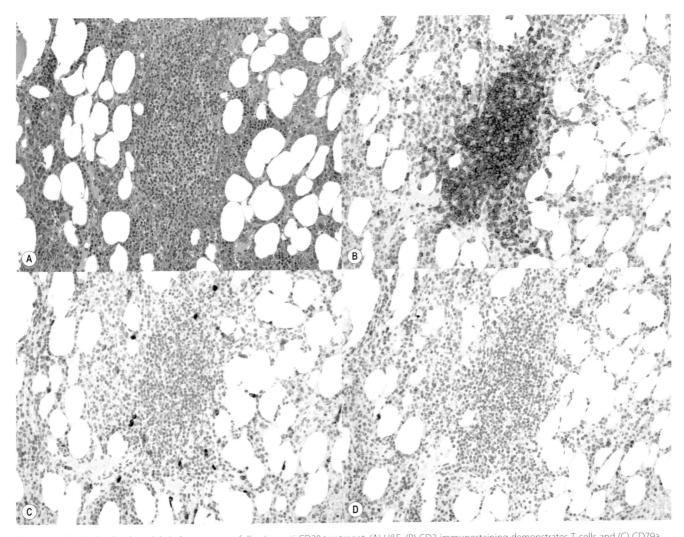

Fig. 29.25 (A–D) T-cell-rich nodule in bone marrow following anti-CD20 treatment. (A) H&E, (B) CD3 immunostaining demonstrates T-cells and (C) CD79a immunostaining demonstrates very few weakly stained B lymphocytes plus positive plasma cells. There was very little demonstrable CD20 expression. (D) Original magnification ×20.

all cases, since immunosuppression associated with the lymphoma and its treatment may predispose patients to primary infection or reactivation.

BMTB sections from patients with classical HL may show granulocytic hyperplasia with an increased proportion of eosinophils as described above.

Differential diagnosis and classification of lymphoma when bone marrow trephine biopsy provides the sole source of tissue for assessment

Occasionally, lymphoma presents with BM as the sole site of disease or as the most accessible site for diagnostic biopsy. As an additional problem, BM aspiration frequently yields no lymphoma cells in patients in whom BMTB sections show definite evidence of lymphoma infiltration, so that FCM data cannot be obtained to support the diagnosis. In these circumstances, BM histology is crucial to diagnosis. The spatial distribution and cellular composition of lymphoma infiltrates, supplemented by judicious use of IHC, permits accurate WHO classification in most cases. The various spatial patterns of lymphoma in different diagnostic categories have been described in earlier sections of this chapter. No single pattern is unique to any lymphoma entity but it is possible to make some helpful generalizations. Paratrabecular infiltration is highly suggestive of FL although it may also be seen in LPL, MCL and SMZL; in the latter conditions, paratrabecular infiltrates are rarely as extensive or linear as in FL and are usually accompanied by other patterns (varying combinations of nodular and interstitial). Paratrabecular infiltration occurs with exceptional rarity in CLL; stromal alterations in treated patients with residual disease at follow-up, or in patients with coincidental marrow pathologies, may occasionally result in formation of focal paratrabecular infiltrates but the dominant pattern remains typical. The typical pattern in CLL is nodular infiltration with greater or lesser degrees of interstitial spread. The presence of scattered or clustered para-immunoblasts in nodular areas of small lymphoid cell infiltration strongly suggests CLL. The presence of scattered blast cells in LPL and SMZL or the rare formation of neoplastic follicles in FL can mimic para-immunoblasts but FL will generally show at least some areas of paratrabecular infiltration while infiltrates of LPL are usually more irregular in shape and less well defined than those of CLL. In SMZL, nodularity is distinctively centered on well preserved nodular clusters of follicular dendritic cells, possibly representing colonized non-neoplastic follicles and readily demonstrated by CD21 or CD23 staining. There is often an additional component of intrasinusoidal infiltration, but a pure intrasinusoidal pattern should raise suspicion of persistent polyclonal B lymphocytosis mimicking SMZL.[159] The presence of numerous plasma cells and formation of Dutcher bodies supports a diagnosis of LPL, both features being rare in CLL; an increased number reactive mast cells typically accompany LPL infiltrates and this feature is less common in CLL. Nodular infiltration is also a frequent pattern in MCL but the nodules in this disease appear monotonous cytologically, without blast cells or plasma cells.

IHC for CD5, CD10, CD23, BCL6 and cyclin D1 (plus CD20 or CD79a and CD3 to assess overall T- and B-cell numbers) usually distinguishes between these various small B-cell lymphomas (see Table 29.1). The 'spaced out' infiltrates of HCL are histologically distinctive and are rarely confused with other small cell subtypes of lymphoma; reticulin staining and IHC for TRAP and annexin A1 provide confirmation, if needed.

Infiltrates of large lymphoid cells require distinction from increased numbers of immature myelomonocytic cells, poorly differentiated plasma cell neoplasms and, rarely, metastatic solid cancers. Diffuse large B cell lymphoma occasionally arises primarily within BM[160] and IHC is highly valuable in this context, as described earlier in this chapter in relation to DLBCL presenting at more usual sites.

As at other sites, recognition and classification of peripheral T-cell lymphomas in the BM can be very difficult. A high index of suspicion and careful assessment of any clinical or laboratory findings suggesting T-cell lymphoma are important. Unexplained or disproportionate histologic features of myelodysplasia in this context should prompt a detailed search for lymphoma infiltrates, including IHC. BM infiltrates in T-cell lymphomas, other than those presenting as

PB lymphocytoses, are generally randomly distributed and contain abundant reactive cells (macrophages, endothelium, fibroblasts, plasma cells, etc.) as well as neoplastic T-cells. Differential diagnosis from HL, T-cell/histiocyte-rich large B-cell NHL and polymorphous forms of PTLD necessitates IHC and sometimes also *IGH* and *TCR* clonality analyses by PCR, as described in the relevant sections above. Infiltrates of classical HL generally form obvious, macrophage-rich, fibrotic patches but characteristic HRS cells may be few and difficult to identify, even with imunohistochemistry. In the absence of other diagnostic tissue, the presence of such cells must be confirmed to establish a diagnosis of classical HL; this may involve examination of H&E- and CD30-stained sections from multiple levels. Subtyping should not be undertaken on the basis of BM histology as it is highly unreliable.

Conclusions

Examination of blood, BM aspirate and trephine biopsy specimens provides complementary information in the assessment of patients with known or suspected lymphoma. BM sampling is important, predominantly in contributing to the planning of treatment and monitoring of disease response to treatment. It may be essential for diagnosis if disease at other sites is inaccessible, the patient is too frail to undergo lymph node biopsy or BM is the only site of disease. Trephine biopsy has a particularly important role in this context; since histologic patterns of BM involvement in trephine biopsy sections permit most lymphomas to be assigned to their WHO categories, especially if supplemented by FCM or IHC immunophenotyping. However, morphologic discrimination between reactive lymphoid nodules and minimal involvement by lymphoma in BM remains difficult in some instances. Application of molecular genetic techniques such as FISH and PCR improves the accuracy of this distinction and aids the assessment of minimal residual disease following treatment.

References

1. Bairey O, Shpilberg O. Is bone marrow biopsy obligatory in all patients with non-Hodgkin's lymphoma? Acta Haematol 2007;118:61–4.

2. Bartl R, Frisch B, Burkhardt R, et al. Assessment of bone marrow histology in the malignant lymphomas (non-Hodgkin's): correlation with clinical factors for diagnosis, prognosis, classification and staging. Br J Haematol 1982;51:511–30.

3. Bartl R, Frisch B, Burkhardt R, et al. Assessment of bone marrow histology in Hodgkin's disease: correlation with clinical factors. Br J Haematol 1982; 51:345–60.

4. Caulet S, Delmer A, Audouin J, et al. Histopathological study of bone marrow biopsies in 30 cases of T-cell lymphoma with clinical, biological and survival correlations. Hematol Oncol 1990; 8:155–68.

5. Chung R, Lai R, Wei P, et al. Concordant but not discordant bone marrow involvement in diffuse large B-cell lymphoma predicts a poor clinical outcome independent of the International Prognostic Index. Blood 2007;110:1278–82.

6. Dufau JP, Le TA, Molina T, et al. Intravascular large B-cell lymphoma with bone marrow involvement at presentation and haemophagocytic syndrome: two Western cases in favour of a specific variant. Histopathology 2000;37:509–12.

7. Fraga M, Brousset P, Schlaifer D, et al. Bone marrow involvement in anaplastic large cell lymphoma. Immunohistochemical detection of minimal disease and its prognostic significance. Am J Clin Pathol 1995;103:82–9.

8. Khoury JD, Jones D, Yared MA, et al. Bone marrow involvement in patients with nodular lymphocyte predominant Hodgkin lymphoma. Am J Surg Pathol 2004;28:489–95.

9. Skinnider BF, Connors JM, Gascoyne RD. Bone marrow involvement in T-cell-rich B-cell lymphoma. Am J Clin Pathol 1997;108:570–8.

10. Bain BJ, Clark DM, Wilkins B. Bone marrow pathology. Oxford: Blackwell Wiley; 2010.

11. Sallah S, Smith SV, Lony LC, et al. Gamma/delta T-cell hepatosplenic lymphoma: review of the literature, diagnosis by flow cytometry and concomitant autoimmune hemolytic

anemia. Ann Hematol 1997;74: 139–42.

12. Schmid C, Isaacson PG. Bone marrow trephine biopsy in lymphoproliferative disease. J Clin Pathol 1992;45:745–50.

13. Schmidt B, Kremer M, Gotze K, et al. Bone marrow involvement in follicular lymphoma: comparison of histology and flow cytometry as staging procedures. Leuk Lymphoma 2006;47:1857–62.

14. Weinberg OK, Seo K, Arber DA. Prevalence of bone marrow involvement in systemic anaplastic large cell lymphoma: are immunohistochemical studies necessary? Hum Pathol 2008;39:1331–40.

15. Audouin J, Le TA, Molina T, et al. Patterns of bone marrow involvement in 58 patients presenting primary splenic marginal zone lymphoma with or without circulating villous lymphocytes. Br J Haematol 2003;122:404–12.

16. Auger MJ, Nash JR, Mackie MJ. Marrow involvement with T cell lymphoma initially presenting as abnormal myelopoiesis. J Clin Pathol 1986;39:134–7.

17. Dogan A, Morice WG. Bone marrow histopathology in peripheral T-cell lymphomas. Br J Haematol 2004;127:140–54.

18. Franco V, Florena AM, Ascani S, et al. CD27 distinguishes two phases in bone marrow infiltration of splenic marginal zone lymphoma. Histopathology 2004;44:381–6.

19. Gaulard P, Kanavaros P, Farcet JP, et al. Bone marrow histologic and immunohistochemical findings in peripheral T-cell lymphoma: a study of 38 cases. Hum Pathol 1991;22:331–8.

20. Grogg KL, Morice WG, Macon WR. Spectrum of bone marrow findings in patients with angioimmunoblastic T-cell lymphoma. Br J Haematol 2007;137:416–22.

21. Vega F, Medeiros LJ, Bueso-Ramos C, et al. Hepatosplenic gamma/delta T-cell lymphoma in bone marrow. A sinusoidal neoplasm with blastic cytologic features. Am J Clin Pathol 2001;116:410–9.

22. Parrens M, Dubus P, Agape P, et al. Intrasinusoidal bone marrow infiltration revealing intravascular lymphomatosis. Leuk Lymphoma 2000;37:219–23.

23. Wong KF, Chan JK, Ng CS, et al. Anaplastic large cell Ki-1 lymphoma involving bone marrow: marrow findings and association with reactive hemophagocytosis. Am J Hematol 1991;37:112–9.

24. Wong KF, Chan JK, Cheung MM, So JC. Bone marrow involvement by nasal NK cell lymphoma at diagnosis is uncommon. Am J Clin Pathol 2001;115: 266–70.

25. Ya-In C, Brandwein J, Pantalony D, Chang H. Hairy cell leukemia variant with features of intrasinusoidal bone marrow involvement. Arch Pathol Lab Med 2005;129:395–8.

26. Wilkins BS, Clark DM. Making the most of bone marrow trephine biopsy. Histopathology 2009;55:631–40.

27. Wickham CL, Sarsfield P, Joyner MV, et al. Formic acid decalcification of bone marrow trephines degrades DNA: alternative use of EDTA allows the amplification and sequencing of relatively long PCR products. Mol Pathol 2000;53:336.

28. Wickham CL, Boyce M, Joyner MV, et al. Amplification of PCR products in excess of 600 base pairs using DNA extracted from decalcified, paraffin wax embedded bone marrow trephine biopsies. Mol Pathol 2000;53:19–23.

29. Faulkner-Jones BE, Howie AJ, Boughton BJ, Franklin IM. Lymphoid aggregates in bone marrow: study of eventual outcome. J Clin Pathol 1988;41:768–75.

30. Krober SM, Horny HP, Greschniok A, Kaiserling E. Reactive and neoplastic lymphocytes in human bone marrow: morphological, immunohistological, and molecular biological investigations on biopsy specimens. J Clin Pathol 1999; 52:521–6.

31. Thiele J, Zirbes TK, Kvasnicka HM, Fischer R. Focal lymphoid aggregates (nodules) in bone marrow biopsies: differentiation between benign hyperplasia and malignant lymphoma – a practical guideline. J Clin Pathol 1999;52:294–300.

32. Brinkmann R, Kaufmann O, Reinartz B, Dietel M. Specificity of PCR-based clonality analysis of immunoglobulin heavy chain gene rearrangements for the detection of bone marrow involvement by low-grade B-cell lymphomas. J Pathol 2000;190:55–60.

33. Bain BJ. Bone marrow aspiration. J Clin Pathol 2001;54:657–63.

34. Bishop PW, McNally K, Harris M. Audit of bone marrow trephines. J Clin Pathol 1992;45:1105–8.

35. Campbell JK, Matthews JP, Seymour JF, et al. Optimum trephine length in the assessment of bone marrow involvement in patients with diffuse large cell lymphoma. Ann Oncol 2003;14:273–6.

36. Lee SH, Erber WN, Porwit A, et al. ICSH guidelines for the standardization of bone marrow specimens and reports. Int J Lab Hematol 2008;30:349–64.

37. Bain BJ, Clark DM, Wilkins B. Bone marrow pathology. Oxford: Blackwell Wiley; 2010.

38. Harris NL, Jaffe ES, Diebold J, et al. World Health Organization classification of neoplastic diseases of the hematopoietic and lymphoid tissues: report of the Clinical Advisory Committee meeting – Airlie House, Virginia, November 1997. J Clin Oncol 1999;17:3835–49.

39. Harris NL, Jaffe ES, Stein H, et al. A revised European-American classification of lymphoid neoplasms: a proposal from the International Lymphoma Study Group. Blood 1994;84:1361–92.

40. Swerdlow SH, Campo E, Harris NL, et al. WHO Classification of Tumours of Haematopoietic and Lymphatic Tissues. Lyon: IARC; 2008.

41. Camacho FI, Algara P, Rodriguez A, et al. Molecular heterogeneity in MCL defined by the use of specific VH genes and the frequency of somatic mutations. Blood 2003;101:4042–6.

42. Dunn-Walters D, Thiede C, Alpen B, Spencer J. Somatic hypermutation and B-cell lymphoma. Philos Trans R Soc Lond B Biol Sci 2001;356:73–82.

43. Klein U, Goossens T, Fischer M, et al. Somatic hypermutation in normal and transformed human B cells. Immunol Rev 1998;162:261–80.

44. Lossos IS, Alizadeh AA, Eisen MB, et al. Ongoing immunoglobulin somatic mutation in germinal center B cell-like but not in activated B cell-like diffuse large cell lymphomas. Proc Natl Acad Sci USA 2000;97:10209–13.

45. Ottensmeier CH, Thompsett AR, Zhu D, et al. Analysis of VH genes in follicular and diffuse lymphoma shows ongoing somatic mutation and multiple isotype transcripts in early disease with changes during disease progression. Blood 1998;91:4292–9.

46. Zhu D, Orchard J, Oscier DG, et al. V(H) gene analysis of splenic marginal zone lymphomas reveals diversity in mutational status and initiation of somatic mutation in vivo. Blood 2002;100:2659–61.

47. Bain B, Gilliland DG, Vardiman J, Horny HP. Chronic eosinophilic leukaemia, not otherwise specified. World Health Organization Classification of Tumours of Haematopoietic and Lymphoid Tissue. Lyon: IARC Press; 2008. p. 51–3.

48. Amen F, Horncastle D, Elderfield K, et al. Absence of cyclin-D2 and Bcl-2 expression within the germinal centre type of diffuse large B-cell lymphoma identifies a very good prognostic subgroup of patients. Histopathology 2007;51:70–9.

49. Martinez N, Camacho FI, Algara P, et al. The molecular signature of mantle cell lymphoma reveals multiple signals favoring cell survival. Cancer Res 2003;63:8226–32.

50. Dave SS, Fu K, Wright GW, et al. Molecular diagnosis of Burkitt's lymphoma. N Engl J Med 2006;354: 2431–42.

51. de Leval L, Rickman DS, Thielen C, et al. The gene expression profile of nodal peripheral T-cell lymphoma demonstrates a molecular link between angioimmunoblastic T-cell lymphoma

(AITL) and follicular helper T (TFH) cells. Blood 2007;109:4952–63.

52. Hans CP, Weisenburger DD, Greiner TC, et al. Confirmation of the molecular classification of diffuse large B-cell lymphoma by immunohistochemistry using a tissue microarray. Blood 2004;103:275–82.

53. Lamant L, de RA, Duplantier MM, et al. Gene-expression profiling of systemic anaplastic large-cell lymphoma reveals differences based on ALK status and two distinct morphologic ALK+ subtypes. Blood 2007;109:2156–64.

54. Lenz G, Wright G, Dave SS, et al. Stromal gene signatures in large-B-cell lymphomas. N Engl J Med 2008;359: 2313–23.

55. Monti S, Savage KJ, Kutok JL, et al. Molecular profiling of diffuse large B-cell lymphoma identifies robust subtypes including one characterized by host inflammatory response. Blood 2005;105:1851–61.

56. Rosenwald A, Wright G, Chan WC, et al. The use of molecular profiling to predict survival after chemotherapy for diffuse large-B-cell lymphoma. N Engl J Med 2002;346:1937–47.

57. Rosenwald A, Wright G, Wiestner A, et al. The proliferation gene expression signature is a quantitative integrator of oncogenic events that predicts survival in mantle cell lymphoma. Cancer Cell 2003;3:185–97.

58. Wright G, Tan B, Rosenwald A, et al. A gene expression-based method to diagnose clinically distinct subgroups of diffuse large B cell lymphoma. Proc Natl Acad Sci USA 2003;100:9991–6.

59. Zettl A, Rudiger T, Konrad MA, et al. Genomic profiling of peripheral T-cell lymphoma, unspecified, and anaplastic large T-cell lymphoma delineates novel recurrent chromosomal alterations. Am J Pathol 2004;164:1837–48.

60. Morton LM, Wang SS, Devesa SS, et al. Lymphoma incidence patterns by WHO subtype in the United States, 1992–2001. Blood 2006;107:265–76.

61. Muller AM, Ihorst G, Mertelsmann R, Engelhardt M. Epidemiology of non-Hodgkin's lymphoma (NHL): trends, geographic distribution, and etiology. Ann Hematol 2005;84: 1–12.

62. Vijay A, Gertz MA. Waldenstrom macroglobulinemia. Blood 2007;109: 5096–103.

63. de Sanjose S, Benavente Y, Vajdic CM, et al. Hepatitis C and non-Hodgkin lymphoma among 4784 cases and 6269 controls from the International Lymphoma Epidemiology Consortium. Clin Gastroenterol Hepatol 2008;6: 451–8.

64. Viswanatha DS, Dogan A. Hepatitis C virus and lymphoma. J Clin Pathol 2007;60:1378–83.

65. Martyak LA, Yeganeh M, Saab S. Hepatitis C and lymphoproliferative disorders: from mixed cryoglobulinemia to non-Hodgkin's lymphoma. Clin Gastroenterol Hepatol 2009;7:900–5.

66. Wilkins BS, Buchan SL, Webster J, Jones DB. Tryptase-positive mast cells accompany lymphocytic as well as lymphoplasmacytic lymphoma infiltrates in bone marrow trephine biopsies. Histopathology 2001;39:150–5.

67. Ho AW, Hatjiharissi E, Ciccarelli BT, et al. CD27-CD70 interactions in the pathogenesis of Waldenstrom macroglobulinemia. Blood 2008; 112:4683–9.

68. Tournilhac O, Santos DD, Xu L, et al. Mast cells in Waldenstrom's macroglobulinemia support lymphoplasmacytic cell growth through CD154/CD40 signaling. Ann Oncol 2006;17:1275–82.

69. Banham AH, Turley H, Pulford K, et al. The plasma cell associated antigen detectable by antibody VS38 is the p63 rough endoplasmic reticulum protein. J Clin Pathol 1997;50:485–9.

70. Iida S, Rao PH, Nallasivam P, et al. The t(9;14)(p13;q32) chromosomal translocation associated with lymphoplasmacytoid lymphoma involves the PAX-5 gene. Blood 1996;88:4110–7.

71. Ocio EM, Schop RF, Gonzalez B, et al. 6q deletion in Waldenstrom macroglobulinemia is associated with features of adverse prognosis. Br J Haematol 2007;136:80–6.

72. Walsh SH, Laurell A, Sundstrom G, et al. Lymphoplasmacytic lymphoma/ Waldenstrom's macroglobulinemia derives from an extensively hypermutated B cell that lacks ongoing somatic hypermutation. Leuk Res 2005;29: 729–34.

73. Wilkins B, Wright DH. Illustrated pathology of the spleen. Cambridge, UK: Cambridge University Press; 2000.

74. Bain B. Blood cells. A practical guide. Oxford: Blackwell Publishing; 2006.

75. Verhoef GE, de Wolf-Peeters C, Zachee P, Boogaerts MA. Regression of diffuse osteosclerosis in hairy cell leukaemia after treatment with interferon. Br J Haematol 1990;76:150–1.

76. VanderMolen LA, Urba WJ, Longo DL, et al. Diffuse osteosclerosis in hairy cell leukemia. Blood 1989;74:2066–9.

77. Sun T, Grupka N, Klein C. Transformation of hairy cell leukemia to high-grade lymphoma: a case report and review of the literature. Hum Pathol 2004;35:1423–6.

78. Hoyer JD, Li CY, Yam LT, et al. Immunohistochemical demonstration of acid phosphatase isoenzyme 5 (tartrate-resistant) in paraffin sections of hairy cell leukemia and other hematologic disorders. Am J Clin Pathol 1997;108: 308–15.

79. Went PT, Zimpfer A, Pehrs AC, et al. High specificity of combined TRAP and DBA.44 expression for hairy cell leukemia. Am J Surg Pathol 2005; 29:474–8.

80. Chen YH, Tallman MS, Goolsby C, Peterson L. Immunophenotypic variations in hairy cell leukemia. Am J Clin Pathol 2006;125:251–9.

81. Hounieu H, Chittal SM, al Saati T, et al. Hairy cell leukemia. Diagnosis of bone marrow involvement in paraffin-embedded sections with monoclonal antibody DBA.44. Am J Clin Pathol 1992;98:26–33.

82. Parnes JR, Pan C. CD72, a negative regulator of B-cell responsiveness. Immunol Rev 2000;176:75–85.

83. Falini B, Tiacci E, Liso A, et al. Simple diagnostic assay for hairy cell leukaemia by immunocytochemical detection of annexin A1 (ANXA1). Lancet 2004;363: 1869–70.

84. Johrens K, Stein H, Anagnostopoulos I. T-bet transcription factor detection facilitates the diagnosis of minimal hairy cell leukemia infiltrates in bone marrow trephines. Am J Surg Pathol 2007;31: 1181–5.

85. Cawley JC. The pathophysiology of the hairy cell. Hematol Oncol Clin North Am 2006;20:1011–21.

86. Galiegue-Zouitina S, Delestre L, Dupont C, et al. Underexpression of RhoH in hairy cell leukemia. Cancer Res 2008; 68:4531–40.

87. Cessna MH, Hartung L, Tripp S, et al. Hairy cell leukemia variant: fact or fiction. Am J Clin Pathol 2005;123: 132–8.

88. Matutes E, Wotherspoon A, Catovsky D. The variant form of hairy-cell leukaemia. Best Pract Res Clin Haematol 2003; 16:41–56.

89. Brito-Babapulle V, Matutes E, Oscier D, et al. Chromosome abnormalities in hairy cell leukaemia variant. Genes Chromosomes Cancer 1994;10:197–202.

90. Mollejo M, Menarguez J, Lloret E, et al. Splenic marginal zone lymphoma: a distinctive type of low-grade B-cell lymphoma. A clinicopathological study of 13 cases. Am J Surg Pathol 1995;19: 1146–57.

91. Isaacson PG, Matutes E, Burke M, Catovsky D. The histopathology of splenic lymphoma with villous lymphocytes. Blood 1994;84:3828–34.

92. Algara P, Mateo MS, Sanchez-Beato M, et al. Analysis of the IgV(H) somatic mutations in splenic marginal zone lymphoma defines a group of unmutated cases with frequent 7q deletion and adverse clinical course. Blood 2002 ;99:1299–304.

93. Corcoran MM, Mould SJ, Orchard JA, et al. Dysregulation of cyclin dependent kinase 6 expression in splenic marginal zone lymphoma through chromosome

7q translocations. Oncogene 1999;18: 6271–7.

94. Novara F, Arcaini L, Merli M, et al. High-resolution genome-wide array comparative genomic hybridization in splenic marginal zone B-cell lymphoma. Hum Pathol 2009;40:1628–37.

95. Ruiz-Ballesteros E, Mollejo M, Rodriguez A, et al. Splenic marginal zone lymphoma: proposal of new diagnostic and prognostic markers identified after tissue and cDNA microarray analysis. Blood 2005;106:1831–8.

96. Traverse-Glehen A, Baseggio L, Bauchu EC, et al. Splenic red pulp lymphoma with numerous basophilic villous lymphocytes: a distinct clinicopathologic and molecular entity? Blood 2008;111: 2253–60.

97. Baro C, Salido M, Domingo A, et al. Translocation t(9;14)(p13;q32) in cases of splenic marginal zone lymphoma. Haematologica 2006;91:1289–91.

98. Armitage JO, Weisenburger DD. New approach to classifying non-Hodgkin's lymphomas: clinical features of the major histologic subtypes. Non-Hodgkin's Lymphoma Classification Project. J Clin Oncol 1998;16:2780–95.

99. Griesser H, Kaiser U, Augener W, et al. B-cell lymphoma of the mucosa-associated lymphatic tissue (MALT) presenting with bone marrow and peripheral blood involvement. Leuk Res 1990;14:617–22.

100. Rosenwald A, Ott G, Stilgenbauer S, et al. Exclusive detection of the t(11;18) (q21;q21) in extranodal marginal zone B cell lymphomas (MZBL) of MALT type in contrast to other MZBL and extranodal large B cell lymphomas. Am J Pathol 1999;155:1817–21.

101. Brynes RK, Almaguer PD, Leathery KE, et al. Numerical cytogenetic abnormalities of chromosomes 3, 7, and 12 in marginal zone B-cell lymphomas. Mod Pathol 1996;9: 995–1000.

102. Dierlamm J, Rosenberg C, Stul M, et al. Characteristic pattern of chromosomal gains and losses in marginal zone B cell lymphoma detected by comparative genomic hybridization. Leukemia 1997;11:747–58.

103. Walsh SH, Rosenquist R. Immunoglobulin gene analysis of mature B-cell malignancies: reconsideration of cellular origin and potential antigen involvement in pathogenesis. Med Oncol 2005;22:327–41.

104. Du M, Diss TC, Xu C, et al. Ongoing mutation in MALT lymphoma immunoglobulin gene suggests that antigen stimulation plays a role in the clonal expansion. Leukemia 1996;10: 1190–7.

105. Arcaini L, Lucioni M, Boveri E, Paulli M. Nodal marginal zone lymphoma: current knowledge and future directions of an heterogeneous disease. Eur J Haematol 2009;83:165–74.

106. Traverse-Glehen A, Felman P, Callet-Bauchu E, et al. A clinicopathological study of nodal marginal zone B-cell lymphoma. A report on 21 cases. Histopathology 2006;48:162–73.

107. Henrique R, Achten R, Maes B, et al. Guidelines for subtyping small B-cell lymphomas in bone marrow biopsies. Virchows Arch 1999;435:549–58.

108. Arcaini L, Lucioni M, Boveri E, Paulli M. Nodal marginal zone lymphoma: current knowledge and future directions of an heterogeneous disease. Eur J Haematol 2009;83:165–74.

109. Ott G, Katzenberger T, Lohr A, et al. Cytomorphologic, immunohistochemical, and cytogenetic profiles of follicular lymphoma: 2 types of follicular lymphoma grade 3. Blood 2002;99: 3806–12.

110. Raynaud P, Caulet-Maugendre S, Foussard C, et al. T-cell lymphoid aggregates in bone marrow after rituximab therapy for B-cell follicular lymphoma: a marker of therapeutic efficacy? Hum Pathol 2008;39:194–200.

111. Landgren O, Tilly H. Epidemiology, pathology and treatment of non-follicular indolent lymphomas. Leuk Lymphoma 2008;49(Suppl. 1):35–42.

112. Cheuk W, Wong KO, Wong CS, Chan JK. Consistent immunostaining for cyclin D1 can be achieved on a routine basis using a newly available rabbit monoclonal antibody. Am J Surg Pathol 2004;28:801–7.

113. Ruchlemer R, Parry-Jones N, Brito-Babapulle V, et al. B-prolymphocytic leukaemia with t(11;14) revisited: a splenomegalic form of mantle cell lymphoma evolving with leukaemia. Br J Haematol 2004;125:330–6.

114. Conlan MG, Bast M, Armitage JO, Weisenburger DD. Bone marrow involvement by non-Hodgkin's lymphoma: the clinical significance of morphologic discordance between the lymph node and bone marrow. Nebraska Lymphoma Study Group. J Clin Oncol 1990;8:1163–72.

115. Kluin PM, van Krieken JH, Kleiverda K, Kluin-Nelemans HC. Discordant morphological characteristics of B-cell lymphomas in bone marrow and lymph node biopsies. Am J Clin Pathol 1990;94:59–66.

116. Kremer M, Spitzer M, Mandl-Weber S, et al. Discordant bone marrow involvement in diffuse large B-cell lymphoma: comparative molecular analysis reveals a heterogeneous group of disorders. Lab Invest 2003;83:107–14.

117. Heyning FH, Hogendoorn PC, Kramer MH, et al. Primary non-Hodgkin's lymphoma of bone: a clinicopathological investigation of 60 cases. Leukemia 1999;13:2094–8.

118. Alizadeh AA, Eisen MB, Davis RE, et al. Distinct types of diffuse large B-cell lymphoma identified by gene expression profiling. Nature 2000;403:503–11.

119. El Weshi A, Akhtar S, Mourad WA, et al. T-cell/histiocyte-rich B-cell lymphoma: clinical presentation, management and prognostic factors: report on 61 patients and review of literature. Leuk Lymphoma 2007;48:1764–73.

120. Fan Z, Natkunam Y, Bair E, et al. Characterization of variant patterns of nodular lymphocyte predominant Hodgkin lymphoma with immunohistologic and clinical correlation. Am J Surg Pathol 2003;27:1346–56.

121. Quintanilla-Martinez L, de Jong D, de Mascarel A, et al. Gray zones around diffuse large B cell lymphoma. Conclusions based on the workshop of the XIV meeting of the European Association for Hematopathology and the Society of Hematopathology in Bordeaux, France. J Hematop 2009;2:211–36.

122. Bennett JM, Catovsky D, Daniel MT, et al. Proposals for the classification of the acute leukaemias. French-American-British (FAB) co-operative group. Br J Haematol 1976;33:451–8.

123. Howell WM, Leung ST, Jones DB, et al. HLA-DRB, -DQA, and -DQB polymorphism in celiac disease and enteropathy-associated T-cell lymphoma. Common features and additional risk factors for malignancy. Hum Immunol 1995;43:29–37.

124. Obermann EC, Diss TC, Hamoudi RA, et al. Loss of heterozygosity at chromosome 9p21 is a frequent finding in enteropathy-type T-cell lymphoma. J Pathol 2004;202:252–62.

125. Weidmann E. Hepatosplenic T cell lymphoma. A review on 45 cases since the first report describing the disease as a distinct lymphoma entity in 1990. Leukemia 2000;14:991–7.

126. Cooke CB, Krenacs L, Stetler-Stevenson M, et al. Hepatosplenic T-cell lymphoma: a distinct clinicopathologic entity of cytotoxic gamma delta T-cell origin. Blood 1996;88:4265–74.

127. Macon WR, Levy NB, Kurtin PJ, et al. Hepatosplenic alphabeta T-cell lymphomas: a report of 14 cases and comparison with hepatosplenic gammadelta T-cell lymphomas. Am J Surg Pathol 2001;25:285–96.

128. Lai R, Larratt LM, Etches W, et al. Hepatosplenic T-cell lymphoma of alphabeta lineage in a 16-year-old boy presenting with hemolytic anemia and thrombocytopenia. Am J Surg Pathol 2000;24:459–63.

129. Wlodarska I, Martin-Garcia N, Achten R, et al. Fluorescence in situ hybridization study of chromosome 7 aberrations in hepatosplenic T-cell lymphoma: isochromosome 7q as a common

abnormality accumulating in forms with features of cytologic progression. Genes Chromosomes Cancer 2002;33: 243–51.

130. Abouyabis AN, Shenoy PJ, Lechowicz MJ, Flowers CR. Incidence and outcomes of the peripheral T-cell lymphoma subtypes in the United States. Leuk Lymphoma 2008;49:2099–107.

131. Benharroch D, Meguerian-Bedoyan Z, Lamant L, et al. ALK-positive lymphoma: a single disease with a broad spectrum of morphology. Blood 1998;91:2076–84.

132. Falini B, Pileri S, Zinzani PL, et al. ALK+ lymphoma: clinico-pathological findings and outcome. Blood 1999;93: 2697–706.

133. Stein H, Foss HD, Durkop H, et al. CD30(+) anaplastic large cell lymphoma: a review of its histopathologic, genetic, and clinical features. Blood 2000;96: 3681–95.

134. Falini B, Pulford K, Pucciarini A, et al. Lymphomas expressing ALK fusion protein(s) other than NPM-ALK. Blood 1999;94:3509–15.

135. Pulford K, Lamant L, Morris SW, et al. Detection of anaplastic lymphoma kinase (ALK) and nucleolar protein nucleophosmin (NPM)-ALK proteins in normal and neoplastic cells with the monoclonal antibody ALK1. Blood 1997;89:1394–404.

136. Dogan A, Attygalle AD, Kyriakou C. Angioimmunoblastic T-cell lymphoma. Br J Haematol 2003;121:681–91.

137. Ree HJ, Kadin ME, Kikuchi M, et al. Angioimmunoblastic lymphoma (AILD-type T-cell lymphoma) with hyperplastic germinal centers. Am J Surg Pathol 1998;22:643–55.

138. Rodriguez-Justo M, Attygalle AD, Munson P, et al. Angioimmunoblastic T-cell lymphoma with hyperplastic germinal centres: a neoplasia with origin in the outer zone of the germinal centre? Clinicopathological and immunohistochemical study of 10 cases with follicular T-cell markers. Mod Pathol 2009;22:753–61.

139. Roncador G, Garcia Verdes-Montenegro JF, Tedoldi S, et al. Expression of two markers of germinal center T cells (SAP and PD-1) in angioimmunoblastic T-cell lymphoma. Haematologica 2007;92:1059–66.

140. Dorfman DM, Brown JA, Shahsafaei A, Freeman GJ. Programmed death-1 (PD-1) is a marker of germinal center-associated T cells and angioimmunoblastic T-cell lymphoma. Am J Surg Pathol 2006;30:802–10.

141. Yamane A, Awaya N, Shimizu T, et al. Angioimmunoblastic T-cell lymphoma with polyclonal proliferation of plasma cells in peripheral blood and marrow. Acta Haematol 2007;117:74–7.

142. Smith JL, Hodges E, Quin CT, et al. Frequent T and B cell oligoclones in histologically and immunophenotypically characterized angioimmunoblastic lymphadenopathy. Am J Pathol 2000;156:661–9.

143. Thorns C, Bastian B, Pinkel D, et al. Chromosomal aberrations in angioimmunoblastic T-cell lymphoma and peripheral T-cell lymphoma unspecified: a matrix-based CGH approach. Genes Chromosomes Cancer 2007;46:37–44.

144. Marafioti T, Hummel M, Anagnostopoulos I, et al. Origin of nodular lymphocyte-predominant Hodgkin's disease from a clonal expansion of highly mutated germinal-center B cells. N Engl J Med 1997;337:453–8.

145. Wlodarska I, Stul M, de Wolf-Peeters C, Hagemeijer A. Heterogeneity of BCL6 rearrangements in nodular lymphocyte predominant Hodgkin's lymphoma. Haematologica 2004;89:965–72.

146. Marafioti T, Hummel M, Foss HD, et al. Hodgkin and Reed-Sternberg cells represent an expansion of a single clone originating from a germinal center B-cell with functional immunoglobulin gene rearrangements but defective immunoglobulin transcription. Blood 2000;95:1443–50.

147. Deacon EM, Pallesen G, Niedobitek G, et al. Epstein–Barr virus and Hodgkin's disease: transcriptional analysis of virus latency in the malignant cells. J Exp Med 1993;177:339–49.

148. Hinz M, Loser P, Mathas S, et al. Constitutive NF-kappaB maintains high expression of a characteristic gene network, including CD40, CD86, and a set of antiapoptotic genes in Hodgkin/Reed-Sternberg cells. Blood 2001;97:2798–807.

149. Calvo KR, Traverse-Glehen A, Pittaluga S, Jaffe ES. Molecular profiling provides evidence of primary mediastinal large B-cell lymphoma as a distinct entity related to classic Hodgkin lymphoma: implications for mediastinal gray zone lymphomas as an intermediate form of B-cell lymphoma. Adv Anat Pathol 2004; 11:227–38.

150. Swinnen LJ. Diagnosis and treatment of transplant-related lymphoma. Ann Oncol 2000;11(Suppl. 1):45–8.

151. Thomas JA, Crawford DH, Burke M. Clinicopathologic implications of Epstein–Barr virus related B cell lymphoma in immunocompromised patients. J Clin Pathol 1995;48:287–90.

152. Harris NL, Ferry JA, Swerdlow SH. Posttransplant lymphoproliferative disorders: summary of Society for Hematopathology Workshop. Semin Diagn Pathol 1997;14:8–14.

153. Oyama T, Ichimura K, Suzuki R, et al. Senile EBV+ B-cell lymphoproliferative disorders: a clinicopathologic study of 22 patients. Am J Surg Pathol 2003;27: 16–26.

154. Evens AM, David KA, Helenowski I, et al. Multicenter analysis of 80 solid organ transplantation recipients with post-transplantation lymphoproliferative disease: outcomes and prognostic factors in the modern era. J Clin Oncol 2010;28:1038–46.

155. Foran JM, Norton AJ, Micallef IN, et al. Loss of CD20 expression following treatment with rituximab (chimaeric monoclonal anti-CD20): a retrospective cohort analysis. Br J Haematol 2001; 114:881–3.

156. Chetty R, Echezarreta G, Comley M, Gatter K. Immunohistochemistry in apparently normal bone marrow trephine specimens from patients with nodal follicular lymphoma. J Clin Pathol 1995;48:1035–8.

157. Douglas VK, Gordon LI, Goolsby CL, et al. Lymphoid aggregates in bone marrow mimic residual lymphoma after rituximab therapy for non-Hodgkin lymphoma. Am J Clin Pathol 1999; 112:844–53.

158. Hanson CA, Brunning RD, Gajl-Peczalska KJ, et al. Bone marrow manifestations of peripheral T-cell lymphoma. A study of 30 cases. Am J Clin Pathol 1986;86: 449–60.

159. Feugier P, De March AK, Lesesve JF, et al. Intravascular bone marrow accumulation in persistent polyclonal lymphocytosis: a misleading feature for B-cell neoplasm. Mod Pathol 2004; 17:1087–96.

160. Alvares CL, Matutes E, Scully MA, et al. Isolated bone marrow involvement in diffuse large B cell lymphoma: a report of three cases with review of morphological, immunophenotypic and cytogenetic findings. Leuk Lymphoma 2004;45:769–75.

CHAPTER 30

Abnormalities in immunoglobulin synthesizing cells

FE Davies, KC Anderson

Chapter contents

©2011 Elsevier Ltd
DOI: 10.1016/B978-0-7020-3147-2.00030-4

Disease phases

MGUS

Myeloma

Leukemic

Genetic events

↓ Immortalization   ↓ Independent growth of malignant plasma cell
  ↓ Chromosomal translocations   ↓ Change in adhesion molecules
     ↓ Increasing genetic instability   ↓ p53, RAS mutation

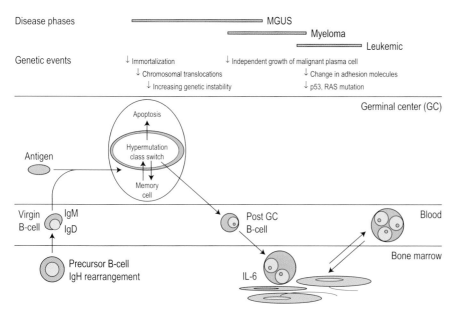

Fig. 30.1 A model of myeloma pathogenesis. After encountering cognate antigen, a virgin B-cell transforms to form a germinal center (GC). The initial event in the development of MGUS is immortalization of such a cell, which is then at an increased risk of developing chromosomal translocations into the IgH switch region and of increased genetic instability. In MGUS there is a continual passage of clonally related cells through the GC, where the cells continue to acquire mutations within their clonally related IgH regions. These cells subsequently migrate to the bone marrow where they differentiate into plasma cells. The development of myeloma is associated with the independent growth of one such clone that proliferates within the bone marrow. During the early phases of myeloma, plasma cells pass into the blood and subsequently home back to the marrow. In the later stages of the disease, changes in adhesion molecules result in a leukemic phase that is associated with the acquisition of p53 and RAS mutations.

Multiple myeloma

Multiple myeloma (MM) is a clonal B-cell neoplasm that affects terminally differentiated plasma cells. The clinical picture involves a combination of bone destruction, immune deficiency, bone marrow (BM) failure and renal failure. A paraprotein or monoclonal immunoglobulin (Ig) is usually present in the blood and/or the urine and the BM is infiltrated by malignant plasma cells (PC). Myeloma-related organ or tissue impairment may also be present. The current median survival is approximately 6–7 years which has increased by at least a year during the last decade due to the introduction of targeted therapies.

Epidemiology and etiology

MM represents 10–15% of all hematologic malignancies and 1% of all cancers, with an incidence of 2/100 000.[1] The incidence increases with age, with approximately 40% of patients presenting under the age of 60 years and only 2% of cases occurring before the age of 40 years. There is a moderate excess in males. Geographic and racial differences play an important role, as the disease is more common in black people than Caucasians and has a low incidence in Chinese people. These rates are retained after migration to new countries, suggesting an inherited rather than an environmental explanation for the differences. Epidemiological studies have been carried out to identify environmental risk factors.[2,3] An association with radiation exposure is seen in survivors of the World War II atomic bombs, as well as in occupationally and therapeutically exposed groups. There is also a suggestion of an association with farming, paper production, woodwork and exposure to a variety of chemicals including petroleum, benzene and materials associated with plastic and rubber manufacture. In addition to traditional epidemiology studies, there is much interest in determining whether inherited polymorphic variation can influence the development of MM or a patient's response to treatment.[2,3] To date

most studies have been small and have concentrated on single nucleotide polymorphisms (SNPs) that affect the function of genes already known to be important in MM pathogenesis (e.g. immune response and cytokine genes). The introduction of newer high-throughput technologies with near complete genome coverage will enable this important area to be investigated further over the next few years.

Biology

The cell of origin

The main phenotypic features of myeloma PC include abnormal localization within the BM, replacement of normal BM elements, and dysregulation of Ig secretion. Normal PC in BM are derived from cells that have passed through a germinal center in a lymph node or other organ. Within the germinal center, cells undergo somatic hypermutation, class switching of the Ig gene, and selection by antigen-binding affinity; only cells with high binding affinity survive to become PC. In myeloma the Ig genes from individual plasma cells show the same pattern of somatic hypermutation, consistent with the clonal expansion of a single postgerminal center B-cell.[4,5] The high incidence of translocations involving the switch region on chromosome 14 would also indicate that the final molecular oncogenic event occurs late in B-cell development. This contrasts with monoclonal gammopathy of unknown significance (MGUS) where there is intraclonal variation in the pattern of mutation, suggesting transformation of a virgin or memory B-cell with progeny which continue to pass through the normal process of germinal center selection before becoming plasma cells (Fig. 30.1).

Biology and growth signaling

Following the transformation of the proliferative 'plasmablastic' cell located in the germinal centre, adhesion molecules mediate homing of the immortalized progeny of this

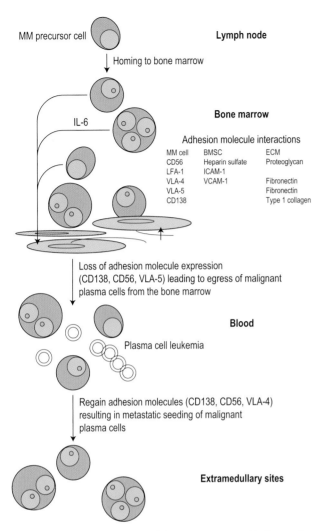

Fig. 30.2 Adhesion molecules and disease progression. Myeloma cells (MM) home to the bone marrow where they adhere to bone-marrow stromal cells and extracellular matrix proteins, resulting in an increase in IL-6 secretion and myeloma cell growth and survival. In the terminal phase of disease and plasma-cell leukemia changes in adhesion molecule profile lead to the egression of myeloma cells into the peripheral blood and extravascular sites.

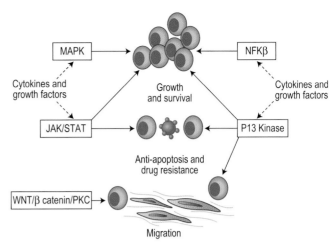

Fig. 30.3 Key myeloma signaling pathways. A number of signaling pathways are responsible for the increase in proliferation, survival, cell cycle and migration of myeloma cells.

cell from the lymph node to specialized niches within the BM, where maturation into a malignant PC occurs (Fig. 30.2). Further genetic hits lead to loss of tumor suppressor genes, expression of oncogenes and alteration in cell cycle control, resulting in a proliferative advantage for the MM cell and disease progression. Binding of myeloma cells to the BM stroma occurs and localizes tumor cells within the BM microenvironment. This binding to stroma results in an increase in the paracrine transcription and secretion of cytokines (particularly interleukin (IL)-6, insulin-like growth factor 1 (IGF1) and vascular endothelial growth factor (VEGF)), mediating myeloma cell growth and survival, and protection from drug-induced apoptosis (Fig. 30.3).[6,7]

The cytokines IL6, IGF1 and VEGF together with direct myeloma cell to cell contact trigger signaling via the Ras/MEK/MAPK pathway resulting in myeloma cell growth, survival and drug resistance.[7–9] Mutations affecting these pathways result in cytokine independent myeloma cell growth,

the development of drug resistance and extramedullary disease. IL6 and IGF1 also signal via the PI3kinase-AKT-mTOR pathway, mediating myeloma growth, cell cycle and apoptosis.[7–9] Activation of mTOR results in phosphorylation of P70S6 and 4E-BP1, which plays a key role in regulating the translation of cyclin D and c-myc, two proteins known to be central to myeloma pathogenesis. IL6 also triggers signaling via the JAK/STAT3 pathway and triggers drug resistance via activation of RAFTK and the mitochondrial release of Smac.

Nuclear factor kappa B (NFκB) signaling is important in B-cell biology and most myeloma cell lines demonstrate activation of NFκB leading to increased myeloma cell growth and survival. The pathway is also the target of multiple mutational events with 20% of cases harboring mutations or deletions of key inhibitory members of both the canonical and non-canonical pathways.[10,11] A further key pathway is the TNFα superfamily (SDF1, CD40, BAFF, APRIL). Although the direct effect of TNFα on cell proliferation is modest, it markedly up-regulates the secretion of IL6 from BM stromal cells leading to dramatic increases in myeloma cell growth. TNFα also induces NFκB dependent expression of adhesion molecules increasing binding between myeloma cells and stromal cells resulting in protection from drug-induced apoptosis. In addition, CD40 mediates a p53 dependent increase in myeloma cell growth and PI3kinase/AKT/NFκB dependent migration.

Cytogenetic and molecular abnormalities

Translocations occurring as a result of aberrant class switch recombination events are the earliest known genetic events in MM (Fig. 30.4).[12] The molecular characterization of the common recurrent translocations, t(4;14), t(11;14), t(14;16) and t(6;14), has identified a number of deregulated oncogenes including FGFR3/MMSET, cyclin D1, c-MAF and cyclin D3, respectively. In addition to switch translocations, secondary events such as chromosomal copy number alterations are common and genetic instability occurs resulting in deletions (e.g. 13q-, 17p-/p53, 1p-/CDKN2C, 16q-/CYLD/

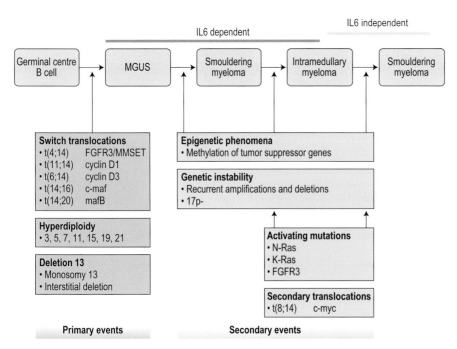

IL6 dependent

IL6 independent

Germinal centre B cell → MGUS → Smouldering myeloma → Intramedullary myeloma → Smouldering myeloma

Switch translocations
- t(4;14)   FGFR3/MMSET
- t(11;14) cyclin D1
- t(6;14)   cyclin D3
- t(14;16) c-maf
- t(14;20) mafB

Hyperdiploidy
- 3, 5, 7, 11, 15, 19, 21

Deletion 13
- Monosomy 13
- Interstitial deletion

Epigenetic phenomena
- Methylation of tumor suppressor genes

Genetic instability
- Recurrent amplifications and deletions
- 17p-

Activating mutations
- N-Ras
- K-Ras
- FGFR3

Secondary translocations
- t(8;14)   c-myc

Primary events

Secondary events

Fig. 30.4 Key genetic events in the transformation of MGUS to myeloma. Genetic events in myeloma can be characterized as primary or secondary events. Switch translocations occur early and result in the overexpression of a number of key oncogenes including the D group cyclins and maf. Later events include genetic instability methylation and activating mutations.

Table 30.1 Genetic abnormalities in myeloma[12–21]

Abnormality	Feature	Frequency	Significance
IgH translocations			
t(11;14)	Over-expression of cyclin D1	15%	Favorable prognosis
t(4;14)	Over-expression of FGFR3, MMSET and cyclin D2	10–15%	Adverse prognosis
t(6;14)	Over-expression of IRF4/MUM1 and cyclin D3	2%	Adverse prognosis
t(14;16)	Dysregulation of c-maf	<5%	Adverse prognosis
t(14;20)	Dysregulation of maf B	1–2%	Adverse prognosis
Copy number abnormalities			
del(13q)	Usually monosomy. Strong association with t(4;14). Effect due to Rb1 loss	45–50%	Neutral prognosis. Adverse if associated with t(4;14)
del(17p)	Effect due to TP53 loss	5–10%	Adverse prognosis
del 1p	CDKN2C/FAF1	10%	Adverse prognosis
amp 1q	Often linked with del 1p	30–40%	Adverse prognosis
del 16q	WWOX and CYLD	20%	Adverse prognosis
Hyperdiploid	Odd numbered chromosomes	45–50%	Favorable prognosis

WWOX, NFκB inactivation/BIRC/TRAF3), activating mutations (e.g. NRas, FGFR3) and secondary translocations (e.g. t(8;14)). This has led to a molecular classification of myeloma based on the presence of switch translocations, hyperdiploidy and deregulation of the D group cyclins (Table 30.1).[13] Two broad groups of patients can be recognized: a hyperdiploid group where there is a low incidence of switch translocations (<30%) and a non-hyperdiploid group where the incidence is high (>85%). Chromosome 1 abnormalities, usually 1q gain and 1p loss, are among the most prevalent cytogenetic abnormalities. The majority involve rearrangements located in the pericentromeric regions of the chromosomes and form jumping translocations. The actual gene responsible for the biological effects is uncertain although CSK1B and CDKN2C have been suggested as candidates. Recent studies have also suggested epigenetic changes contribute to the disease phenotype with patients showing overexpression of MMSET, a protein with histone methyl transferase activity and mutations in UTX, a histone demethylase.[15]

Advances in technology have now enabled the correlation of these genetic features with clinical outcome and has identified a series of distinct clinical subgroups. One such group are patients with the t(4;14)(p16.3;q32), which is present in 10–15% of myeloma cases.[16,17] The translocation leads to dysregulation of two potential oncogenes, fibroblast growth factor receptor 3 (FGFR3) and multiple myeloma SET domain (MMSET). Myeloma carrying t(4;14) has a distinct gene expression profile and clinical profile with a short duration of response to chemotherapy, resistance to conventional alkylating agents and poor overall prognosis compared with other translocation groups. Patients with a t(11;14), present in 15% of cases, also have a distinct clinical phenotype. This translocation results in the up-regulation of cyclin D1, is associated with lymphoplasmacytic morphology, CD20 expression, λ light chain usage and low CD56.[18] In addition, rare IgM myeloma often carry t(11;14).[19] The prognostic significance depends on the series examined but ranges from neutral to favorable.

Patients with deletion of 17p also have a distinct clinical phenotype with a high incidence of extramedullary disease and aggressive course, short remissions and a short overall survival.[20,21] Abnormalities of both the long and short arm of chromosome 1 have been linked with short survival, and gene expression profiles identifying patients with high risk disease are highly enriched for genes located on this chromosome. The prognostic significance of chromosome 13 deletion is more controversial with some studies showing a strong prognostic significance whereas other studies demonstrate little effect. This appears to depend on the detection method used to determine the presence of the abnormality, chromosome banding versus interphase FISH. In addition, all patients with a t(4;14) demonstrate deletion of chromosome 13, and as t(4;14) patients tend to have a poor prognosis this 'linked effect' may account for some of the differences.

Gene expression profiling has enabled a number of groups to determine prognostic signatures containing between 15 and 70 genes that identify high risk or poor prognostic patients. It is important to note, however, that there is minimal overlap between the different signatures and validation is ongoing as to whether these signatures can be used in different treatment contexts or different stages of disease.

Bone disease

Bone destruction in MM is a prominent feature and causes considerable morbidity. Bone remodeling is a continuous process of resorption by osteoclasts and the subsequent formation of new bone by osteoblasts. In myeloma there is an increase in the number of osteoclasts and bone resorption in areas of the marrow adjacent to abnormal PC, but not in those areas adjacent to normal BM cells. New bone formation is also reduced when the tumor burden in the BM is high, and the combination of increased resorption and decreased formation leads to an uncoupling of normal bone remodeling.[22,23] The central players involved in this process include: the receptor activator of NFκB (RANK); RANKL, the ligand for RANK; and osteoprotegerin (OPG) (Fig. 30.5). RANKL exists in a membrane and soluble form and via its receptor RANK increases bone resorption by increasing osteoclast formation and activity. OPG prevents bone resorption by acting as a decoy receptor preventing the binding of RANKL to RANK thereby inhibiting the up-regulation

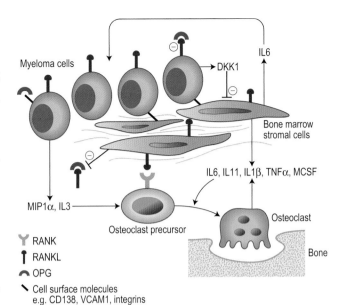

Fig 30.5 Pathogenesis of myeloma bone disease. Osteolytic bone lesions are characteristically seen in myeloma due to an uncoupling of the osteoclastic and osteoblastic activity within the bone marrow. Osteoblasts are derived from mesenchymal lineage, while osteoclasts arise from myeloma hematopoietic precursors. Binding of myeloma cells to the bone marrow stroma results in an increase in the production of RANKL, MCSF and other osteoclast activating factors (OAFs). In addition myeloma cells express MIP1α and IL3. All of these factors contribute to enhanced proliferation and differentiation of osteoclast precursors leading to bone resorption. OPG acts as a decoy receptor for RANKL and prevents the binding of RANKL to RANK hence inhibiting osteoclast development and bone resorption. Dickkop1 (DKK1) is also expressed by myeloma cells. This inhibits WNT signaling reducing osteoblast development.

proliferation and fusion of osteoclast precursors to produce mature osteoclasts. A number of other cytokines and chemokines modify the BM microenvironment leading to an upregulation of RANKL by both stroma and osteoblasts including IL6, IL1β, IL11, lymphotoxin, Tumor necrosis factor (TNF)-α, and macrophage inflammatory protein 1α (MIP-1α), further perpetuating the cycle of bone destruction. In addition the increased osteoclast activity results in the secretion of tumor growth factor (TGF)-β, IL-6, β-fibroblast growth factor (FGF) and IGF-1 from the BM matrix in turn leading to further myeloma cell growth.

Diagnostic criteria

An international classification system has recently replaced a number of different diagnostic criteria to aid in the classification of the monoclonal gammopathies.[24] Due to overlapping features, myeloma must be distinguished from the other disorders characterized by the presence of a monoclonal protein including MGUS, Waldenström's macroglobulinemia, non-Hodgkin lymphoma, light-chain amyloid, idiopathic cold agglutinin disease, essential cryoglobulinemia, and heavy-chain disease. Some of these disorders are discussed later in this chapter, while non-Hodgkin lymphomas are discussed in Chapter 29. The majority of MM patients will have an M protein in the serum >30 g/l and/or BM clonal plasma cells >10% (Table 30.2). Patients are then classified depending on the presence or absence of end organ

Table 30.2 Monoclonal (M) protein incidence and type[24]

	Type	Incidence
Serum M protein	Detectable in over 90% of patients using immunofixation	
Urinary M protein	Present in over 75% of patients	
M protein type	IgG	>50%
	IgA	20%
	IgD	2%
	IgE	1%
	Light chain only	20%
	Non-secretory disease	3%

Table 30.3 Myeloma-related organ or tissue impairment (end organ damage)[24]

*Calcium	>0.25 mmol/l above the upper limit of normal or >2.75 mmol/l
*Renal insufficiency	Creatinine >173 mmol/l
*Anemia	Hemoglobin 2 g/dl below the lower limit of normal or hemoglobin <10 g/dl
*Bone lesions	Lytic lesions or osteoporosis with compression fractures
Other	Symptomatic hyperviscosity, amyloidosis recurrent bacterial infections (>2 episodes in 12 months)

*CRAB, calcium, renal insufficiency, anemia or bone lesions.

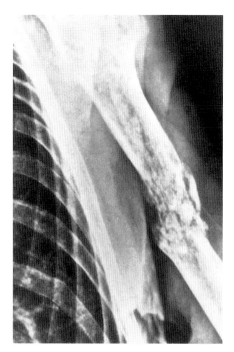

Fig. 30.6 Bone disease in myeloma. Radiograph showing a typical osteolytic lesion and pathologic fracture of the left humerus.

damage related to the plasma cell proliferative process (Table 30.3). Symptomatic patients have evidence of related organ or tissue impairment (end organ damage) (ROTI). Examples include raised calcium levels, renal insufficiency, anemia and bone lesions. Generally these patients require urgent therapy. Asymptomatic patients have no evidence of ROTI and usually undergo close monitoring with treatment initiated at disease progression. The term asymptomatic myeloma tends to include patients previously classified as having smoldering myeloma or Durie–Salmon stage I disease.

Clinical features

The clinical picture of myeloma both at presentation and during its clinical course is complex involving bone destruction leading to pain or fracture with hypercalcemia; infection due to immune deficiency; BM failure leading to anemia and less commonly thrombocytopenia; and renal failure due to hypercalcemia, direct damage from paraprotein or precipitation of light chain in renal tubules. In addition, these features may also be associated with plasmacytoma, hyperviscosity and biochemical disturbances.

Bone disease

The accumulation of myeloma cells within the cavity of bones in the axial skeleton produces bone pain and destruction. The pain arises in the axial skeleton, and loss of height due to collapse of vertebrae and kyphosis are common. Although bone pain may be gradual in onset, pathologic fractures are frequent and usually indicated by the sudden onset of local tenderness and pain. Seventy per cent of patients will have evidence of bone disease at presentation and in almost all cases the bone lesions are osteolytic (Fig. 30.6), but a minority of patients (2%) have osteosclerotic lesions. The majority of patients also have diffuse osteopenia. Bone resorption leads to increased calcium in 20–40% of patients.

Hyperviscosity

Hyperviscosity syndrome occurs in 5–10% of patients and is usually associated with an IgA paraproteinemia, due to the tendency of the IgA paraprotein to polymerize. Clinical features include a predisposition to bleeding from mucosal surfaces, dilatation and segmentation of retinal and conjunctival veins, and central nervous system disturbances including headache, drowsiness, weakness and confusion which may progress to epileptic fits, paralysis and coma. Symptoms improve with vigorous plasmapheresis to reduce both the paraprotein concentration and serum viscosity. Specific therapy to control the underlying disease should be undertaken simultaneously.

Recurrent infections

Susceptibility to infection is a prominent feature of myeloma and the mechanisms responsible for the failure of the immune response are complex. Streptococcal pneumonia and *Hemophilus* infections usually occur early in the disease course. Gram-negative infections occur in refractory disease or in the setting of previous antibiotic therapy, medical intervention and hospitalization. An increase in viral infections, particularly herpes zoster, has been seen following the introduction of the novel therapies. The role of prophylactic antibiotics is controversial.

Renal failure

Twenty per cent of patients have renal insufficiency at the time of diagnosis with 50% of patients developing some form of renal impairment during their illness. The specific renal lesions are due to the formation of intratubular casts of paraprotein or the diffuse precipitation of paraprotein in renal tissue. Many other factors also contribute to the development of renal failure including infection, hypercalcemia, hyperuricemia, direct plasma cell infiltration of the kidneys, dehydration, antibiotic therapy and amyloidosis. Free light chains (Bence Jones proteins) are inherently nephrotoxic, with lambda light chains more nephrotoxic than kappa. The most important aspect of the management of renal failure in myeloma is preventative by the maintenance of a high fluid throughput. Acute episodes of renal failure may be reversible, and even the clinical syndrome of chronic renal failure can be improved by vigorous hydration and reduction of the myeloma cell mass by chemotherapy.

Neurological features

Disorders of the central and peripheral nervous system may also play a prominent part in the clinical presentation and disease course. Nonspecific higher cerebral dysfunction can result from hypercalcemia, hyperviscosity, anemia or uremia and requires urgent treatment. Spinal cord or nerve root compression occurs in 10% of patients usually due to compression by a plasmacytoma. A symmetrical distal sensory or sensorimotor neuropathy may also occur, associated with axonal degeneration with or without amyloid deposition. In some cases this is associated with monoclonal antibodies directed against peripheral nerve myelin. Myelomatous meningitis is rare and is usually associated with rapidly progressive, widespread disease.

Staging and prognostic factors

The international staging system (ISS) reliably separates patients into prognostic groups using simple laboratory measurements.[25] The system is widely used in the clinic to determine which patients should receive therapy, although few physicians would use it to direct specific choice of therapy. The system was derived from clinical and laboratory data from over 10 000 newly diagnosed patients and highlighted beta 2 microglobulin, serum albumin, platelet count, serum creatinine and age as powerful predictors of survival (Table 30.4). In addition to the cytogenetic abnormalities already discussed, other factors with prognostic significance include the extent and type of BM infiltration and measures of tumor-cell proliferation such as the plasma cell labeling index (PCLI). Patients with a plasmablastic morphology have a median survival of 16 months, compared to a median

Table 30.4 International staging system[25] for myeloma patients

	Factors	Median survival
Stage I	β2m <3.5 mg/l albumin >3.5 g/dl	62 months
Stage II	Neither I or III	44 months
Stage III	β2m >3.5 mg/l albumin <3.5 g/dl	29 months

β2m, serum β2 microglobulin.

survival of 35 months for patients with other morphologic subtypes. PCLI is usually low (<1%) at diagnosis, higher at relapse, and lower in patients with MGUS. In addition, a high PCLI correlates with a shorter survival time independent of tumor-cell mass. The percentage of circulating PC at diagnosis has also been shown to be an independent prognostic variable.[26] Some of the newer targeted therapies may be able to overcome the negative prognostic effects of the genetic abnormalities. This highlights the importance of performing FISH/gene array analysis at diagnosis, and suggests that making treatment decisions based on these results is a real option in the near future.

Pathology

A normochromic normocytic anemia is often present, with rouleaux formation and a high nonspecific background staining on the blood smear due to the presence of circulating paraprotein. In patients with more advanced disease, thrombocytopenia and neutropenia may also be present. Occasional circulating PC with a phenotype similar to those within the marrow can be demonstrated. In the majority of cases, PC will exceed 10% of the nucleated cells within the BM. PC usually appear moderately to severely dysplastic with large eccentrically placed nuclei, which may be either multiple or cleaved (Fig. 30.7A, B). Nucleoli are prominent and nuclear inclusions may be present, including Dutcher bodies. Cytoplasm may be sparse or foamy or vacuolated and show Ig inclusions such as Russell bodies (Fig. 30.7C). Plasma cells from IgA myeloma often have a characteristic flame-cell appearance (Fig. 30.7D). Approximately 8% of myeloma cases demonstrate plasmablastic features, with more than 2% of cells having a plasmablastic morphology (Fig. 30.7E). Plasmablasts have a fine reticular chromatin pattern, large nucleoli and less abundant cytoplasm (less than half of the nuclear area). This morphologic subset is associated with a high PCLI, more advanced and aggressive disease, and a worse prognosis (Fig. 30.7F). A reactive plasmacytosis due to chronic inflammation or infection may also present with an increase in BM plasma cells. This can be readily distinguished from MM by the normal morphology as well as polyclonal phenotype of the plasma cells and an increase in eosinophils, mast cells and megakaryocytes.

Plasma cells are terminally differentiated B-cells and hence express a number of B-cell antigens as well as myeloma-associated antigens. Both normal and malignant plasma cells express CD38 and CD138, but usually lack CD10,

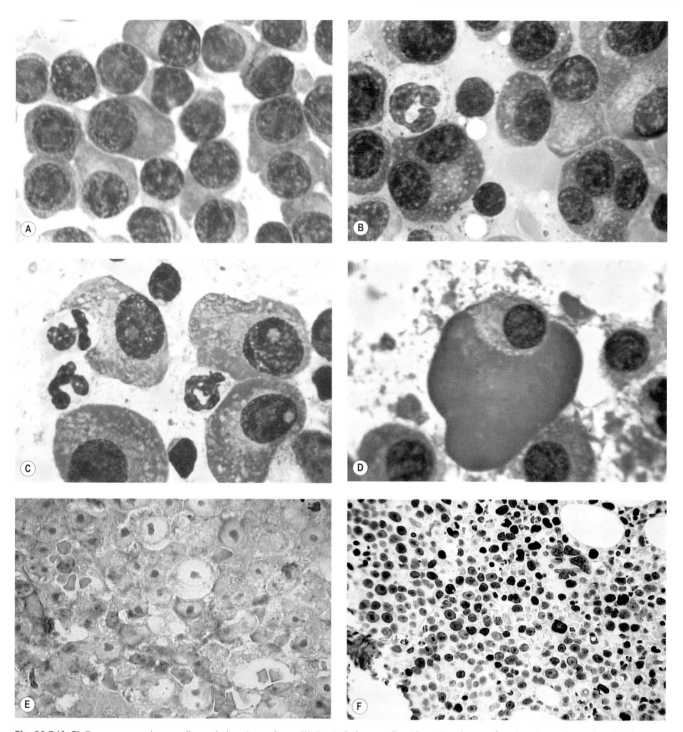

Fig. 30.7 (A–F) Bone-marrow plasma cell morphology in myeloma. (A) Atypical plasma cells with varying degree of nuclear size and cytoplasmic volume. (B) Large multinucleated plasma cells. (C) Plasma cells with inclusion bodies. (D) Flame cell from a patient with IgA myeloma. (E) Plasmablastic cells. (F) Plasmablastic cells with high Ki67 expression.

CD20, CD23, CD34 and CD45RO. The most reliable antibodies used to detect plasma cells by flow cytometry are therefore CD38, CD138 and CD45RO. It is possible to distinguish myeloma plasma cells from their normal counterparts, since the former usually express significantly higher levels of the important adhesion molecules CD56 and CD138 and significantly lower levels of CD19, CD38 and CD45 than the latter. Plasma cells from normal individuals are consistently CD19$^+$ CD56 low; whereas 65% of myeloma cases have a plasma cell phenotype of CD19$^-$ CD56$^+$, 30% CD19$^-$ CD56 low, and 5% CD19$^+$ CD56$^+$.[26] Other immunophenotypic features allowed stratification of patients with MM into three risk categories: poor risk (CD28$^+$ CD117$^-$), intermediate (either both markers negative or both positive), and good risk (CD28$^-$ CD117$^+$).[27] Immunocytochemical studies confirm the monoclonality of the plasma cells, and the type of secreted Ig should correlate with the serum paraprotein and urinary light chain.

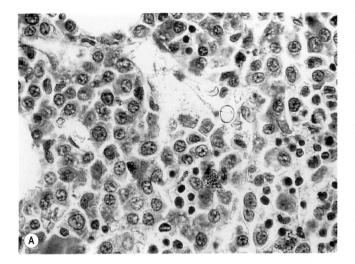

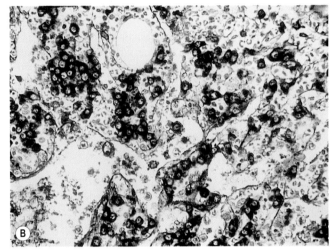

Fig. 30.8 (A, B) Bone marrow biopsy in myeloma. (A). Heavily infiltrated marrow. (B). Immunohistochemistry demonstrating monoclonal kappa positive plasma cells.

Table 30.5 Mechanisms of action of commonly used antimyeloma drugs[29–35]

Drug	Mechanism of action
Alkylating agents (melphalan, cyclophosphamide, BCNU)	Cross-linking DNA strands in resting and dividing cells
Glucocorticoids (dexamethasone, prednisolone)	Increased apoptosis of myeloma plasma cells with associated phosphorylation of RAFTK
Vinca alkaloids (vincristine)	Inhibition of microtubule formation resulting in the arrest of dividing cells in metaphase
Anthracyclines (adriamycin)	Binds to nucleic acids by intercalation with base pairs of the DNA double helix interfering with DNA synthesis
Bisphosphonates (clodronate, pamidronate, zoledronic acid)	Reduced osteoclastic activity and decreased bone absorption Myeloma plasma cell and bone-marrow apoptosis Decreased production of IL-6 and metalloproteinases Activation of $\gamma\delta$ T-cells
Immunomodulatory drugs – IMiDs (thalidomide and lenalidomide)	Growth arrest or increased apoptosis of myeloma plasma cells Alteration in adhesion molecule profile Alteration in cytokine secretion and/or bioavailability (IL6 and VEGF) Decreased angiogenesis Altered immune response
Proteasome inhibitors	Decreased myeloma cell growth and survival signaling (e.g. NFκB) Decreased expression of key anti-apoptotic molecules Dysregulation of intracellular calcium metabolism Down-regulation of genes involved in mismatch repair and DNA double strand break repair Decreased myeloma cell adhesion Stimulation of osteoblast activity

BCNU, carmustine (bis-chloronitrosourea); IL6, interleukin 6; RAFTK, related adhesion focal tyrosine kinase; VEGF, vascular endothelial growth factor.

On BM biopsy, plasma cells normally accumulate around blood vessels. However, in MM this pattern is lost and the myeloma cells are found as single cells or small clusters between adipocytes. As the disease progresses, diffuse marrow replacement occurs, resulting in a packed marrow with complete loss of normal architecture (Fig. 30.8A, B). Occasionally, there is a paratrabecular distribution similar to follicular center lymphoma, and in some patients with aggressive disease tumor nodules containing abnormal PC may be seen. Assessing the degree of marrow infiltration is often difficult due both to the patchy nature of the disease and the presence of either hypoplastic or hyperplastic areas. There may be a discrepancy between the percentage of PC in the aspirate compared to the biopsy, due either to the presence of fibrosis or nodular infiltration resulting in a low number of PC on the smear.

Treatment

Myeloma has a relapsing remitting course that requires serial courses of treatment, with periods of durable remissions in between. With each successive relapse, the treatment free period often becomes shorter and eventually the myeloma cells become resistant to therapy and the disease rapidly progresses leading to death. During the last decade the introduction of a number of targeted therapies for myeloma has resulted in a significant increase in the number of patients achieving a response to therapy, an improvement in quality of life and increased survival. In view of the increased response rates seen with these targeted therapies the response criteria have been standardized and updated.[28] The targeted therapies include the immunomodulatory drugs, thalidomide and lenalidomide, and the proteasome inhibitor bortezomib.[29–35] These now form the backbone of therapy to which corticosteroids or conventional chemotherapy are often added. The mechanisms of action of the commonly used drugs are summarized in Table 30.5. A number of other novel biologically based treatment approaches are currently being evaluated which will be used either alone or in combination with existing treatments to further improve response and outcome. Importantly, *in vitro* and *in vivo* studies of the mechanisms of action of these novel approaches are also providing new insights into the biology of myeloma.

Monoclonal gammopathy of undetermined significance

Monoclonal gammopathy of undetermined significance (MGUS) describes a condition characterized by the presence of a low level of paraprotein in the absence of other clinical features of MM, Waldenström's macroglobulinemia or other B-cell lymphoproliferative disorders.[24] The previous term 'benign monoclonal gammopathy' is a misleading description of the disease, since a proportion of patients will develop a more aggressive plasma cell disorder.

Clinical features

The incidence of MGUS increases with age, with 1% of the population under the age of 60 years and between 4–5% of the population over the age of 80 years being affected. The prevalence in African Americans and Africans is approximately double that in white people.[36,37] The demonstration of a paraprotein in the serum or urine is often an incidental finding and patients are typically asymptomatic. A recent prospective study indicated that MM is always preceded by MGUS.[38] The serum paraprotein is usually less than 3 g/dl, with little or no urinary component, and may be present despite normal total protein or globulin levels. Immune paresis may occur in 30% of cases. There should be no evidence of end organ damage; the presence of bone lesions, hypercalcemia, renal impairment, lymphadenopathy or organomegaly should suggest a diagnosis of myeloma or Waldenström's macroglobulinemia. There is an association of MGUS with a number of disorders including chronic lymphocytic leukemia, polyneuropathy and myopathy, connective tissue disorders, dermatologic disorders, hepatitis C and immunosuppression (AIDS and transiently post bone marrow or renal transplantation).

Biology

The main features of the biology of the disease have been discussed in detail above. Immunoglobulin heavy chain sequence analysis demonstrates an intraclonal variation in the pattern of mutation, suggesting transformation of a virgin or memory B-cell with progeny continuing to pass through the normal process of germinal center selection before becoming plasma cells.[5] Cytogenetic analysis reveals findings similar to myeloma, including a complex karyotype with trisomies and monosomies, structural abnormalities, and translocations involving chromosome 14, although the prognostic significance is not known at present.[12]

Pathology

The peripheral blood picture is normal, with no evidence of circulating plasma cells or anemia. Clonal plasma cells are present within the bone marrow in an interstitial distribution and represent less than 5–10% of the total nucleated cells. Using flow cytometry it is possible to identify plasma cells with both a normal and 'myeloma' phenotype (CD38++, CD19+ and CD56− vs. CD38+, CD19− and CD56+).[26]

Treatment/management/disease progression

There is no specific treatment for patients with MGUS. Long-term surveillance is recommended since approximately 25% of cases will develop an overt plasma cell disorder. Data regarding disease progression have been derived from a cohort of 241 patients with MGUS at the Mayo Clinic who have been followed for 24–38 years.[36,37] The risk of progression was approximately 1% per year with the majority of patients developing myeloma, although some show symptoms or signs of amyloidosis or Waldenström's macroglobulinemia. There are currently no predictive factors to determine which patients will progress. Cases with M proteins of IgA or IgM type are associated with an increased risk of progression, as are patients with higher M protein levels or an abnormal serum free light chain ratio.[39] Overall, 50% of patients with MGUS will die from an unrelated cause; the remaining 25% of patients will continue with stable paraprotein levels, but may develop disease over a longer follow-up period.

Plasma cell leukemia

Plasma cell leukemia (PCL) is a rare plasma cell disorder characterized by the presence of more than $2 \times 10^9/1$ circulating plasma cells which constitute at least 20% of all PB cells.[1] The majority (60%) of cases are *de novo* or primary, in which a leukemic picture develops in the absence of a documented preceding plasma cell disorder. Forty per cent of cases are secondary and occur in a minority of myeloma patients (1%) with terminal disease.

Clinical features

The median age at diagnosis of primary PCL is 55 years, approximately 10 years younger than for myeloma.[40] Although patients with primary PCL present with symptoms similar to those of myeloma, the disease course is often more aggressive with symptoms relating to extramedullary disease including plasmacytomas and hepatosplenomegaly. Anemia, hypercalcemia and renal failure are also more common. Patients with secondary disease usually have advanced myeloma that is refractory to treatment and may present with worsening symptoms related to bone marrow failure including anemia, infections, bleeding or plasmacytomas.

Biology

The adverse biological prognostic factors usually associated with end-stage myeloma are invariably present at diagnosis in cases of primary PCL. These include a high PCLI; frequent translocations involving 11q (cyclin D1); complex cytogenetic abnormalities including amplification of c-myc; as well as mutations of RAS and p53; and changes in adhesion-molecule profile.[41,42]

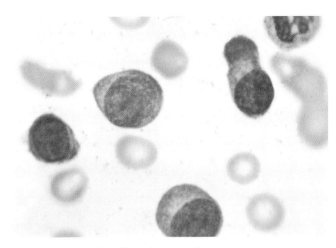

Fig. 30.9 Peripheral blood film of plasma cell leukemia.

Pathology

The peripheral blood is characterized by the presence of a large number of circulating PC, which may be morphologically normal or have blastic features (Fig. 30.9). Anemia is invariably present, and both neutropenia and thrombocytopenia are common. Rouleaux formation is usually also present with a high nonspecific background staining, especially in secondary PCL cases where the level of paraprotein is often high. The BM is heavily infiltrated with plasma cells morphologically similar to those within the PB. Other normal hematopoietic elements are reduced. Occasionally cells can be of lymphocyte size without obvious evidence of plasma cell morphology. In these cases other phenotypic features of plasma cell differentiation must be sought, such as loss of B-cell markers and high expression of CD38 and CD138.

Treatment/management/disease progression

There are few clinical trials addressing the best treatment approaches for patients with PCL. Due to the aggressive nature of the disease combination chemotherapy followed by autologous transplantation seems the most appropriate strategy, although good results have also been obtained with bortezomib and lenalidomide therapy. A number of groups also use more traditional acute leukemia regimens. Patients with underlying myeloma who have developed PCL tend to have end-stage disease resistant to conventional therapy, therefore more experimental treatment approaches are appropriate. The median survival for these patients is extremely poor.

Solitary bone plasmacytoma

Some patients present with a single solitary painful bone lesion due to a plasma cell infiltrate, and further studies reveal no evidence of systemic disease.

Clinical features

The bone lesions are commonly in the axial skeleton, particularly in the vertebrae. The median age at presentation is 60 years and a monoclonal protein may be present, although at a level lower than is usual in myeloma.[1,24,43] Full clinical staging is required in order to differentiate solitary plasmacytoma from MM and reveals a negative skeletal survey, absence of clonal plasma cells on BM examination, and lack of anemia, hypercalcemia or renal involvement.

Pathology

Biopsy of the lesion demonstrates an infiltration of clonal PC. Histologic examination of the PB or BM should reveal no evidence of plasmacytosis, although more sensitive techniques such as flow cytometry and PCR may detect low levels of abnormal clonal cells.

Treatment/management/disease progression

The treatment of choice is radiotherapy. Local control is achieved in 90% of patients, with an accompanying fall in paraprotein level. The majority of patients do develop myeloma over time, with projected 5- and 10-year probabilities of 50% and 75% respectively. Magnetic resonance imaging (MRI) has revealed unsuspected bone lesions in approximately 30% of patients, and there is a suggestion that this technique may be able to distinguish patients who will progress to MM from patients with a more benign clinical course.[44] Other potential prognostic markers include an abnormal serum free light chain ratio and the persistence of the serum monoclonal band for more than a year post radiotherapy.[45,46] There is no definitive evidence that systemic treatment delays the onset of myeloma.

Extramedullary plasmacytoma

Clinical features

Isolated extramedullary plasmacytoma may also occur.[1,47,48] Over 80% of lesions are in the upper respiratory tract and present with epistaxis, nasal discharge, hoarseness or sore throat. Lesions may also occur in the gastrointestinal tract, thyroid, thymus and skin (Fig. 30.10A, B). Twenty-five per cent of patients will have a monoclonal protein present in the serum or urine. It is important to distinguish patients with solitary extramedullary plasmacytoma from patients with soft tissue spread of advanced myeloma due to differences in the clinical disease course.

Pathology

Lesions are characteristically submucosal and contain a neoplastic clonal PC infiltrate. Some lesions reflect marginal cell lymphoma which have undergone extensive plasma cell differentiation.

Treatment/management/disease progression

For solitary extramedullary plasmacytoma, radiotherapy is the treatment of choice and is associated with a less than 5% risk of local recurrence. This risk is further decreased if adjacent lymph nodes are included in the radiation field. Disease progression may occasionally occur either to myeloma with

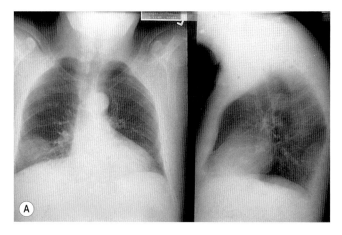

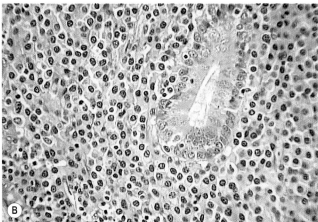

Fig. 30.10 (A, B) (A) Soft tissue plasmacytoma in a patient with end-stage disease with corresponding PA and lateral chest radiograph. (B) Isolated plasmacytoma of small intestine.

typical bone lesions, plasmacytosis and monoclonal protein, or to a disease characterized by multiple extramedullary lesions with no bone marrow plasmacytosis.

POEMS syndrome

The acronym polyneuropathy (P), organomegaly (O), endocrinopathy (E), M-protein (M) and skin changes (S) describes a syndrome associated with plasma cell disorders, particularly but not exclusively osteosclerotic myeloma.[1,49,50] Although extremely rare, it is most frequently reported in Japanese males. A monoclonal protein is demonstrable in the plasma or urine in 75% of patients, usually of IgAl isotype. Clinical features include a demyelinating and axonal mixed neuropathy (more motor than sensory); hepatomegaly, splenomegaly and lymphadenopathy; diabetes mellitus, primary gonadal failure, hypothyroidism and Addison's disease; and skin hyperpigmentation, thickening and hypertrichosis. Sixty per cent of patients will have pathologic changes consistent with multiple myeloma, although the extent of BM infiltration by plasma cells may be low. The increase in PC is usually associated with osteosclerosis. Lymph node involvement is common, and pathologic features resemble the hyaline-vascular variant of Castleman's

disease with follicular hyperplasia, vascular proliferation and an interfollicular infiltration of lymphocytes, plasma cells and immunoblasts. The pathogenesis is not well understood but the overproduction of VEGF secreted by PC is likely to be responsible for the characteristic symptoms. The median survival depends on the pattern of organ involvement and ranges from 2 to 10 years. Treatment is of the underlying plasma cell disorder.

Lymphoproliferative disorders associated with an IgM paraprotein

Waldenström's macroglobulinemia (WM) is a chronic B-cell lymphoproliferative disorder in which most of the clinical manifestations are due to the presence of an IgM paraprotein. The disorder is characterized by bone marrow infiltration with small lymphocytes, lymphoplasmacytoid cells and plasma cells, and a high level of IgM paraprotein. The World Health Organization (WHO) classification considers WM as a clinical syndrome associated with the diagnosis of lymphoplasmacytoid lymphoma/immunocytoma.[1] The morphologic and immunophenotypic features are described in Chapter 29. However, the presence of an IgM paraprotein is not specific for WM. The differential diagnosis includes other indolent lymphoproliferative disorders, for example chronic lymphocytic leukemia (CLL) with IgM paraprotein, splenic lymphoma with villous lymphocytes (SLVL), and splenic marginal zone lymphoma (SMZL).[51,52] Differences in the level of paraprotein, lymphocytic morphology, and degree of marrow involvement in relation to spleen size may help to distinguish WM from SLVL and SMZL, since the malignant cells within these disorders share the same phenotype. Other conditions associated with an IgM paraprotein include MGUS and, rarely, true IgM myeloma.

Biology

Sequence analysis of the immunoglobulin heavy-chain gene demonstrates the presence of somatic mutations within the variable region without intraclonal diversity, suggesting that the malignant cell of origin has traversed the germinal center. Complex abnormal karyotypes have been described, including structural aberrations of 6q and 11q. Although there is no characteristic translocation, a t(9;14)(p13;q32) has been described in which the *PAX-5* gene, which encodes for a B-cell-specific transcription factor, is juxtaposed to the immunoglobulin heavy-chain locus.

Clinical features

WM is 10–20% less common than multiple myeloma. It is predominantly a disease of the elderly, with a median age at presentation of 65 years. It is more common in white people than black people, with a slight male predominance. Symptoms may occur due to tumor cell infiltration of BM (cytopenia, increased infections and bleeding), splenomegaly, hepatomegaly and lymphadenopathy.[51] Other clinical features include hyperviscosity in 20% of patients and type 1 cryoglobulinemia, although clinically relevant cryoglobulinemia causing Raynaud's phenomenon, purpura and glomerulonephritis occurs in less than 5% of patients. Cold

Table 30.6 Types of systemic amyloid

Amyloid type	Association with plasma cell disorder	Precursor protein	Clinical presentation
Light chain (AL)	Yes	Kappa or lambda light chains	Cardiac, renal, hepatic, GI, PNS, soft tissue
Transthyretin (ATTR)	No	Mutant transthyretin	Cardiac, PNS
Senile systemic (SAA)	No	Wild type transthyretin	Cardiac, pulmonary, PNS
Amyloid A (AA)	No	Serum amyloid A	Renal
Fibrinogen (A Fib)	No	Mutant fibrinogen A alpha	Renal, hepatic
Apolipoprotein A1 (Apo-A1)	No	Apolipoprotein A1	Cardiac, renal, hepatic, GI, PNS, skin

GI, gastrointestinal; PNS, peripheral nervous system.

agglutinin anemia may occur in 10% of patients when the monoclonal IgM behaves as a cold reactive antibody that interacts with erythrocyte antigens at low temperatures and results in the development of acrocyanosis, Raynaud's phenomenon, and episodic or chronic hemolysis. Neurological manifestations are present in 10% of patients related to infiltration of peripheral nerves with paraprotein, antibodies against various glycoproteins and glycolipids of the peripheral nerves, and amyloid deposition. In contrast to other plasma cell disorders, there is an absence of bony changes and lytic lesions. Occasionally, renal involvement may be present, due either to glomerular abnormalities or to amyloid deposition resulting in a non-selective proteinuria. Diagnosis requires the presence of an IgM paraprotein in the serum and the infiltration of characteristic cells within the BM (see Chapter 29). As in myeloma, the presence of an IgM paraprotein may be an incidental finding, and the distinction between MGUS and WM is often controversial. MGUS is defined as IgM paraprotein <3 g/dl associated with no constitutional symptoms, organomegaly or anemia. Approximately 10% of patients with MGUS will develop WM at a median follow-up of 8 years.[52] The International Prognostic Staging System for WM (IPSSWM) defines three prognostic groups for patients based on five adverse features (age, hemoglobin, platelets, β2m and level of monoclonal protein).[53] The low risk group is characterized by age less than 65 years and the presence of one adverse feature, whereas the high risk group is characterized by two or more adverse features. The 5-year survival rates are 87%, 68% and 38% respectively.

Treatment/management

Patients with disease related symptoms require treatment. The initiation of therapy should not be based on the level of serum paraprotein alone and asymptomatic patients should be observed. The appropriate choice of therapy depends on a number of patient-related factors including the presence of cytopenias, need for rapid disease control, age and comorbidities.[54,55] Initial management includes the correction of the raised plasma viscosity using plasmapheresis. This treatment is offered as a short-term measure while concomitant chemotherapy to reduce the tumor burden becomes effective. Combination chemotherapy includes the use of alkylating agents, nucleoside analogs and/or rituximab. Patients in resistant relapse are candidates for treatment with novel therapeutic agents.

Disease progression

The majority of patients die from infection, bone marrow failure or progressive disease that has become resistant to treatment. Approximately 20% of patients will die from an incidental cause. In a minority of patients, WM may transform into a high-grade B-cell lymphoma (similar to Ritcher's syndrome in CLL), characterized by unexplained fever, weight loss, rapidly enlarging lymph nodes, extranodal involvement and a reduction in IgM consistent with tumor dedifferentiation. The outcome for these patients is extremely poor.

Light-chain-associated amyloidosis

Amyloidosis is a spectrum of diseases associated with the deposition of extracellular protein in major organs to form characteristic fibrillar sheets that disrupt organ structure and function. Light-chain amyloid (AL), previously called primary amyloid, is characterized by the extracellular deposition of fibrillar protein derived from monoclonal light chains. The light chains are cleaved into fragments that consist of the whole or part of the variable domain of the molecule, although occasionally intact light chains may also be deposited. The fragments form beta-pleated sheets which become insoluble and resistant to degradation following the deposition of glycosaminoglycans and the normal protein serum amyloid P component (SAP). A number of other types of proteins may also be deposited; however, these types of amyloid are not associated with plasma cell abnormalities. The proteins deposited include mutant or wild type transthyretin, the circulating acute phase reactant protein serum amyloid A, and apolipoprotein A1 (Table 30.6).[1,56–58]

Biology

The exact reason for the deposition of protein is unknown, although it is thought that the aberrant structure of the light chain confers the amyloidogenic potential. Mouse studies demonstrate that repeated injections of immunoglobulin from amyloid patients lead to the development of amyloid deposits within the mouse, whereas injections of immunoglobulins from myeloma patients result in no deposits. Many of the genetic abnormalities seen in myeloma are also present in AL amyloid, although the incidence of t(11;14) is higher (30–40%) and is associated with the production of clonal free light chains without the production of intact immunoglobulin.

Clinical features

This is a rare disorder with an annual incidence of 3000 cases in the US. The clinical features depend on the spectrum of organ involvement, with the most commonly affected organs being the heart, kidneys and peripheral nerves. At diagnosis 30% of patients will have more than three organs involved whereas the majority will have only one or two organ involvement. Cardiac features are present in one-third of patients at diagnosis and include cardiomegaly, restrictive cardiomyopathy, cardiac failure and arrhythmias. Renal features include nephrotic syndrome and renal failure. Forty per cent of patients have carpal tunnel syndrome, and peripheral neuropathy is present in 20%. Other features include macroglossia (infrequent but pathognomonic), gastrointestinal malabsorption, hepatosplenomegaly, and skin involvement including papular and nodular lesions and characteristic purpura around the eyes. Rarely, deficiency in factor IX and X may be present, resulting in bleeding disorders due to the binding of calcium-dependent clotting factors to the amyloid deposits. A monoclonal component is present in the serum or urine in 65% and 86% of cases respectively. Immunofixation or serum free light chain assessment is often required to demonstrate the presence of the clone. The monoclonal component may be either κ or λ light chains, although the majority are λ (4:1). Amyloid may occur as a long-term complication of most clonal B-cell disorders, especially myeloma (15%) and less commonly WM.

Pathology

The peripheral blood picture is usually normal, although Howell–Jolly bodies are present in 25% of cases suggesting hyposplenism due to amyloid infiltration of spleen. A low-level plasmacytosis is present on the BM aspirate, and in some cases PC may account for more than 20% of the total nucleated cells. Even if the PC number is normal there is often an imbalance in κ:λ ratio suggesting the presence of abnormal cells, and immunoglobulin heavy chain PCR will confirm a clonal picture. When amyloid occurs in association with WM, lymphoplasmacytoid cells will be present. The bone biopsy reveals similar findings to those in the aspirate, but in addition demonstrates amyloid deposits within the small blood vessel walls or extravascularly. Examination with bipolarized light following staining with Congo red demonstrates apple green birefringence. This is pathognomonic for light-chain amyloid and is the standard for diagnosis. Amyloid also stains metachromically with crystal violet, fluoresces after staining with thioflavine-T, and is pink and homogenous on H&E staining (Fig. 30.11 A–D). Immunohistochemistry staining for fibrinogen may also be useful. Light-chain amyloid may be distinguished from other types of amyloid immunochemically using type-specific

anti-light-chain sera, although this may be negative since a number of antibodies react with parts of the molecule that have been degraded during formation of the protein deposit. It may also be distinguished from other types of amyloid, as there is no abolition of Congo red staining by prior treatment with potassium permanganate. As immunohistochemistry staining for amyloid typing is unreliable immunogold electron microscopy may be required. The characteristic amyloid deposition can be demonstrated in all affected organs on biopsy (Fig. 30.11E). If biopsy of the primary organ is dangerous, then a fine-needle aspirate of abdominal fat, or a gingiva or rectal biopsy are less invasive ways to demonstrate the presence of disease and are commonly positive (80% of cases). Scintigraphy using radio-labeled SAP is useful to determine the extent of disease and organ involvement.

Treatment/management

Supportive therapy is directed toward alleviating symptoms and improving the function of affected organs (i.e. controlling heart failure, renal failure). Specific treatment is also required to reduce or eliminate the plasma cell clone, as the amyloid deposition may regress when the primary source of protein is removed. Oral melphalan and dexamethasone or high dose melphalan and stem cell transplant are considered the standard therapies for AL amyloid.[58,59] Owing to an increased risk of peri-transplant related mortality (10–25%), current guidelines suggest that this therapy should be offered only to patients with less than three-organ involvement and reasonable cardiac function. Given the impressive improvement in response rates and survival with the introduction of novel therapies in myeloma, ongoing studies are investigating the potential use of thalidomide, lenalidomide and bortezomib in amyloid.[60,61] Splenectomy may be helpful in ameliorating coagulation deficiencies and patients with predominantly cardiac or renal involvement should be considered for organ transplantation.

Disease progression

Because amyloid is deposited in key viscera, such as the heart and liver, the disease may progress rapidly. The median survival of untreated patients is 12–15 months, with 50% of deaths occurring from a cardiac cause. The two critical determinants in survival are the presence and extent of heart involvement and response to therapy. With minimal organ involvement and a good response to therapy median survivals of up to 5 years have been reported; however, if the heart is the main affected organ then the median survival is only 6 months. Other poor prognostic variables include renal failure, jaundice and large total body amyloid deposition demonstrated by SAP scintigraphy.

Heavy-chain disorders

This group of rare plasma cell disorders is characterized by the production of a monoclonal Ig that is formed from truncated heavy chains with no associated light chains.[1,62–64] The diagnosis depends on the detection of structurally abnormal immunoglobulin in patient serum or urine which

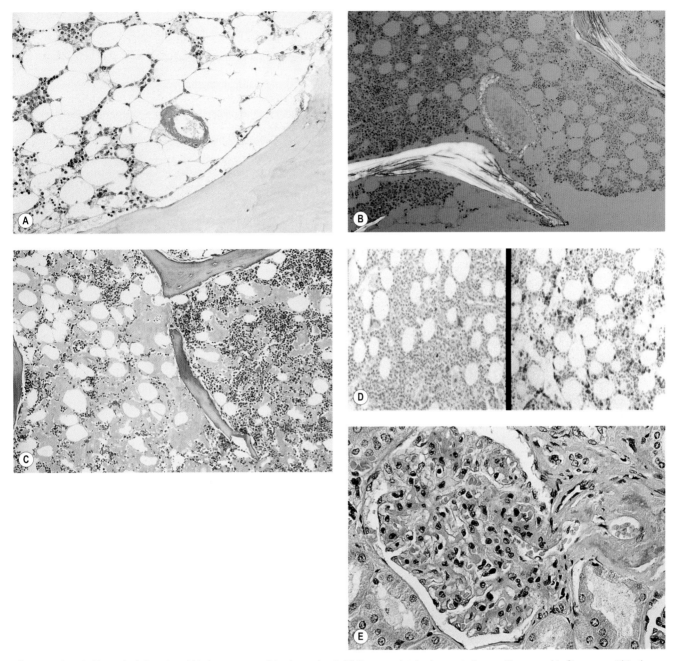

Fig. 30.11 (A–E) (A) Amyloid deposits within bone marrow blood vessel wall. (B) Congo red stain demonstrating positive green birefringence within the blood vessel wall. (C) Interstitial amyloid. (D) Immunohistochemistry demonstrating monoclonal lambda positive plasma cells. (E) Renal amyloid.

consists mainly of the Fc region of the molecule. The actual length of the chain varies between patients but is usually one-half to three-quarters of the normal counterpart, with the majority of cases having complete deletion of the $C_{H}1$ domain. The mechanisms leading to the production of the abnormal protein are not clearly understood. The analysis of rearranged gene sequences demonstrates a high level of somatic mutation with deletions and insertions of sequences of unknown origin. This suggests that cells producing the abnormal heavy chains arise during somatic hypermutation in the germinal center, and that further genetic alterations are required at a later stage in the developmental process for malignant transformation to occur. The abnormal Ig is not evident by serum electrophoresis in a high proportion of cases, and identification may therefore require more sensitive techniques. The presenting clinical features depend on the type of heavy chain involved.

α-Heavy-chain disease

α-Heavy-chain disease predominantly affects the bowel and is associated with the production of the heavy chain of IgA, usually α1 subtype that forms polymers that are secreted into the serum and bowel lumen. It is a variant of extranodal marginal zone lymphoma of mucosal associated lymphoid tissue (MALT).

Clinical features

Over 400 cases have been reported to date with the majority from the Mediterranean or the Middle East.[65] Presentation is usually in the third decade of life with a slight male predominance. Environmental factors in early infancy are important in the etiology of the disease, especially low socioeconomic status and poor hygiene leading to the development of recurrent infectious diarrhea and chronic parasitic infections. The main clinical features include diarrhea, weight loss, abdominal pain, vomiting and evidence of malabsorption. Abdominal masses may also be present. Occasionally, the disease may present with respiratory symptoms due to infiltrations in the respiratory tract.

Pathology

Intestinal lesions characteristically affect segments of the duodenum and the jejunum with no intervening normal mucosa. Initially a plasmacytic or lymphoplasmacytic infiltrate involving the mucosal lamina propria is present (stage A). With disease progression atypical cells extend to the submucosa, and villous atrophy may occur (stage B). Some cases evolve into large cell lymphoma of immunoblastic type (stage C) which may present as discrete ulcerating tumors or extensive infiltrates of long segments of bowel wall. The mesenteric lymph nodes are usually involved. Infiltration of the BM, liver and spleen is rare, but may occur with stage C disease. A mild to moderate anemia may be present due to the malabsorption of iron, folate and vitamin B_{12}.

Treatment/management/disease progression

In the absence of therapy, the disease is generally progressive with the initial benign lesions evolving into immunoblastic lymphoma. In early stage disease treatment with antibiotics (metronidazole and ampicillin) results in complete clinical, histologic and immunologic remission in about 40% of patients, supporting the hypothesis of an underlying infectious etiology. CHOP-based chemotherapy regimens are recommended for more advanced disease, although the median overall survival is poor.

γ-Heavy-chain disease

γ-Heavy-chain disease (γHCD) is a heterogeneous group of disorders and presents with a variety of clinical and pathologic features that are characterized by the secretion of abnormal IgG heavy chains. It is an extremely rare disorder with only 100 cases reported in the literature.

Clinical features

γHCD predominantly occurs in black and Asian people with a median age at presentation of 60 years, although a number of cases have been reported in children. The clinical features include lymphadenopathy, hepatomegaly and splenomegaly with associated constitutional symptoms such as weight loss and fever. Autoimmune disorders occur frequently and include rheumatoid arthritis, systemic lupus erythematosus, vasculitis and myasthenia gravis.

Pathology

There is no consistent morphologic pattern corresponding to the serologic diagnosis of γHCD.[66] The BM is usually infiltrated with lymphocytes, lymphoplasmacytoid cells or plasma cells. Lymph node biopsy may show evidence of a lymphoplasmacytic proliferation, a PC infiltrate, or non-Hodgkin's lymphoma. Unusual pathologic features include eosinophils or multinucleated giant cells, suggesting the presence of an atypical granulomatous lesion. The PB may show evidence of a moderate normochromic normocytic anemia, lymphocytosis with atypical lymphoplasmacytoid cells or plasma cells, and eosinophilia.

Treatment/management/disease progression

The clinical disease course varies. If the abnormal heavy chain is an incidental finding, then no therapy is required. For symptomatic patients therapy with agents that are active in other plasma cell disorders should be utilized.

μ-Heavy-chain disease

This type of heavy-chain disease is extremely rare, with only 29 cases reported worldwide. It is characterized by the secretion of abnormal heavy chains of IgM and is usually associated with the presence of other lymphoproliferative disorders, particularly CLL and less commonly WM and myeloma.

Clinical features

Presenting features include hepatomegaly, splenomegaly and abdominal lymphadenopathy. Unlike other types of heavy-chain disorders, light-chain secretion may also occur and give rise to an amyloid-like picture.

Pathology

The majority of patients have morphologic and phenotypic features indistinguishable from CLL on peripheral blood smear. A lymphocytosis or plasmacytosis is present within the BM. If present, PC are characteristically vacuolated.

Treatment/management/disease progression

The mainstay of treatment is therapy directed at the underlying lymphoproliferative disorder.

Cryoglobulinemia

The presence of an underlying plasma cell disorder may lead to the development of cryoglobulinemia. In type I cryoglobulinemia the paraprotein secreted, usually IgG or IgM, has the characteristics of a cryoglobulin. In type II and type III cryoglobulinemia the paraprotein, usually IgM, has antibody activity against another immunoglobulin, often polyclonal IgG, and results in immune complex formation. In 75% of patients, no pathologic manifestations other than those due to the characteristic of the immunoglobulin are present at the time of diagnosis and the term 'essential cryoglobulinemia' is appropriate.[67] Over a 10-year period of follow-up, approximately 25% of patients will develop symptoms and signs associated with a lymphoproliferative disorder. In the remaining 25% of cases, the cryoglobulinemia is a manifestation of an overt lymphoproliferative disorder including myeloma, WM, immunocytoma, MALT lymphoma and follicular lymphoma. In this subset of patients 25% will have type I, 70% type II and 5% type III cryoglobulinemia.

Clinical features

The clinical features depend on the type of cryoglobulin formed and result from either the precipitation of the Ig at reduced body temperatures or to the deposition of immune complexes in major organs or the periphery. The most common presenting features include vasculitis of the skin, arthralgia, peripheral neuropathy, proliferative glomerulonephritis and hepatitis.

Pathology

The peripheral blood film is usually normal. In a minority of cases a cryoglobulin precipitate is present, usually demonstrable as a weakly basophilic globular mass, less often as crystals or a fibrillar deposit. Occasionally, cryoglobulin precipitates are ingested by neutrophils or monocytes and are seen as globular, variably basophillic intracytoplasmic inclusions. Within the BM a lymphocytosis is common in essential cryoglobulinemia, and in up to 40% of cases clonality can be demonstrated using either immunohistochemistry or flow cytometry. In cases associated with an underlying lymphoproliferative disorder, the histologic features of that disorder will dominate. On biopsy of the kidney, membranoproliferative glomerulonephritis (60%) and mesangial proliferative glomerulonephritis (20%) can be demonstrated. Chronic active hepatitis with periportal lymphoid infiltrates is often present on liver biopsy.

Treatment/management/disease progression

Cytotoxic therapy including cyclophosphamide and steroids, along with plasmapheresis is the mainstay of treatment for symptomatic essential cryoglobulinemia. More recently rituximab has been shown to be effective for resistant cases. If an underlying lymphoproliferative disorder is present, then therapy must be directed at reducing tumor-cell burden.

Acknowledgments

We are extremely grateful to Dr Arthur Skarin (Dana Farber Cancer Institute, Boston, USA), Dr Carl O'Hara, (Boston, Boston Medical Center, USA), Dr Andrew Jack (Hematological Malignancy Diagnostic Service, Leeds General Infirmary, Leeds, UK), Dr Neil Rabin, (University College Hospital, London, UK) and Dr Brian Walker (Institute of Cancer Research, London, UK) for the illustrations.

References

1. McKenna RW, Kyle RA, Khuel WM, et al. cell neoplasms. In: Swerdlow SH, Campo C, Harris NL, et al, editors. WHO classification of tumours of haematopoietic and lymphoid tissues. Lyon: IARC; 2008. p. 194–5.

2. Morgan GJ, Davies FE, Linet M. Myeloma aetiology and epidemiology. Biomedicine and Pharmacotherapy 2002;56:223–34.

3. Davies FE, Avet-Loiseau H, Bergsagel PL. Epidemiology, etiology and molecular pathogenesis. In: Richardson P, editor. Multiple Myeloma: State of the Art. Remedica, London; 2010.

4. Bakkus, MHC, Heirman C, Van Riet I, et al. Evidence that multiple myeloma Ig heavy chain VDJ genes contain somatic mutations but show no intraclonal variation. Blood 1992;80:2326–35.

5. Sahota SS, Leo R, Hamblin TJ, et al. Ig VH gene mutational patterns indicate different tumour cell status in human myeloma and monoclonal gammopathy of undetermined significance. Blood 1996;87:746–55.

6. Teoh G, Anderson KC. Interaction of tumour and host cells with adhesion and extracellular matrix molecules in the development of multiple myeloma. Hematology and Oncology Clinics of North America 1997;11:27–42.

7. Podar K, Chauhan D, Anderson KC. Bone marrow microenvironment and the identification of new targets for myeloma therapy. Leukemia 2009;23:10–24.

8. Hideshima T, Mitsiades C, Tonon G, et al. Understanding multiple myeloma pathogenesis in the bone marrow to identify new therapeutic targets. Nature Cancer Reviews 2007;7:585–98.

9. Podar K, Hideshima T, Chauhan D, et al. Targeting signaling pathways for the treatment of mulitple myeloma. Expert Opinions in Therapeutic Targets 2005; 9:359–81.

10. Annunziata CM, Davis RE, Demchenko Y, et al. Frequent engagement of the classical and alternative NFkappaB pathways by diverse genetic abnormalities in multiple myeloma. Cancer Cell 2007;12:115–30.

11. Keats JJ, Fonesca R, Chesi M, et al. Promiscuous mutations activate the noncanonical NFkappaB pathways in multiple myeloma. Cancer Cell 2007; 12:131–44.

12. Fonseca R, Bergsagel PL, Drach J, et al. International Myeloma Working Group molecular classification of multiple myeloma: spotlight review. Leukemia 2009;23:2210–21.

13. Bergsagel PL, Kuehl WM, Zhan F, et al. Cyclin D dysregulation: an early and unifying pathogenic event in multiple myeloma. Blood 2005;106:296–303.

14. Walker BA, Morgan GJ. Use of single nucleotide polymorphism-based mapping arrays to detect copy number changes and loss of heterozygosity in multiple myeloma. Clinical Lymphoma and Myeloma 2006;7:186–91.

15. Smith E, Boyd K, Davies FE. The potential role of epigenetic therapy in multiple myeloma. British Journal of Haematology 2010;148:702–13.

16. Chesi M, Nardini E, Brents LA, et al. Frequent translocation t(4;14) (p16.3;q32.3) in multiple myeloma: association with increased expression and activating mutations of fibroblast growth factor receptor 3. Nature Genetics 1997;16:260–4.

17. Dring AM, Davies FE, Fenton JAL, et al. A global expression based analysis of the consequences of the t(4;14) in myeloma. Clinical Cancer Research 2004;10: 5692–701.

18. Robillard N, Avet-Loiseau H, Garand R, et al. CD20 is associated with a small mature plasma cell morphology and t(11;14) in multiple myeloma. Blood 2003;102:1070–1.

19. Feyler S, O'Connor SJ, Rawstron AC, et al. IgM myeloma: a rare entity characterised

by a CD20-CD56-CD117- immunophenotype and the t(11;14). British Journal of Haematology 2008;140:545–51.

20. Avet-Loiseau H, Attal M, Moreau P, et al. Genetic abnormalities and survival in multiple myeloma: the experience of the Intergroupe Francophone du Myélome. Blood 2007;109:3489–95.

21. Avet-Loiseau H, Li C, Magrangeas F, et al. Prognostic significance of copy-number alterations in multiple myeloma. Journal of Clinical Oncology 2009;27:4585–90.

22. AJ Ashcroft, FE Davies, GJ Morgan. Aetiology of bone disease and the role of bisphosphonates in multiple myeloma. Lancet Oncology 2003;4:284–92.

23. Lentzsch S, Ehrlich LA, Roodman GD. Pathophysiology of multiple myeloma bone disease. Hematology and Oncology Clinics of North America 2007;21: 1035–49.

24. Kyle RA, Child JA, Anderson KC, et al. Criteria for the classification of monoclonal gammopathies, multiple myeloma and related disorders: a report of the International Myeloma Working Group. British Journal of Haematology, 2003;121:749–57.

25. Greipp PR, San Miguel Dure BGM, et al. International staging system for multiple myeloma. Journal of Clinical Oncology 2005;23:3412–20..

26. Rawstron AC, Owen RG, Davies FE, et al. Circulating plasma cells in multiple myeloma: characterisation and correlation with disease status. British Journal of Haematology 1997;97:46–55.

27. Mateo G, Montalban MA, Vidriales MB, et al. Prognostic value of immunophenotyping in multiple myeloma: a study by the PETHEMA/GEM cooperative study groups on patients uniformly treated with high-dose therapy. Journal of Clinical Oncology 2008;26:2737–44.

28. Durie BGM, Harousseau JL, Miguel JS, et al. International uniform response criteria for multiple myeloma. Leukemia 2006;20(9):1467–73.

29. Raab MS, Podar K, Breitkreutz I, et al. Multiple myeloma. Lancet 2009;374: 324–39.

30. Weber DM, Chen C, Niesvizky R, et al. Lenalidomide plus dexamethasone for relapsed multiple myeloma in North America. New England Journal of Medicine 2007;357:2133–42.

31. Dimopoulos M, Spencer A, Attal M, et al. Lenalidomide plus dexamethasone for relapsed or refractory multiple myeloma. New England Journal of Medicine 2007; 357:2123–32.

32. Richardson PG, Sonneveld P, Schuster MW, et al. Bortezomib or high-dose dexamethasone for relapsed multiple myeloma. New England Journal of Medicine 2005;352:2487–98.

33. Singhal S, Mehta J, Desikan R, et al. Antitumor activity of thalidomide in refractory multiple myeloma. New England Journal of Medicine 1999; 18:1565–71.

34. Hideshima T, Chauhan D, Shima Y, et al. Thalidomide and its analogues overcome drug resistance of human multiple myeloma cells to conventional therapy. Blood 2000;96:2943–50.

35. Hideshima T, Richardson P, Chauhan D, et al. The proteasome inhibitor PS-341 inhibits growth, induces apoptosis, and overcomes drug resistance in human multiple myeloma cells. Cancer Research 2001;61:3071–6.

36. Kyle RA, Therneau TM, Rajkumar SV, et al. Prevalence of monoclonal gammopathy of undetermined significance. New England Journal of Medicine 2006;354:1362–9.

37. Kyle RA, Rajkumar SV. Monoclonal gammopathy of undetermined significance. British Journal of Haematology 2006;134:573–80.

38. Landgren O, Kyle RA, Pfeiffer RM, et al. Monoclonal gammopathy of undetermined significance (MGUS) consistently precedes multiple myeloma: a prospective study. Blood 2009;113: 5412–7.

39. Rajkumar SV, Kyle RA, Therneau TM, et al. Serum free light chain ratio is an independent risk factor for progression in MGUS. Blood 2005;106:812–7.

40. Ramsingh G, Mehan P, Luo J, et al. Primary plasma cell leukemia: a surveillance, epidemiology, and end results database analysis between 1973 and 2004. Cancer 2009;115:5734–9.

41. Garcia-Sanz R, Orfao A, Gonzalez M, et al. Primary plasma cell leukemia: clinical, immunophenotypic, DNA ploidy and cytogenetic characteristics. Blood 1999; 93:1032–7.

42. Tiedemann RE, Gonzalez-Paz N, Kyle RA, et al. Genetic aberrations and survival in plasma cell leukemia. Blood 2008;22: 1044–52.

43. British Committee for Standards in Haematology. Guidelines on the diagnosis and management of solitary plasmacytoma of bone and solitary extramedullary plasmacytoma. British Journal of Haematology 2004;124: 717–26.

44. Moulopouos LA, Dimopoulos MA, Weber D, et al. Magnetic resonance imaging in the staging of solitary plasmacytoma of bone. Journal of Clinical Oncology 1993;11:1311–5.

45. Dingli D, Kyle RA, Rajkumar S, et al. Immunoglobulin free light chains and solitary plasmacytoma of bone. Blood 2006;108:1979–83.

46. Ozsahin M, Tsang R, et al. Outcomes and patterns of failure in solitary plasmacytoma. International Journal of Radiation Oncology 2006;64:210–7.

47. Dimopoulos MA, Kiamouris C, Moulopoulos LA. Solitary plasmacytoma of bone and extramedullary plasmacytoma. Hematology and Oncology Clinics of North America 1999;13:1249–57.

48. Knowling MA, Harwood AR, Bergsagel DE. Comparison of extramedullary plasmacytomas with solitary and multiple plasma cell tumors of bone. Journal of Clinical Oncology 1983;1:255–62.

49. Dispenzieri A, Kyle RA, Lacy MQ, et al. POEMS syndrome: definitions and long term outcome. Blood 2003;101: 2496–506.

50. Dispenzieri A. POEMS syndrome. Blood Reviews 2007;21:285–99.

51. Dimopoulos MA, Panayiotidis P, Moulopoulos LA, et al. Waldenstroms macroglobulinemia: clinical features, complications and management. Journal of Clinical Oncology 2000;18:214–26.

52. Kyle RA, Garton JP. The spectrum of IgM monoclonal gammopathy in 430 cases. Mayo Clinic Proceedings 1987;62: 719–1.

53. Morel P, Duhamel A, Gobbi P, et al. International prognostic scoring system for Waldenström macroglobulinemia. Blood 2009;113:4163–70.

54. Dimopoulos MA, Gertz MA, Kastritis E, et al. Update on treatment recommendations from the fourth international workshop on Waldenström's macroglobulinemia. Journal Clinical Oncology 2009;27:120–6.

55. Treon SP. How I treat Waldenström macroglobulinemia. Blood 2009;114: 2375–85.

56. Gilmore JD, Hawkins PN, Pepys MB. Amyloidosis: a review of recent diagnostic and therapeutic developments. British Journal of Haematology 1997;99: 245–56.

57. Falk RH, Comenzo RL, Skinner M. The systemic amyloidoses. New England Journal of Medicine 1997;337:898–909.

58. Comenzo RL. How I treat amyloidosis. Blood 2009;114:3147–51.

59. Jaccard A, Moreau P, Leblond V, et al. High dose melphalan versus melphalan plus dexamethasone for AL amyloidosis. New England Journal of Medicine 2007;357:1083–93.

60. Dispenzieri A, Lacy MQ, Zeldenrust SR, et al. The activity of lenalidomide with or without dexamethasone in patients with primary systemic amyloidosis. Blood 2007;109:465–70.

61. Kastritis E, Enagnostopoulos A, Roussou M, et al. Treatment of light chain AL amyloidosis with the combination of bortezomib and dexamethasone. Haematologica 2007;92:135–1358.

62. Cogne M, Silvain C, Khamlichi AA, et al. Structurally abnormal immunoglobulins in human immunoproliferative disorders. Blood 1992;79:2181–95.

63. Fermand JP, Brouet JC. Heavy chain diseases. Hematology and Oncology Clinics of North America 1999;13: 1281–94.

64. Seligmann M, Mihaesco E, Preud'homme JL, et al. Heavy chain diseases: current findings and concepts. Immunology Reviews 1979;48:145–67.

65. Rambaud JC, Brouet JC Seligmann M, et al. Alpha chain disease and related lymphoproliferative disorders. In: Ogra P, Mestecky J, Lamm ME, et al, editors. Handbook of Mucosal Immunology. San Diego: Academic Press; 1994. p. 425.

66. Wester SM, Banks PM, Li CY. The histopathology of gamma heavy chain disease. American Journal of Clinical Pathology 1982;78:427–36.

67. Monti G, Galli M, Invernizzi F, et al. Cryoblobulinaemias: a multicentre study of the early clinical and laboratory manifestations of primary and secondary disease. Q J M 1995;88:115–26.

Section E

Abnormalities of hemostasis

CHAPTER 31

Hemostasis: principles of investigation

DH Bevan, B Sørensen

Chapter contents

Introduction

The hemostatic system, a complex defense against bleeding, is critical to survival. Its integrity is compromised by inherited or acquired failure of its individual components, or by deregulation of the entire system provoked by organ failure, the inflammatory response, or exposure to cancer cell surfaces. Hemostasis also acts (in the wrong place, at the wrong time) as thrombosis. Bleeding is always a threat, while thrombosis increases due to age-related changes in coagulation factors and blood vessels to become the dominant hemostatic risk in later life.

The extreme complexity of hemostasis revealed by scientific scrutiny induces a degree of alienation in many clinicians practicing at the bedside and in the operating theatre.

The hematologist must be their translator of basic knowledge into clinically useful advice, and guide to the increasing menu of potent drugs and biological agents available for the therapy of bleeding and thrombosis.

To do this work a reliable toolkit of investigational methods is essential. These include a focused approach to the patient's personal and familial medical history, a set of rapid laboratory tests to indicate the presence and general nature of any hemostatic malfunction, and the ability to extend this inquiry to measurement of specific proteins and analysis of DNA if required. The principle underlying these 'nested' methods of investigation is common to all disciplines in clinical pathology: provide data that increases (or decreases) the likelihood that a particular pathologic state – a diagnosis – is present and needs specific therapy or other intervention.

©2011 Elsevier Ltd
DOI: 10.1016/B978-0-7020-3147-2.00031-6

Hemostatic tests retain unique features and problems in interpretation. Even coagulation screening tests (the only commonly requested tests that require explicit coreporting of control experiments) are complex bioassays in miniature. An abnormal value can have diametrically opposed meanings for patient care depending on the clinical context. Expressing clinical pretest probability in an intelligible way and using test results to modify this probability is the best way of avoiding potential confusion and error.[1]

The application of meta-analysis of randomized studies ('evidence-based medicine') to diagnostic laboratory testing has been limited,[2] and hemostatic testing is no exception. It is therefore not possible yet to claim evidence-based validation, in its strict sense, for many of the principles discussed below. However, the writings of many expert clinician–scientists over the years are the best guide we have to these principles, and should certainly form a starting-point for further analyses.

Physiology of hemostasis applied to diagnosis

The clinical approach to the patient who may have a hemostatic disorder is informed by knowledge of the physiology of hemostasis. Hemostatic reactions operate in a clock-like sequence, the first two phases being termed 'primary' and 'secondary' hemostasis.

A careful clinical history and examination (see below) can tentatively locate the potential defect in one of these phases, guiding the selection of initial investigations. The pretest probability of a defect involving primary hemostasis rises if abnormal bleeding follows a 'mucosal' pattern (see below), while a history of muscle or joint bleeding increases the likelihood of a coagulation deficiency. Disorders of the regulatory protein C pathway tend to manifest as venous thromboembolism. Abnormalities of the final phase of hemostasis, fibrinolysis, tend to contribute to bleeding in specific clinical settings, for example disseminated intravascular coagulation (DIC) and hepatic failure.

To assist this diagnostic thinking, it helps to keep in mind a simplified map of the hemostatic system, whatever knowledge of its complexity one possesses (or not, as the case may be). These simple maps are caricatures: readers are referred to fuller versions[3,4] and to other chapters in this volume.

Primary hemostasis: formation of the platelet plug[5] (Fig. 31.1)

Platelets, highly structured and excitable anucleate cellular bodies, circulate in the blood at a concentration of $150–400 \times 10^9/l$.

Platelet adhesion

Vessel wall damage provokes a variety of signals from damaged or activated vascular endothelial cells and/or exposure of the underlying subendothelial matrix. Platelets first adhere to the signaling site via adhesive ligands. The dominant interaction is between platelet membrane receptor glycoprotein Ib-IX and the giant polymer von Willebrand factor (vWF), particularly its most adhesive high molecular weight forms.

Platelet aggregation

Adherent platelets flatten and activate membrane fibrinogen receptors (glycoprotein IIb-IIIa) that bind plasma fibrinogen (Fb). The resulting syncytial platelet aggregate provides a reactive surface composed of platelet membranes. This activated membrane flips inside out, exposing the negatively charged phospholipid, phosphatidylserine (PS). By binding the tenase and prothrombinase complexes, PS allows coagulation reactions to proceed. This altered ('activated') platelet membrane is sometimes termed platelet factor 3.

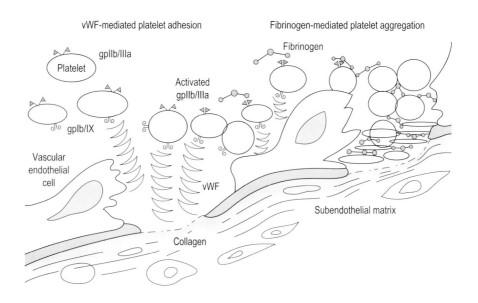

Fig. 31.1 Platelet adhesion and aggregation at sites of vascular damage (schematic).

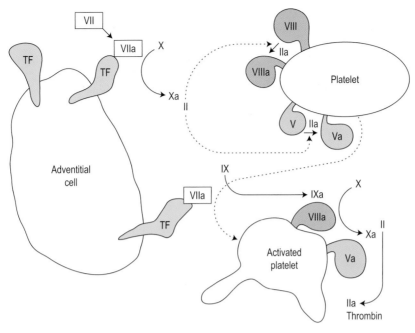

Fig. 31.2 Thrombin generation *in vivo*: coagulation factor interactions mediated by cell surfaces (schematic).

Secondary hemostasis: generation of fibrin clot by the coagulation pathway (Fig. 31.2)

Unless underpinned by a fibrin net, primary platelet plugs disintegrate under the shear stress of flowing blood. The complex coagulation pathway that generates fibrin can be divided into three substages:

Clot initiation: the tissue factor/factor VIIa complex

The receptor tissue factor (TF), exposed on adventitial cells, activated endothelial cells and leukocytes in the damage zone, then binds and activates factor VII. TF/VIIa complexes bind and activate factor X. Resulting FXa moves to the platelet surface.

This is a regulatory 'decision point'. If this burst of FXa cleaves sufficient thrombin from its precursor (prothrombin), thrombin-mediated activation of the co-factors factor VIII and factor V, and the enzyme factor IX – together with recruitment of more thrombin-activated platelets – assemble a 'critical mass' that allows coagulation to proceed. If thrombin generation falls short, tissue factor pathway inhibitor (TFPI) suppresses the TF/VIIa/Xa complex and coagulation is stalled.

Clot amplification: the 'tenase' complex

If the 'decision' is positive, sufficient FVIIIa and FIXa are formed to make the intrinsic tenase complex, in which FVIIIa acts as a rate-enhancing co-factor in the cleavage of FX to FXa by FIXa, providing a sustained source of FXa. The location of this FXa on the platelet surface enables it to move to the nascent prothrombinase complex.

Clot propagation: the prothrombinase complex

The surge of FXa forms prothrombinase complexes with FVa on platelet surfaces, speeding thrombin generation from prothrombin. Thrombin cleaves fibrinogen to form a durable fibrin clot, and binds to it, promoting further clot growth. This is a secure barrier against bleeding.

Clot regulation and removal: the protein C and fibrinolytic pathways

Two further systems regulate and eventually remove the clot (in the context of tissue repair and neoangiogenesis) (also see Chapter 28):

Clot regulation: the protein C system[6] and antithrombin

Thrombin formed around healthy vascular endothelial cells puts a brake on coagulation by binding to a receptor, thrombomodulin, which retargets it to protein C. Thrombin/thrombomodulin activates PC, which inactivates FVa and FVIIIa, slowing thrombin formation. To target FVa and FVIIIa in their membrane complexes, aPC needs a co-factor, protein S.

Thrombin activity is restricted to the platelet surface and the fibrin matrix of the clot by a conformation-dependent inhibitor, antithrombin (AT)[7] that inactivates fluid-phase thrombin. To work efficiently, AT must bind to heparin-like proteoglycans on healthy endothelial cells.

Fibrinolysis: the plasmin system[8]

Clots contain the seeds of their own destruction in the form of a clot-bound protein, plasminogen. This is cleaved by tissue plasminogen activator (tPA) secreted by healthy vascular endothelial cells, or urokinase on the surface of macrophages, to the fibrinolytic enzyme plasmin. Plasmin cleaves fibrin into fibrin degradation products, notably the D-dimer fragment specific to cleavage of cross-linked fibrin.[9] This removes the clot, and activates matrix metalloproteinases that initiate remodeling of vessels (angiogenesis).

One problem in the investigation of coagulation is the artificial nature of available laboratory tests, which commence by separating plasma from the very cell surfaces crucial to *in vivo* hemostasis, particularly platelets. These absent membranes are then simulated by adding back tissue extracts or recombinant proteins with properties similar (but rarely identical) to the physiologic substrates. In addition, as is seen below, the coagulation 'screen' – the crucial bridge between the clinical perception that something is wrong and its laboratory definition – invokes an obsolete model of hemostasis. A clear mental distinction must be made between the current model of *in vivo* hemostasis and the older model applied *in vitro*.

The clinical approach to the patient with a possible hemostatic disorder

> *If you prick us, do we not bleed?*
>
> William Shakespeare, 'The Merchant of Venice', III.i.

The question of a possible hemostatic disorder occurs in two main settings. An individual is referred because they have presented with, or self-reported, clinical phenomena suggesting excess bleeding. Investigation can proceed in a structured elective style. In the second case, excess bleeding occurs acutely in a patient undergoing treatment in the hospital, emergency department or surgical theater. The tempo, urgency and completeness of the diagnostic work-up (before recourse to therapeutic action) are then different, but the principles are shared.

Experts writing about the investigation of possible bleeding disorders unanimously stress the importance of a carefully taken history.[10-12] They also recommend specific questions, answers to which alter the pretest probability of a bleeding disorder. The discussion below draws on this consensus. Similarly, key findings on clinical examination may aid the diagnostic process, although they are less frequent than narrative clues.

It must be conceded that these narrative and clinical signs have not been formally tested, either singly or in clusters, for their relative value in predicting the presence of hemostatic disorders. Such testing has refined and simplified the use of clinical clues in other contexts,[13] and may be of future benefit in hemostasis. Until such clarification becomes available, the shared insight of experienced clinicians is our best guide.

History

The role of the history-taker is to determine if the patient's account is consistent with excessive bleeding. After initial open questioning related to the presenting complaint, a systematic inquiry is made with the help of key questions intended to elicit quantitative information about the bleeding in question. People (including doctors) tend to

1. Q: How much did you bleed?
   A: Loads. A cupful … the pillow was red …
   Q: The whole pillow?
   A: Well, where my mouth was, you know …
2. Q: When was the tooth pulled?
   A: About 3 p.m.
   Q: How long did the bleeding last?
   A: Still going lunchtime the next day.
   Q: What did you do?
   A: I had to go back to the dentist. She put stitches in, but she wasn't happy, so she sent me to hospital …

overestimate, by eye, volumes of blood lost from the body, so it is more informative to focus questioning on the duration of a bleeding episode and what had to be done about it.

Key questions

Surgical challenges

Dental surgery

Surgical trauma to the incompressible tooth socket sitting in the fibrinolytic milieu of the oral cavity is a stiff challenge to the hemostatic system. Useful questions about the effect of extractions focus on the duration of bleeding and the actions compelled by it. Compare the two accounts in Box 31.1. The second account gives a much clearer indication of excessive blood loss. Most people (in the UK, at least) are disinclined to make an early return to the dentist without a pressing reason.

Other types of surgery

Questions about blood loss after circumcision and tonsillectomy are traditional, but the timing and selectivity of the former, and decreasing popularity of the latter, mean that only a small minority of individuals (or their parents) will give a useful response. As in the case of dental extraction, questions should focus on duration of bleeding and subsequent medical actions.

Many individuals are referred for investigation of a possible bleeding disorder as a result of excess blood loss after major surgery, although the commonest cause of this is purely 'surgical' – a transected blood vessel evading the hemostat. Large and/or late wound hematomata or generalized 'oozing' from a tissue surface or organ bed are more likely to indicate a hemostatic disorder. The patient's own recall of these events is likely to be hazy, and documentation of the amount, duration and clinical reaction to peri- and postoperative bleeding should be sought in the patient's medical records.

Epistaxis

Nosebleeds are a universal experience in childhood, so the usefulness of enquiring about them (nearly everyone will recall some) depends on the questions asked. In bleeding disorders, epistaxes tend to run 'like a tap' rather than to drip; require a bowl to catch the blood rather than a tissue; and resist arrest (or reroute via the mouth) on pinching the nares. Frequently recurring epistaxes that provoke multiple nasal cauterizations also increase the possibility of a bleeding disorder.

Gastrointestinal or urogenital bleeding

Rectal bleeding compels a search for colorectal disease even if a systemic bleeding disorder is present. Coumarin-induced rectal bleeding has led to the early detection and cure of cancers. Similar action must follow hematemesis, hematuria or vaginal bleeding. Occasional prolonged episodes of spontaneous hematuria occur in hemophilia, sometimes in mildly affected individuals.

Menstruation

As with other perceptions of bleeding symptoms by both sexes, women accustomed only to their own menstrual loss may not regard it as abnormally heavy. Bleeding for >7 days per month, bleeding that regularly 'breaks through' sanitary protection, the need to wear both tampons and pads (or double pads), and the need to protect the bed with a towel, or to cancel social engagements due to bleeding, are reliable indications of menorrhagia. Questioning should be sensitive and preceded by an explanation of its relevance.

Bruising

A sizeable minority of the population will answer 'yes' to 'do you bruise easily?' and many older people bruise the sun-thinned skin of their hands and forearms, so this question is not helpful. A semi-quantitative approach is useful: the bruises can be compared to some common object (in the UK the 50 pence coin, about 2 cm in diameter). Having frequent bruises larger than this is significant. Most normal ('simple') bruises occur on the outer surfaces of the upper arms and thighs, 'bumpers' in contact with the environment: bruises on the trunk, neck or face, or on the inner aspects of limbs are more significant, as are palpable bruises (hematomata). Solar or simple bruises are rarely pathologic.

A patient complaining of easy bruising who cannot show a single bruise at the time of the consultation, or one who agrees that there are fewer days with bruises than days without,[11] is less likely to have a bleeding disorder. Thrombocytopenic purpura crop around the ankles, where venous pressure is highest, and are more likely to be perceived as 'a rash' than as bruises.

'Third space' bleeds

In the hemophilias (inherited and acquired), over-anticoagulation with heparins or coumarins, and other systemic bleeding disorders, the presenting complaint may be hemorrhage into joints, muscles, or other deep tissue compartments. These events may not be perceived as bleeds by the patient or even by the attending clinical team, since they present with pain, swelling, nerve entrapment or other space-occupying features rather than with evident blood loss. By mimicking tumors, or presenting as acute monoarthritis, they may provoke biopsy or drainage attempts with potentially catastrophic results. In the context of anticoagulant therapy, failure to recognize such bleeds, and consequent 'pushing on' with heparin or warfarin, is equally dangerous.

The first-line clinicians called upon to deal with these events are rarely experienced in their recognition, so the best protection lies in local in-service education and guidelines, together with constant availability of hematologic advice and the freedom to access it.

Summation and duration of bleeding episodes

All types of blood loss should be summated. A patient with a credible history of significant bruising and epistaxis is more likely to have a bleeding disorder than one with bruising alone. Bleeding symptoms that go back to childhood or adolescence are likely to be inherited, and prompt a family history, while if recently developed they point to an acquired cause and a general enquiry for systemic disease.

Pattern of bleeding

A 'mucosal' pattern of bleeding episodes (epistaxis, menorrhagia, bleeding after dental surgery) may guide the initial investigation towards platelet and vWF analysis since it suggests a problem with primary hemostasis. Presentation with hemarthrosis or other third-space bleeds is classical in hemophilia. However, this is hardly a clear distinction, since hemophilia also causes mucosal hemorrhage and dental disasters: stating that menorrhagia is more likely in primary bleeding disorders than in hemophilia is tautologic. In general, it is necessary to perform at least screening tests (see below) of both primary hemostasis and coagulation in people who bleed too much.

Drug history

A full list of all prescribed or over-the-counter medication (including herbal and other complementary medicines) taken by the individual should be compiled. Aspirin remains the most prevalent agent causing bleeding symptoms and abnormal platelet function test results: in addition to being prescribed widely for its antithrombotic effect, it is a component of many preparations on sale to the public. Some of these preparations have names that advertize the presence of aspirin (e.g. Aspro®) while others (e.g. Nurse Sykes' Powders®) do not: a full list of such products is given in the British National Formulary.[14] Other non-steroidal anti-inflammatory agents share the aspirin effect. Antibiotics, major tranquillizers and antidepressive agents may all be associated with bleeding via antiplatelet function effects. Platelet function testing should be performed first with the patient taking the drug, then 2 weeks after stopping, in order to demonstrate its effect.

Family history

A reliable family history entails documenting a pedigree chart including all known family members with their names and dates. The key questions illustrated above are asked about each member in turn, seeking confirmation of any said to have a bleeding tendency. Any described as having hemophilia should, if possible, be traced to the Hemophilia

Center carrying out their care: a relative famous for 'hemophilia' often turns out to have no evidence of the disorder at all.

Taking a family history of this quality is time-consuming, may take more than one session, and suits the elective better than the emergency setting. It often extends the individual's historical knowledge of their family beyond its limit. Furthermore, a negative family history excludes nothing, since many bleeding disorders, including severe hemophilia, occur sporadically.

Clinical examination

Skin

The whole skin surface should be inspected for purpura and bruising, documenting the distribution, size and age of lesions and correlating them with the clinical history. Palpation of bruises will detect hematomata, while palpable purpura suggests vasculitis. Close attention should be paid to the ankles, where venous and capillary pressure is highest: petechiae first appear here in thrombocytopenia, and signs of venous or arterial insufficiency may be evident. Large bruises (ecchymoses) typical of hemophilia or anticoagulant overdose may be found tracking into dependent parts of the body such as the scrotum.

The surface of lesions should be inspected. Edema may indicate the urticarial component of anaphylactoid purpura. Lesions of hereditary hemorrhagic telangiectasia may be seen in finger pulps and ear lobes, spreading over the face in later life. Bruises with abrasions or thermal trauma, that follow the outline of a blunt object, or are associated with other signs of abuse or self-harm may indicate non-accidental injury or factitious bruising.

Scars should be examined. Keloid formation might rule out a skin bleeding time. In Ehlers–Danlos syndrome they pucker like tissue paper on sideways compression, and may show central breakdown with fresh exudation. Poor scar quality may also be seen in hypo- or afibrinogenemia.

Non-hemorrhagic lesions mistaken for signs of bleeding include cherry-red Campbell de Morgan spots, stretch marks, livedo reticularis and Majocchi's purpura or other 'dermatological' purpuras.

Mucosae

The oral cavity should be inspected for the petechiae or 'blood blisters' of 'wet' thrombocytopenia. Gingival bleeding is usually associated with gingivitis. Oral hemorrhage in the hemophilias occurs at sites of minor trauma or dental surgery, and may consist of a small but persistent bleeding point, a friable oozing clot, or a tumor-like sublingual swelling.

Musculoskeletal system

Joints should be examined for warmth, effusion, synovitis, reduced range of movement and misalignment. Muscle groups should be examined for wasting and contractures. These signs of cumulative damage due to hemarthrosis and intramuscular hematomas are characteristic of the hemophilias, but are also seen in rare disorders such as type 3 von Willebrand disease (vWD), deficiency or severe recessive

disorders such as homozygous factor XIII, factor VII or factor X deficiency. Intramedullary hemorrhage of the long bones is a feature of afibrinogenemia and α2-antiplasmin deficiency, both very rare: it mimics lytic bone disease.[15]

Nervous system

Evidence of nerve compression injuries may be evident combined with damage to the musculoskeletal system identified above. Retinoscopy should be performed in all patients with purpura, particularly involving the oral mucosa: retinal hemorrhages indicate active CNS bleeding and the need for urgent therapy.

Active bleeding

The postoperative or traumatized patient with excessive bleeding should be examined for the signs itemized above, but sites of blood loss should be directly observed if possible. External losses, including those via surgical drains, should be assessed: dilution with tissue exudate can exaggerate blood losses. Similar overestimation can occur in hematuria. If in doubt in either of these situations, a hemoglobin estimate on the drain fluid or urine can be helpful. Tracking hematomata should be sought. All intravascular access points, together with other skin incisions pre- or postdating the main episode of blood loss, should be inspected for evidence of bleeding or rebleeding after earlier closure. Fresh bleeding from such sites is a sign of DIC in its consumptive phase.

On defining the pretest probability of a bleeding disorder

Using information from the history and examination the clinician can work out a broad pretest probability (e.g. low, moderate or high) that the patient has a clinical bleeding disorder. The accuracy and precision of the history and examination described above in defining this pretest probability have not been tested by methods that have provided such information in other contexts.[13] Such studies are feasible and desirable in bleeding disorders, but even in their absence, a rational estimate of pretest probability is a crucial step towards interpreting the results of laboratory testing. Without it, tests of hemostasis can be frankly misleading.

Screening tests of hemostasis: two warnings

Armed with an estimate of pretest probability, the next step is to perform screening tests of hemostasis to generate further data capable of increasing or decreasing it.

On venipuncture

This requires a blood sample, which should be taken by an expert venipuncturist – especially in the case of a child – from a peripheral vein with minimal venous stasis. On no account should the jugular, subclavian or femoral veins be approached if there is any possibility of a bleeding disorder. Many inexperienced clinicians seem drawn to perform a 'femoral stab' on patients covered in bruises: this can result in a massive compartment bleed in the femoral triangle.

Multiple attempts to obtain samples from the antecubital fossa can likewise result in severe bleeds. An expert hand is vital.

On screening tests

These tests 'screen' hemostasis, not people – a source of considerable misunderstanding and futile testing. They do not meet the epidemiological standard of true screening tests because they are not sensitive or specific enough to screen a population for bleeding disorder. They only work in concert with the history and examination as described above.

The 250 'clotting screen' requests typically made every day in a large teaching hospital represent educational failure. This futile attempt to screen the population entering hospital for surgery (or other intervention) for bleeding risk depends partly on misinterpretation of the ambiguous term 'screen'. Even more misleading – and potentially wasteful – is the lazy application of the term 'thrombophilia screen' to detailed testing for inherited and acquired thrombophilia. When the term 'screen' is unavoidable, it is used below strictly to refer to tests performed as the result of a clinical history of bleeding or thrombosis.

Initial screening tests, usually applied whatever the pattern of abnormal bleeding, consist of a multiparameter blood count including the platelet count, and coagulation tests: a prothrombin time (PT), activated partial thromboplastin time (APTT), and sometimes a thrombin clotting time (TT).

If the pretest probability of a bleeding disorder is possible or probable, normal results in these initial tests should be followed by a skin bleeding time estimation or whole blood platelet function analysis. The need for further platelet function tests, specific assays of hemostatic proteins or genes, or further clinical tests for systemic disorders depends in part on the results of 'global' tests of hemostasis, but should also proceed if the full history is convincing, even if initial tests are normal. Below, tests of primary hemostasis and coagulation are grouped together for coherency, but they are also ranked into 'screening' and 'diagnostic' categories.

Laboratory investigation of hemostasis

Tests of primary hemostasis

Screening tests

The platelet count

Methods. In the current laboratory, platelet counting is performed on an anticoagulated venous blood sample as part of the multiparameter 'full blood count' generated by automated cytometers. Current systems count particles of platelet-like size (2–37 μm^3) by electrical aperture impedence or laser light scattering. To censor 'noise' at the low end and red cells at the high end of this range, devices fit a lognormal distribution curve to this raw count or otherwise manipulate it to calculate the reported platelet count.

The validity of the platelet count accordingly depends on instrument standardization, calibration and quality control: details of these procedures can be found elsewhere.[15] Because instruments count particles by size, blast cell fragments (in acute leukemia) or schistocytic red cells (in thrombotic thrombocytopenic purpura) may lead to overestimation, and large platelets (in immune thrombocytopenia or myelofibrosis) to underestimation, of the true platelet count.

A commoner source of error in platelet counting is ethylenediaminetetraacetic acid (EDTA)-induced platelet clumping, an *in vitro* artifact confirmed by microscopy of a blood film of EDTA-anticoagulated blood and a recount in citrate-anticoagulated blood. A low platelet count should also be checked by examining the specimen tube for clot formation.

Normal and abnormal platelet counts. The normal ('Gaussian') reference range for the concentration of platelets in venous blood ('the platelet count') is 150–400 × 10^9/l. By definition, 5% of normal individuals have platelet counts outside this range. To regard and investigate asymptomatic individuals with isolated, stable, mild thrombocytopenia (100–150 × 10^9/l) as if they had a disease may be to confound 'Gaussian' and 'diagnostic' concepts of normality.[1] However, evidence to justify abandoning this seemingly unproductive practice is lacking.

By contrast, in a sick patient, falling platelet counts in the range 150–400 × 10^9/l, or even from >400 × 10^9/l into the normal range, may indicate the early, reversible stages of dangerous hemostatic disorders (e.g. DIC or heparin-induced thrombocytopenia). A falling platelet count in the normal range may also be a clue to the presence of sepsis, falciparum malaria or other systemic diseases. Any fall of >50 × 10^9/l in a 24-h period should alert the hematologist and be communicated to the clinical team.

Correlating the platelet count with the clinical situation. The action taken in response to the finding of a low platelet count depends on the presence or risk of bleeding, since the two are not always correlated. In many patients with immune thrombocytopenia (ITP), clinical bleeding may be minor or absent even at very low counts (<10 × 10^9/l), and precipitant therapy may not be necessary. However, the presence of mucosal bleeding in ITP indicates early therapy.

Lesser degrees of thrombocytopenia (20–50 × 10^9/l) are dangerous when combined with reduced platelet function (e.g. antiplatelet agents, myelodysplasia, myelofibrosis); abnormal coagulation (e.g. DIC); leukemia (e.g. acute promyelocytic leukemia); cerebral vasculopathy in sickle cell anemia, or with severe anemia of any cause. In these situations, aggressive therapy including intensive platelet transfusion support is often needed.

When confronting a reduced platelet count, an apparently simple variable, potential laboratory error or artifact must be sought, and the platelet count must be placed firmly in the clinical context. These are core principles in all hemostatic testing.

Platelet function testing

If a history of excess bleeding suggests a defect in primary hemostasis but the platelet count is normal, or insufficiently reduced to account for it (>100 × 10^9/l), tests of platelet function are indicated. Recent technological developments have changed the range and sequence of tests applied for this purpose. It is logical first to perform 'global' tests of platelet function: skin bleeding time and whole blood platelet function analysis. If either or both give results consistent with abnormal platelet function, further definition of the defect by platelet aggregometry and other tests should be attempted.

The limited sensitivity of these methods, and the myriad defects that can occur in the platelet's parallel activation, transduction and secretion systems,[16] often mean that no definitive diagnosis can be made outside a research laboratory. A degree of diagnostic uncertainty is tolerable, however, because therapeutic modalities for disorders of primary hemostasis tend to be broadly applicable across them all.

Whole blood platelet function analysis. Many workers have attempted to develop devices that mimic (and therefore test) the linked phases of platelet adhesion and aggregation in uncentrifuged whole blood.[17] Recent automated devices appear to accomplish this in a valid and reproducible way. By eliminating the need to prepare platelet-rich plasma, they reduce both sample volume and the time needed to do the test. These methods appear to be more sensitive to subtle platelet function defects, possibly because they eliminate *ex vivo* platelet activation during centrifugation.

The most widely used device is the PFA-100® (Dade-Behring)[18] which draws a citrated blood sample through paired filters impregnated with platelet agonists and measures the time taken by resulting platelet aggregates to occlude them, providing two numerical end-points. One filter contains collagen and adenosine diphosphate (ADP): occlusion of this (at the high shear rate achieved by the device) is dependent on vWF–platelet gpIb/IX interaction and therefore the vWF content of the blood sample. The second filter combines collagen with epinephrine, and the rate of occlusion tests platelet granule function and signal transduction. Occlusion of the collagen/epinephrine filter is also very sensitive to the effect of aspirin and other antiplatelet agents. Use of this device is now widespread in laboratories testing for vWD and platelet function disorders. PFA-100 analysis, where available, is also tending to replace the skin bleeding time for evaluating the response of primary bleeding disorders to therapy with desmopressin, sources of vWF, or platelet concentrates.[18]

The skin bleeding time (SBT)

Previously a major criterion for the diagnosis of defects in primary hemostasis, prolongation of the skin bleeding time (even in its most reliable form, the Ivy template method) lost some of this status after being shown to lack sensitivity, reproducibility and operator-independence[19] in general use. In expert hands it can still produce useful evidence in equivocal cases,[11] and it remains part of the constellation of tests helpful in the diagnosis of vWD, although PFA-100 analysis is probably more sensitive.[18]

The Ivy method is recommended. A sphygmomanometer cuff is applied above the elbow and kept inflated to 40 mmHg to increase distal capillary pressure uniformly. Using a disposable device (e.g. Simplate®), a 5 mm long × 1 mm deep incision is made on the volar surface of the forearm, and a stopwatch started. Emerging blood is traditionally lifted off with the edge of a Whatman® filter paper, without applying pressure to the incision. The watch is stopped when the cut stops bleeding, and the time recorded as the SBT. Using this technique, an SBT >10 min is abnormal, indicating a primary bleeding disorder.

Measuring the size of the blots or further observation of the cut for rebleeding are no longer thought to add useful data. The procedure is uncomfortable for many patients, especially children, and leaves a small scar even if properly dressed with skin closures. Patients should be warned about this before giving valid consent to the procedure. After one instance of reflex withdrawal of the forearm that extended the cut from 5 mm to 3 cm, the author always keeps one hand gently but firmly on the patient's wrist when doing this test.

Diagnostic tests

Classical platelet aggregometry

This elegant but demanding technique was introduced by Born.[20] Platelet-rich plasma (PRP) prepared by centrifugation of citrated blood is subsampled into warmed plastic cuvettes, stirred, and exposed to platelet agonists in doses that provoke aggregation of normal platelets. Consequent aggregation (or the lack of it) is detected by increasing light transmission through the cuvette, the time-course and extent of which are recorded on paper in the form of a curve. Interpretation combines inspection of the shape of this curve with a value for % aggregation, 100% being taken as the difference in light transmission between stirred PRP and buffer solution ('blank').

Platelet agonists (collagen, thrombin, epinephrine, arachidonate) cause aggregation by binding to receptors on the platelet surface and provoking the platelet release reaction, or by serendipitous interaction with the gpIb/IX receptor and vWF in the patient plasma (ristocetin). The combined response of an individual's platelets to a panel of these reagents may form a pattern characteristic of a specific disorder (e.g. Glanzmann's thrombasthenia), a narrow differential diagnosis (e.g. Bernard–Soulier disease versus vWD), or a broad class of disorders (e.g. δ- and α-storage-pool disorders). Aggregometry is therefore indispensable in the diagnosis of severe platelet function disorders, but requires expert performance and interpretation.

In practice, the investigation of individuals with convincing histories of excess bleeding is often frustrated by normal findings using classical aggregometry. This suggests that the technique is relatively insensitive to mild platelet function disorders. In about half such cases, PFA-100® analysis (see above) detects a prolonged closure time, usually of the collagen–epinephrine filter.

Investigations of platelet granule structure and function

Measurement of the release of effector molecules from δ-granules (e.g. ADP by the luciferase method, or ^{14}C-serotonin release) or α-granules (e.g. β-thromboglobulin by ELISA) after platelet stimulation by agonists may further define disorders with findings on aggregometry or whole blood analysis consistent with storage pool disorders.

Transmission electron microscopy of platelets may demonstrate abnormal granule number or ultrastructure.

Fluorescence-activated cell sorting (FACS) analysis of platelets labeled with monoclonal antibodies specific for cell membrane epitopes (e.g. glycoproteins Ib/IX and IIb/IIIa) are useful in the diagnosis of Bernard–Soulier disease and Glanzmann's thrombasthenia respectively.

These techniques straddle the boundary between diagnostic and research laboratory methods. They are appropriate

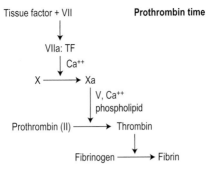

Fig. 31.3 Sequence of reactions in the prothrombin time (PT) test.

only for reference laboratories that have sufficient expertise, technical resources and experience to correctly interpret their results.

Coagulation tests

Coagulation screening tests

This venerable set of simplified bioassays is performed on platelet-poor plasma centrifuged from a citrated sample of blood. In the modern laboratory, coagulometers detect the assay end-point of fibrin clot formation by mechanical or optical means.

Prothrombin time (PT) and the international normalized ratio

As invented by Quick,[21] a source of tissue factor ('thromboplastin': an aqueous extract of mammalian brain or, increasingly, a recombinant version)[22] is added to citrated test plasma at 37°C and the mixture recalcified. Maximal stimulation of the clot initiation ('extrinsic') pathway results in clot formation in 12–15 s.

The PT depends on: 1) concentrations and activity of coagulation factors VII, X, V, II and fibrinogen in the test plasma; and 2) the sensitivity of the chosen thromboplastin to these activities and their inhibition. The PT is more sensitive to early-acting factors, particularly FVII, than to FII and fibrinogen (Fig. 31.3).

The end-point (clot formation) is timed and compared to the mean result obtained testing normal plasmas. If the PT (performed for diagnosis) is prolonged, a 50:50 mixing test (see below for the APTT) can be performed to indicate whether factor deficiency or inhibition is more likely to be responsible, although inhibitors affecting the PT alone are rare.

The PT is reported as a time (the control time coreported) or, increasingly, as a ratio (PT test plasma: PT normal plasma). Ratios obtained with different thromboplastins are transformed ('normalized') by the international sensitivity index (ISI) assigned to the test thromboplastin to correct for its sensitivity to factors VII, X and II by comparing its performance to that of an international reference thromboplastin.[23] The transformed ratio is reported as the international normalized ratio (INR):

$$INR = (PTpatient/MNPT)^{ISI}$$

where MNPT = the geometric mean PT of the population (in practice, 20 normal plasma samples).

The INR was introduced to harmonize coumarin anticoagulation, but it also functions as the prothrombin time for diagnosis ratio (PTDr) if a suitably sensitive thromboplastin is used. The closer the ISI of a thromboplastin to 1.0, the more likely it is to be reliable in both settings.

Interactions between thromboplastins and automated coagulometers performing the PT introduce more complexity. A large laboratory should not only determine its own reference range for the INR/PTDr, but also the 'system ISI' of its coagulometer/thromboplastin combination(s).[24]

INR >1.2 indicates a defect in the TF/VII clot initiation pathway to thrombin. This could be due to deficiency or inhibition (anticoagulant or antibody) of any or all of factors VII, X, V, II, or fibrinogen (if <1 g/l) (Box 31.2). Coumarin therapy rapidly reduces FVII levels and the INR is sensitive to FVII. The INR is therefore used to monitor coumarin therapy (therapeutic range 2–4).

Activated partial thromboplastin time (APTT)

This mini-assay of the clot amplification ('intrinsic') pathway was introduced by Langdell et al.[25] A phospholipid reagent that mimics the activated platelet surface (i.e. rich in PS,[26] although to supraphysiologic levels)[27] is incubated with test plasma at 37°C. Erratic contact activation is over-ridden by adding a strong activator such as kaolin, and the mixture recalcified. Sequential reactions provoked by contact activation in the presence of PS result in clot formation in 30–40 s.

The clotting end-point is measured by a coagulometer and expressed as the APTT in seconds, compared to the locally derived reference range. The APTT is also expressed as a ratio (APTTr) when used as a monitoring test for therapy with unfractionated heparin (UFH), and the use of this ratio in diagnostic work is acceptable.

This end-point depends on: 1) the concentrations and activities of contact factors prekallikrein, high-molecular-weight kininogen (HMWK) and factor XII; 2) the concentrations and activities of coagulation factors XI, IX, VIII, X, V, II and fibrinogen; and 3) the sensitivity of the whole test system to these activities and their inhibition. The APTT is more sensitive to contact and early-acting coagulation factors than to prothrombin and fibrinogen (Fig. 31.4). Elevated acute-phase proteins (factor VIII and fibrinogen) shorten the APTT and may obscure the effect of mild deficiencies and inhibitors in pregnancy and sepsis.

The APTT is an important test in three clinicopathologic situations. First, it detects inherited and acquired

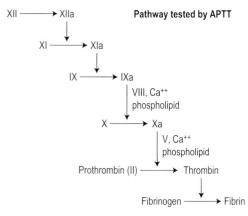

Pathway tested by APTT

Fig. 31.4 Sequence of reactions in the activated partial thromboplastin time (APTT) test.

hemophilia A and B because of its sensitivity to factors VIII and IX, and their inhibition, in plasma. Second, it detects the presence of 'lupus-like' (phospholipid-dependent) inhibitors because of its sensitivity to PS in the test reagent. Third, it detects the presence and concentration of heparin in plasma, and is therefore used to monitor unfractionated (but not low-molecular-weight) heparin therapy.

A reagent/coagulometer system sensitive to all three of these variables should be employed if possible, but the key function of the APTT – its role in the coagulation screen – is to detect hemophilia. Sensitivity to factor VIII and IX (i.e. the ability to detect levels of either factor below 45 IU/dl) is paramount, the practical convenience of a multifunctional APTT notwithstanding. A reference laboratory might opt for different APTT systems for different roles, rather than compromise any of them.

APTT correction tests

The sensitivity of the APTT to inhibitors of coagulation dictates that further information is gained by repeating the APTT on a 50:50 mixture of test plasma and normal pooled plasma. This correction test should be performed in most instances of prolonged APTT or APTTr not due to heparin therapy or contamination (see below).

A prolonged APTT due to contact or coagulation factor deficiency corrects on addition of an equal volume of pooled normal plasma to the test sample. For example, the factor IX content of a normal pool suffices to bring the mixture up to a level giving a near-normal APTT, even if the test plasma has <1% normal factor IX. In contrast, an inhibitor in the test plasma will inactivate coagulation factors in the added normal plasma, preventing correction.

'Correction' has been defined as the APTT of the mixture 'being near to that of normal'[28] but using current reagents, most authors imply that correction of the APTT in a 50:50 mix means 'to normal'[12,29,30] (i.e. APTTr <1.2). As with all coagulation tests, local criteria based on the performance of reagents and coagulometers and the experience of expert laboratory staff should be determined and applied. Since full, partial or absent correction (i.e. all possible results of the test) will all lead to more sensitive assays of coagulation factors and inhibitors, correction tests only indicate where to start.

If the clinical situation and/or screening tests suggest a possible factor VIII inhibitor, a modified method reflects inhibitor kinetics and identifies mild but clinically significant inhibitors. Unlike phospholipid-dependent antibodies, allo- and autoimmune anti-FVIII antibodies may need incubation with the target proteins for up to 2 h at 37°C to inhibit them. Extended incubation of the mixture therefore avoids illusory correction of a slow-acting inhibitor. An extra control (test and normal plasmas incubated separately and mixed just before testing) corrects for loss of factor VIII activity due to incubation alone.[31]

Classic mixing experiments

Correction studies employing absorbed plasma reagents, aged serum, or plasmas from patients with severe deficiencies, are popular thought experiments in practical examinations in hematology. Laboratories that have the time, staff and expertise to prepare, store, and maintain stringent quality control of a library of such reagents still find their differential correction of patient APTT a rapid route to specific diagnosis.[11] However, these requirements, and incompatibility with the automated coagulometers used to confirm the specific diagnosis of coagulation factor deficiencies, mean that they are no longer part of current routine practice. In any event, findings in classic mixing experiments must always be confirmed by specific factor assays.

Diagnostically misleading APTT prolongation

APTT sensitivity extends to components of the test plasma that are clinically irrelevant (prekallikrein, HMWK and factor XII) and the frequent contamination of coagulation samples with heparin from intravenous lines. The APTT is therefore prone to diagnostic false positives when used as an indiscriminate screening test in hospital practice, potentially causing delay and cost while the cause of a long APTT is tracked down. For these reasons, and its sensitivity both to states causing severe bleeding (hemophilia) and dangerous thrombosis (lupus anticoagulant), the APTT can only be interpreted in the light of the clinical history (Box 31.3).

APTT detects UFH but not low-molecular-weight heparins (LMWH). APTTr monitors UFH therapy (therapeutic range APTTr 1.5–2.5). Samples taken via heparin-flushed lines are useless: heparin cannot be flushed out.

Thrombin time (TT)

This simple test (Fig. 31.5) adds thrombin to test plasma and times the resulting clot end-point. TT is expressed in seconds and compared to a normal control range (e.g. TT 15 s,

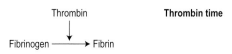

Fig. 31.5 The thrombin time (TT) test reaction.

Box 31.4 Causes of ↑ TT (>3s >control)

Afibrinogenemia

Hypofibrinogenemia

Dysfibrinogenemia

Inhibitors of fibrin polymerization: paraproteins, fibrin–fibrinogen degradation products (FDPs)

Heparin (unfractionated)

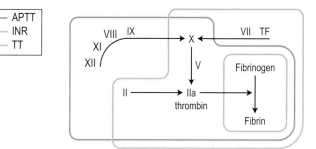

Fig. 31.6 The coagulation screen as a 'circuit tester'.

control = 11 s). An abnormal TT (>15 s) is due to: 1) deficiency of fibrinogen; 2) an inhibitor capable of inhibiting exogenous thrombin (e.g. heparin, hirudin); or 3) inhibition of fibrinogen polymerization due to an abnormal fibrinogen molecule (dysfibrinogenemia) or interfering substances (fibrin/fibrinogen degradation products, paraproteins) (Box 31.4). Some laboratories add calcium to the thrombin solution used in the TT to narrow the normal range and improve reproducibility, but this entails a loss of sensitivity to dysfibrinogens and is not recommended.

Heparin interference with coagulation screening tests: the reptilase time

Heparin contamination is common in samples from wards, theaters and intensive care units – anywhere that intravenous access devices are used for blood sampling. It is therefore reasonable to exclude it before pursuing a diagnosis of DIC (see below), which it mimics. Reptilase (the venom of *Bothrops atrox*) clots fibrinogen in a heparin-insensitive way while retaining sensitivity to other abnormalities that prolong the TT. A reptilase time (normal 10–12 s) is therefore a helpful and necessary adjunct to the coagulation screen.

Fibrinogen assay

Measuring the concentration of fibrinogen in plasma can be regarded as an extension of the initial coagulation screen: the PT and APTT are relatively insensitive to moderate hypofibrinogenemia and a prolonged TT requires explanation if heparin contamination has been excluded by a reptilase time. The most reliable method for the automated routine laboratory is the Clauss method,[32] a parallel-line bioassay based on the TT performed on serial dilutions of patient plasma and control. Fibrinogen estimates 'derived' from automated PT or APTT analysis can be misleading in the very states (e.g. DIC) in which fibrinogen assay is most useful, and are not recommended.

Fibrin–fibrinogen degradation products (FDPs) and D-dimer assay

In several clinical situations it is helpful to detect the presence of plasmin-digested cleavage products of cross-linked fibrin and fibrinogen termed fibrin–fibrinogen degradation products (FDP). An elevated FDP concentration

(>100 mg/ml) suggests DIC (see below) or rarer primary fibrinolytic states.

A variety of commercial immunoassays use polyclonal antibodies to detect and quantify molecules expressing fibrinogen epitopes, for example by coated latex bead agglutination. These include native fibrinogen and its direct plasmin cleavage products, as well as fragments that signify plasmin digestion of intravascular fibrin. This lack of specificity necessitates testing serum produced by *ex vivo* clotting in the presence of an inhibitor of fibrinolysis (e.g. aprotinin) to prevent *ex vivo* generation of FDP, requiring a separate and specific FDP sample tube.

Recently developed assays employ monoclonal antibodies that recognize the D-dimer fragment produced by plasmin digestion of cross-linked fibrin (i.e. thrombus).[11] The increased sensitivity and specificity of this assay allows detection of the relatively low levels of D-dimer circulating in the presence of deep vein thrombosis and pulmonary embolism (venous thromboembolic disease, VTED). D-dimer assay combined with the pretest probability estimate derived from a clinical scoring system is useful in the diagnosis of VTED.[33] Since the D-dimer assay retains sensitivity to DIC and uses the citrated coagulation screen sample it has largely replaced older polyspecific assays for serum FDP.

Logical use of the coagulation screen

Combining the results of the PT, APTT and TT tests, and using them as a logical 'circuit tester' (see Fig. 31.6) maximizes the information provided by the coagulation screen, particularly when considered with the platelet count. The logic of the coagulation screen combined with platelet testing has been expressed in algorithmic form[34] and as a web-based interactive computer program,[35] but is probably straightforward enough to keep in one's head.

For example, if the APTT ratio is increased and corrects to normal with 50:50 normal plasma, but the INR, TT and platelet count are normal, the probable deficiency is restricted to one of the factors tested only by the APTT: FXII, FXI, FIX or FVIII. The exact deficiency is determined by specific assays of single factors, starting with a factor VIII assay because this is the commonest cause of severe hemophilia (see Box 31.5).

A single gene lesion typically reduces the function of a single coagulation factor, and therefore usually prolongs a single coagulation screen test. Exceptions to this rule of thumb are, in the first case, genetic disorders causing combined factor deficiencies (e.g. FV + FVIII deficiency),[36] and in the second case, severe FX, FV, prothrombin or fibrinogen deficiencies; these are all rarities.

A 66-year-old male bled for 48 h after surgery. Excess bleeding was noted from surgical drains and as a wound hematoma. Pretest probability of a bleeding disorder (from history and examination)

$\therefore$ = high

Platelet count = 245×10^9/l

APTTr $\uparrow$ (1.9) corrects with 50 : 50 normal plasma.

INR and TT normal.

$\therefore$ There is a deficiency (it corrects) of one or more factors tested only by the APTT: a contact factor, or clotting factors VIII, IX or XI.

Pretest probability suggests FVIII, FIX or FXI deficiency: all can cause excess bleeding after surgery. Contact factor deficiencies do not cause excess bleeding.

Specific activity assays of these factors are performed, starting with FVIII-C (the commoner of the two potentially severe deficiencies).

Result: FVIII:C = 190 IU/dl (normal 50–150 IU/dl)

FIX:C = 13 IU/dl (normal 50–150 IU/dl)

$\therefore$ The patient has mild hemophilia B (Christmas disease). This may not become manifest as bleeding until a major surgical challenge occurs, perhaps for the first time in later life. In the context of surgery no hemophilia is 'mild'.

$\therefore$ therapy is needed to raise the FIX level.

Box 31.6 Final words on screening tests of hemostasis

If the clotting screen or full blood count is abnormal, refocus the history and examination (e.g. to look for malignancy or hepatic disease).

Clinical findings always take precedence over negative laboratory screening.

If there is moderate or high pretest probability of a bleeding disorder, ignore negative screening tests and proceed to assays of specific coagulation factors and platelet function.

If these in turn find nothing, refer the problem to an expert in the field of hemostasis.

Disorders of hemostasis that may not affect screening tests

von Willebrand disease (vWD). This common disorder may prolong the APTT, but this depends on a secondary effect on FVIII/vWF binding. Clinically significant type I vWD is often associated with a normal APTT. If the pretest probability of a bleeding disorder is moderate or high, whole blood platelet function (see above) should be measured. This procedure will also ensure that platelet function disorders, also 'silent' in the coagulation screen, are not missed. vWF assays should be done if whole blood platelet function analysis is not available.

Mild but clinically significant deficiencies of coagulation factors. Depending on reagent/coagulometer system sensitivities, mild deficiencies (i.e. factor levels 10–40 IU/dl) may not be detected by the APTT. When normal coagulation screening tests and platelet function are found in the context of a high pretest likelihood of a clinical bleeding disorder, exclusion of factor VIII, factor IX and factor XI deficiencies finally depends on specific assays (see Box 31.6).

Factor XIII deficiency. This transglutaminase stabilizes fibrin polymer by catalyzing fibrin cross-linking. Factor XIII deficiency, a rare autosomal recessive disorder, presents classically as bleeding from the umbilical cord stump or delayed bleeding after surgical challenge.

Clots formed from the plasma of individuals with severe factor XIII deficiency (<0.03 units/ml) differ from normal by dissolving in 5M urea, monochloroacetic acid or 2% acetic acid. This simple screening test should be applied to individuals with a high pretest probability of a bleeding disorder who give negative results with all other tests, supplemented by more sensitive immunoassays for factor XIII.

In contrast, systemic diseases or drugs alter the synthesis, postsynthetic processing or function of several clotting factors and may reduce the platelet count. They are therefore reflected by abnormalities of several screening tests. For example, hepatocellular failure: 1) reduces the plasma concentration of all coagulation factors; 2) induces a hyperfibrinolytic state further consuming them; and 3) is often associated with portal hypertension causing splenic pooling of platelets.

The dangerous clinical disorder of hemostasis designated DIC also causes abnormalities in several screening tests because coagulation factors and platelets are consumed by chaotic activation of the whole hemostatic system. The APTTr may be misleadingly low in DIC, either because DIC is occurring on the background of an acute phase response (in sepsis or pregnancy) or due to circulating activated coagulation factors. Whenever the clinical situation and/or the pattern of abnormalities seen in the coagulation screen are consistent with DIC, an FDP or D-dimer assay (see above) should be added to the screen to detect the high levels of fibrin/fibrinogen degradation products characteristic of DIC. A fibrinogen assay should also be done to guide supportive transfusion therapy.

Heparin, by blocking the function of several clotting factors, mimics the effect of these serious global disorders of hemostasis by prolonging all three coagulation screening tests. It mainly confounds when samples for coagulation screening are drawn from vascular access devices flushed with heparin to keep them patent. Although such contamination can be partly excluded by performing a reptilase time test (see above), this causes delay in critical situations. It is better to establish a general rule that all coagulation samples must be taken by direct venipuncture.

Diagnostic coagulation tests

Specific assays of individual clotting factors

The final diagnostic step in the investigation of an individual with a potential bleeding disorder is assay of the biological activity and/or molecular concentration of individual coagulation factors in their plasma. Knowledgeable interpretation of the results of screening tests will narrow the range of likely defects and the first assays performed should follow this logic. This is preferable to 'shotgun' analyses because coagulation assays are expensive tests that consume the scarce resource of expert technical attention. Clearly, the labeling of an individual as having an inherited severe coagulation disorder has such profound implications for them, their family and the healthcare system that the investigation must attain the highest possible degree of certainty at this stage.

Functional bioassays

The most clinically relevant assay of a coagulation factor tests its ability to promote clot formation in human plasma – its 'activity'. Testing function in a biological system (e.g. human plasma) is termed bioassay. In exchange for clinical relevance, the complexity of bioreagents imposes limits on accuracy and reproducibility. To keep these limits within tolerable bounds the use of a hierarchy of plasma standards to calibrate and control assays is essential, as is constant participation in quality control exercises. These are discussed in the next section.

The activity of a coagulation factor is determined by bioassay, in which the potency of the patient's plasma – its ability to correct the prolonged clotting time of plasma missing the factor in question – is compared to that of a plasma standard. Since the plasma standard has a known content of the factor, the unknown content of the patient's plasma can be calculated by comparison. The resulting activity is indicated by the suffix [:C], for example factor VIII:C.

If the calibration trail of the assay standard leads eventually to the current International Standard, the result can be expressed in international units (IU). Strictly, the activity of a coagulation factor in plasma should be expressed as IU/ml (normal 0.5–1.5 IU/ml), but is often expressed as IU/dl (normal 50–150 IU/dl) in order to match the intuitive convention of 'per cent normal'.

One-stage assays. The simplest assay design is the one-stage method which depends on correction of the clotting time (e.g. using the APTT as the 'marker system' in a FVIII:C assay) of a plasma from which the factor in question is absent. This reagent is termed the substrate plasma. Individuals with severe inherited deficiencies remain a major source of substrate plasma (which accordingly is a potential infection risk), although the availability of commercial reagents reliably depleted of single coagulation factors by immunoadsorption has broadened the applicability of one-stage assays. As a result, because of their conceptual simplicity, adaptability to automation, and use of everyday (i.e. APTT, PT) reagents, one-stage assays are commoner in practice than more complex designs, except in special situations.

All one-stage assays share the same design apart from their marker system, which may be the PT (for prothrombin, FV:C, FVII:C and FX:C assays) the APTT (for FVIII:C, FIX:C, FXI:C or contact factor assays) or snake venom clotting times (Taipan for prothrombin (not in the context of coumarin therapy), Russell's viper for FX:C).

Serial dilutions (at least three) of patient plasma are added to substrate plasma. The same is done with the assay standard. Clot end-points are measured for each dilution.

The manual method plots clotting times on the vertical axis against dilution on the horizontal axis, using logarithmic graph paper. This results in two 'curves' (which should form parallel straight lines) – a standard curve and an unknown (patient) curve. From the standard curve, a horizontal line ('of equal potency') is drawn to where it intercepts the unknown curve: a vertical line dropped to the horizontal axis from this point marks the potency of the

patient plasma relative to the standard. Full descriptions of this method, including the requirements for parallelism on which its validity rests, can be found elsewhere.[37–39]

Even when controlled and standardized, it remains a bioassay with irreducible limits on precision and reproducibility. A single assay can only be relied upon to give an answer within 20% of the 'true' value (the idealized mean value of an infinite number of tests). This is one basis (the other being the variation of plasma FVIII levels in individuals) of the common rule that at least three assays (reducing the error to ± 10%) are required to define the severity of hemophilia. To reduce the error to ± 2.5% would theoretically require 64 assays.[37] These sources of within-laboratory error are compounded by inter-laboratory variance, which in external quality control exercises can give a CV (coefficient of variation) of 30–50%.[40]

In modern routine laboratories the potency is calculated mathematically by computer modules linked to automated coagulometers.

Two-stage assays. This form of assay differs by eliminating the substrate plasma and phospholipid reagent of the APTT-based assay: instead, a reaction mixture is prepared (containing excess FIX and FX) in which the formation of factor Xa is proportionate to the concentration of FVIII:C or FIX:C in dilutions of unknown and assay standard plasmas as above. FXa thus generated is measured by its action in a second reaction mixture (using a clot end-point) or directly by its action on a chromogenic substrate (see below). Potency calculations are then carried out as for one-stage assays.

Chromogenic assays. Rather than using a clotting end-point in a two-stage assay as above, the availability of synthetic amidolytic substrates sensitive to factor Xa enable the use of a color reaction detectable and quantifiable by spectrophotometry. This chromogenic method has been adapted to measure several hemostatic enzymes and their inhibitors, and is highly compatible with automation.[41] One theoretical advantage of the chromogenic method is that it directly measures the first product (FXa) of the FVIII/FIX interaction, rather than requiring the participation of several other factors in the production of a clotting end-point. This increases the precision and reproducibility of the assay. In addition, lack of dependence on phospholipid reagents makes the chromogenic method more reliable in the assay of therapeutic concentrates, both in the vial and in the patient.[27]

Immunoassays

Immunoassays use poly- or monoclonal antibodies to detect and quantify coagulation proteins. Except in the special case of 'functional' epitopes (i.e. immunologic determinants linked so closely to the functional site of a molecule that they are assumed to act as a reliable marker of its activity), immunoassays detect the presence of a protein rather than its function. Immunoassays may therefore give normal results in disorders due to loss-of-function mutations that result in normal or slightly reduced amounts of protein (e.g. type 2A vWD). However, immunoassay remains a cornerstone of diagnosis in vWD because of the continued lack of a reliable non-surrogate functional assay of vWF.

The ability to stick purified monoclonal antibodies to plastic or latex surfaces, together with ubiquitous chromogenic reactions derived from the alkaline phosphatase/

anti-alkaline phosphatase (APAAP) method, have transformed immunoassay technology. Enzyme-linked immunosorption assay (ELISA) and recent latex agglutination assays are rapidly supplanting the older radiometric and immunoelectrophoretic methods (e.g. Laurell electroimmunoassay).[42] Such immunoassays are most often used in the diagnosis of vWD and thrombophilia.

Molecular diagnosis in disorders of hemostasis

The diagnostic chain may now be continued to DNA sequencing and the direct detection of gene mutations or deletions affecting genes encoding coagulation proteins, particularly carrier detection and antenatal diagnosis in the hemophilias. However, gene analysis has not yet become part of the standard clinical diagnostic criteria for coagulation and platelet disorders as it has for some types of thrombophilia.

The problem of testing the fibrinolytic system

The fibrinolytic system is of vital importance to the organism, and scientific investigation and exploitation of its components has led to important therapeutic agents with major impact in common life-threatening thrombotic disorders. None the less, it remains the 'Cinderella' of hemostatic testing.[43] Partly, this is due to the evanescent nature of most clinical disturbances of fibrinolysis. Compared to chronic disorders of coagulation, the fibrinolytic system rarely 'sits still' for long enough to study it. In addition, a fibrinolytic equivalent to the coagulation screen does not really exist: the euglobulin clot lysis time (ECLT) is insensitive and poorly reproducible. Immunoassays of key fibrinolytic enzymes and inhibitors are available, but interpreting their results in thrombotic syndromes is difficult and currently unproductive.[43] In acute clinical situations fibrinogen and D-dimer assays will give clues to the presence of hyperfibrinolysis. α2-Antiplasmin deficiency, the only well-documented inherited bleeding disorder attributed to chronic excess plasmin activity, does not declare itself in any screening test: clinical suspicion should lead to measurement of α2-antiplasmin by ELISA.[44]

Monitoring hemostasis using global tests

The tests discussed above (except the PFA-100 system) require separation of citrated plasma or platelet-rich plasma from venous blood samples, resulting in an *ex vivo* derivative that differs in two crucial ways from the circulating *in vivo* blood.

Firstly, key cellular messengers, calcium ions, are removed from the milieu. Secondly, the complex interactions between coagulation factors and the cell membranes of platelets, leukocytes and red cells are negated and substituted by a phospholipid reagent that is unphysiological in both composition and dose.

Given these test features, it is perhaps fortunate that generally reliable, clinically useful inferences can be based on their use. However, it is widely perceived that validated test systems capable of measuring events in whole blood, complete with its cellular elements, could generate information that correlates better with clinical reality. Such test systems are referred to as *global tests of hemostasis*.

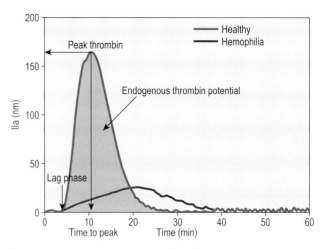

Fig. 31.7 A quantitative dynamic profile of thrombin generation.

The ideal coagulation test

The ideal global assay would measure the dynamics of thrombin generation, detect whole blood clot formation and/or fibrin formation, and evaluate the structure and stability of the formed clot.

Such an assay should improve determination of the baseline phenotype, and therapeutic monitoring in an individual with a bleeding disorder. It should also help in diagnosis when conventional tests have given normal or equivocal results, as happens in up to 20% of individuals with a credible history of excess bleeding on challenge.

This ideal test does not yet exist, but automated methods for measuring (a) thrombin generation, and (b) whole blood coagulation with thromboelastography/thromboelastometry are currently the most promising candidates for the role.

Calibrated automated thrombin generation measurement

In the calibrated automated thrombin (CAT) assay, a fluorogenic thrombin substrate is incubated with test plasma and coagulation is activated by tissue factor. After recalcification, a computer converts automated continuous measurements of fluorescence into a quantitative dynamic profile of thrombin generation (Fig. 31.7).

Thrombin generation measurements are hypersensitive to pre-analytic variables, so meticulous blood sampling procedures are vital. Many laboratories add corn trypsin inhibitor (CTI – a direct and potent inhibitor of coagulation factor XIIa) to the blood sampling tubes in order to avoid or minimize spontaneous contact activation. This step reduces assay variability.

Interpretation and clinical feasibility. Three informative variables can be measured from the thrombin generation curve: *lag time, time to peak thrombin* and *endogenous thrombin potential* (Fig. 31.7). The course of thrombin generation comprises an initiation phase before the first thrombin is detected (the *lag time*), and an amplification phase during which the maximum rate of thrombin generation occurs.

Thrombin generation then reaches a peak and the time required to reach this point is described as *time-to-peak thrombin*. The total amount of thrombin generation (= area under the curve) is frequently called the *endogenous thrombin potential* (ETP).

In principle, abnormal thrombin generation curves are characterized by 1) a prolonged or shortened lag time, 2) reduced or increased peak thrombin, or 3) reduced or elevated ETP.

The lag time is primarily determined by: levels of free tissue factor, tissue factor pathway inhibitor, factor VII, factor IX and fibrinogen. The amplification phase of thrombin is highly dependent on the number and function of platelets. Hence, the higher the platelet count in the sample, the higher the maximum rate and acceleration of thrombin generation.

Males seem to have a lower [ETP]thrombin production than females. In addition, thrombin generation increases with age and decreases as a result of low temperature.

Thrombin generation has been used for laboratory phenotyping a variety of bleeding disorders. The best characterized hemostatic dysfunction described by thrombin generation profiles is hemophilia A.

The current categories of mild, moderate and severe hemophilia A are based simply on the assayed level of factor VIII in plasma. They are not an absolute guide to an individual's bleeding severity and need for therapy. The rate specific characteristics of thrombin generation have been reported to more accurately reflect the clinical heterogeneity of hemophilia. In particular, thrombin generation has been documented as predictive in distinguishing milder phenotypes of severe hemophilia despite similar low levels of factor VIII (e.g. less than 1% of normal).

Thrombin generation profiles have also been used for monitoring the hemostatic response to treatment. Hemophilia A is treated by substitution with a factor VIII concentrate, but about 20% of patients consequently develop alloantibody inhibitors against factor VIII. These patients can be treated with inhibitor 'bypassing agents' such as recombinant factor VIIa or plasma-derived activated prothrombin complex concentrates (FEIBA), but conventional assays cannot measure the hemostatic effect of these bypassing agents. Thrombin generation measurement has been used to monitor substitution with these agents. The overall experience with thrombin measurements as a surrogate of hemostatic efficacy is still rather limited, but preliminary results appear promising.

Outside hemophilia, thrombin generation has proven advantageous for illustrating the hemostatic potential of prothrombin complex concentrates compared with fresh frozen plasma for reversal of vitamin K antagonist therapy.

Finally, thrombin generation is an elegant method for illustrating the impact of various types of anticoagulation. Heparin, direct thrombin inhibitors and indirect or direct factor Xa inhibitors compromise thrombin generation by prolonging the lag phase and reducing peak thrombin and ETP.

Whole blood thromboelastometry

Thrombelastography (TEG®) and thromboelastometry (ROTEM®) provide a visualization of continuous viscoelastic changes occurring during whole blood clot formation. Both devices consist of a cup into which the sample (whole blood,

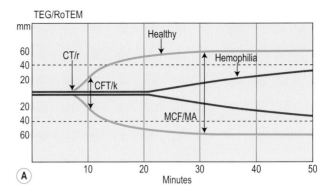

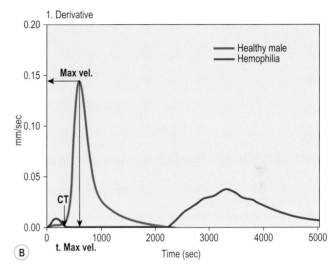

Fig. 31.8 (A, B) (A) Standard whole blood thromboelastometry profiles and parameters. The clotting time (CT/r) reflects the initiation of clot formation, whereas the clot formation time (CFT/k) illustrate the dynamic of clot formation. The maximum amplitude is the maximum clot formation (MCF). As illustrated, in a condition of severe Hemophilia A, patients have a delayed and slot clotting process. (B) Illustrate the first derivative of the standard whole blood thromboelastometry profile. The velocity profile enhance the dynamic abnormality of hemophilia as illustrated by a reduced maximum velocity (MaxVel) of clot formation.

platelet-rich or -poor plasma) and reagents are placed and a pin which sits in the centre of the cup when the device is running. Reduced movement of the pin during clot formation is registered with specialized computer software and visualized on a computer providing a coagulation signal similar to that of traditional thrombelastography (Fig. 31.8A).

Interpretation and clinical feasibility. Traditional thrombelastographic parameters include clotting time (r, CT), clot formation time (k, CFT), and maximal clot formation (MA, MCF) as depicted in Fig. 31.8. Thromboelastometry also assesses clot strength and fibrinolysis levels of MA/MCF (Fig. 31.8).

In principle, abnormal thromboelastographic/thromboelastometry profiles are characterized by 1) a prolonged or shortened r or CT, 2) prolonged k or CFT, or 3) a compromised or elevated MA or MCF.

The digital raw signal from the TEG or ROTEM analyzers can be differentiated to velocity profiles of whole blood clot formation and dynamic coagulation parameters illustrating the propagation phase of clotting can be derived (Fig. 31.8B) such as the maximum velocity (MaxVel) of clot formation and the time until the occurrence of the maximum value (t, MaxVel).

TEG® and ROTEM® have been validated as bedside monitoring tools for diagnosing perioperative coagulopathies and guiding optimal hemostatic intervention. Recent studies have documented that routine use of TEG or ROTEM can reduce unnecessary transfusion of allogeneic blood products and optimize goal-directed hemostatic intervention with coagulation factor concentrates. Several commercial standard assays are available providing activation of the intrinsic pathway (e.g. with kaolin) or extrinsic pathway (with tissue factor) as well as fibrinogen sensitive assays and assays to neutralize heparin.

In addition to the standard assays, sensitive assays have been developed that employ activation with minute (physiological) amounts of tissue factor (as little as 1/50 000th of the concentration used to measure the prothrombin time).

The low tissue factor assay reveals heterogeneity in whole blood coagulation patterns among patients with factor VIII levels <1%, those with less abnormal blood clotting profiles tending to have a less severe bleeding phenotype.

The low tissue factor assay has also been used to illustrated different response patterns to various levels of coagulation factor VIII concentrate. In addition, both *in vitro* and *in vivo* studies have demonstrated the ability of thromboelastography to predict the clinical response to bypassing agents in patients with inhibitors.

In the near future, it is possible that thromboelastography may be used to help design individual treatment regimens for patients with hemophilia, with or without inhibitors. This will become increasingly more important as new therapeutic agents become available.

Minimizing error in hemostatic testing, interpretation and process

The hematologist must identify potential sources of imprecision, error or misinterpretation in laboratory testing that could impede correct diagnosis and patient safety. Tests of hemostasis are fertile ground for such errors: no hematologist can afford to be a passive consumer of their results. Areas that require constant vigilance are:

The pre-analytical phase. Traumatic venipuncture, stop-flow blood drawing and suboptimal mixing or filling of sodium citrate-containing coagulation sample tubes are all potential sources of error. Polycythemia (by decreasing the plasma : citrate ratio) and anemia (the reverse effect) can alter results. Coagulation samples should be tested as soon as possible: any sample waiting more than 3 h (>2 h for FVIII:C assays) for analysis will give misleading results. Coagulation bioassays should preferably be done on fresh rather than frozen-thawed plasma, although pressures on the modern laboratory often prevent observance of this rule.

Test methodology. Written standard operating procedures (SOPs) for every test in its repertoire must be held in the laboratory – and used. SOPs must be regularly updated and externally peer-reviewed as part of an inspection by an accrediting agency. Training must ensure observation of SOPs by all workers performing or validating tests during the laboratory 24 h cycle, and by operators of any point-of-care devices under supervision by the laboratory.

Test reagents and calibration: the hierarchy of standards. Bioassays impose a requirement for reference materials, including thromboplastin reagents, assay standards[40] and drugs. Plasma or concentrate standards are freeze-dried aliquots of plasma or concentrate with a certified content of the factor in question. These secondary standards are in turn assayed (calibrated) against primary International Standard materials held by national biological standards agencies such as the National Institute for Biological Standards and Controls in the UK, and ultimately the World Health Organization and other international bodies.[45] Tracing a calibration trail through this hierarchy of standards ensures that results obtained in different laboratories and in different countries are comparable.

Internal quality control and external quality assurance. Laboratories must perform regular internal quality control procedures, particularly after introducing new tests, methods or machines or when established versions give cause for concern. They must also participate in external quality assurance schemes commensurate with their function: a Hemophilia Center laboratory would be expected to participate in an extended scheme that focused on assays of single coagulation factors, the detection and quantification of coagulation inhibitors, etc. Regular participation in the exercises provided by such a scheme registers a 'running score' of the performance of a laboratory that indicates the reliability of its results. This cumulative performance indicator must be available for inspection by the users of these results. The collated results of such exercises, published among users as surveys, provide useful information on the performance of current tests.

Potential confounding effects. The influence of age on hemostatic variables must always be considered and age-specific reference ranges consulted, particularly interpreting results obtained in infants and children, whose levels of vitamin K-dependent factors and natural anticoagulants differ from those in adults. Pregnancy, particularly during the third trimester and in the peripartum, is associated with marked changes in the levels of both procoagulant and anticoagulant proteins, with potential under- or over-diagnosis of hemostatic abnormalities. The ABO blood group status of an individual must be considered when interpreting vWF levels, which can also be affected by age, exercise, the acute-phase response, or needle-phobia. vWF levels may also change throughout the menstrual cycle, although this is not a universal finding.

Maximizing the clinical utility of hemostatic testing

New responsibilities: multidisciplinary audit and clinical governance. It is no longer enough for the laboratory simply to issue a reliable test result. An additional responsibility is to provide the result to the end-user as rapidly as required and with all the interpretation required to maximize its utility.

A frequent practical problem, particularly in the investigation of mild bleeding disorders, is failure to provide a diagnostic decision even after a lengthy series of tests and repeat measurements. This situation arises most often when vWD or platelet function disorders are in question, and results in frustration for the patient and referring clinician. A patient left in diagnostic limbo may be subjected to delays in surgical or other treatment, or even unnecessarily exposed to blood products.

To minimize this problem, the diagnostic process (including confirmatory testing) should be planned and carried out as a single sequence, preferably under the supervision of a single clinician (nurse or doctor), rather than as a piecemeal affair subject to the vagaries of clinic appointments and changing staff. An experienced clinician should evaluate the resulting evidence, including personal and family histories, make a clear probabilistic judgment on the presence or absence of a hemostatic disorder, explain it to the patient and document it. In addition, a clear plan of action in the event of surgery should be formulated, even if this is merely to observe blood loss carefully, and communicated to the surgical team. By these means even patients in whom no objective cause can be found despite credible histories of excess bleeding can be helped.

The performance of the diagnostic pathway for disorders of hemostasis should be continually evaluated and improved by the multidisciplinary team, using the methods of clinical audit. In this way it is possible to avoid leaving patients and their physicians uncertain of the outcome of the diagnostic process.

Combining test results with clinical scoring systems. Clinical scoring systems can be used to refine the crude pretest probability estimate described above. The most striking example of this in current practice is the combination of a simple but validated clinical risk assessment with laboratory measurement of the D-dimer concentration in a blood sample. The predictive power of this combination allows secure diagnosis and treatment of venous thromboembolic disease.[33] It is likely that similar combinations of clinical and laboratory methods would be valuable in other contexts. Validated clinical decision rules have great potential value in medicine,[1] and hemostatic testing stands to gain considerable value by inclusion in similar models.

References

1. Sackett DL, Straus SE, Richardson WS, et al. Diagnosis and screening. In: Sackett DL, Straus SE, Richardson WS, et al, editors. Evidence-Based Medicine. 2nd ed. Edinburgh: Churchill Livingstone; 2000. p. 67–93.

2. Deeks JJ. Systematic reviews of evaluations of diagnostic and screening tests. British Medical Journal 2001;323:157–62.

3. Mann KG. Biochemistry and physiology of blood coagulation. Thrombosis and Haemostasis 1999;82(2):165–74.

4. Hoffman M, Monroe DM. A cell-based model of haemostasis. Thrombosis and Haemostasis 2001;85:958–65.

5. Ruggeri ZM. Mechanisms initiating platelet thrombus formation. Thrombosis and Haemostasis 1997;78(1): 611–6.

6. Esmon CT. Protein C, protein S, and thrombomodulin. In: Colman RW, Hirsh J, Marder VJ, et al, editors. Hemostasis and Thrombosis: Basic Principles and Clinical Practice. 4th ed. Philadelphia: Lippincott Williams & Wilkins; 2001. p. 335–53.

7. Carrell RW, Huntington, JA, Mushunje A, Zhou A. The conformational basis of thrombosis. Thrombosis and Haemostasis 2001;86:14–22.

8. Bachmann F. Plasminogen–plasmin enzyme system. In: Colman RW, Hirsh J, Marder VJ, et al, editors. Hemostasis and Thrombosis: Basic Principles and Clinical Practice. 4th ed. Philadelphia: Lippincott Williams & Wilkins; 2001. p. 275–320.

9. Bounameaux H, de Moerloose P, Perrier A, Reber G. Plasma measurement of D-dimer as a diagnostic aid in suspected venous thromboembolism: an overview. Thrombosis and Haemostasis 1994;71: 1–6.

10. Nilsson I-M. Assessment of blood coagulation and general haemostasis. In: Bloom AL, Thomas DP, editors.

Haemostasis and Thrombosis. 2nd ed. Edinburgh: Churchill Livingstone; 1987. p. 922–32.

11. Bowie EJW, Owen CA. Clinical and laboratory diagnosis of hemorrhagic disorders. In: Ratnoff OD, Forbes CD, editors. Disorders of Hemostasis. 3rd ed. Philadelphia: WB Saunders; 1996. p. 53–78.

12. Greaves M, Preston FE. Approach to the bleeding patient. In: Colman RW, Hirsh J, Marder VJ, et al, editors. Hemostasis and Thrombosis: Basic Principles and Clinical Practice. 4th ed. Philadelphia: Lippincott Williams & Wilkins; 2001. p. 783–93.

13. Richardson WS, Wilson MC, Guyatt GH, et al. Users' guides to the medical literature: XV. How to use an article about disease probability for differential diagnosis. Journal of the American Medical Association 1999;281: 1214–9.

14. Tossetto A, Castaman G, Rodighiero F. Assessing bleeding in von Willebrand disease with bleeding score. Blood Reviews 2007;21(2):89–97.

14. British National Formulary 42. London: British Medical Association and Royal Pharmaceutical Society of Great Britain; 2001. p. 210.

15. Groner W, Simson E. Standardization. In: Groner W, Simson E, editors. Practical Guide to Modern Hematology Analyzers. Chichester: John Wiley; 1995. p. 95–117.

16. Rao AK. Congenital disorders of platelet secretion and signal transduction. In: Colman RW, Hirsh J, Marder VJ, et al, editors. Hemostasis and Thrombosis: Basic Principles and Clinical Practice. 4th ed. Philadelphia: Lippincott Williams & Wilkins; 2001. p. 893–904.

17. Salzman EW. Measurement of platelet adhesiveness: a simple in vitro technique demonstrating an abnormality in von Willebrand's disease. Journal of

Laboratory and Clinical Medicine 1963; 62:724–35.

18. Jilma B. Platelet function analyser (PFA-100): a tool to quantify congenital or acquired platelet dysfunction. Journal of Laboratory and Clinical Medicine 2001;138:152–63.

19. Rodgers RPC, Leven J. A critical reappraisal of the bleeding time. Seminars in Thrombosis and Hemostasis 1990;16:1–20.

20. Born GVR, Cross MJ. The aggregation of blood platelets. Journal of Physiology (London) 1963;168:178–95.

21. Quick AJ. The thromboplastin reagent for the determination of prothrombin. Science 1940;92:113–4.

22. Tripodi A, Arbini A, Chantarangkul V, Mannucci PM. Recombinant tissue factor as a substitute for conventional thromboplastin in the prothrombin time test. Thrombosis and Haemostasis 1992;67:42–5.

23. WHO Expert Committee on Biological Standardization (1999) Guidelines for thromboplastins and plasma used to control oral anticoagulant therapy. Technical Report Series 889, forty-eighth report, Geneva, Switzerland.

24. Chantarangkul V, Tripodi A, Mannucci PM. The effect of instrumentation on thromboplastin calibration. Thrombosis and Haemostasis 1992;67:588–9.

25. Langdell RD, Wagner RH, Brinkhous KM. Effect of antihemophilic factor in one-stage clotting tests. A presumptive test for hemophilia and simple one-stage hemophilic factor assay procedure. Journal of Laboratory and Clinical Medicine 1953;41(4):637–47.

26. Kelsey PR, Stevenson KG, Poller L. The diagnosis of lupus anticoagulants by the activated partial thromboplastin time – the central role of phosphatidyl serine.

Thrombosis and Haemostasis 1984;52: 172–5.

27. Mikaelson M, Oswaldson U, Jankowski MA. Measurement of Factor VIII activity of B-domain deleted recombinant Factor VIII. Seminars in Haematology 2001; 38(2) (suppl 4):13–23.

28. Austen DEG, Rhymes IL. Laboratory diagnosis of blood coagulation disorders. In: Biggs R, Rizza CR, editors. Human Blood Coagulation, Haemostasis and Thrombosis. 3rd ed. Oxford: Blackwell Scientific; 1984. p. 175.

29. Giddings JC. The investigation of hereditary coagulation disorders. In: Thompson JM, editor. Blood Coagulation and Haemostasis: A Practical Guide. 2nd ed. Edinburgh: Churchill Livingstone; 1980. p. 48–116.

30. Greaves M, Cohen H, Machin SJ, Mackie I. Guidelines on the investigation and management of the antiphospholipid syndrome. British Journal of Haematology 2000;109:704–15.

31. Kaspar CK, Ewing NP. Measurement of inhibitor to factor VIIIC (and IXC). In: Bloom AL, editor. The Hemophilias. Edinburgh: Churchill Livingstone; 1982. p. 39–50.

32. Clauss A. Gerrinnungsphysiologische schnellmethode zur bestimmung des fibrinogens. Acta Haematologica 1957;17:237–46.

33. Wells PS, Anderson DR, Rodger M, et al. Excluding pulmonary embolism at the bedside without diagnostic imaging: management of patients with suspected pulmonary embolism presenting to the emergency department by using a simple clinical model and D-dimer. Annals of Internal Medicine 2001;135:98–107.

34. Favoloro EJ. Assessment of haemostatic function: follow up evaluation of abnormal screening coagulation tests and possible outcomes. Australian Journal of Medical Science 1994;15:39–45.

35. Nguyen AND, Uthman MO, Johnson KA. A web-based teaching program for laboratory diagnosis of coagulation disorders. Archives of Pathology and Laboratory Medicine 2000;124: 588–93.

36. Seligsohn U, Zivelin A, Zwang E. Combined factor V and factor VIII deficiency among non-Ashkenazi Jews. New England Journal of Medicine 1982;307:1191–5.

37. Rizza CR, Rhymes IL. Coagulation assay of VIIIC and IXC. In: Bloom AL, editor. The Hemophilias. Edinburgh: Churchill Livingstone; 1982. p. 18–38.

38. Barrowcliffe TW, Curtis AD. Principles of bioassay. In: Bloom AL, Thomas DP, editors. Haemostasis and Thrombosis. 2nd ed. Edinburgh: Churchill Livingstone; 1987. p. 996–1004.

39. Mannucci PM, Tripodi A. Factor VIII clotting activity. In: Jespersen J, Bertina RN, Haverkate F, editors. E.C.A.T. Assay Procedures. 2nd ed. London: Kluwer Academic; 1999. p. 107–19.

40. Barrowcliffe TW. Standardization of assays of factor VIII and factor IX. Ricerca in Clinica e in Laboratorio 1990;20(2): 155–65.

41. Hutton L. Chromogenic substrates in haemostasis. Blood Reviews 1987;1:201–6.

42. Giddings JC. Immunoanalysis of haemostatic components. In: Bloom AL, Thomas DP, editors. Haemostasis and Thrombosis. 2nd ed. Edinburgh: Churchill Livingstone; 1987. p. 982–95.

43. Bauer KA. Conventional fibrinolytic assays for the evaluation of patients with venous thrombosis: don't bother. Thrombosis and Haemostasis 2001;85:377–8.

44. Favier R, Aoki N, de Moerloose P. Congenital α2-antiplasmin deficiencies: a review. British Journal of Haematology 2001;114:4–10.

45. Hubbard AR, Rigsby P, Barrowcliffe TW. Standardization of factor VIII and von Willebrand factor in plasma: callibration of the 4th International Standard (97/586). Thrombosis and Haemostasis 2001;85(4):634–8.

CHAPTER 32

Disorders affecting megakaryocytes and platelets: inherited conditions

JG White

Chapter contents

Introduction

The blood platelet is a deceptively simple cell. Though the smallest of the circulating blood elements, it derives from the largest cell in bone marrow, the megakaryocyte. Its diminutive appearance, lack of a nucleus and clear hyaloplasm (cytoplasm) made it difficult for early microscopists to recognize the platelet as a distinct entity.[1–4] As a result it was the last of the circulating cellular elements to be identified.[5] Anonymity, however, suited the platelet well. The cell prefers to remain nondescript, and seeks its refuge as far from the center of the column of flowing blood as possible.[6] Other blood cells carry oxygen, remove carbon dioxide,

supply nutrients, transport waste, and leave the circulation to participate in immune and inflammatory reactions as required, but not the platelet. It remains as quiet as possible for its 10–12 day life span. If the cell can retire in the spleen without becoming involved in any of the useful activities served by other blood elements, the platelet's life can be considered a complete success.

Thus the platelet has no function in the circulation, except one: to keep blood flowing. It is the sentinel on guard at all times to react immediately with sites of vascular injury as soon as subendothelium is exposed. Within seconds platelets fill an injured site with a hemostatic plug that prevents further loss of blood and ultimately, with other cell systems, restores the integrity of the vascular system for normal blood flow.[7–10]

The platelet serves its function as the silent sentinel of the circulation very well, but, unfortunately, it does have a blind side. It does not distinguish its role in hemostasis from involvement in thrombosis. As a result participation of platelets in vaso-occlusive events leading to heart attacks, strokes or other ischemic phenomena often overshadows its value as the basic cellular unit of hemostasis.[11]

While normal platelets contribute significantly to hemostasis and thrombosis, abnormal platelets cause bleeding disorders that may express mild symptoms or life-threatening hemorrhage. The study of individuals with platelet-related bleeding disorders has been very important. Not only has it helped to provide appropriate treatment for the bleeding patient, but it has also greatly improved our knowledge of normal hemostasis and the mechanisms of thrombosis. The present chapter focuses on the inherited disorders of platelets and their parent megakaryocytes.

Structure

Before discussing pathology, aspects of normal megakaryocyte and platelet morphology will be considered. The megakaryocyte develops in human bone marrow from the same stem cell as do other cellular elements.[12] However, its transformation from a megakaryoblast into a multinucleated giant cell is unique. The nucleus undergoes a process of endoreduplication without cell division. As a result the cell enlarges dramatically and contains many unseparated nuclear lobes (Fig. 32.1). The final number of lobes is variable, but is usually 16–32. During this process of maturation the megakaryocyte begins to form organelles including alpha granules, dense bodies and lysosomes. The surface of the giant cell invaginates into the cytoplasm forming demarcation membranes, and converts the matrix into incomplete, platelet-sized subunits. Megakaryocytes may rest at stages during maturation, but ultimately complete their development and move to endothelial cells of the bone marrow sinuses. There they extend pseudopods between endothelial cells and deliver platelets to the circulation.

The product of this beautiful developmental sequence is rather unimpressive. It is the smallest of the cellular elements in blood and on peripheral smears resembles a speck of dirt rather than a cell. Yet, closer examination in the electron microscope reveals that the platelet is a disc similar in appearance to the discus hurled by athletes. At high magnification in the low-voltage high-resolution scanning microscope the plasma membrane is furrowed, resembling the surface of the brain[13] (Fig. 32.2). Dimples appearing on the exposed surface and in replicas of freeze-fractured platelets are openings of the surface-connected open canalicular system (OCS). Thin sections in the equatorial plane reveal a circumferential coil of microtubules supporting platelet discoid form lying just below the surface membrane[14] (Fig. 32.3). A large number of alpha granules, a few dense bodies and occasional lysosomes are randomly dispersed in the cytoplasm, along with mitochondria and masses of glycogen particles. Elements of the dense tubular system (DTS) of channels are also scattered randomly with two exceptions. One channel is closely associated with the circumferential

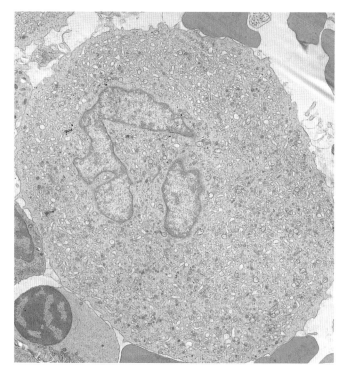

Fig. 32.1 Megakaryocyte. Human megakaryocyte from a trephine sample fixed immediately after removal from the needle. The large cell in thin section has a relatively spherical shape and smooth surface contours. Internal membranes and organelles are randomly distributed throughout the cytoplasm, but are separated from the surface by a thin margin. The appearance suggests a mature cell in the resting state, and not in the process of proplatelet formation or platelet shedding. × 4350.

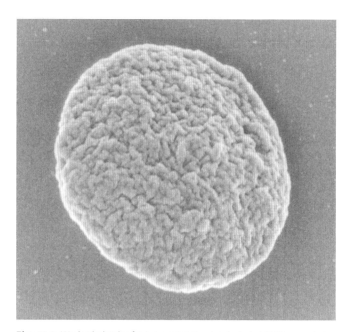

Fig. 32.2 Washed platelet from a suspension incubated at 37°C mounted on a 4 × 8 mm glass slide fragment, fixed with glutaraldehyde and dried by the critical point method for study in the low-voltage, high-resolution scanning electron microscope (LVHR-SEM). The cell has retained its characteristic discoid form. Convolution of the rugose surface membrane resembles the gyri and sulci on the brain. × 25 000.

coil of microtubules (Fig. 32.4). Other DTS channels are interwoven with elements of the OCS to form membrane complexes (MC). The similarity of this organization to the sarcoplasmic reticulum of embryonic muscle cells has been noted.[15] Cytoplasm surrounding the organelles and other formed structures is a featureless protein matrix in thin section, but even in the resting state contains some actin filaments. Alpha granules are the most numerous of the formed organelles. They vary somewhat in size and shape, but are generally round. A nucleoid, more dense than the matrix of the alpha granule, is often seen in thin sections. Cross-sections of a few tubular elements in the matrix are von Willebrand factor concentrated in alpha granules. Dense bodies often have a typical bull's eye appearance with the inherently opaque central core separated from the enclosing membrane by a clear space. The morphology of dense bodies, however, is extremely variable (Fig. 32.5). Some dense bodies have long, tail-like extensions or appear to be localized in alpha granules. The basis for the structural variation in dense bodies is unknown.

Disorders of megakaryocytes

In a very real sense, all of the conditions affecting the parents are visited on the progeny. Thus, except for immune thrombocytopenias, all platelet abnormalities are found in megakaryocytes. It has been easier in the past, however, to characterize the problems in platelets from circulating blood than on megakaryocytes from bone marrow. Defects in such conditions as the TAR (thrombocytopenia and absent radii) syndrome,[16] therefore, remain ill defined.

Congenital megakaryocyte hypoplasia

Amegakaryocytic thrombocytopenia and congenital megakaryocyte hypoplasia are rare conditions in newborn infants.[17] The cause for inability to promote conversion of stem cells into megakaryocytes is unknown, since some cases

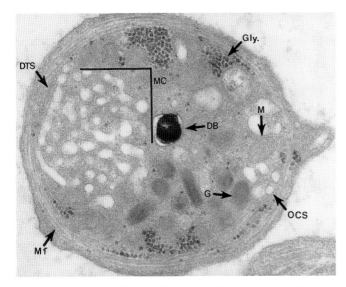

Fig. 32.3 Thin section of a discoid human platelet. A circumferential microtubule (MT) lying just under the cell wall supports the lentiform shape. Elements of the open canalicular system (OCS) and channels of the dense tubular system (DTS) are randomly dispersed in the cytoplasm and also closely associated in some areas to form membrane complexes (MC). Organelles, including alpha granules (G), dense bodies (DB) and mitochondria (M) are evenly spread throughout the cell. Gly, glycogen. × 37 000.

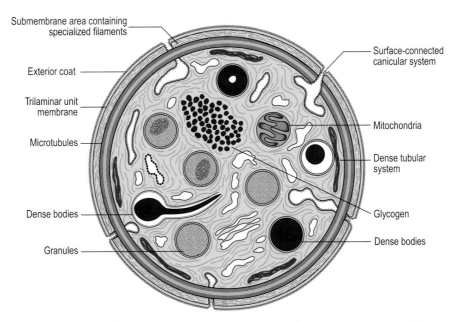

Fig. 32.4 The diagram summarizes ultrastructural features observed in thin sections of discoid platelets cut in the equatorial plane. Components of the peripheral zone include the exterior coat (EC), trilaminar unit membrane (CM) and submembrane area containing specialized filaments (SMF) which form the wall of the platelet and line channels of the surface-connected canalicular system (CS). The matrix of the platelet interior is the sol-gel zone containing actin microfilaments, structural filaments, the circumferential band of microtubules (MT) and glycogen (Gly). Formed elements embedded in the sol-gel zone include mitochondria (M), granules (G) and dense bodies (DB). Collectively, they constitute the organelle zone. The membrane systems include the surface-connected canalicular system (OCS) and the dense tubular system (DTS), which serve as the platelet sarcoplasmic reticulum.

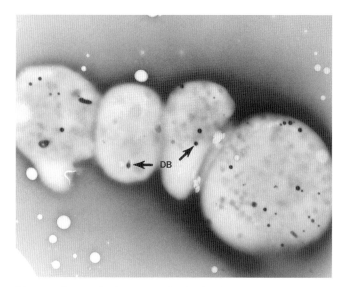

Fig. 32.5 Human platelets examined unfixed and unstained in the transmission electron microscope. Dense bodies (DB) inside the cytoplasm are inherently electron opaque, permitting visualization and enumeration by this technique. × 10 000.

have had normal levels of thrombopoietin. Hemorrhagic complications may be mild or life-threatening. Steroids appear to be of little value, but supportive care and platelet transfusion may be successful in some cases until megakaryocyte production begins.

Thrombocytopenia and absent radii (TAR) syndrome[16–18]

Megakaryocyte hypoplasia is a characteristic feature of the TAR syndrome. The basis for the hypoplasia is unknown. Occasional patients will have a leukemoid blood picture, but this eventually disappears and megakaryocyte production increases. Chromosomal abnormalities have not been reported, but are undoubtedly present in this disorder. Circulating platelets in patients with the TAR syndrome appear normal.

Fanconi anemia

Most interest has focused on the anemia in this disorder, but it should be realized that Fanconi anemia is a major cause of heritable thrombocytopenia due to megakaryocytic hypoplasia.[19] It is characterized by the association of bone marrow failure and pancytopenia with other congenital anomalies affecting the musculoskeletal and genitourinary systems. While the congenital anomalies are evident at birth, the pancytopenia may be delayed for several years. Thrombocytopenia and megakaryocytic hypoplasia may be the first signs of impending bone marrow failure in Fanconi anemia.

Disorders of platelets

Inherited platelet disorders are, in reality, megakaryocyte disorders, as indicated above. The platelets have been studied intensively in these conditions while the megakaryocytes

remain a mystery. Therefore our efforts in this chapter are focused on platelets and megakaryocytes are introduced where possible.

Platelet organelle defects

Dense bodies – general aspects

In 1951, Rand and Ried[20] found that 5-hydroxytryptamine (5-HT, serotonin) was a normal constituent of platelets, and Baker et al.[21] were able to demonstrate that subcellular particles separated from platelets were rich in this amine, as well as in adenosine triphosphate (ATP). Many workers subsequently confirmed the observation of Baker et al.[21] and added the findings that serotonin, ATP, and ADP were located either in vacuoles or the granule fraction.[22] The subcellular localization of 5-HT at the ultrastructural level, utilizing methods which had been successful in differentiating catecholamine-containing organelles in the adrenal gland, was reported by Wood.[23] Employing an initial fixation in glutaraldehyde followed by exposure to potassium dichromate at low or high pH, he was able to identify organelles rich in different amines, including 5-HT. One of the cells in his report which demonstrated localization of serotonin in very dense organelles was the blood platelet. The association of serotonin with dense bodies was confirmed by ultrastructural autoradiography[24] and by chemical determinations on isolated platelet subcellular organelles prepared by density gradient centrifugation.

An examination of thin sections of glutaraldehyde-osmic acid-fixed platelets in our laboratory revealed a different frequency of serotonin storage organelles.[25] An average of 1–1.4 dense bodies per thin sectioned platelet was found in counts on 100 cells from five normal human donors (see Fig. 32.3). Some sectioned platelets had no dense bodies in their cytoplasm. This deficiency, however, was compensated for by a significant number of cells containing 4–8 opaque organelles.

Evaluation of platelets by the whole-mount technique supported the findings made in thin-sectioned material.[26] Inherently electron-opaque dense bodies were easily counted in the unstained whole mounts (see Fig. 32.5). An average of 6.15 dense bodies per platelet was found with a range of 0–24 per cell in platelets from 10 donors.

The origin of platelet dense bodies has not been specifically defined. Early work had suggested that formation of the organelles was directly related to the uptake of serotonin.[23,27] Dense bodies were found only in circulating platelets, never in megakaryocytes. Later, however, it was shown that dense bodies are present in megakaryocytes from normal human bone marrows. If dense bodies are present in megakaryocytes, then some mechanism must exist for their development in the parent cell. Ultrastructural studies have suggested that such a mechanism does exist. Employing the uranaffin reaction introduced by Richards and Da Prada,[28] Daimon and Gotoh[29] confirmed the presence of dense bodies in megakaryocytes.

Hermansky–Pudlak syndrome (HPS)

The Hermansky–Pudlak syndrome (HPS) is a recessively inherited autosomal disease in which the triad of

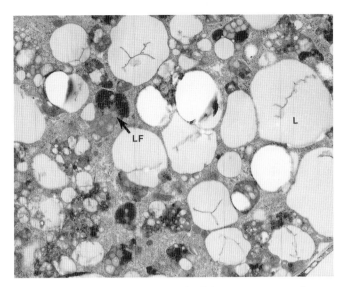

Fig. 32.6 Hermansky–Pudlak syndrome (HPS). Bone marrow macrophage from a patient with HPS. Erythrocytes and other cells are in various stages of digestion. Products resulting from their destruction include lipid droplets (L) and inclusions resembling ceroid-lipofuchsin (LF). The appearance is similar to that of the 'sea blue histiocyte' observed in various storage diseases. × 11 000.

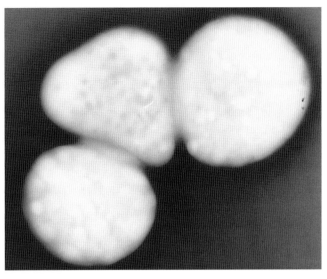

Fig. 32.7 Hermansky–Pudlak syndrome (HPS). Unstained, unfixed, whole-mount preparation of platelet from an HPS patient reveal complete absence of dense bodies. × 13 500.

tyrosinase-positive oculocutaneous albinism, accumulation of ceroid-like material in reticuloendothelial cells of bone marrow (Fig. 32.6) and other tissues, and a hemorrhagic diathesis due to defective platelets are constantly associated.[30] HPS occurs in patients of diverse ethnic extraction. It has been observed in American Caucasian and black populations, Argentinians, Belgians, Canadians, Czechs, Dutch, English, Finns, Germans, East Indians, Irish, Italians, Japanese, Hasidic and Ashkenazi Jews, Mexicans, Poles, Puerto Ricans, Swiss and Ukrainians.[31] HPS occurs in isolates in Holland, Switzerland and Chennai, India. It is estimated that HPS occurs in approximately 1 in 2000 Puerto Ricans in the northwestern quarter of the island. The pigmentary phenotype of Puerto Rican and non-Puerto Rican HPS patients is extremely variable. Some resemble tyrosinase-negative albinos with no clinically detectable pigment in skin, hair and eyes. Most have some pigment in skin, hair and eyes and resemble tyrosinase-positive, oculocutaneous albinos. A few have deeply pigmented skin and hair, but depigmented ocular fundi, and resemble ocular albinos. However, all phenotypes include nystagmus, hypoplasia of the fovea, albinotic fundi, and decreased visual acuity.

Ceroid storage has been associated with restrictive lung disease, kidney failure and cardiomyopathy. However, not all HPS patients develop these problems. The youngest patient we have seen with storage disease was a 6-year-old boy with restrictive lung disease and granulomatous colitis, while the oldest patient without clinical evidence of storage disease was 54 years of age.

The major cause of death in patients with HPS is fibrotic restrictive lung disease, which occurred in 43% of deceased subjects.[32] All deaths from this cause occurred between 35 and 46 years of age. The second leading cause of death is hemorrhage in the perinatal period or in mothers at delivery. Sixteen per cent died from this cause. While morbidity data show that 21.6% of HPS patients have evidence of

granulomatous colitis, sequelae of this condition resulted in death in only 8.1% of the deceased subjects. Thus, 67.6% died from causes directly associated with the syndrome, while 32.4% died from causes unrelated to HPS.

A granular, yellow, autofluorescent material which resembles ceroid-lipofuchsin histochemically and ultrastructurally accumulates in tissues of HPS patients. The amount of accumulation is age dependent, and the tissues in which it accumulates vary in different patients. The organs most frequently affected and in which the largest amounts of material accumulate are initially the epithelium of proximal renal tubules and later the distal tubules with little in glomeruli or the collecting tubules, bone marrow macrophages (Fig. 32.6), spleen and liver, predominantly in the portal area and in Kupfer cells. Ceroid was stored in lysosome-like structures as a granular amorphous material or occasionally with a tendency to form curvilinear or fingerprint patterns. The amount of ceroid in tissues did not always correlate with the amount of tissue damage. Tissue damage was primarily limited to gut and lung, tissues normally associated with active macrophages.

As a result of their platelet defects, HPS patients usually have a mild bleeding diathesis with ease of bruising, epistaxis and prolonged bleeding following injury, delivery or tooth extraction.[30–32] Fatal hemorrhagic episodes have occurred and are often associated with the use of cyclooxygenase inhibitors such as acetylsalicylic acid. In previous reviews of ultrastructural defects in congenital disorders of platelet function it was suggested that HPS was the first disorder in which an abnormality detectable in the electron microscope could be correlated directly with a specific biochemical deficiency, impaired platelet function in vitro, and clinical bleeding problems in patients.[33] The population of electron-dense bodies in HPS platelets was greatly reduced and in some cases virtually absent (Fig. 32.7). Biochemical analysis revealed that HPS platelets had very low levels of serotonin and a marked reduction in the non-metabolic pool of adenine nucleotides. However, earlier studies had shown that neither serotonin nor adenine nucleotides were responsible for the inherent opacity of platelet dense bodies, but that a concentration of heavy metal, such as calcium, impaired passage of the electron beam.[26] Subsequent studies have shown that normal platelet dense bodies are rich in calcium, and that HPS platelets contain significantly less calcium than do normal cells.

HPS platelets develop the same sequential changes as normal platelets when stimulated by aggregating agents, including shape change, internal transformation, and molding of cell surfaces together in tightly packed, small aggregates. Owing to the marked deficiency in ADP, the amount of nucleotide secreted by activated HPS cells is insufficient to bring uninvolved platelets into large aggregates and sustain the platelet–platelet association long enough to establish irreversible aggregation. As a result, HPS platelets do not develop second waves of aggregation when exposed to concentrations of ADP, epinephrine and thrombin, which cause biphasic, irreversible aggregation of normal cells on the aggregometer. However, they will form irreversible aggregates if exposed to a high concentration of exogenous ADP. In addition, they can form irreversible aggregates, in some instances, even when stirred with epinephrine alone.

Other defects reported in HPS platelets may be partly responsible for the elevated threshold of activation. Abnormalities in prostaglandin synthesis and formation of thromboxane A$_2$ have been noted. These have been related to defective malondialdehyde formation or decreased liberation of arachidonic acid from membrane phospholipids. The abnormalities may influence the aggregation response to arachidonate, although some patients have a normal response to this agent. Some have noted that secretion of acid hydrolases is delayed in HPS platelets, and the defect can be corrected by adding back ADP, a product normally stored in dense bodies. Thus, the defective function of HPS platelets may not be due to storage pool deficiency alone, but to other facets of platelet regulatory physiology that may be directly or indirectly involved.

Storage pool deficiency (SPD)

Patients with mild bleeding problems seemingly related to abnormal platelet secretion were recognized before the HPS was reported.[34] Weiss et al.[35] described six members of a family in whom secretable ADP was decreased. They postulated that their aggregation defects might be due to a specific deficiency in the non-metabolic pool of ADP. Subsequent studies of this family and other patients with a similar history and laboratory findings confirmed that defective platelet function was due to platelet storage pool deficiency (SPD). The platelet abnormality in SPD is very similar, if not identical, to that observed in HPS, even though SPD patients have normal pigmentation and no evidence of ceroid-lipofuchsin storage. As a result, it is difficult to relate the absence of dense bodies in HPS platelets to defects in melanosome formation or storage of aging pigment.

Platelets from patients with SPD are normal in size and number. Structural features of their platelets are normal, other than the marked deficiency (Fig. 32.8) or absence of dense bodies. Weiss et al.[36] pointed out that the deficiency of adenine nucleotides and serotonin is less profound in SPD than in HPS platelets, and often quite variable. The

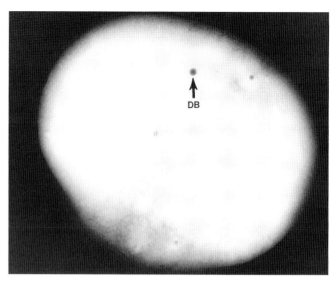

Fig. 32.8 Storage pool deficiency (SPD). Unstained, unfixed, whole-mount preparation reveal a single dense body (DB) in one platelet. The frequency in this patient was one dense body for every 20 platelets. × 16 000.

bleeding in SPD patients has been found to correlate inversely with the dense body content of ATP and ADP, but appears more closely tied to the ADP level. Incubation of normal platelets with ^{14}C-serotonin results in rapid uptake of the amine and concentration in dense bodies. In patients with SPD, the initial rate of uptake is normal, but saturation levels are decreased.[36] Normal platelets retain ^{14}C-serotonin in dense bodies for many hours, while SPD platelets lacking dense bodies rapidly lose the radioactive amine. The lost serotonin is quickly converted to 5-hydroxyindolacetic acid and 5-hydroxytryptophal by monoamine oxidases.

Failure of SPD platelets to retain serotonin has been attributed to a failure to form metal–nucleotide complexes necessary to bind 5-HT. The reason they are unable to develop metal–nucleotide complexes, however, is unknown. The origin of dense bodies in the parent megakaryocyte was discussed above. It is possible that HPS and SPD megakaryocytes fail to generate vesicles from the Golgi apparatus destined to become dense bodies. If they do make them, the vesicles may be defective and unable to transport calcium, nucleotides, or both to their interior. Since a variable number of dense bodies are present in platelets from many patients with SPD, it is probable that they make the membrane precursor, but it does not function properly. The nature of the defect remains unknown.

Platelet storage disease (SPD) has been reported to be less frequent than HPS.[36] However, it may be more common. Since bleeding symptoms are mild and the pseudoalbinism and ceroid-lipofuchsin accumulation characteristic of HPS are absent, individuals with SPD may not come to the attention of physicians. Also, the degree of adenine nucleotide and serotonin deficiency in SPD platelets is variable and usually not as severe as in the HPS, resulting in further moderation of the disease. As a result, many patients with SPD may go undetected during their lifetimes.

Weiss et al.[36] have provided an excellent analysis of this condition. Of 18 patients with various granule disorders,

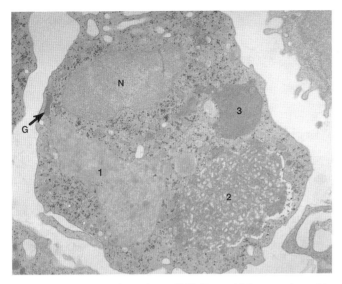

Fig. 32.9 Chediak–Higashi syndrome (CHS). Neutrophil from a patient with CHS. A nuclear lobe (N) and normal-sized granule (G) are dwarfed by greatly enlarged lysosomes (1, 2, 3). × 16 000.

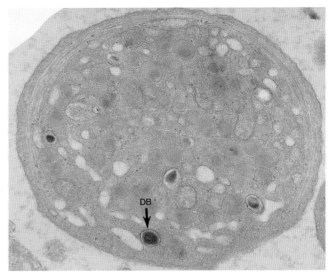

Fig. 32.10 Chediak–Higashi syndrome (CHS). Platelets from most patients with CHS are storage-pool deficient. However, some patients are only mildly abnormal. The cell in this illustration is from a patient with all of the features of CHS. However, his platelets contain about half the normal number of dense bodies (DB). × 30 000.

four were found to have dense body deficiency without other clinical features of HPS. In at least one family the disorder appeared to be inherited as an autosomal dominant. The hemorrhagic symptoms in SPD patients were generally mild, and they lacked the severe gastrointestinal bleeding seen in some patients with HPS. Depletion of dense body contents and electron-opaque organelles was less in SPD platelets compared to individuals with HPS. Weiss et al.[36] noted that serotonin levels in SPD platelets were reduced in proportion to the reduction in platelet ADP. SPD platelets may also be deficient in their ability to synthesize intermediates of prostaglandin biosynthesis. After stimulation by collagen, SPD platelets produced less than 20% of the PGE_2 and PGF_2 synthesized by normal cells.

The decrease in dense bodies in SPD correlates with the deficiency in serotonin and adenine nucleotides, the impaired response of the cells to aggregating agents, and the clinical symptoms of the patient. Thus, SPD is the second disorder in which impaired platelet function can be directly associated with an ultrastructural defect in the cells. However, the normal pigmentation of individuals with this disorder and the absence of an unusual accumulation of ceroid or lipofuchsin in macrophages suggest that the cause is basically different than that responsible for platelet storage pool deficiency in HPS. The genetic basis for the SPD found in other inherited disorders, such as Wiskott–Aldrich syndrome[37] and TAR syndrome[38] remains to be determined.

Chediak–Higashi syndrome (CHS)

The Chediak–Higashi syndrome (CHS)[39,40] is a rare, autosomally inherited disorder characterized clinically by photophobia, nystagmus, pseudoalbinism, marked susceptibility to infection, hepatosplenomegaly, lymphadenopathy and malignancy.[41] Laboratory diagnosis is based on the presence of giant organelles in nearly all leukocytes on Wright-stained peripheral blood smears[42] (Fig. 32.9; see also Chapter 17). The massive granules have been found in neutrophils,

eosinophils, lymphocytes and monocytes from blood and in their bone marrow precursors.[43]

Despite the presence of thrombocytopenia, which develops during the accelerated phase of CHS, and an early report describing two patients with markedly decreased platelet serotonin,[44] blood platelets have not been considered a major problem in this disease. However, several studies have shown that platelets express the genetic fault of the disorder.[45-47] Platelets from patients with CHS are biochemically, physiologically and functionally abnormal.[45] The defect has been related to a marked reduction in platelet-dense bodies.[48,49] Elevated levels of cyclic 3′,5′-adenosine monophosphate (cAMP) were noted in platelets from one infant with CHS.[45] However, the level of cAMP was corrected to normal by treatment with ascorbate without apparent improvement in platelet function.[50] Thus, the platelet appears to be involved in the expression of the CHS along with other blood cells containing cytoplasmic granules.

As attractive as these findings were when first reported, there is little enthusiasm for them at present. Elevations in levels of cAMP or decreased concentrations of cGMP were not found in blood cells of other patients with CHS.[51] Reversal of clinical symptoms by treatment with large amounts of vitamin C has not been found in most patients with the disease. Observations of a decrease in microtubule numbers in CHS cells[52] that led to the studies of cyclic nucleotides and the suggestion to use ascorbate[50] to treat the disease were not confirmed.[51]

Involvement of platelets in CHS appears variable. A patient with characteristic clinical and laboratory features of the disease has been followed in this laboratory for 20 years.[53] His platelets are functionally, biochemically and morphologically very close to normal (Fig. 32.10). We have studied several other patients with CHS who have storage pool deficiency, and their platelets are almost, but not completely, devoid of dense bodies.

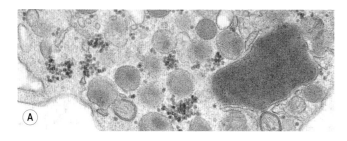

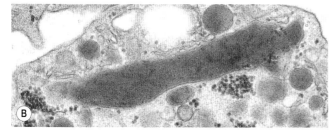

Fig. 32.11 (A, B) Chediak–Higashi syndrome (CHS). About 5% of platelets from patients with CHS contain giant granules. Incubation for acid phosphatase activity has shown that the giant granules in CHS platelets are lysosomes. A, B × 44 000.

In addition to storage pool deficiency, platelets from patients with CHS have been found to contain the giant granule anomaly.[46] Giant granules of a type not seen in normal platelets or in other platelet disorders were found in platelets from our patient with CHS in a ratio of about 1:100 cells in thin sections (Fig. 32.11A, B). Parmley et al.[47] have confirmed this observation in another patient and have shown that the giant granules in CHS platelets are acid phosphatase positive. The relationship of the giant granule anomaly to the storage pool deficiency of CHS platelets has not been defined.

Alpha granules

Alpha granules are the most numerous of the three types of platelet storage organelles destined for secretion[14,54] (see Fig. 32.3). They vary in size from 0.2 to 0.3 µm in diameter, but an occasional large granule is not uncommon in normal platelets. Alpha granules are round to oval in shape when viewed in thin sections. However, rod- and spindle-shaped alpha granules are not rare. Two zones of differing opacity are evident in the matrix of the organelle. The nucleoid is the more electron dense, and frequently has the opacity of a platelet dense body.

The lighter zone of the alpha-granule matrix usually appears unorganized. However, an occasional spindle- or rod-shaped granule can have a periodic substructure, suggesting an orderly arrangement of constituent proteins.[55] Since fibrinogen is present in alpha granules, the periodicity has been related to this protein.[56] Direct evidence for this, however, is lacking. Periodicity is far more apparent in whole-mount preparations than in thin sections of human and animal platelet alpha granules. For example, whole mounts of bovine platelets reveal periodicity in the substructure of every alpha granule. Tubular elements resembling microtubules in cross-section are present in alpha granules.[57] Ultrastructural immunocytochemistry has shown that the tubular structures are von Willebrand factor (vWF) or that vWF is very closely associated with them.[58]

Biochemical studies together with evaluation of platelets from patients who lack alpha granules have provided a long list of proteins concentrated within them.[59] Fibrinogen and vWF have been mentioned. Beta-thromboglobulin (β-TG), platelet factor 4 (PF-4), thrombospondin, platelet-derived growth factor (PDGF), factor V, and high-molecular-weight kininogen are also present. The list grows longer each year. Some of the alpha-granule proteins are synthesized by megakaryocytes, while others may be taken up from blood into either megakaryocytes or platelets. The ability of platelets to take up foreign particulates from plasma and transfer them to apparently intact alpha granules was reported several years ago.[60] Recently, megakaryocytes have been shown to take up transfused horseradish peroxidase into alpha granules and the organelles can be detected subsequently in circulating platelets by cytochemical techniques. Recognition of this pathway is important because it appears to resolve a long-standing argument concerning the origin of platelet fibrinogen. Defibrination of animal models, followed by histochemical and cytochemical studies of bone marrow and platelets, has shown that platelet fibrinogen originates from blood.[61,62]

Secretion of alpha-granule contents is a characteristic feature of the platelet response to potent aggregating agents. The process of secretion has been characterized as a transfer of chemical substances confined in storage organelles of resting platelets to the exterior plasma without simultaneous loss of cytoplasmic constituents.[63] Platelet release is highly selective, involving some organelles and not others, and physiologic, since it does not result from nonspecific injury.[64,65]

Several mechanisms have been proposed to explain how substances confined to the storage organelles in resting platelets are discharged to the exterior during the platelet release reaction. One theory suggests that organelles move to the periphery of activated platelets, fuse with the cell membrane at any point, and extrude their contents to the outside. A similar sequence of events has been observed during the process of secretion in many endocrine systems.[66] However, the evidence advanced to support this mechanism in platelets is quite meager.

Ginsberg et al.[67] have suggested a different mechanism for secretion of products from platelet organelles. Based on immunocytochemical and ultrastructural studies of PF$_4$ secretion, they suggested that platelet alpha granules fuse together in the activated platelet, resulting in the formation of a large compound granule or sealed vacuole. Their evidence indicated that the sealed vacuole formed by granule fusion moves to the periphery of activated cells and fuses with the plasma membrane, resulting in release.

Small vacuoles do develop in thrombin-activated platelets.[68] Yet the actual fusion of granules to form a compound vacuole and its movement to the cell surface as proposed by Ginsberg et al. have not been observed in activated samples. There is a swelling of the OCS and dilatation of granule membranes after communication and discharge of contents into the OCS. Granule fusion is rarely seen under these conditions, but can occur under others.[69] It has been noted in platelets from patients with certain leukemias[70] (Fig. 32.12), and regularly develops in platelets during long-term

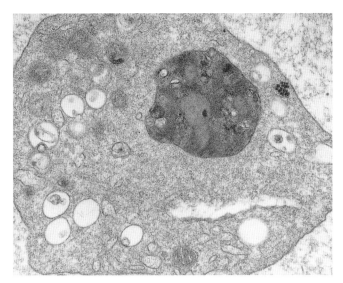

Fig. 32.12 Giant alpha granules. Alpha-granule fusion resulting in the formation of giant organelles is common in patients with myeloproliferative syndromes or myelomonocytic leukemia. × 29 000.

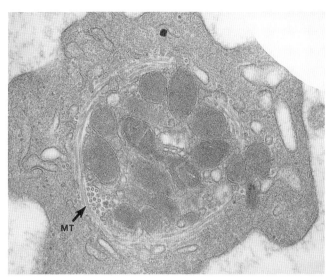

Fig. 32.14 Internal transformation. Shape change and pseudopod formation following exposure to agonists are accompanied by internal changes. Organelles move from random positions and concentrate in platelet centers. The closely associated granules are encircled by constricted rings of the circumferential microtubule (MT) and microfilaments not visible in this thin section. × 45 000.

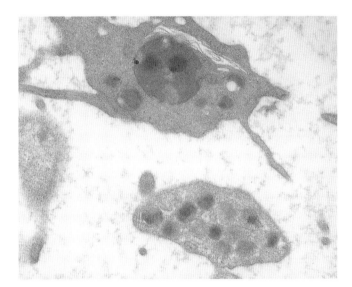

Fig. 32.13 Giant alpha granules. Platelets from a sample of platelet-rich plasma (PRP) stored under mildly alkaline conditions for 2 weeks. Fusion of alpha granules to form giant organelles is common during long-term storage. × 23 000.

storage under mildly alkaline conditions[71] (Fig. 32.13). Granule fusion in leukemic platelets or during storage, however, does not appear related to the release reaction.

In recent studies we have examined the release reaction in bovine platelets[72] and re-evaluated the secretory pathway in human cells.[73] Tannic acid, often used as an electron-dense stain, was employed to delineate the process of secretion. The chemical dye was found in a preliminary investigation to precipitate fibrinogen and selectively deposit osmic acid on fibrinogen and fibrin. Samples of citrate platelet-rich plasma (C-PRP) and washed human platelets stimulated by thrombin in the presence of ethylenediaminetetraacetic acid (EDTA) develop dramatic changes in their morphology. The

cells lose their lentiform appearance, become irregular in form, and extend numerous pseudopods. Platelet organelles become concentrated in cell centers and enclosed within rings of constricted microtubules (Fig. 32.14). Higher concentrations of thrombin cause rapid discharge of granule contents and reduction in their number. As a result, dense spots of actomyosin, in which centrally concentrated organelles are enclosed in less activated platelets, appear more prominent in strongly stimulated cells.[74]

Tannic-acid-stained platelet aggregates from C-PRP were identical in appearance to unstained control aggregates, except for the presence of osmium black precipitate. Amorphous black material surrounded the aggregates and was deposited between the cells. Electron-dense material was also present in normal-sized and swollen granules in many platelets. Connections between channels and granules and direct communication between canaliculi and the surrounding plasma were evident.

Amorphous precipitate was not present outside the thrombin-activated cells from samples of washed platelets resuspended in the presence of EDTA, and aggregates were absent. The platelets, however, revealed the same physical changes observed in thrombin-aggregated cells from platelet-rich plasma (PRP). Many granules were stained intensely by tannic acid-osmium. Other granules were swollen and their content of amorphous stained material appeared diluted. Channels of the OCS were also delineated by electron-dense stain. Some channels were tortuous and narrow and contained little tannic acid. Others were filled by electron-dense material and widely dilated. Communications between granules and OCS channels were evident in many platelets (Fig. 32.15). The connection appeared to foster swelling of the granules and dilation of the channels, so that recognition of the site of fusion was often obscured. More than one granule was frequently in communication

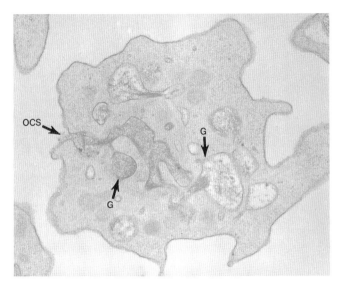

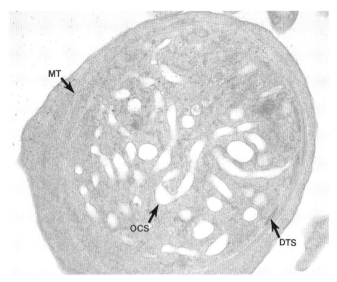

Fig. 32.15 Platelet secretion. Platelet from a sample of washed cells suspended in a buffer containing EDTA and stimulated by 3 U/ml of thrombin. The sample was fixed in glutaraldehyde containing tannic acid 3 min after exposure to the agonist without stirring. Tannic acid acts as a selective mordant, binding osmic acid to fibrin and fibrinogen under these conditions, permitting ultrastructural identification of the secretory process. In this example at least two granules (G) have fused with one channel of the open canalicular system (OCS) and their content of fibrinogen–fibrin is in the process of extrusion from the platelet. × 33 000.

Fig. 32.16 Gray platelet syndrome (GPS). Alpha granules are absent in this platelet from a patient with GPS. Channels of the open canalicular system (OCS) are the dominant feature. DTS, dense tubular system; MT, microtubule. × 15 000.

with the same OCS channel. This relationship often resulted in extensive dilation of the OCS and granules fused to it. Occasionally, channel openings on to the surface were dilated, but usually remained constricted as in resting platelets. In some examples a single channel opened in more than one place on to the surface membrane of an activated platelet. The electron-dense material present in channels frequently appeared in the process of extrusion into the surrounding medium.

The difference in the mechanism of secretion in bovine compared to human cells may seem confusing. Bovine platelets do not have a well-defined OCS. As a result, they use the surface membrane as the primary route for discharge of products from secretory granules. Human platelets have an extensive system of internalized surface membrane formed into channels of the OCS. It is used as the primary route of secretion in human cells. Bovine platelets can develop primitive canaliculi following activation and granule products can leave the cell through these conduits. Yet it employs the cell surface as a preferential route for exocytosis. The basis for the species variations in platelet structure resulting in different preferred routes for secretion of granule products remains unknown. However, it is clear that there are significant differences in bovine and human platelet shape change, pseudopod formation, spreading on surfaces, and internal transformation. Differences, therefore, in the mode of platelet secretion are not surprising.

Gray platelet syndrome

The gray platelet syndrome (GPS) is a rare disorder.[75] Since description of the first case, two other patients have been reported in the United States.[59,76] In France, two siblings, a

brother and sister, have been characterized with GPS.[77] Recently, a patient from New Zealand, two in Australia, another living in England, and a family in Japan have been found to have GPS.

The original patient[75] was evaluated for thrombocytopenia as a child and found to have large, nearly agranular platelets which appeared gray or blue–gray on Wright-stained blood smears. Splenectomy improved, but did not correct the platelet count to normal. It remained between 100 000 and 125 000/mm³. Most of his platelets retained the large agranular appearance noted before splenectomy, but a small percentage were of normal size and contained some granules. Since his mean platelet volume was increased (11.1 μm³), the thrombocytopenia was probably relative, as it is in other giant platelet syndromes, and the circulating platelet biomass (platelet number × mean platelet volume) was normal.[78]

Aggregation studies revealed an essentially normal response to most aggregating agents. However, the reaction of gray platelets to collagen and thrombin was less than normal.[59] Increasing concentrations of these reagents restored the full response. Levels of serotonin and adenine nucleotides were normal. PF4, β-TG, fibrinogen, thrombomodulin and PDGF were markedly reduced. Lysosomal enzymes and catalase were within normal limits. Ultrastructural studies revealed wide variations in platelet size and morphology. Most platelets were relatively large, vacuolated, and nearly devoid of organelles (Fig. 32.16). Dense bodies, occasional mitochondria, and a few granules were present in the cells.[76] Cytochemical studies with the uranaffin reaction confirmed the presence of dense bodies. A few small granules were positive for catalase and larger granules revealed reaction products for acid phosphatase and β-glucuronidase. The percentage of alpha granules was less than 15% of control platelets. Many cells were filled with elements of the dense tubular system (Fig. 32.17), while others principally contained channels of the OCS. Dilated vacuoles communicating with the OCS were common, and

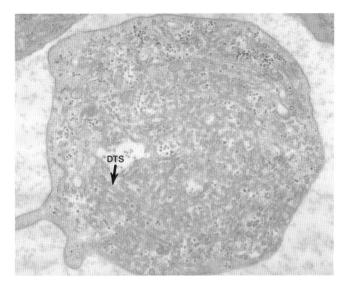

Fig. 32.17 Gray platelet syndrome (GPS). The GPS platelet in this illustration is filled with channels from the dense tubular system (DTS). × 24 000.

appeared to be sites usually occupied by alpha granules. This observation was important because megakaryocytes in patients with GPS can synthesize the proteins missing in alpha granules, but the products are lost before the large platelets reach circulating blood.

The problem in this disorder appears to be related to packaging.[79] Proteins destined for concentration in alpha granules either do not reach the developing organelles or are lost after inclusion within their membranes. The latter seems to be more likely. Breton-Gorius et al.[80] have shown that loss of granule contents and release of PDGF from megakaryocytes may be a major, but not the only, factor involved in development of marrow fibrosis in the GPS, in patients with megakaryocytic leukemia and in myeloproliferative disorders.

In addition to proliferation of reticulin or fibrosis, the marrow of patients with GPS reveals one other abnormal feature. Emperiopolesis, the uptake of other blood cells into the demarcation membrane systems of megakaryocytes, is not a rare finding.[79] Originally, it was considered to be an indication of malignant disease, but it does occur in normal individuals. In GPS it is a striking feature.[79] Some megakaryocytes contain 10–12 neutrophils and occasional monocytes. The loss of chemotactic proteins from defective granules through the OCS of developing platelets and demarcation membranes of the parent cell may attract leukocytes to the evolving channel system.

Our second patient with GPS also has Goldenhar's syndrome.[81] Examination of the literature and two other patients with Goldenhar's syndrome failed to reveal gray platelets. Since other patients with GPS do not have the second syndrome, there does not appear to be any direct link between them.

A Japanese family with GPS[82] appears to have a more severe problem with bleeding than the American patients. Also, the response of their platelets to ADP and collagen was abnormal, whereas platelets from both of our patients with GPS aggregated in a normal manner when stirred with these agents. The alpha-granule deficiency and reduction in levels of granule-associated products were significantly less in Japanese kindred compared to the patients studied here. In view of the less-severe platelet alpha-granule deficiency, a plethora of other morphologic defects, reduced production of thromboxane A_2, severe deficiency of platelet factor 3 activity, and low levels of factor VIII subunits, it is possible that the disorder presented by the Japanese family may be a variant of the GPS reported by Raccuglia.[75] The Japanese workers have suggested that the condition found in their kindred may more likely represent a release-type defect[83] than an organelle deficiency disorder. Since other patients with GPS are profoundly deficient in alpha granules compared to the Japanese kindred, the suggestion may be appropriate for their family.

Alpha-granule, dense-body deficiency

Although intermediate forms appear to exist, only one case of combined alpha-granule, dense-body deficiency has been defined.[36] The patient with combined deficiency has hemorrhagic symptoms. No other stigmata are evident in this patient. As a result, there is nothing else to suggest the presence of platelet alpha-granule dense-body deficiency. Since there is only a single case of combined defect, the pattern of inheritance is uncertain. The morphology of platelets with deficiency in both alpha granules and dense bodies is very different from that of gray platelets. Though variable in size, the cells missing both secretory organelles are not significantly increased in mean platelet volume. The large vacuoles commonly observed filling the cytoplasm of gray platelets are virtually absent from cells with the combined defect.[84] This observation suggests that the abnormality responsible for failure to form granules in the combined deficiency disorder differs from that in the GPS. No basis for the decrease in dense bodies was detected in thin sections of platelets from the patient with combined deficiency.

Heterogeneous storage organelle deficiency

Weiss et al.[36] have described two families with diminution of dense bodies and partial deficiency of alpha granules. One of the families also had platelets with an increased lecithin to phosphatidyl ethanolamine ratio, increased glycoprotein IV, and decreased adhesion to subendothelium. The inheritance of the combined partial deficiencies of alpha granules and dense bodies in the two families appears to be autosomal dominant.

Enlarged alpha granules

Jacobsen–Paris–Trousseau syndrome

A novel genetic thrombocytopenia with platelet inclusion bodies, dysmegakaryopoiesis, mild congenital anomalies and mental retardation associated with chromosome 11 deletion at 11q23 was recently reported.[85–87] platelet inclusion bodies were found to be giant alpha granules present in 15% of the cells in peripheral blood (Fig. 32.18). This condition had not been described previously, and as a result the authors termed it the Paris–Trousseau syndrome. However, the Jacobsen syndrome is also associated with deletion of chromosome 11 at q23.3.[88–90] Typical anomalies

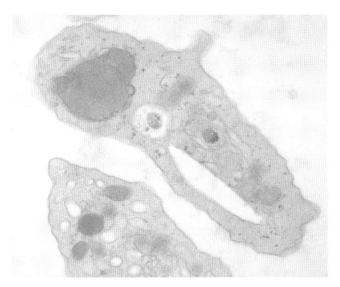

Fig. 32.18 Jacobsen, Paris–Trousseau syndrome. Platelet is from a patient with Jacobsen syndrome whose platelets contain the giant alpha granules identical to those in patients with the Paris–Trousseau syndrome. × 45 000.

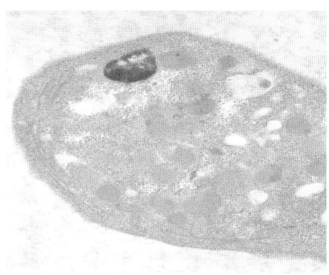

Fig. 32.20 Platelet lysosomes. Cell from a sample of washed platelets incubated for acid phosphatase activity in medium containing cerium as the capture agent. Reaction product is confined to a single organelle. × 35 000.

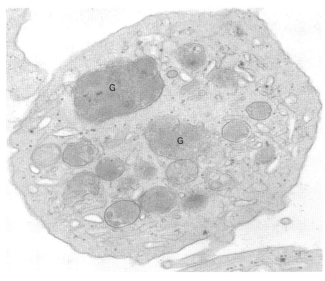

Fig. 32.19 Platelet from another patient with the Jacobsen syndrome containing several giant alpha granules (G) identical to those found in platelets from Paris–Trousseau syndrome patients. × 38 000.

include trigonocephaly, facial dysmorphism, cardiac defects, syndactyly and psychomotor retardation, although none of these features is invariably present.[88] Approximately 47% of the patients with Jacobsen syndrome were found to be thrombocytopenic,[85] but investigation of their platelets by electron microscopy was not reported. Recently, we have evaluated platelets from two patients with Jacobsen syndrome.[91] Both individuals have the same giant alpha granules in their platelets observed in cells from patients with the Paris–Trousseau syndrome (Fig. 32.19). Since patients with the Paris–Trousseau syndrome and Jacobsen syndrome share the same chromosomal defect, we have suggested that the two disorders are the same. The only difference may

be that dense bodies were virtually absent in platelets from the two patients with Jacobsen syndrome. Reports on the Paris–Trousseau syndrome have not mentioned the state of platelet dense bodies.[85–87]

Lysosomes

Platelets are known to contain and secrete a variety of hydrolytic enzymes, including acid phosphatase, aryl sulfatase, β-N-acetylgalactoseaminidase, α-arabinosidase, and others.[92] For many years it was believed that hydrolases were confined to alpha granules, but subcellular fractionation suggested they were localized at a different site in the cell.[22] Platelet lysosomes have been difficult to characterize cytochemically, although an early study suggested that acid phosphatase was localized to an organelle similar in size to the alpha granules.[93] Bentfield and Bainton[94] studied the localization of acid phosphatase and aryl sulfatase in rat megakaryocytes and platelets. Their investigations suggested that lysosomes arose as variably-sized vesicles from the Golgi cisternae. The lysosomal vesicles ranged from 175 to 250 nm in diameter and were much smaller than alpha granules.[95]

Recently we have used cerium as the capture ion for phosphate liberated by acid phosphatase, rather than lead phosphate (Fig. 32.20). Results of our experiments support the concept that hydrolytic enzymes are localized to a form of granule in platelets rather than to vesicles. The concept that platelet lysosomes are granules rather than vesicles is supported by other observations. Platelets contain very few, if any, vesicles. Those present are usually covered by barbs typical of clathrin-coated endocytic vesicles.[96] The rest are in reality part of the tortuous open canalicular system, as demonstrated by electron-dense tracers. Thus, the multiple proteins making up the acid hydrolase complement of platelet lysosomes appear to be packaged in organelles similar to those found in phagocytic cells.

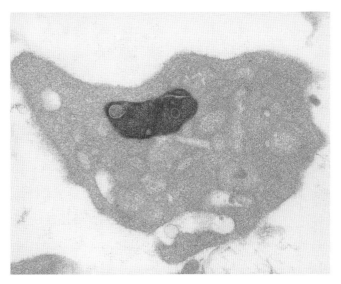

Fig. 32.21 Chediak–Higashi syndrome (CHS). Platelet from patient with CHS reacted for acid phosphatase with cerium as the capture agent. A giant lysosome in the cell cytoplasm is positive for the hydrolytic enzyme activity. × 35 000.

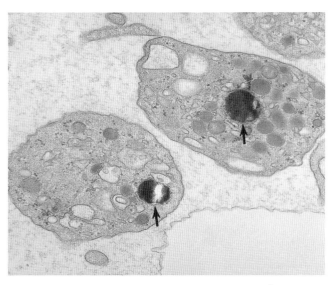

Fig. 32.22 Giant dense body disorder (GDBD). Dense bodies (↑) in two platelets from one of our patients with the GDBD are huge compared to adjacent alpha granules and mitochondria. × 26 000.

Chediak–Higashi syndrome

Characteristic features of the Chediak–Higashi syndrome (CHS) were discussed earlier in this chapter. Most of the circulating leukocytes, including neutrophils, eosinophils, basophils, monocytes and lymphocytes, contain various forms of giant lysosomes (see Fig. 32.9). It was this feature that suggested that CHS is a form of lysosomal disease.[97]

Most of the interest in platelets from patients with CHS has focused on the storage pool deficiency and virtual absence of dense bodies discussed above. Yet, dense bodies are not lysosomes. Why they are absent rather than enlarged like abnormal organelles in other cells in this disorder[98] is unknown. The fact that CHS platelets do contain giant lysosomes has received less attention.[46] Enlarged organelles are present in 1–5% of their platelets (see Figs 32.11A, B). A cytochemical study has shown that the giant granules contain acid phosphatase, demonstrating that they are lysosomes[47] (Fig. 32.21). The relationship of the giant lysosomes in CHS platelets to the absence of dense bodies has not been defined. However, the platelet in CHS is the only cell in this disorder shown to have abnormalities in two distinctly different types of organelles.[46,98]

Giant dense body disorder

Recently, we have evaluated an impressive giant-platelet dense body disorder.[84] The child was found to have thrombocytopenia shortly after birth. During the course of evaluating him we found that his mother had a normal platelet count, but the same platelet defects as her child. Platelets from both contain excessive numbers of giant electron-opaque organelles (Fig. 32.22). Despite their increased number and size, the platelets from mother and child contained normal levels of serotonin and adenine nucleotides. Concentrated platelet samples from the child and C-PRP from his mother responded normally to aggregating agents.

Siblings and relatives of the propositi had normal platelets. Immunocytochemistry revealed that the giant dense bodies contained peroxidase and were, therefore, lysosomes. The reason why these giant lysosomes are inherently electron opaque is unclear.

Disorders of platelet membranes and membrane organization

Platelet membranes and membrane systems are unique.[99] Surface membranes enclosing all other circulating blood cells develop through a process of maturation and cell division. Platelet membranes are formed within the confines of a single cell which does not undergo division into daughter cells.[100] The mechanism involved in the formation of platelets within the parent megakaryocyte has been of great interest for many years, but has not been resolved. Behnke[101,102] used electron-dense tracers to demonstrate that the surface of maturing rat megakaryocytes undergoes invagination, resulting in sequestration of the cytoplasm into subunits about the size of platelets (Fig. 32.23). As beautiful as that work was, it did not reveal how tube-like channels from the parent cell surface could develop into flat sheets that form the outer membranes of discoid platelets.[103] Also, it could not be determined in thin sections whether or not individual platelets were completely formed or were parts of membrane-demarcated chains[104] (Fig. 32.23).

Wright[100] was the first to suggest that megakaryocytes in bone marrow produce cytoplasmic processes resembling chains that penetrate into the intravascular compartment and fragment to produce platelets. The *in vitro* study of Thiery and Bessis[105] gave substance to this concept. They demonstrated that future platelets in the cytoplasm of megakaryocytes became arranged in long, ribbon-like structures. The projections elongated progressively, giving the megakaryocyte an octopus-like appearance in the phase contrast

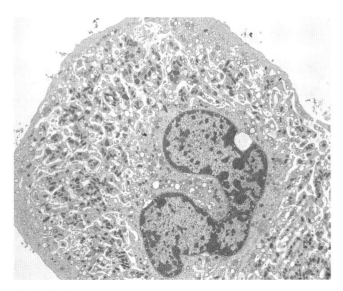

Fig. 32.23 Megakaryocyte. Platelet-forming cell from human marrow. Areas on the left and right sides of the cell appear to be breaking up into platelets or proplatelets. × 4300.

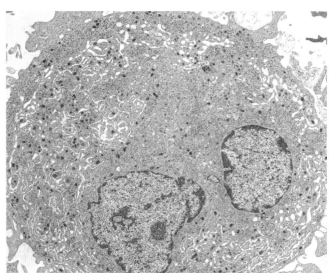

Fig. 32.24 Thin section of a megakaryocyte from a patient with Wiskott–Aldrich syndrome (WAS). The cell is of normal size and all structures, including the demarcation membrane system, resemble similar structures in normal megakaryocytes. × 4500.

microscope. In time, the long processes developed alternating swellings and constrictions. If the cell at this stage was disturbed, platelets would break loose from their attachment threads to the chain, adhere to glass, and spread in a normal manner.

Support for the observations of Thiery and Bessis was provided by Becker and deBruyn[106] and subsequently by Scurfield and Radley,[107] on fixed samples of bone marrow examined in scanning and transmission electron microscopes. Platelets were derived from long intrasinusoidal extensions originating from extravascularly located megakaryocytes. Release into the circulation was probably initiated by local constrictions in the long processes, yielding either single cells or long segments of proplatelet cytoplasm. Incompletely segmented platelets resembling extended pieces of proplatelet cytoplasm have been recovered from human blood. Thus, the literature provides considerable support for the concept that platelets are delivered from bone marrow matrix to the sinusoids via long processes which constrict segmentally to provide single cells or chains of incompletely separated platelets to circulating blood.[108]

It is hoped that a clear understanding of platelet formation will develop soon. We need the clarification in order to understand why circulating platelets have a nearly identical size, with a mean platelet volume (MPV) of 7–10 fl. It almost seems that platelets are stamped out in a mold and then delivered to blood. Yet the megakaryocyte is no mold. It is a dynamic membrane-forming system and understanding how it works is the key to understanding normal and abnormal platelet membranes and membrane organization.[109]

Small platelets

Wiskott–Aldrich syndrome

The Wiskott–Aldrich syndrome (WAS) is an X-linked, recessively inherited disorder characterized by thrombocytopenia, eczema and recurrent infections.[110,111] Immunologic

defects include reduced levels of IgM, reduced or absent isoagglutinins to blood groups A and B, reduced lymphocyte counts, impaired lymphocyte responses to certain mitogens, and markedly elevated IgE.[37,112] Platelets, in addition to being present in reduced numbers, are one-half to two-thirds normal size and have been reported to be deficient in granules, dense bodies, mitochondria, adenine nucleotides and serotonin.[37] However, our findings suggest that organelles are normal, even though the cell is small (Fig. 32.24).

After splenectomy, platelet counts may return to normal in many patients, and increase in the number of cells is associated with restoration of normal size and ultrastructural appearance.[113] The results suggest that the platelet defect in WAS may be due to extrinsic factors influencing maturation of megakaryocytes in the bone marrow.[114] Wiskott–Aldrich syndrome is not ordinarily considered to result from an intrinsic membrane defect, although a surface-membrane glycoprotein deficiency was reported.[115] Most workers consider a metabolic abnormality[116] in oxidative phosphorylation to underlie the small size and defective function.[117] However, it is possible that WAS is caused by a membrane maturation defect in the megakaryocyte.

Development of specific zones in cytoplasm destined to become individual platelets follows a definite sequence of events. Deoxyribonucleic acid synthesis and endoreduplication of the nucleus take place first.[118] This is followed by a laying down of a huge system of rough endoplasmic reticulum (RER) for synthesis of proteins.[119] Transfer of synthesized proteins to the Golgi zone is followed by delivery to three different types of storage organelles that fill the cytoplasm of the huge cell. The final event involves invagination of the surface to form demarcation membranes, which delineate a general outline of individual cells.[101] If, for some reason, the process of maturation were interrupted, what might be expected to occur? For example, in idiopathic thrombocytopenic purpura or severe hemorrhage the demand for platelets in circulating blood causes early release of large, young platelets, some of which contain residual elements of RER. The result suggests that the demarcation membranes are incompletely developed before platelets are released, resulting in larger size.

If, on the other hand, maturation is delayed in the marrow by 1 or 2 days, demarcation membranes would have time to overdevelop. As a result, the platelet zones may be one-half normal size. Because the platelets would be 2 or 3 days older than normal cells before leaving the parent cell in the marrow, energy reserves would be decreased and life span shortened.[117] The short life span of platelets and delayed development of megakaryocytes would cause thrombocytopenia. All of these features are characteristics of WAS. Thus, although the hypothesis is speculative, WAS may represent a postmature disorder owing to protracted membrane formation in the megakaryocyte. The observation that splenectomy often restores numbers, size, biochemistry and function to normal[113] supports the possibility that WAS platelets are not intrinsically abnormal, but become so if maturation is delayed.

Giant platelet disorders

Mediterranean macrothrombocytopenia

Large platelets, moderate thrombocytopenia, and splenomegaly have been described in a significant percentage of persons originating from the Italian and Balkan peninsulas and is therefore referred to as Mediterranean macrothrombocytopenia.[78] Erythrocyte stomatocytosis is also observed in high frequency in the population. Individuals with this problem do not have a bleeding tendency. There is an inverse correlation between platelet counts and mean platelet volume, so that individuals with Mediterranean macrothrombocytopenia have the same platelet biomass in circulating blood as individuals with normal platelet counts. Thus, thrombocytopenia is not due to bone marrow failure. Platelet ultrastructure appears to be normal. The mode of inheritance has not been clearly established. Therefore, Mediterranean macrothrombocytopenia is a benign morphologic variant, reflecting a tendency within every species for the circulating platelet biomass to vary within defined limits.[78]

May–Hegglin anomaly (MHA)

May–Hegglin anomaly (MHA) has an autosomal dominant pattern of inheritance.[120,121] Platelet counts are reduced to about 50 000/mm³ in these patients, but the MPV is 5–7 times that of normal cells (Fig. 32.25). If one multiplies the platelet number by MPV to obtain the platelet mass in circulating blood, there is little difference between the values obtained in MHA and normal individuals.[78] Thus, patients with MHA are not really thrombocytopenic. The number of megakaryocytes present in bone marrow of MHA patients is not increased, and their mean volume is similar to that of normal megakaryocytes.

A characteristic feature of MHA, in addition to giant platelets, is the presence of spindle-shaped bodies in all types of granulocytes and in monocytes[122] (Figs 32.25–32.27). The inclusions are referred to as Dohle bodies, but are not to be confused with the enlarged azurophilic granules in neutrophils of patients with severe infections[123]

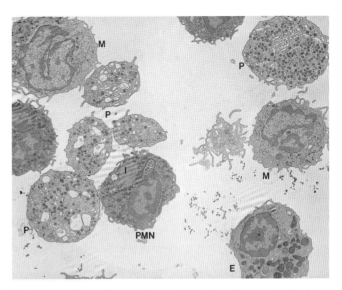

Fig. 32.25 Buffy coat from a patient with May–Hegglin anomaly. Platelets (P) in this thin section are as large as monocytes (M), eosinophils (E), and polymorphonuclear leukocytes (PMN). One PMN contains a May–Hegglin inclusion (I). × 4000.

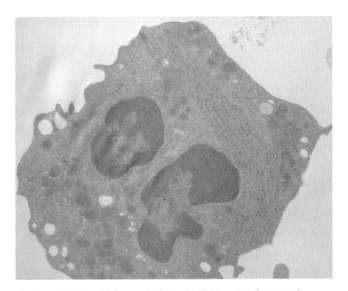

Fig. 32.26 Neutrophil from an individual with May–Hegglin anomaly (MHA) containing a spindle-shaped inclusion typical of the MHA. × 13 000.

(Fig. 32.28), even though they are referred to by the same name. Dohle bodies in MHA leukocytes are basophilic on Wright-stained blood smears and react positively when stained with methylgreen pyronine.[124] The immature nature of the inclusions suggested by these staining reactions is borne out in ultrastructural studies.[125] Short segments of RER, clusters of ribosomes, and a framework of parallel filaments are the principal constituents of May–Hegglin inclusions viewed in thin section[126] (Fig. 32.27). The filaments are 8–9 nm in diameter and resemble intermediate filaments found in many cell types.[127] Light and electron microscopic studies suggest that MHA inclusions result from a failure to completely disassemble and resorb the RER and ribosome clusters characteristic of early states in the development of mature circulating cells.

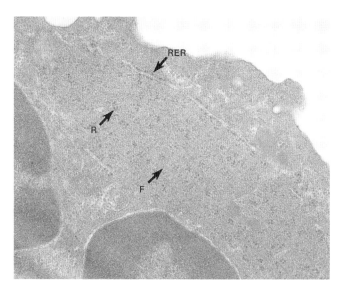

Fig. 32.27 May–Hegglin inclusion. Fragments of rough endoplasmic reticulum (RER) are associated with May–Hegglin anomaly (MHA) inclusions, but the predominant structures are rows of ribosomes (R) dispersed between intermediate filaments (F). The inclusion is not enclosed within a membrane. × 20 000.

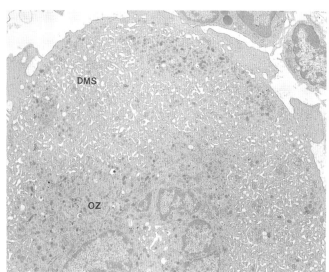

Fig. 32.29 Megakaryocyte from bone marrow of a patient with May–Hegglin anomaly (MHA). The large cells are similar in size to those from normal individuals. However, their internal organization is different. Areas of intense demarcation membrane system (DMS) formation in MHA megakaryocytes are separated from organelle zones (OZ), whereas they are intermixed in normal platelet-forming cells. × 3800.

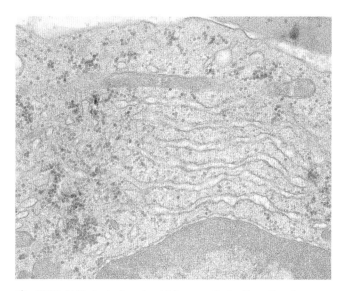

Fig. 32.28 Dohle body. A neutrophil from a patient with septicemia. Parallel stacks of rough endoplasmic reticulum present in this cell give the impression of being a distinct inclusion (Dohle body) when viewed in the light microscope on Wright-stained blood smears. × 33 000.

MHA inclusions may also be related in some way to giant platelet formation in the megakaryocyte[128] (Fig. 32.29). Although channels of the demarcation membrane system (DMS) derived from the surface membrane may appear in primitive megakaryocytes, the tortuous mass of membrane does not reach its full stage of development in the form of platelet-sized fields until protein synthesis is virtually complete.[118] At this stage the channels of RER have ordinarily been converted to smooth endoplasmic reticulum (SER), and are distributed evenly throughout the cytoplasm. Only by removal or drastic modification of the massive membrane

barrier imposed by the RER is it possible for the surface-derived DMS to penetrate into and subdivide the deepest recesses of megakaryocyte cytoplasm.

Yet the mere disappearance of one membrane system and development of another does not explain the fine balance of interaction between the DMS and SER. In every platelet, close associations between the surface-derived channels and residual elements of SER can be identified. We have called these specialized associations membrane complexes (MC).[53] Since MCs are intrinsic features of normal platelet anatomy, it is clear that their development in the parent megakaryocyte requires a balanced distribution of elements from the two channel systems throughout the cytoplasm.

What would happen if the timing of these events leading to sequestration of megakaryocyte cytoplasm was thrown off? If demand for platelets was greatly increased so they had to be delivered from immature megakaryocytes to circulating blood before completion of protein synthesis, what would they look like? One would expect their cytoplasm to be less mature and to contain at least some RER. Indeed, the platelets in the peripheral blood of patients with idiopathic thrombocytopenic purpura (ITP) often have this appearance. Also, on the basis of the rationale given above, one would expect ITP platelets to be large. Indeed they are, and the name 'megathrombocyte' was coined to describe them.[129] Thus, shortening of the time interval for development and interaction of the DMS and SER can result in large platelets with immature features.

MHA platelets, despite their large size, do not resemble the megathrombocytes of ITP (Fig. 32.30). The giant MHA thrombocytes are almost uniformly huge, while ITP platelets are irregular in size, with only a few large cells present in peripheral blood.[130] Characteristics of immaturity are lacking in the MHA platelets. Organelles, including alpha granules, lysosomes, dense bodies, mitochondria and peroxisomes, are present in normal numbers and distribution. The

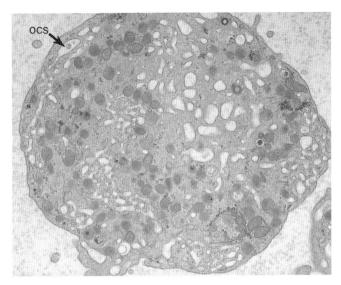

Fig. 32.30 May–Hegglin anomaly (MHA) platelet. Aside from their large size, the morphology of MHA platelets is very similar to that of normal cells. However, they are relatively spherical, rather than discoid in shape, and the open canalicular system (OCS) is more prominent. × 18 000.

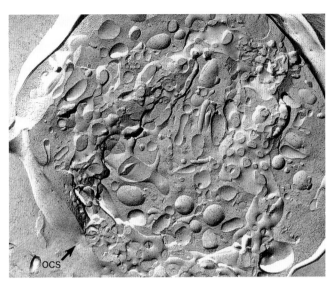

Fig. 32.31 Replica of a freeze-fractured platelet from a patient with May–Hegglin anomaly. The open canalicular system (OCS) is prominent. Channels communicating with the cell surface join each other and pursue tortuous courses throughout the cytoplasm. In some areas they form close associations with elements of the dense tubular system in membrane complexes. × 27 000.

basophilia and occasional segments of RER found in left-shifted ITP[129] platelets are absent in MHA cells.

In fact, the only apparent difference between huge MHA platelets and normal-sized cells is the increased amount of internalized membrane and the size of the membrane complexes (Figs 32.30 and 32.31). Clearly, there is no defect in the ability of MHA megakaryocytes to invaginate the surface membranes and form the DMS; nor does there appear to be a problem of interaction between DMS and SER to form membrane complexes. These intricate mazes formed by the two channel systems in MHA megakaryocytes are very prominent in circulating platelets. Thus, the membrane systems and their interactions appear to be involved in some way in the pathogenesis of the giant platelets of the MHA.[131]

The precise mechanism is still uncertain. Since both the DMS and SER are fully developed in MHA megakaryocytes, an imbalance of some form in their interaction would seem to be a likely possibility.[132] The inclusions in MHA leukocytes may provide a clue to the defective process in the megakaryocytes. MHA inclusions appear to represent collections of RER, ribosomes, and filaments which have failed to disappear during the maturation sequence. Their tendency to remain in aggregates into mature stages may be reflected in developing MHA megakaryocytes. If channels of RER remain associated for prolonged periods during conversion to SER, the interaction with the wave of advancing DMS could be perturbed. As a result, excessive interaction may occur between the two types of channels to form large membrane complexes with a consequent reduction in the interactions of DMS to form sequestration zones. The imbalance could result in giant platelets and increased membrane complex formation, precisely the characteristic features of circulating MHA platelets.

There is a second way in which persistence of channels of RER or clusters of SER could result in giant platelet formation. As mentioned above, the RER during the stage of

protein formation presents a formidable barrier to penetration by DMS pushing in from the cell surface. If it fails to disassemble, even though conversion to SER takes place, barriers may remain, and result in a decreased number of very large sequestration zones.[132]

There may be other possible ways in which an imbalance of membrane interaction could result in evolution of the giant MHA platelets. However, the two suggested have the advantage of bringing together the pathogenesis of the MHA inclusions in leukocytes and the development of giant platelets in megakaryocytes. Some of the individuals with MHA have prolonged bleeding times and hemorrhagic symptoms which cannot be explained on the basis of reduced platelet numbers alone. However, tests of platelet function and aggregation have, in general, been normal and the platelet defect responsible for excessive bleeding in MHA has not been defined.[127]

Epstein's syndrome (ES)

Interstitial or mixed nephritis and nerve deafness[133] (Alport's syndrome) represent a well-known and not very rare hereditary disease. Epstein et al.[134] were first to note that some families with this autosomal dominant disorder were also thrombocytopenic and had giant, abnormal platelets. Affected members had prolonged bleeding times, defective platelet adhesion, and abnormal aggregation in response to collagen and epinephrine. Another family with hereditary deafness, renal disease and thrombocytopenia reported by Eckstein et al.[135] had large platelets with normal ultrastructural morphology and *in vitro* function. Eckstein's family was considered a variant of the syndrome reported by Epstein,[134] but the basis for the differences in platelet function and clinical bleeding problems in the separate families has not been explained. More recently Hansen et al.[136] reported that giant platelets from a family with Epstein syndrome lack

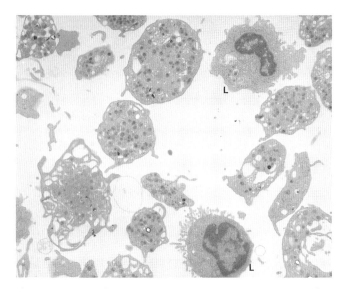

Fig. 32.32 Platelets from a patient with Epstein's syndrome (ES). Most of the platelets in this thin section are as large as the two lymphocytes (L). × 6000.

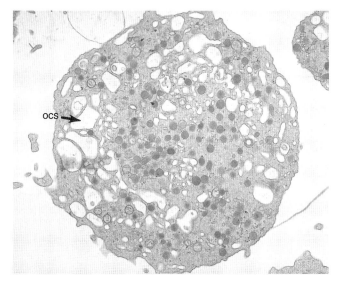

Fig. 32.33 Platelet from patient with Epstein's syndrome (ES). The cell is large, but basic morphologic features are similar to those of normal platelets. Channels of the open canalicular system (OCS) are as prominent in ES cells as they are in May–Hegglin anomaly (MHA) platelets. × 13 000.

microtubules and dense bodies. Neither defect was recorded in previous studies of platelet ultrastructure in patients with ES,[134,137] and we have not encountered these additional defects in our patients.

Platelets from these patients with ES are usually not quite as large as those from individuals with MHA, but are nearly indistinguishable from them in all other respects[138] (see Fig. 32.30). The enlarged platelets are frequently the size of lymphocytes, monocytes and neutrophils, and, like nucleated blood cells, are spherical in shape, rather than discoid (Figs 32.32 and 32.33). Immunofluorescence studies with specific antibodies against tubulin, the subunit protein of microtubules, have shown that the large cells have markedly increased numbers of microtubule coils which are highly disorganized

compared to normal platelets.[139] Instead of forming a marginal band consisting of 8–12 closely associated coils lying just inside the surface membrane along its greatest circumference, the ES platelet has 50–100 coils organized like a ball of yarn, rather than a marginal bundle. It is not certain whether the disorganized microtubule coils cause the spherical shape of ES platelets or are the result of it.

The OCS is prominent in ES platelets, as it is in MHA cells.[138] The association of OCS channels with elements of the dense tubular system results in the formation of large membrane complexes in ES and MHA platelets. Membrane complexes are part of normal anatomy, and therefore are not inherently abnormal in giant platelets. However, the large size of membrane complexes in ES and MHA platelets has suggested that the huge complexes may be the cause of macrothrombocytopenia.[131,134] Since the precise mechanisms of normal platelet membrane formation and organization in megakaryocytes have not been clearly defined, it is uncertain what the formation of giant membrane complexes has to do with the genesis of giant platelets.

Hereditary nephritis associated with May–Hegglin syndrome

The giant platelets observed in patients with MHA and ES are virtually identical. What separates the syndromes are other features of the hereditary disorders. ES patients are characterized by all of the features of Alport's syndrome[133] in addition to giant platelets, but lack the leukocyte inclusions characteristic of MHA.[140] MHA patients have spindle-shaped inclusions in circulating granulocytes and monocytes, but do not have high-frequency hearing loss, congenital cataracts or interstitial nephritis.

Brivet et al.[141] have described a family in whom features of MHA and ES appeared together. Basophilic inclusion bodies, referred to as Dohle bodies in their report, were found in granulocytes of three affected family members studied. Clinical deafness and congenital cataracts were not found. Proteinuria, intermittent hematuria and mild elevation in blood pressure were presenting features of the nephritis in an 11-year-old female member of the family. A paternal grand-aunt had died while on periodic hemodialysis and the father had proteinuria.

In contrast to the family reported from France, our kindred has characteristic features of Alport's syndrome.[133] High-frequency deafness and congenital cataracts were found in affected members in four generations. Renal biopsies revealed interstitial nephritis typical of ES and Alport's syndrome.[142] One family member has undergone renal transplantation.

Platelets were large, but their light microscopic and ultrastructural appearance was not significantly different from that of normal platelets (Fig. 32.34). Platelet aggregation in response to epinephrine, arachidonate, thrombin, adenosine diphosphate, collagen and restocetin was normal. Levels of nucleotides and serotonin were normal in proportion to cell volume. The concentration of adenosine triphosphate secreted and the percentage of arachidonic acid converted to thromboxane B_2 were also proportional to cell number. Thus, this family represents a variant of Alport's syndrome with cataracts and leukocyte inclusions that, because of the associated macrothrombocytopenia, may be confused with MHA or ES.[143]

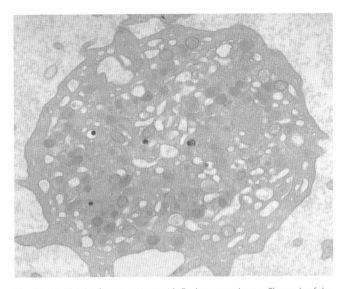

Fig. 32.34 Platelet from a patient with Fechtner syndrome. Channels of the open canalicular system are a prominent feature, but otherwise the morphology is identical to that found in normal platelets. × 16000.

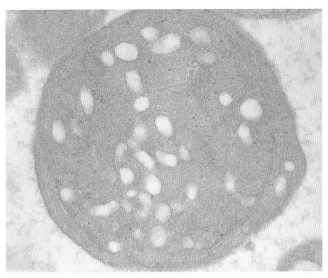

Fig. 32.35 Pseudo-gray platelets. This cell is from a patient with transient leukemia of childhood and Down syndrome. The cells are of normal size, but devoid of alpha granules. As a result, they strongly resemble platelets from patients with gray platelet syndrome. × 36000.

Gray platelet syndrome (GPS)

General features and specific details of GPS were discussed above. Platelets from patients with GPS are very large and often bizarre.[75] Therefore, the syndrome is classified as a giant platelet disorder, as well as a disorder of platelet organelles. The choice of GPS as the appellation for this disorder was based on the appearance of the cells on Wright-stained blood smears. Absence of alpha granules and relative immaturity provided a grayish cast to the cells when observed in the light microscope. The other main feature was their large size. As a result, Raccuglia felt it necessary to distinguish gray platelets from the large cells found in other giant platelet disorders. Although GPS platelets are big, they are not as large as the cells from patients with MHA or ES.[132,138] As a result, platelet counts are usually higher in GPS patients than in patients with other giant platelet disorders. The morphology of gray platelets is also strikingly different from that of ES and MHA cells.[76] The virtual absence of alpha granules in most platelets is a characteristic feature. Gray platelets are found in other disorders, such as the transient leukemia of infancy in Down syndrome (Fig. 32.35), in myeloproliferative syndromes, and in certain leukemic states in adults, but usually involve only a small percentage of the cells.

Absence of alpha granules permits the gray platelet to manifest a wide range of morphologic appearances.[76] Sometimes the cytoplasm is a monotonous matrix with a few mitochondria and dense bodies. In other GPS platelets the cytoplasm may be dominated by elements of the DTS, channels of the OCS, or a combination of the two, and the membrane complexes that result from their interaction. Vacuoles similar in size or larger than alpha granules were a common feature of the large gray platelets. The presence in megakaryocytes[109] as well as in platelets and the absence of alpha granules suggested that these structures might have been destined to enclose alpha granules.[76] Studies with electron-dense tracers demonstrated that the empty, sac-like

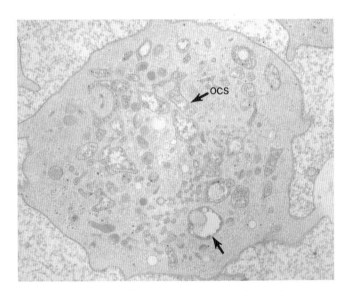

Fig. 32.36 Gray platelets fixed in the presence of an electron-dense tracer, tannic acid. Channels of the open canalicular system (OCS) and putative alpha granules (↑) connected to the OCS are filled with the stain. × 20000.

structures were in direct continuity with surrounding plasma through channels of the OCS (Fig. 32.36).

Recent immunocytochemical studies have confirmed the suggestion that the vacuoles are putative alpha-granule membranes.[144] An antibody, GMP-140, specific for alpha-granule membranes was localized in resting gray platelets to the vacuole membranes by immunogold techniques. Activation of gray platelets by thrombin resulted in redistribution of GMP-140 to the plasma membrane, just as in normal platelets. Endogenously synthesized PF4 was undetectable in gray platelets, but plasma-derived proteins, albumin and IgG were present in normal amounts and secreted in a normal manner after exposure to thrombin. Therefore, the fundamental defect in GPS appears to be transfer of the endogenously synthesized alpha-granule proteins to their appropriate target, or loss of these proteins to the outside due to premature connection of the organelles to demarcation membranes or channels of the OCS.[109] Our studies favor the latter hypothesis.

Cramer et al.[145] used an immunogold method to localize fibrinogen and vWF in platelets from three patients with GPS. Both vWF and fibrinogen were distributed homogeneously in the rare normal alpha granules and also in small, abnormal alpha granules. The small structures were similar in size to immature granules present in normal megakaryocytes. Stimulation of GPS platelets by thrombin resulted in the release of fibrinogen from the small organelles to channels of the OCS. These findings add further support to the concept that GPS megakaryocytes make the proteins destined for alpha granules and do target them appropriately. However, the putative alpha granules, for the most part, are unable to retain the proteins and lose them to the surrounding plasma.

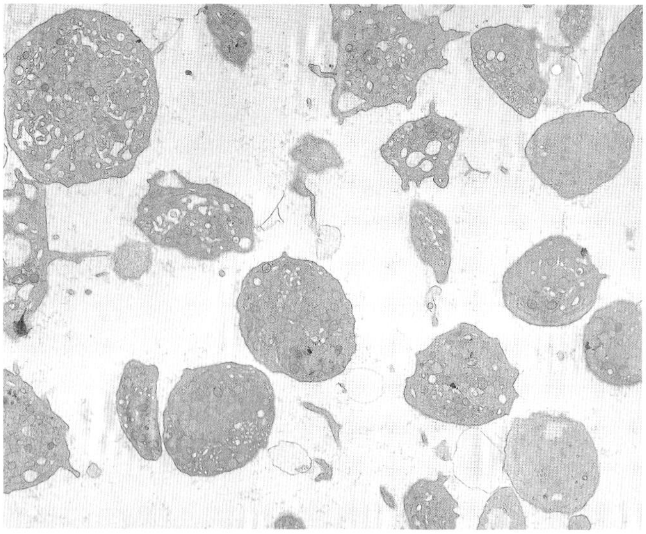

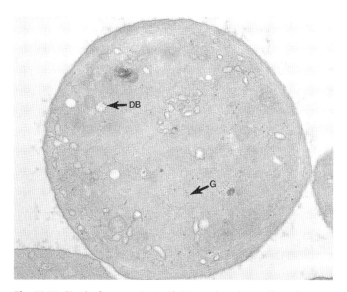

Fig. 32.37 Platelets from a patient with Montreal platelet syndrome (MPS). Except for their large size, MPS platelets resemble normal platelets. × 6000.

Montreal platelet syndrome (MPS)

A giant platelet disorder affecting three generations of a Canadian family has been studied extensively by Frojmovic and his colleagues[146] since it was first reported by Lacombe and d'Angelo.[147] The syndrome is characterized by autosomal dominant inheritance, the presence of giant platelets on peripheral blood smears with absence of leukocyte inclusions, a prolonged bleeding time, greatly reduced platelet counts (<10000–15000/mm³), spontaneous platelet aggregation and normal clot retraction. At first the family members were thought to have the Bernard–Soulier syndrome, but ristocetin-induced platelet aggregation was normal and studies of surface membrane glycoproteins revealed no abnormality. The basis for the spontaneous aggregation of patient platelets was studied in detail without resolving the problem.[148] There may be an undescribed abnormality in MPS cell membranes resulting in the binding of fibrinogen and a calcium-independent form of spontaneous platelet aggregation.

Electron microscopy of MPS platelets revealed increased volume, but nowhere near the size of MHA or ES platelets (Figs 32.37 and 32.38). There was an increased frequency of large alpha granules in these cells, but the difference from normal platelets was not significant. MPS platelets contained elements of the OCS and DTS, as well as membrane complexes, but they were not unusual in size or frequency in comparison to MHA or ES cells. This is of interest because Frojmovic has shown that shape-changing agents produce unusually large platelets when stirred with cells from the family with MPS.[146] The rationale offered to explain hypervolumetric shape change is based on the assumption that MPS platelets contain an excessively well-developed OCS. Stimulation by potent agonists was speculated to cause evagination of the overdeveloped OCS on to the surface, greatly expanding its total surface area. The microscopic studies showing a normal frequency of OCS channels in MPS platelets suggest that the hypothesis may be incorrect. It is possible that the hypervolumetric shape change may be due to other factors influencing MPS platelet membrane resistance to deformation.[149]

Fig. 32.38 Platelet from a patient with Montreal syndrome. The cell contains a normal component of alpha granules (G) and dense bodies (DB). × 19000.

Bernard–Soulier syndrome (BSS)

BSS[150] is an autosomal recessively inherited hemorrhagic disorder resulting from platelet inability to adhere to vascular subendothelium as a consequence of a surface membrane defect.[151]

At least three of the major glycoproteins, GPIb, GPIX, and GPV, are modified or absent from the surface membranes of BSS platelets.[152] Patients with BSS are thrombocytopenic and most reports suggest that a significant proportion of their platelets are markedly enlarged (Fig. 32.39). However, Frojmovic has suggested that BSS platelets are not increased in size.[153] Rather, they appear large compared to normal platelets on peripheral blood smears because of a proposed tendency to spread into thin films on contact with glass. The

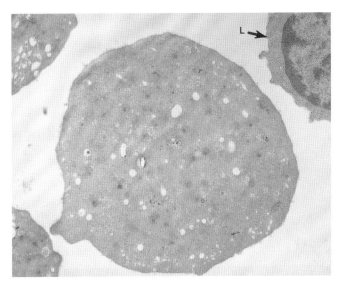

Fig. 32.39 Bernard–Soulier syndrome. Most patients with this disorder have very large platelets. This cell is larger than the adjacent lymphocyte (L). × 15 000.

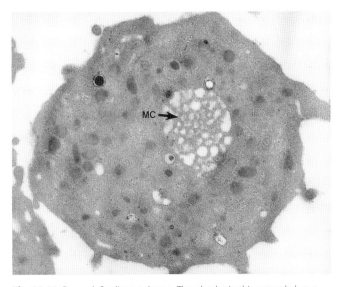

Fig. 32.40 Bernard–Soulier syndrome. The platelet in this example has a membrane complex (MC), but channels of the open canalicular system are not especially prominent in cells from these patients. × 22 000.

volume of BSS platelets in suspension was found to be normal. Abnormal spreading was related to an increased content of intracellular membrane extruded on to the cell surface during the spreading process (Fig. 32.40).

Characteristic ultrastructural defects have not been observed in thin sections of BSS platelets, but a report based on evaluation of replicas from freeze-fractured BSS platelets has indicated a distinct difference in the size and distribution of intramembranous particles (IMP) compared to normal platelets.[154] IMP are exposed on both the P-face (PF) and the E-face (EF) of freeze-fractured normal platelets and vary in size from about 5 to 13 nm. Approximately 1000 IMP/μm^2 are present on the EF compared to 500 IMP/μm^2 on the PF of human cells, yielding a PF/EF ratio of 0.5. Chevalier

et al.[154] reported an increase in larger IMP in both fracture faces of BSS platelets and a greater concentration of particles on the PF than on the EF, resulting in reversal of the normal PF/EF ratio. Other recent reports have suggested that BSS platelets contain increased numbers of dense bodies, the storage pool of adenine nucleotides.[155] The increase in dense bodies is associated with a fivefold increase in the capacity of BSS platelets to store serotonin.

GPIb, one of the glycoproteins missing from the surface membranes of BSS platelets,[152] is the receptor for vWF. As a result, BSS platelets do not aggregate with ristocetin or bovine factor VIII, which must interact with vWF and platelet GPIb to cause aggregation. BSS platelets also respond less well than normal cells to thrombin, possibly due to their deficiency in another surface-membrane glycoprotein, GPV or GPIX. Thus, the surface-membrane glycoprotein defects in BSS platelets have been closely linked to functional impairment *in vitro* and *in vivo*.

Other studies have raised questions about some of these findings. Examination of platelets from numerous patients with BSS by electronic sizing, ultrastructural and morphometric techniques has revealed that all are enlarged, though there is considerable variation. Some BSS patients have platelets about twice normal size, while others reveal cells as large as those from families with MHA or ES. Thus, BSS is a giant platelet disorder as originally described, despite the suggestion that BSS platelets were of normal size in suspension.[153]

Frojmovic et al. proposed that the hypervolumetric shape change and tendency to spread into thin films on glass slides were due to an excessive amount of internalized surface membrane in the form of channels of the open canalicular system.[153] However, careful study of platelets from several BSS patients in the electron microscope after incubation of their cells with electron-dense tracers has failed to reveal an increase in the OCS (Figs 32.39 and 32.40). If anything, the extent of the OCS in BSS platelets is less than in normal cells. Thus, the suggestion that evagination of an overdeveloped OCS is the basis for excess spreading or hypervolumetric shape change observed in BSS platelets appears unwarranted.

Investigations employing the technique of micropipette elastimetry[156] may offer a better explanation for observations described by Frojmovic et al. Micropipette elastimetry has been used extensively to evaluate mechanical properties of erythrocyte membranes, but platelets seemed too small to study by this procedure. However, the problems have been overcome, and the technique extended to the investigation of normal and abnormal platelets.[156] Under the same conditions of negative pressure, membrane segments aspirated from BSS platelets are two to three times longer than those drawn from normal cells or other inherited disorders. Deformability of thrombasthenic platelets was normal, indicating that deficiency in a different glycoprotein than that missing on BSS platelets is not sufficient to affect deformability. Other giant platelet disorders, including MHA, ES and GPS, were also as resistant to aspiration as normal platelets, showing that large size is not a significant factor influencing resistance to micropipette aspiration.

A biochemical basis for the marked softness of BSS platelet membranes has been found to be a transmembrane protein.[157] It is connected on the inside surface to a

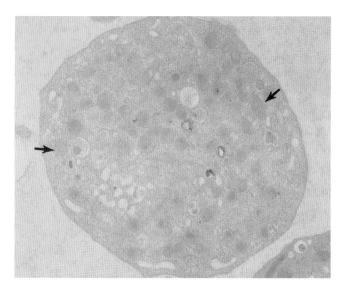

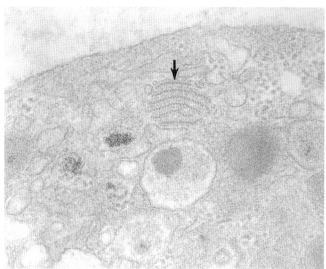

Fig. 32.41 Enyeart anomaly (EA). A platelet from one of our first two patients with this disorder. General features of platelet morphology are normal. However, there are two inclusions (↑) in the cytoplasm that are not found in normal platelets. × 16 000.

Fig. 32.42 Enyeart anomaly (EA). The EA inclusion (↑) is not membrane enclosed. However, it may resemble stacked membranes separated by amorphous, dense material on some occasions. A peculiar variation is shown here. It resembles a helix formed by a light and a dark string twisted tightly together. The linear helices appear stacked, but the precise nature of their organization and derivation remain obscure. × 60 000.

cytoskeletal protein, actin-binding protein. Evaluation of the effects of chilling, cytochalasin B and vincristine on platelet-membrane deformability in micropipettes had shown that the cytoskeleton is very much involved in resistance to deformation.[156] Therefore, the absence of GPIb and its transmembrane link to actin-binding protein of the internal cytoskeleton is the likely explanation for the increased spreading on glass and hypervolumetric shape change of BSS platelets.

The freeze-fracture study that suggested intramembranous particles are larger and distributed differently in a split lipid bilayer of BSS platelets compared to normal cells involved only a single patient with the disorder.[154] In an attempt to confirm this observation, platelets from nine patients with BSS have been evaluated by freeze-fracture. This experience suggests that IMP on both the E-face and P-face of BSS platelets are of normal size and that their distribution yields the same E-face to P-face ratio as on replicas of normal platelet membranes.

Membrane inclusion disorders

Enyeart anomaly (EA)

The literature contains many references to single patients or families with giant platelets, thrombocytopenia and mild to severe bleeding problems. We have tried to characterize as many giant platelet disorders as possible in order to define the mechanism of their formation in megakaryocytes. The Enyeart anomaly (EA) is one of these. A mother and her teenaged daughter were referred to us several years ago with lifelong histories of mild bleeding symptoms and congenital thrombocytopenia. Both have giant platelets (Fig. 32.41). The large cells are relatively unresponsive to stimulation by most aggregating agents, but evaluation of membrane glycoproteins failed to reveal deficiencies in GPIb, GPIIb-IIIa, or other surface receptors. A small inclusion was found in a

small but significant number of their platelets which had not been reported previously (Figs 32.41 and 32.42).

We held our results on two patients, hoping others would appear, and they have. Dr John O'Brien of Portsmouth, England, sent us samples from a patient with giant platelets and both clinical and laboratory findings similar to those for the two women described above. Her platelets were found to contain the same inclusion as in those of the other two. A fourth patient from California with giant platelets also has a small, but significant, number of the inclusions in her cells. Thus, EA appears to represent a distinct giant platelet disorder characterized by the presence of a small inclusion body. The nature of the defect leading to giant platelets, defective function, and formation of the inclusion body remains obscure.

Medich giant inclusion disorder

The young woman with this problem has a lifelong history of mild to severe bleeding.[132] She bruises easily and has had severe menorrhagia, requiring transfusion therapy on two occasions. The patient had macrothrombocytopenia. Her platelet count varies from 30 000 to 60 000/mm^3, and her mean platelet volume is 28–35 fl. The platelets are big, but not as large as those from patients with MHA and ES. They are, however, very abnormal. The principal defects are found in the membrane systems and their organization (Fig. 32.43). Channels of the DTS are arranged in stacks in some cells and in linear arrangements in others. Membrane complexes formed by interaction of channels from the OCS and DTS are often condensed and sometimes enclosed within membranes resembling antophagic vacuoles. The most unusual feature of her platelets, however, is the presence of membranous inclusions not observed previously in human cells (Fig. 32.44). The inclusions are tube-like

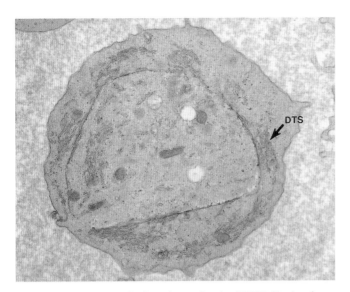

Fig. 32.43 Medich giant platelet inclusion disorder (MGPID). Platelets from this patient are large and reveal considerable variation in morphology. The example shown in this illustration contains primarily elements of the dense tubular system (DTS). One channel appears to encircle the cytoplasm, and has linear and curvilinear segments. × 24 000.

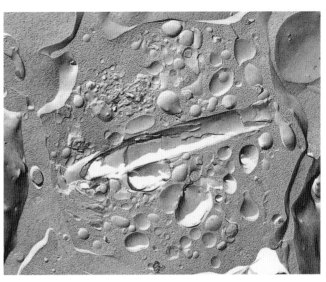

Fig. 32.45 Replica of freeze-fractured Medich giant platelet inclusion disorder cell. The inclusion revealed in the cytoplasm resembles a cigar with several membrane layers. × 17 000.

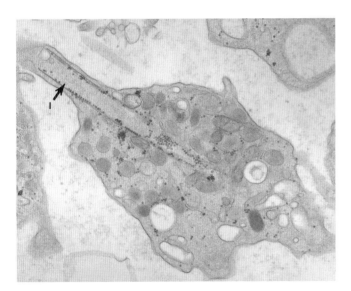

Fig. 32.44 Medich giant platelet inclusion disorder. A membrane inclusion (I) is present in the cytoplasm of this platelet. Glycogen particles are prominent inside the inclusion and along its membranous surfaces. Both ends of the inclusion are open to the cytoplasm. × 20 000.

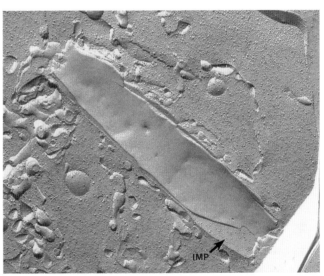

Fig. 32.46 Freeze-fractured platelet from a patient with Medich giant inclusion disorder. Intramembranous particles (IMP) can be seen on one of the exposed membrane faces, but the major membrane lacks IMP. × 32 000.

or cigar shaped, and are composed of membranes wrapped like onion-skin layers around cores of cytoplasm. The inclusion is best seen in freeze-fractured platelets (Fig. 32.45) which reveals another facet of their unusual structure. They are the only membranes in human blood cells and other cell systems which lack intramembranous particles (Fig. 32.46). Our studies suggest that the tubular inclusions result from defective formation of membrane complexes.

At the time we first observed these structures, we considered them unique to the patient and human platelets. However, similar structures are present in platelets from all species of rats we have thus far observed, including the Wistar, Sprague–Dawley and Long–Evans hooded rat and in the giant platelets of the Wistar–Furth rat.[158] Precisely why the inclusions should be a normal constituent of rat platelets and only found in the giant abnormal cells of a single human patient is unknown.

In addition to the morphologic abnormalities, the patient's platelets are relatively unresponsive to aggregating agents, have low baseline calcium levels, and flux calcium poorly when stimulated by thrombin. The defects in calcium metabolism may be directly related to the abnormal organization of the DTS and OCS in her giant platelets.

Platelet microtubule disorders

Inherited conditions affecting the organization or assembly of the circumferential coil of microtubules supporting platelet discoid shape are virtually unknown. In several giant platelet syndromes the microtubules do not form a circumferential coil.[139] Rather, they resemble a ball of yarn. It is not known whether the failure to form a circumferential coil is responsible for the spherical shape of most giant platelets, or that the huge size of the cells prevents their organization into coils. Further confusion is created by the observation that some giant platelets do have circumferential microtubule coils.[76] The subject will require further study.

Absence of circumferential microtubule coils in normal sized platelets

Nearly complete absence of microtubule coils in human platelets is a very rare condition. The phenomenon was first reported in a patient with the Lesch–Nyhan syndrome, a disorder characterized by neurological and behavioral problems, metabolic disturbances and hematological symptoms due to a specific deficiency in hypoxanthine-guanine phosphoribosyl transferase (HGPRT).[159–161] The authors suggested that the spherical or irregular shape of the patient's platelets was due to disassembly of the microtubule coils, and breakdown of microtubules could be involved in the pathogenesis of the complex syndrome. However, it should be noted that an earlier report of three patients with Lesch–Nyhan syndrome whose platelets were studied in the electron microscope failed to reveal any structural abnormality.[162]

The second individual with absent platelet microtubules and microtubule coils was reported in an abstract and no publication ensued.[163] A 49-year-old male was found to have a bleeding diathesis and structurally abnormal platelets which were spherical in form and devoid of circumferential coils of microtubules. The abnormal cells failed to aggregate in response to stirring with several agents that clumped normal platelets, and did not undergo shape change.

The third patient was a 13-year-old male whose platelets were sent to the author of this chapter for evaluation.[164] Differential interference phase contrast light microscopy (DIC) revealed that his platelets were uniformly spherical in form, in contrast to the discoid shape of normal thrombocytes (Figs 32.47 and 32.48). The spherocytes, however, did attach to surfaces and spread as well as normal platelets. Immunofluorescence microscopy employing an anti-tubulin antibody followed by fluorescein-conjugated anti-immunoglobulin antibody revealed tubulin was present in the patient spherocytes (Fig. 32.49), but dispersed throughout the cytoplasm. In resting normal platelets tubulin was concentrated in rings at peripheral margins of the cells (Fig. 32.50). If the normal platelets were chilled to 4°C for 30 minutes to dissolve the circumferential coils, then stained for tubulin, the protein became completely dispersed throughout the cytoplasm and the cells appeared identical to patient spherocytes in the fluorescence microscope. Thin

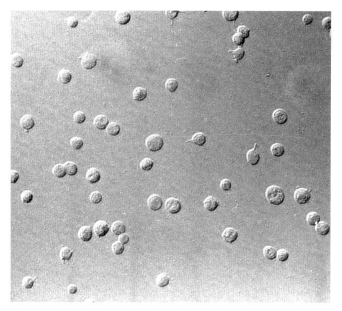

Fig. 32.47 Differential interference phase contrast (DIC) microscopy of normal human platelets fixed prior to mounting on glass. The flattened appearance is typical for discoid cells viewed in this manner. Original magnification × 800.

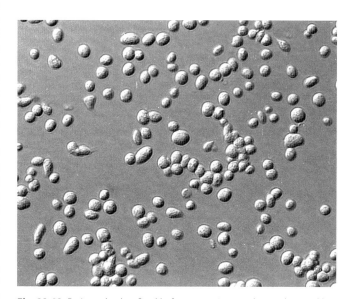

Fig. 32.48 Patient platelets fixed before mounting on glass and viewed by DIC. The round or oval spherocytes resemble balls. Original magnification × 650.

sections of patient platelets examined in the transmission electron microscope also revealed their spherical form and the absence of microtubule coils (Figs 32.51–32.54). Exposure to the thrombin before fixation showed that the spherocytes could undergo internal transformation resulting in the concentration of organelles in platelet centers without undergoing significant shape change or pseudopod extension (Figs 32.55 and 32.56). The failure to extend pseudopods and undergo shape change may be responsible for the patient's bleeding symptoms.

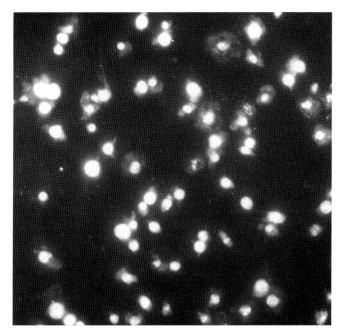

Fig. 32.49 Patient platelets stained for tubulin in the same manner as the normal cells in Fig. 32.53. The spherocytes appear as brightly stained for tubulin as chilled normal platelets, but are devoid of microtubules and microtubule coils. Original magnification × 800.

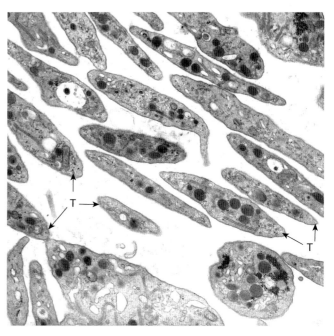

Fig. 32.51 Thin sections of resting normal platelets. A circumferential coil of microtubules (T) evident at the polar ends of each cell supports the discoid shape. Original magnification × 13 000.

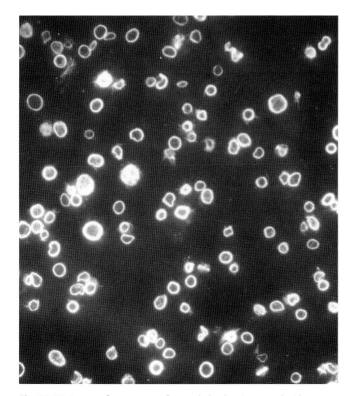

Fig. 32.50 Immunofluorescence of normal platelets interacted with an anti-tubulin antibody followed by fluorescein coupled to anti-IgG. Microtubules are concentrated in coils at the periphery of every platelet. Original magnification × 800.

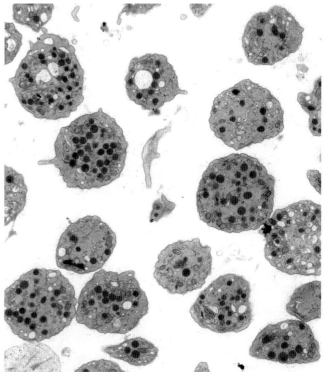

Fig. 32.52 Thin sections of patient's resting spherocytic platelets. Microtubules and microtubule coils are not present in his platelets. Original magnification × 3600.

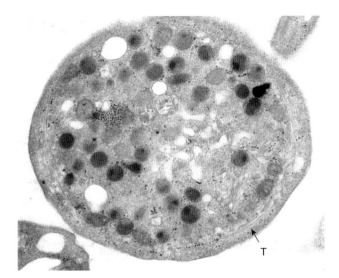

Fig. 32.53 Thin section of normal human platelet cut in the equatorial plane. The discoid shape is supported by a circumferential coil of microtubules (T) lying just under the surface membrane. Original magnification × 30 000.

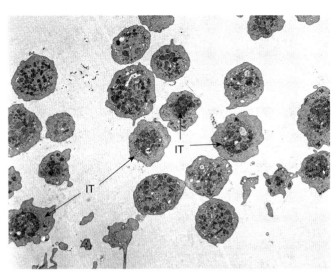

Fig. 32.55 Patient spherocytes treated with 0.2 unit thrombin per ml and fixed after 2 min without stirring. Platelets are only slightly more irregular than in resting state, and very few have developed pseudopods. Internal transformation (IT) has occurred in some cells where organelles are concentrated in cell centers. (↑) Original magnification × 6000.

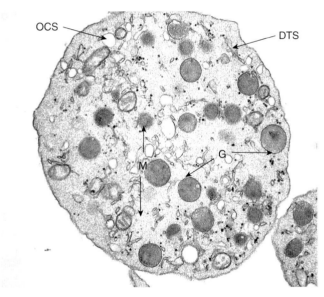

Fig. 32.54 Platelet spherocyte from patient's PRP. The cell contains normal numbers of alpha granules (G) and mitochondria (M). Elements of the open canalicular system (OCS) and dense tubular system (DTS) are also present. Microtubules and microtubule coils are absent. Original magnification × 28 000.

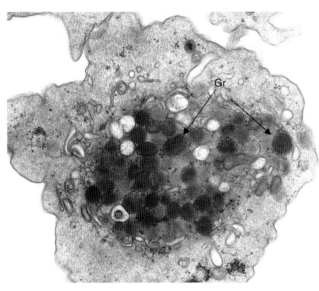

Fig. 32.56 Patient spherocyte treated with thrombin as in the previous illustration. The cell is irregular in form, but has not developed long filapodia. Granules (Gr) are concentrated in and moving toward the platelet center. Original magnification × 30 000.

The presence of normal amounts of tubulin in patient spherocytes suggested the possibility that it might be possible to cause it to assemble into microtubules under certain conditions. Taxol derived from *Taxus brevifolia* has been shown to stabilize microtubules in normal platelets, and cause reassembly of microtubules in chilled platelets whose microtubules had completely dissolved.[165] Microtubules did form in patient spherocytes after incubation with Taxol. They were present in 82% of the cells, and, in many examples the newly assembled microtubules had formed circumferential coils under the surface membrane (Fig. 32.57). That event was associated with conversion of the spherocytes to discocytes (Figs 32.58 and 32.59). The study has shown how important circumferential coils are to platelet discoid shape,[166,167] but further studies will be required to find out why this patient cannot form them normally.

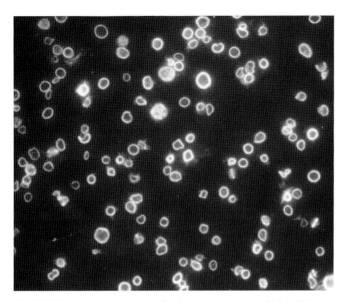

Fig. 32.57 Immunofluorescence of patient spherocytes treated with Taxol, then exposed to anti-tubulin antibody followed by fluorescein coupled to anti-IgG. Microtubule coils are present in the Taxol treated cells and are located just under the surface membrane in most cells. Original magnification × 800.

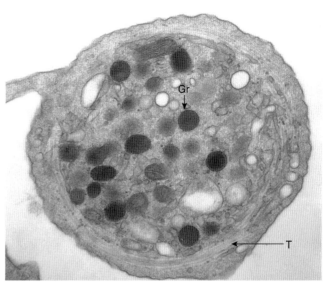

Fig. 32.59 Patient spherocyte treated with Taxol. The cell has formed a complete circumferential coil of microtubules (T) and is almost certainly a disc. Granules (Gr) are randomly dispersed. Original magnification × 36 000.

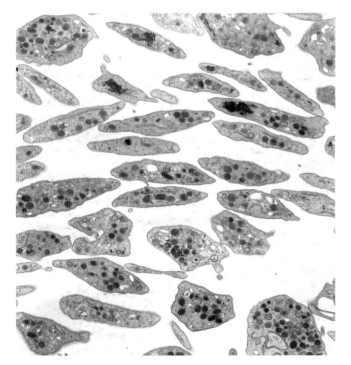

Fig. 32.58 Thin section of patient spherocytes fixed after exposure to Taxol. Nearly all of the spherocytes have developed a discoid form and microtubule coils are apparent at the polar ends of each cell. Original magnification × 13 000.

Summary

As diverse as the group of inherited structural defects and giant platelet disorders presented in this chapter may seem, there is a common thread that ties them together. All appear to represent some form of membrane aberration. Sometimes only a small inclusion identifies the membrane defect, sometimes a massive increase in size. In others, whole populations of organelles are missing or surface membranes lack specific glycoproteins essential for their function. All of them are born in the deep recesses of the bone marrow megakaryocyte. Getting the megakaryocyte out into the light of day, or at least into a culture medium, should certainly lead to the solution of many, if not all, of the disorders of platelet membranes.

References

1. Clay RS, Court TH. The History of the Microscope. London: Charles Griffin; 1932. p. 20–436.

2. van Leeuwenhoek A. Microscopical observations. Philosophical Transactions of the Royal Society of London; 1674. p. 121–8.

3. Hewson W. Experimental Inquiries: Part 1. Containing an Inquiry into the Properties of the Blood. 2nd ed. London: J Johnson; 1774.

4. Donné A. De l'origine des globules du sang, de leur mode de formation et de leur fin. Comptes Rendus Seances de l'Academie des Sciences. Paris 1842;14: 366–8.

5. Bizzozero J. Ueber Einen Neuen Formbestandheil des Bleetes und Dessen Rolle Bei der Thrombose und der Blutgerinnung. Archives in Pathological Anatomy and Physiology 1882;90: 261–332.

6. Tocantins LM. The mammalian blood platelet in health and disease. Medicine 1938;17:155–260.

7. Roth GJ. Developing relationships: arterial platelet adhesion, glycoprotein Ib, and leucine-rich glycoproteins. Blood 1991;77:5–19.

8. Saelman EUM, Nieuwenhuis HK, Hese KM, et al. Platelet adhesion to collagen types I through VIII under conditions of stasis and flow is mediated by GPIa/IIa ($\alpha_2\beta_1$-integrin). Blood 1994;83: 1244–50.

9. Sixma JJ, Wester J. The haemostatic plug. Seminars in Hematology 1977;14: 265–99.

10. Sixma JJ, van Zanten GH, Banga JD, et al. Platelet adhesion. Seminars in Hematology 1995;32:1–6.

11. White JG. Platelet structural physiology: the ultrastructure of adhesion, secretion and aggregation in arterial thrombosis. In: Mehta JL, Conti CR Brest AN, editors. Thrombosis and platelets in myocardial ischemia. Cardiovascular Clinics 1987; 18:13–33.

12. Breton-Gorius J, Levin J, Nurden AT, editors. Molecular Biology and Differentiation of Megakaryocytes. Progress in Clinical and Biological Research, vol. 356. New York: Wiley-Liss; 1990. p. 1–372.

13. White JG, Escolar G. Current concepts of platelet membrane response to surface activation. Platelets 1993;4:176–89.

14. White JG, Gerrard JM. The cell biology of platelets. In: Weissman G, editor. Handbook of Inflammation (The Cell Biology of Inflammation). New York: Elsevier/North Holland; 1980. p. 83–143.

15. White JG. Is the canalicular system the equivalent of the muscle sarcoplasmic reticulum? Hemostasis 1975;4:185.

16. Dignan PSJ, Maular AM, Frantz C. Phocomelia with congenital hypoplastic thrombocytopenia and myeloid leukemoid reactions. Journal of Pediatrics 1967;70:561–73.

17. O'Gorman-Hughes DW. Neonatal thrombocytopenia: assessment of aetiology and prognosis. Australian Paediatric Journal 1967;3:276.

18. Hall JG, Levin J, Kuhn JP, et al. Thrombocytopenia with absent radius. Medicine 1969;48:411.

19. Fanconi G. Familiare infantile perniziosa: artige Anamie (Pernizioses Blutbild und Konstitution). Jahrbuch Kinderheilkund 1927;117:257.

20. Rand M, Ried G. Source of serotonin in serum. Nature 1951;168:385–6.

21. Baker RV, Blaschko H, Born GVR. The isolation from blood platelets of particles containing 5-hydroxytryptamine and adenosine triphosphate. Journal of Physiology (London) 1959;149:55–61.

22. Siegel A, Luscher EF. Non-identity of the granules of human blood platelets with typical lysosomes. Nature 1967;215: 745–6.

23. Wood JG. Electron microscopic localization of 5-hydroxytryptamine (5-HT). Texas Reports of Biology and Medicine 1965;23:828–37.

24. Davis RB, White JG. Localization of 5-hydroxytryptamine in blood platelets: an autoradiographic and ultrastructural study. British Journal of Haematology 1968;15:93–9.

25. White JG. The origin of dense bodies in the surface coat of negatively stained platelets. Scandinavian Journal of Haematology 1968;5:371–82.

26. White JG. The dense bodies of human platelets: inherent electron opacity of serotonin storage particles. Blood 1969;33:598–606.

27. Tranzer JP, Da Prada M, Pletscher A. Letter to the editor. Ultrastructural localization of 5-hydroxytryptamine in blood platelets. Nature 1966;211: 1547–75.

28. Richards JG, Da Prada M. Uranaffin reaction: a new cytochemical technique for the localization of adenine nucleotides in organelles storing biogenic amines. Journal of Histochemistry and Cytochemistry 1977; 25:1322–36.

29. Daimon T, Gotoh Y. Cytochemical evidence of the origin of the dense tubular system in the mouse platelet. Histochemistry 1982;76:189–96.

30. Witkop CJ Jr, Hill CW, Desnick SJ, et al. Ophthalmologic, biochemical, platelet and ultrastructural defects in various types of oculocutaneous albinism. Journal of Investigative Dermatology 1973;60:443–56.

31. Witkop CJ Jr. Inherited disorders of pigmentation. Clinical Dermatology 1985;3:70–134.

32. Witkop CJ, White JG, Townsend D, et al. Ceroid storage disease in Hermansky–Pudlak syndrome: induction in animal models. In: Nagy ZS, editor. Lipofuchsin-1987: State of the Art. Amsterdam: Elsevier; 1988. p. 413–36.

33. White JG. Ultrastructural defects in congenital disorders of platelet function. Annals of the New York Academy of Science 1972;201:205–33.

34. Weiss HJ. Platelet aggregation, adhesion and ADP release in thrombopathia (platelet factor 3 deficiency) – a comparison with Glanzmann's thrombasthenia and von Willebrand's disease. American Journal of Medicine 1967;43:570–8.

35. Weiss HJ, Chervenick PA, Zalusky R. A familial defect in platelet function associated with impaired release of adenisone diphosphate. New England Journal of Medicine 1969;281:1264–8.

36. Weiss HJ, Witte LD, Kaplan KL, et al. Heterogeneity in storage pool deficiency: studies on granule-bound substances in 18 patients including variants deficient in alpha granules, platelet factor-4, beta-thromboglobulin and platelet-derived growth factor. Blood 1979;54: 1296–308.

37. Grottum KA, Hovig T, Holmsen H, et al. Wiskott–Aldrich syndrome: qualitative platelet defects and short platelet survival. British Journal of Haematology 1969;17:373–88.

38. Day HJ, Holmsen H. Platelet adenine nucleotide 'storage pool deficiency' in thrombocytopenia absent radii syndrome. Journal of the American Medical Association 1972;221:1053.

39. Chediak M. Nouvelle anomalie leukocytaire de caractere constitutionnel et familial. Reviews Hematologic Paris 1952;7:362–72.

40. Higashi O. Congenital gigantism of peroxidase granules: the first case ever reported of qualitative abnormality of peroxidase. Tohoku Journal of Experimental Medicine 1954;59:315–21.

41. Wolff SM, Dale DC, Clark RA, et al. The Chediak–Higashi syndrome: studies of host defenses. Annals of Internal Medicine 1972;76:293–306.

42. Bequez-Cesar A. Neutropenia cronica maligna familiar con granulaciones atipicas de los leucocitos. Boletin Society Cubana Pediatrica 1943;15:900–2.

43. White JG, Clawson CC. Development of giant granules in platelets during prolonged storage. American Journal of Pathology 1980;101:635–46.

44. Page AR, Berendes H, Warner J, Good RA. The Chediak–Higashi syndrome. Blood 1962;20:330–8.

45. Boxer GJ, Holmsen H, Robkin L, et al. Abnormal platelet function in Chediak–Higashi syndrome. British Journal of Haematology 1977;35:521–33.

46. White JG. Platelet microtubules and giant granules in the Chediak–Higashi syndrome. American Journal of Medical Technology 1978;44:273–8.

47. Parmley RT, Poon MC, Crist WM, Molluk A. Giant platelet granules in a child with the Chediak–Higashi syndrome. American Journal of Hematology 1979;6:51–60.

48. Bell TG, Myers KM, Prieur DJ, et al. Decreased nucleotide and serotonin storage associated with defective function in Chediak–Higashi syndrome platelets. Blood 1976;48:175–84.

49. Buchanan GR, Handin RI. Platelet function in the Chediak–Higashi syndrome. Blood 1976;47:941–7.

50. Boxer LA, Watanabe AM, Rister M, et al. Correction of leukocyte function in Chediak–Higashi syndrome by ascorbate. New England Journal of Medicine 1976;295:1041–5.

51. Gallin JI, Elin RJ, Hubert RT, et al. Efficacy of ascorbic acid in Chediak–Higashi syndrome (CHS): studies in humans and mice. Blood 1979;53:226–34.

52. Oliver JM. Impaired microtubule function correctable by cyclic GMP and cholinergic agonists in the Chediak–Higashi syndrome. American Journal of Pathology 1976;85:395–418.

53. White JG. Ultrastructural defects in congenital disorders of platelet function. Annals of the New York Academy of Science 1972;201:205–33.

54. White JG. Platelet morphology. In: Johnson SA, editor. The circulating platelet. New York: Academic Press; 1971. p. 45–121.

55. White JG, Krivit W. The ultrastructural localization and release of platelet lipids. Blood 1966;27:167–86.

56. Rodman NF, Mason RG, McDevitt NB, Brinkhous KM. Morphological alterations of human blood platelets during early phases of clotting. American Journal of Pathology 1961;40:271–83.

57. White JG. Tubular elements in platelet granules. Blood 1968;32:148–56.

58. Cramer EM, Meyer D, LeMenn R, Breton-Gorius J. Eccentric localization of von Willebrand factor within tubular structure of platelet alpha granules resembling that of Weibel Palade bodies. Blood 1985;66:710–5.

59. Gerrard JM, Phillips DR, Rao GHR, et al. Biochemical studies of two patients with the gray platelet syndrome – selective deficiency of platelet alpha granules. Journal of Clinical Investigation 1980;66:102–9.

60. White JG. Transfer of thorium particles from plasma to platelets and platelet granules. American Journal of Pathology 1968;53:567–75.

61. Handagama PJ, George JN, Schuman MA, et al. Incorporation of a circulating protein into megakaryocyte and platelet granules. Proceedings of the National Academy of Sciences USA 1987;84:861–5.

62. Handagama PJ, Schuman R, Schuman MA, Bainton DF. In vivo defibrination results in markedly decreased levels of fibrinogen in megakaryocytes and platelets in rats. Abstract, San Antonio, Texas: American Society of Hematology Annual Meeting; 1988.

63. Grette K. Studies on the mechanism of thrombin-catalyzed hemostatic reaction in blood platelets. Acta Physiological Scandinavian 1962;56(Suppl. 195):1–93.

64. Holmsen H. Platelet secretion. In: Colman RW, Hirsh J, Marder VJ, editors. Hemostasis and thrombosis. Philadelphia: Lippincott; 1987. p. 390–403.

65. Kaplan K, Brockman MJ, Chernoff A, et al. Platelet alpha granule proteins: studies on release and subcellular organization. Blood 1979;53:604–18.

66. Stormorken H. The release reaction of secretion. Scandinavian Journal of Haematology 1969;9:(Suppl.):3–24.

67. Ginsberg MH, Taylor L, Painter RG. The mechanisms of thrombin-induced platelet factor 4 secretion. Blood 1980;55:661–9.

68. White JG. The morphology of platelet function. In: Harker LA, Zimmerman TS, editors. Methods in Hematology, series 8L. Measurements of Platelet Function. New York: Churchill-Livingstone; 1983. p. 1–25.

69. David-Ferreira JF. The blood platelet: electron-microscopic studies. International Reviews of Cytology 1964;17:99–148.

70. Maldonado JE. Giant platelet granules in refractory anemia (preleukemia) and myelomonocytic leukemia: a cell marker? Blood Cells 1975;1:129–35.

71. White JG, Clawson CC. Development of giant granules in platelets during prolonged storage. American Journal of Pathology 1980;101:635–46.

72. White JG. The secretory pathway of bovine platelets. Blood 1987;69:878–85.

73. White JG, Krumwiede M. Further studies of the secretory pathway in thrombin stimulated human platelets. Blood 1987;69:1196–203.

74. White JG, Krivit W, Vernier R. The platelet-fibrin relationship in human blood clots: an ultrastructural study utilizing ferritin conjugated anti-human fibrinogen antibody. Blood 1965;25:241–9.

75. Raccuglia G. Gray platelet syndrome: a variety of qualitative platelet disorder.

American Journal of Medicine 1971;51:818–28.

76. White JG. Ultrastructural studies of the gray platelet syndrome. American Journal of Pathology 1979;95:455–62.

77. Levy-Toledano S, Caen JP, Breton-Gorius J, et al. Gray platelet syndrome: alpha-granule deficiency, its influence on platelet function. Journal of Laboratory and Clinical Medicine 1981;98:831–49.

78. Von Behrens WE. Evidence of phylogenelic canalization of the circulating platelet mass in man. Thrombosis Diathesis Haemorrhagica 1972;27:159–63.

79. Breton-Gorius J. On the alleged phagocytosis by megakaryocytes. British Journal of Haematology 1981;47:635–6.

80. Breton-Gorius J, Bizet M, Reyes F. Myelofibrosis and acute megakaryoblastic leukemia in a child: topographic relationship between fibroblasts and megakaryocytes with an alpha-granule defect. Leukemia Research 1982;6:97–110.

81. Goldenhar M. Association malformatives de l'oeil et de l'oreille, en perticulier le syndrome dermoide epibulbaire-appendices appendices auriculaires-fistula auris congenita et ses relations avec la dysostose mandibulofaciale. Journal de Genetique Humaine 1952;1:243–82.

82. Mori K, Suzuki S, Sugai K. Electron microscopic and functional studies on platelets in gray platelet syndrome. Tohoku Journal of Experimental Medicine 1984;143:261–87.

83. Rao AK, Holmsen H. Congenital disorders of platelet function. Seminars in Hematology 1986;23:102–18.

84. White JG. Platelet granule disorders. Critical Reviews of Oncology/Hematology 1986;4:337–77.

85. Breton-Gorius J, Favier R, Guichard J, et al. A new congenital dysmegakary-opoietic thrombocytopenia (Paris–Trousseau) associated with giant platelet alpha-granules and chromosome 11 deletion at 11q23. Blood 1995;85:1805–14.

86. Favier R, Douay L, Esteva B et al: A novel genetic thrombocytopenia (Paris–Trousseau) associated with platelet inclusions, dysmegakaryopoiesis and chromosome deletion at 11q23. Comptes Rendus de l'Academie des Sciences (Paris) 1993;316:698–701.

87. Favier R. Paris–Trousseau thrombocyto-penia: a new entity and a model for understanding megakaryocytopoiesis (editorial). Pathologie et Biologie (Paris) 1997;45:693–6.

88. Jacobsen P, Hauge M, Henningsen K, et al. An (11;21) translocation in four generations with chromosome 11 abnormalities in the offspring. A clinical, cytogenetical, and gene marker study. Human Heredity 1973;23:568–85.

89. Michaelis RC, Velagaleti GV, Jones C, et al. Most Jacobsen syndrome deletion breakpoints occur distal to FRA11B. American Journal of Medical Genetics 1998;76:222–8.

90. Penny LA, Dell' Aquila M, Jones MC, et al. Clinical and molecular characterization of patients with distal 11q deletions. American Journal of Human Genetics 1995;56:676–83.

91. Krishnamurti L, Neglia JP, Nagarajan R, et al. Paris-Trousseau syndrome platelets in a child with Jacobsen's syndrome. Am. J, Hematol 2001;66:295–9.

92. Holmsen H, Day HJ, Stormorken H. The blood platelet release reaction. Scandinavian Journal of Haematology 1969;(Suppl. 8):326.

93. White JG. The ultrastructural cytochemistry and physiology of blood platelets. In the Platelet: Mostafi FK, Brinkhous KM, editors. Baltimore: William and Wilkins; 1971. p. 873–915.

94. Bentfield ME, Bainton DF. Cytochemical localization of lysosomal enzymes in rat megakaryocytes and platelets. Journal of Clinical Investigation 1975;56:1635–49.

95. Stenberg PE, Bainton DF. Storage organelles in platelets and megakaryocytes In: Phillips DR, Shuman M, editors. Biochemistry of Platelets. New York: Academic Press; 1986. p. 257–94.

96. Morgenstern E. Coated membranes in blood platelets. European Journal of Cell Biology 1982;26:315–8.

97. White JG. The Chediak–Higashi syndrome: a possible lysosomal disease. Blood 1966;28:143–56.

98. White JG, Clawson CC. The Chediak–Higashi syndrome: spectrum of giant organelles in peripheral blood cells. Henry Ford Hospital Medical Journal 1979;27:286–98.

99. White JG. Platelet membrane ultrastructural and its changes during platelet activation. In: Harris H, Hirschorn K, editors. Platelet Membrane Receptors: Molecular Biology, Immunology, Biochemistry, and Pathology. New York: Alan R Liss; 1988. p. 1032.

100. Wright JH. The origin and nature of the blood platelets. Boston Medical Surgical Journal 1906;154:643–5.

101. Behnke O. An electron microscope study of the megakaryocyte of the rat bone marrow. I. The development of the demarcation membrane system and the platelet surface coat. Journal of Ultrastructure Research 1968;24:412–33.

102. Behnke O. An electron microscope study of the rat megakaryocyte. II. Some aspects of platelet release and microtubules. Journal of Ultrastructure Research 1969;26:111–29.

103. Tavassoli M. Megakaryocyte–platelet axis and the process of platelet formation and release. Blood 1980;55:537–45.

104. Radley JM, Haller CJ. The demarcation membrane system of the megakaryocyte: a misnomer? Blood 1982;60:213–9.

105. Thiery JP, Bessis M. Mecanisme de la plaquettogenese. Etude in vitro par la microinematographie. Reviews Hematologie 1956;11:162–74.

106. Becker RP, deBruyn PPH. The transmural passage of blood cells into myeloid sinusoids and the entry of platelets into the sinusoidal circulation: a scanning electron microscopic investigation. American Journal of Anatomy 1976;145:183–206.

107. Scurfield G, Radley JM. Aspects of platelet formation and release. American Journal of Hematology 1981;10:285–96.

108. Radley JM, Scurfield GT. The mechanism of platelet release. Blood 1980;56:996–9.

109. Breton-Gorius J, Vainchenker W, Nurden A, et al. Defective alpha-granule production in megakaryocytes from gray platelet syndrome: ultrastructural studies of bone marrow cells and megakaryocytes growing in culture from blood presursors. American Journal of Pathology 1981;102:10–9.

110. Wiskott A. Familiarer angeborener morbus werlhofii? Monatsschrif Kinderheilkunde 1937;68:212–5.

111. Aldrich RA, Steinberg AG, Campbell DC. Pedigree demonstrating a sex-linked recessive condition characterized by draining ears, eczematoid dermatitis and bloody diarrhea. Pediatrics 1954;13:133–41.

112. Prchal JT, Carroll AJ, Prchal JF, et al. Wiskott–Aldrich syndrome: cellular impairments and their implication for carrier detection. Blood 1980;56:1048–53.

113. Lum LG, Tubergen DG, Carash L, Blaese RM. Splenectomy in the management of thrombocytopenia of the Wiskott–Aldrich syndrome. New England Journal of Medicine 1980;302:892–6.

114. Ochs HD, Slichter SJ, Harker LA, et al. The Wiskott–Aldrich syndrome: studies of lymphocytes, granulocytes and platelets. Blood 1980;55:243–52.

115. Parkman R, Kenney D, Remold-O'Donnell E, et al. Surface protein abnormalities in lymphocytes and platelets from patients with Wiskott–Aldrich syndrome. Lancet 1981;II:1387–4.

116. Baldinni MG. Nature of the platelet defect in Wiskott–Aldrich syndrome. Annals of the New York Academy of Science 1972;201:437–44.

117. Krivit W, Yunis E, White JG. Platelet survival studies in Wiskott–Aldrich syndrome. Pediatrics 1966;37:339–41.

118. Levine RF. Old and new aspects of megakaryocyte development and function. In: Levine RF, Williams N, Levin J, et al, editors. Megakaryocyte development and function. New York: Alan R Liss; 1986. p. 1–20.

119. Breton-Gorius J, Vainchenker W. Expression of platelet proteins during the in vitro and in vivo differentiation of megakaryocytes and morphological aspects of their maturation. Seminars in Hematology 1986;23:43–67.

120. May R. Leukocyteneinschlusse. Deutsch Archiv fur Klincal Medingin 1909;96:1–6.

121. Hegglin R. Gleichzertge Konstitutionelle Veranderungen on Neutrophilen und Thrombocyten. Helvetica Medica Acta 1945;12:439–40.

122. Volpe E, Cuccurullo L, Valente A, et al. The May–Hegglin: further studies on leukocytes inclusions and platelet ultrastructure. Acta Haematologica 1974;52:238–47.

123. Dohle V. Leukocyteneinschulusee bei scharlach. Zentralblatt fur Bakteriologie 1912;61:63–8.

124. Jenis EH, Takeuchi A, Dillon DE, et al. The May–Hegglin anomaly: ultrastructure of the granulocytic inclusion. American Journal of Clinical Pathology 1971;55:187–96.

125. White JG, Gerrard JM. Ultrastructural features of abnormal blood platelets. American Journal of Pathology 1976;83:590–632.

126. Jordon SW, Larsen WE. Ultrastructural studies of the May–Hegglin anomaly. Blood 1965;25:921–32.

127. Luscher JM, Schneider J, Mizukami I, Evans RK. The May–Hegglin anomaly: platelet function, ultrastructure and chromosome studies. Blood 1968;32:950–61.

128. Godwin HA, Ginsburg AD. May–Hegglin anomaly: a defect in megakaryocyte fragmentation? British Journal of Haematology 1974;26:117–28.

129. Karpatkin S. Autoimmune thrombocytopenic purpura. Seminars in Hematology 1985;22:260–88.

130. Firkin BG, Wright R, Miller S. Splenic macrophages in thrombocytopenia. Blood 1969;33:240–8.

131. Breton-Gorius J. Development of two membrane systems associated in giant complexes in pathological megakaryocytes. Series Hematologica 1975;8:49–67.

132. White JG. Inherited abnormalities of the platelet membrane and secretory granules. Human Pathology 1987;18:123–39.

133. Alport AC. Hereditary familial congenital hemorrhagic nephritis. British Medical Journal 1927;i:504–6.

134. Epstein CJ, Sahud MA, Piel CA, et al. Hereditary macrothrombocytopathia, nephritis and deafness. American Journal of Medicine 1972;52:299–310.

135. Eckstein JD, Filip DJ, Watts JC. Hereditary thrombocytopenia, deafness and renal disease. Annals of Internal Medicine 1975;82:639–45.

136. Hansen MS, Behnke O, Pedersen NT, Videbaek A. Megathrombocytopenia associated with glomerulonephritis, deafness and aortic cystic medianecrosis. Scandinavian Journal of Haematology 1978;21:197–205.

137. Bernheim J, Dechavanne M, Bryon PA, et al. Thrombocytopenia, macrothrombocytopathia, nephritis and deafness. American Journal of Medicine 1976; 61:145–50.

138. White JG. Membrane abnormalities in congenital disorders of human blood platelets. In: Sheppard JR, Anderson VE, Eaton JW, editors. Membranes and Genetic Disease. New York: Alan R Liss; 1982. p. 351–70.

139. White JG, Sauk JJ. The organization of microtubules and microtubule coils in giant platelet disorders. American Journal of Pathology 1984;116:514–22.

140. Cawley JC, Hayhoe FGJ. The inclusions of the May–Hegglin anomaly and Dohle bodies of infection: an ultrastructural comparison. British Journal of Haematology 1972;22:491–6.

141. Brivet F, Girot R, Barbanel C, et al. Hereditary nephritis associated with May–Hegglin anomaly. Nephron 1981;29:59–62.

142. Peterson LC, Rao KV, Crosson JT, White JG. Fechtner syndrome – a variant of Alport's syndrome with leukocyte inclusions and macrothrombocytopenia. Blood 1985;65:397–406.

143. Rao AK, Holmsen H. Congenital disorders of platelet function. Seminars in Hematology 1986;23:102–18.

144. Rosa JP, George JN, Bainton DF, et al. Gray platelet syndrome: demonstration of alpha granule membrane that can fuse with the cell surface. Journal of Clinical Investigation 1987;80:1138–46.

145. Cramer EM, Meyer D, LeMenn R, Breton-Gorius J. Eccentric localization of von Willebrand factor within a tubular structure of platelet alpha granules resembling that of Weibel Palade bodies. Blood 1985;66:710–5.

146. Milton JG, Frojmovic MM. Shape-changing agents produce abnormally large platelets in a hereditary 'giant platelets syndrome (MPS)'. Journal of Laboratory and Clinical Medicine 1979;93:154–61.

147. Lacombe M, d'Angelo G. Etudes sur une thrombopathie familiare. Neuvo Revue Franc Hematologie 1963;3:611–4.

148. Milton JG, Frojmovic MM, Tang SS, White JG. Spontaneous platelet aggregation in a hereditary giant platelet syndrome (MPS). American Journal of Pathology 1984;114:336–45.

149. White JG, Burris SM, Tukey D, et al. Micropipette aspiration of human platelets: influence of microtubules and actin filaments on deformability. Blood 1984;64:210–4.

150. Bernard J, Soulier JP. Sur une nouvelle variété de dystrophie thrombocytaire hemorragipare congenitale. Semaine des Hôpitaux de Paris 1948;24:317–21.

151. Bernard J. History of congenital hemorrhagic thrombocytopathic dystrophy. Blood Cells 1983;9:179–93.

152. Nurden AT. Glycoprotein defects responsible for abnormal platelet function in inherited disorders. In: George JN, Nurden AT, Phillips DR, editors. Platelet Membrane Glycoproteins. New York: Plenum Press; 1985. p. 357–87.

153. Frojmovic MM, Milton JG, Caen JP. Platelets from 'giant platelet syndrome (BSS)' are discocytes and normal sized. Journal of Laboratory and Clinical Medicine 1978;91:109–13.

154. Chevalier J, Nurden AT, Thiere JM. Freeze-fracture studies on the plasma membranes of normal human, thrombasthenia and Bernard–Soulier platelets. Journal of Laboratory and Clinical Medicine 1979;94:232–45.

155. Rendu F, Nurden AT, Lebret M, Caen JP. Further investigations on Bernard–Soulier platelet abnormalities. A study of 5-hydroxytryptamine uptake and mepacrine fluorescence. Journal of Laboratory and Clinical Medicine 1981; 97:689–97.

156. White JG, Burris SM, Hasegawa D, Johnson M. Micropipette aspiration of human blood platelets: a defect in the Bernard–Soulier's syndrome. Blood 1984;63:1249–52.

157. Fox JEB. Identification of actin-binding protein as the protein linking the membrane skeleton to glycoproteins on platelet plasma membranes. Journal of Biological Chemistry 1985;260:11970–7.

158. Davis RB. Glycogen distribution in rat platelets. American Journal of Pathology 1973;72:241–52.

159. Schneider W, Morgenstern E, Reimers HJ. Disassembly of microtubules in the Lesch–Nyhan syndrome? Klin Wochesnschr 1979;57:181–6.

160. Nyhan WL. Clinical features of the Lesch–Nyhan syndrome. Arch Intern Med 1972;130:186–92.

161. Nyhan WL. The Lesch–Nyhan syndrome. Ann Rev Med 1973;24:41–60.

162. Rivard GE, Izadi P, Lazerson J, et al. Functional and metabolic studies of platelets from patients with Lesch–Nyhan syndrome. Br J Haematol 1975;31:245–53.

163. Dixon RE, Davis WE, Benbow JB, Kremer WB. Spherical platelet syndrome: absent microtubules and a bleeding diathesis. Clin Res 1974;22:338A.

164. White JG, de Alarcon P. Platelet spherocytosis: a new bleeding disorder. Am J Hemotol 2002 Jun;70(2):158–66.

165. White JG. Ultrastructural physiology of platelets with randomly dispersed rather than circumferential band microtubules. Am J Pathol 1983;110:55–63.

166. Winokur R, Hartwig J. Mechanism of shape change in chilled human platelets. Blood 1995;85:1796–804.

167. White JG, Rao GHR. Microtubule coils versus the surface membrane cytoskeleton in maintenance and restoration of platelet discoid shape. Am J Pathol 1998;152:597–609.

CHAPTER 33

Acquired disorders affecting megakaryocytes and platelets

D Provan, AC Newland, PK MacCallum

Chapter contents

Introduction

Platelets play a pivotal role in primary hemostasis, and bleeding may arise through a large number of different pathologies including those that reduce platelet numbers (thrombocytopenia) or render the platelets functionally defective. Therefore, for simplicity we have divided our dis-cussion into those disorders causing quantitative abnormalities of platelets before later discussing qualitative defects that affect the function of platelets. Before examining the pathologic basis of platelet diseases it is useful to review the mechanics of platelet production, as well as the structure and normal function of platelets.

©2011 Elsevier Ltd
DOI: 10.1016/B978-0-7020-3147-2.00033-X

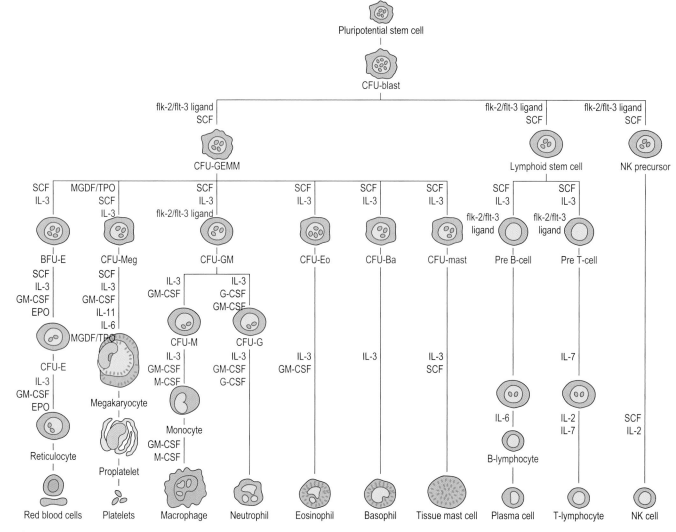

Fig. 33.1 Hematopoietic lineages, showing megakaryocyte development and platelet production. *(From Provan D, Gribben JG 2000 (eds), Molecular Haematology. Blackwell Science, Oxford, with permission.)*

Structure and function of megakaryocytes and platelets

Human platelets

Thrombopoiesis, the generation of platelets from megakaryocytes in the bone marrow, is complex and incompletely understood. Megakaryocytes are large end-stage cells from which platelets bud. The earliest recognized committed progenitor is the burst-forming unit (BFU)-Meg.[1] Fig. 33.1 shows megakaryocyte development from stem cell stage through to platelet production. BFU-Megs develop into colony-forming unit (CFU)-Megs in the presence of growth factors thrombopoietin (TPO), interleukin-3 (IL-3) and IL-11. Megakaryocyte nuclei are large polyploid structures with chromosome contents between diploid (2N) to 64N. Such polyploid status is achieved through a process termed nuclear endoduplication: that is, successive doubling of chromosome content in the absence of cell division. Platelets are produced from megakaryocytes that are 8N or

greater.[2] A single megakaryocyte can generate around 3000 platelets of which 20–30% are pooled in the spleen. In health the peripheral blood platelet count is $150–400 \times 10^9/l$ but this fluctuates, for example, following heavy exercise, 'stress', and around the menstrual cycle. This transient rise in platelet count may be caused by mobilization of platelets pooled in the spleen. There are also racial differences in the 'normal' platelet count and some Mediterranean populations have platelet counts as low as $80 \times 10^9/l$ in health. Platelets are produced at a rate of 35 000–44 000 per microliter per day[3] and have a lifespan of 9–10 days.

Platelet structure and function

Normal platelet function requires the presence of key membrane proteins and two major types of cytoplasmic granules. Because of their limited metabolic activity, and the presence of polymorphic glycoproteins on their exterior surface, platelets are vulnerable to attack by many agents including drugs, toxins, viruses and the immune system. In addition, drugs

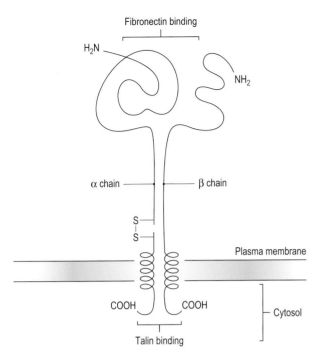

Fig. 33.2 Fibronectin receptor on mammalian fibroblasts: the platelet integrins share homology with the fibronectin receptor.

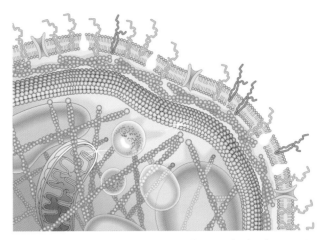

Fig. 33.3 Cartoon of platelet membrane, showing platelet glycoproteins. *(Courtesy of Peg Berrity, Science Photo Library.)*

or diseases that interfere with platelet function do so for the lifetime of the platelet and it may take several days for the effects of any interfering drugs to diminish once the offending agent is stopped.

Platelet membrane constituents

The platelet plasma membrane contains a variety of polymorphic glycoprotein molecules which interact with ligands such as coagulation factors, vessel wall components and other molecules in order to generate the primary hemostatic plug.

The integrin family of proteins

Integrins are key platelet membrane proteins and have been characterized on a large number of leukocytes and many other cells. For example, the fibronectin receptor on mammalian fibroblasts is one of the best characterized matrix receptor proteins[4] (Fig. 33.2). This receptor, in common with all other integrins, is a heterodimer consisting of a noncovalently associated complex of two distinct high-molecular-weight polypeptides, α and β. The receptor functions as a transmembrane linker which mediates the interaction between the intracellular actin cytoskeleton and fibronectin in the extracellular matrix. Like all integrins, the fibronectin receptor recognizes so-called RGD (Arg-Gly-Asp) sequences in matrix components. In platelets, integrins recognize and bind a variety of proteins in order to form a hemostatic plug through a complex mechanism of platelet adhesion, shape change and activation of the clotting pathway.

Platelet integrins and related proteins

Platelets contain five integrin α subunits and two β subunits producing: $\alpha_{IIb}\beta_3$, $\alpha_v\beta_3$, $\alpha_2\beta_1$, $\alpha_5\beta_1$ and $\alpha_6\beta_1$.[5,6,7] These are

shown in Fig. 33.3. Further detail is provided by Table 33.1. These proteins are essential for normal platelet function, and are often the target of immunological attack in disorders such as idiopathic thrombocytopenic purpura (ITP).

Platelet alloantigens

These can be platelet-specific or shared with other cells. Important shared antigens include HLA class I and ABH (blood group A and B) antigens. Platelet-specific antigens fall into five well-defined human platelet antigen (HPA) groups (Table 33.2; see also Chapter 37): HPA-1, HPA-2, HPA-3, HPA-4 and HPA-5, each of which has an α and β allele. Each platelet allotype represents a single amino acid substitution in the platelet glycoprotein molecule. Because some platelet glycoproteins carry epitopes that play a major role in platelet function, platelet alloantibodies may not only cause thrombocytopenia but also affect primary hemostasis.

Cytoplasmic platelet constituents

Platelets contain two principal types of granule: dense bodies and α granules (Fig. 33.4). Dense bodies contain ADP, ATP, 5-HT, calcium and pyrophosphate. The α granules contain more than 300 releasable proteins including adhesion molecules, chemokines, cytokines, coagulation factors, fibrinolytic regulators, growth factors and pro- and anti-angiogenic factors such as PF4, β-thrombospondin, PDGF, vWF, fibrinogen, factor V and fibronectin. The contents of these granules are integral components of the platelet's biological activities.

Biological function of platelets

The primary role of the platelet is the prevention of blood loss from damaged tissues and vessels, i.e. primary hemostasis. This is achieved through platelet activation, adhesion, shape change and aggregation. Platelets may also play a role in the maintenance of vascular integrity by the constitutive release of cytokines and growth factors from their granules that bind to endothelial cell surface receptors resulting

Table 33.1 Platelet integrins and related proteins

Glycoprotein		Ligand	Function
Integrins			
Ia/IIa	$\alpha_2\beta_1$, VLA-5, CD49e/CD29	Collagen	Platelet–collagen adhesion
Ic/IIa	$\alpha_5\beta_1$, CD49b/CD29, VLA-2	Fibronectin	
IIb/IIIa	$\alpha_{IIb}\beta_3$, CD41/CD61	Fibrinogen, vWF, vitronectin	Platelet–platelet aggregation
Non-integrin proteins			
Ib/IX	CD42	vWF	Platelet–endothelial microfibril adhesion
IV		Thrombospondin	Platelet aggregation
V			

vWF, von Willebrand factor.

Table 33.2 **Human platelet alloantigen system.** *(Modified from Waters AH 1999, The immune thrombocytopenias. In: Hoffbrand AV, Lewis SM, Tiddenham EGD (eds), Postgraduate Haematology, 4th edn. Butterworth-Heinemann, Oxford, 597–611)*

System	Antigen	Antigen frequency (%)	Glycoprotein (GP)
HPA-1	HPA-1a	97.46	IIIa
	HPA-1b	30.80	
HPA-2	HPA-2a	99.79	Ib(α)
	HPA-2b	11.81	
HPA-3	HPA-3a	86.14	IIb
	HPA-3b	62.92	
HPA-4	HPA-4a	>99.9	IIIa
	HPA-4b	<0.1	
HPA-5	HPA-5a	989.79	Ia (α)
	HPA-5b	20.65	

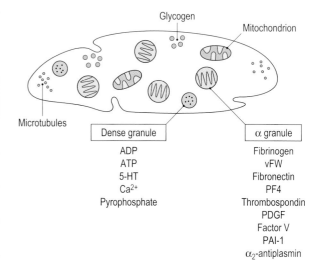

Fig. 33.4 Schematic representation of the platelet showing dense granules and alpha granules, with details of the contents of each.

in intracellular signaling that stabilizes the molecular complexes that form the junctions between adjacent endothelial cells.[8]

Platelet adhesion (Fig. 33.5A)

This process involves interaction between the platelet integrins and the subendothelium. The main integrin involved in platelet adhesion is GPIIb/IIIa which can be activated via a number of signals including exposure to extracellular matrix components such as collagen, in addition to other key activators such as adenosine diphosphate (ADP). Known ligands for platelet integrins include molecules such as fibrinogen, fibronectin and von Willebrand factor (vWF).

Platelet activation

If there is damage to the endothelial lining of blood vessels, platelets become exposed to subendothelial structures. Platelets release a variety of attractants and other chemicals and recruit other platelets which are attracted to the site of injury.

Important platelet activators include ADP, thromboxane A_2 and thrombin. The activated platelets provide a strong procoagulant surface on which the main clotting cascade is amplified, with the final product being the generation of thrombin and the production of a fibrin clot, composed of platelets enmeshed within a fibrin network.

Platelet shape change

After adhesion to the subendothelium, platelets undergo a major shape change, from a discoid shape to one which is irregular, with projections (Fig. 33.6). This process is initially reversible but ultimately becomes irreversible.

Platelet aggregation (Fig. 33.5B)

There are a number of compounds that can induce platelet aggregation, including ADP, collagen, thrombin, adrenaline, vasopressin and others. Aggregation occurs following the shift of GPIIb/IIIa, the dominant integrin on the platelet surface, from a low affinity to a high affinity state and is

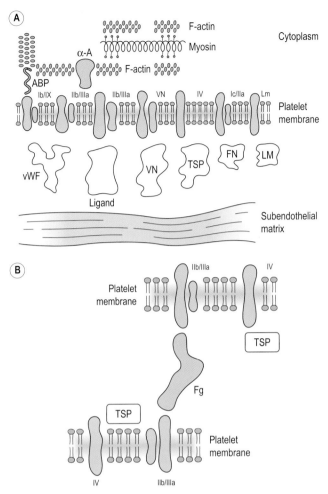

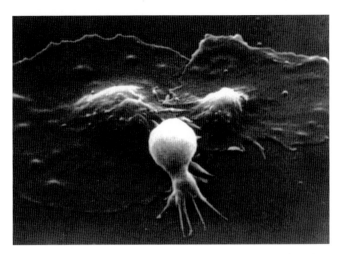

Fig. 33.6 Platelet shape change. Scanning electron micrograph of platelet shape transformation during adhesion to the arterial wall. Assemblies of actin filaments create spike-like attachment points and arrange themselves in an expansive webwork that mantles the neighboring space. *(From Roth GJ. Developing relationships: arterial platelet adhesion, glycoprotein Ib, and leucine-rich glycoproteins. Blood. 1991;77:5–19, with permission.[143])*

Fig. 33.5 (A, B) (A) Platelet adhesion to subendothelium: the platelet membrane contains a variety of glycoprotein receptors to adhesive proteins. VN, vitronectin; Lm laminin receptor; ABP, actin-binding protein; a-A, a-actin; vWF, von Willebrand factor; TSP, thrombospondin; FN, fibronectin. (B) Platelet aggregation: the terminal event in platelet aggregation is thought to be the binding of fibrinogen to GPIIb/IIIa receptors on adjacent platelets. The fibrinogen bridge may be stabilized by thrombospondin bound to its receptor (GPIV). *(From Mackie IJ. The biology of hemostasis and thrombosis. In: Ledingham JGG, Warrell DA, editors. Concise Oxford Textbook of Medicine. Oxford: Oxford University Press; 2000, with permission.[142])*

mediated through the binding of fibrinogen or von Willebrand factor to adjacent platelets.

Quantitative platelet abnormalities: thrombocytopenia

Thrombocytopenia, a reduction in platelet count, may be caused by:

- impaired production
- increased destruction
- altered distribution
- a combination of these.

Pseudothrombocytopenia

This describes patients in whom the peripheral blood platelet count is found to be spuriously low, and is caused by a variety of mechanisms. Platelet clumping caused by the anticoagulant ethylenediaminetetraacetic acid (EDTA) is the commonest cause, with an incidence of around 0.1%. EDTA-induced pseudothrombocytopenia is easily excluded by examination of a blood film which will confirm the presence of numerous large platelet clumps.[9,10] Other causes of pseudothrombocytopenia include the presence of giant platelets, which are not counted as platelets by modern automated counters, and platelet satellitism (platelets attach themselves to monocytes or granulocytes) (Fig. 33.7).

Pooling of platelets in the spleen

This accounts for the thrombocytopenias seen in patients with hepatic cirrhosis and portal hypertension. The term hypersplenism is used for patients in whom there is thrombocytopenia through excessive splenic pooling of platelets.

Mechanism involved

In health, the spleen may pool up to one third of the total platelet mass, and in disease states this may rise to 90%.[11] Although the peripheral blood platelet count may only be a fraction of the normal range, the patient generally has an overall normal platelet mass since production is entirely normal but the low peripheral counts simply reflect a larger than normal mass of platelets pooled in the spleen.

Thrombocytopenia due to failure of platelet production

Acquired amegakaryocytic thrombocytopenia

This describes severe thrombocytopenia caused by a selective reduction in megakaryocytes in an otherwise normal bone

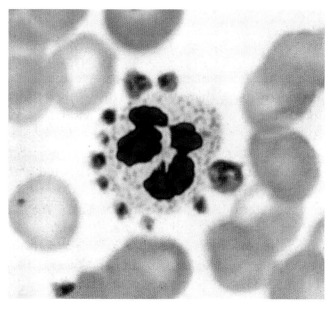

Fig. 33.7 Platelet satellitism. The figure shows a neutrophil surrounded by adherent platelets. *(From Lewis SM, Bain B, Bates I, Dacie J 2000 (eds), Practical Haematology, 9th edn. Churchill Livingstone, Edinburgh, with permission.)*

Table 33.3 Acquired bone marrow failure syndromes

Idiopathic (majority)			
Secondary	Drugs	Predictable	Cytotoxics
			Benzene
		Idiosyncratic	Chloramphenicol
	Viruses	EBV	Gold
		Hepatitis	
		HIV	
		Parvovirus	
	Immune disease		
	Thymoma		
	Pregnancy		
	PNH		
	Radiation		

EBV, Epstein–Barr virus; HIV, human immunodeficiency virus; PNH, paroxysmal nocturnal hemoglobinuria.

marrow, and is the result of damage to the megakaryocyte stem cell. The disorder is analogous to acquired pure red-cell aplasia (PRCA). Acquired amegakaryocytic thrombocytopenia may be caused by drugs, toxins and connective tissue disorders.[12–14]

Drug-induced megakaryocyte hypoplasia

All drugs that are myelosuppressive will inhibit megakaryocyte stem cells. Agents that are cell cycle phase-specific have the most profound effects on megakaryocytes (e.g. methotrexate and cytosine arabinoside). Other drugs may selectively 'poison' megakaryocytes, and induce profound hypoplasia, for example thiazide diuretics, ethanol and estrogens.

Bone marrow failure syndromes

The bone marrow failure (BMF) disorders are those in which there is a failure of bone marrow precursor (stem) cells in contrast to those disorders such as myelodysplastic syndromes in which normal or increased numbers of abnormal cells are produced, or those in which the survival of the cells is reduced. The BMF syndromes are a diverse groups of disorders with a common endpoint in which there is loss of hematopoietic stem cells. BMF can be acquired or inherited (see Table 33.3).

Aplastic anemia

This is discussed in Chapter 13.

Thrombocytopenia due to increased platelet destruction

Causes may be immunologic or non-immunologic.

Non-immunologic causes of thrombocytopenia

Disseminated intravascular coagulation (DIC)

DIC is characterized by excessive activation of the coagulation cascade (see also Chapter 35). In most cases DIC is an acute event, but chronic DIC is well described, although clinically less important. The main problem faced in patients with DIC is bleeding, which may be mild but is often severe with generalized oozing from venepuncture sites, central lines and other indwelling cannulae, gastrointestinal and genitourinary tracts. Microthrombi are found in 5–10% of cases, often affecting digits, with resulting peripheral gangrene.

Pathogenesis

DIC is triggered by the release or exposure of tissue thromboplastins which contain a high concentration of phospholipids following trauma, surgery, mismatched blood transfusion and a variety of other triggers (Table 33.4). In addition to systemic activation of coagulation (leading to fibrin clot formation, organ failure and consumption of platelets and coagulation factors that may cause bleeding), there is dysregulation of natural anticoagulant systems and fibrinolysis.

Laboratory diagnosis

No single laboratory test is diagnostic of DIC. The blood count will usually show thrombocytopenia. Coagulation tests are the most important assays for the detection of DIC, and will show prolongation of prothrombin time (PT), activated partial thromboplastin time (APTT) and thrombin time with reduced fibrinogen and elevated D-dimers.

Table 33.4 Triggers for disseminated intravascular coagulation (DIC)

Trauma	Including surgical
Dissemination of cancer cells	Malignancy, following administration of chemotherapy
Massive hemolysis	Post mismatched blood transfusion
Venoms	e.g. snake venoms
Endothelial injury	Gram-negative sepsis
Infections	
Burns	
Septicemia	

Table 33.5 Classification of thrombocytopenic purpura and hemolytic uremic syndrome. *(Modified from George JN, El-Harake M 1995. Thrombocytopenia due to enhanced platelet destruction by non-immunologic mechanisms. In: Beutler E, Lichtman MA, Coller BS, Kipps TJ (eds), Williams Hematology, 5th edn. McGraw-Hill, New York, 1290–1315)*

Idiopathic TTP/HUS	Classic adult TTP and childhood non-verotoxin-associated HUS-TTP	
Secondary TTP-HUS	Pregnancy-related	TTP, postpartum HUS
	Verotoxin-induced	*Escherichia coli* and *Shigella dysenteriae* I
		Childhood HUS
		Epidemic adult TTP-HUS
	Malignant disease	Especially metastatic carcinomas
	Drug-induced	Chemotherapy agents, e.g. mitomycin C, cisplatin, and other drugs
		Immunosuppressive agents, e.g. cyclosporin, quinine, ticlopidine
	Post-marrow/stem cell transplantation	Especially in conjunction with total body irradiation or high-dose (intensive) chemotherapy

HUS, hemolytic uremic syndrome; TTP, thrombocytopenic purpura.

Management

Supportive care can be given with fresh-frozen plasma (FFP), cryoprecipitate and platelet transfusions but the most effective treatment is removal of the cause.[15]

Thrombotic thrombocytopenic purpura and hemolytic uremic syndrome

Thrombotic microangiopathy refers to a state that is characterized pathologically by occlusive microvascular thrombosis and clinically by profound thrombocytopenia, microangiopathic hemolytic anemia and variable signs and symptoms of organ ischemia.[16] The term primarily refers to two discrete but overlapping syndromes, thrombotic thrombocytopenic purpura (TTP) and hemolytic uremic syndrome (HUS).

TTP is a disseminated microangiopathy, first described by Moschowitz in 1924.[17] It is uncommon, occurring primarily in adults and with an annual incidence in the US of 4–11 cases per million people. HUS has clinical and laboratory features that often overlap with those of TTP. However, HUS is more common in children, the renal abnormalities are more marked than in TTP (Table 33.5; see also Chapter 10) and the underlying pathogenetic mechanisms of the two conditions differ.

Clinical features of TTP

TTP is characterized by the pentad:

- thrombocytopenia
- microangiopathic hemolysis
- neurologic symptoms and signs (typically fluctuating)
- renal function abnormalities
- fever.

TTP can affect any organ system but it is the involvement of the hematopoietic, renal and central nervous systems that leads to the typical clinical features.

The previously high mortality rate has been reduced through effective treatment and good supportive care. The disorder is sporadic, but appears to be more common in people of black origin and in obese individuals. It may develop in pregnancy and in this setting must be differentiated from pre-eclampsia, eclampsia and the HELLP (hemolysis, elevated liver enzymes and low platelets) syndrome.

TTP typically has a sudden onset, with fever and neurologic symptoms including paralysis, coma, fits and psychiatric disturbance. There is usually purpura and the clinical picture is one of a fluctuating course. The causes of TTP can be subclassified into: 1) congenital; 2) idiopathic; and 3) non-idiopathic.[16]

Laboratory investigations

A full blood count and blood film will show anemia (hemoglobin ~ 8–9 g/dl) with polychromasia and other evidence of hemolysis. The film will usually show red-cell fragments and thrombocytopenia (Fig. 33.8). There is usually evidence of hemoglobinemia reflecting the presence of intravascular hemolysis. Lactate dehydrogenase will be elevated. Clotting tests are generally normal although occasionally there may be features of DIC. The direct Coombs test is negative. Renal failure is uncommon but elevated serum creatinine is seen in about a third of cases.

Pathogenesis

Failure to cleave large von Willebrand factor (vWF) multimers is thought to be crucial in the pathogenesis of TTP. Von

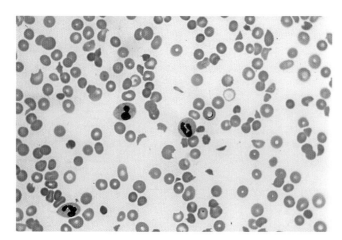

Fig. 33.8 Peripheral blood film from a patient with thrombotic thrombocytopenic purpura (TTP). Note the many fragmented red cells, characteristic of this disorder. *(Figure kindly provided by Dr John Amess, Barts & The London NHS Trust.)*

Willebrand factor is synthesized in vascular endothelial cells and megakaryocytes and assembles into multimers linked by disulfide bonds which are stored in the Weibel–Palade bodies of endothelial cells and α-granules of platelets. A small proportion of these multimers is constitutively secreted by endothelial cells into the circulation, stabilizing factor VIII and mediating both platelet adhesion to sites of vascular injury and platelet aggregation in conditions of high shear. Endothelial cell stimulation causes unusually large vWF multimers to be secreted and these attach to the endothelial cell surface.[16]

A key recent discovery to understanding the pathogenesis of TTP has been the recognition of the role of a deficiency of a von Willebrand factor-cleaving protease, termed ADAMTS 13 (an acronym for a disintegrin and metalloprotease with thrombospondin-1-like domains). ADAMTS 13 cleaves the large vWF multimers secreted by endothelial cells to generate the range of multimer sizes that normally circulate in the blood. This function appears to be critical in preventing thrombosis in the microvasculature because hereditary or acquired deficiency of ADAMTS 13, resulting in an inability to cleave newly secreted von Willebrand factor multimers, leads to increased binding of vWF to platelets and to the disseminated platelet thrombi that are characteristic of TTP.

More than 50 mutations of the ADAMTS 13 gene have been described in patients with the rare congenital or familial form of TTP. About half of these patients present during childhood but the remainder present in adulthood when the acute event may be triggered by conditions such as infection or pregnancy.

In contrast, in the more common idiopathic TTP, ADAMTS 13 deficiency is caused by autoantibodies that inhibit its activity or enhance its clearance from the circulation. Mostly the antibodies are IgG.

There are a number of causes of non-idiopathic thrombotic microangiopathy. These include cancer, pregnancy (see below), certain drugs (quinine, mitomycin, ciclosporin, ticlopidine and clopidogrel) and hemopoietic progenitor cell transplantation.

The characteristic histological features include hyaline thrombi in terminal arterioles and capillaries. The thrombi are composed of platelets and are rich in von Willebrand factor but contain little fibrinogen or fibrin. Immunoglobulins and complement are also often present consistent with the autoimmune origin of TTP.

Diagnosis

There is no specific diagnostic test for TTP and in practice for management purposes the diagnosis is based on laboratory confirmation of thrombocytopenia and microangiopathic hemolytic anemia without an apparent alternative cause and with or without the characteristic clinical features described above.

Management

Plasma exchange with cryosupernatant or FFP is now regarded as the treatment of choice for TTP and should be instituted as soon as possible after diagnosis and continued on a daily basis with replacement of 1.0 to 1.5 times the predicted plasma volume of the patient. Plasma exchange should continue until there is normalization of the neurological state, the platelet count has been $>150 \times 10^9/l$ for at least 2 days, the LDH is normal and the hemoglobin rising.[18] The disease is highly variable in its course and it is difficult to predict the clinical outcome at the outset. Patients require intensive care nursing, and may require ventilation. Hemodialysis may be required along with plasma exchange. A short course of high dose corticosteroids has also been recommended along with aspirin when the platelet count has recovered to $50 \times 10^9/l$.[18] Platelet transfusions should be avoided except in cases of severe hemorrhage. Remission is achieved when the platelet count remains normal for 30 days after discontinuation of plasma exchange.[19] Patients with severe deficiency of ADAMTS 13 appear to have an increased risk of relapse, most within a year. Rituximab has been used to try to reduce the risk of relapse.[20,21]

Hemolytic uremic syndrome

The disorder was first described in 1955 by Gasser,[22] who reported on five patients (all infants) with acute renal failure, who died of renal cortical necrosis. HUS is classified into D+HUS and D-HUS.[16] D+HUS accounts for >90% of cases and is caused by enteric infection with Shiga toxin-producing bacteria, most commonly *Escherichia coli* O157:H7 or occasionally *Shigella dysenteriae* I.[22] It can occur at all ages but is seen typically in young children.[22-24] HUS usually develops 4–6 days after the onset of diarrhea. There is a seasonal incidence, with the highest number of new cases reported in the summer months.[25,26]

D-HUS is uncommon and clinically heterogeneous. These individuals do not have an antecedent enteric infection with a Shiga toxin-producing organism and have a relatively poor prognosis with a mortality rate of about 25%.[16]

The histopathological features of HUS are different from those of TTP. The kidneys are preferentially involved and the thrombi are composed primarily of fibrin with few platelets and little vWF.[16] Endothelial damage is pronounced in childhood D+HUS. Marked destruction of the renal cortex may occur and glomerular thrombosis is characteristic with an appearance suggesting capillary congestion rather than ischemia.[16] D-HUS has been little studied but the renal lesions appear to differ with more pronounced mesangial involvement and less glomerular thrombosis than in D+HUS.[16]

Pathogenesis. Most D+HUS results from *E. coli* O157 infections caused by food-borne outbreaks from cattle. Unwashed fruit is another source of some outbreaks. Subunits of Shiga toxin produced by the bacteria bind to microvascular endothelial cells particularly in the kidney and on monocytes and platelets. The toxin is subsequently internalized and inhibits protein synthesis leading to cell death. Cytokine release is stimulated further increasing Shiga toxin binding. Resulting endothelial cell damage has prothrombotic consequences that lead to the histopathological changes described above.[16]

D-HUS in contrast is associated with complement dysregulation and mutations in one of the complement regulatory proteins (factor H, factor I, membrane cofactor protein (MCP) and factor B) have been described in about 50% of these patients.[16] In some patients an autoantibody against factor H has been recognized and in about 5% of cases mutations that impair thrombomodulin function have been identified.[27]

Clinical features. Children typically present with diarrhea (often bloody), vomiting and abdominal pain. Because of the large volume of fluid loss, patients are often oliguric or anuric at presentation. Fever, hypertension and fits are also features.

Laboratory findings. There is evidence of acute renal failure and features of microangiopathic hemolysis.[28] The blood count will generally show an elevated WBC, most usually neutrophilia; the prognosis is worst for patients with total neutrophil counts exceeding 20×10^9/l.[25]

Management. Around half of the children affected will require hemodialysis for between 1 and 2 weeks. Unlike in adult TTP, plasma exchange using FFP replacement is not often required in children.

Outlook. Unlike adult TTP, childhood D+HUS is rarely fatal and the mortality is around 3–5%. The outlook is less favorable in D-HUS. In cases with end-stage renal failure that have undergone renal transplantation, the outcome appears to correlate with the cause of the complement dysregulation. Recurrence of HUS has not been seen in transplanted kidneys in patients with MCP mutations whereas the condition did recur following renal transplantation in patients with factor H or factor I mutations, perhaps because these latter two factors are made in the liver. Combined liver and kidney transplants may be successful in some of these cases.[16]

Pre-eclampsia and HELLP syndrome

In addition to TTP and HUS there are a number of causes of thrombotic microangiopathy that can occur during pregnancy, in particular pre-eclampsia/eclampsia and the HELLP syndrome. Differentiation between these different conditions can be problematic. Pre-eclampsia occurs after 20 weeks of pregnancy and is associated with hypertension, edema, sodium retention, proteinuria and DIC. It may progress to eclampsia which is characterized by convulsions.[29] Previously, pre-eclampsia/eclampsia and HELLP have been considered distinct disorders but it seems more likely that they represent a spectrum of a pathologic process.

HELLP syndrome

This disorder, characterized by hemolysis, elevated liver enzymes and low platelet count, occurs in 0.5–0.9% of all pregnancies,[30,31] and is associated with a mortality rate of 1–4%.[32] It occurs in up to 10% of cases of severe pre-eclampsia. Perinatal mortality is high and may reach 10–20%.[32]

Clinical features. HELLP is associated with generalized weakness, nausea and vomiting, right upper quadrant pain, headache and visual upset.[33] In some cases HELLP may occur following delivery.[36]

Pathophysiology. There may be abnormalities of the placental vessels with resulting placental ischemia. This is associated with the systemic release of a thromboxanes, angiotensin, tumor necrosis factor-α (TNF-α) and other procoagulant proteins.[31,33] DIC may result leading to thrombi which threaten major end-organs including placenta, renal, hepatic and central nervous systems. The thrombi lead to endothelial damage and there is microangiopathic hemolytic anemia (MAHA) and failure of the organs affected by the thrombotic process. Liver failure and occasionally liver rupture may result.[34]

Management. Prompt delivery, and control of the hypertension are required, in addition to correcting the factor deficiencies caused by the DIC. Corticosteroids have been used as well as plasma exchange and plasmapheresis.[35] Maternal deaths, where these occur, are usually due to uncontrolled DIC. Cases in which thrombotic microangiopathy persists post-partum should be considered for plasma exchange.[18]

Thrombocytopenia caused by massive blood transfusion

Massive transfusion whereby a patient's total blood volume is replaced over a short time period (24 h or less) may lead to thrombocytopenia, and although the degree of thrombocytopenia is largely related to the amount of blood transfused, the mechanism is not purely dilutional. Patients receiving 15 units of red cells within a 24-hour period develop mild thrombocytopenia, with platelet counts between 47 and 100×10^9/l, whereas patients transfused with 20 units of red cells over the same period develop more pronounced thrombocytopenia $(25–61 \times 10^9$/l).[36,37]

Management

Severe thrombocytopenia can be prevented by administering platelet concentrates prophylactically to patients receiving more than 20 units of red cells within a 24-hour time period.

Liver disease

Thrombocytopenia secondary to alcohol

Thrombocytopenia occurring in alcoholic patients may be caused by a variety of mechanisms including cirrhosis, splenomegaly and folic acid deficiency. However, thrombocytopenia may be found in the absence of any or all of these pathologies, and is probably due to the direct toxic effects of alcohol on the bone marrow itself, since ethanol is a poison and can suppress the production of platelets by the marrow.[38,39]

Thrombocytopenia in hepatocellular failure

In addition to the other coagulopathies induced by liver failure, thrombocytopenia is often present and generally reflects the hypersplenism that occurs in portal hypertension. In fulminant hepatic failure, there are abnormalities of both platelet structure and function. On laboratory testing there may be evidence of mild DIC, although this is not generally of major clinical importance.[40] In addition, patients with chronic liver disease often have elevated levels of fibrin degradation products which interfere with platelet aggregation.

Thrombocytopenia caused by infection

There are numerous infections caused by a wide variety of pathogenic bacteria, fungi, viruses and protozoa that result in thrombocytopenia in humans. The mechanism underlying the thrombocytopenia is variable. In many cases there is suppression of marrow function, and this is particularly the case with viral infections and accounts for most cases of mild thrombocytopenia. Implicated viruses include mumps,[41] varicella,[42] EBV,[43] rubella[44] and many others.

Mechanism of thrombocytopenia

There is a variety of mechanisms involved in thrombocytopenia induced by infection. Following measles infection in children, there is a reduction in marrow megakaryocytes and by day 3 of the infection many of the megakaryocytes have vacuoles within the nucleus and cytoplasm.[45]

Thrombocytopenia induced by HIV infection

HIV infection probably induces thrombocytopenia through a variety of mechanisms, including immune-mediated thrombocytopenia with reduced platelet life span,[46–48] and through direct infection of megakaryocytes themselves. This may occur at any stage in the course of HIV infection, and 40% of HIV positive individuals develop thrombocytopenia at some point in the illness.[49–51] Unlike classical idiopathic thrombocytopenic purpura (ITP), males and females are affected equally and thrombocytopenia may be the presenting feature in 10% of HIV positive people.[52]

Thrombocytopenia due to hematinic deficiencies

Thrombocytopenia may be a feature of vitamin B_{12} or folate deficiency, and mild thrombocytopenia is found in 20% of patients with megaloblastic anemia caused by vitamin B_{12} deficiency.[53]

Immunologic causes of thrombocytopenia

Here we have restricted our discussion to the more important immune-mediated causes of thrombocytopenia, namely neonatal alloimmune thrombocytopenia (NAIT), post-transfusion purpura (PTP), ITP, drug-induced thrombocytopenia and heparin-induced thrombocytopenia (HIT) (Table 33.6). Since the targets involved in several of these disorders are human platelet alloantigens we outline briefly their salient features.

Table 33.6 Disorders associated with immune-mediated thrombocytopenia. *(From Chong BH 1998, Diagnosis treatment and pathophysiology of autoimmune thrombocytopenias. Critical Reviews in Oncology Hematology 20(3):271–296)*

Autoimmune	Idiopathic (ITP)
	Secondary immune
	Autoimmune disorders, e.g. SLE, rheumatoid, thyroid disease
	Lymphoproliferative disorders, e.g. CLL, NHL
	Cancer, e.g. solid tumors
	Miscellaneous, e.g. post-BMT, chemotherapy
	Viral infection
	e.g. HIV, measles, mumps, rubella, EBV, varicella
	Drug-induced
Alloimmune	Post-transfusion purpura
	Neonatal alloimmune thrombocytopenia

BMT, bone-marrow transfer; CLL, chronic lymphocytic leukemia; EBV, Epstein–Barr virus; HIV, human immunodeficiency virus; ITP, idiopathic thrombocytopenic purpura, SLE, systemic lupus erythematosus; NHL, Non-Hodgkin lymphoma.

Molecular basis of HPA antigens

Platelets have a variety of cell surface antigens, some of which are shared by other cells, such as HLA class I, and blood groups A and B. Others are platelet-specific and are not found on any other type of cell. To date there are 19 alloantigen systems described on platelets, all of which map to membrane proteins (Table 33.2). Eleven of the 19 are carried on GPIIb/IIIa ($\alpha_{IIb}\beta_3$ integrin heterodimer), three are on GPIb/IX/V, two on GPIa/IIa ($\alpha_2\beta_1$), and one on each of GPIV, GPV and CD109. The molecular basis for most of these is now elucidated (see Chapter 37).

Antibody response to non-self HPA antigens

The difference between self and non-self HPAs is determined by a single amino acid substitution, and for this reason HPAs are not particularly immunogenic, in comparison with, for example, Rh(D) and HLA class I antigens. The most clinically important HPAs are HPA-1a and HPA-5a, since antibodies to these antigens account for 95% of cases of NAIT. Alloantibodies to the other HPAs also occur but at much lower frequency.

Alloimmunization against platelet-specific antigens is associated with three major clinical syndromes: neonatal alloimmune thrombocytopenia, post-transfusion purpura and refractoriness to platelet transfusions. Only the first two are discussed here.

Alloantibody-mediated thrombocytopenia

Neonatal alloimmune thrombocytopenia

Antibodies to HPA occur in 1 in 365 pregnancies and cause severe thrombocytopenia in 1 in 1100 neonates at term, accounting for around 20% of cases of thrombocytopenia in neonates. NAIT occurs when there is feto-maternal incompatibility for HPA. The condition was first described by van Loghem et al in 1959.[54]

During pregnancy, or following a blood transfusion, the mother becomes sensitized and produces alloantibodies against HPA. Maternal IgG anti-HPA crosses the placenta resulting in premature destruction of fetal platelets.

Antigens involved in NAIT

In Caucasian females NAIT is most commonly due to anti-HPA-1a (98% of the population are HPA-1a$^+$). Other implicated antigens include HPA-1b,[55] 101 HPA-2a,[56] HPA-3a,[57] HPA-3b,[58] HPA-4a,[59] HPA-4b,[60] HPA-5b[61] and HPA-5a.[62]

Diagnosis of NAIT

In contrast to maternal ITP, the mother in NAIT has a normal platelet count and is completely well. The neonate is generally asymptomatic at birth, apart from a low platelet count. In cases where neonates are symptomatic the platelet count is generally $<30 \times 10^9$/l. If no treatment is given, the baby's platelet count may remain low for up to 2 weeks, and occasionally longer.

Maternal serum is tested against the father's platelets in addition to normal control platelets. Occasionally, the maternal antibody titer is low at delivery and difficulty to detect using the above techniques. However, there are techniques available for the detection of low-titer maternal antibodies.[63]

Clinical features

Unlike hemolytic disease of the newborn where the firstborn child is unaffected, in NAIT the firstborn child may be affected. Recurrence in subsequent pregnancies is common, if there is feto-maternal incompatibility. The newborn infant is usually normal at birth but most will have some degree of bleeding due to the marked thrombocytopenia.

Management

The NAIT may be very mild and require no therapy apart from close monitoring of the neonate's platelet count. If treatment is required there are a variety of options available including:

1. Corticosteroids, although it is uncertain whether corticosteroids reduce the period of thrombocytopenia.[64]
2. Platelet transfusions, which are useful if there is serious bleeding. These can be random donor platelets but more ideally should be antigen-negative (HPA-1a and HPA-5a negative). The mother's platelets may be used, but these should be washed to remove antibody which is present in the mother's plasma.[65]
3. Intravenous immunoglobulin.[66]
4. Exchange transfusion, which removes antibody and reduces the period of thrombocytopenia.[67]

Future pregnancies

This depends on the father's genotype for the particular HPA. For example, if he is homozygous then each pregnancy will be affected. In cases where the father is heterozygous, 50% of pregnancies will be affected and the fetus can be typed using DNA obtained from chorionic villus sampling.[68]

Post-transfusion purpura (PTP)

This rare disorder occurs 7–10 days following a red-cell transfusion in recipients who possess alloantibodies against platelet antigens of the donor. In addition to destroying the incoming platelets, the alloantibody also mediates destruction of the recipient's own platelets (i.e. lacking the target antigen).[69]

Pathogenetic basis

Platelet alloantibodies may be present in the recipient against any one of the six major platelet antigens: anti-HPA-1a, anti-HPA-1b,[70] anti-HPA3a,[71] anti-bak-b,[72] anti-HPA-4a or anti-HPA-5b.[73] In most cases the antibody has specificity for HPA-1a (2% of the population is HPA-1a–).[74]

Clinical features

PTP affects multiparous women, although it has been reported in males,[70] between the ages of 16 and 80 years. Patients have usually been exposed to platelet antigens through either pregnancy or transfusion or both. The platelet antigen most commonly involved is HPA-1a.

Laboratory features

Patients usually have a platelet count less than 10×10^9/l and the bone marrow will show normal or increased numbers of megakaryocytes. Diagnosis of PTP requires the demonstration of the presence of platelet-specific alloantibodies in the serum of the affected patient. Most patients with PTP are HPA-1a$^-$ and the presence of HPA-1a platelets in the transfused blood boosts the primary response.[70,72,75,76] The antiplatelet antibodies produced are mainly of IgG1 and IgG3 class. Why patients destroy their own platelets which are HPA-1a$^-$ is unclear but is believed to involve IgG3. Possibly HPA-1a$^+$ platelets release HPA-1a which combines with the newly-formed anti-HPA-1a. This complex is absorbed on to the surface of the patient's HPA-1a$^-$ platelets.

Management

Corticosteroids may help the purpura but do not appear to be effective in increasing the platelet count. Intravenous immunoglobulin (IVIg) is the mainstay of treatment.[69] Occasionally, plasma exchange may be required. If platelet are required these should be HPA-1a$^-$. Fatal intracranial hemorrhage occurs in 10% but most patients recover within 1–6 weeks.[69]

Autoantibody-mediated thrombocytopenia

This includes acute and chronic ITP, in addition to thrombocytopenia secondary to other autoimmune disorders, lymphoproliferative diseases or drugs.

Immune thrombocytopenic purpura (ITP)

In ITP platelets are opsonized with antiplatelet autoantibodies and removed prematurely by the reticuloendothelial system (RES) leading to a reduced peripheral blood platelet count. In addition, in many patients platelet production is reduced. ITP is therefore a disorder of platelet destruction and relative failure of production.[77] The etiology of ITP is obscure and the clinical course is variable and unpredictable. ITP has an incidence of 5.8–6.6 new cases per million population per year in the US,[78] with a similar incidence in the UK. Childhood ITP is generally seasonal and typically

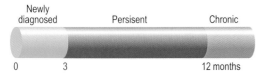

Newly
diagnosed   Persistent   Chronic

0   3   12 months

Fig. 33.9 This schematic shows the new terminology used for the phases of ITP. The disease begins as *newly diagnosed* ITP which may last beyond 3 months after which it is called *persistent* ITP. If ITP lasts longer than 12 months it is known as *chronic* ITP.

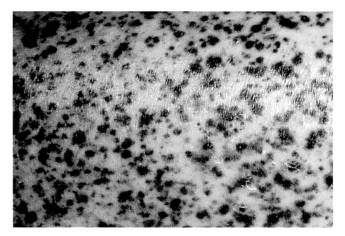

Fig. 33.10 Petechial hemorrhages on the shin of a patient with severe chronic ITP.

follows a trivial viral infection or vaccination, and in most cases is transient, requiring no treatment with spontaneous recovery in 80% of cases. In the adult (generally chronic) form there is usually no obvious antecedent illness and most patients have chronic thrombocytopenia; spontaneous recovery is uncommon.[79] In most cases of adult ITP the platelet glycoprotein (GP) antigen targets are GPIIb/IIIa and GPIb/IX.[80]

The terminology used in ITP has been updated following a consensus meeting of international experts. The term 'acute ITP' is no longer in use, and chronic ITP, which used to define ITP persisting longer than 6 months, now refers to ITP lasting beyond 12 months[81] (Fig. 33.9).

Self-limiting ITP is the most common form of ITP found in children, with an annual incidence of between 3 and 8 per 100 000 per year.[82,83]

Pathophysiology

It is believed that this type of ITP is most likely due to an inappropriate immune response to an environmental trigger; the nature of this trigger is not yet identified.[84,85] The disorder may represent an abnormality of antigen-presenting cells, with an increase in the numbers of CD4+ and CD8+ cells. The platelets are rapidly destroyed by the immune complexes that bind to the Fc receptors on the platelets, or due to autoantibodies that bind to the antigenic site on the platelets. Platelets that are coated with antibody or immune complexes are rapidly cleared by the reticuloendothelial system.

Clinical features

The children affected by ITP are, in general, well. The disorder is commonest in children between the ages of 2 and 5 years and, unlike adult chronic ITP, there is no sex predominance. A viral illness predates the development of ITP in most cases of childhood ITP. Physical signs of thrombocytopenia usually take the form of bruising or petechial hemorrhage. Splenomegaly, hepatomegaly and lymphadenopathy are not features of newly diagnosed ITP. A recent UK study reported that in some 76% of children with ITP the disorder was mild with bruising and occasional epistaxis.[82] Around 4% had no bleeding symptoms and only 3% had severe bleeding from the gastrointestinal tract, nose or vagina requiring hospitalization. In around 15% of children the disease persisted longer than 6 months and fell into the 'chronic ITP' group. The chronic form was found to be commoner in older children and in females.

Laboratory investigation

The blood count will show an isolated thrombocytopenia but should otherwise be normal. The platelet count is often less than $10 \times 10^9/l$.[82] Anemia may be present in cases in which there has been significant bleeding.

Bone marrow aspirates

The need to carry out a bone marrow aspirate is debatable, but when this is carried out there tends to be normal or increased numbers of megakaryocytes confirming that the thrombocytopenia is due to peripheral destruction rather than a failure of production. However, if there is any suspicion regarding the presence of underlying disease accounting for the thrombocytopenia or the child has features not typical of ITP then performing a bone marrow aspirate may be indicated.

Thrombopoietin (TPO) levels

These are not measured routinely, but in cases where TPO has been assayed in ITP the levels tend not to be elevated.[86–88]

Management

Most children with ITP need no therapy. There is no set threshold for medical intervention and what constitutes a 'safe' platelet count is not known.[89] From studies of the natural history of patients with newly diagnosed ITP, we know that patients with this disorder have far fewer bleeding problems than those patients with comparable platelet counts caused by other diseases, such as acute leukemia or aplastic anemia. This, in part, reflects the fact that platelet function in ITP is extremely good, with a large proportion of reticulated (young) platelets in the peripheral blood.[90] If therapy is required to elevate the platelet count then the options comprise oral corticosteroids, intravenous immunoglobulin and splenectomy.

Chronic immune thrombocytopenic purpura (ITP)

Clinical features of ITP

This is the most common form of ITP in adults. Patients may be asymptomatic or may have purpura, bruising or mucosal bleeding including gum bleeding, retinal hemorrhage, epistaxis, melena or menorrhagia (Fig. 33.10). The degree of

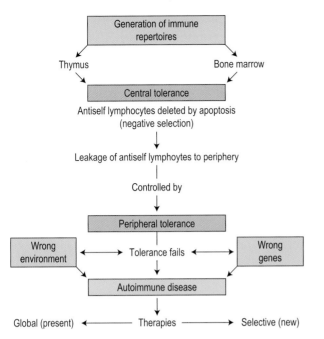

Fig. 33.11 Possible mechanism involved in the development of autoimmune disease such as ITP. Self-reactive lymphocytes are generated during B-cell development. These are normally eliminated but some may 'leak' into the periphery. This, by itself, is probably insufficient to lead to autoimmunity, and requires a specific genetic predisposition in addition to the 'wrong environment' (e.g. viral infection) to produce the autoimmune phenotype. *(From Mackay IR. Tolerance and autoimmunity. British Medical Journal. 2000;321:93–96, with permission.[93])*

bleeding is largely dependent on the platelet count, and patients with platelet counts below $10 \times 10^9/l$ are at greatest risk of bleeding. Splenomegaly is not a feature of ITP and if present, tends to suggest a diagnosis other than ITP.

Pathophysiology of ITP

ITP is an autoimmune disease characterized by increased platelet destruction due to the presence of antiplatelet antibodies. This results in increased platelet clearance by the RES. Several investigators have demonstrated specific autoantibodies against platelet membrane antigens, thus confirming the autoimmune nature of the disorder.[91,92] The cause is unknown but it appears likely that in a genetically predisposed individual, a trigger such as infection leads to loss of self-tolerance[93] (Fig. 33.11).

Glycoprotein (GP)-specific autoantibodies may be important in the pathogenesis of chronic ITP;[94] from available data GPIIb/IIIa appear to play a major role in the development of chronic ITP in 30–40% of cases.[62,95] Fig. 33.12 illustrates the structure of GPIIb/IIIa schematically. Previous investigators have looked for autoantigenic epitopes on the GPIIb/IIIa molecule using competitive binding between human autoantibodies and mouse monoclonal antibodies (MoAbs).[96,97]

Implicated epitopes

Kekomaki et al. have shown that the 33kDa chymotryptic core fragment of IIIa is a frequent target in chronic ITP.[98] Fujisawa and colleagues have used synthetic peptides

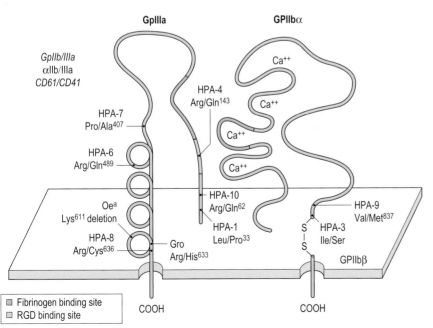

Fig. 33.12 Schematic representation of GPIIb/IIIa. *(From Provan D, Gribben JG (eds) 2000, Molecular Haematology. Blackwell Science, Oxford, with permission.)*

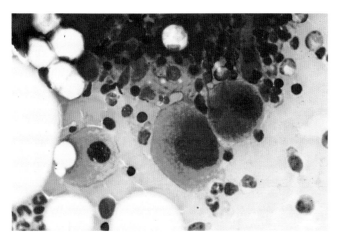

Fig. 33.13 Bone-marrow aspirate in patient with ITP showing increased numbers of megakaryocytes, some of which are young with fewer nuclei than mature megakaryocytes. *(Figure kindly provided by Dr John Amess, Barts & The London NHS Trust.)*

corresponding to IIIa sequences and have shown that in five of 13 sera from patients with chronic ITP binding was to residues 721–744 or 742–762, corresponding to the carboxy terminal of IIIa.[97]

GP-specific human MoAbs have been developed as important tools in the search for GP autoepitopes in chronic ITP.[94,99] Some investigators have localized certain autoantigenic epitopes to regions of IIb or IIIa but blocking experiments using murine MoAbs have produced contradictory data in terms of homogeneity of the IIb/IIIa antigenic repertoire.[96] Only a few cryptic epitopes on IIb/IIIa have been recognized using GP-specific human MoAbs.

Antibody class

The autoantibodies involved in ITP are generally IgG, but IgA and IgM autoantibodies have also been reported.[62]

Diagnosis

Despite advances in serologic and other techniques the diagnosis of ITP remains largely clinical, and one of exclusion. Secondary causes include systemic lupus erythematosus (SLE), lymphoproliferative disease, HIV infection and others. Standard investigative tests include full blood count which will confirm the presence of isolated thrombocytopenia, blood film to ensure there are no red cell fragments or other diseases such as leukemia or parasitic infections, and an autoimmune profile, to exclude a secondary cause for the thrombocytopenia. A bone marrow aspirate is often carried out in adults, but not usually in children, and will usually show normal or increased numbers of megakaryocytes in an otherwise normal marrow (Fig. 33.13).

Standard first-line therapy

Therapy is seldom necessary for patients whose platelet counts exceed 20–30 × 10⁹/l and in whom there are few spontaneous bleeding episodes[47] unless they are undergoing any procedure likely to induce blood loss.[100] Standard treatments, including oral prednisolone,[32] IVIg,[79,101,102] and splenectomy, will elevate the platelet count sufficiently in the

majority of adults. However, some 20–25% of adults with ITP are refractory to first-line therapy.

Chronic ITP failing to respond to therapy

This defines those patients who fail to respond to first-line treatment or require unacceptably high doses of corticosteroids to maintain a safe platelet count. A number of agents have been used as second-line therapy for ITP including high-dose steroids, high-dose IVIg, intravenous anti-D, vinca alkaloids, danazol, azathioprine, combination chemotherapy and dapsone. An excellent summary is provided by McMillan.[78]

Experimental therapies

For those who fail to respond to standard first- and second-line therapy and who require treatment the options are limited and include: interferon-α,[79] cyclosporin A, CAMPATH 1H, and protein A columns.[103]

Thrombopoietin receptor agonists (TPO-mimetics)

Traditionally anti-platelet autoantibodies accelerating platelet clearance from the peripheral circulation have been recognized as the primary pathophysiologic mechanism in chronic immune thrombocytopenia (ITP). Recently, increasing evidence supports the coexistence of insufficient megakaryopoiesis. Inadequate low thrombopoietin (TPO) levels are associated with insufficient proliferation and differentiation of megakaryocytes, decreased proplatelet formation and subsequent platelet release.[104] The successful isolation and cloning of thrombopoietin (TPO) in the mid-1990s and identification of its key role in platelet production was a major breakthrough, rapidly followed by the development of the recombinant thrombopoietins, recombinant human TPO and a pegylated truncated product, PEG-rHuMGDF. Both agents increased platelet counts but development was halted because of the development of antibodies that cross-reacted with native TPO, resulting in prolonged treatment-refractory thrombocytopenia. Second generation thrombopoietin receptor agonists were developed with no sequence homology to native TPO and these have now been extensively used with no significant side-effects.[105] Two agents are currently available and have been used in early clinical studies and are licensed in some countries at the time of writing. Romiplostim (AMG 531, Nplate®; Amgen, Thousand Oaks, CA, USA) is a novel recombinant thrombopoiesis-stimulating Fc-peptide fusion protein ('peptibody') and eltrombopag, a non-peptide, synthetic TPO-receptor agonist (GSK, London, UK; marketed as Promacta in the US and Revolade in the UK). These two novel activators of thrombopoietin receptors have been used in several phase III studies and both agents demonstrate increase of platelet counts in about 80% of chronic ITP patients within 2–3 weeks. These agents substantially broaden the therapeutic options for patients with chronic ITP although long-term results are still pending.[106,107]

Secondary immune thrombocytopenia

Immune-mediated thrombocytopenia, similar to ITP, may occur in patients with other underlying autoimmune diseases such as systemic lupus erythematosus (SLE). Table 33.7 summarizes the main causes of immune-mediated thrombocytopenia caused by autoantibodies.

Drug-induced thrombocytopenia

Drugs may induce thrombocytopenia through a variety of mechanisms, both immune and non-immune. Only drug-induced immune thrombocytopenia is discussed here; drug-induced qualitative abnormalities are discussed later in the chapter. In drug-induced immune-mediated thrombocyto-penia, drug-dependent antibodies most commonly recognize epitopes of glycoproteins Ib-IX and IIb-IIIa.[108] Fig. 33.14 shows the pathways involved in prostaglandin metabolism highlighting the sites of action of aspirin and non-steroidal anti-inflammatory drugs (NSAIDs).

Clinical features

Thrombocytopenia is an uncommon drug-related side-effect. The predominant features are of bleeding or bruising. The number of drugs suspected of causing thrombocytopenia is quite large but strong evidence is only available for a few of these including: quinine,[109,110] quinidine,[111] sulfona-mides,[112] trimethoprim, abciximab, and gold salts.[113] The incidence of thrombocytopenia in the cases of abciximab is relatively common at 0.5–1% after first exposure rising to 10–14% after second exposure.[114] The incidence is also high with gold at about 1%.[114]

The onset of thrombocytopenia is usually between 5 and 14 days after first exposure to the drug in cases of primary exposure, but in only a few hours if it is a secondary exposure.

Patients present with petechial hemorrhages, bruising and in some cases bleeding from either the gastrointestinal or the

Table 33.7 Causes of thrombocytopenia due to autoantibodies

Idiopathic	ITP (newly diagnosed, peristent and chronic)
Secondary to other autoimmune or inflammatory disorders	SLE Other autoimmune disorders Lymphoproliferative disease, e.g. CLL Post-BMT
Associated with viral infections	e.g. HIV
Drug-induced	e.g. quinine, quinidine, heparin, gold salts

BMT, bone-marrow transfer; CLL, chronic lymphocytic leukemia; HIV, human immunodeficiency virus; ITP, idiopathic thrombocytopenic purpura; SLE, systemic lupus erythematosus.

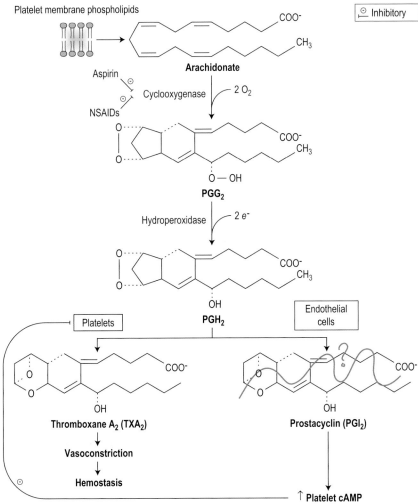

⊖ Inhibitory

Fig. 33.14 Arachidonic acid metabolism and the generation of thromboxane A$_2$ and PGI$_2$. This is inhibited by aspirin and other NSAIDs leading to excessive bleeding.

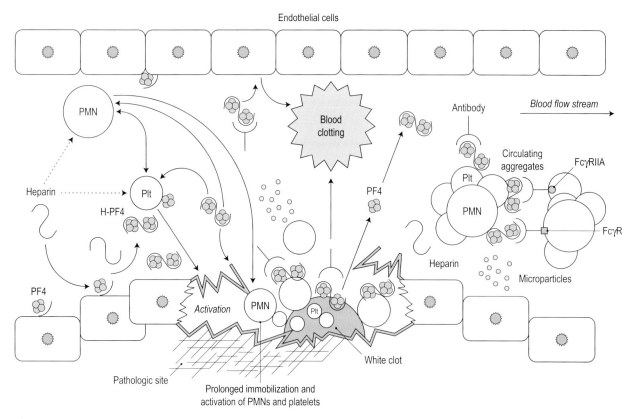

Fig. 33.15 Heparin-induced thrombocytopenia. Generation of heparin-platelet factor 4 complexes (H-PF4) in heparin-treated patients. Development of heparin-dependent antibodies which focus the immune response onto platelets and endothelial cells. Cell activation and cell–cell interactions, a phenomenon which is strongly enhanced at pathologic sites. Formation of a white clot, blood activation and clotting, and release of circulating aggregates and procoagulant microparticles in the blood circulation. PMN, polymorphonuclear cells (neutrophils). *(From Amiral J, Meyer D. Heparin-induced thrombocytopenia: diagnostic tests and biological mechanisms. Baillière's Clinical Haematology. 1998;11:447–460, with permission.*[144]*)*

genitourinary tract. There may be associated hemolysis or neutropenia.

Investigations

Serologic tests may confirm the presence of drug-dependent antibodies. However, there are many patients in whom immune-mediated platelet destruction is believed to be occurring who have no detectable drug-dependent antibodies,[73] and the reverse is also true, whereby patients have drug-dependent antibodies in their plasma but with no accompanying thrombocytopenia.[115] Overall, therefore, the diagnosis of drug-induced thrombocytopenia through the action of drug-dependent antibodies remains largely clinical.

Management

The drug should be stopped and in most cases complete recovery will result in a few days. In cases of life-threatening bleeding therapeutic options include: plasma exchange, platelet transfusions, IVIg or corticosteroids.

Predictable (non-immune) thrombocytopenia

There are many drugs that will induce thrombocytopenia in a predictable fashion. These include anticancer (chemotherapy) drugs, which inhibit growth of stem cells, resulting in a reduction in all three cell lines (i.e. induce pancytopenia).

Drug-induced immune thrombocytopenia

Despite many reports of agents capable of inducing immune-mediated platelet destruction, there is good evidence for only a handful of these, namely heparin (see below), quin(id)ine, gold and trimethoprim-sulfamethoxazole. Heparin-induced thrombocytopenia represents a serious drug-induced platelet disorder and is discussed in detail below.

Heparin-induced thrombocytopenia (HIT)

Heparin-induced thrombocytopenia (HIT) is a common and serious complication of heparin therapy. It has an immunologic basis that is not yet fully understood and, in contrast to other drug-induced causes of thrombocytopenia, is associated with a thrombotic rather than a bleeding tendency. This condition was previously called type II HIT to distinguish it from the mild and clinically benign type I HIT which is sometimes observed early in the course of heparin administration, is non-immune mediated and self-limiting, and is not associated with a bleeding or clotting tendency (Fig. 33.15).

Pathogenesis

PF4 is a chemokine produced by megakaryocytes and released from platelet α-granules upon platelet activation.

Released PF4 binds cell-surface glycosaminoglycans and heparin. Formation of the PF4-heparin complex causes a conformational change in the protein leading to exposure of cryptic epitopes to which the antibodies in HIT are usually generated. The anti-PF4/heparin antibodies, which are of IgG isotype, bind to PF4 through their F(ab) domains. Serial PF4 molecules align on the platelet surface and several IgG molecules bind, leading to the formation of large immune complexes that cross-link the platelet FcγIIa receptors, and resulting in platelet aggregation and an associated platelet procoagulant response.[116] HIT antibodies also bind to endothelial cells and monocytes resulting in additional procoagulant effects through increased expression of tissue factor and formation of platelet-monocyte aggregates leading to thrombin generation. Therefore in HIT the clinical manifestations are the result of both FcγIIa-dependent platelet activation and activation of the coagulation system through tissue factor expression and platelet activation.

Clinical features

The risk of HIT is greater with 5 or more days of exposure to unfractionated heparin (1–3%) than to low-molecular-weight heparin (0–0.8%).[117] The risk is also greater in certain patient groups such as surgical patients than in others, e.g. obstetrics. In HIT the platelet count usually falls by >50% and this typically occurs 5–14 days after the start of therapeutic or prophylactic heparin administration (the first day of heparin administration is day 0). The platelet count generally reaches a nadir in the range $20–100 \times 10^9/l$ and it is very unusual for it to drop below $10–15 \times 10^9/l$ in contrast to some other drug-induced thrombocytopenias. HIT can also be of rapid onset, developing within 24 hours in patients who have had heparin exposure within the previous 3 months. Occasionally delayed-onset HIT can occur beginning several days to weeks after heparin exposure and caused by antibodies that activate platelets independently of heparin. Although hemorrhage is uncommon, because of the enhanced thrombin generation as described above, there is a high rate of thrombotic events affecting major vessels. In patients treated with heparin for ischemic vascular disease, arterial thrombosis is common, and in those receiving heparin for thrombotic diseases such as deep vein thrombosis (DVT), the associated thrombus is usually venous. Even in the presence of heparin there may be considerable extension of the DVT, which may prove fatal. The mortality rate is high at 30%. Other manifestations of HIT occasionally occur, for example skin lesions (erythema with or without central necrosis) at sites of heparin injections or acute systemic reactions after intravenous heparin administration. DIC may also be seen in some patients. Thus the development of any of these features, new or recurrent thrombosis, or the development of thrombocytopenia during or following heparin administration should always prompt consideration of HIT.

Diagnosis

The differential diagnosis of HIT is wide and includes sepsis, multi-organ failure, malignancy, the antiphospholipid syndrome and other drugs that cause thrombocytopenia. HIT is a clinicopathological syndrome and the diagnosis is based on a combination of clinical and laboratory features.

The laboratory tests are of two types, measurement of antibody binding to PF4/heparin complexes or detection of heparin-dependent activation by patient serum.[116] The former is performed by enzyme-immunoassay (EIA) and is highly sensitive but with a specificity that ranges from 50% to 90%. The strength of the assay correlates with the probability of HIT – the diagnosis is likely in those that are strongly positive (>1.0 optical density (OD)) but unlikely in those that are weakly positive (0.4–1.0 OD).[116] In the functional assays, aggregation of donor platelets by patient serum or plasma plus heparin is assessed. The optimal assays of heparin-dependent platelet activation use washed platelets. The sensitivity of the functional assays for HIT is generally lower than the EIAs but the specificity is higher and can reach 95–99% with assays that use washed platelets. The specificity of both types of assay is further enhanced by the finding that a positive result at low heparin concentration is inhibited at high heparin concentration due to disruption of PF4/heparin complexes.

Combining clinical assessment and appropriate laboratory testing is essential in the diagnosis of HIT.[116] The first stage is estimation of the pretest probability, for example, using the so-called 4Ts scoring system which takes account of: 1) degree of thrombocytopenia; 2) timing of thrombocytopenia; 3) presence of thrombosis or other clinical manifestations of HIT; 4) other potential causes of thrombocytopenia. In patients with a low pretest probability no laboratory testing is required and heparin can be continued. If the EIA is negative HIT is very unlikely and heparin can be continued. If the EIA is weakly positive at low heparin concentration and reactivity is not inhibited at high concentration, HIT is unlikely and heparin can be continued. A strongly positive IgG EIA indicates an increased risk of platelet activating antibodies and a platelet activation assay should be performed. If this is positive, HIT is extremely likely. Finally the clinical situation should be reassessed to support or exclude the diagnosis.

Management

In HIT the heparin should be stopped immediately and a non-heparin anticoagulant should be substituted. Stopping heparin alone is insufficient as the risk of thrombosis approaches 50% even in those who have isolated thrombocytopenia and are clinically asymptomatic at the time of diagnosis. Cross-reactivity between unfractionated and low-molecular-weight heparin approaches 100% and therefore the latter should not be used when HIT occurs in patients receiving the former. Since initiation of vitamin K antagonists may worsen the thrombosis associated with HIT, these should be stopped and vitamin K administered. The main agents that are used instead of heparin are two direct thrombin inhibitors, lepirudin and argatroban, and the heparinoid danaparoid. Other agents that are sometimes used, though not approved in this setting, are the direct thrombin inhibitor bivalirudin, and the synthetic pentasaccharide and factor Xa inhibitor fondaparinux. The main disadvantage of these agents is that they all carry a significant risk of bleeding and none has an antidote. They each have advantages and disadvantages in different clinical settings and expert advice should be sought when considering their use. If oral anticoagulants are required they should be initiated at low doses after the platelet count has recovered to

Table 33.8 Drugs and disorders interfering with platelet function

Systemic disorders	Uremia
	Cardiac by-pass surgery
Hematologic disorders	Myeloproliferative diseases
	Leukemia
	Myelodysplasia
	Paraproteinemias, including multiple myeloma
Drugs	Aspirin
	Antibiotics
	Anticoagulants
	Others

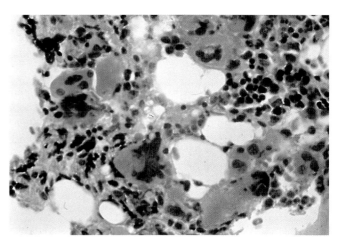

Fig. 33.16 Trephine biopsy in patient with essential thrombocythemia, one of the myeloproliferative disorders, showing greatly increased numbers of megakaryocytes with clustering. *(Figure kindly provided by Dr John Amess, Barts & The London NHS Trust.)*

>150 × 10^9/l and overlapped with one of the agents mentioned above for a minimum of 5 days and until the INR has been in the therapeutic range for 48 hours. Platelet transfusions are contraindicated in HIT.

Although exposure to heparin is usually avoided following the diagnosis of HIT, the antibodies do not usually persist beyond 100 days and re-exposure to heparin after this time does not generally lead to recurrence of HIT.

Other drugs causing immune-mediated platelet destruction

There are many drugs implicated in immune-mediated thrombocytopenia. The evidence is strongest for quinine, quinidine, heparin and gold salts,[113] as already discussed. Other implicated agents, though with fewer reports to date, include: α-methyldopa,[118] diclofenac,[119] rifampin,[120] carbamazepine[121] and sulfonamides. Readers are referred to George et al. for an excellent review of the topic.[122]

Acquired functional abnormalities of platelets

Bleeding problems may arise through either inadequate numbers of platelets or functional abnormalities of the platelets themselves. This section discusses disorders in which there are abnormalities of platelet function along with their pathogenetic basis (Table 33.8).

Uremia in renal failure

Bleeding may be a feature of either acute or chronic renal failure,[123,124] with spontaneous bleeding into the skin, mucous membranes including the gastrointestinal or genitourinary tracts, central nervous system and other sites (see also Chapter 35).

Pathogenesis

Platelet function, in the presence of uremia, is abnormal,[123,125-127] and a variety of laboratory studies have shown that all aspects of platelet activity are affected, including platelet adhesion, aggregation and procoagulant activity.[128-130]

The normal process of platelet adhesion has been shown to involve contact of platelets to endothelial structures. This is dependent on the binding of vWF to GP Ib/IX.[124] In the presence of uremia there may be a qualitative or quantitative abnormality of vWF or GPIb/IX itself.

Management

The most important factor to consider is whether the patient is actively bleeding, rather than abnormalities detected using bleeding time, and other coagulation assays. Hemodialysis itself will help correct the bleeding induced by the uremia.[127] Desmopressin (DDAVP) which promotes the release of vWF from vascular endothelial cells may reduce the bleeding time in some uremic patients.[126]

Myeloproliferative disorders

The myeloproliferative diseases (MPDs) are neoplastic hematologic stem cell disorders and include essential thrombocythemia (ET) (Fig. 33.16), polycythemia rubra vera (PRV), idiopathic myelofibrosis (IMF) and chronic myeloid leukemia (CML). These disorders are associated with both bleeding and thrombosis.

Pathophysiology

In PRV there is a rise in whole blood viscosity through elevation of the hematocrit which may contribute to thrombosis.[133,134] Abnormalities in platelet function have been reported in MPDs, and the bleeding time is prolonged in a minority of patients. However, bleeding may occur even if the template bleeding time is normal.[133]

Platelet abnormalities in the myeloproliferative disorders

Platelets may be larger than normal, although in some cases they are smaller. Their survival may be reduced, especially in essential thrombocythemia. Platelet aggregation is abnormal with the standard aggregants including ADP and collagen, though this is not a feature of thrombocytosis when the underlying cause is reactive, thereby excluding thrombocytosis per se as a cause of the abnormal aggregation.[134] It may, in fact, be a secondary consequence of the conversion of arachidonic acid to prostaglandin endoperoxides or lipooxygenase products,[135] or a decrease in platelet responsiveness to thromboxane A$_2$.[136]

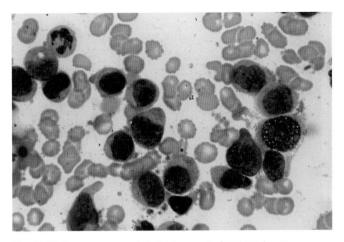

Fig. 33.17 Bone-marrow aspirate (high power) of AML M4 (acute myelomonocytic leukemia), showing large myeloblasts. *(Figure kindly provided by Dr John Amess, Barts & The London NHS Trust.)*

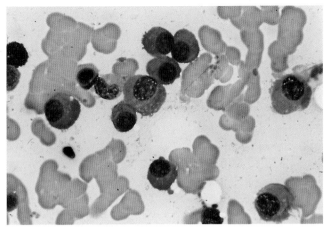

Fig. 33.18 Bone-marrow aspirate in multiple myeloma showing large numbers of plasma cells. The paraprotein may cause platelet dysfunction through a variety of mechanisms including hyperviscosity, development of uremia and other mechanisms. *(Figure kindly provided by Dr John Amess, Barts & The London NHS Trust.)*

Management

For PRV, a reduction in hematocrit, aiming for a level less than 0.45 (45%) is an approach adopted by most hematologists.[137] Ongoing clinical trials may help determine the optimal level of hematocrit. The bone marrow may be suppressed effectively using hydroxyurea or busulfan with an overall reduction in platelet count in patients with essential thrombocythemia.[138,139] However, even though the peripheral platelet count is lowered, this does not necessarily correct the associated platelet abnormalities. The management of the patient who is actively bleeding is more complex.

Platelet abnormalities in leukemia and myelodysplastic syndromes

Bleeding is common in both types of disease, and is often due to thrombocytopenia. However, functional abnormalities of platelets are also recognized. In acute myeloid leukemia (AML) for example, platelets may be larger than usual, with abnormalities of shape and the appearance of their granules (Fig. 33.17).

Management

Patients with functional platelet abnormalities generally respond to platelet transfusion. Correction of the underlying malignancy with definitive therapy will also improve the acquired bleeding diathesis. Similar abnormalities are also seen in MDS and treatment generally consists of regular platelet transfusions[140,141] (Fig. 33.18).

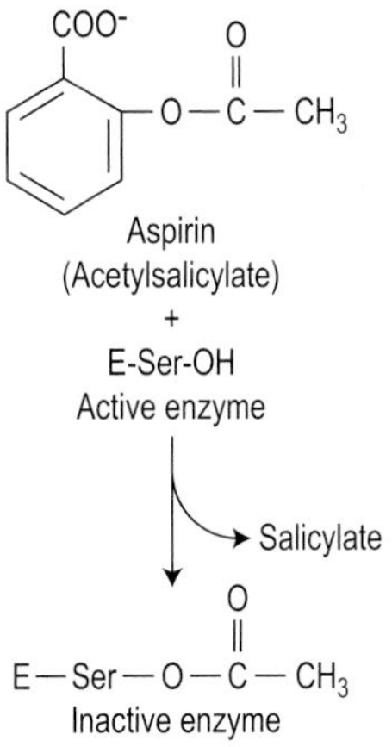

Drugs that interfere with platelet function

Drugs may cause bleeding through the induction of profound thrombocytopenia. In addition, there are numerous agents that may induce bleeding through the interference with the normal function of platelets. Thus, although the platelet count may be entirely normal, the platelets are rendered functionally defective. Aspirin and non-steroidal anti-

Fig. 33.19 Aspirin (acetylsalicylic acid) inhibits cyclooxygenase irreversibly by acetylation of a serine within the active site of the enzyme (E).

inflammatory agents (NSAIDs) are the most common cause of acquired platelet dysfunction (Table 33.9). Their effects are mediated through irreversibly inhibiting cyclooxygenase activity in the platelet resulting in impairment of the granule release reaction and defective aggregation. Aspirin, in particular, acetylates the serine residue at position 530 of prostaglandin synthase, the enzyme responsible for converting arachidonate to prostaglandin cyclic endoperoxides, and thereby inhibits the synthesis of prostacyclin and thromboxane A_2 (Fig. 33.19). These effects are seen in both the platelet and endothelium, but the effect of aspirin on platelet function is detectable for several days after the drug is stopped since there is a lag phase before new platelets lacking the drug enter the circulation. Endothelial cells, on the other hand, are able to generate prostaglandin synthase much more rapidly.

Aspirin is widely used in the secondary prevention of arterial thrombotic events such as acute coronary syndromes and strokes. Dipyridamole is a pyrido-pyrimidine derivative

Table 33.9 Drugs interfering with platelet function

NSAIDs	Aspirin Diclofenac Mefenamic acid Others	Cyclooxygenase inhibitors
Antibiotics	Penicillins Cephalosporins Nitrofurantoin	In high doses, particularly in ill patients, many antibiotics may interfere with platelet aggregation
Anticoagulants	Heparin Epsilon aminocaproic acid	
Drugs that increase platelet cAMP	Dipyridamole Iloprost	Dipyridamole is a phosphodiesterase inhibitor
Cardiovascular system drugs	Diltiazem Isosorbide dinitrate Nifedipine Propranolol	
Psychotropics	Tricyclic antidepressants such as imipramine and amitriptyline Phenothiazines, e.g. chlorpromazine, promethazine	
Anesthetics	Local and general anesthetics (e.g. halothane)	
Anticancer drugs	Chemotherapeutic agents such as mithramycin, BCNU and daunorubicin	
Anticoagulants	Heparin and coumadin	
Miscellaneous	Dextrans Ticlopidine Lipid-lowering drugs, e.g. clofibrate Quinidine Ethanol	

NSAIDs, non-steroid anti-inflammatory drugs. *(Modified from Rao AK, Carvalho ACA 1994. In: Colman RW et al (eds), In Hemostasis and Thrombosis: Principles and Practice, 3rd edn. JB Lippincott, Philadelphia.)*

that vasodilates coronary microvessels and inhibits platelet activation by increasing levels of cyclic AMP and cyclic GMP. It is used along with aspirin in the secondary prevention of stroke.

Clopidogrel is a thienopyridine which irreversibly blocks the ADP receptor P2Y12 on platelets. It requires a two-step activation process involving a series of cytochrome P450 isoenzymes. Like aspirin its effect on platelets is irreversible and it is widely used in the secondary prevention of arterial disease but it has a delayed onset of action and there is significant inter-individual variability in platelet response. Other P2Y12 antagonists that differ in their pharmacological properties and have been more recently developed include prasugrel and ticagrelor. None of these agents completely prevents platelet activation. However, the consequences of the latter can be inhibited by the parenteral administration of GP IIb/IIIa inhibitors such as abciximab, eptifibatide and tirofiban.

References

1. Long MW, Gragowski LL, Heffner CH, Boxer LA. Phorbol diesters stimulate the development of an early murine progenitor cell. The burst-forming unit-megakaryocyte. J Clin Invest 1985;76:431–8.

2. Jackson CW. Megakaryocyte endomitosis: a review. Int J Cell Cloning 1990;8:224–6.

3. Harker LA, Finch CA. Thrombokinetics in man. J Clin Invest 1969;48:963–74.

4. Hynes RO. Integrins: a family of cell surface receptors. Cell 1987;48:549–54.

5. Kasirer-Friede A, Kahn ML, Shattil SJ. Platelet integrins and immunoreceptors. Immunol Rev 2007;218:247–64.

6. Kieffer N, Phillips DR. Platelet membrane glycoproteins: functions in cellular interactions. Annu Rev Cell Biol 1990;6:329–57.

7. Kunicki TJ, Newman PJ. The molecular immunology of human platelet proteins. Blood 1992;80:1386–404.

8. Nachman RL, Rafii S. Platelets, petechiae, and preservation of the vascular wall. N Engl J Med 2008;359:1261–70.

9. Payne BA, Pierre RV. Pseudothrombocytopenia: a laboratory artifact with potentially serious consequences. Mayo Clin Proc 1984;59:123–5.

10. Savage RA. Pseudoleukocytosis due to EDTA-induced platelet clumping. Am J Clin Pathol 1984;81:317–22.

11. Aster RH. Pooling of platelets in the spleen: role in the pathogenesis of

'hypersplenic' thrombocytopenia. J Clin Invest 1966;45:645–57.

12. Gewirtz AM, Hoffman R. Transitory hypomegakaryocytic thrombocytopenia: aetiological association with ethanol abuse and implications regarding regulation of human megakaryocytopoiesis. Br J Haematol 1986;62:333–44.

13. Manoharan A, Williams NT, Sparrow R. Acquired amegakaryocytic thrombocytopenia: report of a case and review of literature. Q J Med 1989;70:243–52.

14. Boggs DR. Amegakaryocytic thrombocytopenia. Am J Hematol 1985;20:413–6.

15. Levi M, ten Cate H, van der Poll T, van Deventer SJ. Pathogenesis of disseminated intravascular coagulation in sepsis. JAMA 1993;270:975–9.

16. Zheng XL, Sadler JE. Pathogenesis of thrombotic microangiopathies. Annu Rev Pathol 2008;3:249–77.

17. Moschowitz E. Hyaline thrombosis of the terminal arterioles and capillaries: a hitherto undescribed disease. Proceedings of the New York Pathological Society 1924;24:21–4.

18. Allford SL, Hunt BJ, Rose P, Machin SJ. Guidelines on the diagnosis and management of the thrombotic microangiopathic haemolytic anaemias. Br J Haematol 2003;120:556–73.

19. George JN. Clinical practice. Thrombotic thrombocytopenic purpura. NEJM, 2006;354(18):1927–35

20. Schleinitz N, Ebbo M, Mazodier K, et al. Rituximab as preventive therapy of a clinical relapse in TTP with ADAMTS13 inhibitor. Am J Hematol 2007;82:417–8.

21. Scott SM, Szczepiorkowski ZM. Rituximab for TTP. Am J Hematol 2005;80:87–8.

22. Gasser C, Gautier E, Steck A, et al. [Hemolytic-uremic syndrome: bilateral necrosis of the renal cortex in acute acquired hemolytic anemia.] Schweiz Med Wochenschr 1955;85:905–9.

23. Ashkenazi S. Role of bacterial cytotoxins in hemolytic uremic syndrome and thrombotic thrombocytopenic purpura. Annu Rev Med 1993;44:11–8.

24. Neill MA, Agosti J, Rosen H. Hemorrhagic colitis with Escherichia coli 0157:H7 preceding adult hemolytic uremic syndrome. Arch Intern Med 1985;145:2215–7.

25. Martin DL, MacDonald KL, White KE, et al. The epidemiology and clinical aspects of the hemolytic uremic syndrome in Minnesota. N Engl J Med 1990;323:1161–7.

26. Milford DV, Taylor CM, Guttridge B, et al. Haemolytic uraemic syndromes in the British Isles 1985–8: association with verocytotoxin producing Escherichia coli. Part 1: Clinical and epidemiological aspects. Arch Dis Child 1990;65:716–21.

27. Delvaeye M, Noris M, De Vriese A, et al. Thrombomodulin mutations in atypical hemolytic-uremic syndrome. N Engl J Med 2009;361:345–57.

28. Rowe PC, Orrbine E, Wells GA, McLaine PN. Epidemiology of hemolytic-uremic syndrome in Canadian children from 1986 to 1988. The Canadian Pediatric Kidney Disease Reference Centre. J Pediatr 1991;119:218–24.

29. Brenner BM. Vascular injury to the kidney. In: Fauci AS, Braunwald E, Isselbacher KJ, editors. Principles of Internal Medicine. New York: McGraw–Hill; 1998.

30. Ishibashi M, Ito N, Fujita M, et al. Endothelin-1 as an aggravating factor of disseminated intravascular coagulation associated with malignant neoplasms. Cancer 1994;73:191–5.

31. Jones SL. HELLP! A cry for laboratory assistance: a comprehensive review of the HELLP syndrome highlighting the role of the laboratory. Hematopathol Mol Hematol 1998;11:147–71.

32. Portis R, Jacobs MA, Skerman JH, Skerman EB. HELLP syndrome (hemolysis, elevated liver enzymes, and low platelets) pathophysiology and anesthetic considerations. AANA J 1997;65:37–47.

33. Stone JH. HELLP syndrome: hemolysis, elevated liver enzymes, and low platelets. JAMA 1998;280:559–62.

34. Sheikh RA, Yasmeen S, Pauly MP, Riegler JL. Spontaneous intrahepatic hemorrhage and hepatic rupture in the HELLP syndrome: four cases and a review. Journal of Clinical Gastroenterology 1999;28:323–8.

35. Hamada S, Takishita Y, Tamura T, et al. Plasma exchange in a patient with postpartum HELLP syndrome. J Obstet Gynaecol Res 1996;22:371–4.

36. Counts RB, Haisch C, Simon TL, et al. Hemostasis in massively transfused trauma patients. Ann Surg 1979;190:91–9.

37. Leslie SD, Toy PT. Laboratory hemostatic abnormalities in massively transfused patients given red blood cells and crystalloid. Am J Clin Pathol 1991;96:770–3.

38. Lindenbaum J, Hargrove RL. Thrombocytopenia in alcoholics. Ann Intern Med 1968;68:526–32.

39. Post RM, Desforges JF. Thrombocytopenia and alcoholism. Ann Intern Med 1968;68:1230–6.

40. Kelly DA, Summerfield JA. Hemostasis in liver disease. Semin Liver Dis 1987;7:182–91.

41. Ninomiya N, Maeda T, Matsuda I. Thrombocytopenic purpura occurring during the early phase of a mumps infection. Helv Paediatr Acta 1977;32:87–9.

42. Espinoza C, Kuhn C. Viral infection of megakaryocytes in varicella with purpura. Am J Clin Pathol 1974;61:203–8.

43. Angle RM, Alt HL. Thrombocytopenic purpura complicating infectious mononucleosis. Blood 1050;5:499.

44. Bayer WL, Sherman FE, Michaels RH, et al. Purpura in congenital and acquired rubella. N Engl J Med 1965;273:1362–6.

45. Oski FA, Naiman JL. Effect of live measles vaccine on the platelet count. N Engl J Med 1966;275:352–6.

46. Ballem PJ, Belzberg A, Devine DV, et al. Kinetic studies of the mechanism of thrombocytopenia in patients with human immunodeficiency virus infection. N Engl J Med 1992;327:1779–84.

47. Yang R, Zhong CH. Pathogenesis and management of chronic idiopathic thrombocytopenic purpura: an update. International Journal of Hematology 2000; 71:1824.

48. Walsh CM, Nardi MA, Karpatkin S. On the mechanism of thrombocytopenic purpura in sexually active homosexual men. N Engl J Med 1984;311:635–9.

49. Abrams DI, Chinn EK, Lewis BJ, et al. Hematologic manifestations in homosexual men with Kaposi's sarcoma. Am J Clin Pathol 1984;81:13–8.

50. Frontiera M, Myers AM. Peripheral blood and bone marrow abnormalities in the acquired immunodeficiency syndrome. West J Med 1987;147:157–60.

51. Treacy M, Lai L, Costello C, Clark A. Peripheral blood and bone marrow abnormalities in patients with HIV related disease. Br J Haematol 1987; 65:289–94.

52. Rossi G, Gorla R, Stellini R, et al. Prevalence, clinical, and laboratory features of thrombocytopenia among HIV-infected individuals. AIDS Res Hum Retroviruses 1990;6:261–9.

53. Stabler SP, Allen RH, Savage DG, Lindenbaum J. Clinical spectrum and diagnosis of cobalamin deficiency. Blood 1990;76:871–81.

54. van Loghem JJ, Dorfmeyer H, van de Hart M, Schreuder F. Serological and genetical studies on the platelet antigen (Zw). Vox Sanguinis 1959;4:161–9.

55. Mueller-Eckhardt C, Becker T, Weisheit M, et al. Neonatal alloimmune thrombocytopenia due to fetomaternal Zwb incompatibility. Vox Sang 1986;50:94–6.

56. Bizzaro N, Dianese G. Neonatal alloimmune amegakaryocytosis. Case report. Vox Sang 1988;54:112–4.

57. von dem Borne AE, von Riesz E, Verheugt FW, et al. Baka, a new platelet-specific antigen involved in neonatal allo-immune thrombocytopenia. Vox Sang 1980;39:113–20.

58. McGrath K, Minchinton R, Cunningham I, Ayberk H. Platelet anti-Bakb antibody associated with neonatal alloimmune thrombocytopenia. Vox Sang 1989;57:182–4.

59. Friedman JM, Aster RH. Neonatal alloimmune thrombocytopenic purpura and congenital porencephaly in two siblings associated with a 'new' maternal antiplatelet antibody. Blood 1985;65:1412–5.

60. Shibata Y, Matsuda I, Miyaji T, Ichikawa Y. Yuka, a new platelet antigen involved in two cases of neonatal alloimmune thrombocytopenia. Vox Sang 1986;50:177–80.

61. Kaplan C, Morel-Kopp MC, Kroll H, et al. HPA-5b (Br(a)) neonatal alloimmune thrombocytopenia: clinical and immunological analysis of 39 cases. Br J Haematol 1991;78:425–9.

62. Kiefel V, Shechter Y, Atias D, et al. Neonatal alloimmune thrombocytopenia due to anti-Brb (HPA-5a). Report of three cases in two families. Vox Sang 1991;60:244–5.

63. Mueller-Eckhardt C, Kayser W, Forster C, et al. Improved assay for detection of platelet-specific PlA1 antibodies in neonatal alloimmune thrombocytopenia. Vox Sang 1982;43:76–81.

64. Katz J, Hodder FS, Aster RS, et al. Neonatal isoimmune thrombocytopenia. The natural course and management and the detection of maternal antibody. Clin Pediatr (Phila) 1984;23:159–62.

65. Adner MM, Fisch GR, Starobin SG, Aster RH. Use of 'compatible' platelet transfusions in treatment of congenital isoimmune thrombocytopenic purpura. N Engl J Med 1969;280:244–7.

66. Suarez CR, Anderson C. High-dose intravenous gammaglobulin (IVG) in neonatal immune thrombocytopenia. Am J Hematol 1987;26:247–53.

67. Pearson HA, Shulman NR, Marder VJ, Cone TE. Isoimmune neonatal thrombocytopenic purpura: clinical and therapeutic considerations. Blood 1964;23:154.

68. McFarland JG, Aster RH, Bussel JB, et al. Prenatal diagnosis of neonatal alloimmune thrombocytopenia using allele-specific oligonucleotide probes. Blood 1991;78:2276–82.

69. Mueller-Eckhardt C. Post-transfusion purpura. Br J Haematol 1986;64:419–24.

70. Taaning E, Morling N, Ovesen H, Svejgaard A. Post transfusion purpura and anti-Zwb (-P1A2). Tissue Antigens 1985;26:143–6.

71. Keimowitz RM, Collins J, Davis K, Aster RH. Post-transfusion purpura associated with alloimmunization against the platelet-specific antigen, Baka. Am J Hematol 1986;21:79–88.

72. Kickler TS, Ness PM, Herman JH, Bell WR. Studies on the pathophysiology of posttransfusion purpura. Blood 1986;68:347–50.

73. Christie DJ, Pulkrabek S, Putnam JL, et al. Posttransfusion purpura due to an alloantibody reactive with glycoprotein Ia/IIa (anti-HPA-5b). Blood 1991;77:2785–9.

74. Seidenfeld AM, Owen J, Glynn MF. Post-transfusion purpura cured by steroid therapy in a man. Can Med Assoc J 1978;118:1285–6.

75. Simon T, Collins J, Kunicki T. Post-transfusion purpura with antiplatelet antibody specific for the platelet antigen Pena. Blood 1986;68:117a.

76. Waters AH. Post-transfusion purpura. Blood Rev 1989;3:83–7.

77. Nugent D, McMillan R, Nichol JL, Slichter SJ. Pathogenesis of chronic immune thrombocytopenia: increased platelet destruction and/or decreased platelet production. Br J Haematol 2009;146:585–96.

78. McMillan R. Therapy for adults with refractory chronic immune thrombocytopenic purpura. Ann Intern Med 1997;126:307–14.

79. George JN, Woolf SH, Raskob GE, et al. Idiopathic thrombocytopenic purpura: a practice guideline developed by explicit methods for the American Society of Hematology. Blood 1996;88:3–40.

80. Warner MN, Moore JC, Warkentin TE, et al. A prospective study of protein-specific assays used to investigate idiopathic thrombocytopenic purpura. Br J Haematol 1999;104:442–7.

81. Rodeghiero F, Stasi R, Gernsheimer T, et al. Standardization of terminology, definitions and outcome criteria in immune thrombocytopenic purpura of adults and children: report from an international working group. Blood 2009;113:2386–93.

82. Bolton-Maggs PH, Moon I. Assessment of UK practice for management of acute childhood idiopathic thrombocytopenic purpura against published guidelines. Lancet 1997;350:620–3.

83. Buchanan GR. The nontreatment of childhood idiopathic thrombocytopenic purpura. Eur J Pediatr 1987;146:107–12.

84. Imbach P. Immune thrombocytopenia in children: the immune character of destructive thrombocytopenia and the treatment of bleeding. Semin Thromb Hemost 1995;21:305–12.

85. Imbach PA, Kuhne T, Hollander G. Immunologic aspects in the pathogenesis of immune thrombocytopenic purpura in children [published erratum appears in Curr Opin Pediatr 1997 Jun;9(3):298]. Curr Opin Pediatr 1997;9:35–40.

86. Baatout S. Thrombopoietin. A review. Haemostasis 1997;27:1–8.

87. Kaushansky K. The molecular mechanisms that control thrombopoiesis. J Clin Invest 2005;115:3339–47.

88. Kaushansky K. Thrombopoietin and the hematopoietic stem cell. Ann N Y Acad Sci 2005;1044:139–41.

89. Lilleyman JS. Intracranial haemorrhage in idiopathic thrombocytopenic purpura. Paediatric Haematology Forum of the British Society for Haematology. Arch Dis Child 1994;71:251–3.

90. Kienast J, Schmitz G. Flow cytometric analysis of thiazole orange uptake by platelets: a diagnostic aid in the evaluation of thrombocytopenic disorders. Blood 1990;75:116–21.

91. Woods VLJ, Kurata Y, Montgomery RR, et al. Autoantibodies against platelet glycoprotein Ib in patients with chronic immune thrombocytopenic purpura. Blood 1984;64:156–60.

92. Woods VLJ, Oh EH, Mason D, McMillan R. Autoantibodies against the platelet glycoprotein IIb/IIIa complex in patients with chronic ITP. Blood 1984;63:368–75.

93. Mackay IR. Science, medicine, and the future: tolerance and autoimmunity. BMJ 2000;321:93–6.

94. Hou M, Stockelberg D, Kutti J, Wadenvik H. Glycoprotein IIb/IIIa autoantigenic repertoire in chronic idiopathic thrombocytopenic purpura. Br J Haematol 1995;91:971–5.

95. McMillan R, Tani P, Millard F, et al. Platelet-associated and plasma anti-glycoprotein autoantibodies in chronic ITP. Blood 1987;70:1040–5.

96. Varon D, Karpatkin S. A monoclonal anti-platelet antibody with decreased reactivity for autoimmune thrombocytopenic platelets. Proc Natl Acad Sci USA 1983;80:6992–5.

97. Fujisawa K, Tani P, O'Toole TE, et al. Different specificities of platelet-associated and plasma autoantibodies to platelet GPIIb-IIIa in patients with chronic immune thrombocytopenic purpura. Blood 1992;79:1441–6.

98. Kekomaki R, Dawson B, McFarland J, Kunicki TJ. Localization of human platelet autoantigens to the cysteine-rich region of glycoprotein IIIa. J Clin Invest 1991;88:847–54.

99. Nugent DJ, Kunicki TJ, Berglund C, Bernstein ID. A human monoclonal autoantibody recognizes a neoantigen on glycoprotein IIIa expressed on stored and activated platelets. Blood 1987;70:16–22.

100. Young NS, Barrett AJ. The treatment of severe acquired aplastic anemia. Blood 1995;85:3367–77.

101. Provan A. Management of adult idiopathic thrombocytopenic purpura. Prescribers' Journal 1992;32:193–200.

102. Provan D, Newland A. Idiopathic thrombocytopenic purpura in adults. J Pediatr Hematol Oncol 2003;25(Suppl. 1):S34–8.

103. Cahill MR, Macey MG, Cavenagh JD, Newland AC. Protein A immunoadsorption in chronic refractory ITP reverses increased platelet activation but fails to achieve sustained clinical benefit. Br J Haematol 1998;100:358–64.

104. Provan D, Stasi R, Newland AC, et al. International consensus report on the

investigation and management of primary immune thrombocytopenia. Blood 2010;115:168–86.

105. Newland A. Thrombopoietin receptor agonists in the treatment of thrombocytopenia. Curr Opin Hematol 2009;16:357–64.

106. Bussel JB, Provan D, Shamsi T, et al. Effect of eltrombopag on platelet counts and bleeding during treatment of chronic idiopathic thrombocytopenic purpura: a randomised, double-blind, placebo-controlled trial. Lancet 2009;373:641–8.

107. Molineux G, Newland A. Development of romiplostim for the treatment of patients with chronic immune thrombocytopenia: from bench to bedside. Br J Haematol. 2010 150(1): 9–20.

108. Garratty G. Drug-induced immune cytopenia. Transfus Med Rev 1993;7: 213–4.

109. Connellan JM, Deacon S, Thurlow PJ. Changes in platelet function and reactivity induced by quinine in relation to quinine (drug) induced immune thrombocytopenia. Thromb Res 1991;61:501–14.

110. Kunicki TJ, Christie DJ, Aster RH. The human platelet receptor(s) for quinine/ quinidine-dependent antibodies. Blood Cells 1983;9:293–301.

111. Salom IL. Purpura due to inhaled quinidine. JAMA 1991;266:1220.

112. Curtis BR, McFarland JG, Wu GG, et al. Antibodies in sulfonamide-induced immune thrombocytopenia recognize calcium-dependent epitopes on the glycoprotein IIb/IIIa complex. Blood 1994;84:176–83.

113. Coblyn JS, Weinblatt M, Holdsworth D, Glass D. Gold-induced thrombocytopenia. A clinical and immunogenetic study of twenty-three patients. Ann Intern Med 1981;95:178–81.

114. ASTER AND BORIGIE, NEJM, 2007

115. Warkentin TE, Chong BH, Greinacher A. Heparin-induced thrombocytopenia: towards consensus. Thromb Haemost 1998;79:1–7.

116. Greinacher A. Heparin-induced thrombocytopenia. J Thromb Haemost 2009;7(Suppl. 1):9–12.

117. Shantsila E, Lip GY, Chong BH. Heparin-induced thrombocytopenia. A contemporary clinical approach to diagnosis and management. Chest 2009;135:1651–64.

118. Manohitharajah SM, Jenkins WJ, Roberts PD, Clarke RC. Methyldopa and associated thrombocytopenia. Br Med J 1971;1:494.

119. Epstein M, Vickars L, Stein H. Diclofenac induced immune thrombocytopenia. J Rheumatol 1990;17:1403–4.

120. Burnette PK, Ameer B, Hoang V, Phifer W. Rifampin-associated thrombocytopenia secondary to poor compliance. DICP 1989;23:382–4.

121. Casasin T, Allende A, Macia M, Guell R. Two episodes of carbamazepine-induced severe thrombocytopenia in the same child. Ann Pharmacother 1992;26: 715–6.

122. George JN, El-Harake M. Thrombocytopenia due to enhanced platelet destruction by non-immunologic mechanisms. In: Beutler E, Lichtman MA, Coller BS, Kipps TJ, editors. Williams Hematology. New York: McGraw-Hill; 1995.

123. Rabiner SF. Uremic bleeding. Prog Hemost Thromb 1972;1:233–50.

124. Remuzzi G. Bleeding disorders in uremia: pathophysiology and treatment. Adv Nephrol Necker Hosp 1989;18: 171–86.

125. Castaldi PA, Rozenberg MC, Stewart JH. The bleeding disorder of uraemia. A qualitative platelet defect. Lancet 1966; 2:66–9.

126. Livio M, Benigni A, Remuzzi G. Coagulation abnormalities in uremia. Semin Nephrol 1985;5:82–90.

127. Remuzzi G, Livio M, Marchiaro G, et al. Bleeding in renal failure: altered platelet function in chronic uraemia only partially corrected by haemodialysis. Nephron 1978;22:347–53.

128. Castillo R, Lozano T, Escolar G, et al. Defective platelet adhesion on vessel subendothelium in uremic patients. Blood 1986;68:337–42.

129. Zwaginga JJ, Ijsseldijk MJ, Beeser-Visser N, et al. High von Willebrand factor concentration compensates a relative adhesion defect in uremic blood. Blood 1990;75:1498–508.

130. Zwaginga JJ, Ijsseldijk MJ, de Groot PG, et al. Defects in platelet adhesion and aggregate formation in uremic bleeding disorder can be attributed to factors in plasma. Arterioscler Thromb 1991;11: 733–44.

131. Weiss HJ, Turitto VT, Baumgartner HR. Effect of shear rate on platelet interaction with subendothelium in citrated and native blood. I. Shear rate – dependent decrease of adhesion in von Willebrand's disease and the Bernard–Soulier syndrome. J Lab Clin Med 1978;92: 750–64.

132. Murphy S. Polycythemia vera. Dis Mon 1992;38:153–212.

133. Schafer AI. Essential thrombocythemia. Prog Hemost Thromb 1991;10:69–96.

134. Ginsburg AD. Platelet function in patients with high platelet counts. Ann Intern Med 1975;82:506–11.

135. Schafer AI. Deficiency of platelet lipoxygenase activity in myeloprolifera-tive disorders. N Engl J Med 1982;306: 381–6.

136. Okuma M, Takayama H, Uchino H. Subnormal platelet response to thromboxane A2 i$_n$ a patient with chronic myeloid leukaemia. Br J Haematol 1982;51:469–77.

137. Kaplan ME, Mack K, Goldberg JD, et al. Long-term management of polycythemia vera with hydroxyurea: a progress report. Semin Hematol 1986;23:167–71.

138. Kessler CM, Klein HG, Havlik RJ. Uncontrolled thrombocytosis in chronic myeloproliferative disorders. Br J Haematol 1982;50:157–67.

139. Murphy S, Iland H, Rosenthal D, Laszlo J. Essential thrombocythemia: an interim report from the Polycythemia Vera Study Group. Semin Hematol 1986;23:177–82.

140. Cowan DH, Haut MJ. Platelet function in acute leukemia. J Lab Clin Med 1972;79: 893–905.

141. Meschengieser S, Blanco A, Maugeri N, et al. Platelet function and intraplatelet von Willebrand factor antigen and fibrinogen in myelodysplastic syndromes. Thromb Res 1987;46:601–6.

142. Mackie IJ. The biology of haemostasis and thrombosis. In: Ledingham JGG, Warrell DA, editors. Concise Oxford Textbook of Medicine. Oxford: Oxford University Press; 2000.

143. Roth GJ. Developing relationships: arterial platelet adhesion, glycoprotein Ib, and leucine-rich glycoproteins. Blood 1991;77:5–19.

144. Amiral J, Meyer D. Heparin-induced thrombocytopenia: diagnostic tests and biological mechanisms. Baillière's Clinical Haematology 1998;11:447–60.

CHAPTER 34

Inherited disorders of coagulation

NS Key, JC Boles

Chapter contents

Introduction

This chapter will focus on the inherited disorders of coagulation, ranging from the more common disorders such as von Willebrand disease and hemophilia A and B to a number of the so-called 'rare congenital bleeding disorders'. Inherited and acquired disorders affecting platelets, acquired hemorrhagic disorders and the thrombophilias will be discussed elsewhere (Chapters 32, 33, 35 and 36 respectively).

Hemophilia

Hemophilia, from the Greek *haima* for blood and *philia* for friend or friendship, is a term that encompasses two X-linked

inherited clotting factor deficiency states, namely factor VIII (hemophilia A or 'classical hemophilia'), or factor IX (hemophilia B or 'Christmas disease'). In older literature, factor XI deficiency is sometimes referred to as hemophilia C, but that term is now essentially obsolete. Therefore, for the purpose of this discussion, hemophilia will be used in reference to hemophilia A and B only.

Inheritance

Hemophilia A and B are X-linked recessive disorders and thus affect males almost exclusively. Mothers and daughters of affected males are, by definition, obligate carriers. Rarely a female may manifest symptomatic hemophilia through one of the following mechanisms: 1) homozygous female

©2011 Elsevier Ltd
DOI: 10.1016/B978-0-7020-3147-2.00034-1

offspring of an affected male and a carrier female; 2) high degree of lyonization (skewed X-chromosome inactivation) of alleles in a carrier; and 3) hemizygosity of females with concomitant Turner syndrome.[1] Females who appear phenotypically hemophilic should also undergo evaluation to exclude von Willebrand disease and testicular feminization syndrome.

The molecular basis of hemophilia A and B (FVIII and FIX genes)

Hemophilia A is more common than hemophilia B possibly because the factor VIII (FVIII) gene is considerably larger and thereby more susceptible to spontaneous mutation. The cloning of the FVIII gene and the sequencing of the cDNA was reported in landmark papers in 1984.[2–4] The FVIII gene comprises around 186 000 base pairs, compared to the FIX gene which has approximately 34 000 base pairs. In fact, the FVIII gene is one of the larger genes in the human genome, accounting for about 0.1% of the X chromosome. It contains three identifiable domain types in the sequence A1-A2-B-A3-C1-C2. This sequence comprises a heavy chain (A1 and A2 domains), a connecting region (B domain) and a light chain (A3, C1, and C2 domains). Some of these domains have specific functions, such as binding to factor IXa (A2 domain with A1/A3-C1-C2 dimer) while different epitopes of the C2 domain bind to phosphatidylserine (a procoagulant phospholipid expressed on the surface of activated platelets and endothelium) as well as von Willebrand factor, thrombin, and factor Xa. The B-domain is not required for procoagulant activity. The FVIII gene possesses 26 exons; within intron 22 are the start points for two further genes, one entirely contained within the intron and apparently expressed in most tissues (F8A) and a second beginning within the intron and utilizing exons 23–26 of the FVIII gene itself (F8B).[5]

After the FVIII gene was cloned, it became apparent that there was not a uniform genotypic abnormality that accounted for all cases of hemophilia A, and a variety of responsible mutations has now been described. The reader is referred to an online resource for the known mutations of factor VIII known as HAMSTeRS (Hemophilia A Mutation, Structure, Test, and Resource Site), which can be found at http://hadb.org.uk (see also Table 34.1). The most common mutation resulting in severe hemophilia A involves one of several inversions within intron 22 that collectively account for approximately 45–50% of cases. These mutations result in failure of transcription across this intron due to inversion of a section of the X chromosome at the tip of the long arm, resulting in the separation of the factor gene into two parts (Fig. 34.1). Recognition of this mutation has had a significant impact on carrier detection, as it is usually the first and most rapidly identifiable mutation sought.[6] Failure to identify an intron 22 inversion in severe hemophilia is an indication to evaluate for a much less common defect in intron 1 (present in <5% of cases) and then complete gene sequencing. In contrast to severe hemophilia A, moderate and mild hemophilia A are usually due to missense mutations in the FVIII gene.[6]

Hemophilia B is an X-linked deficiency of FIX and clinically behaves in an identical fashion to hemophilia A. The FIX protein consists of 454 amino acids. The FIX gene is

Table 34.1 Available online resources for documented mutations in coagulation factor deficiency states

Fibrinogen	www.hgmd.org www.geht.org/databaseang/fibrinogen/
Prothrombin	www.coagMDB.org/
Factor V	An up-to-date database on FV mutations has been complied by Dr. Hans L. Vos and is available upon request (email: H.L.Vos@lumc.nl)
Factor VII	www.coagMDB.org/
Factor VIII	http://hadb.org.uk
Factor IX	www.kcl.ac.uk/ip/petergreen/haemBdatabase.html; www.coagMDB.org/
Factor X	www.coagMDB.org/
Factor XI	www.FactorXI.org/
FXIII	www.f13-database.de/(xhgmobrswxgori45zk5jre45)/index.aspx
VWF	www.ragtimedesign.com/vwf/mutation www.vwf.group.shef.ac.uk/

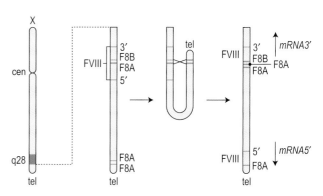

Fig. 34.1 How the tip flips: the mechanism of inversion through intron 22. cen, centromere; tel, telomere. *(Reproduced with permission from Hoffbrand AV, Mitchell Lewis S, Tuddenham EGD, eds. Postgraduate Haematology. Butterworth Heinemann, Oxford, 1999).*

contained on the long arm of the X chromosome and contains eight exons. The complete sequence of the gene has been determined. Since the FIX gene is a simple gene it has been possible to perform detailed analysis using polymerase chain reaction (PCR)-based analysis. In this way, a plethora of hemophilia B point mutations have been established. In some cases of severe hemophilia B, affected individuals may have a large (or even total) deletion of the FIX gene.

The FIX point mutations and smaller deletions typically result in production of a nonfunctioning but immunologically detectable, FIX protein ('cross-reacting material positive' or CRM+). Hemophilia resulting from large to complete deletions or nonsense mutations is more likely to be CRM−. Patients that are CRM− are more susceptible to the development of FIX alloantibodies, which overall are relatively uncommon in hemophilia B compared to hemophilia A.[7] The Hemophilia B Mutation Database can be found online at http://www.kcl.ac.uk/ip/petergreen/haemBdatabase.html (Table 34.1).

As alluded to above, inhibitory alloantibodies that develop in a proportion of patients with hemophilia A and B following replacement therapy correlate to some extent with factor VIII and factor IX mutation type and location;[8] this aspect is discussed in greater detail below.

Diagnosis of hemophilia carrier state

The initial step in an evaluation for hemophilia carrier status involves a thorough family history. While factor activity levels are usually low in carriers of hemophilia, they may remain in the normal range. Therefore, direct molecular detection of the hemophilic gene is now considered the gold standard.

Incidence and clinical manifestations

The incidence of hemophilia A is estimated at 1 : 5000 live male births (Table 34.2). Factor VIII deficiency accounts for approximately 80% of hemophilia. Hemophilia B is much less common, with an estimated incidence of 1 : 30 000 live male births. Notably, the hemophilias have equal incidence across racial and ethnic groups.

Throughout this chapter we will refer to factor activity levels. We will reference activity as international units/ deciliter (IU/dl). As a point of information, 100% activity $= 100$ IU/dl $= 1$ IU/ml.

The clinical severity of the disorder is variable but correlates well with endogenous factor levels. It is possible to differentiate three degrees of clinical severity: 1) severe hemophilia where there is spontaneous hemorrhage into joints and muscles (<1 IU/dl factor activity); 2) moderate hemophilia where bleeding occurs after minor trauma (1–5 IU/dl factor activity); and 3) mild hemophilia when prolonged bleeding only occurs with trauma of after operative procedures (5–50 IU/dl factor activity). In general, related males will have identical factor activity levels since they will have inherited the same genetic defect.

Of all patients with hemophilia, approximately $\frac{1}{3}$-$\frac{1}{2}$ will have severe disease. In general, hemophilia A and B of a corresponding severity manifest a similar clinical picture. It is estimated that approximately 50% of severe and 30% of mild/moderate hemophilia cases are without significant family history and are considered the result of a spontaneous mutation.[9]

Some patients with severe hemophilia may have a milder clinical course. For example, patients with the Leyden phenotype of hemophilia B have severe disease in childhood that becomes mild after puberty. This is thought to be secondary to a mutation in the promoter region that disrupts the binding site for hepatocyte nuclear factor-4 (HNF-4) but not an overlapping site for an androgen response element. This responsiveness to male sex hormones may explain the milder clinical course that emerges after puberty.[10–12]

Patients with severe hemophilia may also co-inherit a hereditary prothrombotic condition such as a prothrombin G20210A gene mutation or factor V Leiden that may partially offset their hemophilia and result in fewer or less severe hemorrhagic episodes.[13–16]

Bleeding may occur in any part of the body, but most commonly affects the joints, followed by muscles and the gastrointestinal tract. The joints most commonly involved are listed in decreasing order of incidence: knees (50% of all bleeding episodes), elbows, ankles, shoulders and wrists.[17,18]

Recurrent joint bleeds represent significant morbidity for hemophiliacs as they ultimately result in degeneration of cartilage and progressive joint space narrowing and destruction accompanied by chronic pain and decreasing range of motion. Clinically, recurrent joint hemorrhage is usually manifest as pain, swelling and loss of range of motion of the affected joint. The pattern of intra-articular and intramuscular bleeding in hemophilia is distinct from the typical mucosal pattern of bleeding noted in patients with von Willebrand disease or platelet disorders.

Intramuscular hemorrhage represents the second most common site of bleeding. The location of bleeding dictates morbidity. Hemorrhage into large, unconfined muscles may result in significant blood loss and anemia. However, hemorrhage into tightly confined spaces may lead to compartment syndrome, such as in the forearm, where if not adequately treated, it may result in a Volkmann's ischemic contracture, or into the iliopsoas muscle where it may acutely result in femoral nerve compression.

Severe hemophiliacs may develop a pseudotumor. These are chronically unresolved hematomas produced by repetitive bleeding episodes into muscle that slowly enlarge and become encapsulated and organized over time. The accompanying inflammatory process may eventually encroach or destroy surrounding structures, frequently including bone. Unfortunately pseudotumors are more common in areas of the world where there is often inadequate treatment of hemophilia. Immediate and appropriate treatment of acute bleeding episodes theoretically minimizes the risk of pseudotumor formation. Even with appropriate factor replacement, surgical removal of large pseudotumors is associated with up to a 20% mortality.[19]

Bleeding into the central nervous system is a particularly ominous complication, and is an all too frequent cause of death.[20] In children, particularly in the neonatal period, intracranial hemorrhage (ICH) may occur with minimal or no recognized trauma. In adults, 50% of cases of ICH appear to be spontaneous. HIV infected hemophiliacs treated with protease inhibitors may be at higher risk for spontaneous intramuscular or ICH.[21] Of patients who experience an ICH, approximately 50% will develop permanent neurologic sequelae, and up to 30% will die.

Treatment of hemophilia

The care of patients with hemophilia is complicated and requires multidisciplinary care. Hemophilia treatment centers (HTC) exist to provide comprehensive medical and psychosocial services to patients and their families. Soucie et al. described a survival advantage for patients with hemophilia treated at an HTC compared to those treated in alternative systems in the United States.[22]

The general approach to treatment of both hemophilia A and B is similar. Management focuses on replacement of FVIII or FIX to levels sufficient to prevent or limit existing hemorrhage. The clinical scenario dictates the target factor activity level. For example, a target activity level of 100 IU/ dl is desired during episodes of life threatening hemorrhage such as ICH, whereas levels of 30–40 IU/dl may be sufficient for minor events, such as joint bleeds.

Table 34.2 Features of selected inherited disorders of coagulation

Disorder		Inheritance pattern	Incidence	Phenotype	Diagnostics			Treatment
					PT	PTT	TCT	
Abnormality in fibrinogen	Dysfibrinogenemia	Autosomal	1 in 1 million	Variable bleeding and/or clotting	Prolonged	Prolonged	Prolonged or shortened	Fibrinogen concentrate, cyropreciptiate, or FFP
	Afibrinogenemia	Autosomal		Severe	Infinite	Infinite	Infinite	Fibrinogen concentrate, cyropreciptiate, or FFP
Prothrombin deficiency (factor II deficiency)		Autosomal	1 in 2 million	Generally correlates with FII levels	Prolonged	Prolonged	Normal	PCC or FFP
Factor V deficiency		Autosomal	1 in 1 million	Mild–moderate	Prolonged	Prolonged	Normal	FFP, or exchange transfusion
Combined factor V and VIII deficiency		Autosomal	1 in 2 million	Moderate-severe	Prolonged	Prolonged	Normal	Combination of FVIII concentrate and FFP
Factor VII deficiency		Autosomal	1 in 500 000	Moderate–severe	Prolonged	Normal	Normal	Recombinant-activated factor VII or FVII concentrate
Hemophilia A (factor VIII deficiency)		X-linked Recessive	1 in 5000 male births	Variable, depending on factor VIII level	Normal	Prolonged	Normal	Factor VIII concentrates
Hemophilia B (factor IX deficiency)		X-linked Recessive	1 in 30000 male births	Variable, depending on factor IX level	Normal	Prolonged	Normal	Factor IX concentrates
Factor X deficiency		Autosomal	1 in 1 million	Variable, depending on factor X level	Prolonged	Prolonged	Normal	PCC
Factor XI deficiency		Autosomal	1 in 1 million	Variable, not dependent on factor XI levels	Normal	Prolonged	Normal	Factor XI concentrate
Factor XIII deficiency		Autosomal	1 in 2 million	Severe	Normal	Normal	Normal	Factor XIII concentrate or FFP
Vitamin K dependent factor deficiency		Autosomal	1 in 2 million	Severe	Prolonged	Prolonged	Normal	High dose vitamin K, FFP or PCC
α_2-Plasmin inhibitor deficiency		Autosomal		Severe	Normal	Normal	Normal	Antifibrinolytics

Plasma-derived and recombinant factor products

The discovery in the 1960s that factor VIII is concentrated about tenfold in cryoprecipitate, and the subsequent description of the production of antihemophilic globulin in a closed-bag system made more specific replacement therapy for people with hemophilia possible. Unfortunately, however, prior to the application of effective virucidal methods to such concentrates in the 1980s, a significant proportion of hemophilia patients contracted hepatitis C and HIV/AIDS. All factor concentrates, whether plasma derived or recombinant are now virucidally treated through viral inactivation, attenuation or elimination which has eradicated lipid-enveloped viruses such as HIV, hepatitis B and C and West Nile virus. There have been no documented cases of transmission of these diseases since 1985 for FVIII concentrates and 1990 for FIX concentrates. However, routine virucidal treatment does not reliably eradicate some nonlipid-enveloped viruses such as parvovirus B-19 and hepatitis A and outbreaks related to factor concentrate have been reported.[23,24] The recommendation remains that all infants who receive factor replacement are vaccinated against hepatitis A and B during infancy. Recently, a concern has been raised that plasma derived concentrates, and even possibly recombinant factor concentrates stabilized with human albumin could theoretically transmit prions associated with Creutzfeldt–Jakob disease (CJD) or variant CJD.[25]

Factor VIII and FIX products are often classified based on their final purity, which is defined by specific activity (international units (IU) of factor activity per milligram (mg) of protein (IU/mg)). Products with low specific activities (<50 IU/mg) are considered intermediate purity because they are contaminated with additional plasma proteins such as vWF and fibronectin. High purity products (>50 IU/mg) and ultra high purity products (>3000 IU/mg for FVIII products and >160 IU/mg for FIX) have little to no protein contamination.

Table 34.3 shows the main blood-borne viruses with their genomic and physicochemical characteristics. It can be seen that the risk of HIV infection in virally inactivated concentrates is miniscule.[26] The risk of transmission of hepatitis B and C has also been essentially erradicated. However, as mentioned, there remains the problem of possible transmission of hepatitis A and parvovirus in solvent detergent treated plasma-derived clotting factors; for this reason, many inactivation processes include more than one virucidal method. For FIX concentrate the process of nanofiltration has been used to prevent transmission of hepatitis A and parvovirus.

All of the currently available commercial products, both plasma-derived and recombinant, appear to have similar efficacy as determined by post-administration recovery levels. In general, the dosing of these products is based upon the desired factor activity level, plasma volume of distribution, and half-life of the product used.

Although the FIX gene was cloned in 1982 the development of recombinant FIX was considerably more difficult because of the post-translational modifications required for full activity.[27]

The choice of clotting factor to be used should be individualized for each patient. The cost, age of patient, alloantibody status and presence/absence of HIV/hepatitis should be considered. A general rule is that the cost of the final product increases proportionately to its purity. Another consideration for FIX products involves the thrombogenic potential for intermediate-purity products, which in fact are rarely used any longer for replacement in hemophilia B in developed countries. Disseminated intravascular coagulation, stroke and myocardial infarction have been associated with repeated use of these products. It has been argued that this effect may be related to the activated clotting factors such as Xa and IIa present in these products. The ultra high purity products have been associated with little or no associated thrombosis, and they are now routinely the product of choice for primary prophylaxis, surgery and immune tolerance induction.

A recent article provides a review of contemporary coagulation factor products and their uses in inherited disorders or coagulopathy.[28]

1-Deamino-8-D-arginine vasopressin (DDAVP) or desmopressin

DDAVP or desmopressin is a synthetic analog of vasopressin which lacks the vasopressor effects. It has played an important role in the treatment of mild hemophilia A and type 1 von Willebrand disease (vWD) for several decades.[29] In the mid 1970s, it was demonstrated that an infusion of DDAVP

Table 34.3 Main blood-borne viruses transmitted by coagulation factor concentrates (reproduced with permission from Mannucci 1996[12])

Virus	Genome	Lipid-enveloped	Size (nm)	Solvent/detergent resistant	Heat resistant
Human immunodeficiency virus, type I	RNA	Yes	80–100	No	No
Hepatitis A virus	RNA	No	27	Yes	No
Hepatitis B virus	DNA	Yes	42	No	No
Hepatitis C virus	RNA	Yes	35–65	No	No
Hepatitis D virus	RNA	Yes	35	No	No
B19 parvovirus	DNA	No	20	Yes	Yes

increased the plasma concentrations of FVIII:C, vWF and tissue plasminogen activator (tPA) when infused into normal volunteers.[30,31] The increase in plasma FVIII:C and vWF is generally two- to sixfold baseline levels. The increased plasma levels of vWF are secondary to release from Weibel–Palade bodies located in endothelial cells and perhaps also from platelet α-granules.[31] The source of the FVIII store released upon treatment with DDAVP is not established.

Lethagen et al demonstrated the effectiveness of intranasal administration, which is an ideal choice for home administration.[32] Intranasal DDAVP approximates the effect obtained with intravenously or subcutaneously administered product.[33] For adults with mild hemophilia A the recommended dose of 0.3 µg/kg (IV or SQ), or 300 µg intranasally, can be repeated at intervals of 12–24 hours. However, tachyphylaxis (depletion of FVIII/vWF from repeated endothelial exocytosis into plasma) may develop, as well as flushing and/or hypotension. Mannucci et al. reported that the response to a second dose of DDAVP is approximately 30% less than that obtained with the first.[34] It was also demonstrated that a full response to DDAVP is usually recovered within 3–4 days after a break in treatment. Since DDAVP also stimulates the release of tPA (a profibrinolytic enzyme), consideration should be given to concurrent administration of an antifibrinolytic agent with DDAVP for the management of bleeding in the oropharynx or gastrointestinal tract. DDAVP is an antidiuretic which may promote excessive free water retention and subsequent hyponatremia. It is usually therefore avoided in younger children and the elderly. It has also been suggested that DDAVP may rarely cause angina pectoris, stroke and coronary artery thrombosis in the elderly population where caution is advised.[35]

DDAVP is not recommended when baseline FVIII and/or VW antigen levels are <5 IU/dl (i.e. in severe or moderate hemophilia A, or in type 3 vWD), since in these patients, no clinically useful response is likely. In candidate patients, a formal trial of DDAVP, with monitoring of FVIII and vW antigen levels for up to 6 hours is recommended, since there is considerable inter-individual variability in responsiveness and half-life of the secreted factors.

Antifibrinolytic agents

Antifibrinolytic agents are an often underutilized adjunctive therapy in the management of bleeding in hemophilia. These agents, ε-aminocaproic acid and tranexamic acid, act by inhibiting fibrinolysis mediated by plasmin thereby enhancing clot stability. Given their mechanism of action, they are particularly helpful in anatomic areas subject to increased fibrinolysis such as the oro- and nasopharynx and often also in menorrhagia.[36]

These agents may be used alone or in combination with DDAVP especially in the management of dental extractions. They may be administered intravenously, orally or topically (such as in the form of a mouthwash).

Inhibitors

Alloantibody formation against FVIII or FIX in response to treatment is now considered to be the most significant complication of hemophilia care. One of the earliest references recording inhibitors was that of Davidson et al. in 1949.[37]

The development of inhibitors is more common in patients with hemophilia A than in those with hemophilia B. Inhibitors are more common in patients with severe forms of hemophilia A or B. More recent studies have suggested that up to 20–30% of patients with severe hemophilia A and up to 3% of severe hemophilia B patients will develop a clinically significant inhibitor at some time in their life.[38–40] Inhibitors are significantly less common in mild to moderate hemophilia A, at 3–15%.[38,41,42]

Prospective clinical trials evaluating recombinant FVIII products in previously untreated patients (PUP) provided invaluable insight into the incidence of inhibitors with these products in hemophilia A. Notably, these prospective trials performed frequent laboratory surveillance, which as discussed below may account for the higher incidence of inhibitors than was previously appreciated. In the Kogenate™ PUP study, 20% of patients developed an inhibitor after a median of 9 exposure days. Of those with severe disease, 25% developed an inhibitor, while less than 10% with mild or moderate disease did so. In patients who developed an inhibitor, approximately 50% had spontaneous resolution or persistently low titers despite continued treatment. The authors described these as 'transient' inhibitors. The cumulative probability of inhibitor development was 36% after 18 days of treatment.[38] This incidence rate is similar to that reported in the Recombinate™ PUP study with a cumulative probability of 38% at a median 25 days exposure.[43] As would be expected, lower rates of inhibitor development were reported in trials that enrolled previously treated patients (PTP).[44,45]

Inhibitors are typically IgG subclass 4 or 1, appear at a median of 9–12 days after exposure to factor concentrate, and do not naturally occur prior to factor exposure. Presumably the higher incidence of inhibitor development in patients with severe hemophilia A is explained by the almost complete absence of circulating endogenous FVIII. The absence of in utero exposure to FVIII is thus associated with a failure to develop tolerance to this antigen, such that patients remain predisposed to antibody formation upon exposure to exogenous factor later in life. Data available in the international electronic databases suggest that patients with large deletions (>200 bp) or stop mutations are more likely to develop inhibitors, while those with smaller deletions or missense mutations are less likely to do so.[6,46] Patients with moderate or mild hemophilia A may synthesize FVIII that has an abnormal tertiary or quaternary structure. Epidemiologically, these individuals appear to be especially prone to develop inhibitors later in life, and particularly at times of intensive exposure to FVIII replacement, such as after surgery.[47] It is hypothesized that at such times, the immunologic system, which is in a state of activation, is more likely to perceive the normal wild type FVIII as a 'foreign' antigen.

Patients with hemophilia B are at much lower risk of inhibitors. These tend to occur in individuals with significant deletions in the FIX gene. Development of an inhibitor in these patients is often accompanied by allergic reactions to FIX-containing products, which may be severe. Because of their relative rarity, less is known about the epidemiology of inhibitors in hemophilia B, although many of the risk factors that predispose to FVIII inhibitors in hemophilia A are believed also to be relevant.

One such risk factor is subject race/ethnicity, which appears to influence inhibitor formation. The Malmo International Brother Study (MIBS) reported the incidence of inhibitors in Caucasian and black people to be 27% and 56% respectively.[48] Hispanic people also appear to be at higher risk of inhibitor formation. A recent study has suggested that this disparity may be at least partially explained by the types of recombinant products used in these populations and their underlying FVIII haplotypes. On the basis of four single nucleotide polymorphisms (SNPs) within the FVIII protein, six wild-type haplotypes, designated H1 through H6, can be discerned. However, only the H1 and H2 haplotypes match the available recombinant factor products approved for clinical use. Viel et al. reported the background haplotypes for 78 black patients with hemophilia. Patients with H3 or H4 haplotypes (which were more prevalent in African-Americans) had a significantly higher incidence of inhibitor development than those with H1 or H2 (odds ratio, 3.6; 95% confidence interval, 1.1 to 12.3; $P = 0.04$).[49] This study suggests that a mismatch between patient haplotype and replacement product haplotype may predisopose to development of an inhibitor. If confirmed, this study suggests that 'individualized' forms of FVIII replacement therapy could in theory mitigate the risk of inhibitor formation in the future.

There also appears to be a familial predisposition to inhibitor development. Siblings of patients with hemophilia and an inhibitor are at increased risk of inhibitor development.[41] The results of the CANAL (Concerted Action on Neutralizing Antibodies in severe hemophilia A) cohort study led to the development of a risk stratification score that predicted the development of inhibitory antibodies in untreated patients with severe hemophilia A.[50,51] The risk factors that were proposed in this scoring system were family history of inhibitors, presence of a high risk gene mutation and intensive treatment at first episode.

It has been suggested that switching between FVIII products and use of recombinant factor products is associated with higher incidence of inhibitor development. Although results from the CANAL cohort study do not support the latter association,[52] a great deal of circumstantial evidence continues to raise this concern.[53,54]

Management of inhibitors

Currently, the most serious complication of factor replacement therapy in hemophilia is the development of FVIII antibodies. An inhibitor should be suspected when administration of factor concentrate at quantities historically sufficient to raise the deficient factor level to an adequate hemostatic level does not result in improvement in bleeding and/or the expected target plasma factor level. Once an inhibitor is suspected, the Bethesda assay (or the Nijmegen modification of the Bethesda assay) may be used to measure its strength. This assay incubates dilutions of patient plasma with pooled normal plasma at 37°C for 2 hours. Residual FVIII activity is then measured in each dilution. The reciprocal of the dilution of patient plasma to pooled normal plasma that results in a residual 50% FVIII activity is the Bethesda unit titer. The greater the dilution titer, the stronger the inhibitor.

Patients with a peak historical Bethesda titer of <5 BU/ml are defined as being low responders and those >5 BU/ml as high responders. The classification into low responders and high responders is clinically important as it provides the rationale for management. The treatment goals in patients with inhibitors are twofold, namely: 1) to achieve adequate hemostasis; and 2) to eradicate the antibody using an immune tolerance induction strategy. Bleeding in low-responder patients can be treated with human or porcine FVIII concentrates (when available) at a dose and frequency sufficient to overwhelm the antibody and therefore obtain therapeutic plasma levels of FVIII. Although there have been no documented cases of transmitted blood-borne infectious agents, porcine FVIII was removed from production in 2004 because of contamination by porcine parvovirus. However, clinical trials evaluating recombinant porcine FVIII are currently enrolling subjects.[55]

Bleeding in high-responder patients is more difficult to treat as the inhibitor cannot be simply overwhelmed using higher doses of factor concentrates. These patients are therefore treated with so-called 'bypassing agents'. These bypassing agents include prothrombin complex concentrates (PCCs) – either unactivated or activated (aPCC) – as well as recombinant factor VIIa concentrate (rFVIIa). Bypassing agents are believed to work by activating the coagulation cascade at levels below the action of the inhibitor.

Immune tolerance induction

Immune tolerance induction (ITI) regimens are used in an effort to eradicate alloantibody inhibitors. ITI is a process whereby prolonged daily exposure to factor concentrates, with or without adjunctive immunosuppression, is aimed at desensitizing the immune system to the presence of factor and therefore suppresses production of inhibitor antibodies. Several international registries have reported that the overall success rate with inhibitor eradication in severe hemophilia A is about 70%. It has been noted that ITI is more successful in patients with lower titer inhibitors (peak titer <200 BU/ml). ITI is generally less successful in hemophilia B and may be associated with development of the nephrotic syndrome or anaphylaxis to FIX containing products in some patients. In general, once the inhibitor resolves, the patients are placed on indefinite prophylaxis regimens. There is a low but finite risk of relapse.

Prophylaxis

As replacement products have become safer, regimens aimed at preventing hemarthroses and subsequent hemophilic arthropathy have been developed and are known as primary prophylaxis when initiated early in childhood. In hemophilia, the difference between <1% factor activity and 2–3% factor activity is clinically significant. Primary prophylaxis regimens were devised to maintain trough factor activity levels of at least 2–3% at all times, which has been shown to reduce the incidence of spontaneous hemarthrosis in severe hemophilia. These regimens are often initiated prior to or after the first episode of hemarthrosis, generally around 14–18 months of age.[56] In severe hemophilia A, the superiority of the primary prophylaxis strategy compared to the traditional 'on demand' strategy (in which factor concentrate is administered at the onset of hemarthrosis) has been convincingly demonstrated, and it is now considered the

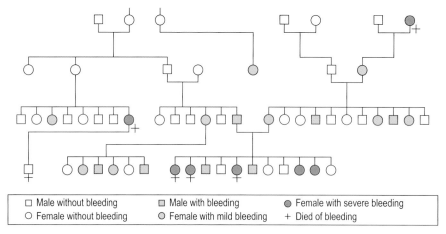

Fig. 34.2 From the original family described by von Willebrand in 1926. *(Reproduced with permission from Lee CA. Women and von Willebrand disease. May 1999. Haemophilia 5(suppl 2): 38–45).*

standard of care in wealthier economies that are able to bear the higher cost.[57]

von Willebrand disease

von Willebrand disease (vWD) is the most common of the inherited bleeding disorders. It was initially described by Erik von Willebrand in 1926. The proband and her family members, many of whom were affected, lived in the Åland Islands in the Gulf of Bothnia. Dr von Willebrand named the disorder hereditary pseudohemophilia when he recognized a distinctive autosomal pattern of inheritance rather than the typical X-linked recessive pattern noted in hemophilia. Figure 34.2 is a partial representation of the original family tree described by Dr von Willebrand in 1926.

vWD results from a quantitative or qualitative defect of von Willebrand factor (vWF). vWF is a high-molecular-weight glycoprotein with two major functions: 1) it promotes platelet adhesion to the sub-endothelium and platelet aggregation under high shear conditions during primary hemostasis; and 2) it is the carrier of FVIII in plasma thereby preventing proteolysis of FVIII within the circulation. Thus, a deficiency or a qualitative defect of vWF will result in defects in both the primary phase of hemostasis and of coagulation/secondary hemostasis. vWD is most often inherited in an autosomal dominant fashion, but an autosomal recessive pattern is noted in some subtypes of type 2 disease as well as type 3 disease, as described below. Patients with vWD may have a mild, moderate or severe bleeding tendency, which is lifelong and is usually proportional to the vWF level.

In a large epidemiologic study in Italian children, Rodeghiero et al. found the prevalence of vWD to be 0.82%.[58] Only a fraction of these individuals were symptomatic, estimated at approximately 5% of those with the disorder.[59]

vWD has been divided into three subtypes according to the pathophysiology. Types 1 and 3 are the result of a partial or virtually complete quantitative deficiency of vWF respectively, while type 2 refers to a qualitative defect in vWF. Type 1 is the most common form, accounting for approximately

70%, while type 2 accounts for 15–20% and type 3 for 2–5% of vWD patients (see Fig. 34.4, below).

The diagnosis of vWD should be suspected in any patient who experiences excessive mucocutaneous bleeding, particularly if the family history suggests an autosomal pattern of inheritance. The most common bleeding symptoms are epistaxis, bleeding after dental extractions and menorrhagia. However, the bleeding tendency can be quite variable and also depends on the type and the severity of the disease. A validated bleeding score has been developed to elucidate and quantify bleeding in patients with vWD.[60] However, laboratory tests are essential in establishing the diagnosis of vWD, because of the variable bleeding history.

Screening tests

In general, patients with vWD have platelet counts that are normal, but thrombocytopenia may occur in patients with the type 2B variant. The bleeding time is usually prolonged, but can be normal in patients with milder forms of vWD, particularly type 1. The prothrombin time (PT) is normal, but the APPT may be prolonged, depending on the FVIII:C levels. Platelet function analyzer (PFA-100™) closure times or bleeding time are most frequently used to screen for defective primary hemostasis in vWD. A number of laboratory tests are helpful in establishing a diagnosis of vWD, as well as clarifying the subtype. These include: vWF antigen, vWF activity (risocetin co-factor activity and/or collagen-binding activity), FVIII activity, ristocetin-induced platelet aggregation, and vWF multimer studies. These are listed below followed by a brief individual description.

Platelet function analyzer (PFA-100™) closure time and bleeding time

Both of these assays are used as global screens of the adequacy of primary hemostasis. Neither is specific to any defined entity, and they vary in their sensitivity to the two major categories of abnormality being sought, namely vWD and intrinsic platelet function defects.[61] The PFA-100™ is a tabletop instrument that measures the ability of platelets in whole blood to occlude an aperture in a membrane and form a plug under flow. It requires adequate vWF and platelet function. Its sensitivity in diagnosing vWD is debated, but it is clearly superior to the bleeding time in this regard.[62] One advantage of this instrument is that it does measure the ability of endogenous platelets to adhere to a membrane consisting of collagen and either epinephrine or ADP under physiological flow conditions. This is important since arterial shear stresses contribute to unfolding and consequent activation of vWF as an adhesive target for platelets.

The bleeding time is principally a measure of the interaction between vascular endothelium, platelets and plasma factors such as fibrinogen and vWF. If the bleeding time is prolonged it may be useful in the diagnosis of vWD, but in mild and moderate disease it may remain normal. The bleeding time is invasive, time consuming and operator dependent, which has led to its fall from favor as a screening test. While it is classically prolonged in the more severe variants of vWD, it is no longer commonly employed in clinical practice.

vWF antigen

vWF antigen (vWF:Ag) is most often measured in plasma using an enzyme-linked immunoadsorbent assay (ELISA), although immuno-radiometric assays may be utilized. More recently, an automated turbidometric test has been described that utilizes latex beads coated with antibodies against vWF. The results of this assay appear to compare favorably to those obtained by ELISA; however, rheumatoid factors may falsely impact the assay.[63] vWF:Ag is usually unmeasurable in type 3, may be low in type 1 and low or normal in type 2 vWD.

vWF activity (ristocetin co-factor activity)

vWF activity is generally measured as the ristocetin co-factor activity (vWF:RCo). This assay measures the interaction of vWF with the platelet glycoprotein 1b/IX/V complex. It is based on the ability of the antibiotic ristocetin to agglutinate normal human platelets in the presence of vWF (present in the test plasma). In patients with normal von Willebrand structure (type 1 vWD), vWF:RCo values are reduced in proportion to the vWF antigen. Levels of vWF:RCo lower than those of vWF antigen (i.e. if the ratio of vWF:RCo to vWF:Ag is <0.7) are characteristic of type 2 vWD. While ristocetin co-factor activity is considered by many to be the 'gold standard' it is labor-intensive and difficult to standardize among laboratories.[64]

vWF activity (collagen-binding activity)

A second assay to measure vWF activity is the collagen-binding activity (vWF:CB). In this assay, dilutions of normal or patient plasma are added to an ELISA plate coated with collagen. Bound vWF is measured with an antibody.[65] vWF:CB is often measured in conjunction with vWF:RCo and vWF:Ag. Rare cases of vWD associated with alterations in the collagen binding site could be missed if vWF activity is assessed solely via an assessment of vWF:RCo.

Factor VIII activity (FVIII:C)

As discussed above, normal vWF acts as a carrier protein for FVIII in plasma and thereby protects it from proteolytic inactivation. Therefore, if a patient has a vWF level that is sufficiently low, or the vWF contains a mutation in its binding site for FVIII (type 2N), a decreased FVIII:C and prolongation of the APTT may result. FVIII:C is very low (1–5 IU/dl) in patients with type 3 vWD while it may be normal or mildly decreased in patients with type 1 or type 2 vWD. Patients with type 2N vWD have variably low FVIII:C levels, but most often mimic the phenotype of mild hemophilia A, with levels >5 IU/dl.

Ristocetin-induced platelet aggregation (RIPA)

The RIPA is measured by adding ristocetin to test platelet-rich plasma. Most vWD types have a low response to ristocetin, but the principal value of the RIPA is in the differential diagnosis of type 2 vWD variants. Specifically, patients with type 2A vWD manifest a profoundly reduced response to ristocetin added to their platelet rich plasma, due to the lack of more functional higher molecular weight multimers in their plasma. On the other hand, patients with type 2B vWD are characterized by increased response to low concentrations of ristocetin, because of an increased affinity of the larger multimers of vWF for the platelet GP1b/IX/V complex (due to a 'gain of function' mutation). Type 2B vWD also should be distinguished from the rare 'pseudo vWD', which is due to a gain of function mutation in the GP1b/IX/V complex. Affected individuals similarly show an increase in ristocetin responsiveness in the RIPA assay, but they can be differentiated from type 2B vWD by repeating the RIPA assay using mixtures of normal platelets and test plasma, and vice versa.

vWF multimeric analysis

This is performed on high-resolution agarose gels. These gels are used to detect the presence, absence or decrease in the high molecular weight multimers that may be used to differentiate between type 1 (where there is a global decrease in all multimers) and some of the type 2 subtypes. In types 2A and 2B vWD (as well as psudo-vWD), the higher molecular weight multimers are selectively absent or severely reduced.

Factor VIII binding assay

This assay measures the affinity of test vWF for FVIII. It is used to evaluate for type 2N vWD in which there is a qualitative abnormality in the FVIII binding domain of vWF that results in decreased FVIII levels in plasma secondary to increased proteolytic cleavage.

The subtypes of vWD

The diagnosis of vWD should be made on the basis of three components, namely: 1) a history of excessive bleeding, either spontaneous mucocutaneous or post-surgical (or both); 2) a family history of excessive bleeding; and 3) confirmatory laboratory testing. The National Heart Lung and Blood Institute have published guidelines for the diagnosis, evaluation and management of vWD (see Figs 34.3 and 34.4).[66,67]

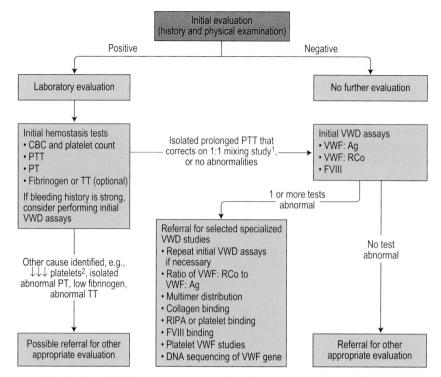

Fig. 34.3 National Heart Lung and Blood Institute (NHLBI) recommended algorithm for Laboratory Assessment for vWD.

	Normal	Type 1	Type 2A	Type 2B	Type 2M	Type 2N	Type 3	PLT-VWD
VWF:Ag	N	L, ↓ or ↓↓	↓ or L	↓ or L	↓ or L	N or L	absent	↓ or L
VWF:RCo	N	L, ↓ or ↓↓	↓↓ or ↓↓↓	↓↓	↓↓	N or L	absent	↓↓
FVIII	N	N or ↓	N or ↓	N or ↓	N or ↓	↓↓	1-9 IU/dL	N or L
RIPA	N	often N	↓	often N	↓	N	absent	often N
LD-RIPA	absent	absent	absent	↑↑↑	absent	absent	absent	↑↑↑
PFA-100® CT	N	N or ↑	↑	↑	↑	N	↑↑↑	↑
BT	N	N or ↑	↑	↑	↑	N	↑↑↑	↑
Platelet count	N	N	N	↓ or N	N	N	N	↓
VWF multimer pattern	N	N	abnormal	abnormal	N	N	absent	abnormal

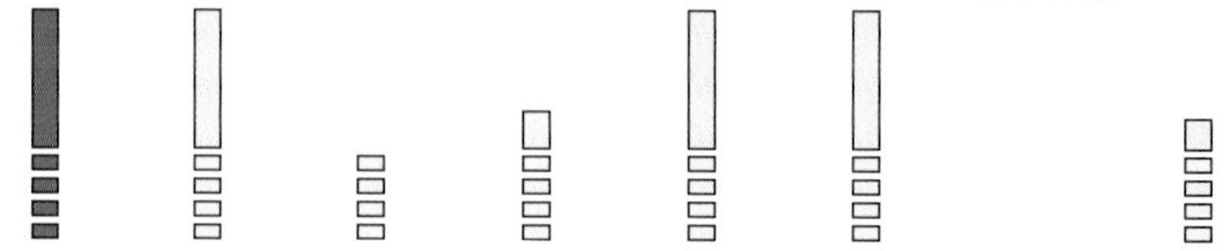

Fig. 34.4 Expected laboratory values in vWD (from NHLBI guidelines[66]). The symbols and values represent prototypical cases. In practice, laboratory studies in certain patients may deviate slightly from these expectations. L, 30–50 IU/dl; ↓, ↓↓, ↓↓↓, relative decrease; ↑, ↑↑, ↑↑↑, relative increase; BT, bleeding time; FVIII, factor VIII activity; LD-RIPA, low-dose ristocetin-induced platelet aggregation (concentration of ristocetin ≤0.6 mg/ml); N, normal; PFA-100® CT, platelet function analyzer closure time; RIPA, ristocetin-induced platelet aggregation; vWF, von Willebrand factor; vWF:Ag, vWF antigen; vWF:RCo, vWF ristocetin co-factor activity.

Type 1 vWD

Inheritance is autosomal dominant and patients typically manifest mild to moderate symptoms, with normal or variably prolonged PFA-100 closure times/bleeding time and concordantly decreased levels of vWF:Ag and vWF:RCo. FVIII:C is reduced in proportion to the reduction in vWF:Ag, and vWF multimeric structure is normal. The vWF plasma levels are dependent on ABO blood group and vWF may be 25% lower in persons with blood type O. However, it has been found that when the range for vWF:RCo and vWF:Ag are adjusted for this variable to two standard deviations below the population mean, about half the individuals still have an abnormal family history and an abnormal bleeding history.[68,69] Thus, the diagnosis of type 1 vWD needs to take into account the clinical bleeding history. There have been trends to sub-classify type 1 vWD according to pathophysiologic basis; for example, depending on the platelet vWF content, three subtypes have been identified, platelet normal, platelet low and platelet discordant.[70] More recently, subtypes have been defined on the basis of whether accelerated plasma clearance of vWF accounts for the disorder.[71]

Type 2 vWD

Type 2A is mainly inherited as autosomal dominant, but recessive inheritance has also been described. Patients with type 2A vWD have normal to low vWF:Ag levels with disproportionately lower vWF:RCo and an abnormal multimer pattern characterized by loss of high-molecular-weight multimers. The reduction in high-molecular weight-multimers may be the result of abnormal biosynthesis of the larger multimers of vWF or alternatively, increased susceptibility of these multimers to proteolysis.[72] There is reduced responsiveness to ristocetin in the RIPA test.

Type 2B can be identified because of increased response to ristocetin in the RIPA test despite the absence of large multimers in plasma. It is most commonly inherited in an autosomal dominant manner. There may be mild thrombocytopenia as the large multimers bind to platelets spontaneously in plasma and the subsequent aggregates may be cleared from the circulation. The degree of baseline thrombocytopenia may be exaggerated during periods of stress (for example, after surgery or during pregnancy).

2M vWD is usually an autosomal dominant disorder with a reduced vWF:RCo to vWF:Ag ratio but normal vWF multimer distribution (differentiating it from type 2A), and reduced binding of abnormal vWF to GP1b/V/IX on platelets.

Type 2N (N for Normandy) vWD is characterized by normal levels of vWF:Ag and vWF:RCo, normal multimeric structure but low plasma FVIII:C levels. The inheritance is autosomal recessive, in contrast to hemophilia A, which is inherited in a sex-linked recessive manner. It is due to a decreased plasma half-life of FVIII, which has reduced binding affinity to vWF.[73]

Type 3 vWD, or severe vWD, is a rare disorder that is inherited as a homozygous or double heterozygous genetic disorder with an estimated incidence of 1–5 : 1 000 000. It is characterized by a near or complete absence or vWF and severely diminished levels of FVIII. (1–5 IU/dl). Therefore, patients with type 3 vWD clinically manifest symptoms of mucocutaneous hemorrhages as well as the hemarthroses and hematomas that are reminiscent of severe hemophilia.[74]

Platelet type or pseudo-vWD is a primary platelet disorder characterized by an increased affinity of the platelet GP1b/IX/V complex for normal vWF.[75] These patients have clinical and laboratory features similar to those of type 2B vWD. It can be distinguished from type 2B vWD in the RIPA test, as already described.

Management of vWD

In general, treatment is dictated primarily by the vWD type, and therefore a thorough laboratory evaluation is warranted prior to initiation of treatment. The goals of treatment are to correct quantitative or qualitative deficiencies in vWF, platelets and FVIII. Treatment options include DDAVP, clotting factor concentrates, platelet transfusions and/or antifibrinolytics (Table 34.4).

1-Deamino-8-D-arginine vasopressin (DDAVP) or desmopressin

DDAVP, as discussed above, increases both the FVIII:C and vWF plasma concentrations.[30,31] The mechanism whereby it achieves this effect is still not completely elucidated. Advantages of DDAVP include its relative inexpense (compared to clotting factor concentrate), ease of administration (it is often administered by patients at home as a nasal spray), and the absence of risk of blood-borne virus transmission. Dosing is similar to that used in mild hemophilia at 0.3 µg/kg.[32,33] When given intravenously, the FVIII and vWF levels are usually increased three- to fivefold above basal levels within 30 minutes. DDAVP is most effective in type 1 vWD, especially in the platelet normal type and in those without

Table 34.4 Management of different types and subtypes of vWD

	Subtype distribution		Inheritance pattern	Treatment
Type 1	70%		Autosomal dominant	DDAVP, factor VIII concentrates rich in VWF
Type 2	15–20%	2A	Autosomal dominant	Factor VIII concentrates rich in VWF
		2B	Autosomal dominant	Factor VIII concentrates rich in VWF
		2N	Autosomal recessive	Factor VIII concentrates rich in VWF
		2M	Autosomal dominant	DDAVP, factor VIII concentrates rich in VWF
Type 3	2–5%		Autosomal recessive	Factor VIII concentrates rich in VWF

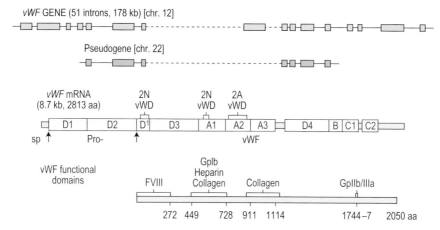

Fig. 34.5 The vWF gene, mRNA and protein. *(Reproduced with permission from Ginsburg D. The molecular biology of von Willebrand disease. May 1999. Haemophilia 5(suppl 2): 19–27).*

accelerated clearance of vWF from plasma. It is contraindicated in type 2B vWD because of the transient induction of thrombocytopenia.[76] Patients with type 3 vWD are usually unresponsive to DDAVP.

Antifibrinolytics

Both tranexamic acid and aminocaproic acid are antifibrinolytic agents that can be used alone or as adjunctive treatments in vWD. These agents promote clot stabilization by inhibiting plasmin-mediated fibrinolysis. A recent randomized study compared tranexamic acid to intranasal DDAVP in a group of women with menorrhagia and abnormal laboratory hemostasis that included patients with vWD. This study showed that both tranexamic acid and intranasal DDAVP improved menstrual blood loss and quality of life but that tranexamic acid was more effective.[77] Anti-fibrinolytic agents are relatively contraindicated in patients with an underlying prothrombotic condition, because of the risk of thrombosis. They are also contraindicated in the management of gross hematuria from the upper urinary tract as resultant ureteral obstruction by insoluble clot has been described.

Clotting factor concentrates

Replacement therapy with products containing vWF is often necessary in patients with more severe vWD or in situations when prior therapies have failed to control bleeding. For patients who are unresponsive to DDAVP, blood products containing FVIII and vWF are the treatment of choice. Cryoprecipitate was the mainstay of vWD treatment for many years. However, since virucidal methods cannot be applied to cryoprecipitate, this option has largely been replaced in the well-resourced world with plasma-derived clotting factor concentrates. There are several products available that contain vWF and FVIII. These are available as intermediate-purity FVIII products that have been licensed in many countries for the treatment of both hemophilia A (where they are dosed in FVIII units) and vWD (dosed in ristocetin co-factor units). A recombinant vWF product is currently in pre-clinical development.

Estrogens

Estrogen therapy has for many years been regarded as a useful adjunctive therapy in women with vWD. It is believed that estrogens increase the rate of endothelial vWF synthesis; however, the clinical effect is variable and its efficacy in vWD and menorrhagia may be mediated through changes in the endothelium that make severe bleeding less likely.[78]

The molecular basis of vWD

vWF cDNA was first cloned in 1985 by four independent groups.[79–82] It was then possible to deduce the structure of the protein which was later confirmed by direct amino acid sequencing.[83] Fig. 34.5 illustrates the specific functional domains within vWF. In addition to the large and complex vWF gene, there is a conserved partial pseudogene which may complicate genotyping analysis.[80] The vWF gene spans 178 kb on the short arm of chromosome 12 and is composed of 52 exons.

The first genetic defects identified in patients with vWD were large deletions associated with type 3 vWD.[84] Following the introduction of PCR techniques, it was possible to amplify and sequence small amounts of vWF mRNA from peripheral blood platelets which led to the identification of the first point mutations in type 2A vWD pedigrees.[85]

The International Society on Thrombosis and Hemostasis has established a database on mutations in vWF which can be found at www.ragtimedesign.com/vwf/mutation (Table 34.1).

The identification of specific genetic defects has enabled an understanding of the molecular basis of the different vWD subtypes. For example, mutations in the A1 domain of vWF, the location responsible for binding to platelet GP1b alpha, are usually found in patients with type 2B vWD.[86]

Rare inherited bleeding disorders

Hemophilia A and B and vWD represent approximately 85% of the inherited bleeding disorders. The other 15% of congenital disorders of hemostasis comprises deficiencies in fibrinogen, prothrombin, factor V, combined V/VIII, VII, X,

XI, XIII. and α_2-plasmin inhibitor (α_2-PI). Many of these disorders are inherited in an autosomal recessive fashion, and they are therefore more prevalent in societies in which consanguinity is a cultural norm, and/or where a founder effect has arisen (see Table 34.1 for available online mutation databases and Table 34.2 for features of coagulation factor deficient states).

Disorders of fibrinogen

Congenital disorders of fibrinogen may result from absent production (afibrinogenemia) or synthesis of a dysfunctional protein (dysfibrinogenemia). Fibrinogen is a 340 kD homodimer composed of two identical pairs of three chains, α, β and γ, that are connected by three disulfide bonds. These chains are encoded on three genes (FGA, FGB, FGG) located on chromosome 4 and synthesized by hepatocytes.[87] A list of reported FGA, FGB and FGG mutations is available online at www.hgmd.org (Table 34.1). Afibrinogenemia may result from a mutation in any of these genes. However, defects in the FGA gene are the most common cause of afibrinogenemia.[88,89]

Congenital afibrinogenemia can result in a bleeding disorder of variable severity.[90] It is inherited in an autosomal recessive fashion with an incidence of 1–2 : 1 000 000. It is encountered more commonly in countries where consanguinity is practiced. Heterozygotes are usually asymptomatic. Symptoms often manifest in the neonatal period as umbilical stump bleeding or bleeding after circumcision.[90] In older individuals, bleeding can occur at any site and can be quite catastrophic – in particular there is a risk of spontaneous splenic rupture and intracranial hemorrhage.[91] There is an increased rate of miscarriage in the first trimester in women with afibrinogenemia.[92] There appears to be a paradoxical increased risk of thrombosis in afibrinogenemia, probably due to an absence of the inhibitory effect that is exerted on thrombin by fibrin. In this situation, thrombosis (particularly arterial) is believed to be explained by thrombin-mediated platelet activation.

Congenital dysfibrinogenemias, like the afibrinogenemias, are the result of defects in FGA, FGB, or FGG. The vast majority are due to missense point mutations that result in a dysfunctional protein. The congenital dysfibrinogenemias may lead to an asymptomatic (55%), hemorrhagic (25%) or thrombotic (10–20%) phenotype. Rarely, the disorder may result in both a hemorrhagic and thrombotic condition (1–2%).[93]

As there is considerable variability in the clinical presentation of the fibrinogen disorders, treatment should be individualized, but in general replacement therapy in patients with a hemorrhagic phenotype and/or fetal loss in pregnancy is given to increase the fibrinogen level to 50–100 mg/dl.[94]

Replacement therapy should be in the form of a specific fibrinogen concentrate when available. Failing this, cryoprecipitate and, less commonly, fresh frozen plasma (FFP) are used.[94] Recombinant fibrinogen is in pre-clinical development.

Prothrombin deficiency

Congenital prothrombin deficiency is extremely rare, with an estimated incidence of 1 : 2 000 000. It is inherited in an autosomal recessive manner. It is characterized by a concordant decrease in both prothrombin antigen and activity.[95] Aprothrombinemia has not been reported and is thought to be incompatible with life.

In the reported cases of hypoprothrombinemia, severe hemorrhage including intracranial hemorrhage, mucus membrane bleeding and deep-tissue bleeding have been reported. Although heterozygous individuals are usually asymptomatic, bleeding following tooth extraction and tonsillectomy has been reported.[96] There have also been reports of a bleeding disorder with congenital dysprothrombinemia with a reduced level of prothrombin activity compared to antigen.[97] The treatment for prothrombin deficiency is replacement with FFP or prothrombin complex concentrates (PCCs). A minimum target prothrombin level of 30 IU/dl has been suggested for hemostasis.[98]

Factor V deficiency

Congenital factor V (FV) deficiency is an autosomal recessive disorder, occurring in an estimated 1 : 1 000 000 of the population. FV deficiency may be mild, moderate or severe and is associated with mucus membrane bleeding, bruising and possibly intracranial hemorrhage.[99] The bleeding noted in severe (<1 IU/dl) deficiency is often less severe than would be predicted. Spontaneous hemarthroses are uncommon in comparison to severe deficiencies in FVIII and FIX. Combined deficiencies of FV and FVIII, discussed in greater detail below, should be considered in the differential diagnosis.[100] There are no FV concentrates available so the mainstay of treatment for FV deficiency is FFP at a dose of 15–20 ml/kg. Plasma exchange can be used preoperatively in patients who are unable to tolerate the required volume of transfusion.[101] Platelet transfusions may be used as a source of FV, even in patients who have developed neutralizing inhibitors to FV.[102] There are also case reports of rVIIa use in the treatment of patients with severe FV deficiency with inhibitors.[101]

The use of bovine thrombin contaminated with bovine FV during cardiac and other surgeries has been associated with the appearance of cross-reacting acquired anti-human FV inhibitors.[103] However, with the availability of newer topical human thrombin products, this should be regarded as an avoidable complication.

Combined factor V and VIII deficiency

The overall incidence of combined FV and FVIII deficiency (F5F8D), an autosomal recessive disorder, is approximately 1 : 2 000 000, although it is much more common in Middle Eastern Jews and Iranians of non-Jewish descent (1 : 100 000). Patients have detectable, but low antigen and activity levels of both factors in the 5–15 IU/dl range. In the more than 30 kindreds reported, affected subjects experience excessive postoperative bleeding, mucosal bleeding and hemarthrosis. Two mutations appear to be associated with all known cases of F5F8D and both involve secretory pathway proteins (LMAN-1 and MCFD2).[104] These patients require a combination of a FVIII concentrate and FFP to manage bleeding events.

Factor VII deficiency

FVII deficiency occurs at a rate of 1 : 500 000 individuals. Patients with less than 1 IU/dl FVII activity manifest a severe bleeding disorder. Those individuals with more than 5 IU/dl have relatively mild symptoms, with bleeding most commonly affecting mucus membranes; affected women may suffer severe menorrhagia. Factor VII activity correlates rather poorly with bleeding severity, but in general, only relatively modest amounts of circulating FVII are required for adequate hemostasis, and bleeding is uncommon – even with surgery – in individuals with FVII:C levels >15–20 IU/dl.[105,106]

Plasma-derived clotting factor concentrates of FVII are available in Europe but not in the United States. Recombinant human activated FVII (rFVIIa) is approved for use in the US and Europe for patients with FVII deficiency.[107,108] Prothrombin complex concentrates or FFP can be used to correct FVII deficiency when FVII concentrate or rFVIIa is unavailable.

Factor X deficiency

Congenital FX deficiency has an estimated incidence of 1 : 1,000,000 and is an autosomal recessive disorder.[109] Bleeding severity appears to correlate with FX activity, and it may be very severe. In a series of 32 Iranian patients with congenital FX deficiency, the most common bleeding symptoms were epistaxis, menorrhagia, hemarthrosis and spontaneous hematomas.[109] The preferred treatment of FX deficiency is with prothrombin complex concentrates. Acquired FX deficiency associated with amyloidosis is due to binding of FX to amyloid fibrils, and treatment of the underlying amyloidosis and/or splenectomy has been shown to improve the circulating FX level.[110]

Factor XI deficiency

FXI deficiency, also sometimes referred to as Rosenthal syndrome or hemophilia C, was originally described in three related individuals in an American Jewish family who presented with significant bleeding after dental procedures and tonsillectomy.[111] FXI deficiency is particularly common among Ashkenazi Jews where the gene frequency approaches 8–9%.[112] The inheritance is autosomal but not necessarily in a classical recessive fashion, as some heterozygotes are symptomatic, and some mutations in FXI are associated with an autosomal dominant inheritance pattern. Severe FXI deficiency, <15–20 IU/dl (normal range: 70–150 IU/dl), occurs in homozygous or compound heterozygous individuals and a partial deficiency, 20–70 IU/dl, occurs in heterozygous individuals.[113]

Jewish population studies have provided the majority of clinical and physiologic data on FXI deficiency. In 1989 Asakai et al. described the first three mutations resulting in severe FXI deficiency in six Jewish patients (types I, II, III).[114] Two years later, a fourth mutation (type IV) was described. Type II and III mutations are point mutations that occur with equal frequency in the Jewish population and are much more common than types I or IV. The majority of all Jewish patients with severe FXI deficiency are homozygotes (II/II, III/III) or compound heterozygotes (II/III).[115]

Severely affected individuals are at risk of bleeding after surgery, particularly in areas prone to fibrinolysis such as the oral cavity and the urogenital system. Bleeding is likely to occur after tonsillectomy, after dental extractions and after genitourinary procedures such as prostatectomy. Bleeding patterns, however, are often unpredictable and some patients with severe deficiency remain asymptomatic. An analysis of 247 bleeding histories in 50 kindreds showed that 30–50% of heterozygotes bled excessively, including some with levels of 50–70 IU/dl. Many of the affected women suffered with menorrhagia.[116]

Mild bleeding episodes may not require treatment. Several strategies for replacement have been described and include FFP, antifibrinolytic agents,[117] FXI concentrates (available in the UK and France),[118] and rFVIIa (not FDA approved for this purpose).[119]

FXI concentrates appear to be hemostatically effective, but disseminated intravascular coagulation and arterial thrombosis have been reported in up to 10% of recipients. The thrombotic potential has been addressed by the addition of heparin to the concentrate and by the recommendation that the dose should preferably be controlled to maintain levels no greater than 70 IU/dl. It has been suggested that such concentrates should be used with caution in individuals with pre-existing cardiovascular disease.[120]

Inhibitors to FXI are uncommon but may occur in patients with severe FXI deficiency after exposure to plasma infusions. Salomon et al. reported on 118 unrelated Israeli patients with severe FXI deficiency. Of the seven who developed an inhibitor, all were homozygous for the type II mutation and all had received replacement therapy with FFP.[121] These patients can be treated successfully with rFVIIa.[119]

Factor XIII deficiency

Congenital FXIII deficiency is a rare autosomal recessive condition with an incidence of 1 : 2 000 000 individuals in most societies.[122] Homozygous individuals have a level of <1 IU/dl, while heterozygous individuals who have levels of approximately 50 IU/dl do not experience abnormal bleeding. The most common presentation is bleeding from the umbilical stump.[123] Other bleeding symptoms include intracranial hemorrhage, hemarthrosis, menorrhagia and bleeding following trauma.[124] Delayed wound healing and spontaneous abortion may also result from FXIII deficiency.[125] Replacement therapy as FXIII concentrate, FFP or cryoprecipitate can be used. FXIII has a very long half-life of 8–12 days and the levels required to maintain hemostasis are only in the range of 2–5%. Factor concentrate can be used on a prophylactic basis.[126] A phase I trial of recombinant FXIII product has recently been described in patients with congenital deficiency.[126]

Vitamin K-dependent factor deficiencies

The vitamin K-dependent coagulation factors are factors II, VII, IX, X, proteins C and S. Combined deficiency of the vitamin K-dependent factors may result from missense mutations in the genes for vitamin K reductase (VKORC-1) or gamma-glutamyl carboxylase.[127–129] These rare autosomal recessive disorders have an estimated incidence of 1 : 2 000 000. Factor activity levels are variable and can range from 1% to 30%. Clinically patients may present with severe umbilical stump bleeding or intracranial hemorrhage.[130] Partial correction of the vitamin K-dependent factors may be accomplished by providing supplemental vitamin K at high doses in the majority of patients. In the setting of hemorrhagic symptoms, FFP or PCC may be used.

α_2-Plasmin inhibitor deficiency (aka α_2-antiplasmin deficiency)

α_2-Plasmin inhibitor deficiency is a rare autosomal recessive disorder that requires a high index of suspicion for diagnosis as screening tests are often unremarkable or only slightly abnormal. Homozygous patients typically present with menorrhagia, hematuria, epistaxis and hemarthrosis, while heterozygous patients may only demonstrate increased hemorrhagic symptoms following surgery or trauma. Bleeding relating to surgery is often temporally delayed. Antifibrinolytics are the cornerstone of treatment.

References

1. Lusher JM, McMillan CW. Severe factor VIII and factor IX deficiency in females. Am J Med 1978 Oct;65(4):637–48.

2. Gitschier J, Wood WI, Goralka TM, et al. Characterization of the human factor VIII gene. Nature 1984 Nov 22–28; 312(5992):326–30.

3. Toole JJ, Knopf JL, Wozney JM, et al. Molecular cloning of a cDNA encoding human antihaemophilic factor. Nature 1984 Nov 22–28;312(5992):342–7.

4. Vehar GA, Keyt B, Eaton D, et al. Structure of human factor VIII. Nature 1984 Nov 22–28;312(5992):337–42.

5. Tuddenham EG, Laffan MA. Inherited bleeding disorders. In: Hoffbrand AV, Mitchell Lewis S, Tuddenham EGD, editors. Postgrauate Haematology. Oxford: Butterworth Heinermann; 1999.

6. Kemball-Cook G, Tuddenham EG, Wacey AI. The factor VIII structure and mutation resource site: HAMSTeRS version 4. Nucleic Acids Res 1998 Jan 1; 26(1):216–9.

7. Lollar P. Pathogenic antibodies to coagulation factors. Part one: factor VIII and factor IX. J Thromb Haemost 2004 Jul;2(7):1082–95.

8. Goodeve AC, Peake IR. The molecular basis of hemophilia A: genotype-phenotype relationships and inhibitor development. Semin Thromb Hemost 2003 Feb;29(1):23–30.

9. Kasper CK, Lin JC. Prevalence of sporadic and familial haemophilia. Haemophilia 2007 Jan;13(1):90–2.

10. Crossley M, Ludwig M, Stowell KM, et al. Recovery from hemophilia B Leyden: an androgen-responsive element in the factor IX promoter. Science 1992 Jul 17; 257(5068):377–9.

11. Reijnen MJ, Peerlinck K, Maasdam D, et al. Hemophilia B Leyden: substitution of thymine for guanine at position-21 results in a disruption of a hepatocyte nuclear factor 4 binding site in the factor IX promoter. Blood 1993 Jul 1;82(1): 151–8.

12. Kurachi S, Huo JS, Ameri A, et al. An age-related homeostasis mechanism is essential for spontaneous amelioration of hemophilia B Leyden. Proc Natl Acad Sci U S A 2009 May 12;106(19): 7921–6.

13. Lee DH, Walker IR, Teitel J, et al. Effect of the factor V Leiden mutation on the clinical expression of severe hemophilia A. Thromb Haemost 2000 Mar;83(3): 387–91.

14. Shetty S, Vora S, Kulkarni B, et al. Contribution of natural anticoagulant and fibrinolytic factors in modulating the clinical severity of haemophilia patients. Br J Haematol 2007 Aug;138(4): 541–4.

15. van Dijk K, van der Bom JG, Fischer K, et al. Do prothrombotic factors influence clinical phenotype of severe haemophilia? A review of the literature. Thromb Haemost 2004 Aug;92(2): 305–10.

16. Escuriola Ettingshausen C, Halimeh S, Kurnik K, et al. Symptomatic onset of severe hemophilia A in childhood is dependent on the presence of prothrombotic risk factors. Thromb Haemost 2001 Feb;85(2):218–20.

17. Rodriguez-Merchan EC. Pathogenesis, early diagnosis, and prophylaxis for chronic hemophilic synovitis. Clin Orthop Relat Res 1997 Oct;(343):6–11.

18. Avina-Zubieta JA, Galindo-Rodriguez G, Lavalle C. Rheumatic manifestations of hematologic disorders. Curr Opin Rheumatol 1998 Jan;10(1):86–90.

19. Rodriguez Merchan EC. The haemophilic pseudotumour. Int Orthop 1995;19(4): 255–60.

20. Rizza CR, Spooner RJ, Giangrande PL. Treatment of haemophilia in the United Kingdom 1981–1996. Haemophilia 2001 Jul;7(4):349–59.

21. Wilde JT. Protease inhibitor therapy and bleeding. Haemophilia 2000 Sep;6(5): 487–90.

22. Soucie JM, Nuss R, Evatt B, et al. Mortality among males with hemophilia: relations with source of medical care. The Hemophilia Surveillance System Project Investigators. Blood 2000 Jul 15; 96(2):437–42.

23. Mannucci PM, Gdovin S, Gringeri A, et al. Transmission of hepatitis A to patients with hemophilia by factor VIII concentrates treated with organic solvent and detergent to inactivate viruses. The Italian Collaborative Group. Ann Intern Med 1994 Jan 1;120(1):1–7.

24. Wu CG, Mason B, Jong J, et al. Parvovirus B19 transmission by a high-purity factor VIII concentrate. Transfusion 2005 Jun;45(6):1003–10.

25. Ludlam CA, Powderly WG, Bozzette S, et al. Clinical perspectives of emerging pathogens in bleeding disorders. Lancet 2006 Jan 21;367(9506):252–61.

26. Busch MP, Glynn SA, Stramer SL, et al. A new strategy for estimating risks of transfusion-transmitted viral infections based on rates of detection of recently infected donors. Transfusion 2005 Feb; 45(2):254–64.

27. Choo KH, Gould KG, Rees DJ, Brownlee GG. Molecular cloning of the gene for human anti-haemophilic factor IX. Nature 1982 Sep 9;299(5879): 178–80.

28. Key NS, Negrier C. Coagulation factor concentrates: past, present, and future. Lancet 2007 Aug 4;370(9585): 439–48.

29. Party UK von Willebrand Working Party. Guidelines for the diagnosis and management of von Willebrand disease. Haemophilia 1997;3(Suppl. 2):1–25.

30. Cash JD, Gader AM, da Costa J. Proceedings. The release of plasminogen activator and factor VIII to lysine vasopressin, arginine vasopressin, 1-desamino-8-d-arginine vasopressin, angiotensin and oxytocin in man. Br J Haematol 1974 Jun;27(2):363–4.

31. Mannucci PM, Ruggeri ZM, Pareti FI, Capitanio A. 1-Deamino-8-d-arginine vasopressin: a new pharmacological approach to the management of haemophilia and von Willebrand's diseases. Lancet 1977 Apr 23;1(8017): 869–72.

32. Lethagen S, Ragnarson Tennvall G. Self-treatment with desmopressin intranasal spray in patients with bleeding disorders: effect on bleeding symptoms and socioeconomic factors. Ann Hematol 1993 May;66(5):257–60.

33. Rodeghiero F, Castaman G, Mannucci PM. Prospective multicenter study on subcutaneous concentrated desmopressin for home treatment of patients with von Willebrand disease and mild or moderate hemophilia A. Thromb Haemost 1996 Nov;76(5):692–6.

34. Mannucci PM, Bettega D, Cattaneo M. Patterns of development of tachyphylaxis in patients with haemophilia and von Willebrand disease after repeated doses of desmopressin (DDAVP). Br J Haematol 1992 Sep;82(1):87–93.

35. Bond L, Bevan D. Myocardial infarction in a patient with hemophilia treated with DDAVP. N Engl J Med 1988 Jan 14; 318(2):121.

36. Djulbegovic B, Marasa M, Pesto A, et al. Safety and efficacy of purified factor IX concentrate and antifibrinolytic agents for dental extractions in hemophilia B. Am J Hematol 1996 Feb;51(2): 168–70.

37. Davidson CS, Epstein RD, Miller GF, Taylor FHL. Hemophilia, a clinical study of 40 patients. Blood 1949 Feb;4(2): 97–119.

38. Lusher JM, Arkin S, Abildgaard CF, Schwartz RS. Recombinant factor VIII for the treatment of previously untreated patients with hemophilia A. Safety, efficacy, and development of inhibitors. Kogenate Previously Untreated Patient Study Group. N Engl J Med 1993 Feb 18; 328(7):453–9.

39. Hoyer LW, Scandella D. Factor VIII inhibitors: structure and function in autoantibody and hemophilia A patients. Semin Hematol 1994 Apr;31(2 Suppl. 4): 1–5.

40. Rasi V, Ikkala E. Haemophiliacs with factor VIII inhibitors in Finland: prevalence, incidence and outcome. Br J Haematol 1990 Nov;76(3):369–71.

41. Hay CR, Ludlam CA, Colvin BT, et al. Factor VIII inhibitors in mild and moderate-severity haemophilia A. UK Haemophilia Centre Directors Organisation. Thromb Haemost 1998 Apr;79(4):762–6.

42. Fijnvandraat K, Turenhout EA, van den Brink EN, et al. The missense mutation Arg593→Cys is related to antibody formation in a patient with mild hemophilia A. Blood 1997 Jun 15; 89(12):4371–7.

43. Lee C. Recombinant clotting factors in the treatment of hemophilia. Thromb Haemost 1999 Aug;82(2):516–24.

44. McMillan CW, Shapiro SS, Whitehurst D, et al. The natural history of factor VIII:C inhibitors in patients with hemophilia A: a national cooperative study. II. Observations on the initial development of factor VIII:C inhibitors. Blood 1988 Feb;71(2):344–8.

45. Sultan Y. Prevalence of inhibitors in a population of 3435 hemophilia patients in France. French Hemophilia Study Group. Thromb Haemost 1992 Jun 1; 67(6):600–2.

46. Goodeve AC, Williams I, Bray GL, Peake IR. Relationship between factor VIII mutation type and inhibitor development in a cohort of previously untreated patients treated with recombinant factor VIII (Recombinate).

Recombinate PUP Study Group. Thromb Haemost 2000 Jun;83(6):844–8.

47. Eckhardt CL, Menke LA, van Ommen CH, et al. Intensive peri-operative use of factor VIII and the Arg593→Cys mutation are risk factors for inhibitor development in mild/moderate hemophilia A. J Thromb Haemost 2009 Jun;7(6):930–7.

48. Astermark J, Berntorp E, White GC, Kroner BL. The Malmo International Brother Study (MIBS): further support for genetic predisposition to inhibitor development in hemophilia patients. Haemophilia 2001 May;7(3):267–72.

49. Viel KR, Ameri A, Abshire TC, et al. Inhibitors of factor VIII in black patients with hemophilia. N Engl J Med 2009 Apr 16;360(16):1618–27.

50. ter Avest PC, Fischer K, Mancuso ME, et al. Risk stratification for inhibitor development at first treatment for severe hemophilia A: a tool for clinical practice. J Thromb Haemost 2008 Dec;6(12): 2048–54.

51. Gouw SC, van der Bom JG, Marijke van den Berg H. Treatment-related risk factors of inhibitor development in previously untreated patients with hemophilia A: the CANAL cohort study. Blood 2007 Jun 1;109(11):4648–54.

52. Gouw SC, van der Bom JG, Auerswald G, et al. Recombinant versus plasma-derived factor VIII products and the development of inhibitors in previously untreated patients with severe hemophilia A: the CANAL cohort study. Blood 2007 Jun 1; 109(11):4693–7.

53. Mannucci PM, Gringeri A, Peyvandi F, Santagostino E. Factor VIII products and inhibitor development: the SIPPET study (survey of inhibitors in plasma-product exposed toddlers). Haemophilia 2007 Dec;13(Suppl. 5):65–8.

54. Goudemand J, Rothschild C, Demiguel V, et al. Influence of the type of factor VIII concentrate on the incidence of factor VIII inhibitors in previously untreated patients with severe hemophilia A. Blood 2006 Jan 1; 107(1):46–51.

55. Giangrande PL, Kessler CM, Jenkins CE, et al. Viral pharmacovigilance study of haemophiliacs receiving porcine factor VIII. Haemophilia 2002 Nov;8(6): 798–801.

56. van den Berg HM, Fischer K, Mauser-Bunschoten EP, et al. Long-term outcome of individualized prophylactic treatment of children with severe haemophilia. Br J Haematol 2001 Mar;112(3):561–5.

57. Manco-Johnson MJ, Abshire TC, Shapiro AD, et al. Prophylaxis versus episodic treatment to prevent joint disease in boys with severe hemophilia. N Engl J Med 2007 Aug 9;357(6):535–44.

58. Rodeghiero F, Castaman G, Dini E. Epidemiological investigation of the prevalence of von Willebrand's disease. Blood 1987 Feb;69(2):454–9.

59. Sadler JE, Mannucci PM, Berntorp E, et al. Impact, diagnosis and treatment of von Willebrand disease. Thromb Haemost 2000 Aug;84(2):160–74.

60. Rodeghiero F, Castaman G, Tosetto A, et al. The discriminant power of bleeding history for the diagnosis of type 1 von Willebrand disease: an international, multicenter study. J Thromb Haemost 2005 Dec;3(12):2619–26.

61. Hayward CP, Harrison P, Cattaneo M, et al. Platelet function analyzer (PFA)-100 closure time in the evaluation of platelet disorders and platelet function. J Thromb Haemost 2006 Feb;4(2):312–9.

62. Quiroga T, Goycoolea M, Munoz B, et al. Template bleeding time and PFA-100 have low sensitivity to screen patients with hereditary mucocutaneous hemorrhages: comparative study in 148 patients. J Thromb Haemost 2004 Jun; 2(6):892–8.

63. Veyradier A, Fressinaud E, Sigaud M, et al. A new automated method for von Willebrand factor antigen measurement using latex particles. Thromb Haemost 1999 Feb;81(2):320–1.

64. Favaloro EJ, Smith J, Petinos P, et al. Laboratory testing for von Willebrand's disease: an assessment of current diagnostic practice and efficacy by means of a multi-laboratory survey. RCPA Quality Assurance Program (QAP) in Haematology Haemostasis Scientific Advisory Panel. Thromb Haemost 1999 Oct;82(4):1276–82.

65. Riddell AF, Jenkins PV, Nitu-Whalley IC, et al. Use of the collagen-binding assay for von Willebrand factor in the analysis of type 2M von Willebrand disease: a comparison with the ristocetin cofactor assay. Br J Haematol 2002 Jan;116(1):187–92.

66. Nichols WL, Hultin MB, James AH, et al. von Willebrand disease (vWD): evidence-based diagnosis and management guidelines, the National Heart, Lung, and Blood Institute (NHLBI) Expert Panel report (USA). Haemophilia 2008 Mar;14(2):171–232.

67. The National Heart, Lung, and Blood Institute. The Evaluation and Management of Von Willebrand Disease, National Heart, Lung, and Blood Institute, National Institutes of Health, Bethesda 2007. Bethesda; 2007 [updated 2007; cited 2009 9/1/2009]; Available from: www.nhlbi.nih.gov/guidelines/vwd.

68. Nitu-Whalley IC, Lee CA, Griffioen A, et al. Type 1 von Willebrand disease – a clinical retrospective study of the diagnosis, the influence of the ABO blood group and the role of the bleeding history. Br J Haematol 2000 Feb;108(2): 259–64.

69. Sadler JE. A revised classification of von Willebrand disease. For the Subcommittee on von Willebrand Factor of the Scientific and Standardization

Committee of the International Society on Thrombosis and Haemostasis. Thromb Haemost 1994 Apr;71(4):520–5.

70. Weiss HJ, Meyer D, Rabinowitz R, et al. Pseudo-von Willebrand's disease. An intrinsic platelet defect with aggregation by unmodified human factor VIII/von Willebrand factor and enhanced adsorption of its high-molecular-weight multimers. N Engl J Med 1982 Feb 11;306(6):326–33.

71. Haberichter SL, Castaman G, Budde U, et al. Identification of type 1 von Willebrand disease patients with reduced von Willebrand factor survival by assay of the vWF propeptide in the European study: molecular and clinical markers for the diagnosis and management of type 1 VWD (MCMDM-1VWD). Blood 2008 May 15;111(10):4979–85.

72. Lyons SE, Bruck ME, Bowie EJ, Ginsburg D. Impaired intracellular transport produced by a subset of type IIA von Willebrand disease mutations. J Biol Chem 1992 Mar 5;267(7):4424–30.

73. Mazurier C, Dieval J, Jorieux S, et al. A new von Willebrand factor (vWF) defect in a patient with factor VIII (FVIII) deficiency but with normal levels and multimeric patterns of both plasma and platelet vWF. Characterization of abnormal vWF/FVIII interaction. Blood 1990 Jan 1;75(1):20–6.

74. Lak M, Peyvandi F, Mannucci PM. Clinical manifestations and complications of childbirth and replacement therapy in 385 Iranian patients with type 3 von Willebrand disease. Br J Haematol 2000 Dec;111(4):1236–9.

75. Miller JL, Castella A. Platelet-type von Willebrand's disease: characterization of a new bleeding disorder. Blood 1982 Sep;60(3):790–4.

76. Holmberg L, Nilsson IM, Borge L, et al. Platelet aggregation induced by 1-desamino-8-D-arginine vasopressin (DDAVP) in type IIB von Willebrand's disease. N Engl J Med 1983 Oct 6;309(14):816–21.

77. Kouides PA, Byams VR, Philipp CS, et al. Multisite management study of menorrhagia with abnormal laboratory haemostasis: a prospective crossover study of intranasal desmopressin and oral tranexamic acid. Br J Haematol 2009 Apr;145(2):212–20.

78. Harrison RL, McKee PA. Estrogen stimulates von Willebrand factor production by cultured endothelial cells. Blood 1984 Mar;63(3):657–64.

79. Ginsburg D, Handin RI, Bonthron DT, et al. Human von Willebrand factor (vWF): isolation of complementary DNA (cDNA) clones and chromosomal localization. Science 1985 Jun 21;228(4706):1401–6.

80. Sadler JE, Shelton-Inloes BB, Sorace JM, et al. Cloning and characterization of two cDNAs coding for human von

Willebrand factor. Proc Natl Acad Sci USA 1985 Oct;82(19):6394–8.

81. Verweij CL, de Vries CJ, Distel B, et al. Construction of cDNA coding for human von Willebrand factor using antibody probes for colony-screening and mapping of the chromosomal gene. Nucleic Acids Res 1985 Jul 11;13(13):4699–717.

82. Lynch DC, Zimmerman TS, Collins CJ, et al. Molecular cloning of cDNA for human von Willebrand factor: authentication by a new method. Cell 1985 May;41(1):49–56.

83. Titani K, Kumar S, Takio K, et al. Amino acid sequence of human von Willebrand factor. Biochemistry 1986 Jun 3;25(11):3171–84.

84. Shelton-Inloes BB, Chehab FF, Mannucci PM, et al. Gene deletions correlate with the development of alloantibodies in von Willebrand disease. J Clin Invest 1987 May;79(5):1459–65.

85. Ginsburg D, Konkle BA, Gill JC, et al. Molecular basis of human von Willebrand disease: analysis of platelet von Willebrand factor mRNA. Proc Natl Acad Sci USA 1989 May;86(10):3723–7.

86. Grainick HR, Williams SB, McKeown LP, et al. Von Willebrand's disease with spontaneous platelet aggregation induced by an abnormal plasma von Willebrand factor. J Clin Invest 1985 Oct;76(4):1522–9.

87. Tennent GA, Brennan SO, Stangou AJ, et al. Human plasma fibrinogen is synthesized in the liver. Blood 2007 Mar 1;109(5):1971–4.

88. Neerman-Arbez M, Honsberger A, Antonarakis SE, Morris MA. Deletion of the fibrinogen [correction of fibrogen] alpha-chain gene (FGA) causes congenital afibrogenemia. J Clin Invest 1999 Jan;103(2):215–8.

89. Duga S, Asselta R, Santagostino E, et al. Missense mutations in the human beta fibrinogen gene cause congenital afibrinogenemia by impairing fibrinogen secretion. Blood 2000 Feb 15;95(4):1336–41.

90. al-Mondhiry H, Ehmann WC. Congenital afibrinogenemia. Am J Hematol 1994 Aug;46(4):343–7.

91. Shima M, Tanaka I, Sawamoto Y, et al. Successful treatment of two brothers with congenital afibrinogenemia for splenic rupture using heat- and solvent detergent-treated fibrinogen concentrates. J Pediatr Hematol Oncol 1997 Sep–Oct;19(5):462–5.

92. Evron S, Anteby SO, Brzezinsky A, et al. Congenital afibrinogenemia and recurrent early abortion: a case report. Eur J Obstet Gynecol Reprod Biol 1985 May;19(5):307–11.

93. Haverkate F, Samama M. Familial dysfibrinogenemia and thrombophilia. Report on a study of the SSC

Subcommittee on Fibrinogen. Thromb Haemost 1995 Jan;73(1):151–61.

94. Mannucci PM, Duga S, Peyvandi F. Recessively inherited coagulation disorders. Blood 2004 Sep 1;104(5):1243–52.

95. Akhavan S, Mannucci PM, Lak M, et al. Identification and three-dimensional structural analysis of nine novel mutations in patients with prothrombin deficiency. Thromb Haemost 2000 Dec;84(6):989–97.

96. Girolami A, Scarano L, Saggiorato G, et al. Congenital deficiencies and abnormalities of prothrombin. Blood Coagul Fibrinolysis 1998 Oct;9(7):557–69.

97. Poort SR, Michiels JJ, Reitsma PH, Bertina RM. Homozygosity for a novel missense mutation in the prothrombin gene causing a severe bleeding disorder. Thromb Haemost 1994 Dec;72(6):819–24.

98. Bolton-Maggs PH, Perry DJ, Chalmers EA, et al. The rare coagulation disorders – review with guidelines for management from the United Kingdom Haemophilia Centre Doctors' Organisation. Haemophilia 2004 Sep;10(5):593–628.

99. Salooja N, Martin P, Khair K, et al. Severe factor V deficiency and neonatal intracranial haemorrhage: a case report. Haemophilia 2000 Jan;6(1):44–6.

100. Peyvandi F, Tuddenham EG, Akhtari AM, et al. Bleeding symptoms in 27 Iranian patients with the combined deficiency of factor V and factor VIII. Br J Haematol 1998 Mar;100(4):773–6.

101. Sallah AS, Angchaisuksiri P, Roberts HR. Use of plasma exchange in hereditary deficiency of factor V and factor VIII. Am J Hematol 1996 Jul;52(3):229–30.

102. Chediak J, Ashenhurst JB, Garlick I, Desser RK. Successful management of bleeding in a patient with factor V inhibitor by platelet transfusions. Blood 1980 Nov;56(5):835–41.

103. Rapaport SI, Zivelin A, Minow RA, et al. Clinical significance of antibodies to bovine and human thrombin and factor V after surgical use of bovine thrombin. Am J Clin Pathol 1992 Jan;97(1):84–91.

104. Zhang B, McGee B, Yamaoka JS, et al. Combined deficiency of factor V and factor VIII is due to mutations in either LMAN1 or MCFD2. Blood 2006 Mar 1;107(5):1903–7.

105. Barnett JM, Demel KC, Mega AE, et al. Lack of bleeding in patients with severe factor VII deficiency. Am J Hematol 2005 Feb;78(2):134–7.

106. Giansily-Blaizot M, Verdier R, Biron-Adreani C, et al. Analysis of biological phenotypes from 42 patients with inherited factor VII deficiency: can biological tests predict the bleeding risk? Haematologica 2004 Jun;89(6):704–9.

107. Scharrer I. Recombinant factor VIIa for patients with inhibitors to factor VIII or

IX or factor VII deficiency. Haemophilia 1999 Jul;5(4):253–9.

108. Mariani G, Testa MG, Di Paolantonio T, et al. Use of recombinant, activated factor VII in the treatment of congenital factor VII deficiencies. Vox Sang 1999; 77(3):131–6.

109. Peyvandi F, Mannucci PM, Lak M, et al. Congenital factor X deficiency: spectrum of bleeding symptoms in 32 Iranian patients. Br J Haematol 1998 Jul; 102(2):626–8.

110. Furie B, Voo L, McAdam KP, Furie BC. Mechanism of factor X deficiency in systemic amyloidosis. N Engl J Med 1981 Apr 2;304(14):827–30.

111. Rosenthal RL, Dreskin OH, Rosenthal N. Plasma thromboplastin antecedent (PTA) deficiency; clinical, coagulation, therapeutic and hereditary aspects of a new hemophilia-like disease. Blood 1955 Feb;10(2):120–31.

112. Seligsohn U. Factor XI deficiency. Thromb Haemost 1993 Jul 1;70(1): 68–71.

113. Bolton-Maggs PH, Young Wan-Yin B, McCraw AH, et al. Inheritance and bleeding in factor XI deficiency. Br J Haematol 1988 Aug;69(4):521–8.

114. Asakai R, Chung DW, Ratnoff OD, Davie EW. Factor XI (plasma thromboplastin antecedent) deficiency in Ashkenazi Jews is a bleeding disorder that can result from three types of point mutations. Proc Natl Acad Sci USA 1989 Oct;86(20):7667–71.

115. Asakai R, Chung DW, Davie EW, Seligsohn U. Factor XI deficiency in Ashkenazi Jews in Israel. N Engl J Med 1991 Jul 18;325(3):153–8.

116. Bolton-Maggs PH, Patterson DA, Wensley RT, Tuddenham EG. Definition of the bleeding tendency in factor XI-deficient kindreds – a clinical and laboratory study. Thromb Haemost 1995 Feb; 73(2):194–202.

117. Berliner S, Horowitz I, Martinowitz U, et al. Dental surgery in patients with severe factor XI deficiency without plasma replacement. Blood Coagul Fibrinolysis 1992 Aug;3(4):465–8.

118. Mannucci PM, Bauer KA, Santagostino E, et al. Activation of the coagulation cascade after infusion of a factor XI concentrate in congenitally deficient patients. Blood 1994 Aug 15;84(4): 1314–9.

119. O'Connell NM. Factor XI deficiency. Semin Hematol 2004 Jan;41(1 Suppl. 1): 76–81.

120. Bolton-Maggs PH, Colvin BT, Satchi BT, et al. Thrombogenic potential of factor XI concentrate. Lancet 1994 Sep 10; 344(8924):748–9.

121. Salomon O, Zivelin A, Livnat T, et al. Prevalence, causes, and characterization of factor XI inhibitors in patients with inherited factor XI deficiency. Blood 2003 Jun 15;101(12):4783–8.

122. Eshghi P, Abolghasemi H, Sanei-Moghaddam E, et al. Factor XIII deficiency in south-east Iran. Haemophilia 2004 Sep;10(5): 470–2.

123. Kitchens CS, Newcomb TF. Factor XIII. Medicine (Baltimore) 1979 Nov;58(6): 413–29.

124. Abbondanzo SL, Gootenberg JE, Lofts RS, McPherson RA. Intracranial hemorrhage in congenital deficiency of factor XIII. Am J Pediatr Hematol Oncol 1988 Spring;10(1):65–8.

125. Rodeghiero F, Castaman GC, Di Bona E, et al. Successful pregnancy in a woman with congenital factor XIII deficiency treated with substitutive therapy. Report of a second case. Blut 1987 Jul;55(1): 45–8.

126. Brackmann HH, Egbring R, Ferster A, et al. Pharmacokinetics and tolerability of factor XIII concentrates prepared from human placenta or plasma: a crossover randomised study. Thromb Haemost 1995 Aug;74(2):622–5.

127. Darghouth D, Hallgren KW, Shtofman RL, et al. Compound heterozygosity of novel missense mutations in the gamma-glutamyl-carboxylase gene causes hereditary combined vitamin K-dependent coagulation factor deficiency. Blood 2006 Sep 15; 108(6):1925–31.

128. Rost S, Fregin A, Ivaskevicius V, et al. Mutations in VKORC1 cause warfarin resistance and multiple coagulation factor deficiency type 2. Nature 2004 Feb 5;427(6974):537–41.

129. Wu SM, Stanley TB, Mutucumarana VP, Stafford DW. Characterization of the gamma-glutamyl carboxylase. Thromb Haemost 1997 Jul;78(1):599–604.

130. Brenner B, Tavori S, Zivelin A, et al. Hereditary deficiency of all vitamin K-dependent procoagulants and anticoagulants. Br J Haematol 1990 Aug;75(4):537–42.

CHAPTER 35

Acquired bleeding disorders

DJ Perry, C Grove

Chapter contents

©2011 Elsevier Ltd
DOI: 10.1016/B978-0-7020-3147-2.00035-3

Table 35.1 Disorders associated with an acquired hemostatic defect

Physiological deficiencies Neonates	*Vitamin K deficiency* Neonates Gastrointestinal disease Vitamin K antagonists Biliary obstruction Liver disease Miscellaneous, e.g. cephalosporins, parenteral nutrition
Liver disease	*Disseminated intravascular coagulation*
Drug induced bleeding Anticoagulants Thrombolytic agents Anti-platelet agents Miscellaneous	*Renal disease and renal failure*
Massive blood transfusion	*Cardiopulmonary bypass and extracorporeal circuits*
Acquired inhibitors of coagulation Factor VIII inhibitors Other factor inhibitors Anti-phospholipid antibodies	*Miscellaneous* Snake venoms and other toxic agents Myeloproliferative disorders Malignancy Paraproteinemias

Introduction

Acquired disorders of hemostasis are significantly more common than inherited disorders of hemostasis and as such are frequently encountered in routine clinical practice. Acquired disorders of coagulation may be physiological such as those that are seen in pregnancy, the newborn and with advancing age or they may be pathological. The latter often arise as a complication of multi-system disease and may therefore be associated with multiple clotting abnormalities (Table 35.1).

Physiological deficiencies

Neonates

The coagulation system of the newborn infant is complex and reflects hepatic immaturity. Most of the clotting factors are present in reduced concentration in the newborn infant apart from factors V, VIII and fibrinogen.[1-3] These physiological deficiencies in clotting factors result in prolongation of the prothrombin time (PT) and activated partial thromboplastin time (APTT) and as a consequence of this, reference ranges reflecting both gestational and neonatal age must be used to assess coagulation in the neonate.[1-3] The platelet count is normal in the neonate although there may be a qualitative platelet abnormality. Fibrinolysis in the neonate is similar to that of adults.

The pattern of bleeding seen in neonates – umbilical bleeding, cephalohematomas, bleeding after circumcision, oozing after venepuncture and bleeding into the skin – is different from that seen in adults.

Drug-induced bleeding disorders

Drugs are a common cause of an acquired bleeding disorder. In many cases the drug may be obvious, e.g. an anticoagulant, but in other cases it may be less clear, as with the inhibitory effect on vitamin K metabolism observed with some cephalosporins.[4]

Heparin

Unfractionated heparin (UFH), the low molecular weight heparins (LMWHs) and fondaparinux (a synthetic pentasaccharide) are anticoagulants that potentiate the action of antithrombin by increasing its inhibitory activity.[5] The inhibitory activity of UFH is directed against both thrombin (IIa) and factor Xa whereas that of the LMWH is primarily against factor Xa.[5] Fondaparinux has exclusively anti-Xa activity. Bleeding in patients receiving heparin is usually secondary to excessive anticoagulation. Heparin is metabolized by the liver and excreted by the kidneys and LMWHs may accumulate in patients with impaired renal function[6] and a dosage adjustment may be required if the creatinine clearance is less than 30 ml/min.

In patients receiving unfractionated heparin intravenously the rate of major hemorrhage ranges from 0%–7%. Fatal bleeding with a 5–14 day course of heparin ranges from 0%–2%. The risk of hemorrhage is significantly increased if there is concomitant use of other anticoagulants particularly anti-platelet agents such as aspirin or clopidogrel. Other patient-specific factors, including impaired renal function, disordered liver function, thrombocytopenia and invasive procedures, significantly increase the risk of bleeding. In individuals who are actively bleeding, unfractionated heparin can be effectively neutralized by protamine sulphate, a strongly basic drug that binds to the heparin. A dose of 1 mg of protamine sulphate will neutralize approximately 100 units of heparin. In overdose, protamine sulphate can function as an anticoagulant and no more than 50 mg of protamine sulphate should be administered at any one time. Protamine sulphate neutralizes only 60% of the anti-Xa activity of the low molecular weight heparins and is, therefore, less effective in correcting the bleeding problems associated with their use.[7] Protamine sulphate does not bind to fondaparinux and is, therefore, of no value in the management of patients on fondaparinux who are bleeding.

Laboratory monitoring[8]

1. *Unfractionated heparin*: therapeutic anticoagulation with UFH is monitored by means of the APTT aiming to maintain the APTT at 1.5–2x the mid-point of the reference range. In patients in whom the APTT is prolonged prior to the initiation of anticoagulation therapy, e.g. factor XII deficiency or a lupus anticoagulant, the measurement of anti-Xa levels may be necessary.

2. *LMWH and fondaparinux*: LMWHs have primarily anti-Xa activity and have little effect upon the APTT unless given in overdose. For patients receiving

therapeutic LMWHs, routine monitoring is not usually indicated but may be in children, obese or underweight patients, or those with renal disease, pregnancy or unexpected bleeding or thromboses while on treatment. In patients receiving thromboprophylaxis with a LMWH, routine monitoring is not usually necessary. Fondaparinux inhibits exclusively Xa and so its activity, when necessary, is monitored using an anti-Xa assay. The elimination of fondaparinux from the body is reduced in individuals with renal impairment as the drug is primarily excreted in the urine. The clearance of fondaparinux from the body is reduced by approximately 25%, 40%, and 55% in patients with mild, moderate, and severe kidney impairment, respectively.

Hirudin and bivalirudin

Hirudin was originally isolated from the medicinal leech *Hirudo medicinalis* but now is available in a recombinant form (r-hirudin or lepirudin). Bivalirudin is a small (MW 2180 Da) synthetic peptide modeled after hirudin, which contains 20 amino acids and two thrombin-binding domains. Bivalirudin and lepirudin are direct thrombin inhibitors and bind to both the catalytic site and the anion-binding exosite of circulating and clot-bound thrombin but do not require antithrombin for their anticoagulant activity.[9–11] Lepirudin and bivalirudin inhibit the conversion of fibrinogen to fibrin but also other thrombin-catalyzed reactions, for example activation of clotting factors and thrombin-induced platelet aggregation.

Lepirudin is a potent anticoagulant but has a very narrow therapeutic window and plasma levels of lepirudin show high levels of inter-individual variability even when the dose is adjusted for body weight. Over-anticoagulation with lepirudin can lead to severe bleeding problems. Lepirudin has a short half-life and its natural clearance through the kidneys may be sufficiently rapid such that in cases of overdose, specific neutralization is not required. In bleeding patients rVIIa or prothrombin complex concentrates may be of value or alternatively plasmaphoresis or exchange transfusion may remove lepirudin from the circulation.

Newer anticoagulants

Dabigatran etexilate is a pro-drug that is converted to dabigatran by esterase-catalyzed hydrolysis in the liver and the plasma. Dabigatran is a direct thrombin inhibitor which inhibits both clot-bound and free thrombin. Dabigatran is cleared primarily by the kidneys (85%) and a smaller amount (6%) is excreted in the feces.

Dabigatran is licensed for the primary prevention of venous thromboembolism in adult patients who have undergone elective total hip or knee replacement surgery. Laboratory monitoring of dabigatran is not routinely indicated although it is possible that in some cases, for example in the bleeding patient, this may be of value. The APTT shows a non-linear response to increasing doses of dabigatran and appears less sensitive and less precise than an ecarin clotting time (ECT). The ECT may provide a method for monitoring patients on dabigatran. To date no simple mechanism exists for the rapid reversal of dabigatran in, for example, the bleeding patient.

Rivaroxaban is an oral and highly selective inhibitor of factor Xa which inhibits free Xa and Xa bound to the pro-thrombinase complex. Rivaroxaban is licensed for the primary prevention of venous thromboembolism in adult patients who have undergone elective total hip or knee replacement surgery. A specific antidote to rivaroxaban is not available. Monitoring of rivaroxaban is not generally indicated and although the APTT is prolonged it is not recommended as a method for laboratory monitoring.

Laboratory monitoring

Therapeutic anticoagulation with lepirudin or bivalirudin is commonly monitored by the activated partial thromboplastin time (APTT) but there is considerable inter-individual variability in the degree of prolongation of the APTT at identical plasma levels of these drugs. The 'ecarin' clotting time (ECT) has been suggested as a more accurate test for monitoring individuals receiving direct thrombin inhibitors[12] including dabigatran if needed. Ecarin is isolated from the venom of the saw-scaled viper *Echis carinatus* and in the assay a known amount of ecarin is added to the plasma. Ecarin activates prothrombin to meizothrombin – this activity is inhibited by lepirudin but is unaffected by heparin. The meizothrombin induces clotting via fibrinogen cleavage to fibrin. This prolongation in the clotting time increases in a linear fashion with increasing concentrations of lepirudin but also with bivalirudin, dabigatran and argatroban, another direct thrombin inhibitor. The ecarin chromogenic assay employs a similar approach but the concentration of meizothrombin is measured using a chromogenic substrate.[13]

Warfarin and vitamin K antagonists

Warfarin is a 4-hydroxycoumarin derivative that exerts its action by blocking the regeneration of vitamin K from its epoxide. The major complication of all vitamin K antagonists is bleeding and this risk increases as the intensity of treatment, i.e. the INR, increases.[14,15] Independent risk factors for bleeding during long-term warfarin therapy include age greater than 65 years, a history of past gastrointestinal bleeding, stroke, atrial fibrillation and one or more of three co-morbid conditions: myocardial infarction, renal insufficiency and severe anemia.[16] For any individual the risk of bleeding is related to the duration of anticoagulant therapy although the risk may be higher in the early phase of treatment. Most studies in unselected groups of patients suggest that the risk of major bleeding is ~3% per annum and that CNS hemorrhage occurs at a rate of 0.1% per annum.[17]

The anticoagulant action of warfarin is potentiated by many drugs and these include:

- Drugs that displace warfarin from its plasma protein binding sites, e.g. statins
- Drugs that inhibit the metabolic clearance of warfarin, e.g. cimetidine, omeprazole, amiodarone, allopurinol
- Drugs that interfere with vitamin K metabolism, e.g. cephalosporins, high dose salicylates
- Drugs that independently increase the anticoagulant action, e.g. clofibrate, anabolic steroids, erythromycin.

Minor bleeding episodes in patients receiving oral anticoagulants may be treated with local measures and withdrawal of the drug. In cases of severe or life-threatening hemorrhage, rapid reversal of anticoagulation is required and this is most effectively achieved by the use of a combination of vitamin K and clotting factor concentrates (containing factors II, VII, IX and X) and less effectively by vitamin K and fresh frozen plasma.[18]

Phenindione. Phenindione is a vitamin K antagonist but differs from warfarin in its chemical structure. The degree of anticoagulation induced by phenindione is monitored by the INR although the dosing is different from that of warfarin with a loading dose of 200 mg on day 1, 100 mg on day 2 with subsequent dosing based upon the INR. The normal maintenance dose lies between 50 and 150 mg/day. Phenindione is rarely used because of the higher risk of side-effects including skin rashes and abnormal liver function tests.

Laboratory monitoring

Warfarin and other vitamin K antagonists are monitored by measuring the International Normalised Ratio (INR). The INR is the ratio of the prothrombin time of a patient divided by the mean normal prothrombin time of a normal plasma pool corrected for the sensitivity of the tissue factor used in the test:

$$\left[\frac{\text{Patient Prothrombin time in seconds}}{\text{Normal mean Prothrombin time of a donor plasma pool}} \right]^{ISI}$$

where the ISI (International Sensitivity Index) is a value derived by calibrating the tissue factor used in the assay against an international WHO standard, the ISI of which is 1.0. For an individual who is not on warfarin the INR is 1.0. The target INR for any patient varies depending upon the indication for treatment but is usually 2.5, 3.0 or 3.5. The risk of bleeding on any VKA increases as the INR increases and patients with a target INR of 3.5 have a significantly greater risk of hemorrhage than those with a target INR of 2.5.[17]

Thrombolytic agents

Thrombolytic drugs act by stimulating endogenous fibrinolysis. T-PA or U-PA convert plasminogen to plasmin, a potent proteolytic enzyme which breaks down both cross-linked and non-cross-linked fibrin. The currently available thrombolytic agents include:

- Recombinant human tissue plasminogen activator (rt-PA)
- Urokinase (U-PA)
- Reteplase – a recombinant non-glycosylated form of human t-PA that contains only 357 of the 527 amino acids of the original protein
- Tenecteplase – a recombinant fibrin-specific form of t-PA but engineered at three sites to confer a higher fibrin specificity than native t-PA and a greater resistance to inactivation by endogenous plasminogen activator type I (PAI-1) – the major inhibitor of t-PA
- Staphylokinase
- Streptokinase and its anisolyated derivative APSAC.

T-PA, urokinase, reteplase and tenecteplase produce their pharmacological actions by converting plasminogen to plasmin at the site of fibrin deposition. In contrast staphylokinase and streptokinase bind to free plasminogen in the plasma leading to systemic hyperfibrinolysis. Bleeding occurs in 3–40% of patients receiving thrombolytic therapy and this risk is greatly increased in patients who are also receiving anti-platelet drugs or other anticoagulants.[19] Thrombolytic therapy predisposes to bleeding by depleting the plasma concentration of procoagulant proteins and by the generation of anticoagulant fibrin(ogen) degradation products. Thrombolytic therapy cannot distinguish between a pathological thrombus occluding a critical vessel, e.g. coronary artery, and a physiological thrombus that is preventing bleeding from a critical site, e.g. in the cerebral circulation. Platelet function in patients receiving thrombolytic therapy is also impaired because of inhibition of platelet aggregation by high levels of FDPs and also by impaired platelet adhesion by plasmin-induced proteolysis of glycoprotein Ib (GpIb) and von Willebrand factor (vWF).[20]

For patients receiving thrombolytic therapy and who develop minor bleeding episodes the thrombolytic agent, together with any anticoagulant or anti-platelet agent, must be discontinued. For life-threatening bleeding episodes, a fibrinolytic inhibitor should be given e.g. tranexamic acid. Fresh frozen plasma and/or cryoprecipitate or a fibrinogen concentrate should be given to restore depleted clotting factors.[19]

Laboratory monitoring

Laboratory monitoring of thrombolytic therapy is often unnecessary when its administration is short-term. However, during a more prolonged infusion (>24 hours) sequential monitoring may be of value. Fibrinolytic therapy alters most laboratory tests of coagulation but few tests predict either the efficacy of thrombolysis or the risks of bleeding. The APTT is prolonged in patients receiving thrombolytic therapy because of depletion of fibrinogen, factors V and VIII and the generation of high levels of fibrin(ogen) degradation products. An APTT ratio of 1.5 indicates significant systemic fibrinolysis.[19] Plasma fibrinogen concentration falls during thrombolytic therapy reflecting the presence of free plasmin within the circulation. The fibrinolytic activity of the plasma can be measured by means of the euglobulin clot lysis time (ELT) which is shortened in patients receiving thrombolytic therapy but this is rarely, if ever, used. The thromboelastogram (TEG) may be of value and is considerably easier to perform than the ELT.

Anti-platelet drugs

A wide variety of drugs are in common use that have potent anti-platelet actions and such drugs are often used in combination, for example aspirin and clopidogrel. The risk of hemorrhage is significantly increased when anti-platelet drugs are used in combination with other anticoagulants, for example warfarin and aspirin.

1. Aspirin and non-steroidal anti-inflammatory drugs inhibit platelet function by preferentially inhibiting platelet cyclooxygenase activity while maintaining the

activity of the enzyme within the endothelial cells.[21] In this way, there is a reduction in the production of platelet thromboxane A_2 (TxA_2), a potent inducer of platelet aggregation, but preservation in prostacyclin (PGI_2) synthesis by the endothelial cell. Omega-3 fatty acids can substitute for arachidonic acid in prostaglandin synthesis resulting in the synthesis of thromboxane A_3 (TxA_3), which has little effect upon platelet aggregation. However, within the endothelial cell, synthesis of a novel prostaglandin occurs (PGI_3) which has potent anti-platelet activity.

2. Several drugs such as dipyridamole result in a decrease in platelet intracellular calcium concentration by inhibiting cAMP degradation. Elevated levels of cAMP favor movement of Ca^{2+} into the dense bodies where it is inert and so effectively decreases intracellular Ca^{2+} levels.[21]

3. Drugs such as ticlopidine and clopidogrel selectively inhibit platelet aggregation by binding to and blocking the $P2Y_{12}$ platelet receptor thereby inhibiting ADP-induced aggregation.[22,23]

4. A number of drugs selectively bind to and block the platelet GpIIb/IIIa complex resulting in a loss of activity. These include abciximab, a monoclonal antibody, eptifibatide (a cyclic heptapeptide derived from a protein found in the venom of the southeastern pygmy rattlesnake, *Sistrurus miliarius barbouri*) and tirofiban a synthetic, non-peptide inhibitor. These drugs are potent inhibitors of platelet function that can result in severe bleeding problems.[24] In addition, in a small number of patients their use is associated with a profound thrombocytopenia which may exacerbate the bleeding tendency.[25,26]

5. Platelet function abnormalities can be induced by certain antibiotics, particularly the β-lactam antibiotics.[25,26] Penicillin, particularly penicillin G, ticarcillin and carbenicillin, have been reported to inhibit platelet function and to cause a clinically significant bleeding tendency particularly when administered in high dose.[25,26] Some cephalosporins also appear to interfere with vitamin K metabolism resulting in an additional and additive increased risk of bleeding.[27]

6. Finally, a variety of drugs appear to have nonspecific effects upon platelet function. β-adrenergic agents have a weak but inconsistent effect on platelet function *in vitro* but are rarely if at all associated with a clinical bleeding tendency. Sodium valproate can result in thrombocytopenia but can also result in qualitative platelet abnormalities.[28]

Laboratory monitoring

There is increasing interest in monitoring platelet function in patients receiving anti-platelet drugs to identify those individuals who demonstrate drug 'resistance' and may have a reduced benefit.[29–34] Platelet aggregation studies or the use of the platelet function analyzer 100 (PFA-100™) may be of value in identifying these patients.[35–37]

Hemostatic defects associated with vitamin K deficiency

Vitamin K and vitamin K deficiency

Vitamin K_1 is a fat-soluble vitamin obtained primarily from green leafy vegetables. It is absorbed in the upper part of the small intestine and its absorption is dependent upon the presence of pancreatic lipases and bile. Most of the vitamin K absorbed from the gut is stored in the liver although the stores of vitamin K are only a few days. The normal daily requirement of vitamin K is 0.5–1.0 µg/kg. Vitamin K_2 is synthesized by the gut flora but cannot compensate for a total deficiency of vitamin K_1. Vitamin K_3 is a synthetic form of vitamin K.

Vitamin K oxidation to its epoxide form is essential for the post-translational gamma-carboxylation of the glutamic acid residues present in the N-terminal region of factors II, VII, IX, X, protein C and S. Efficient gamma-carboxylation allows the modified glutamic acid residues to bind calcium and subsequently to the phospholipid receptors on cell membranes allowing coagulation to proceed. In the absence of efficient gamma-carboxylation, partially carboxylated forms of the clotting factors are released into the circulation, co-called 'PIVKAS'. During carboxylation, vitamin K is oxidized to vitamin K epoxide and recycled to its active form by reductases. Oral anticoagulants such as warfarin inhibit vitamin K epoxide reduction and prevent recycling of vitamin K to its active form, thereby limiting the activity of the carboxylase.

Vitamin K deficiency in neonates and young infants

Three types of vitamin K deficiency are seen in the newborn child and young infant:

* *Early form*: an early form of hemorrhagic disease in the new born infant, occurring within the first 24 hours of life, is most commonly seen in infants whose mothers have received anticonvulsant therapy during pregnancy. This condition is prevented by the administration of daily vitamin K to the mother, for the 2 weeks prior to delivery.

* *Hemorrhagic disease of the newborn (HDN)*. HDN is the classic hemorrhagic diathesis associated with a deficiency of vitamin K and arises because of the limited transplacental passage of vitamin K during development; hepatic immaturity particularly in premature infants; the sterile gut of the newborn infant; the poor intake of nutrients in the first few days of life and because human breast milk in comparison to cows' milk contains little vitamin K. Bleeding usually occurs between the second and fifth days of life and commonly presents with intracranial hemorrhage which may be fatal in up to 20% of cases. To prevent this disorder, newborn infants are routinely given 1 mg intramuscular vitamin K_1 at birth.[38,39]

* *Late form*: infants who are not given vitamin K_1 at birth and who are exclusively breastfed may develop a later form of the disorder between 3 and 8 weeks of age. Again such infants frequently present with intracranial

bleeds. Infants who do not receive intramuscular vitamin K should receive oral vitamin K within the first 24 hours of birth, again at 1 week and again at 4 weeks of life. Oral vitamin K is ineffective in infants who have liver disease or malabsorption problems and these children should receive regular doses of parenteral vitamin K.

Vitamin K deficiency in adults

Vitamin K deficiency in adults can occur in a variety of situations including malabsorption, fasting, alcoholism and in association with various drugs particularly coumarins, some antibiotics and salicylates. Vitamin K deficiency may also be seen in patients receiving parenteral nutrition and for these reasons such patients should receive prophylactic vitamin K.

Adults with vitamin K deficiency may present with a wide variety of clinical hemorrhagic problems including gastrointestinal bleeding and recurrent epistaxes.

Laboratory findings

Adults and children with vitamin K deficiency both show a normal platelet count (unless there is an associated pathology such as liver disease or DIC which may result in thrombocytopenia), a prolonged prothrombin time (PT), a prolonged activated partial thromboplastin time (APTT) but a normal thrombin time and fibrinogen level. The functional activity of the vitamin K dependent clotting factors are reduced and dysfunctional forms – PIVKAs – can be detected in the plasma of affected individuals.[40]

Management of vitamin K deficiency

The principles of treatment involve treating the underlying cause, the administration of vitamin K and, in cases of severe hemorrhage, transfusion with fresh frozen plasma or in some cases a plasma-derived clotting factor concentrate containing vitamin K clotting factors (II, VII, IX and X). There were some concerns that the use of parenteral vitamin K, but not oral vitamin K, in the newborn infant was associated with an increased risk of childhood cancer. However, subsequent studies have not confirmed these early findings.[38,41]

Hemostatic defects in liver disease

The liver is responsible for the synthesis of all the coagulation factors apart from von Willebrand factor (vWF). The liver also synthesizes either completely or in part many of the proteins involved in the regulation of coagulation – antithrombin, protein C, protein S, heparin co-factor II and those involved in fibrinolysis – plasminogen and α_2-antiplasmin. The liver is also responsible for the clearance of activated clotting factors that are generated by the clotting cascade and during fibrinolysis. Liver disease is therefore associated with a major disruption of the clotting system resulting in an increased risk of hemorrhage. Factors V and VII are sensitive markers of hepatic function and may be used as an index of severity.[42]

Defective production of clotting factors arises because of a failure in hepatic synthetic function including gamma-carboxylation of the vitamin K-dependent clotting factors although there may also be reduced absorption of the fat-soluble vitamins including vitamin K as a result of cholestasis. Von Willebrand factor is often raised in patients with liver failure reflecting its extra-hepatic site of synthesis (endothelial cells and megakaryocytes) and its acute phase nature.

Thrombocytopenia is a common finding in liver disease and is often due to sequestration of platelets within the spleen – hypersplenism. Thrombocytopenia may also be seen in association with alcohol abuse, folate deficiency, DIC and in some cases of viral hepatitis where the causative virus may have a direct effect upon megakaryopoiesis or accelerate peripheral destruction.[43] A qualitative platelet abnormality is often seen in patients with liver failure which further exacerbates the bleeding tendency.

Fibrinogen is relatively well maintained in liver disease until the terminal stages when the levels may drop dramatically. In addition, as a result of an increased sialic acid content of fibrinogen, patients with liver failure may develop an acquired dysfibrinogenemia resulting in slow fibrin polymerization and a relatively unstable fibrin clot.[44,45] Abnormal fibrinogens and non-carboxylated prothrombin are also synthesized by patients with primary hepatocellular carcinoma and have been used as markers of these disorders.[44]

Many patients with liver disease have evidence of systemic fibrinolysis secondary to reduced synthesis of α_2-antiplasmin, reduced clearance of t-PA and low grade DIC.[46–50] Primary hyperfibrinolysis may result in severe bleeding problems following surgery in patients with liver disease where tissue damage results in the release of large amounts of plasminogen activators which swamp the impaired protective mechanisms of the liver resulting in systemic fibrinolysis.

Chronic low-grade DIC is a common feature of liver disease. This occurs secondary to release of tissue thromboplastin from the damaged hepatocytes, reduced synthesis of the inhibitors of coagulation – antithrombin, protein C and protein S – and reduced clearance of activated clotting factors. Ascitic fluid appears to contain a potent thromboplastin-like material and may result in severe DIC following creation of a peritovenous shunt in which large amounts of ascitic fluid are infused directly into the circulation.[51]

Laboratory findings in liver disease

Individuals with liver disease show a prolongation of the prothrombin time and activated partial thromboplastin time. Von Willebrand factor and protein S may be normal to high reflecting their extra-hepatic sites of synthesis. Features of DIC including raised D-dimers and FDPs, are common in liver disease and this may contribute to the thrombocytopenia observed in such patients although hypersplenism may also result in thrombocytopenia. An acquired qualitative defect platelet may also be present. Fibrinogen levels are often well maintained but patients may show an acquired dysfibrinogenemia resulting in a prolonged thrombin time and reptilase time.

There is increasing evidence that highlights the poor correlation between bleeding and the results of various laboratory tests of hemostasis in patients with liver disease.

Thrombin generation testing and measurement of platelet adhesion are normal in these patients. This has implications for managing patients about to undergo invasive procedures when historically fresh frozen plasma has been administered to these patients to reduce their perceived increased risk of bleeding based upon the results of conventional laboratory tests of hemostasis.[49]

Management of the coagulopathy of liver disease

Patients with liver disease may require no treatment unless they are actively bleeding or about to undergo an invasive procedure. In such cases, patients may require vitamin K, fresh frozen plasma and occasionally cryoprecipitate or fibrinogen concentrates to correct the clotting factor deficiencies and platelet transfusions to maintain the platelet count above $50 \times 10^9/l$. Patients with liver disease may develop catastrophic variceal bleeding and in such cases in addition to local measures, replacing clotting factors and platelets, rVIIa may have some benefit. Prothrombin complex concentrates have been avoided in patients with liver disease because of concerns that they could precipitate a thrombotic event.[52,53] Increasingly, however, they are now being used in such patients as a rapid means for reversing the coagulopathy.

The INR in liver disease

The INR is frequently measured in patients with liver disease and serves as a prognostic factor in both the model for end-stage liver disease (MELD)[54] and Child–Pugh scoring system[55] and in addition to determining the prognosis, is also used to prioritize patients for transplantation. However, the INR is designed to monitor patients on warfarin and not with liver disease[56] and may impact on prioritization for liver transplantation.[57] For these reasons an INR using a tissue factor that has been calibrated for patients with liver disease, 'ISI^{Liver}', has been proposed.[57,58]

Hemostatic defects associated with renal disease and uremia

The coagulopathy associated with renal disease is complex and rarely due to deficiency of a single clotting factor.[59]

Recognized causes of a coagulopathy in patients with renal disease include:

- *Anemia.* The anemia that is often associated with renal disease disrupts normal platelet function. There is an inverse relationship between the template bleeding time and the hematocrit. This arises because of a decrease in the interaction of platelets with the vascular endothelium due to changes in axial blood flow with cells moving from the periphery to the center of the flowing blood. Red cells also release ADP and thromboxane A_2 (TxA_2) which augment platelet function. Hemoglobin has a high affinity for nitric oxide (NO) but in the anemic individual there is less Hb to scavenge NO. As a consequence NO may accumulate, activating guanylyl cyclase, increasing

cGMP levels and impairing platelet aggregation. NO levels may be increased in patients with renal disease[60] due to elevated levels of TNFα and IL-1β which stimulate the synthesis of NO.

- *Thrombocytopenia.* Individuals with uremia often have a mild thrombocytopenia.[61,62] This may arise because of a suppressive effect of the uremic state on megakaryopoiesis.
- *Decreased platelet adhesion.* Patients with uremia often display reduced platelet adhesion. This may reflect disordered platelet function particularly of the GpIb receptor which is important in the binding of von Willebrand factor[63,64] and to a reduction in the levels of the high molecular weight von Willebrand factor multimers.[65] These high molecular forms of vWF are critical for the interaction of platelets with the vascular endothelium.
- *Qualitative platelet defect.* Some patients show an acquired storage pool-like defect with reduced platelet 5-HT and ADP content.[66] In addition, there may be abnormal intracellular calcium mobilization and increased intracellular levels of both cAMP and cGMP.[67] Finally, there may be decreased thromboxane A_2 production – a potent inducer of platelet aggregation.[68]
- *Increased prostacyclin (PGI^2) production.* Individuals with renal disease have higher levels of PGI$_2$ than controls.[69] PGI$_2$ is a potent vasodilator and inhibits platelet aggregation by modulating the production of cAMP through activation of adenylyl cyclase.
- *Increased fibrinolysis.* Antiplasmin complexes, fibrinogen and fibrin degradation products are significantly increased in patients with renal failure and the activity of plasminogen activator inhibitor is slightly reduced, denoting an activation of fibrinolysis.[66]
- *Drugs.* The half-life of heparin is increased in patients with renal failure and its effects following hemodialysis may persist for some time.
- *Uremic toxins.* The cause of many of these problems is unclear but may in part be related to the failure to remove so called 'middle molecules' (300-5000 Da) which accumulate in renal failure such as guanidinosuccinic acid (GSA) and phenols. GSA and phenolic acid are known to inhibit ADP-induced platelet aggregation.

Laboratory diagnosis

The bleeding time is frequently prolonged in patients with renal disease and uremia. Platelet aggregation tests are often abnormal but there is a poor correlation between the abnormality and the risk of bleeding. vWF multimer analysis may show a loss of the high molecular weight forms although the latter is not always a consistent finding. There is usually no specific clotting factor deficiency in renal disease unless there is some other coexisting disease process. However, the thrombin times and reptilase times may be prolonged in patients with renal disease due to an acquired dysfibrinogenemia arising from a low serum albumin.[70] However, these patients do not appear to be at risk of bleeding and may actually be at increased risk of thrombosis due to increased platelet activation.[71]

Treatment

Increasing the frequency of dialysis tends to shorten the bleeding time and reduce the bleeding symptoms in some but not all patients with renal failure. Correction of the anemia and raising the hematocrit by approximately 30% by transfusion of red cells or by the use of erythropoietin results in a reduction in the bleeding time and reduces the symptoms of bleeding.[72,73]

The administration of cryoprecipitate which contains large amounts of the high molecular forms of vWF in addition to FVIII and fibrinogen may correct the bleeding time and may be of value in patients with renal disease who are actively bleeding. The synthetic vasopressin derivative desmopressin has also been shown to be of value in patients with renal disease and works by increasing the release of high molecular weight vWF multimers from the Weibel–Palade bodies.[68] The effects are rapid and usually persist for 3–4 hours and sometimes as long as 8 hours. However, patients exhibit tachyphylaxis with a reduction in the response to treatment. Desmopressin is also associated with water retention and hyponatremia which limits how frequently it can be administered.

Finally, the use of conjugated estrogens has been shown to be of benefit in reducing the bleeding time and decreasing bleeding symptoms in patients with chronic renal disease. Intravenous estrogens given for 4–5 days causes detectable improvement in the bleeding time of most patients after 6 hours with the maximal improvement seen between the first and second week of treatment and with the effects persisting for 10–14 days.[74] Similar effects have been observed with oral conjugated estrogens and with transdermal 17β-estradiol patches.[75]

Hemostatic defects associated with 'massive' blood transfusion

Massive blood transfusion is variously defined as the replacement of more than one blood volume in less than 24 hours, the loss of >4 L of blood in 24 hours, the loss of >2 L of blood in 4 hours or a blood loss of >150 ml/minute. However, most healthy individuals can cope with the replacement of up to 80% of their circulating blood volume with stored blood and suffer no hemostatic defects. Hemostatic defects usually arise when more than one blood volume is lost and replaced within 2 hours. Approximately 30% of severely multiply-injured patients will have a coagulopathy on emergency admission.[76,77]

In a massive transfusion situation factors that may potentiate a coagulopathy include hypothermia, hypocalcemia, hemodilution and acidemia. Hypothermia and hypocalcemia can occur as a complication of the rapid infusion of large amounts of cold blood that contains citrate as an anticoagulant. Blood is commonly separated into its component parts shortly after collection and only concentrated red cells are then available for transfusion. Transfusion of large amounts of concentrated red cells, without adequate replacement of clotting factors or platelets, is likely to result in disordered hemostasis. Similar problems occur when large amounts of colloid are infused. *In vitro* hemodilution with hydroxyethyl starch, gelatin or albumin leads to significant changes in coagulation when assessed by thromboelastography, with the most pronounced effects seen with hydroxyethyl starch.[68,69] However, even when whole blood is administered there are a number of hemostatic defects that arise. Stored blood undergoes a progressive loss of factors V and VIII. After 24 hours at 4°C there is a 50% loss in factor VIII activity and after 14 days there is a 50% loss in the activity of factor V. Platelets stored at 4°C rapidly lose activity and after 48 hours they show virtually no activity.

Laboratory diagnosis

Prolongation of the PT, APTT and TT, reduction in circulating fibrinogen and thrombocytopenia are common features of massive blood transfusion. FDPs and D-dimer may be raised and there may be evidence of systemic fibrinolysis. The thromboelastogram (TEG) is useful in monitoring patients who receive large amounts of blood as it allows a relatively rapid global and dynamic assessment of blood coagulation.

Treatment

The treatment of the coagulopathy arising from massive blood transfusion is dictated by the clinical situation and the results of laboratory tests. Individuals with a prolonged PT and APTT (usually greater than 1.5x control values) but only a borderline reduction in fibrinogen benefit from the use of fresh frozen plasma (FFP). If there is a significant fall in fibrinogen (<1 g/l) then fibrinogen replacement is indicated with cryoprecipitate or fibrinogen concentrates. If the platelet count falls below 75×10^9/l, then platelet concentrates should be given.

A unit of fresh frozen plasma takes 15–20 minutes to thaw and its infusion results in an increase in each of the coagulation factors of about 5%. A unit of cryoprecipitate takes 10–15 minutes to thaw and an infusion of 10–15 bags (each from a single donor) will raise the fibrinogen level in the plasma by approximately 0.5–1 g/l in a 70 kg adult. In a massive transfusion situation treatment is often given empirically, without awaiting laboratory results. Recent experience in trauma situations suggests that early use of FFP in a 1 : 1 ratio with packed red blood cells is associated with improved outcome.[77-79] Treatment should not be unnecessarily delayed in people with massive hemorrhage and such empirical approaches have some value. However, it is important that regular coagulation studies and full blood count are also performed to monitor the efficacy of product replacement and guide subsequent management.

The use of DDAVP is of little value as such patients are already stressed and as a result have elevated vWF levels. In individuals in whom the bleeding cannot be arrested, there have been some encouraging reports of successful treatment with recombinant factor VIIa (rVIIa),[80] although this is not a licensed indication and there is a potential risk of thromboembolic complications.

Hemostatic defects associated with the use of extracorporeal circuits

Patients undergoing cardiopulmonary bypass (CPB) develop a complex coagulopathy that is related to the surgical procedure, to the bypass machine, to the various drugs that they may receive during bypass and finally due to their underlying illness. In some cases bleeding may occur due to defective surgical hemostasis and such patients may require surgical re-exploration.

Quantitative platelet abnormalities

The platelet count falls during CPB often as early as 5 minutes after institution of bypass. The platelet count may remain depressed for several days after the procedure. Hemodilution and platelet adhesion to synthetic surfaces are primary contributors to CPB-induced thrombocytopenia.[81]

The bleeding time is markedly prolonged in patients undergoing hypothermic CPB although it usually normalizes within 24 hours following cessation of bypass.[82] The prolonged bleeding time does not correlate with the fall in platelet count suggesting that it is secondary to impaired platelet function.

Qualitative platelet abnormalities

Circulation through an extracorporeal circuit causes transient morphological changes in platelets that are consistent with primary aggregation and activation.[83] Hypothermia exacerbates this acquired platelet function defect. Platelets have been shown by scanning electron microscopy to adhere to the synthetic surfaces of the circuits. Fibrinogen, a potent co-factor in platelet aggregation is readily adsorbed onto synthetic surfaces and together with small amounts of thrombin also present on such surfaces induce platelet aggregation. When platelets adhere to synthetic surfaces they are activated and the contents of the α-granules are released into the circulation. Other agonists that activate platelets during CPB surgery include heparin, collagen, plasmin and inflammatory mediators.[84]

There is a loss of platelet membrane glycoproteins during CPB that can be demonstrated by the use of specific monoclonal antibodies.[85] Platelets are also subject to significant physical trauma during CPB that can strip the glycoproteins from the surface of the platelet. A loss of platelet membrane glycoproteins results in decreased platelet adhesion and impaired fibrinogen binding.

Clotting factor abnormalities and DIC

Coagulation protein levels decrease rapidly after initiation of cardiopulmonary bypass and enzymatic function may be reduced due to hypothermia. The initial changes are largely due to hemodilution[86] but the fluid used to prime the bypass circuit, cardioplegia fluid and cell salvage systems, which recycle washed concentrated red cells, all contribute to hemodilution.

During CPB blood is pumped over 1.4–6.0 m^2 of nonbiological surfaces and is exposed to high shear stress within the extracorporeal circuit. Contact activation is triggered by factor XII, prekallikrein or high molecular weight kininogen interacting with artificial surfaces, generating thrombin.[87]

The tissue factor (TF) pathway is activated during CPB[88] and is probably more important for thrombin generation. Tissue factor is exposed with vessel wall injury and exposed myocardium, epicardium, adventitia, muscle, fat and bone also express TF. Blood from the pericardial cavity has higher mononuclear cell TF than paired samples from the perfusate[89] and pericardial wound blood is often drained into the cardiotomy reservoir, filtered and returned to the circulation.[84,90] Thrombin generated via the contact and tissue factor pathways during CBP initiates fibrinolysis in the pericardial wound and perfusion circuit. This leads to a consumptive coagulopathy that is mild in most patients.

Fibrinolytic activity

Fibrinolytic activity increases significantly both during and after CPB and this contributes to the increased risk of bleeding.[91] Increased fibrinolysis in patients undergoing CPB may also contribute to the acquired platelet abnormality.[92] Hypothermia has been shown in animal experiments to induce activation of the fibrinolytic pathway and may, therefore, increase the systemic fibrinolytic activity associated with CPB.[93]

Increased fibrinolytic activity is observed shortly after heparinization and before the patient is started on bypass. Heparin appears to induce a rise in systemic plasmin activity that only improves after completion of CPB. The effect is induced by a fall in α_2-antiplasmin that is caused both by heparin and CPB.[91] Levels of t-PA increase during CPB and this suggests that CPB is a stimulus to the release of t-PA from the vascular bed. It is probable that tissue damage may also contribute to this effect.[94] Plasminogen activator inhibitor-1 levels remain unchanged. Plasminogen and antithrombin (III) fall during CPB and remain depressed for 2–3 days postoperatively.[95]

Drugs

Anticoagulation with heparin is fundamental to CPB. Heparin is administered before CPB is commenced as an IV bolus dose usually 250–300 U/kg. Its effect during bypass is monitored by means of the activated clotting time (ACT). At the end of CPB, the heparin is reversed with protamine, given in incremental doses until the ACT returns to normal. Although the anticoagulant effect of heparin mediated through its action on antithrombin may be reversed by protamine, its effects upon fibrinolysis and platelets is not and this may contribute to the bleeding observed following CPB. In addition, increased bleeding after CPB may occur due to 'heparin rebound'.[96–98] This arises for a variety of reasons including: 1) release of heparin from protamine–heparin complexes; 2) the movement of cold heparin-containing extracellular fluid into the periphery following postoperative rewarming; and 3) replacement of antithrombin in plasma which facilities the anticoagulant action of heparin.

Acquired inhibitors

Topical bovine thrombin was frequently used in patients undergoing cardiothoracic surgery and the use of such agents has been associated with the development of factor V inhibitors.[99,100] The mechanism is believed to be the development of an antibody directed against bovine factor V which is capable of cross-reacting with human factor V, resulting in its rapid clearance from the plasma.

Laboratory monitoring

Preoperative screening tests are of little value in predicting those patients who are likely to develop significant postoperative bleeding. A personal and family history to assess the likelihood of a bleeding disorder and a comprehensive drug history are essential before any form of major surgery.

Almost all laboratory tests are abnormal both during and immediately after CPB due to the effects of CPB on coagulation and platelets and the use of heparin to anticoagulate the patient. In the bleeding postoperative patient, laboratory tests including the PT, APTT, fibrinogen and platelet count should be performed. There is often a delay in obtaining the results of these tests and a more global assessment of hemostasis such as that obtained with the thromboelastogram (TEG) may be of value.[101-103] The TEG also provides a rapid method for screening for the presence of heparin (by the use of heparinase-treated cups) and a relatively simple method for assessing fibrinolysis, something that is otherwise difficult to perform.

Treatment

In patients in whom the presence of heparin is demonstrated, the use of small amounts of protamine to neutralize the heparin may be appropriate. Platelet transfusions are often empirically given to patients during or at the end of CPB on the basis of the thrombocytopenia and acquired platelet defects that are commonly seen in such patients. Fresh frozen plasma and cryoprecipitate or fibrinogen concentrate should be used to correct prolongation of the PT and APTT and reductions in fibrinogen in the bleeding patient.

Antifibrinolytic therapies in the form of synthetic lysine derivatives [e.g. tranexamic acid] and aprotinin, a broadspectrum serine protease that inhibits trypsin, kallikrein and plasmin, have been widely used in cardiac surgery. These agents all reduce allogeneic blood transfusion requirements when compared to placebo.[104] A regimen employing aprotinin has been shown to reduce blood loss in patients undergoing cardiac surgery by 80% in addition to shortening operating times.[105,106] However, several recent large observational studies have reported an association between aprotinin use and increased rates of death, vascular events and renal impairment following cardiac surgery.[107-110] The current evidence favors the use of lysine analogs over aprotinin if antifibrinolytic therapy is required, although this is an area of ongoing investigation.[104]

Disseminated intravascular coagulation (DIC)

DIC is a pathological process in which there is systemic activation of coagulation resulting in widespread fibrin deposition within the vascular tree. The activation of coagulation leads to the formation of microthrombi and the consumption of platelets and clotting factors. DIC is always secondary to some process although these are diverse.

Four major pathways can lead to the development of DIC:

1. Tissue damage following, for example trauma, surgery, malignancy or an obstetric complication[111-113] results in the release of procoagulant material into the circulation and activation of the coagulation cascade.
2. Damage to endothelial cells changes the physiological properties of the endothelium, exposing collagen and making it intensely procoagulant. Such damage is seen in immune-mediated causes of DIC, in association with various infections and some metabolic disorders.
3. Direct platelet activation leading to intravascular platelet microaggregates can lead to the development of DIC. This is seen in association with some infections and in some patients with circulating immune complexes.
4. Some malignancies,[114,115] pancreatitis[116] and some snake venoms[117,118] can directly activate the clotting cascade.

Activation of coagulation through any of the above trigger mechanisms leads to excess thrombin generation, platelet activation and the formation of microthrombi within the circulation. Post-mortem data show microthrombi in only 65-75% of patients with documented DIC. It is probable these microthrombi are removed by the fibrinolytic system or that their formation is limited particularly in patients with hypofibrinogenemia as a consequence of their DIC. In patients who develop microthrombi these occlude the microcirculation leading to organ and tissue damage.

In the later stages of DIC, consumption of clotting factors and platelets as well as the effects of fibrinolysis may result in uncontrolled bleeding. Increased fibrinolytic activity is an inevitable consequence of intravascular thrombin formation. Continued activation of the coagulation cascade results in increased thrombomodulin expression on the surface of endothelial cells, which together with thrombin, leads to the activation of protein C. Activated protein C leads to inactivation of factor Va and VIIIa, further increasing the bleeding tendency. Activated protein C also leads to inhibition of PAI-1, the major intravascular inhibitor of t-PA, thereby stimulating fibrinolysis. Damage to endothelial cells results in increased release of t-PA, further stimulating fibrinolysis. In the latter stages of DIC, the natural anticoagulants including antithrombin and protein C are depleted. Depletion of protein C seems particularly severe in patients with DIC secondary to meningococcal septicemia.[119]

Laboratory diagnosis of DIC

The diagnosis of DIC requires an appropriate clinical context and the demonstration of coagulation abnormalities on laboratory testing. Screening assays provide evidence of the level of consumption of clotting factors and platelets. These tests provide a snapshot of abnormalities present at a particular time point and should be regularly repeated.

The tests that are most frequently abnormal in DIC are:

- Platelet count
- Fibrin(ogen) degradation products (FDPs)
- Prothrombin time
- Activated partial thromboplastin time
- Thrombin time
- Fibrinogen concentration.

The precise pattern of coagulation abnormalities is dependent upon the triggering mechanism responsible for the development of DIC. The platelet count is frequently reduced in DIC and is particularly low in patients with DIC

Table 35.2 ISTH Scoring system for overt DIC

1. Risk assessment: Does the patient have an underlying disorder known to be associated with overt DIC?
   If yes: proceed
   If no: do not use this algorithm
2. Order global coagulation tests (prothrombin time, platelet count, fibrinogen, fibrin related marker)
3. Score the test results as shown below
4. Calculate score
   ≥5 compatible with overt DIC: repeat score daily
   <5 suggestive of non-overt DIC: repeat next 1–2 days

	Score		
	0	1	2
Platelet count	>100	<100	<50
Fibrin related marker, e.g. D-dimer, FDP	No increase	Moderate increase	Strong increase
Prolonged prothrombin time	<3 s	3<x<6 s	>6 s
Fibrinogen level	>1 g/l	<1 g/l	<1 g/l

FDP: fibrinogen degradation product.

secondary to sepsis. Examination of the blood film in cases of DIC may show the presence of fragmented red cells although if these are present in high concentration, then other causes of a microangiopathic hemolytic anemia (MAHA) should be considered. Increased fibrinolytic activity results in an increase in the levels of circulating fibrin complexes and fibrin degradation products (FDPs). However, some patients with severe DIC have no elevation in FDPs and such patients tend to have a poor prognosis. Similarly a normal PT, APTT or fibrinogen does not exclude the diagnosis of DIC. The PT and APTT are prolonged in the majority of cases, but may be normal due to the presence of circulating activated clotting factors.[120] Fibrinogen is an acute phase protein and may remain within the normal range, despite increased consumption.

In DIC an abnormal 'biphasic' aPTT waveform is a specific and early indicator of DIC; however, this is only obtainable on certain photo-optical analyzers that display clot formation over time.[121–123]

The International Society of Thrombosis and Hemostasis (ISTH) has developed a scoring system for the diagnosis of DIC[124] (Table 35.2). A score of 5 or greater identifies overt DIC. Increasing scores are strongly correlated with mortality in several studies.[125,126]

Management of acute DIC

The aims of therapy are to treat the underlying disorder and to control the coagulation defect. Aggressive treatment of the underlying disorder is essential. Plasma products and platelet transfusion are generally not indicated on the basis of abnormal laboratory results alone in an asymptomatic patient unless there is a high risk of bleeding. In an actively bleeding patient management is controversial, but maintenance of intravascular volume and plasma products to correct the coagulation defect are generally required. Fresh frozen plasma (FFP) contains all the coagulation factors and the inhibitors of coagulation. The use of prothrombin complex concentrates (PCCs) may be a useful alternative to FFP in patients susceptible to fluid overload, although they contain only selected clotting factors. In individuals with a fibrinogen <1 g/l despite FFP replacement, fibrinogen concentrates or cryoprecipitate may be required. Platelet infusions should be considered in bleeding patients when the platelet count falls to <50×10^9/l. The adequacy of blood component therapy should be monitored clinically and with repeat laboratory tests.

Some cases of DIC are associated with dramatic falls in antithrombin and/or protein C levels. In such situations supplementation with antithrombin or protein C concentrates may be beneficial.[119,127] Improvements in laboratory parameters have been shown with antithrombin concentrate, but a mortality benefit has not been clearly demonstrated in randomized controlled trials and current evidence is insufficient to inform clinical practice.[120,128] Activated protein C has been demonstrated to reduce mortality in severe sepsis in a randomized controlled trial[129] which included patients with overt DIC.[130] Activated protein C increases the risk of major bleeding and patients with severe thrombocytopenia or who were at high risk of bleeding were excluded from this trial. A benefit has not been demonstrated in patients with sepsis and a low risk of death[131] or in patients with DIC from other causes.

The use of heparin in DIC is controversial and treatment doses should probably be reserved for cases in which there is a poor clinical response to conventional treatment or where thrombosis is the predominant clinical problem. Patients with DIC are at high risk of venous thromboembolism (VTE) and the use of VTE prophylaxis is standard care for patients who are not actively bleeding.[120] Inhibitors of fibrinolysis are generally not indicated in patients with DIC but may be of value in patients with primary hyperfibrinolysis. Recombinant factor VIIa is not currently licensed for use in patients with DIC and life-threatening bleeding, although there are published reports of its use.

Chronic DIC

The initiation of DIC is not always a rapid severe clinical event but can occur gradually, allowing compensation for the consumption of clotting factors and platelets. A bleeding diathesis will only become clinically apparent when compensation fails.

The majority of cases of chronic DIC probably occur in patients with an underlying malignancy. It is occasionally seen in women in whom there has been an intrauterine death and there is tissue injury/necrosis with the release of TF into the circulation. Liver disease may also be associated with the development of chronic DIC. Some patients with vascular malformations e.g. Kasabach–Merritt syndrome, a benign tumor in which there is a convoluted mass of vascular channels which consume platelets and clotting factors, may also develop chronic DIC.[132,133]

Laboratory tests in cases of chronic, localized DIC show a reduced or normal platelet count, a normal or prolonged PT and APTT and a reduced, normal or elevated fibrinogen concentration. D-dimer levels and fibrin(ogen) degradation products (FDPs) are raised.

The optimal management of patients with chronic DIC is treatment of the underlying disorder. This may be removal of a dead fetus in cases of intrauterine death, or the surgical repair of an aortic aneurysm. Some benign vascular malformations respond to treatment with anticoagulants such as heparin or occasionally steroids.

Acquired hyperfibrinolysis

This unusual disorder occurs as a consequence of inappropriate or excessive activation of fibrinolysis or a decrease in the inhibitors of fibrinolysis. The result is in an increased risk of hemorrhage. Acquired hyperfibrinolysis can arise for a number of reasons:

- Increased release into the circulation of plasminogen activators, e.g. in prostatic carcinoma and DIC
- Defective clearance of activators, e.g. liver disease
- Secondary to thrombolytic therapy
- Localized systemic release of activator, e.g. prostatectomy
- Defective inhibition of fibrinolysis, e.g. liver disease, DIC (reduced α_2-antiplasmin), congenital or acquired α_2-antiplasmin deficiency.

Laboratory investigation of systemic hyperfibrinolysis

The platelet count in acquired hyperfibrinolysis is usually normal unless this is accompanied by DIC in which case the platelet count may be low. The D-dimer level is frequently normal because the lysis is primarily of fibrinogen rather than cross-linked fibrin. Markers of fibrinolysis such as the euglobulin clot lysis time (ELT), the fibrin plate lysis test and

the TEG are abnormal reflecting the underlying hyperfibrinolytic state. α_2-Antiplasmin levels are often reduced.

Management of systemic hyperfibrinolysis

Patients with hyperfibrinolysis and who are bleeding should be managed by correcting the underlying disorder wherever possible. Correction of the depleted inhibitors, e.g. PAI-1 and α_2-antiplasmin, requires the administration of fresh frozen plasma and cryoprecipitate. In cases in which there is no evidence of DIC, the administration of fibrinolytic inhibitors may be of value.

Bleeding and malignancy

Bleeding associated with malignancy is often secondary to DIC, liver disease or the effects of treatment. Rarely it may be due to the development of specific clotting factor inhibitors.[115,134–136] Many tumors can activate coagulation and fibrinolysis to facilitate their spread.[115] Tumors also stimulate the release of various cytokines including IL-1 and TNF stimulating monocytes and macrophages to increase the expression of tissue factor and thereby initiating coagulation. Hemorrhage as a consequence of DIC in patients with malignancy is rarely a problem unless the platelet count is less that 50×10^9/l or the fibrinogen is <0.5 g/l. High concentrations of FDPs may impair platelet function and fibrin polymerization.

Acute leukemias

DIC can complicate many types of acute leukemia, both lymphoblastic and myeloblastic,[137] and it is well described in acute promyelocytic leukemia (APML), a disorder in which marked fibrinolysis is common. In APML the leukemic cells express abnormally high levels of annexin II[138] and annexin II has high affinity for plasminogen and t-PA and is a co-factor for plasminogen activation by t-PA. Leukemic cells expressing annexin II stimulate the generation of cell-surface plasmin more efficiently than non-leukemic cells. In addition, levels of α_2-antiplasmin are typically reduced in APML.[139] Over-expression of annexin II leading to hyperfibrinolysis may explain the hemorrhagic complications of acute promyelocytic leukemia. Annexin II is expressed by cerebral microvascular endothelial cells in higher amounts than in other endothelial tissues, which may account for the relatively high incidence of intracranial hemorrhage in APML.[139] The early initiation of treatment with a differentiating agent (e.g. ATRA) is essential to reduce bleeding fatalities in APML. Replacement of clotting factors with FFP and cryoprecipitate and the transfusion of platelets are also of value. Routine use of heparin and antifibrinolytic agents are not indicated.

L-aspariginase is an important part of the treatment regime for ALL. It can occasionally cause a bleeding tendency by inhibiting the synthesis of various clotting factors[140,141] although it is more frequently associated with thrombotic complications (through its effects on antithrombin, protein C and S).

Myeloproliferative disorders

The myeloproliferative disorders are a group of diseases that include polycythemia vera (PV), chronic myeloid leukemia (CML), essential thrombocythemia (ET) and myelofibrosis. Thrombocytopenia may occur in such patients either as a consequence of bone marrow replacement/failure or secondary to chemotherapy. A wide variety of acquired platelet defects have been described in patients with myeloproliferative disorders.[142-144] A number of studies have shown specific loss of platelet membrane glycoproteins – IIb/IIIa and GpIb[145,146] although the results of platelet aggregation studies are variable. Myeloproliferative disorders can also be associated with an acquired platelet storage pool deficiency and both dense granule and α-granule deficiency have been reported.[147]

Acquired von Willebrand syndrome (AVWS) has also been associated with the myeloproliferative disorders. Multimeric analysis in such patients usually shows a loss of the high molecular weight forms of the protein and there is a disproportionate decrease in ristocetin co-factor activity resembling type 2A vWD.[148]

Paraproteinemias

Patients with a paraproteinemia such as myeloma or Waldenström macroglobulinemia often have an abnormal clotting profile although bleeding is relatively uncommon. A variety of abnormalities have been described and these usually arise due to the effect the abnormal paraprotein has on platelet and/or clotting factor function. Some patients with myeloma can develop a circulating heparin-like anticoagulant, which can result in a severe, unrelenting bleeding that is often fatal.[149,150]

Amyloidosis may be associated with the development of selective factor X deficiency.[151,152] The mechanisms for this are unclear but it is believed that the factor X is adsorbed from plasma onto the amyloid deposits. Such patients can be difficult to treat and show a poor response to therapy. Treatment with high dose chemotherapy and autologous stem cell transplant can be effective, but there is a high risk of bleeding complications in the peritransplant period. The administration of factor X is of little benefit as the protein is rapidly removed from the circulation. Splenectomy may be of value in some cases.[153]

Acquired inhibitors of coagulation

Acquired inhibitors of coagulation are antibodies directed against various coagulation factors, which rapidly neutralize their procoagulant activity, resulting in a bleeding diathesis or increasing the severity of a pre-existing coagulation disorder. Such antibodies may occur in response to treatment in patients with an inherited coagulation disorder, e.g. hemophilia A or B (alloantibodies) or develop as autoantibodies in individuals with or without an underlying immune disorder (Table 35.3).

The most frequent spontaneous inhibitors or antibodies are directed against the factor VIII molecule, have an equal sex incidence and occur primarily in the elderly (after the

Table 35.3 Acquired coagulation inhibitors

Factor inhibitor	Reported associations
II	SLE, liver cirrhosis, prosthetic cardiac valves, bovine clotting factors, monoclonal gammopathies
V	Bovine clotting factors, β-lactam antibiotics, malignancy, autoimmune disease, postpartum, post-surgery
VII	Malignancy (solid or hematological)
VIII	Solid tumors, lymphoproliferative disorders, autoimmune disease, peripartum, medications (e.g. penicillin, phenytoin)
IX	Postpartum
X	Amyloid
XI	Autoimmune disease, malignancy, infection
XIII	Tuberculosis-isoniazid, penicillin, phenytoin, leukemias, severe liver disease, paraprotein disorders, autoimmune disorders, e.g. SLE
vWF	Monoclonal gammopathies, lymphoproliferative disorders, myeloproliferative disorders, autoimmune disease

7th decade of life). Less frequently, they develop in women postpartum.[154-157]

Factor V inhibitors are occasionally seen following the use of bovine clotting factors or the use of β-lactam antibiotics. Inhibitors directed against factor II (prothrombin) have been reported in association with SLE, liver cirrhosis and in some patients with prosthetic cardiac valves. Factor VII inhibitors, in the absence of factor VII deficiency, are rare but are occasionally seen in patients with an underlying tumor, in some patients with myeloma, chronic lymphocytic leukemia and non-Hodgkin lymphoma. In myeloma the inhibitors frequently resolve as the disease is treated. Inhibitors to factor XIII have been reported in SLE, in association with monoclonal gammopathies and in some patients receiving isoniazid.

Acquired heparin-like anticoagulants have been described in some patients with myeloma and various solid tumors.

Laboratory findings in acquired inhibitors

In patients with an acquired factor VIII inhibitor, the PT is normal but the APTT is prolonged and fails to correct in a mix with normal plasma. Factor VIII coagulant activity is reduced and factor VIII inhibitors are present. The inhibitor in a patient with an acquired factor VIII deficiency is complex. The linear relationship between inhibitor concentration and the amount of factor VIII inhibited observed in hemophilia A patients with inhibitors is not seen in other patient groups.

Management of acquired inhibitors

In patients who are not actively bleeding no treatment may be required. However, any potential cause for the development of the inhibitor should be sought and wherever possible treated. FEIBA – an activated prothrombin complex concentrate (APCC) – may be of value or recombinant activated factor VII (rVIIA) may be useful. Treatment is often combined with immunosuppressive therapy including steroids and in selected cases cyclophosphamide or rituximab may be used.

Acquired von Willebrand syndrome

Acquired von Willebrand syndrome (AVWS) is a rare, but probably under-diagnosed bleeding disorder. The clinical and laboratory features are identical to inherited vWD, but occur in individuals with no personal or family history of bleeding. AVWS most commonly occurs in patients with lymphoproliferative or myeloproliferative disorders and cardiovascular disease.[158] The usual mechanism is increased elimination of von Willebrand factor (vWF), although reduced synthesis is thought to be important in AVWS associated with hypothyroidism.[159] Increased elimination of vWF may occur due to the formation of antibodies to vWF/FVIII, which increase clearance by the reticuloendothelial system and/or impair vWF function. Other mechanisms include adsorption of vWF onto malignant cells, increased proteolysis of vWF multimers or loss of high molecular weight multimers under conditions of high shear stress (e.g. aortic valve disease).

In AVWS, assays for plasma vWF typically show a normal or mildly reduced vWF antigen level, with reduced functional activity (reduced ristocetin co-factor activity or collagen binding). Factor VIII procoagulant activity levels may be normal or low. In contrast to acquired hemophilia, circulating inhibitors to vWF are uncommon.[158]

Treatment options for AVWS include intravenous immunoglobulin, immunosuppression, intermediate purity factor VIII concentrates and high purity vWF concentrates. DDAVP can improve VWF levels, but the effect is usually less durable than in congenital vWD.

Snake venoms and other toxic coagulopathies

Snake venoms can have multiple effects on coagulation.[160] Many snake venoms contain serine proteases with thrombin-like activity, which cleave fibrinogen, resulting in hypofibrinogenemia and some are fibrinolytic.[161] Snake venom thrombin-like enzymes are generally not inhibited by heparin. Snake venoms also commonly contain prothrombin, factor X and factor V activators. Activators of other components of the coagulation pathway, such as factor XIII and plasminogen activators have also been described.[160] Some purified snake venoms are used in the routine diagnostic laboratory, due to their specific effects on coagulation[162] (Table 35.4).

Table 35.4 Snake venoms, mechanisms of action and potential diagnostic laboratory use

Snake	Mechanism of action	Diagnostic use
Bothrops atrox	Thrombin-like enzyme	Reptilase time; an alternative to the thrombin time in heparin contaminated samples
Daboia russelli	Activation of factor X	DRVVT : LAC Factor X assays
Echis carinatus	Phospholipid independent prothrombin activation	Echis time; hirudin monitoring Textarin: ecarin ratio; LAC
Pseudonaja textilis	Phospholipid dependent prothrombin activation	Textarin: ecarin ratio; LAC
Agkistrodon contortrix contortrix	Protein C activator	Protein C and S measurement Activated protein C resistance
Bothrops jararaca	Platelet aggregation in the presence of vWF	Used with ristocetin to differentiate variants of vWD and Bernard–Soulier disease

DRVVT, dilute Russell's viper venom time; LAC, lupus anticoagulant; vWF, von Willebrand factor.

Envenomation by some elapid and viperid snakes containing such hemotoxins results in venom induced consumptive coagulopathy (VICC). The PT and APTT are typically markedly prolonged or unclottable, with low fibrinogen and very high fibrin(ogen) degradation products. Recovery of coagulation lags behind venom neutralization. The role of factor replacement (FFP or cryoprecipitate) in VICC remains controversial.[163–165] A proportion of cases can go on to develop a thrombotic microangiopathy.[166]

A number of other toxic agents may be associated with an acquired hemostatic defect, leading to a bleeding disorder.[161] Pharmacological agents, for example interleukin-2 (IL-2), when used at high concentration can induce a DIC-like syndrome with systemic hyperfibrinolysis.[165] *Lonomia achelous* is a caterpillar with particularly toxic saliva that induces hypofibrinogenemia together with low levels of factors V and XIII. Fibrin degradation products are increased and plasminogen is decreased.[162–164]

References

1. Andrew M, Paes B, Milner R, et al. Development of the human coagulation system in the healthy premature infant. Blood 1988;72(5):1651–7.

2. Andrew M, Vegh P, Johnston M, et al. Maturation of the hemostatic system during childhood. Blood 1992;80(8): 1998–2005.

3. Williams MD, Chalmers EA, Gibson BE. The investigation and management of neonatal haemostasis and thrombosis. Br J Haematol 2002 Nov;119(2):295–309.

4. Sattler FR, Weitekamp MR, Sayegh A, Ballard JO. Impaired hemostasis caused by beta-lactam antibiotics. Am J Surg 1988;155(5A):30–9.

5. Perry DJ. Antithrombin and its inherited deficiencies. Blood Reviews 1994;8: 37–55.

6. Barrowcliffe TW. Low molecular weight heparin(s). Br J Haematol 1995;90(1): 1–7.

7. Hubbard AR, Jennings CA. Neutralisation of heparan sulphate and low molecular weight heparin by protamine. Thromb Haemost 1985;53(1):86–9.

8. Baglin TP, Keeling DM, Watson HG. Guidelines on oral anticoagulation (warfarin): third edition – 2005 update. Br J Haematol 2006 Feb;132(3): 277–85.

9. Bichler J, Fritz H. Hirudin, a new therapeutic tool? Annals of Hematology 1991;63(2):67–76.

10. Kaiser B. Anticoagulant and antithrombotic actions of recombinant hirudin. Seminars in Thrombosis and Hemostasis 1991;17(2):130–6.

11. Kaiser B, Fareed J, Walenga JM, et al. In vitro studies on thrombin generation in citrated, r-hirudinized and heparinized whole blood. Thrombosis Research 1991;64(5):589–96.

12. Potzsch B, Hund S, Madlener K, et al. Monitoring of recombinant hirudin: assessment of a plasma-based ecarin clotting time assay. Thrombosis Research 1997;86(5):373–83.

13. Lange U, Nowak G, Bucha E. Ecarin chromogenic assay – a new method for quantitative determination of direct thrombin inhibitors like hirudin. Pathophysiology of Haemostasis and Thrombosis 2004;33(4):184–91.

14. Panneerselvam S, Baglin C, Lefort W, Baglin T. Analysis of risk factors for over-anticoagulation in patients receiving long-term warfarin. Br J Haematol 1998; 103(2):422–4.

15. Hull R, Hirsh J, Jay R, et al. Different intensities of oral anticoagulant therapy in the treatment of proximal-vein thrombosis. New England Journal of Medicine 1982;307(27):1676–81.

16. Landefeld CS, Goldman L. Major bleeding in outpatients treated with warfarin. American Journal of Medicine 1989;87:144–52.

17. Palareti G, Leali N, Coccheri S, et al. Bleeding complications of oral anticoagulant treatment: an inception-cohort, prospective collaborative study (ISCOAT). Italian Study on Complications of Oral Anticoagulant Therapy. Lancet 1996;348(9025):423–8.

18. Makris M, Greaves M, Phillips WS, et al. Emergency oral anticoagulant reversal: the relative efficacy of infusions of fresh frozen plasma and clotting factor concentrate on correction of the coagulopathy. Thromb Haemost 1997; 77(3):477–80.

19. Ludlam CA, Bennett B, Fox KA, et al. Guidelines for the use of thrombolytic therapy. Haemostasis and Thrombosis Task Force of the British Committee for Standards in Haematology. Blood Coagul Fibrinolysis 1995;6(3):273–85.

20. Bonnefoy A, Legrand C. Proteolysis of subendothelial adhesive glycoproteins (fibronectin, thrombospondin, and von Willebrand factor) by plasmin, leukocyte cathepsin G, and elastase. Thrombosis Research 2000;98(4):323–32.

21. Vane JR, Botting RM. Anti-inflammatory drugs and their mechanism of action. Inflamm Res 1998;47(Suppl 2):S78–87.

22. Easton JD. Clinical aspects of the use of clopidogrel, a new antiplatelet agent. Circulation 1999;100(15):1667–72.

23. Quinn MJ, Fitzgerald DJ. Clopidogrel and ticlopidine – improvements on aspirin? Drug Ther Bull 1999;37(8): 59–61.

24. Nurden AT, Poujol C, Durrieu-Jais C, Nurden P. Platelet glycoprotein IIb/IIIa inhibitors: basic and clinical aspects. Arterioscler Thromb Vasc Biol 1999;19(12):2835–40.

25. Burroughs SF, Johnson GJ. b-Lactam antibiotic-induced platelet dysfunction: evidence for irreversible inhibition of platelet activation *in vitro* and *in vivo* are prolonged exposure to penicillin. Blood 1990;75:1473–80.

26. Brown CH, Natelson EA, Bradshaw MW, et al. The haemostatic defect produced by carbenicillin. New England Journal of Medicine 1974;291:265–70.

27. Shearer MJ, Bechtold H, Andrassy K et al. Mechanism of cephalosporin-induced hypoprothrombinemia: relation of cephalosporin side chain, vitamin K metabolism and vitamin K status. Journal of Clinical Pharmacology 1988; 28:88–95.

28. Loiseau P. Sodium valproate, platelet dysfunction, and bleeding. Epilepsia 1981;22(2):141–6.

29. Zimmermann N, Hohlfeld T. Clinical implications of aspirin resistance. Thromb Haemost 2008 Sep;100(3): 379–90.

30. Gasparyan AY, Watson T, Lip GY. The role of aspirin in cardiovascular prevention: implications of aspirin resistance. J Am Coll Cardiol 2008 May 13;51(19):1829–43.

31. Tseeng S, Arora R. Aspirin resistance: biological and clinical implications. J Cardiovasc Pharmacol Ther 2008 Mar; 13(1):5–12.

32. Patrono C, Rocca B. Aspirin: promise and resistance in the new millennium. Arterioscler Thromb Vasc Biol 2008 Mar; 28(3):s25–32.

33. Fitzgerald DJ, Maree A. Aspirin and clopidogrel resistance. Hematology Am Soc Hematol Educ Program. 2007: 114–20.

34. Michos ED, Ardehali R, Blumenthal RS, et al. Aspirin and clopidogrel resistance. Mayo Clinic Proceedings 2006 Apr;81(4): 518–26.

35. Harrison P. The role of PFA-100 testing in the investigation and management of haemostatic defects in children and adults. Br J Haematol 2005 Jul;130(1): 3–10.

36. Chakroun T, Addad F, Abderazek F, et al. Screening for aspirin resistance in stable coronary artery patients by three different tests. Thrombosis Research 2007;121(3): 413–8.

37. Lordkipanidze M, Pharand C, Schampaert E, et al. A comparison of six major platelet function tests to determine the prevalence of aspirin resistance in patients with stable coronary artery disease. Eur Heart J 2007 Jul;28(14):1702–8.

38. Zipursky A. Prevention of vitamin K deficiency bleeding in newborns. Br J Haematol 1999;104(3):430–7.

39. von Kries R. Oral versus intramuscular phytomenadione: safety and efficacy compared. Drug Saf 1999;21(1):1–6.

40. Fujimura Y, Okubo Y, Sakai T, et al. Studies on precursor proteins PIVKA-II, -IX, and -X in the plasma of patients with 'hemorrhagic disease of the newborn'. Haemostasis 1984;14(2): 211–7.

41. McKinney PA, Juszczak E, Findlay E, Smith K. Which vitamin K preparation for the newborn? Case-control study of childhood leukaemia and cancer in Scotland: findings for neonatal intramuscular vitamin K. Drug Ther Bull 1998;36(3):17–9.

42. Green G, Poller L, Thomson JM, Dymock IW. Factor VII as a marker of hepatocellular synthetic function in liver disease. J Clin Pathol 1976;29(11): 971–5.

43. Nagamine T, Ohtuka T, Takehara K, et al. Thrombocytopenia associated with hepatitis C viral infection. J Hepatol 1996;24(2):135–40.

44. Martinez J, Palascak JE, Kwasniak D. Abnormal sialic acid content of the dysfibrinogenemia associated with liver disease. J Clin Invest 1978;61(2):535–8.

45. Green G, Thomson JM, Dymock IW, Poller L. Abnormal fibrin polymerization in liver disease. Br J Haematol 1976; 34(3):427–39.

46. Pernambuco JR, Langley PG, Hughes RD, et al. Activation of the fibrinolytic system in patients with fulminant liver failure. Hepatology 1993;18(6):1350–6.

47. Caldwell SH, Sanyal AJ. Coagulation and hemostasis in liver disease: controversies and advances. Preface. Clin Liver Dis 2009 Feb;13(1):xv.

48. Tripodi A. Hemostasis in chronic liver disease. J Thromb Haemost 2006 Sep; 4(9):2064–5.

49. Tripodi A, Mannucci PM. Abnormalities of hemostasis in chronic liver disease: reappraisal of their clinical significance and need for clinical and laboratory research. J Hepatol 2007 Apr;46(4): 727–33.

50. Tripodi A, Primignani M, Mannucci PM. Abnormalities of hemostasis and bleeding in chronic liver disease: the paradigm is challenged. Intern Emerg Med. 2010; 5(1):7–12.

51. Tempero MA, Davis RB, Reed E, Edney J. Thrombocytopenia and laboratory evidence of disseminated intravascular coagulation after shunts for ascites in malignant disease. Cancer 1985;55(11): 2718–21.

52. Kohler M. Thrombogenicity of prothrombin complex concentrates. Thrombosis Research 1999;95(4 Suppl 1):S13–7.

53. Marassi A, Manzullo V, di Carlo V, Mannucci PM. Thromboembolism following prothrombin complex concentrates and major surgery in severe liver disease. Thromb Haemost 1978;39(3):787–8.

54. Kamath PS, Weisner RH, Malinchoc M, et al. A model to predict survival in patients with end-stage liver disease. Hepatology 2001;33(2):467–70.

55. Pugh RN, Murray-Lyon IM, Dawson JL, et al. Transection of the oesophagus for bleeding oesophageal varices. British Journal of Surgery 1973;60(8): 646–9.

56. Kovacs MJ, Wong A, MacKinnon K, et al. Assessment of the validity of the INR system for patients with liver impairment [see comments]. Thromb Haemost 1994; 71(6):727–30.

57. Trotter JF, Olson J, Lefkowitz J, et al. Changes in international normalized ratio (INR) and model for endstage liver disease (MELD) based on selection of clinical laboratory. Am J Transplant 2007 Jun;7(6):1624–8.

58. Tripodi A. How to implement the modified international normalized ratio for cirrhosis (INR(Liver)) for end-stage liver disease calculation. Journal of Hepatology 2008;47(4):1424.

59. Mannucci PM, Remuzzi G, Pusineri F, et al. Deamino-8-D-arginine vasopressin shortens the bleeding time in uremia. New England Journal of Medicine 1983; 308(1):8–12.

60. Noris M, Benigni A, Boccardo P, et al. Enhanced nitric oxide synthesis in uremia: implications for platelet dysfunction and dialysis hypotension. Kidney Int 1993;44(2):445–50.

61. Michalak E, Walkowiak B, Paradowski M, Cierniewski CS. The decreased circulating platelet mass and its relation to bleeding time in chronic renal failure. Thromb Haemost 1991;65(1):11–4.

62. Zachée P, Vermylen J, Boogaerts MA. Hematologics aspects of end-stage renal failure. Annals of Hematology 1994; 69:33–40.

63. Sloand EM, Sloand JA, Prodouz K, et al. Reduction of platelet glycoprotein Ib in uraemia. Br J Haematol 1991;77(3): 375–81.

64. Sloand JA, Sloand EM. Studies on platelet membrane glycoproteins and platelet function during hemodialysis. J Am Soc Nephrol 1997;8(5):799–803.

65. Gralnick HR, McKeown LP, Williams SB, et al. Plasma and platelet von Willebrand factor defects in uremia. American Journal of Medicine 1988;85(6): 806–10.

66. Mezzano D, Tagle R, Panes O, et al. Hemostatic disorder of uremia: the platelet defect, main determinant of the prolonged bleeding time, is correlated with indices of activation of coagulation and fibrinolysis. Thromb Haemost 1996; 76(3):312–21.

67. Vlachoyannis J, Schoeppe W. Adenylate cyclase activity and cAMP content of human platelets in uraemia. Eur J Clin Invest 1982;12(5):379–81.

68. Smith MC, Dunn MJ. Impaired platelet thromboxane production in renal failure. Nephron 1981;29(3–4):133–7.

69. Pemuzzi G. Prostacyclin-like activity and bleeding in renal failure. Lancet 1977; 310:1195–7.

70. Gandrille S, Jouvin MH, Toulon P, et al. A study of fibrinogen and fibrinolysis in 10 adults with nephrotic syndrome. Thromb Haemost 1988 Jun 16;59(3): 445–50.

71. Remuzzi G, Mecca G, Marchesi D, et al. Platelet hyperaggregability and the nephrotic syndrome. Thrombosis Research 1979;16(3–4):345–54.

72. Fabris F, Cordiano I, Randi ML, et al. Effect of human recombinant erythropoietin on bleeding time, platelet number and function in children with end-stage renal disease maintained by haemodialysis. Pediatr Nephrol 1991; 5(2):225–8.

73. Vigano G, Benigni A, Mendogni D, et al. Recombinant human erythropoietin to correct uremic bleeding. Am J Kidney Dis 1991;18(1):44–9.

74. Livio M, Mannucci PM, Vigano G, et al. Conjugated estrogens for the management of bleeding associated with renal failure. New England Journal of Medicine 1986;315(12):731–5.

75. Sloand JA, Schiff MJ. Beneficial effect of low-dose transdermal estrogen on bleeding time and clinical bleeding in uremia. Am J Kidney Dis 1995;26(1): 22–6.

76. Brohi K, Singh J, Heron M, Coats T. Acute traumatic coagulopathy. J Trauma 2003 Jun;54(6):1127–30.

77. Maegele M. Frequency, risk stratification and therapeutic management of acute post-traumatic coagulopathy. Vox Sang 2009 Jul;97(1):39–49.

78. Borgman MA, Spinella PC, Perkins JG, et al. The ratio of blood products transfused affects mortality in patients receiving massive transfusions at a combat support hospital. J Trauma 2007 Oct;63(4):805–13.

79. Dann EJ, Michaelson M, Barzelay M, et al. Transfusion medicine during the summer of 2006: lessons learned in northern Israel. Transfus Med Rev 2008 Jan;22(1):70–6.

80. Berkhof FF, Eikenboom JC. Efficacy of recombinant activated factor VII in patients with massive uncontrolled bleeding: a retrospective observational analysis. Transfusion 2009 Mar;49(3): 570–7.

81. Bevan DH. Cardiac bypass haemostasis: putting blood through the mill. Br J Haematol 1999 Feb;104(2):208–19.

82. Harker LA, Malpass TW, Branson HE. Mechanism of abnormal bleeding in individuals undergoing cardiopulmonary bypass: acquired transient platelet dysfunction associated with selective a-granule release. Blood 1980;56:824–34.

83. Rinder CS, Bohnert J, Rinder HM, et al. Platelet activation and aggregation during cardiopulmonary bypass. Anesthesiology 1991;75(3):388–93.

84. Edmunds Jr LH, Colman RW. Thrombin during cardiopulmonary bypass. Ann Thorac Surg 2006 Dec;82(6):2315–22.

85. Kondo C, Tanaka K, Takagi K, et al. Platelet dysfunction during cardiopulmonary bypass surgery. With special reference to platelet membrane glycoproteins. Asaio J 1993;39(3): M550–3.

86. Harker LA, Malpass TW, Branson HE, et al. Mechanism of abnormal bleeding in patients undergoing cardiopulmonary bypass: acquired transient platelet dysfunction associated with selective alpha-granule release. Blood 1980 Nov; 56(5):824–34.

87. Wendel HP, Jones DW, Gallimore MJ. FXII levels, FXIIa-like activities and kallikrein activities in normal subjects and patients undergoing cardiac surgery.

Immunopharmacology 1999;45(1–3): 141–4.

88. Boisclair MD, Lane DA, Philippou H, et al. Mechanisms of thrombin generation during surgery and cardiopulmonary bypass. Blood 1993; 82(11):3350–7.

89. Chung JH, Gikakis N, Rao AK, et al. Pericardial blood activates the extrinsic coagulation pathway during clinical cardiopulmonary bypass. Circulation 1996 Jun 1;93(11):2014–8.

90. Yavari M, Becker RC. Coagulation and fibrinolytic protein kinetics in cardiopulmonary bypass. J Thromb Thrombolysis 2009 Jan;27(1):95–104.

91. Ray MJ, Marsh NA, Hawson GA. Relationship of fibrinolysis and platelet function to bleeding after cardiopulmonary bypass. Blood Coagul Fibrinolysis 1994;5(5):679–85.

92. de Haan J, Schonberger J, Haan J, et al. Tissue-type plasminogen activator and fibrin monomers synergistically cause platelet dysfunction during retransfusion of shed blood after cardiopulmonary bypass. J Thorac Cardiovasc Surg 1993;106(6):1017–23.

93. Yoshihara H, Yamamoto T, Mihara H. Changes in coagulation and fibrinolysis occurring in dogs during hypothermia. Thrombosis Research 1985;37(4): 503–12.

94. Valen G, Eriksson E, Risberg B, Vaage J. Fibrinolysis during cardiac surgery. Release of tissue plasminogen activator in arterial and coronary sinus blood. Eur J Cardiothorac Surg 1994;8(6):324–30.

95. Despotis GJ, Levine V, Joist JH, et al. Antithrombin III during cardiac surgery: effect on response of activated clotting time to heparin and relationship to markers of hemostatic activation. Anesth Analg 1997;85(3):498–506.

96. Kimmel SE, Sekeres MA, Berlin JA, et al. Adverse events after protamine administration in patients undergoing cardiopulmonary bypass: risks and predictors of under-reporting. J Clin Epidemiol 1998;51(1):1–10.

97. Martin P, Horkay F, Gupta NK, et al. Heparin rebound phenomenon – much ado about nothing? Blood Coagul Fibrinolysis 1992;3(2):187–91.

98. Pifarre R, Babka R, Sullivan HJ, et al. Management of postoperative heparin rebound following cardiopulmonary bypass. J Thorac Cardiovasc Surg 1981; 81(3):378–81.

99. Zumberg MS, Waples JM, Kao KJ, Lottenberg R. Management of a patient with a mechanical aortic valve and antibodies to both thrombin and factor V after repeat exposure to fibrin sealant. American Journal of Hematology 2000; 64(1):59–63.

100. Berruyer M, Amiral J, Ffrench P, et al. Immunization by bovine thrombin used with fibrin glue during cardiovascular operations. Development of thrombin and factor V inhibitors. Journal of Thoracic and Cardiovascular Surgery 1993;105(5):892–7.

101. Spiess BD, Tuman KJ, McCarthy RJ, et al. Thromboelastography as an indicator of post-cardiopulmonary bypass coagulopathies. J Clin Monit 1987;3(1): 25–30.

102. Tuman KJ, McCarthy RJ, Djuric M, et al. Evaluation of coagulation during cardiopulmonary bypass with a heparinase-modified thromboelastographic assay. J Cardiothorac Vasc Anesth 1994; 8(2):144–9.

103. Tuman KJ, Spiess BD, McCarthy RJ, Ivankovich AD. Comparison of viscoelastic measures of coagulation after cardiopulmonary bypass. Anesth Analg 1989;69(1):69–75.

104. Henry D, Carless P, Fergusson D, Laupacis A. The safety of aprotinin and lysine-derived antifibrinolytic drugs in cardiac surgery: a meta-analysis. CMAJ 2009 Jan 20;180(2):183–93.

105. Lu H, Du BC, Soria J, et al. Postoperative hemostasis and fibrinolysis in patients undergoing cardiopulmonary bypass with or without aprotinin therapy. Thromb Haemost 1994;72(3):438–43.

106. Orchard MA, Goodchild CS, Prentice CR, et al. Aprotinin reduces cardiopulmonary bypass-induced blood loss and inhibits fibrinolysis without influencing platelets. Br J Haematol 1993;85(3):533–41.

107. Mangano DT, Tudor IC, Dietzel C. The risk associated with aprotinin in cardiac surgery. N Engl J Med 2006 Jan 26; 354(4):353–65.

108. Shaw AD, Stafford-Smith M, White WD, et al. The effect of aprotinin on outcome after coronary-artery bypass grafting. N Engl J Med 2008 Feb 21;358(8):784–93.

109. Schneeweiss S, Seeger JD, Landon J, Walker AM. Aprotinin during coronary-artery bypass grafting and risk of death. N Engl J Med 2008 Feb 21;358(8): 771–83.

110. Mangano DT, Miao Y, Vuylsteke A, et al. Mortality associated with aprotinin during 5 years following coronary artery bypass graft surgery. JAMA 2007 Feb 7; 297(5):471–9.

111. Steiner PE, Lushbaugh CC. Maternal pulmonary embolism by amniotic fluid as a cause of obstetric shock and unexpected deaths in obstetrics. JAMA 1986;255(16):2187–203.

112. Graeff H, Kuhn W. Coagulation disorders in obstetrics. Major Problems in Obstetrics and Gynecology 1980; 13(1):1–157.

113. Bonnar J, McNicol GP, Douglas AS. Coagulation and fibrinolytic systems in pre-eclampsia and eclampsia. Br Med J 1971;2(752):12–6.

114. Higuchi T, Shimizu T, Mori H, et al. Coagulation patterns of disseminated intravascular coagulation in acute promyelocytic leukemia. Hematol Oncol 1997;15(4):209–17.

115. Francis JL, Biggerstaff J, Amirkhosravi A. Hemostasis and malignancy. Seminars in Thrombosis and Hemostasis 1998;24(2): 93–109.

116. Lasson A, Ohlsson K. Consumptive coagulopathy, fibrinolysis and protease-antiprotease interactions during acute human pancreatitis. Thrombosis Research 1986;41(2):167–83.

117. Than T, Hutton RA, Myint L, et al. Haemostatic disturbances in patients bitten by Russell's viper (*Vipera russelli siamensis*) in Burma. British Journal of Haematology 1988;69(4):513–20.

118. Hasiba U, Rosenbach LM, Rockwell D, Lewis JH. DIC-like syndrome after envenomation by the snake, *Crotalus horridus horridus*. New England Journal of Medicine 1975;292(10):505–7.

119. Smith OP, White B, Vaughan D, et al. Use of protein-C concentrate, heparin, and haemodiafiltration in meningococcus-induced purpura fulminans. Lancet 1997;350(9091): 1590–3.

120. Levi M, Toh CH, Thachil J, Watson HG. Guidelines for the diagnosis and management of disseminated intravascular coagulation. British Committee for Standards in Haematology. Br J Haematol 2009 Apr; 145(1):24–33.

121. Downey C, Kazmi R, Toh CH. Novel and diagnostically applicable information from optical waveform analysis of blood coagulation in disseminated intravascular coagulation. Br J Haematol 1997 Jul; 98(1):68–73.

122. Toh CH, Samis J, Downey C, et al. Biphasic transmittance waveform in the APTT coagulation assay is due to the formation of a Ca(++)-dependent complex of C-reactive protein with very-low-density lipoprotein and is a novel marker of impending disseminated intravascular coagulation. Blood 2002 Oct 1;100(7):2522–9.

123. Matsumoto T, Wada H, Nishioka Y, et al. Frequency of abnormal biphasic aPTT clot waveforms in patients with underlying disorders associated with disseminated intravascular coagulation. Clin Appl Thromb Hemost 2006 Apr; 12(2):185–92.

124. Taylor Jr FB, Toh CH, Hoots WK, et al. Towards definition, clinical and laboratory criteria, and a scoring system for disseminated intravascular coagulation. Thromb Haemost 2001 Nov;86(5):1327–30.

125. Bakhtiari K, Meijers JC, de Jonge E, Levi M. Prospective validation of the International Society of Thrombosis and Haemostasis scoring system for disseminated intravascular coagulation. Crit Care Med 2004 Dec;32(12): 2416–21.

126. Angstwurm MW, Dempfle CE, Spannagl M. New disseminated intravascular coagulation score: a useful tool to predict mortality in comparison with Acute Physiology and Chronic Health Evaluation II and Logistic Organ Dysfunction scores. Crit Care Med 2006 Feb;34(2):314–20; quiz 28.

127. Balk R, Emerson T, Fourrier F, et al. Therapeutic use of antithrombin concentrate in sepsis. Seminars in Thrombosis and Hemostasis 1998;24(2):183–94.

128. Wiedermann CJ, Kaneider NC. A systematic review of antithrombin concentrate use in patients with disseminated intravascular coagulation of severe sepsis. Blood Coagul Fibrinolysis 2006 Oct;17(7):521–6.

129. Bernard GR, Vincent JL, Laterre PF, et al. Efficacy and safety of recombinant human activated protein C for severe sepsis. N Engl J Med 2001 Mar 8; 344(10):699–709.

130. Dhainaut JF, Yan SB, Joyce DE, et al. Treatment effects of drotrecogin alfa (activated) in patients with severe sepsis with or without overt disseminated intravascular coagulation. J Thromb Haemost 2004 Nov;2(11):1924–33.

131. Abraham E, Laterre PF, Garg R, et al. Drotrecogin alfa (activated) for adults with severe sepsis and a low risk of death. N Engl J Med 2005 Sep 29; 353(13):1332–41.

132. Watzke HH, Linkesch W, Hay U. Giant hemangioma of the liver (Kasabach–Merritt syndrome): successful suppression of intravascular coagulation permitting surgical removal. J Clin Gastroenterol 1989;11(3):347–50.

133. White CW. Treatment of hemangiomatosis with recombinant interferon alfa. Seminars in Hematology. 1990.

134. Bick RL. Coagulation abnormalities in malignancy: a review. Seminars in Thrombosis and Hemostasis 1992;18(4): 353–72.

135. Kunkel LA. Acquired circulating anticoagulants in malignancy. [Review]. Seminars in Thrombosis and Hemostasis 1992;18(6):416–23.

136. Kunkel LA. Acquired circulating anticoagulants. [Review]. Hematology Oncology Clinics of North America 1992;6(6):1341–57.

137. Sletnes KE, Godal HC, Wisloff F. Disseminated intravascular coagulation (DIC) in adult patients with acute leukaemia. Eur J Haematol 1995;54(1): 34–8.

138. Menell JS, Cesarman GM, Jacovina AT, et al. Annexin II and bleeding in acute promyelocytic leukemia. New England Journal of Medicine 1999;340(13): 994–1004.

139. Stein E, McMahon B, Kwaan H, et al. The coagulopathy of acute promyelocytic leukaemia revisited. Best Pract Res Clin Haematol 2009 Mar;22(1):153–63.

140. Priest JR, Ramsay NK, Bennett AJ, et al. The effect of L-asparaginase antithrombin, plasminogen, and plasma coagulation during therapy for acute lymphoblastic leukemia. Journal of Pediatrics 1982;100(6):990–5.

141. Ramsay NK, Coccia PF, Krivit W, et al. The effect of L-asparaginase of plasma coagulation factors in acute lymphoblastic leukemia. Cancer 1977;40(4):1398–401.

142. Baker RI, Manoharan A. Platelet function in myeloproliferative disorders: characterization and sequential studies show multiple platelet abnormalities, and change with time. Eur J Haematol 1988;40(3):267–72.

143. Boneu B, Nouvel C, Sie P, et al. Platelets in myeloproliferative disorders. I. A comparative evaluation with certain platelet function tests. Scand J Haematol 1980;25(3):214–20.

144. Ginsburg AD. Platelet function in patients with high platelet counts. Ann Intern Med 1975;82(4):506–11.

145. Jensen MK, de Nully Brown P, et al. Increased platelet activation and abnormal membrane glycoprotein content and redistribution in myeloproliferative disorders. Br J Haematol 2000;110(1):116–24.

146. Mazzucato M, De Marco L, De Angelis V, et al. Platelet membrane abnormalities in myeloproliferative disorders: decrease in glycoproteins Ib and IIb/IIIa complex is associated with deficient receptor function. Br J Haematol 1989;73(3): 369–74.

147. Yamamoto K, Sekiguchi E, Takatani O. Abnormalities of epinephrine-induced platelet aggregation and adenine nucleotides in myeloproliferative disorders. Thromb Haemost 1984; 52(3):292–6.

148. Budde U, Dent JA, Berkowitz SD, et al. Subunit composition of plasma von Willebrand factor in patients with the myeloproliferative syndrome. Blood 1986;68(6):1213–7.

149. Tefferi A, Nichols WL, Bowie EJ. Circulating heparin-like anticoagulants: report of five consecutive cases and a review. American Journal of Medicine 1990;88(2):184–8.

150. Chapman GS, George CB, Danley DL. Heparin-like anticoagulant associated with plasma cell myeloma. Am J Clin Pathol 1985;83(6):764–6.

151. Furie B, Greene E, Furie BC. Syndrome of acquired factor X deficiency and systemic amyloidosis in vivo studies of the metabolic fate of factor X. New England Journal of Medicine 1977;297(2):81–5.

152. Furie B, Voo L, McAdam K, Furie BC. Mechanism of factor X deficiency in systemic amyloidosis. New England Journal of Medicine 1981;304:827–30.

153. Greipp PR, Kyle RA, Bowie E. Factor X deficiency in primary amyloidosis. Resolution after splenectomy. New England Journal of Medicine 1979; 301:1050–1.

154. Yee TT, Taher A, Pasi KJ, Lee CA. A survey of patients with acquired haemophilia in a haemophilia centre over a 28-year period. Clinical and Laboratory Haematology 2000;22(5):275–8.

155. Saxena R, Mishra DK, Kashyap R, et al. Acquired haemophilia – a study of ten cases. Haemophilia 2000;6(2):78–83.

156. Michiels JJ. Acquired hemophilia A in women postpartum: clinical manifestations, diagnosis, and treatment. Clin Appl Thromb Hemost 2000;6(2): 82–6.

157. Michiels JJ, Hamulyak K, Nieuwenhuis HK, et al. Acquired haemophilia A in women postpartum: management of bleeding episodes and natural history of the factor VIII inhibitor. Eur J Haematol 1997;59(2):105–9.

158. Federici AB, Rand JH, Bucciarelli P, et al. Acquired von Willebrand syndrome: data from an international registry. Thromb Haemost 2000 Aug;84(2):345–9.

159. Franchini M, Lippi G. Acquired von Willebrand syndrome: an update. Am J Hematol 2007 May;82(5):368–75.

160. Isbister GK. Procoagulant snake toxins: laboratory studies, diagnosis, and understanding snakebite coagulopathy. Semin Thromb Hemost 2009 Feb; 35(1):93–103.

161. Swenson S, Markland FS Jr. Snake venom fibrin(ogen)olytic enzymes. Toxicon 2005 Jun 15;45(8):1021–39.

162. Marsh N, Williams V. Practical applications of snake venom toxins in haemostasis. Toxicon 2005 Jun 15; 45(8):1171–81.

163. Brown SG, Caruso N, Borland ML, et al. Clotting factor replacement and recovery from snake venom-induced consumptive coagulopathy. Intensive Care Med 2009 Sep;35(9):1532–8.

164. Isbister GK, Duffull SB, Brown SG. Failure of antivenom to improve recovery in Australian snakebite coagulopathy. QJM 2009 Aug;102(8):563–8.

165. Jelinek GA, Smith A, Lynch D, et al. FFP after brown snake envenoming: think twice. Anaesth Intensive Care 2005 Aug; 33(4):542–3.

166. Isbister GK, Little M, Cull G, et al. Thrombotic microangiopathy from Australian brown snake (*Pseudonaja*) envenoming. Intern Med J 2007 Aug; 37(8):523–8.

CHAPTER 36

Natural anticoagulants and thrombophilia

E Norström, G Escolar

Introduction

Correct hemostasis is the result of a delicate balance among procoagulant and anticoagulant systems. The ultimate goal of coagulation mechanisms is to prevent excessive bleeding. A series of coordinated events among enzymatic reactions and platelet responses will generate thrombin that will convert soluble fibrinogen into fibrin to help consolidating an initial hemostatic plug formed by platelets at sites of vessel damage. Failure of the coagulation mechanisms results in excessive bleeding. Mechanisms of coagulation are conveniently regulated to limit the extent of the activation once it has been triggered. There is a scientifically based concern that in the next decades thrombotic complications will become the most important contributors to mortality and morbidity in modern societies. Excessive coagulation or deficient regulation by natural anticoagulants are the underlying causes of thrombosis.

This chapter is arranged in four main sections. The first will review the mechanisms leading to blood coagulation. The following section will focus on the description of natural anticoagulants to provide information on the molecular/pathogenic mechanisms that lead to thrombophilia. The third section will place special emphasis in thrombophilic states, their pathophysiology and their clinical implications. The last section will attempt to provide a simplified view of laboratory tests, need to perform screening and a schematic approach to the management of patients with thrombotic complications.

©2011 Elsevier Ltd
DOI: 10.1016/B978-0-7020-3147-2.00036-5

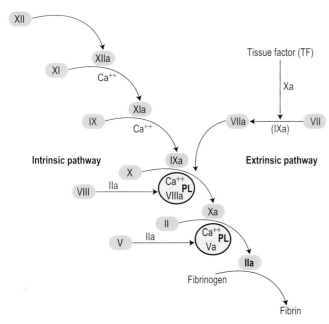

Fig. 36.1 The classic coagulation cascade. The intrinsic coagulation pathway is initiated when blood gets in contact with a foreign surface. The extrinsic pathway is initiated after tissue factor (TF) is exposed at sites of vascular injury. The two pathways converge at the activation of FX to FXa and a common pathway that leads to thrombin formation. Ovals indicate reactions that are accelerated by anionic phospholipids (PL) exposed on activated platelet membranes.

Coagulation

Classic cascade mechanism of coagulation vs. cell-based models of thrombin generation

In the mid 1960s two different investigators conceived an original concept of the coagulation mechanisms triggered as a 'cascade' of proteolytic reactions acting as biological amplifiers.[1,2] According to those classic concepts, coagulation mechanisms were activated through intrinsic and extrinsic pathways converging on a common pathway that will finally activate prothrombin into thrombin that would cause soluble fibrinogen to become polymerized into a solid fibrin clot (Fig. 36.1).

Modern concepts have integrated the classic stepwise cascade into a more comprehensive scheme in which blood coagulation is initiated by cellular components *in vivo*.[3] Actual models contemplate the implication of cellular and enzymatic mechanisms in three differentiated steps: Initial activation, propagation and thrombin generation (Fig. 36.2). Fibroblasts, smooth muscle cells of the vascular wall, activated monocytes or endothelial cells, or even platelets are potential cellular sources of TF.[4,5] According to current knowledge, the activation of the coagulation is initiated at the very moment in which TF is exposed on cellular surfaces. TF is a transmembrane protein that binds plasma factor VII/VIIa. In a first step, the TF exposed on damaged vascular

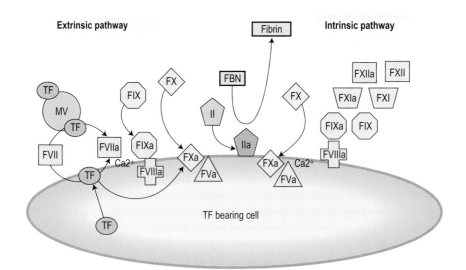

Fig. 36.2 The cell-based model of coagulation emphasizes that tissue factor (TF) exposed on cell surfaces is the key event for the activation of coagulation under physiological circumstances. TF can be provided by fibroblasts, smooth muscle cells of the vascular wall, activated monocytes, endothelial cells, platelets or transported by microvesicles (MV). TF expressed on damaged or activated cellular surfaces forms a complex with FVII-FVIIa. This complex will activate FX to FXa and FIX to FIXa. FXa stays in the vicinity of the TF-bearing cell and, in the presence of FVa, converts a small amount of prothrombin (FII) to thrombin (FIIa) on the cell surface. The small amount of thrombin generated will be sufficient to activate platelets and FVIII, FV, and FXI. FVIIIa, FVa, and FXa occupy sites on the activated cell surface (activated platelets). FIXa, activated by TF-FVIIa, does not remain on the TF cell, but converts FX to FXa on the activated cell surface. FXIa acts to boost FIXa generation on the activated platelet, increasing FXa and subsequent thrombin generation. The intrinsic pathway may also take place on cellular surfaces, but its contribution to physiological coagulation is limited. *(Adapted from references [3–5]).*

areas forms a complex with FVII/FVIIa. FVIIa is present in reduced amounts in circulating blood. The TF:FVIIa complexes will activate FIX and FX. FXa generated will activate small quantities of prothrombin (FII) into thrombin (FIIa). Small amounts of thrombin generated in this short loop will be able to promote further activation of the coagulation by further activating FV and FVIII in the presence of platelet phospholipids and FIX.[3] During the propagation step FIXa bound to FVIIa on the surface of activated platelets form the tenase complex that will further activate FX into FXa. FXa binds to FVa on the phospholipid surface provided by activated platelets and form the prothrombinase complex. During the final step of the cell-based model, the prothrombinase complex will further magnify the generation of thrombin facilitating the conversion of prothrombin into thrombin. Large amounts of thrombin generated during the final step will convert fibrinogen into fibrin. Thrombin itself activates FXIII thus stabilizing the fibrin formed.

Molecular mechanism

The majority of enzymes in the coagulation cascade are members of the same group of proteins called serine proteases (Table 36.1). They exhibit their function by limited proteolysis of peptide bounds of their substrates. The cascade design of the coagulation system allows a great amplification of signal in each step, since the enzymes activate more than one molecule of substrate. However, the enzymes by themselves do not have high catalytic efficiency and therefore the assembly of enzyme complexes is of crucial importance. This is for instance demonstrated by the bleeding diathesis experienced by hemophilia A patients, where the co-factor FVIII is deficient. In the enzyme complexes the activated membrane, exposing negatively charged phosphatidyl-serine plays a key role. Both the substrate and enzyme bind to the membrane concentrating the proteins at the surface. The correct orientation of the proteins on the cell surface facilitates the interaction. The importance of the membrane is shown in studies of the prothrombinase complex where the addition of phospholipid membrane gives an about 1000-fold increase in catalytic efficiency. Addition of co-factor FVa gives an additional increase and thus the prothrombinase complex is 10^6 times more efficient than the enzyme alone.[6]

Vitamin K-dependent proteins and their binding to the membrane

The vitamin K dependent plasma proteins are a group of Gla domain containing proteins that require vitamin K for their synthesis[7] (Table 36.1). The Gla domains contain 9–12 Glu residues that are γ-carboxylated in a post-translational process that require vitamin K. The γ-carboxylated Glu residues (Gla residues) mediate the binding of Ca^{2+} ions and are crucial for the membrane interaction. Thus, in patients on treatment with vitamin K antagonist (coumarin) the γ-carboxylation is impaired leading to loss of calcium and membrane binding. Due to high sequence similarity, the fold and phospholipid binding mechanism are thought to be similar for all the Gla domains. Although the sequence of the Gla domains are very similar for all the vitamin K zymogens, their affinities for the membrane surface vary 100

to 1000-fold. It has been suggested that this is caused by amino acid sequence differences in just a few positions.[8]

Regulatory mechanisms

The main regulators of coagulation are antithrombin (AT), tissue factor pathway inhibitor (TFPI) and the protein C pathway. The different inhibitors regulate different phases in the coagulation. For instance TFPI regulates the initiation phase while the protein C system regulates the propagation phase. Heparin co-factor II (HCII) and protein Z-dependent protease inhibitor are of less importance. Even protein C inhibitor (PCI) and plasminogen inhibitor-1 (PAI-1) have been shown to have some anticoagulant effect by inhibiting thrombin.

Activation of coagulation switches on a series of mechanisms aimed at controlling and correcting fibrin formation. Plasminogen is converted into plasmin to initiate fibrinolysis. Mechanisms of coagulation and fibrinolysis are regulated at different steps by inhibitory mechanisms that maintain an adequate balance. This chapter is mainly focused on the implication of natural anticoagulants in thrombophilia. Certainly genetic or acquired alterations of fibrinolysis may result in delayed cleavage of the fibrin clot formed resulting in an indirect hypercoagulable state or in persistency of the associated symptoms.[9,10] Despite the critical role of the fibrinolytic system in the resolution of thrombotic events, the overall impression is that its contribution to thrombophilia is relatively low when compared with deficiencies of natural anticoagulants.

SERPINs: a family of coagulation inhibitors

An important proportion of the natural anticoagulants exert their inhibitory action through inhibition of the enzymatic action of procoagulant serine proteases. This family of inhibitory proteins is called SERPINs (SERine Protease INhibitors). Antithrombin (SERPINC1), heparin co-factor II (SERPIND1), protein C inhibitor (SERPINA5) and PAI-1 (SERPINE1), are representative members of this family of inhibitors (Table 36.1). Although their primary sequence similarity is low, these proteins have a conserved three-dimensional structure that is crucial for their function in the regulation of hemostasis, thrombosis and fibrinolysis.[11] Their mechanism of action can be compared to a mousetrap, where the serine protease to be inhibited is lured into an irreversible binding leading to a distortion of the enzyme and loss of activity.[12] The inhibition is irreversible and one molecule of serpin can only inhibit one molecule of serine protease.

Antithrombin

Antithrombin (AT) is a α_2-globulin, member of the serpin family of protease inhibitors (SERPINC1), synthesized in the liver and is the major inhibitor of blood coagulation. Human AT is a single chain glycoprotein of 432 aminoacids with a reactive site cleaved by target enzymes located at Arg393-Ser 394. Antithrombin is a very powerful inactivator of thrombin (FIIa) and FXa, but does also inhibit FVIIa, FIXa, FXIa and FXIIa to a lesser extent.[13] Antithrombin has a molecular

Table 36.1 Procoagulant and anticoagulant factors

Inventory of natural procoagulant and anticoagulant factors. Blood coagulation is accomplished through the interaction of several serin protease enzymes. Coagulation reactions are strictly regulated through an organized system of serin-protease inhibitors (serpins). An adequate interplay among coagulant (orange boxes) and anticoagulant factors (blue boxes) maintains a balanced hemostasis.

Factor	Name	Function	Characteristics	Concentration μg/ml	Plasma half-life (hours)	Chromosome
Factor I	Fibrinogen	Generates the final fibrin clot	Structural	2000–4000	72–120	4q23-q32
Factor II	Prothrombin	FIIa activates I, V, VII, VIII, XI, XIII, protein C, platelets	Serin proteases, Gla	100–150	60–70	11p11-q2
Factor III	Tissue factor	Binds to FVII. Initiates *in vivo* coagulation	Cellular	–	–	1p21-p22
Factor V	Proacelerin	Forms the prothrombinase complex with FX	Co-factor	5–10	12	1q21-q25
Factor VII	Proconvertin	Activates IX, X	Serin protease, Gla	0.5	3–6	13q34
Facor VIII	Antihemophilic A	Forms tenase complex with FIX	Co-factor	0.1–0.2	8–12	Xq28
Factor IX	Antihemophilic B Christmas	Activates FX: forms tenase complex with FVIII	Serin protease, Gla	4–5	18–24	Xq27.1-q27.2
Factor X	Stuart–Prower	Activates FII. Forms prothrombinase complex with FV	Serin protease, Gla	8–10	30–40	13q34
Factor XI	Antihemophilic C	Activates IX	Serin protease, non Gla	5	52	4q32-q35
Factor XII	Hageman	Activates factor XI and prekallikrein	Serin protease, non-Gla	30	60	5q33
Factor XIII	Fibrin stabilizer	Consolidates fibrin	Serin protease, non-Gla	10–30	240	6p24-25
AT	Antithrombin	Inhibits serine proteases: FIIa, FXa, but also FVIIa and FIXa	SERPINC1	150–400	72	1q23-q25
Protein C	Protein C (PC)	Inactivates Va and VIIIa	Zymogen, Gla	4–5	6	2q13-q14
Protein S	Protein S	Acts with activated protein C	Co-factor	25	42	3p11.1-q11.2
Protein Z	Protein Z	Facilitates interactions of FIIa with phospholipids and degradation of FXa	Acts with ZPI (SERPINA10)	2–3	60	13q34
Thrombomodulin	Thrombomodulin	Localizes thrombin to endothelial surfaces	Cellular	–	–	20p11.2-cen
TFPI	Tisue factor pathway inhibitor	Inhibits FVIIa/TF complexes and FXa	Kunitz	0.1	8	2q31-q32.1
TAFI	Thrombin activatable-fibrinolysis inhibitor	Reduces formation of plasmin triggered by clot formation	Zymogen	6	N/A	13q34
α₂-AP	α₂-antiplasmin	Inhibits plasmin	SERPINF2	70	60	17p13.3
PAI-1/2	Plasminogen activator inhibitor	Inactivates tPA and Urokinase	SERPINE1	20 ng/ml	1.5	7q21.3-q22
α₁-AT	α₁-antitrypsin	Inhibits FIIa and activated PC	SERPINA1	1.4	100	14q32.1

weight of 58 200 kDa. There are two isoforms, α and β, of circulating AT. The α represents 90–95% and the β, 5–10% of the total. Under physiological conditions AT circulates in a form that expresses low inhibitory affinity. AT possess a binding site for heparin, being the β isoform the fraction with a higher affinity for heparin.[14] Under physiological conditions heparin sulfates present on the surface of endothelium will provide a background level of activation on AT. Interaction of specific glycosaminoglycan sequences with the specific heparin-binding domain induces a conformational change in AT and accelerates by an order of a thousand times its inhibitory action on activated serin proteases.[15] Inactivation of thrombin (FIIa) by AT produces thrombin–antithrombin complexes (TAT) that can be determined and used as a surrogate marker of the activation of the coagulation. The anticoagulant action of conventional heparins, low molecular weight heparins, and pentasaccharide is mediated by AT. Congenital or acquired deficiencies of AT, may reduce the therapeutic action of the previous anticoagulants. In addition to its anticoagulant action AT has an important anti-inflammatory effect that seems closely dependent on its ability to bind to endothelial glycosaminoglycans.

Protein C system

The protein C system restricts the propagation phase of the coagulation by down-regulation of the FV and FVIII. This regulation requires the assembly of the enzyme, activated protein C with the substrate FV or FVIII on membrane surfaces. As for the procoagulant enzymes, full anticoagulant effect of activated protein C requires presence of co-factors. In the case of FVa-degradation, protein S is the co-factor, whereas in the inactivation of FVIII two proteins function as co-factors, protein S and the intact form of FV.

Protein C structure

Protein C is a vitamin K-dependent protein of 62 kDa that circulates in blood as a zymogen in a concentration of about 4 μg/ml. The protein is synthesized in the liver. The mature protein C molecule is composed of a light and a heavy chain, the two chains being disulfide-linked. The light chain consists of a Gla domain and two epidermal growth factor (EGF)-like domains. The heavy chain contains a short activation peptide and a serine protease domain. Similar to the procoagulant co-factors, protein C circulates as an inactive proenzyme and needs to be activated to gain anticoagulant activity. Like for the other vitamin K-dependent proteins, the Gla domain of protein C mediates the membrane binding. Compared to the other vitamin K-dependent coagulation proteins, protein C has a quite low affinity for the membrane.[8]

Protein C activation complex

Protein C is activated by thrombin in complex with thrombomodulin.[16] Thrombomodulin is a transmembrane glycoprotein consisting of a short cytoplasmic tail, a well-conserved membrane spanning region and a serine-threonine rich domain followed by 6 EGF-like repeats.[17] Upon binding to thrombomodulin, thrombin changes its substrate specificity and is able to activate protein C. The efficiency of the thrombomodulin/thrombin complex is low and an additional co-factor, the endothelial receptor EPCR is needed for fully efficient protein C activation.

Protein C function

Activated protein C (APC) down-regulates the blood coagulation by limited proteolytic cleavage of co-factors FVIIIa and FVa. FVa and FVIIIa are homologous co-factors with the same domain structure: A1-A2 (the heavy chain), the B domain (only present in the non-activated FV and FVIII) and A3-C1-C2 (the light chain). APC cleaves at sites in the heavy chains of the proteins, at Arg306, Arg506 and Arg679 in FVa and Arg336 and Arg562 in FVIIIa.[18] For the inactivation of FVa, the Arg506 cleavage is kinetically favored, but leads only to a partial loss of pro-coagulant function, due to decreased affinity for FXa. For complete loss of activity the cleavage at Arg306 is also needed, which leads to dissociation of the fragments. The FVIIIa is by itself an unstable molecule and is spontaneously degraded by dissociation of the A2 domain. Cleavage of FVIIIa at Arg336 is kinetically favored over cleavage at Arg562 in APC-mediated inactivation of FVIIIa. The cleavage at Arg336 does however not lead to complete loss of activity and the additional cleavage at Arg562 is needed.[19]

Protein S

Protein S is a 70 kDa large vitamin K-dependent protein that circulates in the blood in a concentration of 20–25 mg/ml. More than 60% of the protein S circulates in blood bound to a complement regulator protein called C4b-binding protein (C4BP).[20] Protein S is mainly synthesized in the liver but synthesis has also been observed in endothelial cells, by testicular Leydig cells and by osteoclasts.[21] Protein S has the following domain structure: an N-terminal vitamin K-dependent Gla domain, a thrombin-sensitive region (TSR), four EGF-like domains and two laminin G-type (LamG) domains (also called the SHBG-like domain). Like the other vitamin K-dependent blood proteins, the Gla domain of protein S mediates the membrane binding. Of the vitamin K-dependent proteins, protein S has the highest affinity for the membrane surface.[8] The TSR is not found in the other vitamin K-dependent proteins. The region is sensitive to thrombin cleavage and cleavage leads to loss of APC co-factor function.[22] Factor Xa has also been reported to cleave in the TSR, with the same result.

Protein S function

Protein S is an important co-factor for APC both in the inactivation of FVa and FVIIIa. In the FVa-inactivation protein S stimulates the proteolytic cleavage at Arg306 about 20-fold and only minor stimulation of the Arg506-cleavage is observed.[18] However, when FVa participates in the prothrombinase complex protein S also influences the cleavage at Arg506 by counteracting the FXa-mediated inhibition of this cleavage site. It was originally thought that only the free form of protein S stimulates the APC-mediated cleavage of FVa; however, a recent report indicates that protein S in complex with C4BP can also stimulate the cleavage at Arg306.[23] In the inactivation of FVIIIa protein S functions as a co-factor synergistically with the intact form of factor V.[18] Protein S stimulates both the cleavage sites in FVIIIa.

In addition to being a co-factor for APC, protein S has been shown to exhibit an APC-independent anticoagulant activity.[24] It has been demonstrated that the APC-independent anticoagulant function of protein S is an effect on the TFPI inhibition of the extrinsic pathway.[25] As there is covariation of plasma TFPI and protein S levels both in health and in disease, these findings suggest that the risk of DVT associated with protein S deficiency states might be in part explained by the accompanying low plasma TFPI levels.[24]

Tissue factor pathway inhibitor TFPI

TFPI, also known as lipoprotein-associated coagulation inhibitor or extrinsic pathway inhibitor, is a Kunitz-type inhibitor with a molecular weight of 34 kD.[26] The molecule possesses an acidic amino terminus, three Kunitz-type domains and a basic carboxy terminus. Circulating TFPI is synthesized by endothelial cells and smooth muscle cells.[27] Approximately 10% of the blood TFPI is present in platelets. TFPI neutralizes FVIIa-TF complexes, but is also capable of neutralizing FVIIa and FXa, though at a much slower rate. In fact, the inhibitory action of TFPI on FVIIa-TF complexes requires certain levels of FXa. In experimental animals, administration of TFPI reduces mortality in a model of septic shock induced by *Escherichia coli*.[28]

Abnormal levels of TFPI or mutation in the respective gene are not strongly associated with thrombophilia. Treatment with exogenous hormones has a profound lowering effect on TFPI levels in women, with lower levels in oral contraceptive users than in premenopausal non-users. Levels of TFPI are strongly reduced levels in patients with abetalipoproteinemia, though they do not seem to be exposed to an enhanced risk of thrombosis. Recent studies indicate that low levels of TFPI, especially low TFPI-free and total antigen in plasma, may constitute a risk factor for DVT.[29]

Protein Z-dependent protease inhibitor

Protein Z is a vitamin K-dependent protein with a molecular weight of 62 kD, plasma concentration ranging from 2 to 3 µg/ml and with an approximate half-life of 2.5 days. Although the structure of protein Z contains a Gla domain it does not possess protease activating action on other coagulation factors. Protein Z promotes FXa inhibition induced by ZPI.[30] Protein Z-dependent protease inhibitor (ZPI) is another member of the serpin family (SERPINA10) with known inhibitory action on FXa and FXIa.[31] Heparin enhances the interaction of ZPI with FXIa.

The prothrombotic phenotype associated to protein Z-ZPI deficiency is controversial. Knock out mice for the protein Z gene do not seem to develop a thrombotic tendency unless there is another associated condition such as factor V Leiden.[32] It has been postulated that thrombotic potential of the protein Z and ZPI deficiencies studies in humans question the thrombotic relevance of both ZPI and PZ deficiencies except when they act in combination with other prothrombotic factors.[30]

Other inhibitors and co-factors

Heparin co-factor II (HCII) is a member of the serpin family (SERPIND1), serine protease inhibitor molecular weight 66.5 kD and plasma concentration 85 µg/ml with a half life of 2–3 days. HCII inhibits thrombin in the presence of polyanionic molecules such as heparins, chondroitin, heparan and dermatan sulfates. Although HCII is responsible for an almost 20–30% of thrombin (FIIa) inhibition, deficiencies in HCII do not seem to enhance the risk of thrombosis. Low levels of HCII compatible with a heterozygous deficiency state are found in 1% of the general population but are not found more commonly in patients with thrombosis.

Histidine-rich glycoprotein (HRG) seems to promote an enhancement on plasminogen activation. Although high levels of HRG have been identified in some patients with thrombosis as well as some with deficiency, a causal relationship is not established.

Alpha 2 macroglobulin (α2MG) is a large glycoprotein which nonspecifically inhibits a number of plasma proteases. It does this by binding to lysyl residues in the proteases. α2MG exhibits inhibitory activity against kallikrein, thrombin and FXa. Deficiencies in α2MG do not result in severe thrombophilia, though they have been thought to be responsible for some rare thrombotic episodes before puberty.

Alpha-1-antitrypsin is another serpin (SERPINA1) which has activity against enzymes of the coagulation system, in particular factors XIa and Xa (70% and 35% of plasma-neutralizing activity, respectively) although its principal targets are pancreatic and leukocyte elastases.

Thrombophilia

While inherited bleeding disorders have been known and investigated for centuries, we have been aware of inherited abnormalities leading to thrombosis for only the past four decades. The term thrombophilia defines a series of genetically determined conditions with an increased tendency to thrombosis.

Thrombophilic states have been gaining attention as health professionals have realized the epidemiological impact of thrombotic complications on our societies. Venous thromboembolism (VTE), comprising deep-vein thrombosis (DVT) and pulmonary embolism (PE), are becoming a major public health concern since they are bound to a high incidence of major disability and a leading cause of morbidity and mortality for the general population. Comprehensive epidemiological data have been generated from studies on US and EC populations reveal a VTE incidence of ranging from 70 to 180 per 100 000 person-years with slight differences among geographical areas.[33] Similar data are already reported for the European population.[34,35] Rates of recurrence after a primary thrombotic event reach 30%. The mortality related to VTE estimated from one epidemiological analysis in six European countries including 300 million inhabitants predicted more than 350 000 deaths per year.[35] Still these analyses underestimate the total medical and social cost of the disease because they do not include undiagnosed or misdiagnosed clinical thrombotic events, associated complications, unrecognized VTE-related or post-thrombotic syndromes.

Table 36.2 Genetic risk factors in venous thromboembolism

Combinations among previous alterations produce a multiplying effect on the relative risks for any of the single traits. Association of orthopedic surgery, long-term immobilization, pregnancy, hormonal replacement, antiphospholipid syndrome or malignancies with one or two of the previous alterations implies a very high risk for thrombosis, and prophylaxis with anticoagulants should be considered.

		Deficiency or alteration	Healthy	Patients with thrombosis
A	Strong genetic risk	Antithrombin	<1%	2–5%
		Protein C	<1%	2–5%
		Protein S	<1%	2–5%
B	Moderate genetic risk	FV Leiden	2–15%*	18–35%
		Prothrombin G20210A	1–3%	7–10%
		Homocystinemia	5–10%	18–20%
		Dysfibrinogenemia	6%	10%
C	Variable genetic risk	Homocystinemia Elevated levels of FI, FVIII, FIX; FXI	8–10%	15–30%
		ABO group		

*Highly variable among different ethnic groups.

The pathogenesis of thrombosis involves alterations in the blood vessel and a hypercoagulable condition developing in the circulating blood.[36] The hypercoagulable condition is multifactorial and may involve genetic or acquired deficiencies of natural anticoagulants, abnormal function of coagulation factors and often combinations of these.[37-40] Genetic risk factors range from rare anticoagulant deficiencies with high risk of VTE to common genetic polymorphism with moderate risk (Table 36.2). DVT and PE are obvious manifestations of thrombophilia, but miscarriage, repeated abortions and occasional arterial thrombosis should also be considered related to a thrombophilic state. Thrombophilia should also be suspected in patients who present with idiopathic thrombosis of the portal vein. Incidence of thrombotic complications are common in cases of coinheritance of two hereditary factors, especially when they are associated with other acquired risks such as immobilization, pregnancy, hormonal replacement, antiphospholipid syndrome or hyperhomocysteinemia. The following text will attempt to review the contribution of genetic deficiencies of natural anticoagulants, polymorphisms producing coagulant factors with abnormal functions and other conditions known to be associated with elevated risk of thrombotic complications. Emphasis would be placed on those thrombophilic states known to be associated with elevated risk of thrombosis or those with a high prevalence in the population.

Hereditary deficiencies of natural anticoagulants

Antithrombin deficiency

Antithrombin deficiencies are uncommon with prevalence in the general population ranging from 1 in 500 to 1 in 5000 (Table 36.2). Hereditary AT deficiency was first reported by Olav Egeberg in several members of a family with a clear history of thrombotic events.[41] Although plasma levels range from 112 to 140 µg/ml, laboratories usually refer levels as percentages with normality ranging from 80% to 120%.

Most patients with congenital heterozygous AT deficiencies have levels below 60%. Deficiencies are associated with increased risk of VTE and pregnancy loss and rarely with arterial thrombosis. There is no definite relationship between levels and risk of thrombosis.[42]

Inherited quantitative (type I) and qualitative (type II) deficiencies have been described. In type I AT deficiency, functional and antigenic levels are proportionally decreased. Normal antigenic levels and abnormally reduced functional activities are found in type II. Several mutations are responsible for the type II deficiencies that can be further classified into subtypes.[43] Acquired deficiencies of AT are observed in patients with cirrhosis, nephrotic syndrome and patients with sepsis and disseminated intravascular coagulation. Treatments with L-asparginase and heparins may also reduce levels of AT.

Protein C deficiency

The importance of the protein C system is demonstrated by the thrombotic disorders associated with protein C or protein S deficiency.[44] Homozygous protein C deficiency is a rare condition that causes severe and fatal thrombosis already in the neonatal period. The clinical picture is characterized by purpura fulminans, thrombosis in the brain and disseminated intravascular coagulation. Heterozygous protein C deficiency is more common and is estimated to be around 1/300.[45] The condition gives a higher risk for venous thrombosis while the risk for arterial thrombosis seems unaffected. Protein C deficiencies can be classified as type I and type II deficiencies. Type I deficiencies are the most common of the two and results in a reduction in both activity and antigen level whereas in type II deficiency the antigen levels are normal while the activity of APC is decreased. In heterozygous patients a very variable penetrance is observed, probably dependent on the coexistence of other risk factors. For instance, combined heterozygous protein C deficiency and APC resistance gives a high rate of thrombosis.[46]

Protein S deficiency

Homozygous protein S deficiency is very rare and gives a clinical picture similar to that of homozygous protein C deficiency.[47] Heterozygous protein S deficiency is associated with venous thrombosis[48] and late fetal loss. The prevalence of protein S deficiency is difficult to assess because of diagnostic difficulties and the rareness of the disease. The protein S levels are influenced by age, sex, pregnancy, oral contraceptive use, vitamin K intake and polymorphism in the PS gene. Also, the protein S genome is large and a pseudogene, PROSP, exists with about 97% sequence similarity to the protein S gene (PROS1), complicating mutational diagnostics.

Protein S deficiency is divided into three subclasses.[47] Type I is characterized by a decreased amount of total and free protein S in plasma as well as decreased APC-co-factor activity. Type II is a qualitative defect where the protein S levels are normal but the anticoagulant APC co-factor activity is impaired. In type III defects the APC-co-factor activity is impaired and the amount free protein S is decreased; however, the total protein S is normal. There is a debate if the distinction between type I and type III deficiencies has any biological basis. Often type I and type III deficiencies coexist in the same families. An often occurring glycosylation variant, protein S Heerlen, seems, however, to solely be associated with type III deficiency.

Genetic polymorphisms causing abnormal function of coagulant factors

Activated protein C resistance and factor V Leiden

Activated protein C resistance was detected in 1993 and shown to give a predisposition for venous thrombosis.[49] It is characterized by less prolongation of the APTT-based clotting time in the presence of APC compared to normal. The condition is in at least 90% of the cases caused by a point mutation in FV at nucleotide 1691, rendering the amino acid Arg506 to a Gln (FV Leiden),[50] thereby impairing the APC-mediated cleavage at the Arg506 site, the fast phase of the FVa inactivation. It also leads to a loss of anticoagulant co-factor function of FV, since the cleavage at Arg506 is needed for full expression of this activity.[18] The mutation is only present in Caucasians and the prevalence varies between 2% and 15%.[51] In Europe the prevalence is highest in the northern parts. The polymorphism occurred from a common source about 30 000 years ago (founder effect). The most common clinical manifestations of FV Leiden are superficial and deep venous thrombosis. Pulmonary embolism can also occur, though to a lesser extent than for deficiencies of antithrombin, protein S and protein C. No increased risk for arterial thrombosis has been observed in FV Leiden carriers.

The increased risk for venous thrombosis is about 5–10-fold in heterozygous state and 50–100-fold in homozygous individuals. Thus, FV Leiden, especially in its heterozygous form, is quite a low risk factor for venous thrombosis but because of its high prevalence in the Western population it is present in about 20% of patients presenting with a first thromboembolic event.

Two other naturally occurring mutations that affect the Arg306 site have been reported, FV Hong Kong and FV Cambridge.[18] While FV Cambridge is very rare, FV Hong Kong is found in a prevalence of 4.7%, in the Hong Kong population. The association to DVT for FV Cambridge is complicated by the low prevalence. None of the studies performed for FV Hong has convincingly shown any association with increased risk for venous thrombosis.

Another polymorphism in FV gene that has been suggested to be associated with thrombotic disease is the HR2 haplotype.[52] This consists of numerous point mutations in one allele and is found to be frequent in many populations both in Europe, Asia and Africa. Several functional defects have been reported for this polymorphism. The factor V levels are moderately low, it has been suggested to give a mild APC-resistance and the co-factor function of FV in the APC-mediated inactivation of FVIIIa has been reported to be moderately impaired. There is an ongoing debate on the clinical significance of the HR2 haplotype. However, compound heterozygous individuals for FV Leiden and the HR2 haplotype have a higher risk for venous thrombosis compared to individuals heterozygous for FV Leiden.

Prothrombin polymorphism

In 1996 another polymorphism was identified that is associated with venous thrombosis, the prothrombin polymorphism.[53] This is a substitution in the 3′-untranslated region of prothrombin at nucleotide 20210, G to A. Since the mutation is in the untranslated region, the mutation does not give any amino acid substitution. However, it is associated with elevated prothrombin levels, which is thought to be the reason behind the hypercoagulability. The molecular mechanism behind the increased prothrombin levels has been suggested to be an increased process of the pre-mRNA to the ready translatable RNA as well as a higher translation efficiency.[54] Just as for FV Leiden, the 20210 A allele arose from a founder about 20 000–30 000 years ago. Several studies have estimated the prevalence of the 20210 A allele in the white population to around 2%, with an opposite distribution as compared to FV Leiden, with the highest prevalence in southern Europe and a lower prevalence in northern Europe. Studies have confirmed that the 20210 A allele is a risk factor for DVT, including cerebral vein thrombosis. The increased risk for DVT has been estimated to be approximately threefold.

Dysfibrinogenemia

Abnormal fibrinogen molecules (dysfibrinogenemia) are found in some cases of patients presenting with venous thrombosis.[55] Dysfibrinogenemia is caused by many different mutations in all the three different fibrinogen polypeptides, Aα, Bβ and γ. Only some of the known cases (about 20%) are associated with an increased risk of venous thrombosis; the majority of cases (about 55%) are asymptomatic and the rest (25%) are associated with bleeding. An online database exists listing the known fibrinogen variants and their reported association with symptoms (http://www.geht.org). The molecular mechanism behind the association to thrombophilia is often obscure. Proposed mechanisms include resistance to plasmin degradation and decreased thrombin binding affinity with higher thrombin levels.

Alterations of fibrinolytic mechanisms

The investigation of fibrinolysis has an uncertain place in thrombosis. In the Multiple Environmental and Genetic Assessment (MEGA), an association of overall hypofibrinolysis and venous thrombosis was observed (see [56] for review). On the other hand, when the individual components of the fibrinolytic system were assessed only high TAFI showed evidence of being associated with venous thrombosis, while no association was observed for plasminogen, α_2-antiplasmin, tPA or PAI-1. It is uncertain if the association between overall fibrinolytic potential and venous thrombosis reflects the combined effects of all the fibrinolytic components, the effect of TAFI alone or a mechanism other than fibrin clot lysis.

Excess of other procoagulant factors

Much effort has been put into elucidating the role of procoagulant co-factors in thrombophilia. Similar to the association between low anticoagulant activity and venous thrombosis, it has been postulated that high levels of procoagulant zymogens should give a higher risk for thrombosis. As mentioned above, an association between high prothrombin levels, caused by the prothrombin mutation (G20210A), and DVT is established. Also, high prothrombin levels independent of the mutation are associated with thrombosis.

High levels of fibrinogen have been found to confer a slightly increased risk of thrombosis.[57] Several studies have demonstrated an impact of high FVIII levels on the risk for venous thrombosis. Factor XI levels have, in three larger studies, the Leiden thrombophilia study (LETS), the Multiple Environmental and Genetic Assessment (MEGA) and the Longitudinal Investigation of Thromboembolism (LITE), shown a weak association with venous thrombosis. In contrast, in the case of FIX and FX the results of different studies have been conflicting.[58]

Since FXII is involved in fibrinolytic potential, FXII deficiency has been suggested to result in an increased tendency to thrombosis. However, large studies such as the Leiden thrombophilia study have not supported this hypothesis. Factor XIII cross-links fibrin monomers, after activation by thrombin. A Val34Leu polymorphism has in some studies been associated with a protective effect against venous thrombosis. Intriguingly, the mutation seems to give a higher FXIII activation and higher fibrin cross-linking and further investigation is needed to fully elucidate its impact on venous thrombosis.

Acquired thrombophilic states

Lupus anticoagulants and the antiphospholipid syndrome

The antiphospholipid syndrome (APLS) cannot be considered as a single entity but rather as a combination of clinical and laboratory manifestations that are associated with elevated risks of thrombosis. Antibodies against phospholipids are relatively frequent and often detected as a prolongation of routine coagulation tests. Since these prolongations in coagulation tests were initially observed in patients with lupus erythematosus, antiphospholipid antibodies have also been named lupus anticoagulants.[59] Antiphospholipid antibodies (APA) are a heterogeneous family of immunoglobulins that includes lupus anticoagulants and anticardiolipin antibodies. Lupus anticoagulants behave as acquired inhibitors of coagulation, prolonging phospholipid-dependent *in vitro* coagulation tests. Antiphospholipid antibodies can be measured by immunoassay, using cardiolipin or other anionic phospholipids in solid phase.[60] Elevated presence of antibodies against cardiolipin or phosphatidylserine is more frequently associated with thrombosis. Despite their name, APA do not recognize phospholipids, but plasma proteins bound to suitable anionic surfaces. This may explain their interference with routine coagulation tests.

The antiphospholipid syndrome is a clinical condition characterized by enhanced risk of arterial and venous thrombosis, recurrent miscarriage and occasional thrombocytopenia. Although antiphospholipid antibodies have not been conclusively shown to be causal in thrombosis and miscarriage, they are useful laboratory markers for the antiphospholipid syndrome. Alpha2-glycoprotein I, and prothrombin are the most widely investigated antigenic targets.[61]

In case control studies presence on APA increases fivefold the risk of thrombosis, and in association with other thrombophilia conditions these antibodies may dramatically raise the relative single risk of the original condition. Due to the fact that APA can be detected in different clinical situations, and their relevance in the development and recurrence of thrombotic complications, it is important to confirm their persistence in tests performed over several weeks. Confirmation of the presence of APA associated to other causes of thrombophilia may modify the intensity and duration of the anticoagulant therapy.

Hyperhomocysteinemia

Causes of hyperhomocysteinemia are diverse; they include genetic defects in homocysteine metabolism, vitamin deficiency, kidney disease, malabsorption and age. Severe hyperhomocysteinemia (homocystinuria) is a rare autosomal disease with early onset caused by mutations in homocysteine metabolism. The symptoms are many but include DVT and arterial thrombosis. Mild to moderate homocystinemia can be caused by both acquired and genetic defects.[62] A polymorphism (MTHFR C677T) in the gene for methylene tetrahydrofolate reductase (MTHFR), which participates in the homocysteine–methionine cycle, has a frequency of 10–15% in white North Americans and a frequency as high as 25% in the Hispanic American population (homozygous form). Several studies have demonstrated a weak association of mild to moderate hyperhomocysteinemia and venous thrombosis. However, it is not clear if the association is causative.[63]

Malignancies and inflammatory conditions

The overall risk of venous thrombosis increases by a factor of seven in patients with cancer compared with those without malignancy (odds ratio 6.7, 95% confidence interval 5.2 to 8.6). Patients with hematological malignancies had the highest risk of venous thrombosis, adjusted for age and sex, followed by patients with lung cancer and gastrointestinal cancers. Patients with distant metastases are at higher risk than those without and the risk of thrombosis seems to be highest in the first few months after the diagnosis.[64] The association of thrombotic symptomatology with underlying malignancies is straightforward. Thrombotic complications often precede the diagnosis of malignancy. Approximately 10% of patients presenting with VTE will be found to have malignancy in the subsequent year. Despite this fact, extensive search for malignancies in patients who present with idiopathic thrombosis has been found unproductive and should be disregarded. A thrombophilic state has been recognized in hematological malignancies. Myeloproliferative disorders (MPD), especially polycythemia vera (PV) or essential thrombocythemia (ET), are known to be associated with elevated risk of thrombosis.[65] Alteration of platelet function and increased blood viscosity have been classically related to this elevated risk of thrombosis. Recent investigations are exploring the role of the JAK2 V617F mutation modifying the thrombotic risk in these patients.

Inflammatory and metabolic disorders also contribute to an enhanced thrombotic tendency. Tissue factor (TF) expression is up-regulated by multiple inflammatory proteins, and its expression results in activation of both the extrinsic and intrinsic blood coagulation cascades.[66] Elevated levels of C reactive protein (CRP) and cytokines are frequently observed in patients with DVT. Moreover, the acute phase reaction observed in chronic inflammatory disorders results in the elevation of several procoagulant proteins such as fibrinogen and factor VIII that have also been involved in the generation of a thrombophilic state. Underlying inflammatory mechanisms may also explain the increased rate of thrombosis among patients with infections, malignancies or antiphospholipid antibodies.

Endothelial dysfunction initially described in uremic patients has also been reported in cirrhosis, in diabetes and in patients with the metabolic syndrome. Dysfunctional endothelium has been related to alterations of vascular responses, enhanced platelet activation, accelerated atherosclerosis and elevated thrombotic risk.

Associations among congenital and/or acquired conditions

As shown in Table 36.2, although single hereditary deficiencies have been identified as the underlying cause for thrombophilia, the prevalence of these alterations is relatively low in the healthy population.[67] There is considerable evidence that in most instances the thrombophilic state arises from the interaction of a number of different factors, including hereditary or acquired deficiencies in natural anticoagulants and dysfunctional coagulation factors combined simultaneously with a precipitating clinical situation such as orthopedic surgery, trauma or immobilization. Age above 50 years and obesity are both strongly associated with an elevated incidence of thrombotic events.[68]

Coinheritance of the more prevalent heterozygous mutations FV Leiden and the prothrombin G20210A increases four times the initial odds ratio for VTE of the single mutation.[69] Combinations of FV Leiden, antithrombin, protein C or protein S deficiencies and hyperhomocysteinemia,

have been found to result in a five to tenfold increase in the relative risk of thrombosis, but also in enhanced rates of recurrence and its appearance of thrombotic complications at an early age. Hormonal changes resulting from pregnancy, treatment with oral contraceptives and hormone replacement therapy substantially enhance the risk of VTE in women with thrombophilias. Exposure to oral contraceptives of a woman carrying the prothrombin G20210A mutation increases sixfold the risk of thrombosis. Deficiencies of antithrombin, protein C or protein S also significantly enhance the risk of venous thrombosis in women under oral contraceptives.[70]

Carriers of the factor V Leiden or the prothrombin 20210 A mutation who also had cancer are at 12 times the risk of a venous thrombosis compared with those who only had the mutation. But the research team considered that there was little point in screening for these mutations in patients with cancer, because malignancy was itself associated with a greatly increased risk of venous thromboembolism.[64]

Evaluation, diagnosis and treatment

Evaluation and diagnosis: screening for thrombophilias?

Despite its high prevalence, VTE is often clinically silent, frequently misdiagnosed, and may go unrecognized.[35] Advances in the understanding of the biochemistry of the hemostatic mechanism have led to the development of sensitive methods for measuring peptides, enzyme-inhibitor complexes and enzymes that are liberated with the activation of the coagulation system *in vivo*.[71] Prothrombin fragment F1+2, which is released when prothrombin is converted to thrombin, remains in the plasma and can be used to detect that thrombin has been generated. Fibrinopeptide A is the product of the enzymatic cleavage from the N-terminal ends of the α and β chains of the fibrinogen molecule and is an indirect indicator of fibrin generation. Thrombin–antithrombin (TAT) complexes are generated as a result of natural anticoagulant action of antithrombin neutralizing thrombin (FIIa). TAT complexes can be also quantified in the laboratory and used as indirect markers of the activation of coagulation mechanisms. Despite these tests being highly sensitive in the detection of early activation of the coagulation system and very helpful for research purposes, they possess a low diagnostic value in the confirmation of thrombosis.

The D-dimer is a marker of degradation product of polymerized fibrin. D-dimer levels are elevated in the plasma of the majority of patients with DVT or PTE.[72] A combination of a clinical probability score with well defined cut-off values for the D-dimer can be used to rule out patients clinically unlikely to have DVT.[73] Ultrasound testing and further imaging techniques can be safely used to confirm or discard a diagnosis of DVT or PE. It has been proposed that patients with a low clinical suspicion of a PE and a normal D-dimer do not need additional testing to exclude this disease.[74]

Laboratory tests for detection of hereditary or acquired thrombophilia are available. Controversy exists on how these tests should be applied.[75,76] The overall impression is that an extensive screening after a first thrombotic event is not likely to confer a clinical benefit to the patient.

Laboratory testing must be considered after the initial anticoagulant treatment has been completed. Testing for thrombophilia should be performed: 1) in patients younger than 50 years who develop spontaneous VTE; 2) in patients with a family history of venous thrombosis or with recurrent thrombotic events; or 3) in patients who develop thrombosis in unexpected locations or after being exposed to hormonal treatment. Repeated unexplained abortions must be considered as recurrent thrombotic events.

Phenotypic testing should be performed no sooner than 3 months after acute thrombotic events and at least 2–3 weeks after discontinuation of oral anticoagulant treatment. Testing should be based on the phenotype for antithrombin, protein C and protein S; on the phenotype and genotype (factor V Leiden mutation) for activated protein C resistance; and on the genotype (G20210A mutation) for hyperprothrombinemia. If testing for inherited thrombophilia is positive, the study should be extended to other family members even though they were still asymptomatic. The cost-effectiveness of indiscriminate screening of the general population of asymptomatic women before prescribing oral contraceptives is questionable. Due to their relative increased prevalence, some acquired prothrombotic states should be identified. These states include antiphospholipid syndrome, myeloproliferative disorders and cancer.[77] Confirmation of some of these acquired risks may influence the duration and intensity of the anticoagulant therapy.[40]

It is accepted that genetic or biological causes for thrombophilia are identified in only 30% of the patients. The failure to identify a risk factor in many patients and the belief that genetic factors play an important role in the development of venous thrombosis stimulate the search for novel predictive genetic variants. Genome-wide linkage analysis may provide a key tool for future discovery of new thrombophilic conditions.[78]

Prevention and treatment

As mentioned earlier, VTE is a prevalent medical complication associated with elevated morbidity and mortality rates with inherent social and economical costs.[33,35] Medical approaches to prevent and treat VTE derived from thrombophilic conditions imply three well established levels: prophylaxis of thrombotic events, acute treatment of the thrombotic complications and prevention of further recurrence. Although thrombophilic states are evidently the underlying cause for thromboembolic complications VTE is often clinically silent, misdiagnosed and unrecognized. Epidemiological studies reveal that three quarters of all VTE-related deaths were related to hospital-acquired conditions.[35] Hip or knee arthroplasty, surgery after hip fracture, major trauma or surgery in hospitalized patients with associated thrombophilic conditions are at the highest risk for thrombosis. Surgery in in-patients older than 60 or 40–60 years old with additional hypercoagulable states are also at elevated risk for VTE.[33] The incidence of VTE in these patients can be greatly reduced by appropriate prophylaxis with low molecular weight heparins before and after hospital discharge. Extensive evidence-based guidelines exist for prophylaxis of VTE in patients with variable risk profiles.[79]

Patients with a known thrombophilia who present with VTE should be treated with a standard regimen of heparin overlapped with classic oral anticoagulants (vitamin K antagonists) until an international normalized ratio (INR) of 2.0–3.0 is achieved. The main goal of continued treatment with oral anticoagulants is to prevent recurrent venous thromboembolism which occurs in 30% of untreated patients and 50% untreated patients with a preexisting thrombophilia. Treatment with anticoagulants reduces the risk of recurrence by 90–95%, with an annual risk of fatal hemorrhage of 0.25%.[80] Duration of the anticoagulation to prevent recurrence is still an unresolved issue in thrombophilia. Although discrepancies exist among different guidelines, it is recommended that patients with the lowest risks or those who present with distal vein thrombosis after surgery or trauma should be treated with anticoagulants for 3 months. All other patients should receive treatment with oral anticoagulants for at least 6 months. Extension of oral anticoagulation for 6–18 months should be considered for patients with associated thrombophilias. There is increasing evidence that a normal D-dimer level and the absence of residual venous thrombosis after discontinuation of oral anticoagulation could be used as a predictor of a lower risk of recurrent VTE events.[81] Based on the risk of thrombophilia or associated hereditary or acquired conditions (see Table 36.2), anticoagulant treatment should be maintained indefinitely. The coexistence of malignancies, antiphospholipid antibodies and coinheritance of two or more hereditary deficiencies are situations where indefinite anticoagulant therapy should be considered.

Pregnant patients with thrombophilia who develop VTE should be treated similarly to pregnant women without thrombophilia.[82] Classic oral anticoagulants have been related to embryopathy and should be avoided between 6 and 12 weeks' gestation. Low molecular weight heparins may be considered for pregnant patients who require anticoagulant treatment.[83]

New orally active small molecules that directly target FIIa or FXa are being developed.[84] This new generation of oral anticoagulants is expected to circumvent the slow onset of action, narrow therapeutic window, many food and drug interactions and need for monitoring of classic anti-vitamin K agents.[85] Some of these new anticoagulants are already approved for the indication of thromboprophylaxis in surgical patients at elevated risk. Results of several ongoing clinical trials are likely to confirm new indications in the acute and continued treatment of DVT and VTE. The advent of these new anticoagulants is expected to have a dramatic impact on the management of patients who have developed thrombotic complications. The net balance between prevention of thrombotic events vs. bleeding risk of these new anticoagulants is expected to have a profound impact on the therapeutic approach to patients with known thrombophilic conditions.

References

1. MacFarlane RG. An enzyme cascade in the blood clotting mechanism, and its function as a bichemical amplifier. Nature 1964 May 2;202:498–9.

2. Davie EW, Ratnoff OD. Waterfall sequence for intrinsic blood clotting. Science 1964 Sep 18;145:1310–2.

3. Roberts HR, Hoffman M, Monroe DM. A cell-based model of thrombin generation. Semin Thromb Hemost 2006 Apr;32(Suppl. 1):32–8.

4. Mackman N, Tilley RE, Key NS. Role of the extrinsic pathway of blood coagulation in hemostasis and thrombosis. Arterioscler Thromb Vasc Biol 2007 Aug;27(8):1687–93.

5. Lopez-Vilchez I, Escolar G, Diaz-Ricart M, et al. Tissue factor-enriched vesicles are taken up by platelets and induce platelet aggregation in the presence of factor VIIa. Thromb Haemost 2007 Feb;97(2):202–11.

6. Rosing J, Tans G, Govers-Riemslag JW, et al. The role of phospholipids and factor Va in the prothrombinase complex. J Biol Chem 1980 Jan 10;255(1):274–83.

7. Kalafatis M, Swords NA, Rand MD, Mann KG. Membrane-dependent reactions in blood coagulation: role of the vitamin K-dependent enzyme complexes. Biochim Biophys Acta 1994 Nov 29;1227(3):113–29.

8. McDonald JF, Shah AM, Schwalbe RA, et al. Comparison of naturally occurring vitamin K-dependent proteins: correlation of amino acid sequences and membrane binding properties suggests a membrane contact site. Biochemistry 1997 Apr 29;36(17):5120–7.

9. Kluft C. The fibrinolytic system and thrombotic tendency. Pathophysiol Haemost Thromb 2003 Sep 20;33(5–6):425–9.

10. Cesarman-Maus G, Hajjar KA. Molecular mechanisms of fibrinolysis. Br J Haematol 2005 May;129(3):307–21.

11. Rau JC, Beaulieu LM, Huntington JA, Church FC. Serpins in thrombosis, hemostasis and fibrinolysis. J Thromb Haemost 2007 Jul;5(Suppl. 1):102–15.

12. Huntington JA, Read RJ, Carrell RW. Structure of a serpin-protease complex shows inhibition by deformation. Nature 2000 Oct 19;407(6806):923–6.

13. Patnaik MM, Moll S. Inherited antithrombin deficiency: a review. Haemophilia 2008 Nov;14(6):1229–39.

14. Rosenberg RD, Damus PS. The purification and mechanism of action of human antithrombin-heparin cofactor. J Biol Chem 1973 Sep 25;248(18):6490–505.

15. Carrell RW, Huntington JA. How serpins change their fold for better and for worse. Biochem Soc Symp 2003;(70):163–78.

16. Esmon NL, Owen WG, Esmon CT. Isolation of a membrane-bound cofactor for thrombin-catalyzed activation of protein C. J Biol Chem 1982 Jan 25;257(2):859–64.

17. Esmon CT. The protein C pathway. Chest 2003 Sep;124(Suppl. 3):26S–32S.

18. Nicolaes GA, Dahlback B. Factor V and thrombotic disease: description of a Janus-faced protein. Arterioscler Thromb Vasc Biol 2002 Apr 1;22(4):530–8.

19. Gale AJ, Cramer TJ, Rozenshteyn D, Cruz JR. Detailed mechanisms of the inactivation of factor VIIIa by activated protein C in the presence of its cofactors, protein S and factor V. J Biol Chem 2008 Jun 13;283(24):16355–62.

20. Dahlback B, Stenflo J. High molecular weight complex in human plasma between vitamin K-dependent protein S and complement component C4b-binding protein. Proc Natl Acad Sci USA 1981 Apr;78(4):2512–6.

21. Griffin JH, Fernandez JA, Gale AJ, Mosnier LO. Activated protein C. J Thromb Haemost 2007 Jul;5(Suppl. 1):73–80.

22. Brinkman HJ, Mertens K, van Mourik JA. Proteolytic cleavage of protein S during the hemostatic response. J Thromb Haemost 2005 Dec;3(12):2712–20.

23. Maurissen LF, Thomassen MC, Nicolaes GA, et al. Re-evaluation of the role of the protein S-C4b binding protein complex in activated protein C-catalyzed factor Va-inactivation. Blood 2008 Mar 15;111(6):3034–41.

24. Sere KM, Rosing J, Hackeng TM. Inhibition of thrombin generation by protein S at low procoagulant stimuli: implications for maintenance of the hemostatic balance. Blood 2004 Dec 1;104(12):3624–30.

25. Hackeng TM, Maurissen LF, Castoldi E, Rosing J. Regulation of TFPI function by protein S. J Thromb Haemost 2009 Jul;7(Suppl. 1):165–8.

26. Broze GJ Jr. Tissue factor pathway inhibitor. Thromb Haemost 1995 Jul;74(1):90–3.

27. Bajaj MS, Birktoft JJ, Steer SA, Bajaj SP. Structure and biology of tissue factor pathway inhibitor. Thromb Haemost 2001 Oct;86(4):959–72.

28. Lwaleed BA, Bass PS. Tissue factor pathway inhibitor: structure, biology and involvement in disease. J Pathol 2006 Feb;208(3):327–39.

29. Dahm A, van Hylckamavlieg A, Bendz B, et al. Low levels of tissue factor pathway inhibitor (TFPI) increase the risk of venous thrombosis. Blood 2003;101:4387–92.

30. Corral J, Gonzalez-Conejero R, Hernandez-Espinosa D, Vicente V. Protein Z/Z-dependent protease inhibitor (PZ/ZPI) anticoagulant system and thrombosis. Br J Haematol 2007 Apr;137(2):99–108.

31. Han X, Fiehler R, Broze GJ Jr. Characterization of the protein Z-dependent protease inhibitor. Blood 2000 Nov 1;96(9):3049–55.

32. Yin ZF, Huang ZF, Cui J, et al. Prothrombotic phenotype of protein Z deficiency. Proc Natl Acad Sci USA 2000 Jun 6;97(12):6734–8.

33. Heit JA. The epidemiology of venous thromboembolism in the community. Arterioscler Thromb Vasc Biol 2008 Mar;28(3):370–2.

34. Fowkes FJ, Price JF, Fowkes FG. Incidence of diagnosed deep vein thrombosis in the general population: systematic review. Eur J Vasc Endovasc Surg 2003 Jan;25(1):1–5.

35. Cohen AT, Agnelli G, Anderson FA, et al. Venous thromboembolism (VTE) in Europe. The number of VTE events and associated morbidity and mortality. Thromb Haemost 2007 Oct;98(4):756–64.

36. Schafer AI. Hypercoagulable states: molecular genetics to clinical practice. Lancet 1994 Dec 24;344(8939–8940):1739–42.

37. Seligsohn U, Lubetsky A. Genetic susceptibility to venous thrombosis. N Engl J Med 2001 Apr 19;344(16):1222–31.

38. Christiansen SC, Cannegieter SC, Koster T, et al. Thrombophilia, clinical factors, and recurrent venous thrombotic events. JAMA 2005 May 18;293(19):2352–61.

39. Hron G, Kollars M, Binder BR, et al. Identification of patients at low risk for recurrent venous thromboembolism by measuring thrombin generation. JAMA 2006 Jul 26;296(4):397–402.

40. Bezemer ID, Bare LA, Doggen CJ, et al. Gene variants associated with deep vein thrombosis. JAMA 2008 Mar;19;299(11):1306–14.

41. Egeberg O. Inherited antithrombin deficiency causing thrombophilia. Thromb Diath Haemorrh 1965 Jun 15;13:516–30.

42. Abildgaard U. Antithrombin – early prophecies and present challenges. Thromb Haemost 2007 Jul;98(1):97–104.

43. Maclean PS, Tait RC. Hereditary and acquired antithrombin deficiency: epidemiology, pathogenesis and treatment options. Drugs 2007;67(10):1429–40.

44. Marlar RA, Neumann A. Neonatal purpura fulminans due to homozygous protein C or protein S deficiencies. Semin Thromb Hemost 1990 Oct;16(4):299–309.

45. Miletich J, Sherman L, Broze G Jr. Absence of thrombosis in subjects with heterozygous protein C deficiency. N Engl J Med 1987 Oct 15;317(16):991–6.

46. Koeleman BP, Reitsma PH, Allaart CF, Bertina RM. Activated protein C resistance as an additional risk factor for thrombosis

in protein C-deficient families. Blood 1994 Aug 15;84(4):1031–5.

47. Gandrille S, Borgel D, Sala N, et al. Protein S deficiency: a database of mutations – summary of the first update. Thromb Haemost 2000 Nov;84(5):918.

48. Garcia de FP, Fuentes-Prior P, Hurtado B, Sala N. Molecular basis of protein S deficiency. Thromb Haemost 2007 Sep; 98(3):543–56.

49. Dahlback B, Carlsson M, Svensson PJ. Familial thrombophilia due to a previously unrecognized mechanism characterized by poor anticoagulant response to activated protein C: prediction of a cofactor to activated protein C. Proc Natl Acad Sci USA 1993 Feb 1;90(3): 1004–8.

50. Bertina RM, Koeleman BP, Koster T, et al. Mutation in blood coagulation factor V associated with resistance to activated protein C. Nature 1994 May 5;369(6475): 64–7.

51. Dahlback B. Advances in understanding pathogenic mechanisms of thrombophilic disorders. Blood 2008 Jul 1;112(1):19–27.

52. Bernardi F, Faioni EM, Castoldi E, et al. A factor V genetic component differing from factor V R506Q contributes to the activated protein C resistance phenotype. Blood 1997 Aug 15;90(4):1552–7.

53. Poort SR, Rosendaal FR, Reitsma PH, Bertina RM. A common genetic variation in the 3′-untranslated region of the prothrombin gene is associated with elevated plasma prothrombin levels and an increase in venous thrombosis. Blood 1996 Nov 15;88(10):3698–703.

54. Danckwardt S, Hartmann K, Gehring NH, et al. 3′ end processing of the prothrombin mRNA in thrombophilia. Acta Haematol 2006;115(3–4):192–7.

55. Hill M, Dolan G. Diagnosis, clinical features and molecular assessment of the dysfibrinogenaemias. Haemophilia 2008 Sep;14(5):889–97.

56. Meltzer ME, Doggen CJ, de Groot PG, et al. The impact of the fibrinolytic system on the risk of venous and arterial thrombosis. Semin Thromb Hemost 2009 Jul;35(5):468–77.

57. Soria JM, Almasy L, Souto JC, et al. A genome search for genetic determinants that influence plasma fibrinogen levels. Arterioscler Thromb Vasc Biol 2005 Jun; 25(6):1287–92.

58. Cushman M, O'Meara ES, Folsom AR, Heckbert SR. Coagulation factors IX through XIII and the risk of future venous thrombosis: the Longitudinal Investigation of Thromboembolism Etiology. Blood 2009 Oct 1;114(14):2878–83.

59. Greaves M. Antiphospholipid antibodies and thrombosis. Lancet 1999 Apr 17;353(9161):1348–53.

60. Galli M, Luciani D, Bertolini G, Barbui T. Lupus anticoagulants are stronger risk factors for thrombosis than anticardiolipin antibodies in the antiphospholipid syndrome: a systematic review of the literature. Blood 2003 Mar 1;101(5):1827–32.

61. Espinosa G, Cervera R. Antiphospholipid syndrome. Arthritis Res Ther 2008; 10(6):230.

62. Eldibany MM, Caprini JA. Hyperhomocysteinemia and thrombosis: an overview. Arch Pathol Lab Med 2007 Jun;131(6):872–84.

63. den HM, Willems HP, Blom HJ, et al. Homocysteine lowering by B vitamins and the secondary prevention of deep vein thrombosis and pulmonary embolism: a randomized, placebo-controlled, double-blind trial. Blood 2007 Jan 1;109(1):139–44.

64. Blom JW, Doggen CJ, Osanto S, Rosendaal FR. Malignancies, prothrombotic mutations, and the risk of venous thrombosis. JAMA 2005 Feb 9; 293(6):715–22.

65. Tefferi A, Elliott M. Thrombosis in myeloproliferative disorders: prevalence, prognostic factors, and the role of leukocytes and JAK2V617F. Semin Thromb Hemost 2007 Jun;33(4):313–20.

66. Mackman N. Triggers, targets and treatments for thrombosis. Nature 2008 Feb 21;451(7181):914–8.

67. Bezemer ID, Rosendaal FR. Predictive genetic variants for venous thrombosis: what's new? Semin Hematol 2007 Apr; 44(2):85–92.

68. Rosendaal FR. Venous thrombosis: a multicausal disease. Lancet 1999 Apr 3; 353(9159):1167–73.

69. Emmerich J, Rosendaal FR, Cattaneo M, et al. Combined effect of factor V Leiden and prothrombin 20210A on the risk of venous thromboembolism – pooled analysis of 8 case-control studies including 2310 cases and 3204 controls. Study Group for Pooled-Analysis in Venous Thromboembolism. Thromb Haemost 2001 Sep;86(3):809–16.

70. Bloemenkamp KW, Helmerhorst FM, Rosendaal FR, Vandenbroucke JP. Thrombophilias and gynaecology. Best Pract Res Clin Obstet Gynaecol 2003 Jun;17(3):509–28.

71. Bauer KA. Activation markers of coagulation. Baillière's Best Pract Res Clin Haematol 1999 Sep;12(3): 387–406.

72. Adam SS, Key NS, Greenberg CS. D-dimer antigen: current concepts and future prospects. Blood 2009 Mar 26;113(13): 2878–87.

73. Wells PS, Anderson DR, Rodger M, et al. Evaluation of D-dimer in the diagnosis of suspected deep-vein thrombosis. N Engl J Med 2003 Sep 25;349(13):1227–35.

74. Kearon C, Ginsberg JS, Douketis J, et al. An evaluation of D-dimer in the diagnosis of pulmonary embolism: a randomized trial. Ann Intern Med 2006 Jun 6;144(11): 812–21.

75. Tripodi A. A review of the clinical and diagnostic utility of laboratory tests for the detection of congenital thrombophilia. Semin Thromb Hemost 2005 Feb;31(1):25–32.

76. Dalen JE. Should patients with venous thromboembolism be screened for thrombophilia? Am J Med 2008 Jun; 121(6):458–63.

77. Greaves M, Watson HG. Laboratory testing for prothrombotic states: clinical utility. Curr Hematol Rep 2003 Sep;2(5):429–34.

78. Soria JM, Almasy L, Souto JC, et al. A genome search for genetic determinants that influence plasma fibrinogen levels. Arterioscler Thromb Vasc Biol 2005 Jun; 25(6):1287–92.

79. Geerts WH, Bergqvist D, Pineo GF, et al. Prevention of venous thromboembolism: American College of Chest Physicians Evidence-Based Clinical Practice Guidelines (8th Edition). Chest 2008 Jun;133(Suppl. 6):381S–453S.

80. Hirsh J, Kearon C, Ginsberg J. Duration of anticoagulant therapy after first episode of venous thrombosis in patients with inherited thrombophilia. Arch Intern Med 1997 Oct 27;157(19):2174–7.

81. Zhu T, Martinez I, Emmerich J. Venous thromboembolism: risk factors for recurrence. Arterioscler Thromb Vasc Biol 2009 Mar 1;29(3):298–310.

82. Bates SM, Greer IA, Hirsh J, Ginsberg JS. Use of antithrombotic agents during pregnancy: the Seventh ACCP Conference on Antithrombotic and Thrombolytic Therapy. Chest 2004 Sep;126(Suppl. 3): 627S–44S.

83. Brenner B. Clinical management of thrombophilia-related placental vascular complications. Blood 2004 Jun 1;103(11):4003–9.

84. Eriksson BI, Quinlan DJ, Weitz JI. Comparative pharmacodynamics and pharmacokinetics of oral direct thrombin and factor Xa inhibitors in development. Clin Pharmacokinet 2009;48(1):1–22.

85. Weitz JI, Hirsh J, Samama MM. New anticoagulant drugs: the Seventh ACCP Conference on Antithrombotic and Thrombolytic Therapy. Chest 2004 Sep; 126(Suppl. 3):265S–86S.

595

Section F

Immunohematology

CHAPTER 37

Blood groups on red cells, platelets and neutrophils

G Daniels

Chapter contents

Introduction

Blood groups can be defined as inherited allogeneic variation detected on the surface of blood cells. Although the term is often considered to refer exclusively to erythrocytes, it is equally applicable to other blood cells. In this chapter red cell, platelet and neutrophil groups are described. This is approached, first, from the direction of the structures of these antigens and how they relate to their functions and, second, from their associations with disease, including alloimmune disease.

Red cell surface antigens

Red cell blood groups have been recognized for over a century, since Landsteiner's discovery of the ABO system in 1900. Red cell surface antigens are validated and classified by the International Society of Blood Transfusion (ISBT), which currently recognizes 328 antigens, 284 belonging to one of 30 blood-group systems. Each system consists of between one and 52 antigens encoded either by a single gene or by two or three closely linked homologous genes.[1,2] The 30 blood group systems are listed in Table 37.1.

DOI: 10.1016/B978-0-7020-3147-2.00037-7

Table 37.1 The blood group systems

No.	System name CD no.	System symbol	Gene name(s)	Chromosome	No. of antigens
001	ABO	ABO	ABO	9	4
002	MNS CD235	MNS	GYPA, GYPB, GYPE	4	46
003	P1PK	P1PK	A4GALT	22	2
004	Rh CD240	RH	RHD, RHCE	1	32
005	Lutheran CD239	LU	BCAM	19	20
006	Kell CD238	KEL	KEL	7	32
007	Lewis	LE	FUT3	19	6
008	Duffy CD234	FY	DARC	1	5
009	Kidd	JK	SLC14A1	18	3
010	Diego CD233	DI	SLC4AI	17	22
011	Yt	YT	ACHE	7	2
012	Xg CD99*	XG	XG, CD99	X/Y	2
013	Scianna	SC	ERMAP	1	7
014	Dombrock CD297	DO	ART4	12	7
015	Colton	CO	AQP1	7	4
016	Landsteiner-Wiener CD242	LW	ICAM4	19	3
017	Chido/Rodgers	CH/RG	C4A, C4B	6	9
018	H CD173	H	FUT1	19	1
019	Kx	XK	XK	X	1
020	Gerbich CD236	GE	GYPC	2	11
021	Cromer CD55	CROM	CD55	1	16
022	Knops CD35	KN	CR1	1	9
023	Indian CD44	IN	CD44	11	4
024	Ok CD147	OK	BSG	19	3
025	Raph CD151	RAPH	CD151	11	1
026	John Milton Hagen CD108	JMH	SEMA7A	15	6
027	I	I	GCNT2	6	1
028	Globoside	GLOB	B3GALNT1	3	1
029	Gill	GIL	AQP3	9	1
030	RHAG CD241	RHAG	RHAG	6	3

Blood-group antigens may be carbohydrate structures on red cell surface glycoproteins or glycolipids, or they may be determined primarily by the amino acid sequence of polypeptides or glycoproteins. At least 23 red cell surface proteins express blood-group polymorphism. The functions of some of these structures are reasonably well understood, such as transport of biologically important molecules in and out of the cell, protection of the cell from autologous complement, and anchoring the membrane to the membrane skeleton. Functions of many, however, can only be speculated on from structural similarity to proteins and glycoprotein of known function.[3]

Pathology associated with blood-group polymorphism is usually the result of alloimmune destruction of red cells. This might be a hemolytic transfusion reaction following transfusion of red cells to a patient with an alloantibody directed against a determinant present on donor red cells, or hemolytic disease of the fetus and newborn (HDFN), following placental transfer of maternal IgG antibodies into the fetal circulation. Most blood group systems contain a null-phenotype in which the antigens of that system are not expressed. This usually results from an inactivating mutations in the genes encoding the antigen, yet in most cases null-phenotypes are not associated with any pathology, probably due to functional redundancy of cell surface proteins. For reviews on red cell groups see Daniels[4] and Reid and Lomas-Francis.[5]

The ABO and H histo-blood-group systems and other carbohydrate antigens

ABO and H antigens

ABO is the most important blood-group system from the perspective of clinical blood transfusion. The ABO histo-blood-group antigens are present in many tissues throughout the body and, in soluble form, in body fluids.

At its most basic level, there are two ABO antigens, A and B, and four phenotypes, A, B, AB and O. O is a null phenotype in which neither A nor B is expressed. The A and B determinants are carbohydrate structures, present on red cell membrane glycoproteins and glycolipids. The major carriers of A and B on red cells are the abundant N-glycosylated glycoproteins, the anion exchanger (band 3) and the glucose transporter (GLUT1). Carbohydrate chains are synthesized by the action of glycosyltransferases, enzymes that catalyse the transfer of specific monosaccharides from a nucleotide donor substrate to an acceptor substrate. The acceptor substrate for A- and B- transferases, products of the *A* and *B* alleles, is a terminally fucosylated structure called H antigen (Fig. 37.1). The *A* gene product is an N-acetylgalactosaminyltransferase that transfers N-acetylgalactosamine from a uridine diphosphate (UDP)-N-acetylgalactosamine donor substrate to the fucosylated galactosyl residue of the H antigen, to produce an A-active structure (Fig. 37.1). *B* gene product is a galactosyltransferase that transfers galactose from UDP-galactose to the fucosylated galactose of H, to produce B-active structure (Fig. 37.1). The *O* allele produces no active enzyme, so on group O red cells the H antigen remains unconverted. N-acetylgalactosamine and galactose are the immunodominant sugars of A and B blood groups, respectively.

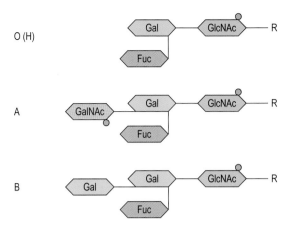

Fig. 37.1 A and B tetrasaccharides and the precursor trisaccharide that expresses H and is abundant on group O cells. R represents the remainder of the molecule.

A- and B-transferases are encoded by a single gene on chromosome 9, cloned by Yamamoto et al[6] in 1990. The *ABO* gene spans about 18–20 kb organized into seven exons of coding sequence. Exons 6 and 7, the two largest, include 77% of the full coding region and encode all of the catalytic domain. The products of the *A* and *B* alleles differ by four amino acid substitutions at residues 176, 235, 266 and 268. Leu266Met and Gly268Ala substitutions are most important in determining whether the gene product has predominantly N-acetylgalactosaminyltransferase (A) or galactosyltransferase (B) activity. The sequence of the most common *O* allele (O^1) is identical to the A sequence, apart from a single nucleotide deletion that is responsible for a reading frame shift after codon 86 and the generation of a translation stop signal at codon 117. This allele encodes a truncated protein lacking the catalytic site. There are two other common *O* alleles: O^{1v}, that, like O^1, has the single nucleotide deletion, but differs from O^1 by nine nucleotide changes within the coding sequence and O^2, that does not have the single nucleotide deletion, but is inactivated by a missense mutation encoding a Gly268Arg substitution (reviewed in [7]).

A antigen is divided into two main subgroups, A_1 and A_2. Red cells of the A_1 and A_2 (and A_1B and A_2B) phenotypes react with anti-A, A_1 cells reacting more strongly than A_2 cells. A_1 cells also react with anti-A_1, an antibody present in the serum of some A_2 and A_2B individuals, so the A antigens of A_1 and A_2 cells differ quantitatively and qualitatively. A_2-transferase is substantially less efficient than A_1-transferase. A_2 DNA has a single base deletion in the codon before the usual translation stop codon, resulting in a reading frameshift and loss of the stop codon. The protein product has an extra 21 amino acid residues at the C-terminus, responsible for reduction in enzyme activity.

About 80% of group A and B people have soluble A and B antigens in their body secretions. The remaining 20% do not secrete A or B substance because their secretions contain no H antigen, the substrate for the A- and B-transferases. This H-deficiency results from inactivity of the fucosyltransferase that is crucial for biosynthesis of H, due to mutations within the fucosyltransferase gene, *FUT2*, active in endodermally-derived tissues. These ABH 'non-secretors' have H and A or B antigens on their red cells because a different fucosyltransferase gene (*FUT1*) is responsible for synthesis of H antigen on mesodermally-derived tissues, including red cells. In the very rare Bombay, phenotype mutations in *FUT1* and *FUT2* result in no H, and consequently no A or B, on red cells or in secretions, regardless of *ABO* genotype. Bombay phenotype individuals usually make a potent anti-H.

HDFN caused by ABO antibodies

Anti-A and -B are predominantly IgM, but may be IgG. Anti-A,B, which reacts with both A and B antigens, is present in the sera of most group O people and is often partly IgG. ABO HDFN is restricted almost exclusively to group A_1 or B fetuses of group O mothers and IgG anti-A,B is generally considered culpable.[8]

About 15% of pregnancies in women of European origin involve a group O mother with a group A or B fetus. This figure does not vary greatly in most other major ethnic groups, yet ABO HDFN requiring clinical intervention is rare, though minor symptoms involving a small degree of red cell destruction may be relatively common. Hydrops due to ABO HDFN is exceedingly rare, but very occasionally exchange transfusion for the prevention of kernicterus is indicated.[8] The main reasons for the low prevalence of clinically significant ABO HDFN is that A and B antigens are present in many tissues. Any antibody crossing the placenta is likely to become bound to placental tissue, reducing the quantity available for destruction of red cells. In addition, immune anti-A,B are mainly IgG2, which does not cause HDFN because there are no Fc receptors for IgG2 on the cells of the mononuclear phagocyte system, and A and B red cell antigens are not fully developed in the fetus or neonate.

Altered expression of ABO antigens in leukemia

The association of weakened expression of A, B and/or H antigens with myeloid malignancies, usually acute myeloid leukemia (AML), is well documented.[4] In some cases all red cells show weakness of the A antigen, whereas in others two populations of red cells are clearly apparent. In a patient with acute monoblastic leukemia, initially only 2% were agglutinated with anti-A, but in remission the proportion of agglutinable cells rose to 65% before falling again shortly before death.[9] Depending on the method used for detection, between 17 and 55% of patients with myeloid malignancies have lower ABH antigenic expression compared with healthy controls.[4] In all cases the changes represent a loss or diminution of antigen strength and never the expression of a new red cell antigen. In some cases loss of A or B was associated with increase in H, in some A or B loss was secondary to loss of H, and in a third group there appeared to be concomitant loss of A/B and H.[10] Modifications of ABH antigens may be detected before diagnosis of malignancy, indicating a preleukemic state. Loss of an ABH antigen in a patient with a hematologic disorder is generally prognostic of AML.

Depression of A or B antigens in AML and in preleukemic states is usually associated with a severe reduction in red cell A- or B-transferase activity, but little or no reduction in red cell H-transferase activity.[11] Although there may be multiple mechanisms underlying the loss of ABH antigens, DNA methylation is significantly associated with silencing of the ABO transcript in patients with myeloid malignancies and the *ABO* transcript can be re-expressed in leukemic cell lines by treating with a demethylating agent.[12]

Lewis antigens

The Lewis antigens, Le^a and Le^b, are not synthesized by erythroid cells, but become incorporated into the red cell membrane from the plasma. Their synthesis from H antigen and from its precursor is catalyzed by an $\alpha 1,3/4$-fucosyltransferase, the product of *FUT3*, a gene on chromosome 19. This fucosyltransferase competes with the H-(*FUT2*), A-, and B-transferases in endodermal tissue for acceptor substrate. The antigens known as Le^x and Le^y, which are not detected on red cells, are isomers of Le^a and Le^b, respectively.[13]

ABH and Lewis antigens on tumors

ABH antigens are often absent from glycoproteins and glycolipids of malignant tissue of the gastrointestinal tract, oral cavity, uterine cervix, lung, prostate, breast and bladder, despite being present in the surrounding epithelium. In many cases loss of ABH antigens preceded formation of distant metastases and hence a poor prognosis.[14,15] Loss of A or B antigens from tumor cells may increase their motility and, consequently, their ability to form metastases. In addition, this absence of A or B antigens generally arises from disappearance of A- or B-transferase activity and results in an accumulation of H, Le^b, Le^y, sialyl-Le^a or sialyl Le^x. Sialyl-Le^a and sialyl Le^x are ligands for selectins, and their presence promotes the metastatic process by facilitating interaction with distant organs.[14,15]

ABO antigen loss results from downregulated transcription of the *ABO* gene, as no A or B mRNA can be detected in high-grade tumors. At least two different mechanisms may be involved, possibly occurring in tumors derived from different souces: 1) loss of heterozygosity (allelic loss) involving deletions within chromosome 9q34, which contain the *ABO* locus in addition to tumor suppressor genes; 2) hypermethylation of the CpG island of the *ABO* promoter region, which down-regulates transcription.[16,17]

Up-regulation of glycosyltransferases in tumors may result in increased levels of certain carbohydrate structures in the plasma.[18] The quantity of circulating sialylated-Le^a, otherwise known as the CA 19-9 antigen, is widely used as a marker to support diagnosis of colorectal, pancreatic and gastric cancer, and as an aid to prognosis after potential curative surgery.[19,20]

Another phenomenon associated with malignancy is the incompatible A antigen occasionally expressed on tumors of group O or B people. About 10% of colonic tumors from group O patients, shown to be homozygous for the O^1 allele, express A antigen and contain A-transferase activity.[21,22] The molecular basis of this O to A conversion is not known, but alternative splicing of *ABO* RNA, resulting in loss of exons 5 and 6, would introduce no frameshift or translation-termination codons, but would eliminate the single nucleotide deletion in exon 6 of O^1 and the putative gene product would be a truncated glycosyltransferase with a potential for A-transferase activity.[14] The higher incidence of gastric and ovarian adenocarcinomas in group A people could be due

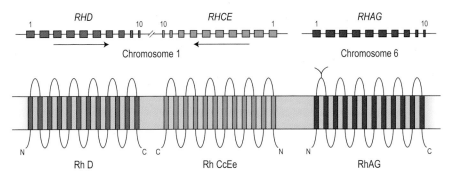

Fig. 37.2 Diagrammatic representation of the 10 exons of the *RHD* and *RHCE* genes and the encoded RhD and RhCcEe proteins, and the 10 exons of *RHAG* and the encoded glycoprotein with its single N-glycan (Y).

to a suppression of development of tumors bearing an A antigen by the anti-A naturally present in group O and B, but not A, patients.[23]

The Rh blood-group system

Rh is the most complex of the human blood-group systems. It has 52 well-defined antigens, the most immunogenic of which is D (RH1). Between 82% and 88% of Caucasians, about 95% of black Africans, and almost 100% of people from the Far East are D-positive. The other main Rh polymorphisms are C/c and E/e, two pairs of antithetical antigens. C has a frequency of 70% and c a frequency of 80% in Europeans. In black Africans the frequency of c is much higher and the frequency of C much lower, whereas in eastern Asia the opposite is the case, with C approaching 100%. In most populations E has a frequency of about 30% and e about 98%.[4,5]

The antigens of the Rh system are encoded by two genes, *RHD* and *RHCE* (reviewed in [24] and [25]). They are highly homologous and have very similar genomic organization, each containing 10 coding exons arranged in opposite orientation on chromosome 1 (Fig. 37.2).[26] *RHCE* encodes the C/c and E/e antigens, plus many others such as C^w, C^x and VS. *RHD* encodes the many epitopes of the D antigen. In Caucasians the D-negative phenotype almost always results from homozygosity for a deletion of *RHD*, whereas about 66% of D-negative Africans have *RHDψ*, an inactive *RHD* gene.[27] The products of the Rh genes are polypeptides that are palmitoylated but, unlike most cell surface proteins, not glycosylated. The D and CcEe proteins differ by only 32–35 amino acids, depending on CcEe phenotype. Hydropathy analysis of the amino acid sequences of the Rh proteins together with immunologic evidence suggests that the Rh proteins span the red cell surface membrane 12 times, with internal termini and six extracellular loops (Fig. 37.2).

In the D-negative phenotype no D protein is present in the membrane, explaining the high immunogenicity of D compared with other Rh antigens. The C/c and E/e polymorphisms represent amino acid substitutions at different positions in the CcEe protein. Rh epitopes are conformational and may be discontinuous; that is, they are very dependent on the shape of the whole molecule and may involve more than one extracellular loop. Studies with monoclonal antibodies have shown that the D antigen consists

of numerous epitopes. There are many variant phenotypes in which some D epitopes are missing, making it possible for a D-like antibody to be produced. Some of these D variants, often referred to as partial D antigens, result from missense mutations in *RHD*, others because a section of *RHD*, ranging from part of an exon to several exons, has been replaced by the equivalent region of *RHCE*. These hybrid *RHD-CE-D* genes are probably the products of gene misalignment and intergenic recombination during meiosis. *RHCE-D-CE* hybrid genes are responsible for some CcEe variants.[24,25]

The Rh proteins are closely associated within the membrane with the Rh-associated glycoprotein (RhAG), probably as a heterotrimer.[28,29] RhAG has sequence and conformational similarities to the Rh proteins, but has a single N-glycan (Fig. 37.2). This complex is part of a larger protein complex in the red cell membrane, which also includes tetramers of band 3 (the anion transporter, AE1), glycophorins A and B, ICAM-4 (the LW blood group antigen), and CD47, the integrin-associated antigen, in addition to ankyrin and protein 4.2 of the cytoskeleton and some cytosolic proteins, including carbonic anhydrase II and hemoglobin (Fig. 37.3).[30] Although the primary function of band 3 is well known – it transfers HCO_3^- ions across the membrane in exchange for Cl^- ions – the function of the Rh protein complex is not known, but there is good evidence that it could act as a gas channel, probably for CO_2 and possibly also for O_2 and NH_3.[29–31] The Rh proteins may also be part of another putative membrane complex that includes the glucose transporter (GLUT1), dimers of band 3, glycophorin C, the Duffy (DARC) and Kell glycoproteins, and Xk, which is attached to the cytoskeleton through protein 4.1R, p55, dematin and adducin.[32–34]

Rh-deficiency syndrome, Rh_{null} and Rh_{mod}

Red cells with the very rare Rh_{null} phenotype have no Rh antigens and lack the Rh proteins. The most usual cause of Rh_{null} is homozygosity for inactivating mutations in *RHAG*. In the absence of RhAG, no Rh proteins are expressed at the red cell surface. Missense mutations in *RHAG* may result in reduced Rh antigen expression, a phenotype called Rh_{mod}. Very rarely Rh_{null} occurs in the presence of RhAG, but with a deletion of *RHD* and inactivating mutations in *RHCE*.[24,25]

Rh_{null} and Rh_{mod} red cells are morphologically and functionally abnormal. Most Rh_{null} individuals have some degree

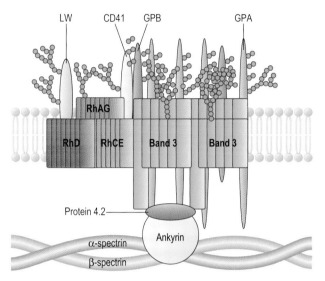

Fig. 37.3 Diagrammatic representation of the band 3/Rh macrocomplex in the red cell membrane and its attachment to the spectrin matrix of the red cell cytoskeleton.

of hemolytic anemia associated with stomatocytosis and spherocytosis, which has been referred to as Rh-deficiency syndrome. Rh$_{null}$ red cells have abnormal organization of their membrane phospholipids, and other anomalies associated with Rh$_{null}$ include increased cation permeability partially compensated by an increase in the number of K^+Na^+ pumps, reduced cation and water contents, and significantly reduced CO_2 permeability.[24,31]

HDFN caused by Rh antibodies

The most common form of HDFN results from IgG anti-D crossing the placenta and facilitating the immune destruction of D+ fetal red cells. The severity of anti-D HDFN is highly variable: the most severely affected fetuses die *in utero* from about the 17th week of gestation onwards; in less severe cases, hydrops fetalis may occur. In those severely affected infants born alive, jaundice may develop rapidly and lead to kernicterus. About 70% of infants who develop kernicterus die within a few days; of those who survive, many have permanent cerebral damage.[8]

Prior to the late 1960s, HDFN caused by anti-D was a relatively common cause of fetal and neonatal mortality and morbidity. Since then the prevalence of severe anti-D HDFN has been dramatically reduced by anti-D immunoglobulin prophylaxis, in which D− women receive an injection of anti-D IgG within 72 h of delivery of a D+ baby. This prevents immunization of the mother by D+ fetal cells at parturition, protecting D+ fetuses in subsequent pregnancies. In order to reduce the risk of immunization during the pregnancy, it is now policy in some countries to offer one or two doses of anti-D IgG to all D− pregnant women, at around 28–30 weeks' gestation.[35]

In Caucasians, only about 60% of fetuses of D− women are D+. When a D− pregnant woman has anti-D, it is beneficial to be able to determine the D phenotype of her fetus in order to determine whether there is any risk from HDFN. Fetal D phenotype can be predicted by polymerase chain

reaction-based tests performed on fetal DNA obtained by amniocentesis, chorionic villus sampling or, non-invasively, from cell-free fetal DNA in maternal plasma.[36] Basically, the tests determine the presence or absence of *RHD* in order to predict whether the fetus is D+ or D−, respectively, though modifications are required to prevent errors that would arise from the presence of certain rare variant genes in Caucasians and the relatively common *RHDψ* in Africans. Where routine antenatal anti-D prophylaxis is offered, it must be offered to all D− pregnant women, as the D type of the fetus is unknown. To prevent unnecessary treatment of pregnant women with blood products, high-throughput technologies suitable for predictng fetal D type from fetal DNA in all D− pregnant women are being developed.[37]

All antibodies to Rh-system antigens should be considered capable of causing HDFN, but the only Rh antibody other than anti-D that regularly causes severe HDFN is anti-c. Anti-C, -E, -e, and -G have all caused HDFN, but the occurrence is rare and the outcome seldom severe. Methods have been developed for predicting fetal C, c and E from fetal DNA in maternal plasma.[36]

The Kell system and Xk

The Kell blood group system comprises 32 determinants, almost all of which represent single amino acid substitutions in the Kell glycoprotein.[38] The Kell glycoprotein crosses the red cell membrane once, but is unique among blood group proteins as its N-terminal is internal and its large, globular C-terminal domain, which contains six potential N-glycosylation sites and 15 cysteine residues, is external.[38] One of the cysteine residues, Cys72, is linked by a disulfide bond to Cys347 of Xk, a multiple membrane spanning protein (see below).[39]

The Kell glycoprotein is an enzyme; part of the neprilysin family of zinc-dependent endopeptidases. The Kell glycoprotein is able to cleave big endothelin-3, a biologically inactive 40-amino acid peptide, to endothelin-3, a 21-amino acid peptide with vasoconstrictor activity.[40] It is not known, however, whether the Kell glycoprotein serves this function *in vivo* and people who lack the Kell glycoprotein, as a result of inactivating mutations in the *KEL* gene (Kell-null phenotype), are apparently healthy.

Anti-K and HDFN

Kell-system antibodies can cause severe HDFN. In Caucasian populations anti-K is often the most common immune red cell antibody outside of the ABO and Rh systems.[8] Most anti-K appear to be induced by blood transfusion and it is becoming common practice for girls and women of childbearing age to be transfused only with K− red cells.

The pathogenesis of HDFN caused by anti-K differs from that due to anti-D. The severity of the anti-K disease is harder to predict than the anti-D disease. This is because there is very little correlation between anti-K titer and severity of disease and because anti-K HDFN is associated with lower concentrations of amniotic fluid bilirubin than in anti-D HDFN. Postnatal hyperbilirubinemia is not prominent in babies with anemia caused by anti-K. There is also reduced reticulocytosis and erythroblastosis in the anti-K disease, compared with anti-D HDFN. These characteristics suggest that there is less hemolysis in HDFN caused by anti-K, compared with HDFN of comparable severity due to anti-D. This has led to speculation that fetal anemia in anti-K HDFN results predominantly from a suppression of erythropoiesis.[41,42] Kell glycoprotein is one of the first erythroid-specific antigens to appear on erythroid progenitors during erythropoiesis, whereas the Rh proteins appear much later.[43-45] Vaughan et al[46] found that *in vitro* proliferation of K+ erythroid blast-forming units (BFU-E) and colony-forming units (CFU-E) was specifically inhibited by monoclonal and polyclonal anti-K. They speculated that the Kell glycoprotein might be involved in regulating the growth and differentiation of erythroid progenitors, possibly by enzymatically modulating peptide growth factors on the cell surface. Consequently, binding of anti-K could block the enzymatic activity of the Kell glycoprotein and suppress erythropoiesis. This theory, however, does not take into account the Kell-null phenotype, in which no Kell glycoprotein is present in erythroid cells, yet erythropoiesis is apparently normal. It is likely, therefore, that anti-K suppresses erythropoiesis through the immune destruction of early erythroid progenitors in the fetal liver. Daniels et al.[45] have used a functional assay to demonstrate that in the presence of anti-K erythroid progenitors, cultured from cord CD34+ cells derived from a K+ RhD+ baby, elicited a strong response from monocytes; no response was obtained with anti-D because Rh antigens do not appear on erythroid cells before they become hemoglobinized erythroblasts.

The Kell–Xk complex and McLeod syndrome

The 444 amino acid Xk polypeptide is unglycosylated and probably spans the membrane 10 times, with internal N- and C-termini.[47] The predicted topographic arrangement is identical to that of members of a family of proteins that cotransport a neurotransmitter together with Na+ and Cl− ions, the amino acid sequence bearing closest resemblance to a Na+-dependent glutamate transporter.[47]

Xk protein expresses Kx antigen and is covalently linked to the Kell glycoprotein as a disulfide-bonded complex in the red cell membrane.[39] The rare absence of Xk gives rise to McLeod syndrome, a multisystem disorder that results from either a gene deletion or from various inactivating mutations within XK, an X-linked gene that encodes the Xk protein.[38,47] McLeod syndrome is characterized by weakness of Kell-system antigens and absence of Kx antigen (McLeod phenotype), acanthocytic red cells and elevated serum creatine kinase; late-onset muscular and neurological defects, including muscle wasting, diminished deep tendon reflex, choreiform movements, cardiomyopathy and psychiatric symptoms are common.[48] It is likely that absence of Xk from the brain, where it is expressed independently of Kell,[49] is responsible for most of the symptoms associated with McLeod syndrome.

A minority of patients with X-linked chronic granulomatous disease (CGD) also have the McLeod phenotype. CGD, an inherited disorder that may be either autosomal or X-linked, impairs the functioning of phagocytes resulting in severe susceptibility to infection. X-linked CGD results from deletion or inactivity of the gene (*CYBB*) for the beta subunit of flavocytochrome b558, or from mutations within that gene.[50] The locus for X-linked CGD and the *XK* locus are discrete and the association of McLeod phenotype with CGD results from deletions of part of the X-chromosome that encompass both genes.[4]

Blood groups on red cell transporters

Membrane transporters facilitate the transfer of biologically important molecules in or out of cells. They are typically polytopic, with an even number of α-helical membrane spanning domains of about 21 amino acids each, and have both termini inside the cytosol. Four red cell membrane transporters have blood group activity: band 3, the anion exchanger is the Diego system antigen; aquaporin 1 (AQP1), a water channel, is the Colton antigen; aquaporin 3 (AQP3), a water and glycerol channel, is the Gill antigen; and HUT11, a urea transporter, is the Kidd antigen.[3]

Band 3 or anion exchanger 1 (AE1), the Diego blood-group antigen, functions as an anion exchanger. It is an antiporter that permits bicarbonate (HCO_3^-) ions to cross the membrane in exchange for Cl− ions, rapidly reversing the accumulation of HCO_3^- in the red cells that would occur when CO_2 in the blood is hydrated to HCO_3^- by carbonic anhydrase located in the red cell cytoplasm. This facilitates transport of HCO_3^- in the plasma, greatly increasing the quantity of CO_2 that the blood can convey to the lungs.[51]

There is only one report of a Diego-null phenotype, a child homozygous for a band 3 mutation, whose red cells had no band 3, and as a consequence no band 4.2, a glycoprotein of the membrane cytoskeleton associated with band 3. The severely hydropic, anemic baby, was delivered by emergency Cesarean section and resuscitated and kept alive by blood transfusion. A cord blood smear revealed dramatic erythroblastosis and poikilocytosis. After 3 years the child was doing reasonably well on a regimen of regular blood transfusions and daily supplements of sodium bicarbonate.[52] So, absence of band 3 is compatible with life, but only with extreme medical intervention.

Tetramers of Band 3 form the core of the band 3/Rh macrocomplex of red cell surface proteins. This complex may also function as a gas channel for CO_2 and/or NH_3 (see section on Rh above).

The Kidd red cell glycoprotein is UT-B, a urea transporter,[53] which is also present in endothelial cells of the vasa recta, the vascular supply of the renal medulla.[54] A urea transporter in red cells has two main functions: 1) transporting urea rapidly in and out the cells to prevent their shrinkage as they pass through the high urea concentration of the renal medulla and subsequent swelling as they leave; and 2) to prevent the red cells from carrying urea away from the renal medulla, which would decrease the urea concentrating efficacy of the kidney.[55] Despite this, a Kidd-null phenotype, resulting from homozygosity for a splice site mutation and exon skipping,[56,57] is relatively common in Polynesians, with an incidence of about 1 in 400.[58] Individuals with the Kidd-null phenotype have no clinical symptoms, but, like UT-B knockout mice, have urine-concentrating ability reduced by about one-third.[59,60] The abundance of UT-A and the water channels AQP2 and AQP3 is increased in the renal medulla of UT-B knockout mice, which could assist in the concentration of urea.[61] This apparent compensation may explain why

Kidd-null individuals have only a modest reduction in urine-concentrating ability. AQP3, but not AQP2, is present on red cells.

Eleven members of the aquaporin family of water channels are found in mammals; two of these, AQP1 (Colton system) and AQP3 (Gill system), are present in human red cells. Aquaporins can be divided into two groups: those like AQP1 that are permeated mostly by water and those like AQP3, known as the aquaglyceroporins, which are permeated by water, but also by other small solutes, especially glycerol.[62] In addition to red cells, the highly water permeable AQP1 is present in kidney, lung, vascular endothelium, brain, and eye. AQP1 deficiency may only become important under stress conditions: individuals homozygous for disrupting mutations in AQP1 have the very rare Colton-null phenotype and about 80% reduction in red cell osmotic permeabilities;[63] they were apparently healthy, but were unable to concentrate urine maximally when deprived of water.[64] In addition to red cells, AQP3 is present in kidney, skin, lung, eye, and colon.[62] The very rare Gill-null phenotype, which results from homozygosity for a splice site mutation in AQP3, is not associated with any obvious clinical syndrome.[65]

Receptors and adhesion molecules

There are some red cell surface proteins that resemble receptor or adhesion molecules, though their precise functions, at least on red cells, are not clear. Cell surface receptors bind specific ligands, often hormones, and then activate an effector that produces an intracellular signal. In addition to functioning as receptors, adhesion molecules are involved in the adhesion of cells to other cells and to the extracellular matrix.[3] It is far from obvious why red cells should display adhesion molecules at their surface and some of these glycoproteins could be vestigial, having served their function during erythropoiesis.

The Duffy antigen receptor for chemokines

The Duffy glycoprotein is DARC, the Duffy antigen receptor for chemokines. It crosses the membrane seven times with a glycosylated extracellular N-terminal domain, which carries Fy^a or Fy^b blood group activity. DARC belongs to the G protein-coupled superfamily of receptors that bind many different ligands, but especially chemokines, proinflammatory cytokines that motivate recruitment of leukocytes. DARC, however, lacks the characteristic Asp-Arg-Tyr (DRY) motif on the second cytoplasmic loop required for G-protein coupling and is, therefore, unlikely to be involved in cell signaling. In addition to being on red cells, DARC is abundant on the endothelium of post-capillary venules and veins of many organs.[66,67]

Chemokines are predominantly secreted chemotactic cytokines, which function primarily to induce the movement of leukocytes along a concentration gradient. DARC is a promiscuous chemokine receptor: it binds with high affinity to 60% of inflammatory chemokines of both CXC and CC classes, but not homeostatic chemokines.[68] DARC on red cells has long been considered to function as a sink, binding excess chemokines to prevent inappropriate activation of neutrophils and disrupting chemokine gradients.[69] Consequently, red cell DARC may support recruitment of leukocytes by removing 'desensitizing' free plasma chemokines and reducing 'background system noise', indirectly enhancing the chemokine-encoded signal on endothelial cells at the sites predestined for leukocyte recruitment.[67,70]

DARC appears to be a negative regulator of growth in prostate, breast, and non-small cell lung carcinoma, probably by the removal of angiogenic CXC chemokines from the tumors and subsequent inhibition of tumor neovascularity.[71–73] In addition, DARC on vascular endothelium interacts directly with CD82, a tetraspanin expressed on cancer cells. CD82 is a suppresser of metastasis: interaction between DARC and CD82 inhibits the spread of the cancer to remote sites and also appears to induce cancer cell senescence.[74]

DARC is exploited by *Plasmodium vivax* as a receptor and is essential for invasion of the red cells by the parasite. *P. vivax* is responsible for tertian malaria, a form of malaria prevalent in Africa, but less severe than that caused by *P. falciparum*.[66] A Duffy-null phenotype, Fy(a–b–), in which DARC is absent from red cells, is common in Africans, the frequency reaching 100% in some regions of West Africa.[4] Fy(a–b–) red cells are refractory to invasion by *P. vivax* merozoites and individuals with the Fy(a–b–) phenotype are resistant to vivax malaria. Fy(a–b–) phenotype in Africans results from homozygosity for a single nucleotide substitution in a GATA-1 erythroid-specific transcription factor binding site in the promoter region of *DARC*.[75] This mutation prevents expression of DARC on erythroid cells, although it is still present in other tissues.[76] The evolutionary advantages of the Fy(a–b–) phenotype in Africans are obvious. However, the promoter mutation associated with the Fy(a–b–) phenotype is associated with lower leukocyte counts and could be responsible for the so-called 'benign ethnic neutropenia' in people of African origin, which could be pertinent to the management of chemotherapy.[77]

Glycoproteins of the immunoglobulin superfamily

The immunoglobulin superfamily (IgSF) is a large collection of glycoproteins abundant on leukocytes (Fig. 37.4). IgSF glycoproteins contain repeating extracellular domains with sequence homology to immunoglobulin domains. Each IgSF domain consists of approximately 100 amino acids and is structured into two β-sheets stabilized by a conserved disulfide bond. IgSF glycoproteins mostly function as receptors and adhesion molecules, and may be involved in signal transduction.[78] IgSF molecules on red cells include the Lutheran (Lu) glycoproteins, ICAM-4 (LW antigen), erythroblast membrane-associated protein (ERMAP, the JMH protein), Scianna antigen, basigin (Ok antigen), and CD47. ICAM-4 and CD47 are part of the band 3/Rh macrocomplex.

The functions of these proteins on red cells are not known, but the Lu-glycoproteins and ICAM-4 may play roles in erythropoiesis. The Lu-glycoproteins bind specifically and with high affinity to LN-10 and -11, isoforms of laminin, a component of the extracellular matrix (ECM) abundant in basement membranes and also present in vascular endothelia.[79] The laminin binding site is formed by Asp312 and a

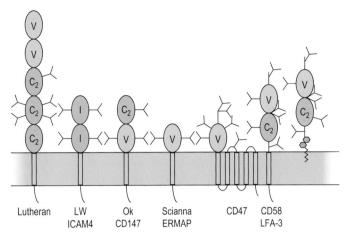

| Lutheran | LW | Ok | Scianna | CD47 | CD58 |
| | ICAM4 | CD147 | ERMAP | | LFA-3 |

Fig. 37.4 Diagrammatic representation of six members of the immunoglobulin superfamily (IgSF) detected in the red cell membrane, including the Lutheran, LW, Ok and Scianna blood group antigens. IgSF domains are shown as V, C2 or I. CD58 is present both as membrane-spanning and glycosylphosphatidylinositol-anchored forms. Y represents N-glycosylation.

surrounding group of negatively charged residues in the region of the flexible linker between IgSF domains 2 and 3 of the Lu-glycoproteins.[80] During *ex vivo* erythropoiesis the Lu-glycoproteins appear on the erythroid cells at about the orthochromatic erythroblast stage.[43,44] The presence of LN-10 and -11 on the bone marrow sinusoidal endothelium has led to speculation that the Lu-glycoproteins are involved in facilitating movement of maturing erythroid cells from the bone marrow, across the sinusoidal endothelium, to the peripheral blood.[43,79]

Like other ICAMs,[78] ICAM-4 is a ligand for integrin adhesion molecules. Although other ICAMs are fairly specific for a single integrin, ICAM-4 interacts with a variety of integrins.[81] Also, unlike other ICAMs, ICAM-4 appears to be restricted to erythroid cells and possibly placenta.[82] During *ex vivo* erythropoiesis, LW antigen is detected around the CFU-E to proerythroblast stage.[43,44] During the latter stages of erythropoiesis, erythroblasts cluster around bone marrow macrophages to form erythroblastic islands, where the erythroblasts extrude their nuclei, which are ingested by the macrophage. Adhesive interactions between ICAM-4 and α4β1 integrin on adjacent erythroblasts and between ICAM-4 on erythroblasts and αV integrins on macrophages may assist in maintaining the stability of the erythroblastic islands.[82,83]

Lu-glycoproteins and ICAM-4 are over-expressed on SS red cells in sickle cell disease. Enhanced binding of the Lu-glycoproteins to LN-10/11 and possibly the α4β1 integrin, and ICAM-4 to αVβ3 integrin on the endothelia of damaged blood vessels could contribute to blockage of the vessels and the painful episodes of vaso-occlusion often suffered by sickle cell patients.[81,84–86] Peptides representing ICAM-4 reduce adhesion and vessel blockage, and may have therapeutic potential.[85]

Raph blood group and CD151

The Raph blood group system contains one antigen, MER2, located on the tetraspanin CD151. Tetraspanins associate

with integrins within basement membranes to generate complexes that bind laminin, and are important in maintaining the integrity of basement membranes. The extremely rare MER2-null blood group phenotype arises from homozygosity for a single nucleotide insertion in exon 5 of the *CD151* gene.[87] The resulting disruption of basement membranes causes hereditary nephritis (all MER2-null patients required dialysis and kidney transplants), epidermolysis bullosa, and neurosensory deafness.[87] The function of CD151 in the red cell membrane, which does not contain integrins, remains unknown.

Complement regulatory glycoproteins

Two red cell surface glycoproteins belong to the complement control protein (CCP) superfamily of complement regulators: 1) decay accelerating factor (DAF, CD55), which is attached to the membrane by a glycosylphosphatidylinositol (GPI) anchor, has four CCP repeating domains, and expresses the 15 antigens of the Cromer blood group system; and 2) complement regulator 1 (CR1, CD35), which has around 30 CCP domains and expresses the nine antigens of the Knops system.

DAF helps to protect red cells from lysis by autologous complement, a role it shares with CD59, another GPI-linked glycoprotein, which is not polymorphic and does not have blood group activity.[88] DAF functions by inhibiting the action of C3-convertases, whereas CD59 prevents assembly of the membrane-attack complex. Patients with paroxysmal nocturnal hemoglobinuria (PNH)[89] have red cells that lack both DAF and CD59 as a result of defective somatic mutations in *PIGA*, an X-linked gene that encodes a subunit of an enzyme essential for the biosynthesis of the GPI anchor.[89] These patients often have severe hemolysis, whereas DAF-deficient, Cromer-null red cells show no signs of hemolysis and individuals with a very rare CD59-deficient phenotype had only mild hemolytic anemia.[4]

The major function of red cell CR1 is to bind and process C3b/C4b-coated immune complexes and transport them to the liver and spleen for removal from the circulation.[90,91] No true Knops-null phenotype has been identified, though red cells of some individuals have very low CR1 copy numbers.[4]

Red cell glycoproteins that anchor the membrane to its skeleton

Band 3, the Diego blood-group antigen, is the red cell anion exchanger, but also has an important structural function. Band 3 has an extended N-terminal domain, which interacts with the red cell membrane cytoskeleton, a submembranous matrix of glycoproteins that is responsible for maintaining the shape and integrity of the red cell. Band 3 interacts with the membrane skeleton through ankyrin and proteins band 4.2 and band 4.1R.[32–34] Heterozygosity for a 27 basepair deletion in the band 3 gene, encoding a nine amino acid deletion, is responsible for Southeast Asian ovalocytosis (SAO), a condition common in the southern Pacific region and among Melanesians. About 20% of cases of hereditary spherocytosis, a common, familial hemolytic anemia characterized by small spheroid red cells, result from mutations within the band 3 gene and an absence or decrease of the mutant protein from the red cell membrane.[51]

The Gerbich blood-group antigens are located on two red cell glycoproteins, glycophorins C and D (GPC and GPD), encoded by a single gene (GYPC) by initiation of translation at two sites.[4,5] The C-terminal cytoplasmic domains of GPC and GPD form a complex with the cytoskeletal protein 4.1R. GPC and GPD may be part of a proposed membrane complex that includes the glucose transporter (GLUT1), dimers of band 3, Rh proteins, the Duffy (DARC) and Kell glycoproteins, and Xk, attached to the cytoskeleton through protein 4.1R, p55, dematin and adducin.[32–34]

In addition there is evidence that RhAG interacts with ankyrin, the Lutheran and Xk proteins with spectrin, and CD44 with protein 4.1R. Red cells lacking RhAG or Xk, or with reduced levels of Lutheran glycoproteins and CD44, have some degree of abnormal morphology.[34]

Associations with infectious disease

Cell surface antigens may be exploited by pathogenic microorganisms for attachment to the cells and subsequent invasion. Many such associations have been reported involving antigens present on red cells, although the targets for the pathogens are often cells other than erythroid cells. Examples of these are associations are Le[b] and *Helicobacter pylori*, P antigen and the Dr[a] antigen of CD55 and *Escherichia coli*, CD35 (Knops antigen) and *Mycobacterium leprae*, and AnWj (an antigen associated with CD44) and *Hemophilus influenzae* (reviewed in [92] and [93]). Mononuclear cells of individuals with the P[k] red cell phenotype, which arises from deficiency of the glycosyltransferase that converts the glycolipid antigen P[k] (Gb3) to P (Gb4), were resistant to HIV-1 infection.[94] P antigen (globoside, Gb4) is a cellular receptor for parvovirus B19, a human pathogen that replicates in erythroid progenitor cells. B19 is the cause of fifth disease, a common childhood illness, and occasionally more severe disorders of erythropoiesis, particularly in immunocompromised patients.[95] Individuals with P deficiency (p phenotype) appear to be naturally resistant to parvovirus B19 infection. Fumagalli et al.[96] concluded that 'blood group antigens have been playing a central role in the host-pathogen arms race during human evolutionary history and no other gene category shows similar levels of widespread selection, with the only exception of loci involved in antigen recognition'.

Red cells of the rare phenotypes in which the sialic acid-rich red cell glycoproteins glycophorins A, B, or C/D are absent are relatively resistant to invasion by *Plasmodium falciparum*.[97] These structures are all exploited as ligands for *P. falciparum* receptors.[98–100] Absence of the Sl[a] antigen of the Knops blood group, which is expressed on CR1 (CD35), and red cells with low expression of CD35, demonstrate reduced rosetting when parasitized with *P. falciparum*, a characteristic associated with severe disease.[101] Sl(a–) phenotype and CD35 deficiency are relatively rare in Caucasians, but are present in about 70% of West Africans and 80% of Papua New Guineans, respectively.[4] The association between the malarial parasite *Plasmodium vivax* and the Duffy antigen is described in a previous section of this chapter.

A major selection pressure responsible for the abundance of O alleles of *ABO*, which almost certainly evolved from A

by a single nucleotide deletion, could be *Plasmodium falciparum* malaria. Despite some apparent discrepancies and contradictions, the overall impression from the literature is that individuals of blood group O are relatively resistant to severe malaria caused by infection with *Plasmodium falciparum*.[102,103] The geographic distribution of group O is consistent with selection by *P. falciparum* in favor of group O individuals in malaria endemic regions.[104]

Platelet antigens

The normal hemostatic function of platelets involves membrane glycoproteins, which function as receptors during platelet adhesion and aggregation. Several of the key platelet glycoproteins are polymorphic. Many of these polymorphisms are alloantigenic and were first recognized because of feto-maternal incompatibility characterized by the production of platelet-specific alloantibodies in the mother and fetal and neonatal alloimmune thrombocytopenia (NAIT). In addition to the well-established role of platelet antigens in the pathogenesis of NAIT, some alloantigenic polymorphisms may affect platelet function and the predisposition to thrombotic disease. Although platelet alloantigens have been identified by many groups around the world, resulting in a variety of different terminologies, the human platelet antigen (HPA) nomenclature has been almost universally adopted.[105,106] Currently, 17 systems are recognized, six containing a pair of alloantigens (1 to 5 and 15) and the remaining 11 containing a single antigen of low frequency (Table 37.2).[125] Unlike the red cell blood group systems, HPA systems represent antithetical antigens, so several different systems can be encoded by the same gene and their antigens present on the same protein. The letters a and b designate the higher and lower frequency antigens, respectively. The letter w (workshop) is added when the antithetical alloantigen has not been identified. Alleles of genes encoding six platelet membrane glycoproteins result in the expression of alloantigens on the cell surface (Table 37.2).

Serological methods for detecting platelet antigens generally involve the use of fluorescent-labeled antibodies. A 10-year review on external quality assessment of these methods was published in 2008.[126] Molecular methods, often involving the application of DNA microarray technology, are also available to predict platelet phenotypes.[127]

Glycoproteins expressing platelet antigens

Antigens on the GPIIb/IIIa (CD41/CD61 or αIIbβ3) complex

GPIIb/IIIa is the most abundant platelet integrin, present at approximately 80 000 copies per platelet. Integrins are a family of hererodimeric proteins, composed of non-covalently associated α- and β-subunits.[128] Upon platelet activation, GPIIb/IIIa is involved in platelet aggregation by binding adhesive proteins such as fibrinogen, fibrin, fibronectin, vitronectin, thrombospondin and von Willebrand factor (vWF).[128,129] Glanzmann's thrombasthenia, a bleeding disorder, results when GPIIb/IIIa is absent or dysfunctional.

Table 37.2 Human platelet antigens (HPAs)

System	Antigen Refs	Former names	Frequency (%)*	Glycoprotein	CD	Amino acid change
1	HPA-1a 107	Zw^a, Pl^{A1}	97.6	GPIIIa	CD61	Leu33
	HPA-1b	Zw^b, Pl^{A2}	26.8			Pro33
2	HPA-2a 108	Ko^b	99.4	GPIbα	CD42b	Thr145
	HPA-2b	Ko^a, Sib^a	14.3			Met145
3	HPA-3a 109	Bak^a, Lek^a	87.7	GPIIb	CD41	Iso843
	HPA-3b	Bak^b	64.1			Ser843
4	HPA-4a 110	Yuk^b, Pen^a	>99.9	GPIIIa	CD61	Arg143
	HPA-4b	Yuk^a, Pen^b	<0.2[†]			Gln143
5	HPA-5a 111,112	Br^b, Zav^b	99.0	GPIa	CD49b	Glu505
	HPA-5b	Br^a, Zav^a, Hc^a	20.0			Lys505
6	HPA-6bw 113	Ca^a, Tu^a	<0.01	GPIIIa	CD61	Gln489Arg
7	HPA-7bw 114	Mo	0.01	GPIIIa	CD61	Ala407Pro
8	HPA-8bw 115	Sr^a	<0.01	GPIIIa	CD61	Cys636Arg
9	HPA-9bw 116	Max^a	<0.01	GPIIb	CD41	Met837Val
10	HPA-10bw 117	La^a	<0.01	GPIIIa	CD61	Gln62Arg
11	HPA-11bw 118	Gro^a	<0.01	GPIIIa	CD61	His633Arg
12	HPA-12bw 119	Iy^a	<0.01	GPIbβ	CD42c	Glu15Gly
13	HPA-13bw 120	Sit^a	<0.01	GPIa	CD49b	Met799Thr
14	HPA-14bw 121	Oe^a	<1.0	GPIIIa	CD61	Lys611del
15	HPA-15a 122	Gov^b	80.0	CD109	CD109	Tyr703
	HPA-15b	Gov^a	60.0			Ser703
16	HPA-16bw 123	Duv^a	<1.0	GPIIIa	CD61	Thr140Ile
17	HPA-17bw 124	Va^a	<0.4	GPIIIa	CD61	Thr195Met

*In white people.

†In Japan.

Three alloantigenic forms of GPIIb have been identified (HPA-3a, -3b, -9bw). Carbohydrate residues on GPIIb appear to contribute to the binding site of HPA-3 antibodies.[130]

GPIIIa is the most polymorphic molecule on the platelet surface apart from HLA class I. The molecular bases of 12 antigens on GPIIIa have been determined (Table 37.2). Ten of the antigens (HPA-1b, -4b, -6bw, -7bw, -8bw, -10bw, -11bw, 14bw, 16bw and 17bw) are encoded by relatively rare single nucleotide substitutions in the common form of GPIIIa. The exception is the HPA-14bw, which results from the deletion of three nucleotides, encoding a single amino acid deletion.

HPA-1a is the most frequent cause of maternal alloimmunization to fetal platelets and is responsible for most cases of NAIT in Caucasians (discussed below). Although only 5–10% of HPA-1a-negative women with HPA-1a-positive fetuses produce anti-HPA-1a, the presence of the *HLA-DRB3*0101* allele increases the risk of alloimmunization by a factor of 140.[131] HPA-1b results from a Leu33Pro substitution. The immune response to HPA-1b does not appear to be HLA restricted.[132] An explanation for this observation was provided when Wu et al.[133] used an *in vitro* peptide-binding assay to show that leucine, but not proline, at position 33 anchors the peptide to the *HLA-DRB3*0101*-encoded molecule.

Antigens on the GPIa/IIa (CD49/CD29 or α2β1)complex

GPIa/IIa, also known as VLA-2 (very late antigen-2), is an integrin expressed at relatively low density on platelets as well as on activated T-lymphocytes. The GPIa/IIa heterodimer comprises a 167 kDa α2 polypeptide and a 130 kDa β1 polypeptide. GPIa/IIa integrin is a receptor for collagen and functions in collagen-mediated platelet activation.[128] A mild bleeding disorder may result when the complex is absent.[134]

Three alloantigens (HPA-5a, -5b and -13w) reside on GPIa; none on GPIIa (Table 37.2). Alloimmunization to the HPA-5b antigen could be responsible for approximately 15% of cases of NAIT in Caucasians (described below). Silent SNPs within codons 224 and 246 of the GPIa gene are associated with up to tenfold variation in expression of the GPIa/IIa complex.[135] Collagen-induced aggregation responses of HPA-13bw-positive platelets were diminished relative to HPA-13bw-negative platelets, indicating that the Met-799Thr substitution affects the function of the GPIa/IIa complex.[120] None of the HPA-13bw-positive individuals studied, however, had any signs of altered hemostasis.

Antigens on the GPIb/IX/V (CD42) complex

GPIb/IX/V binds VWF and mediates the adhesion of platelets to exposed vascular subendothelium surfaces under conditions of high shear stress, and interaction essential for slowing circulating platelets, allowing formation of arterial thrombi. The GPIb-VWF interaction can also activate platelets through intracellular signals.[128] GPIb comprises two disulfide-bonded subunits, GPIbα (CD42b) and GPIbβ (CD42c). GPIb is non-covalently associated with GPIX (CD42a) and GPV (CD42d). There are approximately 25 000 GPb/IX molecules and 12 000 GPV molecules per platelet.

Absence of the complex results in the inherited bleeding disorder Bernard–Soulier syndrome.

Three antigens (HPA-2a, -2b and -12bw) on GPIb have been described (Table 37.2), but none on GPIX or GPV. In addition to these antigenic variations, there are four size variants of GPIbα: A, B, C and D (from largest to smallest). The differences arise from the number of 13-amino acid tandem repeats within the GPIbα (A=4, B=3, C=2, D=1).[136] Only the relatively rare A and B forms of glycoprotein Ibα contain Met145, which is required for the expression of the HPA-2b epitope.[137]

Antigens on CD109

CD109 is a member of the α2-macroglobulin/complement (AMCOM) superfamily, which contains α2-macroglobulin and the complement components C3, C4 and C5. CD109 is a 175 kDa GPI-anchored glycoprotein expressed on platelets, activated T-lymphocytes, cultured endothelial cells and several tumor cell lines.[138-140] CD109 expresses the antithetical alloantigens HPA-15a and -15b (Table 37.2).[141] Antibodies to both antigens may cause NAIT, but they are encountered rarely.

Fetal and neonatal alloimmune thrombocytopenia

A variety of names and acronyms have been used for the condition characterized by thrombocytopenia in a fetus or neonate caused by maternal antibodies crossing the placenta and facilitating the immune destruction of fetal platelets. Because of the analogy with HDFN, the term fetal and neonatal alloimmune thrombocytopenia, but with the more usual acronym NAIT, will be used here. For reviews see.[142-144]

Pathophysiology

In Caucasians, NAIT occurs in about 1 in 1000–2000 births. All the HPAs listed in Table 37.2 have been associated with NAIT. Anti-HPA-1a is the dominant cause of NAIT in Caucasians, responsible for about 80% of cases.[145] After anti-HPA-1a, anti-HPA-5b and -15a are most frequently responsible, followed by anti-HPA-1b, -3a, and -2a/2b.[143,145,146] In people from Africa and eastern Asia HPA-1b is very rare, so anti-HPA-1a antibodies are also rare.[147] In Japanese people, for example, anti-HPA-4a and -4b cause NAIT more frequently than other platelet antibodies.[148]

The natural history of NAIT differs from HDFN in that maternal sensitization to fetal platelet antigens often occurs in the first pregnancy. Approximately 40% of cases of NAIT occur in primiparae. Although the mechanisms involved in immunization remain unclear,[142] GPIIIa, which expresses HPA-1 antigens, is present on placental syncytiotrophoblast microvilli from the first trimester.[149] Syncytiotrophoblasts are naturally shed into the maternal circulation and could be the source of HPA-1a antigen responsible for early immunization of HPA-1a-negative primigravidae.

Maternal HPA antibodies are predominantly IgG1[150] and are transported across the placenta to the fetus. Studies of autoimmune thrombocytopenia in adults suggest that antibody-mediated platelet destruction involves the sequestration of platelets by splenic macrophages in a manner analogous to the extravascular destruction of IgG-sensitized red cells.[151] Fcγ receptor III (FcγRIII) may be involved in the recognition of sensitized platelets: administration of monoclonal anti-FcγRIII to a patient with autoimmune thrombocytopenia was associated with a rise in platelet count.[152]

Clinical features

Fetal thrombocytopenia may start early in pregnancy: almost 50% of affected fetuses have a platelet count of less than $20 \times 10^9/l$.[153] There is no spontaneous remission of the thrombocytopenia *in utero* and, in the absence of therapy, platelet counts usually fall as gestation progresses. In the absence of screening programs, alloimmune thrombocytopenia is usually recognized at birth when the majority of affected cases have petechiae, purpura or overt bleeding. Intracerebral hemorrhage (ICH) occurs in about 20% of affected infants and about one-third of these events are fatal. If non-fatal, mental retardation, cerebral palsy, cortical blindness and seizures often result. Up to 80% of ICH occur prenatally, as early as 16 weeks' gestation, and may lead to structural and metabolic central nervous system abnormalities.[8,143]

Clinically, NAIT is a diagnosis of exclusion. Infants have no signs of disseminated intravascular coagulation, infection, or congenital anomalies that may be associated with thrombocytopenia. The mother has no history of autoimmune disease, thrombocytopenia, or ingestion of drugs that may cause thrombocytopenia. At delivery, standard laboratory tests show that neonatal platelet counts are low. Fetal hemoglobin concentration may be low if bleeding has occurred. Bone marrow biopsy usually reveals normal levels of megakaryocytes. Cranial ultrasound and computerized tomographic scans may reveal dilated cerebral ventricles and evidence of intraventricular hemorrhage.[154] Once suspected on clinical grounds, a provisional diagnosis of NAIT should be confirmed by establishing the presence of platelet-specific alloantibodies in the maternal serum that react with fetal platelets.

Neutrophil antigens

Granulocyte-specific polymorphisms are less well characterized than those on red cells and platelets. Nevertheless, it is well established that some polymorphisms are antigenic and capable of eliciting alloimmune responses resulting in, for example, neonatal alloimmune neutropenia (NAIN). Most neutrophil antigens are expressed on membrane receptors involved in inflammation and the clearance of immune complexes and there is some evidence that these polymorphisms might affect cell function and the risk of some infectious or autoimmune diseases. An HNA terminology, analogous to the HPA terminology for platelets, has been established by the International Society for Blood Transfusion for granulocyte-specific antigens and those shared with a limited number of other cell types (Table 37.3).[161,162]

Glycoproteins expressing neutrophil antigens

Antigens classified in the HNA terminology are located on FcγRIIIb (CD16), CD177, CD11a, CD11b, and CLT2 (SLC44A2) (Table 37.3). Neutrophils also express some antigens with a wide tissue distribution. These include the I and P1 blood group antigens, Le[x] and sialyl-Le[x] (CD15), and HLA class I, and are not discussed here.

Table 37.3 Human neutrophil antigens (HNAs)

System	Antigen Refs	Former names	Frequency (%)*	Glycoprotein	Amino acid change
1	HNA-1a 155	NA1	57–62	FcγRIIIb, CD16	Arg36 Asn65 Ala78 Asp82 Val106
	HNA-1b 155	NA2	88–89		Ser36 Ser65 Ala78 Asn82 Ile106
	HNA-1c 156	SH	5		Ser36 Ser65 Asp78 Asn82 Ile106
2	HNA-2a 157	NB1	87–97	CD177	nk
3	HNA-3a 158, 159	5b	89–96	CLT2 (SLC44A2)	Arg154 (negative Gln154)
4	HNA-4a 160	Mart[a]	99	CD11b	Arg61 (negative His61)
5	HNA-5a 160	Ond[a]	86–92	CD11a	Arg766 (negative Thr766)

*In white people[160]

nk, not known.

Antigens on Fcγ receptor III (FcγRIIIb, CD16)

HNA-1a, -1b and -1c are located on Fcγ RIIIb,[155,156] a low-affinity receptor for complexed IgG, which is selectively expressed on neutrophils.[163] FcγRIIIb has an extracellular region consisting of two disulfide-bonded immunoglobulin-like domains and is linked to the plasma membrane by a GPI-anchor. When subjected to polyacrylamide gel electrophoresis, Fcγ RIIIb migrates as a broad band with a molecular weight between 50 kDa and 80 kDa. The differences in electrophoretic migration arise from amino acid differences between HNA-1a and HNA-1b at positions 65 and 82, which result in two additional glycosylation sites in HNA-1b (Ser65, Asn82).[155] FCGR3B*01 and FCGR3B*02, the alleles encoding HNA-1a and HNA-1b, differ at five SNPs, but only four of these give rise to amino acid changes (Table 37.3). HNA-1c has an identical amino acid sequence to HNA-1b, except for a Ala78Asp substitution.[156] HNA-1c expression is often associated with the presence of an additional Fcγ RIIIb gene, probably as the result of gene duplication and giving rise to an increased quantity of Fcγ RIIIb.[164] Frequencies for HNA-1 alloantigens in Caucasians are shown in Table 37.3. In eastern Asia HNA-1a is more common (88–91%), HNA-1b less common (51–54%) and HNA-1c is relatively rare; in Africans HNA-1c is more common (23–31%) and HNA-1b is less common (46–66%) than in Caucasian, with HNA-1a about the same.[161]

LAN and SAR are high frequency antigens on Fcγ RIIIb, but their molecular genetic bases are unknown.[165,166]

Approximately 0.1% of Caucasians and 4% of black Africans do not have FcγRIIIb as a result of gene deletion. Women with this HNA-1 null phenotype can form isoantibodies causing severe neonatal neutropenia.[167]

Antigens on CD11/CD18

The HNA-4a and -5a alloantigens are located on α chains of β2 integrins: HNA-4a on αMβ2 (CD11b/CD18, Mac-1); HNA-5a on αLβ2 (CD11a/CD18, LFA-1). CD11a is expressed on all leukocytes while CD11b is expressed on granulocytes, monocytes and natural killer cells. Both alloantigens differ from their relatively uncommon, antigen-negative alternatives by a single amino acid (Table 37.3).

Neutrophil antigens on other glycoproteins

HNA-2a is present on granulocytes from between 87% and 99% of Caucasians, Asians, and Africans.[161] Antibodies to HNA-2a recognize CD177, a 56–64 kDa GPI-linked glycoprotein present on the neutrophil surface and secondary granules.[168] HNA-2a-negative phenotype may result from splicing defects in CD177.[169] Expression of HNA-2a is reduced on neutrophils from patients with PNH or chronic myelocytic leukemia, but this appears to be of no clinical relevance.[8] The antibody named NB2 does not appear to be antithetical to anti-HNA-2a (initially named anti-NB1), and may detect human monocyte antigen 1.[125]

HNA-3a is carried on choline transporter-like protein-1 (SLC44A2), a glycoprotein of unknown function with homology to choline transporters. HNA-3-negative phenotype results from Arg154Gln.[158,159]

Clinical syndromes associated with neutrophil antibodies

There are five main clinical syndromes that may be caused by antibodies to HNAs: neonatal alloimmune and isoimmune neutropenia; autoimmune neutropenia; transfusion-related alloimmune neutropenia; transfusion-related acute lung injury; and febrile reactions following transfusion.[8,125]

Neonatal alloimmune neutropenia (NAIN)

NAIN occurs in approximately 1 in 1500 births. It is characterized by neutropenia in a fetus or infant caused by placental transfer of neutrophil IgG antibodies. HNAs are well expressed from before birth and the condition may occur in the first-born infant.[170] Anti-HNA-1a and 2a are the most common causes of NAIN.

NAIN usually has a relatively benign course with infants developing mild infections, predominantly of the skin and mucous membranes. Occasionally, more serious infections resulting in pneumonia and meningitis develop. Hematologic investigation reveals a severe neutropenia, which may persist for up to 6 months.[170] NAIN is probably under-diagnosed as infants are usually asymptomatic at birth and white cell counts might not be performed routinely. Diagnosis is largely one of exclusion. In the absence of disease processes, drugs and environmental factors that can cause neutropenia or impairment of neutrophil function, a provisional diagnosis of NAIN should be confirmed by demonstrating the presence of antibodies in the maternal plasma that react with the infant's neutrophils.

Autoimmune neutropenia of infancy

In addition to their role in the pathogenesis of NAIN, some alloantigenic polymorphisms on neutrophils are also the target of autoantibodies implicated in autoimmune neutropenia of infancy. Disease onset usually occurs between 4 months and 2 years with spontaneous remission in 95% of patients within 7–24 months.[171,172] It is a relatively benign condition associated with infections of the skin, middle ear, throat, and respiratory and digestive tracts. The incidence of autoimmune neutropenia of infancy is approximately 1 in 100 000.[173] Pathogenesis may involve a deficiency of suppresser T-lymphocytes, which results in the production of granulocyte-specific IgG or IgM autoantibodies, usually specific for HNA-1a.[171]

Transfusion-related acute lung injury (TRALI)

Characterized by acute respiratory distress and non-cardiogenic lung edema developing during or within 6 hours of blood transfusion, TRALI is one of the most common causes of transfusion-associated morbidity and death.[174,175] Antibody-mediated TRALI is triggered by leukocyte antibodies, either HLA class I or II antibodies or HNA antibodies.[176,177] In most cases TRALI results from antibodies in transfused plasma, but occasionally the reaction occurs between the recipient's neutrophil antibodies and transfused neutrophils. Neutrophils stimulated by leukocyte antibodies aggregate and release cytotoxic enzymes that damage the endothelial cells of the lung capillaries. Antibodies to HNA-1a, 1b, 2a and 3a have all been incriminated in TRALI.[8] HNA-3a antibodies are rare and difficult to detect, but have been associated with several fatal cases.[178,179]

References

1. Daniels GL, Fletcher A, Garratty G, et al. Blood group terminology 2004. From the ISBT Committee on Terminology for Red Cell Surface Antigens. Vox Sanguinis 2004;87:304–16.

2. Daniels G, Castilho L, Flegel WA, et al. International Society of Blood Transfusion Committee on Terminology for Red Cell Surface Antigens: Macao Report. 3. Vox Sanguinis 2009;96:153–6. Also see online: http://ibgrl.blood.co.uk/.

3. Daniels G. Functions of red cell surface proteins. Vox Sanguinis 2007;93:331–40.

4. Daniels G. Human blood groups. 2nd ed. Oxford: Blackwell Science; 2002.

5. Reid ME, Lomas-Francis C. The blood group antigen facts book. 2nd ed. London: Academic Press; 2004.

6. Yamamoto F, Clausen H, White T, et al. Molecular genetic basis of the histo-blood group ABO system. Nature 1990; 345:229–23.

7. Chester MA, Olsson ML. The ABO blood group gene: a locus of considerable genetic diversity. Transfusion Medicine Reviews 2001;15:177–200.

8. Klein HG, Anstee DJ. Mollison's Blood Transfusion in Clinical Medicine. 11th ed. Oxford: Blackwell Publishing; 2005.

9. Gold ER, Tovey GH, Benney WE, et al. Changes in the group A antigen in a case of leukaemia. Nature 1959;183:892–3.

10. Bianco T, Farmer BJ, Sage RE, Dobrovic A. Loss of red cell A, B, and H antigens is frequent in myeloid malignancies. Blood 2001;97:3633–9.

11. Salmon C, Cartron JP, Lopez M, et al. Level of the A, B and H blood group glycosyltransferases in red cell membranes from patients with malignant hemopathies. Revue Française de Transfusion et Immuno-Hématologie 1984;27:625–37.

12. Bianco-Miotto T, Hussey DJ, Day TK, et al. DNA methylation of the ABO promoter underlies loss of ABO allelic expression in a significant proportion of leukemic patients. PloS ONE 2009; 4:e4788.

13. Henry S, Oriol R, Samuelsson B. Lewis histo-blood group system and associated secretory phenotypes. Vox Sanguinis 1995;69:166–82.

14. Hakomori S. Antigen structure and genetic basis of histo blood groups A, B and O: their changes associated with human cancer. Biochimica et Biophysica Acta 1999;1473:246–66.

15. Le Pendu J, Marionneau S, Cailleau-Thomas A, et al. ABH and Lewis histo-blood group antigens in cancer. APMIS 2001;109:9–31.

16. Dabelsteen E, Gao S. ABO blood-group antigens of oral cancer. Journal of Dental Research 2004;84:21–8.

17. Chihara Y, Sugano K, Kobayashi A, et al. Loss of blood group A antigen expression in bladder cancer caused by allelic loss and/or methylation of the ABO gene. Laboratory Investigation 2005;85: 895–907.

18. Ørntoft TF, Bech E. Circulating blood group related carbohydrate antigens as tumour markers. Glygoconjugate Journal 1995;12:200–5.

19. Steinberg W. The clinical utility of the CA 19-9 tumor-associated antigen. American Journal of Gastroenterology 1990;85:350–5.

20. Grote T, Logsdon CD. Progress on molecular markers of pancreatic cancer. Current Opinion in Gastroenterology 2007;23:508–14.

21. Clausen H, Hakomori S, Graem N, et al. Incompatible A antigen expressed in tumors of blood group O individuals: immunochemical, immunohistologic, and enzymatic characterization. Journal of Immunology 1986;136:326–30.

22. David L, Leitao D, Sobrinho-Simoes M, et al. Biosynthetic basis of incompatible histo-blood group A antigen expression: anti-A transferase antibodies reactive with gastric cancer tissue of type O individuals. Cancer Research 1993;53: 5494–500.

23. Hakomori S. Immunochemical and molecular genetic basis of the histo-blood group ABO(H) and related antigen system. Baillière's Clinical Haematology 1991;4:957–97.

24. Avent ND, Reid ME. The Rh blood group system: a review. Blood 2000;95:375–87.

25. Huang C-H, Liu PZ, Cheng JG. Molecular biology and genetics of the Rh blood group system. Seminars in Hematology 2000;37:150–65.

26. Wagner FF, Flegel WA. The RHD gene deletion occurred in the Rhesus box. Blood 2000;95:3662–8.

27. Singleton BK, Green CA, Avent ND, et al. The presence of an RHD pseudogene containing a 37 base pair duplication and a nonsense mutation in most Africans with the Rh D-negative blood group phenotype. Blood 2000;95:12–8.

28. Conroy MJ, Bullough PA, Merrick M, Avent ND. Modelling the human rhesus proteins: implications for structure and function. British Journal of Haematology 2005;131:543–51.

29. Burton NM, Anstee DJ. Nature, function and significance of Rh proteins in red cells. Current Opinion in Hematology 2008;15:625–30.

30. Bruce LJ, Beckmann R, Ribeiro ML, et al. A band 3-based macrocomplex of integral and peripheral proteins in the RBC membrane. Blood 2003;101:4180–8.

31. Endeward V, Cartron J-P, Ripoche P, Gros G. RhAG protein of the Rhesus complex is a CO_2 channel in the human red cell membrane. FASEB Journal 2008;22: 64–73.

32. Salomao M, Zhang X, Yang Y, et al. Protein 4.1R-dependent multiprotein complex: new insights into the structural organization of the red blood cell membrane. Proceedings of the National Academy of Sciences 2008;105: 8026–31.

33. Khan AA, Toshihiko H, Mohseni M, et al. Dematin and adducin provide a novel link between the spectrin cytoskeleton and human erythrocyte membrane by directly interacting with glucose transporter-1. Journal of Biological Chemistry 2008;238:14600–9.

34. Mohandas N, Gallagher PG. Red cell membrane: past, present, and future. Blood 2008;112:3939–48.

35. Pilgrim H, Lloyd-Jones M, Rees A. Routine antenatal anti-D prophylaxis for RhD-negative women: a systematic review and economic evaluation. Health Technology Assessment 2009;13:1–103.

36. Daniels G, Finning K, Martin P, Massey E. Non-invasive prenatal diagnosis of fetal blood group phenotypes: current practice and future prospects. Prenatal Diagnosis 2009;29:101–7.

37. Finning K, Martin P, Summers J, et al. Effect of high throughput RHD typing of fetal DNA in maternal plasma on use of anti-RhD immunoglobulin in RhD negative pregnant women: prospective feasibility study. British Medical Journal 2008;336:816–8.

38. Lee S, Russo D, Redman C. Functional and structural aspects of the Kell blood group system. Transfusion Medicine Reviews 2000;14:93–103.

39. Russo D, Redman C, Lee S. Association of XK and Kell blood group proteins.

Journal of Biological Chemistry 1998;273:13950–6.

40. Lee S, Lin M, Mele A, et al. Proteolytic processing of big endothelin-3 by the Kell blood group protein. Blood 1999; 94:1440–50.

41. Vaughan JI, Warwick R, Letsky E, et al. Erythropoietic suppression in fetal anemia because of Kell alloimmunization. American Journal of Obstetrics and Gynecology 1994; 171:247–52.

42. Weiner CP, Widness JA. Decreased fetal erythropoiesis and hemolysis in Kell hemolytic anemia. American Journal of Obstetrics and Gynecology 1996;174: 547–51.

43. Southcott MJG, Tanner MJA, Anstee DJ. The expression of human blood group antigens during erythropoiesis in a cell culture system. Blood 1999;93:4425–35.

44. Bony V, Gane P, Bailly P, et al. Time-course expression of polypeptides carrying blood group antigens during human erythroid differentiation. British Journal of Haematology 1999;107: 263–74.

45. Daniels G, Hadley A, Green CA. Causes of fetal anemia in hemolytic disease due to anti-K. Transfusion 2003;43:115–6.

46. Vaughan JI, Manning M, Warwick RM, et al. Inhibition of erythroid progenitor cells by anti-Kell antibodies in fetal alloimmune anemia. New England Journal of Medicine 1998;338:798–803.

47. Ho M, Chelly J, Carter N, et al. Isolation of the gene for McLeod syndrome that encodes a novel membrane transport protein. Cell 1994;77:869–80.

48. Danek A, Rubio JP, Rampoldi L, et al. McLeod neuroacanthocytosis: genotype and phenotype. Annals of Neurology 2001;50:755–64.

49. Clapéron A, Hattab C, Armand V, et al. The Kell and Xk proteins of the Kell blood group are not co-expressed in the central nervous system. Brain Research 2007;1147:12–24.

50. Roos D, de Boer M, Kuribayashi F, et al. Mutations in the X-linked and autosomal recessive forms of chronic granulomatous disease. Blood 1996;87:1663–81.

51. Bruce L. Mutations in band 3 and cation leaky red cells. Blood Cells and Molecular Disease 2006;36:331–6.

52. Ribeiro ML, Alloisio N, Almeida H, et al. Severe hereditary spherocytosis and distal renal tubular acidosis associated with total absence of band 3. Blood 2000;96: 1602–4.

53. Olivès B, Mattei M-G, Huet M, et al. Kidd blood group and urea transport function of human erythrocytes are carried by the same protein. Journal of Biological Chemistry 1995;270: 15607–10.

54. Sands JM. Renal urea transporters. Current Opinions in Nephrological Hypertension 2004;13:525–32.

55. Macey RI, Yousef LW. Osmotic stability of red cells in renal circulation required rapid urea transport. American Journal of Physiology 1988;254:C669–74.

56. Lucien N, Sidoux-Walter F, Olivès B, et al. Characterization of the gene encoding the human Kidd blood group/urea transporter protein. Evidence for splice site mutations in Jk$_{null}$ individuals. Journal of Biological Chemistry 1998; 273:12973–80.

57. Irshaid NM, Henry SM, Olsson ML. Genomic characterization of the Kidd blood group gene: different molecular basis of the Jk(a–b–) phenotype in Polynesians and Finns. Transfusion 2000;40:69–74.

58. Henry S, Woodfield G. Frequencies of the Jk(a–b–) phenotype in Polynesian ethnic groups. Transfusion 1995;35:277.

59. Sands JM, Gargus JJ, Fröhlich O, et al. Urinary concentrating ability in patients with Jk(a–b–) blood type who lack carrier-mediated urea transport. Journal of the American Society of Nephrology 1992;2:1689–96.

60. Yang B, Bankir L, Gillespie A, et al. Urea-selective concentrating defect in transgenic mice lacking urea transporter UT-B. Journal of Biological Chemistry 2002;277:10633–7.

61. Klein JD, Sands JM, Qian L, et al. Upregulation of urea transporter UT-A2 and water channels AQP2 and AQP3 in mice lacking urea transporter UT-B. Journal of the American Society of Nephrology 2004;15:1161–7.

62. King LS, Kozono D, Agre P. From structure to disease: the evolving tale of aquaporin biology. Nature Reviews Molecular Cell Biology 2004;5:687–98.

63. Preston GM, Smith BL, Zeidel ML, et al. Mutations in aquaporin-1 in phenotypically normal humans without functional CHIP water channels. Science 1994;265:1585–7.

64. King LS, Choi M, Fernandez PC, et al. Defective urinary concentrating ability due to a complete deficiency of aquaporin-1. New England Journal of Medicine 2001;345:175–9.

65. Roudier N, Ripoche P, Gane P. AQP3 deficiency in humans and the molecular basis of a novel blood group system, GIL. Journal of Biological Chemistry 2002;48:45854–9.

66. Hadley TJ, Peiper SC. From malaria to chemokine receptor: the emerging physiologic role of the Duffy blood group antigen. Blood 1997;89:3077–91.

67. Rot A. Contribution of Duffy antigen to chemokine function. Cytokine and Growth Factor Reviews 2005;16:687–94.

68. Gardner L, Patterson AM, Ashton BA, et al. The human Duffy antigen binds selected inflammatory but not homeostatic chemokines. Biochemical Biophysical Research Communications 2004;32:306–12.

69. Darbonne WC, Rice GC, Mohler MA, et al. Red blood cells are a sink for interleukin 8, a leukocyte chemotaxin. Journal of Clinical Investigation 1991; 88:1362–9.

70. Pruenster M, Rot A. Throwing light on DARC. Biochemical Society Transactions 2006;34:1005–8.

71. Shen H, Schuster R, Stringer KF, et al. The Duffy antigen/receptor for chemokines (DARC) regulates prostate tumor growth. FASEB Journal 2006; 20:59–64.

72. Wang J, Ou Z-L, Hou Y-F. Enhanced expression of Duffy antigen receptor for chemokines by breast cancer cells attenuates growth and metastasis potential. Oncogene 2006;25:7201–11.

73. Addison CL, Belperio JA, Burdick MD, Strieter RM. Overexpression of the duffy antigen receptor for chemokines (DARC) by NSCLC tumor cells results in increased tumor necrosis. BMC Cancer 2004;4:28.

74. Bandyopadhyay S, Zhan R, Chaudhuri A. Interaction of KAI1 on tumor cells with DARC on vascular endothelium leads to metastasis suppression. Nature Medicine 2006;12:933–8.

75. Tournamille C, Colin Y, Cartron JP, et al. Disruption of a GATA motif in the Duffy gene promoter abolishes erythroid gene expression in Duffy-negative individuals. Nature Genetics 1995;10:224–8.

76. Peiper SC, Wang Z, Neote K, et al. The Duffy antigen/receptor for chemokines (DARC) is expressed in endothelial cells of Duffy-negative individuals who lack the erythrocyte receptor. Journal of Experimental Medicine 1995;181:1311–7.

77. Afenyi-Annan A, Ashley-Koch A, Telen MJ. Duffy (Fy), DARC, and neutropenia among women from the United States, Europe and the Caribbean. British Journal of Haematology 2009;145: 266–7.

78. Isacke CM, Horton MA. The Adhesion Molecule Facts Book. 2nd ed. London: Academic Press; 2000.

79. Parsons SF, Lee G, Spring FA. Lutheran blood group glycoprotein and its newly characterized mouse homologue specifically bind α5 chain-containing human laminin with high affinity. Blood 2001;97:312–20.

80. Mankelow TJ, Burton N, Stefansdottir FO, et al. The laminin 511/521 binding site on the Lutheran blood group glycoprotein is located at the flexible junction of Ig domains 2 and 3. Blood 2007;110:3398–406.

81. Delahunty M, Zennadi R, Telen MJ. LW protein: a promiscuous integrin receptor activated by adrenergic signaling. Transfusion Clinical Biology 2006;13:44–9.

82. Parsons SF, Spring FA, Chasis JA, et al. Erythroid cell adhesion molecules Lutheran and LW in health and disease.

Baillière's Clinical Haematology 1999; 12:729–45.

83. Lee G, Lo A, Short SA. Targeted gene deletion demonstrates that cell adhesion molecule ICAM-4 is critical for erythroblastic island formation. Blood 2006;108:2064–71.

84. Eyler CE, Telen MJ. The Lutheran glycoprotein: a multifunctional adhesion receptor. Transfusion 2006;46:668–77.

85. Kaul DK, Liu X, Zhanmg X. Peptides based on αV-binding domains of erythrocyte ICAM-4 inhibit sickle red cell-endithelial interactions and vaso-occlusion in the microcirculation. American Journal of Physiology and Cell Physiology 2006;291:C922–C930.

86. El Nemer W, Wautier M-P, Rahuel C. Endothelial Lu/BCAM glycoproteins are novel ligands for red blood cell α4β1 integrin: role in adhesion of sickle red blood cells to endothelial cells. Blood 2007;109:3544–51.

87. Karamatic Crew V, Burton N, Kagan A. CD151, the first member of the tetraspanin (TM4) superfamily detected on erythrocytes, is essential for the correct assembly of human basement membranes in kidney and skin. Blood 2004;104:2217–23.

88. Lublin DM. Review: Cromer and DAF: role in health and disease. Immunohematology 2005;21:39–47.

89. Johnson RJ, Hillmen P. Paroxysmal nocturnal hemoglobinuria: nature's gene therapy? Molecular Pathology 2002; 55:145–52.

90. Rao N, Ferguson DJ, Lee S-F, et al. Identification of human erythrocyte blood group antigens on the C3b/C4b receptor. Journal of Immunology 1991;146:3502–7.

91. Moulds JM, Nickells MW, Moulds JJ, et al. The C3b/C4b receptor is recognized by the Knops, McCoy, Swain-Langley, and York blood group antisera. Journal of Experimental Medicine 1991;173: 1159–63.

92. Eder AF, Spitalnik SL. Blood group antigens as receptors for pathogens. In: Blancher A, Klein J, Socha WW, editors. Molecular biology and evolution of blood group and MHC antigens in primates. Berlin: Springer; 1997. p. 268–304.

93. Rios M, Bianco C. The role of blood group antigens in infectious diseases. Seminars in Hematology 2000;37: 177–85.

94. Lund N, Olsson ML, Ramkumar S. The human P^k histo-blood group antigen provides protection against HIV-1 infection. Blood 2009;113:4980–91.

95. Brown KE, Young NS. Parvovirus B19 infection and hematopoiesis. Blood Reviews 1995;9:176–82.

96. Fumagalli M, Cagliani R, Pozzoli U. Widespread balancing selection and pathogen-driven selection at blood group antigen genes. Genome Research 2009; 19:199–212.

97. Pasvol G, Wainscoat JS, Weatherall DJ. Erythrocytes deficient in glycophorin resist invasion by the malarial parasite Plasmodium falciparum. Nature 1982; 297:64–6.

98. Sim BKL, Chitnis CE, Wasniowska K, et al. Receptor and ligand domains for invasion of erythrocytes by Plasmodium falciparum. Science 1994;264:1941–4.

99. Mayer DCG, Jiang L, Achur RN, et al. The glycophorin C N-linked glycan is a critical component of the ligand for the Plasmodium falciparum erythrocyte receptor BAEBL. Proceeding of the National Academy of Science of the United States of America 2006;103: 2358–62.

100. Mayer DCG, Jiang L, Achur RN et al. The glycophorin C N-linked glycan is a critical component of the ligand for the Plasmodium falciparum erythrocyte receptor BAEBL. Proceeding of the National Academy of Science of the United States of America 2006;103: 2358–62.

101. Rowe JA, Moulds JM, Newbold CI, Miller LH. P. falciparum rosetting mediated by a parasite-variant erythrocyte membrane protein and complement-receptor 1. Nature 1997; 388:292–5.

102. Uneke CJ. Plasmodium falciparum malaria and ABO blood group: is there any relationship? Parasitology Research 2007;100:759–65.

103. Loscertales M-P, Owens S, O'Donnell J, et al. ABO blood group phenotypes and Plasmodium falciparum malaria: unlocking a pivotal mechanism. Advances in Parasitology 2007;65:1–50.

104. Cserti CM, Dzik WH. The ABO blood group system and Plasmodium falciparum malaria. Blood 2007;110:2250–8.

105. von dem Borne AEG Kr, Decary F. Nomenclature of platelet specific antigens. British Journal of Haematology 1990;74:239–40.

106. Metcalfe P, Watkins NA, Ouwehand WH, et al. Nomenclature of human platelet antigens. Vox Sanguinis 2003;85: 240–5.

107. Newman PJ, Derbes RS, Aster RH. The human platelet alloantigens, P1A1 and P1A2, are associated with a leucine33/proline33 amino acid polymorphism in membrane glycoprotein IIIa, and are distinguishable by DNA typing. Journal of Clinical Investigation 1989;83: 1778–81.

108. Kuijpers RW, Faber NM, Cuypers HT, et al. NH2-terminal globular domain of human platelet glycoprotein Ibα has a methionine 145/threonine 145 amino acid polymorphism, which is associated with the HPA-2 (Ko) alloantigens. Journal of Clinical Investigation 1992; 89:381–4.

109. Lyman S, Aster RH, Visentin GP, et al. Polymorphism of human platelet membrane glycoprotein IIb associated with the Baka/Bakb alloantigen system. Blood 1990;75:2343–8.

110. Wang R, Furihata K, McFarland JG, et al. An amino acid polymorphism within the RGD binding domain of platelet membrane glycoprotein IIIa is responsible for the formation of the Pena/Penb alloantigen system. Journal of Clinical Investigation 1992;90:2038–43.

111. Santoso S, Kalb R, Walka M, et al. The human platelet alloantigens Br^a and Br^b are associated with a single amino acid polymorphism on glycoprotein Ia (integrin subunit α_2). Journal of Clinical Investigation 1993;92:2427–32.

112. Simsek S, Gallardo D, Ribera A, et al. The human platelet alloantigens, HPA-5(a+, b−) and HPA-5(a−, b+), are associated with a Glu505/Lys505 polymorphism of glycoprotein Ia (the α_2 subunit of VLA-2). British Journal of Haematology 1994;86:671–4.

113. Wang R, McFarland JG, Kekomaki R, et al. Amino acid 489 is encoded by a mutational 'hot spot' on the β3 integrin chain: the CA/TU human platelet alloantigen system. Blood 1993;82: 3386–91.

114. Kuijpers RW, Simsek S, Faber NM, et al. Single point mutation in human glycoprotein IIIa is associated with a new platelet-specific alloantigen (Mo) involved in neonatal alloimmune thrombocytopenia. Blood 1993;81:70–6.

115. Santoso S, Kalb R, Kroll H, et al. A point mutation leads to an unpaired cysteine residue and a molecular weight polymorphism of a functional platelet beta 3 integrin subunit. The Sr^a alloantigen system of GPIIIa. Journal of Biological Chemistry 1994;18:8439–44.

116. Noris P, Simsek S, de Bruijne-Admiraal LG, et al. Max^a, a new low-frequency platelet-specific antigen localized on glycoprotein IIb, is associated with neonatal alloimmune thrombocytopenia. Blood 1995;86:1019–26.

117. Peyruchaud O, Bourre F, Morel-Kopp MC, et al. HPA-10w(b) (La^a): genetic determination of a new platelet-specific alloantigen on glycoprotein IIIa and its expression in COS-7 cells. Blood 1997; 89:2422–8.

118. Simsek S, Folman C, van der Schoot CE, et al. The Arg633His substitution responsible for the private platelet antigen Gro^a unravelled by SSCP analysis and direct sequencing. British Journal of Haematology 1997;97:330–5.

119. Sachs UJ, Kiefel V, Bohringer M, et al. Single amino acid substitution in human platelet glycoprotein Ibbeta is responsible for the formation of the platelet-specific alloantigen Iy^a. Blood 2000;95:1849–55.

120. Santoso S, Amrhein J, Hofmann HA, et al. A point mutation Thr(799)Met on

the α_2 integrin leads to the formation of new human platelet alloantigen Sit[a] and affects collagen-induced aggregation. Blood 1999;94:4103–11.

121. Santoso S. Kiefel V, Richter IG, et al. A functional platelet fibrinogen receptor with a deletion in the cysteine-rich repeat region of the β3 integrin:the Oe[a] alloantigen in neonatal alloimmune thrombocytopenia. Blood 2002;99: 1205–14.

122. Schuh AC, Watkins NA, Nguyen Q, et al. A tyrosine703serine polymorphism of CD109 defines the Gov platelet alloantigens. Blood 2002;99:1692–8.

123. Jallu V, Meunier M, Brément M, Kaplan C. A new platelet polymorphism Duv[a+], localized within the RGD blinding domain of glycoprotein IIIa, is associated with neonatal thrombocytopenia. Blood 2002;99:4449–56.

124. Stafford P, Garner SF, Rankin A, et al. A single-nucleotide polymorphism in the human *ITBG3* gene is associated with the platelet-specific alloantigen Va[a] (HPA-17bw) involved in fetal maternal alloimmune thrombocytopenia. Transfusion 2008;48:1432–8.

125. Allen DL, Lucas GF, Murphy MF, Ouwehand WH. Platelet and neutrophil antigens. In: Murphy MF, Pamphilon DH, editors. Practical Transfusion Medicine. 3rd ed. 2009. p. 44–59.

126. Porcelijn L, van Beers W, Gratama JW, et al. External quality assessment of platelet serology and human platelet antigen genotyping: a 10-year review. Transfusion 2008;48:1699–706.

127. Veldhuisen B, van der Schoot CE, de Haas M. Blood group genotyping: from patient to high-throughput donor screening. Vox Sanguinis 2009;97: 198–206.

128. Kasirer-Friede A, Kahn ML, Shattil SJ. Platelet integrins and immunoreceptors. Immunological Reviews 2007;218: 247–64.

129. Calvete JJ. Platelet integrin GPIIb/IIIa: structure-function correlations. An update and lessons from other integrins. Proceedings of the Society of Experimental Biology and Medicine 1999;222:29–38.

130. Calvete JJ, Muniz-Diaz E. Localization of an O-glycosylation site in the alpha-subunit of the human platelet integrin GPIIb/IIIa involved in Bak[a] (HPA-3a) alloantigen expression. FEBS Letters 1993;328:30–4.

131. Williamson LM, Hackett G, Rennie J, et al. The natural history of fetomaternal alloimmunization to the platelet-specific antigen HPA-1a (PL[A1], Zw[a]) as determined by antenatal screening. Blood 1998;92:2280–7.

132. Kuijpers RWAM, von dem Borne AEG, Kiefel V, et al. Leucine[33]-proline[33] substitution in human platelet glycoprotein IIIa determines HLA-DR52a

(Dw24) association of the immune response against HPA-1a (Zwa/P1A1) and HPA-1b (Zwb/P1A2). Human Immunology 1992;34:253–356.

133. Wu S, Maslanka K, Gorski J. An integrin polymorphism that defines reactivity with alloantibodies generates an anchor for MHC class II peptide binding: a model for unidirectional alloimmune responses. Journal of Immunology 1997;158:3221–6.

134. Nieuwenhuis HK, Akkerman JW, Houdijk WP, et al. Human blood platelets showing no response to collagen fail to express surface glycoprotein Ia. Nature 1985;318:470–2.

135. Kunicki TJ, Kritzik M, Annis DS, et al. Hereditary variation in platelet integrin $\alpha_2\beta_1$ density is associated with two silent polymorphisms in the α_2 gene coding sequence. Blood 1997;89:1939–43.

136. Lopez JA, Ludwig EH, McCarthy BJ. Polymorphism of human glycoprotein Ib$_\alpha$ results from a variable number of tandem repeats of a 13-amino acid sequence in the mucin-like macroglycopeptide region. Structure/ function implications. Journal of Biological Chemistry 1992;267: 10,055–61.

137. Simsek S, Bleeker PM, van der Schoot CE, et al. Association of a variable number of tandem repeats (VNTR) in glycoprotein Ib$_\alpha$ and HPA-2 alloantigens. Thrombosis and Haemostasis 1994;72: 757–61.

138. Smith JW, Hayward CP, Horsewood P, et al. Characterization and localization of the Gova/b alloantigens to the glycosylphosphatidylinositol-anchored protein CDw109 on human platelets. Blood 1995;86:2807–14.

139. Lin M, Sutherland R, Horsfall W, et al. Cell surface antigen CD109 is a novel member of the α_2 macroglobulin/C3, C4, C5 family of thioester-containing proteins. Blood 2002;99:1683–91.

140. Solomon KR, Sharma P, Chan M, et al. CD109 represents a novel branch of the α2-macroglobulin/complement gene family. Gene 2004;327:171–83.

141. Schuh AC, Watkins NA, Nguyen Q, et al. A tyrosine703serine polymorphism of CD109 define the Gov platelet alloantigens. Blood 2002;99:1692–8.

142. Kaplan C. Les thrombopénies foetales et néonatales allo-immunes: problèmes en suspens. Tranfusion Clinique et Biologique 2005;12:131–4.

143. Arnold DM, Smith JW, Kelton JG. Diagnosis and management of neonatal alloimmune thrombocytopenia. Transfusion Medicine Reviews 2008; 22:255–67.

144. van den Akker ESA, Oepkes D. Fetal and neonatal alloimuune thrombocytopenia. Best Practice and Research Clinical Obstetrics and Gynaecology 2008;22: 3–14.

145. Davoren A, Curtis BR, Aster RH, McFarland JG. Human platelet antigen-specific alloantibodies implicated in 1162 cases of neonatal alloimmune thrombocytopenia. Trnafsusion 2004; 44:1220–5.

146. Berry JE, Murphy CM, Smith GA, et al. Detection of Gov system antibodies by MAIPA reveals an immunogenicity similar to the HPA-5 alloantigens. British Journal of Haematology 2000; 110:735–42.

147. Ramsey G, Salamon DJ. Frequency of P1[A1] in blacks. Transfusion 1986; 26:531–2.

148. Shibata Y, Matsuda I, Miyaji T, et al. Yuk[a], a new platelet antigen involved in two cases of neonatal alloimmune thrombocytopenia. Vox Sanguinis 1986; 50:177–80.

149. Kumpel BM, Sibley K, Jackson DJ, et al. Ultrastructural localization of glycoprotein IIIa (GIIIa, β3 integrin) on placental syncytiotrophoblast microvilli: implications for platelet alloimmunization during pregnancy. Transfusion 2008;48:2077–86.

150. Proulx C, Filion M, Goldman M, et al. Analysis of immunoglobulin class, IgG subclass and titre of HPA-1a antibodies in alloimmunized mothers giving birth to babies with or without neonatal alloimmune thrombocytopenia. British Journal of Haematology 1994;87: 813–7.

151. McMillan R, Longmire RL, Tavassoli M, et al. In vitro platelet phagocytosis by splenic leukocytes in idiopathic thrombocytopenic purpura. New England Journal of Medicine 1974;290: 249–51.

152. Clarkson SB, Bussel JB, Kimberley RP, et al. Treatment of refractory immune thrombocytopenic purpura with an anti-Fcγ-receptor antibody. New England Journal of Medicine 1986;314:1236–9.

153. Bussel JB, Zabusky MR, Berkowitz RL, et al. Fetal alloimmune thrombocytopenia. New England Journal of Medicine 1997;337:22–6.

154. Burrows RF, Caco CC, Kelton JG. Neonatal alloimmune thrombocytopenia: spontaneous in utero intracranial hemorrhage. American Journal of Hematology 1988;28:98–102.

155. Ory PA, Clark MR, Kwoh EE, et al. Sequences of complementary DNAs that encode the NA1 and NA2 forms of Fc receptor III on human neutrophils. Journal of Clinical Investigation 1989;84:1688–91.

156. Bux J, Stein E-L, Bierling P, et al. Characterization of a new alloantigen (SH) on the human neutrophil Fcγ receptor IIIb. Blood 1997;89:1027–34.

157. Stroncek DF, Shankar RA, Plachta LB, et al. Polyclonal antibodies against the NB1-bearing 58- to 64-kDa glycoprotein of human neutrophils do not identify an

NB2-bearing molecule. Transfusion 1993;33:399–404.

158. Greinacher A, Wesche J, Hammer E, et al. Characterization of the human neutrophil alloantigen-3a. Nature Medicine 2010;16:45-8.

159. Curtis BR, Cox NJ, Sullivan MJ, et al. The neutrophil alloantigen HNA-3a (5b) is located on choline transporter-like protein 2 and appears to be encoded by an R>Q154 amino acid substitution. Blood 2010;115:2073-76.

160. Simsek S, van der Schoot CE, Daams M, et al. Molecular characterization of antigenic polymorphisms (Ond^a and Marta) of the beta 2 family recognized by human leukocyte alloantisera. Blood 1996;88:1350–8.

161. Bux J. Human neutrophil alloantigens. Vox Sanguinis 2008;94:277–85.

162. Bux J. Nomenclature of granulocyte alloantigens. Transfusion 1999;39:662–3.

163. van de Winkel JGJ, Capel PJA. Human IgG Fc receptor heterogeneity: molecular aspects and clinical implications. Immunology Today 1993;14:215–21.

164. Koene HR, Kleijer M, Roos D, et al. FcγRIIIB genes in NA(1+,2+)SH(+) individuals. Blood 1998;91:673–9.

165. Metcalfe P, Waters AH. Location of the granulocyte-specific antigen LAN on the Fc-receptor III. Transfusion Medicine 1993;2:283–7.

166. Bux J, Hartmann C, Mueller-Eckhardt C. Alloimmune neonatal neutropenia resulting from immunization to a high frequency antigen on the granulocyte Fcγ receptor III. Transfusion 1994;34: 608–11.

167. de Haas M, Kleijer M, van Zwieten R, et al. Neutrophil FcγRIII deficiency, nature and clinical consequences: a study of 21 individuals from 14 families. Blood 1995;86:2403–13.

168. Stroncek DF, Skubitz KM, McCullough JJ. Biochemical characterization of the neutrophil-specific antigen NB1. Blood 1990;75:744–55.

169. Kissel K, Scheffler S, Kerowgan M, Bux J. Molecular basis of NB1 (HNA-2a, CD177) deficiency. Blood 2002;99: 4231–3.

170. Bux J, Jung D, Kauth T, et al. Serological and clinical aspects of granulocyte antibodies leading to alloimmune neonatal alloimmune neutropenia. Transfusion Medicine 1992;2:143–9.

171. Lalezari P, Jiang AF, Yegen L, et al. Chronic autoimmune neutropenia due to anti-NA2 antibody. New England Journal of Medicine 1975;293:744–7.

172. Bux J, Behrens G, Jaeger G, et al. Diagnosis and clinical course of autoimmune neutropenia in infancy: analysis of 240 cases. Blood 1998;91: 181–6.

173. Lyall EGH, Lucas GF, Eden OB. Autoimmune neutropenia of infancy. Journal of Clinical Pathology 1992;45: 431–4.

174. Popovsky MA, Moore SB. Diagnostic and pathogenic considerations in transfusion-related lung injury. Transfusion 1985;25:573–7.

175. Kleinman S, Caulfield T, Chan P, et al. Toward an understanding of transfusion-related lung injury: statement of a consensus panel. Transfusion 2004;44: 1774–89.

176. Bux J. Transfusion-related lung injury (TRALI): a serious adverse event of blood transfusion. Vox Sanguinis 2005;89:1–10.

177. Bux J, Sachs UJH. The pathogenesis of transfusion-related lung injury (TRALI). British Journal of Haematology 2007; 136:788–99.

178. Kopko PM, Marshall CS, MacKenzie MR, et al. Transfusion-related lung injury. Report of a clinical look-back investigation. Journal of the American Medical Association 2002;15:1968–71.

179. Muniz M, Sheldon S, Schuller RM, et al. Patient-specific transfusion-related lung injury. Vox Sanguinis 2008;94:70–3.

CHAPTER 38

Transfusion medicine for pathologists

J McCullough

Chapter contents

©2011 Elsevier Ltd
DOI: 10.1016/B978-0-7020-3147-2.00038-9

Introduction

The discipline of blood transfusion and transfusion medicine at the beginning of the 21st century involves a complex, structured, standardized and regulated production process along with sophisticated hemotherapy. The laboratory techniques used are far different from those of Landsteiner who discovered the ABO blood group system by observing clumps of red cells or hemolysis when the cells from some of his laboratory workers were mixed with the serum from others. Other chapters in this book beautifully describe current extensive knowledge of the structure and function of blood groups[1] and immune hemolytic anemias.[2] In developed countries, virtually all whole blood is collected from unpaid volunteer donors by regional, community-based or individual, hospital-based blood banks. The whole blood is separated into its components shortly following donation; thus each component is available for use for the most appropriate specific clinical condition. This approach, called blood component therapy, places responsibility on the clinician to identify the specific blood deficit of the patient and to choose a specific blood component. In this chapter, we will describe the approaches used to obtain blood, the medical uses of blood components and the complications of transfusion.

Blood supply systems throughout the world

Whole blood

Approximately 75 million units of whole blood are collected worldwide, but this almost certainly does not meet worldwide needs. The organizations and systems that collect and provide blood vary greatly throughout the world. Most developed countries, with the exception of the United States, have some form of a national blood program.[3] The program may be operated by that country's Red Cross or by its government. The extent to which this program is structured, the mechanisms of funding, and the effectiveness of the national blood program in meeting the total blood needs for that country also vary greatly throughout the world. In many developing countries the blood supply may be inadequate to meet the needs, and the blood that is available has a high likelihood of transmitting infectious disease.[4]

The US blood system is operated by multiple organizations.[5] Approximately 15 million units of whole blood are collected each year primarily in regional or community blood centers.[6] Hospitals collect less than 10% of the US blood supply. The American Red Cross is the largest blood collecting organization in the US, accounting for about 45% of the blood supply. Other regional or community blood centers are non-profit organizations governed by local volunteer boards of directors.

It is policy of the International Society for Blood Transfusion and the World Health Organization that blood should be donated voluntarily. The reason for advocating volunteerism in blood donation is not only based on the moral principle of not selling body parts or tissues but also because blood from paid donors has a much higher risk of disease transmission.[7] When a financial payment is involved, there is an incentive for the potential donor to be dishonest about his or her medical history. Despite the increased sophistication of laboratory testing of donated blood, some infectious units of blood will not be detected by present tests.[8] Thus, if the donor is dishonest about his or her medical history, there is more likelihood that the unit may be infectious.

In developed countries, the collection, processing, testing and preparation of blood components is subject to some form of regulation. Although blood is a biological, and thus different from a pharmaceutical, some form of pharmaceutical-type regulation is applied.[5] Thus, there are requirements for donor eligibility, laboratory testing of donated blood, blood preservation and the minimum content of various blood components. Usually these requirements define procedures, records, staff proficiency, specific testing and donor medical requirements that blood banks must follow. In the US, additional standards have been promulgated by the American Association of Blood Banks – a voluntary organization that accredits blood banks as a way of assuring high quality and providing continued education for blood bank professionals.[9,10]

Blood donor recruitment

In developed countries, whether or not there is a national blood program, blood is collected from volunteer donors. The costs that are incurred in collection, testing, production and distribution of blood components are covered in a variety of ways depending on the method of financing healthcare in each country. In some countries, these costs are part of the national health service budget and the funds may be provided to hospitals to purchase blood from the national blood program or the Red Cross. In other countries, the funds may be provided directly to the national blood program or the Red Cross and the blood is then supplied without charge to the hospitals. In many parts of the world, especially in areas without a structured blood system and where individual hospitals must attempt to meet their own blood requirements, patients and their families may be required to obtain a certain number of donors or units of blood before procedures involving blood loss will be undertaken. This requirement may even lead to families paying individuals to donate blood on their behalf. The payment then creates the difficulties of a paid-donor system described earlier.

In developed countries, most people will require a blood transfusion at some time in their lives. The blood supply comes from a small group of dedicated donors. In the US, blood donors differ from the general population in that they are more likely to be male, aged 30–50, more highly educated, employed and Caucasian.[11] Although there have been some studies of the social psychology and motivation of blood donors,[12] the process is not well understood and is likely to vary for different ethnic or cultural groups or countries.[12] A recent developing concern is that with the increasingly stringent donor requirements resulting from the AIDS epidemic, a larger portion of the population is being excluded as potential donors. In addition, as the population in many developed countries ages, there is a decreasing portion of the population available for blood donation. In the US, only about a third of the population meets all the donor requirements.[13]

Plasma

A large number of therapeutic products such as albumin, intramuscular and intravenous immune globulin, and coagulation factor concentrates are prepared from plasma by using large-scale manufacturing processes. The plasma to serve as raw material may be obtained from individual units of whole blood or by plasmapheresis. Worldwide, the demand for these plasma derivatives exceeds that provided from plasma obtained from whole blood donations. Thus, a large amount of the plasma that serves as raw material for the production of derivatives is obtained by plasmapheresis. Plasmapheresis donation requires more time than whole blood donation, and because red cells are not removed from the donor, the donor can donate plasma more frequently than whole blood; in some countries, plasmapheresis donors are paid.

In the US, the plasmapheresis collection and plasma fractionation system is separate from the whole blood collection system. This plasma system is operated by large commercial companies that pay donors and produce plasma derivatives for profit. Thus, it differs in many ways from the whole blood collection system which relies on volunteer donors and is operated by non-profit organizations. In most other developed countries, the plasma system is operated as a not-for-profit system, often as part of the regular, whole blood collection system. Some countries operate their own plasma fractionation plant while others contract with plants operated in other countries. Plasma fractionation involves the processing of up to 10 000 liters of plasma, which may be pooled from as many as 50 000 donors. Thus, the potential for infectivity is substantial. Since the AIDS epidemic, the plasma fractionation industry has introduced pathogen inactivation systems and today most, if not all, plasma derivatives are free of transmission of most viral diseases. Presently many coagulation factor concentrates are manufactured using recombinant DNA technology and thus are free of disease transmission.

The AIDS epidemic has had a major impact on blood banking and transfusion medicine. Although blood bank professionals believe they acted properly, with reasonable speed, and with the public's interest in mind to balance blood safety and blood availability, in many countries the public was not satisfied with this response. The plasma industry was subjected to even more severe criticism, particularly from the hemophilia community. Because plasma derivatives, including coagulation factor concentrates, are prepared from large pools of plasma containing plasma from many donors, a large proportion of these derivatives was contaminated with HIV and many hemophiliacs were infected. Although the plasma industry moved expeditiously to introduce pathogen inactivation steps into the manufacturing process, there was a widely held belief that these companies should have implemented these steps sooner. In addition, in some countries, criminal actions were taken successfully against leaders of the blood programs for failure to take certain actions that might have helped to mitigate the impact of the AIDS epidemic on transfusion recipients. As a result of the AIDS epidemic, there has been a substantial increase in the eligibility requirements for blood donors and increase in the number and specificity of questions about donor's medical history and activities that might place them at risk of being infected with transfusion-transmitted diseases. In addition, the number of tests performed on donated blood has increased and there has also been a fundamental shift in the regulatory philosophy. In most developed countries, the expectation developed that blood donor screening, collection, processing and component production would be carried out much like a pharmaceutical manufacturing process.[5,10] In addition, the use of blood products also changed dramatically. Physicians became much more conservative in prescribing blood and more extensive use of guidelines and monitoring of transfusions has occurred.

Whole blood

Medical history

Selection of blood donors involves ensuring the safety of the donor and obtaining a blood component that is high in quality and has the least possible chance of transmitting disease. This is accomplished by using volunteer blood donors, questioning donors about their general health and medical history, carrying out a brief physical examination of each donor, and laboratory testing the donated blood. The questions used in each country will differ to reflect the kinds of disease exposure donors are most likely to encounter. The general principles will apply, however: questions intended to protect the donor from risks of blood donation and questions (primarily related to infectious diseases) intended to protect the recipient by identifying and excluding donors whose blood might be infectious.

Examples of questions in the medical history designed to protect the donor include whether the donor is under the care of a physician or has a history of cardiovascular or lung disease, seizures, present or recent pregnancy, recent donation of blood or plasma, recent major illness or surgery, unexplained weight loss, unusual bleeding, or is taking medications. Questions about medications help to identify any diseases or illnesses that might make blood donation a risk for the donor.

Most of the questions designed to protect the recipient deal with exposure to infectious diseases. Examples of these questions are the occurrence of or exposure to hepatitis or other liver disease, HIV (or symptoms of AIDS), Chagas disease or babesiosis; use of injected drugs; receipt of growth hormone, coagulation factor concentrates, blood transfusion, recent immunizations, tattoo, acupuncture, ear piercing, or an organ or tissue transplant; travel to areas endemic for malaria; presence of a major illness or surgery; or previous notice of a positive test for a transmissible disease. Examples of questions related to HIV risk behavior include whether the potential donor has had sex with anyone with AIDS, has given or received money or drugs for sex, (for males) has had sex with another male, (for females) has had sex with a male who has had sex with another male.

Physical and laboratory examination of the blood donor

The donor's general appearance is assessed for any signs of illness or the influence of drugs or alcohol. The skin is examined for signs of intravenous drug abuse, lesions suggestive of Kaposi's sarcoma, and local lesions that might make it difficult to decontaminate the skin and thus lead to contamination of the blood unit during venipuncture. Physical examination of the potential donor usually includes the temperature, pulse, blood pressure, weight and blood hemoglobin concentration. The specific requirements for these measures are established by the regulatory agency of each country.

Collection of whole blood

Blood is collected into plastic bags, each of which is sterile and can be used only once. Often combinations of bags are used so that whole blood can be separated into its components in a closed system, thus minimizing the chance of bacterial contamination while making storage of the components for days or weeks possible. The venipuncture site is an area free of skin lesions; it is scrubbed with a soap solution followed by an iodine solution. Because bacterial contamination of blood can be a serious or even fatal complication of transfusion,[14,15] it is important to minimize bacterial contamination by selecting a good venipuncture site and decontaminating it properly.

Venipuncture and blood collection

The blood must flow freely and be mixed with anticoagulant frequently as the blood fills the container to avoid the development of small clots. The actual time for phlebotomy and bleeding is usually about 7 minutes and almost always less than 10 minutes. In much of the world it has been customary to collect 450 ml of blood, although some blood banks are now collecting 500 ml and in some parts of the world less than 450 ml is collected routinely. The anticoagulant is composed of citrate, phosphate and dextrose (CPD) in a ratio of approximately 1 : 15 with whole blood. The amount of blood withdrawn must be within prescribed limits in order to maintain the proper ratio with the anticoagulant; otherwise the blood cells may be damaged and/or anticoagulation may not be satisfactory. The red cells can be stored in the citrate anticoagulant; although in many countries, the anticoagulated plasma is removed and the red cells are resuspended in a solution that allows extended red cell storage.

Adverse reactions to blood donation

Donors have a reaction following approximately 4% of blood donations, but serious reactions are rare. Reactions are more likely to occur in younger, first-time single donors who have a higher pre-donation heart rate and lower diastolic blood pressure.[16,17] The most common reactions include mild weakness, cool skin, diaphoresis, lightheadedness and/or nausea. More extensive reactions involve dizziness, pallor, hypertension, nausea and vomiting, bradycardia and/or hyperventilation which sometimes lead to twitching or muscle spasms. Bradycardia indicates a vasovagal reaction rather than hypotensive or cardiovascular shock, where tachycardia would be expected. Other complications of blood donation include hematoma at the venipuncture site and injury to the bracheal nerve and resulting pain and/or paresthesia due to needle puncture of the nerve or compression from a hematoma.[18–20] Rare but severe donor reactions

involve loss of consciousness, convulsions, serious cardiac difficulties and/or involuntary passage of urine or stool.[16,21]

Donors are advised to drink extra fluids to replace lost blood volume and minimize the chance of fainting and to avoid strenuous exercise for the remainder of the day of donation in order to minimize the possibility that a hematoma will develop at the venipuncture site. Because some donors are subject to lightheadedness or even fainting if they change position quickly, donors in an occupation where fainting would be hazardous to themselves or others are usually advised not to return to work for the remainder of the day.

Special blood donations

Most blood is collected for placement in a 'bank' to provide for the general community and thus may be used by any patient. However, some blood donations are made intentionally to be used by a specific patient. Examples of these include autologous donation, directed donation and patient-specific donation. In some of these situations the usual regulations for blood donation may not apply.

Autologous blood donation

Autologous blood donation can be done in several ways: preoperative donation, acute normovolemic hemodilution, also known as perioperative hemodilution, intraoperative salvage, and/or postoperative salvage.

In the early 1990s, there was great excitement about the potential of autologous blood and it was estimated that in the US autologous blood could account for 20% of all blood used.[22] This has not occurred because much of the autologous blood was collected from patients undergoing procedures with little likelihood of needing blood, surgeons became more skilled at minimizing blood loss, and anesthesiologists became more skilled at managing fluid administration and maintaining patients with lower hemoglobin levels. In 2004, only 3% of donation in the US was autologous.[6]

Preoperative donation. If an elective procedure is scheduled and there is a high likelihood of blood transfusion, the patient can donate blood in advance for his/her own use. Since the donor is actually a patient, they usually do not meet the regulatory requirements for normal blood donation. Thus, the blood is usually not suitable for use by someone else if it is not needed by the original donor/patient. Thus, it is important that autologous blood be collected only for procedures in which there is substantial likelihood that it will be used. Without this type of planning, there is a very high rate of wastage of autologous blood (estimated at 40.4% in the US in 2004).[6] This amount of waste also means that the costs of autologous blood are quite high.[23]

Although there are some contraindications for preoperative autologous blood donation such as bacteremia, symptomatic angina, recent seizures and symptomatic valvular heart lesions, the usual donor requirements do not apply and the final decision whether to withdraw blood from an autologous donor rests with the medical director of the blood bank. This decision may necessitate consultation between the donor's/patient's physician and the blood bank physician.

There are no age or weight restrictions for autologous donation. Pregnant women may donate, but donation is not recommended routinely because these patients rarely require transfusion. The autologous donor's hemoglobin may be lower than that required for routine donors and autologous donors may donate several times within a few weeks prior to the planned surgery. However, usually it is only possible to obtain 2–4 units of blood before the hemoglobin falls to unacceptably low levels.

In most countries, autologous blood must be typed for ABO and D antigen, and at least the first unit must be tested for transmissible diseases. If any of the transmissible disease tests are positive, it may be necessary to label the unit(s) as biohazard in order to alert healthcare personnel to the hazard presented by the potentially infectious blood.

With the discovery of erythropoietin, there was great hope that it could be given to autologous blood donors to increase the number of units they could donate and substantially reduce the use of the general blood supply. Unfortunately this has not occurred because erythropoietin does not result in a meaningful increase in autologous blood units obtained from each patient.

Perioperative hemodilution (acute normovolemic hemodilution).[24] Perioperative hemodilution is carried out in the operating room usually after the patient has undergone general anesthesia. One to two units of whole blood are collected and replaced with an electrolyte solution at three times the volume of blood collected. The patient's hematocrit is maintained at least at 30%. This procedure does not pose unusual risks to patients who are stable and undergoing elective surgery. If it is carried out prior to surgical procedures in which substantial expected blood loss is expected, the 2 units of freshly collected blood are kept in the operating room and can be transfused to the patient during surgery. Theoretical advantages of perioperative hemodilution, in addition to having the blood available, are that blood loss during surgery occurs at a lower hematocrit and thus there is less red cell loss, that surgery is carried out at lower hematocrit which improves blood viscosity and possibly provides better tissue oxygenation, and that the blood that is available for transfusion is fresh. Perioperative hemodilution must be carried out by a committed, knowledgeable anesthesia staff and it appears to have limited but definite value.

Intraoperative blood salvage. In elective, urgent or trauma surgery when substantial blood loss is expected, some of the shed blood can be recovered and returned to the patient. Several devices that combine suction, centrifugation and washing are available for this purpose. Because of the cost of operating these devices, intraoperative blood salvage is usually reserved for situations in which the blood loss is expected to exceed 1000 ml. The device suctions or aspirates blood from the operative site. The collected blood is centrifuged, and, in some cases, a wash solution is added. After processing, the blood is pumped out of the device into a plastic bag so it can be used for transfusion. Contraindications to intraoperative blood salvage are bacterial contamination of the operative site and surgery for malignancy. In both of these situations, transfusion of blood containing bacteria or malignant cells would be undesirable. Examples of situations in which intraoperative blood salvage is used most commonly are vascular surgery, cardiovascular surgery and some major orthopedics procedures.

Postoperative blood salvage. In some situations such as cardiovascular or orthopedic surgery, if there is extensive postoperative bleeding or draining from the surgical site, devices can be used to collect this drainage so that the shed blood can be used for transfusion. This use of postoperative blood salvage has not gained widespread acceptance because the volume of red cells that can be obtained is usually small; if substantial surgical site drainage is occurring, this often indicates a surgical problem that requires intervention. The shed blood usually contains activated coagulation factors, fibrin strands, cellular aggregates and other debris which make transfusion of this material undesirable.

Directed donor blood

Directed donors are friends or relatives who wish to give blood for a specific patient. Usually this is done because the patient hopes those donors will be 'safer' than regular blood donors. In some parts of the world, however, directed donation is a necessity because the general blood supply is not adequate. In the US, data do not indicate that directed donors have a lower incidence of transmissible disease markers,[25] and thus there is no factual rationale for these donations. Directed donors must meet all of the regulatory requirements for routine blood donation. Their blood becomes part of the community's general blood supply if it is not used for the originally intended patient.

Therapeutic bleeding

Blood may be collected as part of the therapy for diseases such as polycythemia vera or hemochromatosis. This blood is not usually used for transfusion because the donors do not meet the FDA requirements. As the genetic basis for hemochromatosis has become known, efforts have begun to gain approval for the use of blood obtained from patients with hemochromatosis.[26,27] Limited experience suggests that a donor program could be effective, but it is not likely that blood from hemochromatosis patients would have a substantial impact on the nation's blood supply.[28]

Preparation, storage, and characteristics of blood components

In developed countries, almost all blood collected is separated into red cells, platelets and plasma. Each component is stored under conditions optimum for that component so that valuable platelets and coagulation factors are recovered and maintained. Plastic bag systems are used for this blood separation, and thus bacterial contamination is avoided. In many parts of the world, blood is not separated into components but is stored as whole blood.

Red blood cells

If whole blood is centrifuged and most of the platelets and plasma are removed, the resulting packed red cells or red cell concentrate is resuspended in a solution to optimize red cell preservation and allow storage of red cells for 42 days at 1–6°C. During the 42 days of storage, there is some loss of viability, adenosine triphosphate, membrane lipid and

2.3-DPG (causing increased affinity of hemoglobin for oxygen), reduced transmembrane transport of sodium and potassium, and accumulation of metabolites. Each unit of red cells has a volume of approximately 300 ml and contains about 200 ml of red cells. Red cells are used to provide oxygen-carrying capacity in anemic patients. The number of units given depends on the degree of anemia or blood loss.

Fresh frozen plasma

In the US, when the unit of whole blood is centrifuged, platelet-rich plasma results. The platelet-rich plasma is then centrifuged and the plasma and platelets are separated, resulting in a unit of plasma and a platelet concentrate. If this plasma is placed at −18°C or colder within 8 hours of collection it is called fresh frozen plasma. Fresh frozen plasma can be stored for up to 1 year at −18°C or colder. The unit of fresh frozen plasma has a volume of approximately 185 ml and contains all the constituents of citrated normal plasma such as the coagulation factors, the components of the complement and fibrinolytic systems, and the plasma proteins that maintain osmotic pressure and modulate immunity.

For transfusion, fresh frozen plasma is thawed in a 37°C water bath for approximately 30 minutes. Microwave ovens usually are not used to thaw fresh frozen plasma because they create hot spots that damage the plasma proteins. Thawed plasma should be transfused as soon as possible, but at the latest within 24 hours. If not used by then, it can be relabeled as thawed plasma and stored for an additional 4 days, although it will have reduced levels of factors V and VIII.

Plasma and source plasma

Plasma can also be removed from whole blood up to 24 hours after collection and stored at −18°C or less and stored for up to 1 year. This 24 hour frozen plasma has reduced levels of factor VIII. Source plasma is collected by plasmapheresis and is intended to serve as the raw material for further manufacture into blood derivatives.

Cryoprecipitate

When previously frozen plasma is thawed at 1–6°C, an insoluble material called cryoprecipitate remains after the liquid plasma is removed. Each bag of cryoprecipitate contains about 100 units of factor VIII and 200 mg of fibrinogen and has a volume of about 10 ml. It can be stored for up to 1 year at −18°C or lower. Cryoprecipitate is thawed in a 37°C water bath, and cryoprecipitate from multiple bags is usually pooled into a single container that is dispensed by the blood bank. Cryoprecipitate is usually given in the same ABO type as the recipient. If there is a shortage, small amounts of ABO-incompatible cryoprecipitate can be given. There is usually little risk of hemolysis from small volumes of ABO-incompatible plasma because the volume of plasma from any individual donor who might have a high-titer antibody is only 10 ml. Because cryoprecipitate contains few red cells, it can be given without regard to Rh type.

Cryoprecipitate was developed originally as a source of factor VIII and was the first concentrated form of this coagulation factor available to treat hemophilia. With the development of coagulation factor concentrates that have undergone viral inactivation, the major use of cryoprecipitate currently is as a source of fibrinogen or as fibrin glue.[29]

Whole blood-derived platelet concentrates – platelet-rich plasma method

Platelets can be produced from units of whole blood or by plateletpheresis. In the US, when platelets are prepared from whole blood, the unit of whole blood is maintained at room temperature and centrifuged, and the platelet-rich plasma is passed into a satellite bag. The platelet-rich plasma is centrifuged again, and the platelet-poor plasma is passed into another satellite bag leaving the platelet concentrate which has a volume of proximately 50 ml. At least 75% of random donor-platelet concentrates contain at least 5.5×10^{10} platelets. Four to six units of random-donor platelets are pooled to provide a therapeutic dose for transfusion. These whole blood-derived platelet concentrates may then be stored for up to 5 days at room temperature (20–24°C). The variables known to be important in platelet preservation are: temperature, method of agitation, volume of suspending plasma and type of storage container. At the end of the storage period, the intravascular recovery and half-life of the stored platelets are approximately 51% and 3.1 days.[30]

Whole blood-derived platelet concentrates – buffy coat method

In some countries, the whole blood is centrifuged and the buffy coat containing leukocytes and platelets is removed.[31] Buffy coats from several units are pooled, the pooled buffy coats are centrifuged, and the platelets are separated from the leukocytes to provide a platelet concentrate. This method provides a therapeutic dose of platelets and no further pooling is necessary. It is thought that this method of preparation provides better platelet function,[31] although it has not been adopted in the US.

Collection and production of blood components by apheresis

Blood components can also be prepared by apheresis.[32] Whole blood is pumped out of one arm, anticoagulant is added, and the blood is passed through an instrument in which it is centrifuged and separated into red cells, plasma, and a leukocyte/platelet fraction. One of the components is removed and the remainder of the blood is returned via the other arm. This process enables a larger number of cells to be obtained than would be available in one unit of whole blood. Several semi-automated instruments are available for the collection of platelets, granulocytes, peripheral blood stem cells, mononuclear cells, plasma or red cells.[32] Some newer instruments allow collection of different combinations of components, such as plasma and platelets.

Platelet concentrates

Plateletpheresis usually takes about 90 minutes during which about 4000–5000 liters of the donor's blood are processed through the blood cell separator. These platelet concentrates have a volume of about 200 ml and contain about 3.5×10^{11} platelets and less than 0.5 ml of red cells. This provides a therapeutic dose of platelets for transfusion. Plateletpheresis has been used increasingly so that in the US about 80% of platelets are produced by plateletpheresis,[6] but plateletpheresis is much less common in many other countries.

Granulocyte concentrates

Because of the small number of circulating granulocytes, it is not practical to prepare granulocyte concentrates from whole blood donations. Instead, leukapheresis is used to process 6.5–8.0 ml of donor blood during about three hours[32] and obtain a granulocyte concentrate. Hydroxyethyl starch is added to the blood cell separator flow system to sediment the red cells and improve the separation of granulocytes from other blood components. To increase the donor's peripheral blood granulocyte count, and thus increase the yield of granulocytes, dexamethasone and recently, granulocyte colony-stimulating factor (G-CSF) has been administered to granulocyte donors.[33]

Mononuclear cell concentrates

Mononuclear cell collection is also done by cytapheresis. This produces a component containing approximately 1×10^{10} mononuclear cells, which are a mixture of lymphocytes and monocytes. These mononuclear cell concentrates may be used for direct transfusion such as in adoptive immunotherapy to prevent relapse of CML following stem cell transplantation or as the starting material for further processing as part of gene therapy or adoptive immunotherapy.

Plasma

Plasmapheresis can be done using sets of multiple attached bags, but this is time-consuming, cumbersome and involves disconnecting the blood bags from the donor to centrifuge and separate the plasma from the red cells. This creates the chance of returning the blood to the wrong donor. Semiautomated instruments are used that require less operator involvement than the bag systems, while producing up to 750 ml of plasma in about 30 minutes depending on the size of the donor. Because few red cells are removed, the procedure can be repeated frequently so that a donor could provide large amounts of plasma.

Peripheral blood stem cells

Hematopoietic stem cells present in the peripheral blood that are capable of providing complete hematopoietic reconstitution in humans stimulated the development of methods to collect peripheral blood stem cells by cytapheresis.[33,34] The number of peripheral blood stem cells (PBSCs) circulating under usual conditions is low but following chemotherapy there is a rebound and a large number of PBSCs can be obtained by apheresis. G-CSF is also given to patients or normal donors to increase the number of circulating PBSCs and provide an adequate dose of cells for successful reconstitution of hematopoiesis.[35,36] Usually approximately $1 \times$ 10^{10} mononuclear cells and 2–6×10^7 CD34+ cells are obtained after processing up to 15 l of the donor's blood during 4–5 hours. The concentrate has a volume of about 200 ml.

Selection of apheresis donors

The criteria and requirements for donors of whole blood apply to the selection of donors for apheresis;[37] however, there are some additional requirements. These may vary in different countries, but they generally define the volume of blood that can be extracorporeal during apheresis, the volume of red cells or plasma that can be removed in a given time, the frequency of donation, and any laboratory tests in addition to those performed for whole blood donation. The laboratory testing of donors for transmissible diseases is the same as that for whole blood donation. Thus, the likelihood of disease transmission from apheresis components is the same as that from components prepared from whole blood.

Reactions in apheresis donors

In general, the types of adverse reactions that occur following cytapheresis are similar to those following whole blood donation. However, some side-effects or reactions unique to cytapheresis occur.[32] These include paresthesias due to the infusion of the citrate used to anticoagulate the donor's blood while it is in the cell separator; myalgia, arthralgia, headache, or flu-like symptoms due to G-CSF in granulocyte donors;[32,37] or headache and/or hypertension from blood volume expansion due to the sedimenting agent hydroxyethyl starch used in the cell separator to improve the granulocyte yield.

Laboratory testing of donated blood

Blood is tested for the ABO and Rh type, and red cell antibody screening (detection) is performed. Tests for cytomegalovirus, HLA antibodies or rare red cell antigens may be done depending on the needs of the blood bank and the patients it serves. Because of the large amount of laboratory and donor data, today's blood center uses pharmaceutical-type manufacturing processes and complex computer and quality control systems in order to ensure accuracy and safety.[5,9,10]

Compatibility testing (crossmatching)

Compatibility testing includes all the steps and procedures involved in providing blood cells that will have an acceptable *in vivo* survival. The crossmatch is only one part of compatibility testing. Other steps in compatibility testing include ABO Rh typing of donor red cells, acquiring a proper sample from the patient, ABO Rh typing of the patient, testing the patient's serum for red cell antibodies, selecting the proper blood component, carrying out the crossmatch, labeling the component with the identity of the recipient and release of the unit from the blood bank. The antibody detection test has become increasingly important during the last few years as it has been established that for patients with no antibodies detectable in this test, the crossmatch can be abbreviated to one that will detect ABO incompatibility. This can be done with a simple saline suspension of red cells and an incubation of approximately 5 minutes at room temperature. Thus, the approach that has developed involves a careful, thorough, sensitive antibody detection test and then the exact method used for the crossmatch depends on the results of the antibody detection test. If no antibodies are found, the simple rapid test to detect ABO incompatibility is used for the crossmatch.[38-40] If antibodies are detected, then the crossmatch uses the longer, more complex methodology used in the antibody detection test.

In the antibody detection test, the patient's serum is reacted with blood cells specially selected from two normal individuals whose cells contain antigens reactive with all of the common clinically significant antibodies. The conditions of this test usually involve incubation of the patient's serum and test red cells suspended either in saline or albumin followed by the anti-human globulin test. Other methods to enhance antibody detection that might be used include treating the red cells with enzymes, changing the serum cell ratio, suspending red cells in low ionic strength solution or the use of chemicals such as polybrene to enhance agglutination.[41] Gel and solid phase test systems are becoming more widely used.

Transfusion therapy

Transfusion of components containing red blood cells

Clinical indications. Red cells are transfused to improve oxygen-carrying capacity or for restoration of blood volume following blood loss. There is no specific hemoglobin value above which patients have a better outcome, feel better, or have improved wound healing. Thus, in making a decision to transfuse a patient to improve oxygen capacity, the patient's overall condition must be considered. For instance, when anemia has developed over a long period of time, the patient adjusts to lower hemoglobin levels and may not require transfusion despite very low hemoglobin levels. Most studies that deal with the physiology of blood loss have been done in normal animals, essentially healthy humans, or military casualties, who are usually young males. Thus, the indications for transfusion in patients with cardiac disease, coronary atherosclerosis or other vascular insufficiency are not established.

In the past, some anesthesiologists and surgeons transfused patients to achieve a hemoglobin level of 10 g/dl prior to surgery. However, there is no scientific basis, nor are there clinical data, to support this practice. Many patients would not be at risk if a transfusion was withheld until the hemoglobin level was approximately 7 g/dl.[42,43]

Transfusion for restoration of blood volume should not be initiated too rapidly because it is clear that in most 'normal' patients the loss of approximately 1000 ml of blood can be replaced by colloid or crystalloid solutions alone. The hemoglobin level may not be of value in this situation because if blood loss has been acute, the patient may have a normal or nearly normal hemoglobin level until equilibration between the intravascular and extravascular space occurs.

Whole blood. Whole blood is rarely used in the developed countries. Instead, it is converted into components to take advantage of the need for plasma and platelets. Acute blood loss is managed by transfusion of red cells and crystalloid or colloid solutions. In developing countries, most transfusions may be of whole blood since facilities for preparation of blood components are often not available.

Red blood cells. Patients with severe anemia usually do not need intravascular volume replacement and thus red cells are the component of choice. In patients with acute massive hemorrhage, who may need both intravascular volume and red cell replacement, crystalloid or colloid solutions, not human plasma, are used with red cells. Crystalloid and colloid solutions have few adverse effects and their use allows the plasma from the original unit of whole blood to be used for the production of coagulation factor concentrate.

Leukocyte reduced red cells. Leukoreduced red cells are being used increasingly throughout the world. In the past, these red cells were used primarily to prevent febrile non-hemolytic transfusion reactions in patients who received multiple transfusions. Leukocyte-reduced red cells reduce the likelihood of HLA alloimmunization and platelet refractoriness[44,45] and may have an immune modulating effect leading to decreased postoperative infection and decreased cancer reoccurrence.[46-48] The availability of filters that remove more than 99% of the leukocytes have made this the method used to prepare leukocyte-depleted red cells.

Washed red cells. When red cells are washed and resuspended in an electrolyte solution, most of the plasma, platelets and leukocytes have been removed. Thus, washed red cells are indicated for patients who have severe reactions caused by plasma. For instance, patients with IgA deficiency can have severe, often fatal, anaphylactic reactions when exposed to plasma containing IgA. Although washed red cells have been used to prevent febrile reactions due to transfused leukocytes, the availability of filters for leukocyte removal has eliminated the use of washed red cells for this purpose.

Frozen deglycerolized red blood cells. Red cells can be protected from injury during freezing by the addition of glycerol. They can then be stored for 20 years or more.[50] Because most of the plasma, platelets and leukocytes have been removed and after thawing and washing these red cells are suspended in an electrolyte solution, they can be used in a similar way to washed red cells. However, the main advantage of frozen deglycerolized red cells is that they can be stored for years, thus allowing development of a depot of red cells of rare types or of autologous red cells. Frozen deglycerolized red cells do not have a reduced likelihood of disease transmission.

Effects of red blood cell transfusion

The effects of red blood cell transfusion on the recipient's hemoglobin and hematocrit levels will be affected by the recipient's blood volume, pretransfusion hemoglobin level, clinical condition (stable, bleeding, etc.), and the hemoglobin content of the donor unit. In general 1 unit of red cells will increase the hemoglobin value 1 g/dl in an average-sized adult.

Transfusion of products containing coagulation factors

Blood components that can be used to replace coagulation factors are fresh frozen plasma and cryoprecipitate. Several plasma derivatives, including factor VIII, factor IX, antithrombin III, and von Willebrand factor concentrates, are available for various coagulation disorders. The plasma derivatives are most useful for single or isolated coagulation factor deficiencies and discussion of this therapy is not within the scope of this book.

Fresh frozen plasma. The most common combined coagulation factor deficiency involves the vitamin K-dependent factors. This deficiency is best managed by treating the underlying condition with or without vitamin K administration. However, if rapid reversal is necessary, fresh frozen plasma or plasma of any age can be used since these coagulation factors do not deteriorate during storage of whole blood at 1–6°C.

Recommended indications for use of fresh frozen plasma are:[49]

1. Replacement of isolated coagulation factor deficiencies when specific components are not available. Examples of this are factors V, VIII, IX, X and XI.
2. Reversal of warfarin effect in patients actively bleeding or who require emergency surgery.
3. Antithrombin III deficiency in patients undergoing surgery or who require heparin for treatment of thrombosis.
4. Treatment of thrombotic thrombocytopenic purpura usually as part of plasma exchange.
5. Replacement of coagulation factors in patients who have depletion of multiple coagulation factors usually due to liver disease and are bleeding or about to undergo surgery. Fresh frozen plasma is not indicated for blood volume replacement or as a nutritional source.
6. Replacement of coagulation factors in massive transfusion is being used more commonly (see section on massive transfusion).

Replacement of immunoglobulins in the treatment of immunodeficiency, such as in patients with protein-losing enteropathy or children or adults with immunodeficiency, is not recommended because of the availability of intravenous immunoglobulin preparations.

Because fresh frozen plasma is usually given to replace multiple plasma proteins, the dose is difficult to determine. The desired level of each protein may be different although for many coagulation factors, a level of 30% is considered adequate to provide hemostasis. In an average-sized adult, 5 units of fresh frozen plasma would be necessary to reach this level. This would involve transfusion of about 1000 ml of plasma; the patient's blood volume and cardiovascular status must be considered.

Coagulation factor concentrates. Deficiency of isolated factor VIII or IX are usually treated with the appropriate factor concentrate. This allows larger doses to be given and the dose can be accurately calculated because each vial of concentrate is assayed for its content of factor.

Cryoprecipitate. Hypofibrinogenemia may occur as an isolated inherited deficiency or in obstetrical complications, disseminated intravascular coagulation, and some forms of cancer. In acquired hypofibrinogenemia, treatment should be directed toward the underlying cause of the disease rather than toward replacement of fibrinogen; however, when the fibrinogen level reaches 50 mg/ml or less, fibrinogen replacement may be necessary.[51,52] Cryoprecipitate is usually used as the source of fibrinogen.[53] The dose of fibrinogen for an adult is 6000–8000 mg, although this varies depending on the patient's fibrinogen level. Usually about 30 bags of cryoprecipitate would be used. A commercially prepared fibrinogen product is now available in Europe.

Transfusion of platelets

Indications for platelet transfusion. Platelet transfusion has increased more than that of other blood components during the past decade.[6] The most common reason for platelet transfusion is to prevent bleeding (prophylactic)[53,54] and prophylactic platelet transfusions are usually given to patients with transient thrombocytopenia due to chemotherapy for malignancy including bone marrow transplantation. Platelets can also be transfused to treat active bleeding, but this accounts for fewer transfusions.

Only a few small controlled studies of prophylactic platelet transfusion have been done, but in the absence of extensive data, it became common practice to transfuse platelets to prevent serious bleeding when the platelet count was less than 20 000/μl.[55] More recent studies have established that prophylactic transfusion can be initiated at platelet count of 10 000/μl without increased bleeding[56,57] and this is the current practice.

The usual dose of platelets for a prophylactic platelet transfusion to an average-sized adult is 1 apheresis unit or a pool of 4–5 whole blood-derived platelet concentrates prepared by either the PRP or buffy coat methods. Frequent transfusions of smaller doses result in less total platelet usage with no increase in bleeding,[54] while others believe that larger doses of platelets are a preferable transfusion strategy.[58]

In a large multi-center trial the likelihood of bleeding was the same in patients who received half or twice the usual platelet dose,[54] although a separate smaller study found higher bleeding when low dose transfusions were used.[59]

The optimum platelet count to achieve in a bleeding patient is not known. The bleeding time increases when the platelet count is less than 100 000/μl[60] which suggests that this number could be the goal of transfusion in actively bleeding patients. However, few studies are available to assist in this decision. It appears that bleeding may be more related to the severity of the surgical procedure than the platelet count[61] and platelet transfusion is recommended for patients undergoing lumbar puncture if the platelet count is less than 20 000/μl.[62] In actively bleeding patients, an attempt to achieve a platelet count of greater than 50 000/μl is recommended.[63]

In patients with autoimmune thrombocytopenic purpura or drug-induced immune thrombocytopenia, platelet antibodies cause shortened survival of transfused platelets, and thus transfusion is recommended only for treatment of severe thrombocytopenia with active hemorrhage.

There is a dose-response effect from platelet transfusion. One to three hours after transfusion, the usual dose of platelets transfused should cause a platelet count increase of about 25 000 µl in an average-sized adult.[64,65] Some patients do not attain the expected post-transfusion increment in platelet count because they are alloimmunized to platelet or leukocyte antigens.[45,65] In addition, platelet survival can be affected by many clinical factors in the patient,[66] such as disseminated intravascular coagulopathy; amphotericin B administration; palpable spleen; presence of HLA antibody, platelet antibody, and fever; and status after marrow transplantation. Prevention of alloimmunization has been accomplished using single-donor (apheresis) platelets, leukocyte-depleted blood components, and UV irradiation.[45]

Because platelet refractoriness is often associated with bleeding and with a poor outcome, this is a major clinical problem in transfusion medicine. Refractoriness is managed by treating clinical factors that might cause refractoriness,[66] the use of ABO-compatible platelets,[67] and the use of platelets as fresh as possible. If these measures fail, an improved response may be obtained by selecting a platelet donor whose HLA type matches that of the recipient,[68–70] although about 30% of HLA-matched transfusions do not provide a satisfactory response. Another approach is to crossmatch the patient's serum with platelets and to select compatible donors based on this laboratory test. This approach is about as effective as the use of HLA-matched donors.[71,72]

Granulocyte transfusion

Many chemotherapy and stem cell transplant regimens cause severe and prolonged granulocytopenia. These patients are at increased risk of infection, which is a major cause of death. The availability of blood cell separators and of donor-stimulation techniques have made it possible to collect large numbers of granulocytes for transfusion, especially with the use of G-CSF stimulated donors. Historically granulocyte transfusions appeared to be helpful,[73] but today most patients respond to antibiotics. Fungal infections, however, continue to be a major problem,[74] and granulocyte transfusions are being used in this setting and for bacterial sepsis unresponsive to antibiotics. No clinical trials have documented the effectiveness of granulocyte transfusion in these situations, but G-CSF stimulation of donors yields very high dose granulocyte concentrates[33] and this has led to a new large-scale clinical trial of granulocyte transfusion.

Blood derivatives

During the late 1930s, the technique was developed for the separation of different plasma proteins. This technique is now used to process thousands of liters of plasma in large batches to produce many plasma proteins, termed plasma derivatives, for therapeutic use. Some of the plasma for production of derivatives is obtained from units of voluntarily donated whole blood separated into components, but most of the plasma is obtained by plasmapheresis of paid donors. This aspect of the blood supply has been extremely effective in producing large amounts of important therapeutic proteins such as albumin, coagulation factor concentrates and immune globulins. However, the risk of disease transmission from paid donors was high[7,75] and this fact was tragically demonstrated with the onset of the AIDS epidemic.[76] Improvements in the manufacturing technique have now made these products free of transmission of most viruses[77,78] and most are now being produced by recombinant DNA methods. The demand for the intravenous form of immune serum globulin is large because if its use in many situations in addition to the FDA-licensed indications of primary congenital immune deficiency and autoimmune thrombocytopenia. A discussion of the use of plasma derivatives is beyond the scope of this chapter.

Transfusion of cytomegalovirus (CMV)-negative blood products

CMV can be transmitted by blood transfusion with a severe, even fatal result. Transfusion-transmitted CMV occurs in immunosuppressed patients and can be prevented by using CMV antibody-negative blood components or blood components filtered to remove the leukocytes that are thought to be the source of latent CMV. These CMV-safe blood components are indicated in neonates,[79] pregnant women,[80] patients undergoing bone marrow transplantation,[81,82] patients with AIDS or severe combined immune deficiency, and patients receiving extensive chemotherapy. There is little information available about the value of CMV-safe blood components in patients who receive solid organ transplants. Most, if not virtually all, of the CMV disease in these patients is due to reactivation of a previous infection, thus CMV-safe blood components are not usually provided to these patients.

Irradiated blood components

Viable lymphocytes contained in blood components can cause fatal graft-versus-host disease (GVHD) in immuno-compromised patients. Transfusion-induced GVHD can be prevented by using blood components that have been gamma irradiated.[83] Irradiation with 1500–5000 Gy interferes with the ability of lymphocytes to proliferate without damaging the cell function.[84] Doses of up to 5000 Gy do not have an adverse effect on red cells, platelets or granulocytes. As the use of irradiated blood components has increased, often it is not possible to transfuse them immediately after they are irradiated. Doses of 2000 or 3000 rads to units of red cells result in potassium levels two and three times normal after storage for 4–5 days which suggests that there is some irradiation damage to the red cell membrane or the sodium-potassium pump. However, the amount of potassium in the supernatant is not considered dangerous, and the normal survival of these cells *in vivo* is the basis for allowing storage of irradiated red cells for the original expiration date or 28 days after irradiation, whichever comes first.

It is difficult to determine which patients should receive irradiated blood components because there are no *in vitro* assays of immunodeficiency that satisfactorily predict which patients are susceptible to transfusion-associated GVHD. However, several kinds of patients are so severely immunocompromised that transfusion-associated GVHD is very likely unless blood components are irradiated. These include: fetuses undergoing intrauterine or exchange transfusion, patients with severe combined immunodeficiency syndrome or Wiskott–Aldrich syndrome, and patients undergoing allogeneic or autologous hematopoietic stem cell transplantation.

Occasionally blood is irradiated for patients who are not immunocompromised. In immunocompetent patients, some cases of transfusion-associated GVHD occurred after transfusion of blood from relatives or unrelated donors who were partially HLA-matched with the patient.[85] Apparent transfusion-associated GVHD has been reported due to fresh blood transfused to two immunocompetent children who underwent cardiac surgery and received blood from donors who were homozygous for an HLA Class I antigen haplotype shared with the recipient. In these cases, the recipient would not have recognized the HLA Class I antigens on the transfused cells as foreign, but lymphocytes in the donated blood would have recognized the recipient's cells as foreign. Because of additional reports of transfusion-associated GVHD in other immunocompetent patients,[86,87] irradiation of the blood components donated by first-degree relatives of the patient has been instituted. Because of the high frequency of certain HLA antigens in the Japanese population and the resulting likelihood that a random, unrelated donor may be partially HLA-matched with the recipient, irradiation may be used more commonly there.

There are several other clinical situations in which isolated cases of transfusion-associated GVHD have been reported and for which a few medical centers use irradiated blood components, but there is no consensus on recommended practice. These include neonates, although there is no evidence that newborns who do not have a congenital immunodeficiency are at increased risk of developing transfusion-associated GVHD; patients with hematologic malignancies, especially those receiving very severe chemotherapy regimens often with radiation; patients with aplastic anemia, although these patients usually do not have defective cellular immunity and there have not been documented cases of transfusion-associated GVHD due to transfusion of normal cells, patients with solid tumors such as neuroblastoma or glioblastoma; and patients with AIDS, although no cases of transfusion-associated GVHD have been reported.

Although irradiation of fresh frozen plasma and cryoprecipitate is probably not necessary, transfusion-associated GVHD has occurred in patients with congenital immune deficiency after transfusion of fresh, liquid plasma. Because previously frozen components contain fragments of leukocytes, but few viable lymphocytes, these components would not be expected to cause transfusion-associated GVHD. Still many blood banks irradiate these plasma components to avoid clerical errors in which a cellular blood component might not be irradiated when necessary.

Fibrin glue

Fibrin glue refers to the use of fibrinogen (in some form) and thrombin as a topical adhesive to control bleeding.[29,88] Fibrin glue is used predominantly by surgeons to stop microvascular bleeding in cardiovascular surgery and to reduce mediastinal drainage, to seal synthetic vascular grafts and bleeding surfaces of the liver or spleen, and in maxillofacial surgery to seal dura and repair peripheral nerves. During the past few years, commercial preparations of fibrin glue have become available.

Transfusion in special situations

Transfusion of blood components in many specific situations is complex hemotherapy and involves considerations that are not appropriate for detailed discussion in this book. Brief examples of a few of these situations will be summarized here.

Massive transfusion

The traditional approach to acute blood loss and massive transfusion was to maintain intravascular volume with crystalloid or colloid and replace platelets, coagulation factors and red cells as needed if depletion of these occurred. This approach accepts that coagulopathy may develop and an attempt is then made to correct this. Contemporary studies have shown results if frozen plasma is used immediately to prevent coagulopathy.[89,90] This has led to the development of standard massive transfusion protocols involving frozen plasma, platelets and red cells in a 4 : 1 : 4 ratio beginning very early in the event of a severe injury with substantial blood loss and use of these protocols is effective in both a military and civilian setting.

Massive transfusion is transfusion equivalent to the patient's blood volume during a 24-hour interval. The effects of massive transfusion upon the recipient are due to the biochemical and functional characteristics of stored blood and include hypothermia, acidosis, hypocalcemia, hyperkalemia, coagulopathy and thrombocytopenia.[91] In patients undergoing acute blood loss and/or massive transfusion, the issues faced are the type of replacement fluid, the kind of blood component to use, the necessity to replace coagulation factors or platelets, the speed with which red cells can be made available, and the blood bank's ability to respond urgently.

Cardiovascular surgery

For patients undergoing cardiovascular surgery, fresh blood and routine platelet transfusions are not necessary. Patients undergoing cardiopulmonary bypass often develop thrombocytopenia and platelet function abnormalities.[92] However, most patients do not experience unusual bleeding and the extent of bleeding is not directly related to these hemostatic abnormalities.[91] Patients who bleed excessively should be managed like any other surgical patients.

Currently there is debate about whether blood stored longer before transfusion is detrimental to these patients.[93,94] This issue is not resolved and several large studies of the effects of red cells stored for different times are underway.

Transplantation

In patients undergoing hematopoietic stem cell transplantation consideration must be given to transfusion strategies before and after transplantation and in ABO- and Rh-incompatible transplants.[95] In solid organ transplantation, routine blood components are usually used for patients receiving kidney and heart transplants, but liver transplant recipients are treated more like patients undergoing massive transfusion.

Neonates

Neonates have special transfusion requirements including pre-transfusion testing, need for CMV-negative blood, and/or irradiated blood components and exchange transfusion. Larger pediatric patients are usually managed similarly to adults. Smaller pediatric patients may require special infusion devices and adjusted doses of components.[96]

Hemophilia

The management of hemophilia patients is a complex subject and will not be covered here.

Provision of red cells in urgent situations

The speed and methods of making blood available are crucial in several clinical situations. Where transfusion is or may be urgent, a blood specimen should be obtained and sent to the blood bank for emergency type and crossmatch. An ABO and Rh type can be performed in about 5 minutes and blood of the same type as the patient selected for transfusion. If necessary, this blood can be released without a full crossmatch. The crossmatch procedure can be shortened to detect only ABO incompatibility since that is usually the most disastrous kind of transfusion reaction. Blood of the patient's ABO type can be available usually in about 15 minutes using this shortened crossmatch. Usually Rh-positive blood would be chosen, but Rh-negative blood may be used if the patient is a young female. When the patient's ABO type is not known, group O red cells are used. This practice has led to the designation of group O, Rh-negative individuals as universal donors because group O, Rh-negative red cells would not be hemolyzed by either anti-A, anti-B, or anti-D if present and would not immunize recipients to D. Group O, Rh-negative (universal donor) red cells do not avoid the potential risk that the recipient may have a red cell antibody other than anti-D or a red cell autoantibody, and hemolysis or transfusion reactions can occur after transfusion of O-negative red cells. Stocking group O, Rh-negative red cells routinely in emergency departments is inappropriate. The red cells may not be stored properly, and there may not be a system of checks for releasing the units; these are practices that can lead to serious problems. Techniques of fluid management and resuscitation are so highly developed today that patients can be maintained for the time required to obtain red cells from the blood bank. Blood bank personnel are aware that there may be situations in which there is an urgent need for blood and each blood bank should have a procedure for the rapid release of red cells.

Exchange transfusion of the neonate

The indications for exchange transfusion in the neonate are: hyperbilirubinemia, sepsis, disseminated intravascular coagulopathy, polycythemia, respiratory distress syndrome, hyperammonemia, anemia, toxin removal, thrombocytopenia and sickle cell disease. The exchange transfusion can be done via the umbilical vein for newborns or a peripheral vein for other neonates or children. Exchange of one blood volume should remove about 65% of the original intravascular constituent, and an exchange of two blood volumes should remove about 85%.[32] Exchange transfusion is usually done with red cells that are only a few days old. If necessary, because of coagulopathy, fresh frozen plasma can be used with the red cells to provide coagulation factors during the exchange transfusion. The potential complications of exchange transfusion are: infection, rebound hypoglycemia, hypocalcemia (due to citrate anticoagulant in the transfused blood), hyperkalemia (if older red cells are used), late onset alkalosis, volume overload, hemolysis, thrombocytopenia, neutropenia, coagulopathy, GVHD and hypothermia. These complications can be avoided or minimized by careful technique and good general patient care, although because many of these patients are quite ill and unstable, exchange transfusion can be a risky procedure.

Autoimmune hemolytic anemia

Patients with autoimmune hemolytic anemia present a special problem for the blood bank because the patient's serum usually reacts with red cells from all donors because of the broad spectrum of reactivity of the autoantibody. This autoantibody reactivity may obscure alloantibodies present in the patient's serum and it may not be possible to obtain red cells for transfusion that are serologically compatible (negative crossmatch). The decision to transfuse a patient with autoimmune hemolytic anemia should be based on the severity of the anemia, whether the anemia is rapidly progressive, and the associated clinical findings.[97] In newly diagnosed patients with autoimmune hemolytic anemia, the hemoglobin should be measured frequently to determine whether the anemia is stable or progressing. Transfusion is not recommended unless the hemoglobin is in the 5–8 g/dl range. Many of these patients will compensate for their anemia, especially on bed rest in the hospital, and transfusion is not necessary. Although autoimmune hemolytic anemia patients are experiencing hemolysis, they usually do not experience signs or symptoms of an acute hemolytic transfusion reaction. In addition to the usual complications associated with transfusion, patients with autoimmune hemolytic anemia may experience increased hemolysis and/or congestive heart failure.

If transfusion is necessary, the two goals of compatibility testing are to select red cells that will survive at least as long as the patient's own cells and to avoid transfusing red cells that are incompatible with any clinically significant alloantibodies the patient may have. There are several serologic strategies to accomplish these goals.[97]

The autoantibodies usually cause the red cells from all donors to have shortened post-transfusion survival. Despite this ongoing hemolysis, patients with autoimmune hemolytic anemia do not require special red cell components. It is advisable to choose units that are in the first week or two of their storage life to obtain the maximum benefit from the transfusion. Packed red cells are satisfactory although leukocyte-depleted red cells are preferable to avoid a possible febrile transfusion reaction, which might be confused with a hemolytic transfusion reaction. There is no reason to use frozen deglycerolized red cells for autoimmune anemia patients.

Pregnant women

Anemia is common during pregnancy; however, transfusion is rarely necessary. If so, it is usually because of some other complicating factor and the choice of blood components should be based on the specific reason for the transfusion (i.e., acute blood loss, sickle cell disease). Pregnant patients receive CMV-safe blood components to prevent acute CMV infection that might cause birth defects in the child.[80]

Autoimmune thrombocytopenia

Most patients with autoimmune thrombocytopenia do not require platelet transfusion despite very low platelet counts. These patients have platelet autoantibodies that severely shorten the intravascular survival of transfused platelets. The transfused platelets survive for only a few minutes or hours[98] and a beneficial effect may not be obtained. If autoimmune thrombocytopenic patients do experience serious hemorrhage, platelet transfusions should be given.

Neonatal alloimmune thrombocytopenia

Neonatal alloimmune thrombocytopenia is the platelet analogue of hemolytic disease of the newborn. That is, the mother becomes immunized to an antigen that she lacks but that the fetus has inherited from the father. Maternal IgG platelet antibodies then cross the placenta and cause thrombocytopenia in the fetus. The antibodies can be detected in the mother;[99] HPA-1 (formerly known as Pl^A1) is the most common. If the neonate requires transfusion, platelets lacking the offending antigen should be used. Alternatively, an exchange transfusion can be done to remove the offending antibody. Alternatively, platelets lacking the antigen can be obtained from the mother, although the plasma containing the antibody should be removed before transfusion and the platelets should be resuspended in saline or group AB plasma. If the mother is not available or cannot donate platelets, most large blood banks have a few HPA-1 negative donors available to provide compatible platelets. The half-life of IgG is approximately 21 days; therefore, more than one platelet transfusion may be necessary in severely affected infants.

Neonatal alloimmune neutropenia

This is the neutrophil analog of hemolytic disease of the newborn and of neonatal alloimmune thrombocytopenia. Patients are usually discovered because they develop an infection at the circumcision site or in the perineal area. Cases due to several different neutrophil-specific antibodies have been reported.[100] Although these infants can be given granulocytes attained from a whole blood donation by the mother, the very short half-life of granulocytes limits the effectiveness of this approach. Thus, exchange transfusion is the recommended for these patients if there is a serious infection.

Rare blood types

There is no universal definition of a rare blood type. This term usually refers to an individual who lacks a blood group antigen that is present in a very high frequency in the normal population (see Chapter 37). This means that the individual will almost certainly be exposed to the antigen if they are pregnant or receive a transfusion. First, it is necessary to determine whether the antibody is clinically significant and likely to cause accelerated destruction of red cells. If the antibody is clinically significant, efforts should be made to obtain red cells that lack the antigen. Most countries have a rare donor registry that can be consulted. Considerable planning may be necessary to obtain the red cells, especially if the donors live in other cities or if the transfusion is to replace blood loss during elective surgery. Red cells from most rare donors may be available only in the frozen state which may create additional problems if the transfusion is for anticipated but uncertain blood loss. If transfusion is needed urgently, close communication is necessary between the blood bank physician and the patient's attending physician to determine a course of action. For instance, if the antibody may cause shortened red cell survival but little or no acute hemolysis, the decision might be made to use incompatible red cells while the search continues for red cells that lack the antigen.

Techniques of blood transfusion

Because complications of transfusion can be caused by improper handling or administration of blood components[101–104] or the administration of the incorrect component to the patient, it is essential that blood transfusions be administered according to clearly defined procedures that are well understood and carried out by qualified personnel.[103] Blood components should be administered only on the written order of a physician. The issues important in administering a transfusion are obtaining consent for transfusion, obtaining the blood sample for compatibility testing, use of blood administration sets and filters, use of venipuncture, procedures for starting the transfusion, use of infusion solutions,[104] identification of the patient and blood component, determination of rate of transfusion, warming of blood and nursing care of patients receiving a transfusion.

Complications of transfusion: recognition and management

Despite its lifesaving role, there are risks associated with blood transfusion. Immunologic complications involve various forms of transfusion reactions while non-immunologic complications are due to the physical effects of the blood component or to transmission of disease. Complications occur during or shortly after about 1–3% of transfusions, although the overall rate of adverse effects is much higher.

In the US, 52 transfusion-related fatalities were reported to the FDA in 2006–2007[102] for a fatality rate of approximately 1/300 000 units of red cells transfused. Since patients receive an average of about 3 units, this would mean a fatality rate of about 1.0–1.2/100 000 patients who received a transfusion (Fig. 38.1).

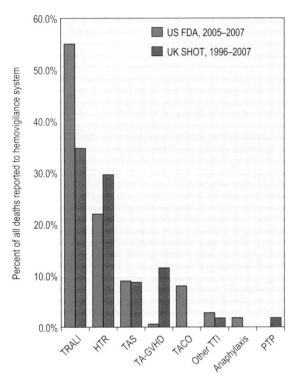

Fig. 38.1 Causes of allogeneic blood transfusion-related deaths as a percentage of all deaths reported to SHOT (1996–2007) or the FDA (2005–2007). *(Adapted from Vamvakas ED, Blajchman MA. Transfusion-related mortality: the ongoing risks of allogeneic blood transfusion and the available strategies for their prevention. Blood 2009; 113:3406–3417.)*

Transfusion reactions

The cause, severity and outcome of a transfusion reaction are difficult to predict from the presenting signs and symptoms. Therefore, all patients who exhibit signs or symptoms during or within several hours after platelet transfusion should be managed initially as if a transfusion reaction was occurring. When a transfusion reaction is suspected, the transfusion should be stopped immediately, the needle should be left in the vein and normal saline should be infused while vital signs are obtained and a brief physical examination is carried out. A new blood sample should be obtained for repeat red blood cell compatibility testing and inspection of the plasma for evidence of hemolysis, and a urine sample should be obtained if the patient can void. If pulmonary symptoms are prominent, a chest X-ray should be obtained. Based on these actions, a preliminary assessment of the situation can be made and definitive treatment initiated.

Hemolytic transfusion reactions. The most dangerous immunologic complication of transfusion is a hemolytic transfusion reaction which responsible for about 22% of fatalities in the US.[102] This means that in the US, about 13 patients/year die, giving an apparent incidence of fatal hemolytic transfusion of about 1/1000000 units of red cells or 1/300000 patients transfused.

ABO incompatibility causes severe hemolytic transfusion reactions because the patient has IgM ABO antibodies that bind complement and cause activation of the complement system release of cytokines and red cell lysis. The signs and symptoms of a hemolytic transfusion reaction are due to complement activation and also to the effects of cytokines.[105,106] The severity of the symptoms does not correlate with the volume of ABO-incompatible red cells transfused or the ultimate outcome of the transfusion reaction.[107,108] The signs of a hemolytic transfusion reaction are well known and include fever, chills, flushing, low back pain, hypotension, dyspnea, abdominal pain, vomiting, diarrhea, chest pain or unexpected bleeding. The most common signs and symptoms are fever, chest pain and hypotension. In a hemolytic transfusion reaction, the coagulation system may be activated and these patients may develop a coagulopathy and/or disseminated intravascular coagulation. Oliguria and renal failure may also be part of a hemolytic transfusion reaction because a variety of factors such as kinens, intravascular coagulation and microthrombi lead to reduced renal blood flow and damage.

There is a classic pattern of alteration in laboratory tests in a hemolytic transfusion reaction. In an acute hemolytic transfusion reaction, the common findings are hemoglobinemia and/or hemoglobinuria, reduced serum haptoglobin, elevated serum bilirubin, a positive direct antiglobulin test and the presence of unexpected red cell antibodies.[107] Laboratory testing should make the diagnosis of hemolysis and identify the red cell antibody involved.

Febrile reactions. These reactions occur in association with about 0.5–1.0% of transfusions. They are due to the patient's leukocyte antibodies, which react with leukocytes present in the transfused components[109] or cytokines contained in the donor blood component.[110] The severity of the reaction is directly related to the number of leukocytes in the blood component[109] or cytokine levels. These febrile reactions can be prevented by removing leukocytes from the blood components. Antipyretics have been used to prevent reactions, but the value is not evidence-based[111] and at most these should be used only in patients who have experienced a reaction. Corticosteroids are used for patients with severe reactions. With the increasing use of leukoreduced components, the problem of febrile transfusion reactions has decreased but continues to be a problem for some patients.

Allergic reactions. Allergic reactions manifested by hives but with no other symptoms occur following 1–2% of transfusions. When this occurs, the transfusion should be stopped; if it is then established that hemolysis is not occurring and there are no other signs or symptoms, the patient can be given an antihistamine and after about 30 minutes the transfusion can be restarted.

Pulmonary reactions. Patients may have several pulmonary reactions to transfusions called transfusion-related acute lung injury (TRALI). TRALI is now the most common cause of transfusion-related fatality,[102] accounting for more than half of the deaths. These reactions are acute, sometimes fatal, usually occur up to 6 hours after the transfusion and are characterized by acute respiratory distress, severe hypoxemia, bilateral pulmonary edema, hypotension, fever and diffuse bilateral infiltrates on chest X-ray.[112,113] Cyanosis may or may not be present. The frequency of these reactions is estimated at between 1/300 and 1/5000 transfusions of plasma-containing components.[113] They are probably more common than previously believed.[112] The reactions are thought to be due to transfusion of HLA- or granulocyte-specific antibodies in the donor unit that react with the patient's leukocytes and also the transfusion of inflammatory mediators.[114] In either situation, it is likely that leukocytes, endothelial cells and lipid and protein inflammatory mediators are involved and lead to endothelial damage, increased cell membrane permeability, increased neutrophil adhesion to endothelium and release of cytokines. These patients can be successfully managed if there is prompt recognition of the reaction and initiation of supportive treatment. The use of plasma products from male donors should decrease the incidence of TRALI.[115–117]

Anaphylactic reactions. Patients who are IgA-deficient and who have IgA antibodies may experience dramatic and rapidly fatal anaphylactic reaction if they receive blood components containing IgA.[118,119] The treatment is the same as for any anaphylactic reaction. The reactions can be prevented by using red cells or platelet concentrates washed to remove plasma IgA and by using plasma components prepared from IgA-deficient donors.

Reactions to platelets

Transfusion reactions can occur during platelet transfusion. These reactions present as chills and fever similar to those seen in a non-hemolytic febrile transfusion reaction. Platelet transfusion reactions are caused by cytokines that accumulate in the platelet concentrate during storage[110] or by the patient's platelet or HLA antibodies that react with leukocytes contained in the platelet concentrates. These reactions can be prevented by removing the leukocytes before storage of platelets.[110] The most common signs and symptoms of a transfusion reaction to platelets are chills, fever and urticaria.

Graft-versus-host disease (GVHD)

Blood components contain viable lymphocytes and can cause GVHD in patients who are severely immunocompromised. Transfusion-associated GVHD can also occur in immunocompetent patients if they receive blood from an HLA-matched (usually homozygous) donor.[85–87] The syndrome characterized by fever, liver dysfunction, skin rash, diarrhea and marrow hypoplasia begins less than 30 days following transfusions and is fatal in approximately 90% of patients. Transfusion-associated GVHD can be prevented by irradiating the blood components prior to transfusions.[83]

Other complications of blood transfusion

Immunization to blood group antigens, iron overload, microemboli, citrate toxicity, hypocalcemia, hyperkalemia, acidosis, alkalosis and cardiac arrhythmias due to cold blood can occur following transfusion.

Transfusion-transmitted diseases

In developed countries, since the AIDS epidemic, the blood supply is safer than ever, but the epidemic and the growing awareness of post-transfusion hepatitis have heightened the public's fears of blood transfusion. In response, physicians have developed more conservative transfusion practices. Several other actions or changes have improved blood safety. These include new donor screening criteria, increased laboratory tests, reduced use of blood because of more conservative transfusion practices, use of autologous blood, and the use of pharmacologic agents to reduce transfusion requirements. Although great visibility and preventative efforts are focused on transfusion-transmitted disease, these account for only about 1% of the transfusion-related fatalities reported to the FDA.[102] The single action that had the largest impact on improving blood safety was the conversion to an all volunteer donor system in the US.[120] While increased laboratory testing of donors is the most visible blood safety step, testing is not done for many transfusion transmissible diseases (see Table 38.1, below) and changes in donor health history have had a major impact.[121] The major transfusion-transmitted diseases are described below.

Post-transfusion hepatitis

Post-transfusion hepatitis is the most common disease transmitted by blood transfusion and it has a major health impact. Post-transfusion hepatitis can be due to hepatitis C virus, hepatitis B virus, hepatitis A virus, CMV or Epstein–Barr virus. The incidence varies in different parts of the world. In the US there are about 90–111 cases of post-transfusion hepatitis C and 66–153 of post-transfusion hepatitis B annually per million units of laboratory tested blood.[122–124]

Hepatitis A usually has a short period of viremia and generally does not involve a carrier state. Thus, post-transfusion hepatitis A is rare, although it can occur if an individual donates blood during the short period of viremia before symptoms develop.[125,126] Donated blood is not tested for hepatitis A because hepatitis A antibodies are not present at this early stage of infection, there is no practical screening test for the virus itself, and post-transfusion hepatitis A is rare.

Most individuals infected with the hepatitis B virus are asymptomatic but about 10% develop persistent viremia and chronic hepatitis B. Thus, an infectious, but apparently healthy, individual may meet all of the donor medical history criteria and donate a unit of infectious blood. Routine screening of blood donors for hepatitis B surface antigen has reduced the previous high incidence of post-transfusion hepatitis B.

In the late 1980s, the hepatitis C virus was discovered[127,128] and this virus accounts for almost all cases of non-A, non-B hepatitis. Testing for antibodies to hepatitis C virus was introduced in the early 1990s and has greatly reduced post-transfusion hepatitis C. Because the screening test for hepatitis C detects antibody to the virus, there is a 'window' period during which the individual has viremia and is infectious, but during which the test for antibodies to hepatitis C virus is negative. Blood donation by asymptomatic individuals during this window period accounts for much of the remaining post-transfusion hepatitis. This delay in antibody production had led to the development of tests to screen donated blood by detection of viral DNA or RNA. This method has been referred to as nucleic acid amplification testing (NAT) and will be discussed later.

Table 38.1 Laboratory testing for transfusion-transmitted disease

Family	Pathogen	Disease	Routinely screened for US	
			Yes	No
Hepatitis viruses	HBV, HCV	Hepatitis	X	
	HEV, HGV	Hepatitis		X
Retroviruses	HIV-1 and -2	AIDS	X	
	HTLV-I and -II	Malignant lymphoproliferative disorders, neuropathy		X
Herpes viruses	CMV	CMV retinitis, hepatitis, pneumonia		X
	EBV	Epstein–Barr syndrome		X
	HHV-8	Kaposi's sarcoma		X
Flaviviruses	WNV	Meningoencephalitis	X	
	Denge	Hemorrhagic fever		X
Parvoviruses	B19	Aplastic anemia		X
Bacteria	Gram (−), gram (+)	Sepsis		X
	Treponema pallidum	Syphilis	X	
	Rickettsia rickettsii	Rocky Mountain spotted fever		X
	Ehrlichia chafeensis	Ehrlichiosis		X
Protozoans	*Trypanosoma cruzi*	Chagas disease		X
	Babesia microti	Babesiosis		X
	Leishmania donovani	Leishmaniasis		X
	Plasmodium spp.	Malaria		X

HIV infection and AIDS

When the epidemiology of HIV infection became known and when it was clear that transfusion-transmitted AIDS did occur, blood banks altered their medical screening practices to defer potential donors from AIDS risk groups; and when the HIV-1 virus was shown to be the cause of AIDS, blood banks initiated routine testing of all donated blood for antibodies to HIV-1 (anti-HIV-1). These two steps greatly improved blood safety and reduced the risk of acquiring HIV infection following transfusion from up to 91% to very low levels. When a blood donor is found to be anti-HIV-1 positive on the initial screening test, confirmatory testing is done by the Western blot method.

Despite the effectiveness of the medical history questioning and laboratory testing of donated blood, there is a remaining risk of acquiring HIV-1 by transfusion. This risk decreased to about 1 in 500 000 units of blood,[129–131] but this meant that up to about 20 people may become infected with HIV-1 annually by transfusion of donated blood which was negative for anti-HIV-1 antibodies. The reasons for the continued risk of transfusion-transmitted HIV-1 are: 1) failure of some infected individuals to develop antibody; 2) lack of representation of variant viral strains of test reagents; 3) laboratory testing errors; and 4) the window phase of infection.[132] Because the window phase accounts for almost all transfusion-transmitted HIV in developed countries, testing

for the HIV antigen itself was attempted. Although it was predicted to shorten the window period and further reduce the likelihood of HIV-1 transmission, the method was not sufficiently sensitive to detect many infectious HIV-1 seronegative donors[133,134] and so it was never adopted. Subsequently, methods that amplify HIV-1 DNA sequences have been applied to blood donor testing, thus making it possible to detect minute amounts of viral DNA or RNA.[135]

Because of the complexity and cost of NAT, sera from multiple donors are tested in a pool, but this technology detects a level of HCV or HIV viral particles/ml at the levels that occur during the window phase of infection. In the US, NAT reduced the HIV-1 window phase period from 22 to 10 days or less and the hepatitis C window phase period from 70 to about 41 days or less.[136] This reduction prevented approximately 2–15 cases of transfusion-transmitted HIV-1 and 40–60 cases of hepatitis C annually in the US.[132]

Other transfusion-transmitted infectious diseases (Table 38.1)

Malaria can be transmitted by transfusion, but this is rare in North America and Western Europe. Most cases involve *Plasmodium malariae*. Donors who might transmit malaria undergo screening by medical history, although this screening method is becoming increasingly difficult as worldwide travel increases. Laboratory testing of donors for malaria is not practical or cost-effective in the US but may be done in parts of the world where malaria is endemic. Transmission of syphilis by blood transfusion was common years ago but now it is extremely rare.[137] The treponema that causes syphilis can survive in refrigerated blood for 48 hours[138] and at room temperature and, thus, can be transmitted from red cell components stored for only a few days or from platelet concentrates stored at room temperature. Although all blood donors are tested for syphilis, this is not a very effective method of preventing transfusion-transmitted syphilis because the serologic tests do not closely coincide with periods of infectivity.

Mosquito borne West Nile virus appeared in the US several years ago and was quickly recognized as a transfusion-transmitted infection.[139] Since deferring donors with a history of mosquito bites is not feasible, a nucleic acid amplification test has been incorporated into the existing NAT systems for HIV and HCV in North America.[140] This has greatly reduced transfusion-transmitted West Nile virus infection but rare cases still occur.[141]

CMV is a herpes virus that is common in the general population and can be transmitted by blood transfusion to both immunocompetent or immunodeficient patients. A large proportion of blood donors have been infected with CMV. There is no practical laboratory test to determine which patients previously infected with CMV but presently healthy enough to donate blood may transmit the virus. Transfusion-transmitted CMV can be prevented by using blood that lacks antibody to CMV or by removing the leukocytes from cellular components.[81,82]

Transmission of HTLV-I via blood transfusion does occur,[142] although no cases of transfusion-transmitted adult T-cell leukemia or tropical spastic parapheresis have been identified in the US. All donated blood in the US is tested for antibodies to HTLV-I. *Trypanosoma cruzi*, the organism that causes Chagas disease, can survive in refrigerated blood and can be transmitted by transfusion. Cases of transfusion-transmitted Chagas disease are rare in North America.[143] Attempts to identify donors potentially infectious for *T. cruzi* by medical history have not been effective.[144] Therefore, a test has been developed[145] and is being implemented to detect carriers of *T. cruzi*. *Babesia microti* can be transmitted by blood donated by asymptomatic infected donors.[146] The ticks that carry this parasite are prevalent in the Northeast, Mid-Atlantic, and Upper Midwest. There is no suitable laboratory screening test for *B. microti*. Some blood banks defer individuals from heavily tick-infested areas during the summer months.

Borrelia burgdorferi, a spirochete transmitted by ticks to humans, can survive in stored blood for up to 45 days.[147] Although transmission of *B. burgdorferi* by transfusion is theoretically possible, it has not been reported. A serologic test is available, but it is not suitable for donor screening. The widespread prevalence of the host tick makes it impractical to defer donors from endemic areas. Parvovirus B19 has been transmitted by blood transfusion.[148,149] No steps are taken to prevent transfusion-transmission of parvovirus B19, but a recent case of transmission by pooled, solvent/detergent-treated plasma[149] led to the screening of lots of this plasma to minimize the likelihood of infection. Theoretically, any disease in which microbes circulate in the blood and survive for a few days in stored blood components could be transmitted by transfusion. However, the diseases of most concern have been discussed. A few other diseases that almost never occur due to transfusions in North America are toxoplasmosis, dengue, chickungunya, leishmaniasis, microfilaria and African trypanosomiasis.

Role of hematopoietic growth factors in transfusion medicine

Erythropoietin

The availability of hematopoietic growth factors opened a new era in transfusion medicine. The first of these, erythropoietin, eliminated the need for red cell transfusions in most patients with end-stage renal failure.[150] It has been estimated nationally that this eliminated as many as 500 000 transfusions in the US. The use of erythropoietin would make these red cell units available for other patients and yet allow patients with renal failure to maintain higher hemoglobin levels and improved quality of life[151] and to avoid the complications of transfusions. Erythropoietin has been used in forms of anemia not due to erythropoietin deficiency, especially cancer which has become the largest use of erythropoietin.

In patients undergoing chemotherapy, erythropoietin is used to increase the hemoglobin to 11 or even 12 g/dl to provide greater stamina and physical energy.[152] However, it has been suggested that use of erythropoietin in these patients may lead to shorter survival due to complications and cancer recurrence.[153,154] Currently, this issue is unresolved.[33] Erythropoietin has also been used to increase autologous blood donation or reduce the homologous blood requirements of patients undergoing elective surgery but is of only limited benefit. This exciting drug has now taken its place in red cell transfusion practices.

Granulocyte-macrophage colony simulating factor (GM-CSF)

G or GM-CSF may decrease the period of chemotherapy-induced leukopenia in patients with malignancy or in those undergoing bone marrow transplantation.[33] Although this reduction may reduce the morbidity and mortality of these procedures, it probably will not greatly alter transfusion therapy in the near future because leukocyte replacement is not widely practiced. However, reducing the incidence and/or severity of infection could modify transfusion therapy if sepsis and disseminated intravascular coagulopathy are avoided with a resulting decline in the use of platelets and fresh frozen plasma. The use of G-CSF to stimulate donors for the collection of peripheral blood stem cells or granulocytes for transfusion has been discussed earlier.

Platelet growth factor

Platelet growth factors shorten the period of thrombocytopenia and elevate the platelet nadir in patients with solid tumors,[33] but these patients do not require many platelet transfusions and so there is little impact on platelet demand.

No beneficial effect on platelet recovery has been found in patients undergoing hematopoietic stem cell transplantation.[33] Thus, despite the exciting development of the availability of platelet growth factors, they have had little impact on transfusion medicine.

Blood substitutes

For years there has been considerable interest in the use of a red cell substitute that would effectively transport oxygen from the lungs to the tissues. The ideal acellular red cell substitute would not require crossmatching or blood typing, could be stored, preferably at room temperature, for a long period, would have a reasonable intravascular life span and thereafter be exited promptly, and would be free of toxicity or disease transmission. The two compounds which have undergone most study are hemoglobin solutions and perfluorocarbons. At ambient oxygen tension, a perfluorocarbon product was not effective, but when patients breathed 100% oxygen, perfluorocarbon provided increased oxygen consumption, increased mixed venous oxygen tension, and increased mixed venous hemoglobin saturation[155] but did not affect patient survival.

In a separate study of severely anemic patients (hemoglobin 1.2–4.5 g/dl) who received the perfluorocarbon product, the amount of oxygen delivered by the perfluorocarbon product was not clinically significant and the patients did not benefit.[156] The major observation in this study was the ability of all the patients to tolerate remarkably low hemoglobin levels and the lack of need for increased arterial oxygen content in control patients who had hemoglobin levels of approximately 7 g/dl.

Work with hemoglobin solutions has progressed slowly. Hemoglobin can be prepared in solution by lysis of red cells but the remaining cell stroma must be removed. However, stroma-free hemoglobin in solution has a short intravascular life span and has a low P^{50} (the point at which 50% is saturated). Thus, research has focused on modifying the structure of the hemoglobin molecule and/or binding the hemoglobin molecule to other molecules to overcome these two problems.[157] At least two stroma-free hemoglobin products have undergone extensive *in vitro* and animal trials and human clinical trials. Unfortunately both of these were associated with an excess of adverse effects or lack of clinical benefit and clinical trials have been discontinued. Thus, after decades of development, there are no ongoing human clinical trials and it does not appear that other products are near human use. The elusive blood substitute does not seem to be close to a reality.

References

1. Daniels G, Hadley A. Blood groups on red cells, platelets, and neutrophils. In: McCullough J, Porwit A, editors. Blood and Bone Marrow Pathology. Harcourt Brace (in press).

2. Kelton J. Acquired hemolytic anemias. In: McCullough J, Porwit A, editors. Blood and Bone Marrow Pathology. Harcourt Brace (in press).

3. McCullough J. National blood programs in developed countries. Transfusion 1996;36:1019–32.

4. Leikola J. How much blood for the world? Vox Sang 1988;54:1–5.

5. McCullough J. The nation's changing blood supply system. JAMA 1993;269:2239.

6. Whitaker BI, Green J, King MR, et al. The 2007 nationwide Blood Collection and Utilization Survey Report. Washington, DC: Department of Health and Human Services; 2008.

7. Eastlund T. Monetary blood donation incentives and the risk of transfusion-transmitted infection. Transfusion 1998;38:881–4.

8. Busch M, Garratty G. Applications of Molecular Biology to Blood Transfusion Medicine. Bethesda, MD: American Association of Blood Banks; 1997. p. 123–76.

9. McCullough J. The continuing evolution of the nation's blood supply system. Am J Clin Pathol 1996;105:689–95.

10. Zuck TF. Current good manufacturing practices. Transfusion 1995;35:95–66.

11. McCullough J. Transfusion Medicine. New York, NY: McGraw Hill; 1998.

12. Giving Blood. In: Piliavin JA, Callero PL, editors. The Development of an Altruistic Identify. Baltimore, Maryland: Johns Hopkins University Press; 1991.

13. Riley W, Schwei M, McCullough J. The United States' potential blood donor pool: estimating the prevalence of donor exclusion factors on the pool of potential donors. Transfusion 2007;47:1180–8.

14. Fuller AK, Uglik KM, Savage WJ, et al. Bacterial culture reduces but does not eliminate the risk of septic transfusion reactions to single-donor platelets. Transfusion 2009;49(12):2588–93.

15. Eder AF, Kennedy JM, Dy BA, et al. Bacterial screening of apheresis platelets and the residual risk of septic transfusion reactions: the American Red Cross experience (2004–6). Transfusion 2007; 47:1134–1142.

16. Kasprisin DO, Glynn SH, Taylor F, Miller KA. Moderate and severe reactions in blood donors. Transfusion 1992;32: 23–6.

17. Eder AF, Dy BA, Kennedy JM, et al. The American Red Cross donor hemovigilance program: complications of blood donation reported in 2006. Transfusion 2008;48:1809–19.

18. Newman BH, Waxman DA. Blood donation-related neurologic needle injury: evaluation of 2 years' worth of data from a large blood center. Transfusion 1996;36:213–5.

19. Berry PR, Wallis WE. Venipuncture nerve injuries. Lancet 1997;1:1236–7.

20. Horowitz SH. Venipuncture-induced causalgia: anatomic relations of upper extremity superficial veins and nerves, and clinical considerations. Transfusion 2000;40:1036–40.

21. Popovsky MA, Whitaker B, Arnold NL. Severe outcomes of allogeneic and autologous blood donation: frequency and characterization. Transfusion 1995; 35:734–7.

22. Brecher ME, Goodnough LT. The rise and fall of preoperative autologous blood donation. Transfusion 2001;41:1459–62.

23. Birkmeyer JD, Goodnough LT, AuBuchon JP, et al. The cost-effectiveness of preoperative autologous blood donation for total hip and knee replacement. Transfusion 1993;33:544.

24. Rottman G, Ness PM. Acute normovolemic hemodilution is a legitimate alternative to allogeneic blood transfusion. Transfusion 1998; 38:477–80.

25. Williams AE, Kleinman S, Gilcher RO, et al. The prevalence of infectious disease markers in directed versus homologous blood donations (abstract). Transfusion 1992;32:45S.

26. Barton JC, Grindon AJ, Baron NH, Bertoli LF. Hemochromatosis probands as blood donors. Transfusion 1999; 39:578–85.

27. Tan L, Khan MK, Hawk JC. Use of blood therapeutically drawn from

hemochromatosis patients. Transfusion 1999;39:1018–26.

28. McDonnell SM, Grindon AJ, Preston BL, et al. A survey of phlebotomy among persons with hemochromatosis. Transfusion 2002;39:651–6.

29. Gibble JW, Ness PM. Fibrin glue, the perfect operative sealant? Transfusion 1990;30(8):741–7.

30. Filip DJ, Aster RH. Relative hemostatic effectiveness of human platelets stored at 4°C and 22°C. J Lab Clin Med 1978; 91(4):618–24.

31. Murphy S, Heaton WA, Rebulla P. Platelet production in the old world – and the new. Transfusion 1996;36: 751–4.

32. McLeod BC, Price TH, Drew MI, editors. Apheresis: Principles and Practice. Bethesda, MD: AABB Press; 1997. p. 27–65.

33. McCullough J, Kahn J, Adamson J, et al. Hematopoietic growth factors – use in normal blood and stem cell donors: clinical and ethical issues. Transfusion 2008;48:2008–25.

34. Anderlini P, Przepiorka D, Champlin R, Korbling M. Biologic and clinical effects of granulocyte colony-stimulating factor in normal individuals. Blood 1996;88: 2819–25.

35. Stroncek DF, Clay ME, Petzoldt ML, et al. Treatment of normal individuals with granulocyte-colony-stimulating factor: donor experiences and the effects on peripheral blood CD34+ cell counts and on the collection of peripheral blood stem cells. Transfusion 1996;36:601–10.

36. Ottinger HD, Beelen DW, Scheulen B, et al. Improved immune reconstitution after allotransplantation of peripheral blood stem cells instead of bone marrow. Blood 1996;88:2775–9.

37. Wiltbank TM, Giordano GF. The safety profile of automated collections: an analysis of more than 1 million collections. Transfusion 2007;47: 1002–5.

38. Heddle NM, O'Hoski P, Singer J, et al. A prospective study to determine the safety of omitting the antiglobulin crossmatch from pretransfusion testing. Br J Haematol 1992;81:579–84.

39. Pinkerton PH, Coovadia AS, Goldstein J. Frequency of delayed hemolytic transfusion reactions following antibody screening and immediate-spin crossmatching. Transfusion 1992;32: 814–7.

40. Oberman HA, Barnes BA, Friedman BA. The risk of abbreviating the major crossmatch in urgent or massive transfusion. Transfusion 1978;18: 137–41.

41. Daniels G. Human Blood Groups. Massachusetts: Blackwell Science Ltd; 1995.

42. Office of Medical Applications of Research, National Institutes of Health.

Perioperative red cell transfusion. JAMA 1988;260:2700.56.

43. Hebert PC, Wells G, Blajchman MA, et al. A multi-center randomized controlled trial of transfusion requirements in critical care. N Engl J Med 1999;340:409–17.

44. Sniecinski I, O'Donnell MR, Nowicki B, Hill LR. Prevention of refractoriness and HLA-alloimmunization using filtered blood products. Blood 1988;71:1402.

45. Trial to Reduce Alloimmunization to Platelets Study Group. Leukocyte reduction and ultraviolet B irradiation of platelets to prevent alloimmunization and refractoriness to platelet transfusions. Authored by the TRAP Study Group, J. McCullough participant. N Engl J Med 1997;337:1861–9.

46. Vamvakas E, Blajchman MA. Transfusion-related immunomodulation (TRIM): an update. Blood Rev 2008;21:327–48.

47. Bilgin YM, van de Watering LMG, Eijsman L, et al. Double-blind, randomized controlled trial on the effect of leukocyte-depleted erythrocyte transfusions in cardiac-valve surgery. Circulation 2004;109:2755–560.

48. van de Watering LMG, Hermans J, Houbiers JGA, et al. Beneficial effect of leukocyte depletion of transfused blood on post-operative complications in patients undergoing cardiac surgery: a randomized clinical trial. Circulation 1998;97:562–8.

49. National Institutes of Health Consensus Conference. Fresh frozen plasma: indications and risks. JAMA 1985;253: 546.

50. Valeri CR, Pivacek LE, Gray AD, et al. The safety and therapeutic effectiveness of human red cells stored at −80°C for as long as 21 years. Transfusion 1989;29: 429–37.

51. Mannucci PM, Federici AB, Sirchia G. Hemostasis testing during massive blood replacement: a study of 172 cases. Vox Sang 1982;42:113.

52. Counts RB, Haisch C, Simon TL, et al. Hemostasis in massively transfused trauma patients. Ann Surg 1979;190:91.

53. Ness PM, Perkins HA. Cryoprecipitate as a reliable source of fibrinogen replacement. JAMA 1979;241:1690.

54. Slichter SJ, Kaufman R, Assmann SF, et al. Dose of prophylactic platelet transfusions and prevention of hemorrhage(the PLADA trial). N Engl J Med 2010;362:600–13.

55. Gaydos LA, Freireich EJ, Mantel N. The quantitative relation between platelet count and hemorrhage in patients with acute leukemia. N Engl J Med 1962; 266:905–9.

56. Rebulla P, Finazzi G, Marangoni F, et al. The Gruppo Italiano Malattie Ematologiche Maligne dell'Adulto: the threshold for prophylactic platelet transfusions in adults with acute myeloid

leukemia. N Engl J Med 1997;337: 1870–5.

57. Heckman KD, Weiner GJ, Davis CS, et al. Randomized study of prophylactic platelet transfusion threshold during induction therapy for adult acute leukemia: 10,000/μL versus 20,000/μL. J Clin Oncol 1997;15:1143–9.

58. Klumpp TR, Herman JH, Gaughan JP, et al. Clinical consequences of alterations in platelet transfusion dose: a prospective, randomized, double-blind trial. Transfusion 1999;37:674–81.

59. Heddle NM, Cook RJ, Tinmouth A, et al. A randomized controlled trial comparing standard- and low-dose strategies for transfusion of platelets (SToP) to patients with thrombocytopenia. Blood 2009; 113:1564–73.

60. Harker LA, Slichter SJ. The bleeding time as a screening test for evaluation of platelet function. N Engl J Med 1972; 287:155.

61. Bishop JF, Schiffer CA, Aisner J, et al. Surgery in acute leukemia: a review of 167 operations in thrombocytopenic patients. Am J Hematol 1987;26:147.

62. Edelson RN, Chernik NL, Posner JB. Spinal subdural hematomas complicating lumbar puncture. Arch Neurol 1974;31:134–7.

63. Schiffer CA, Andrson KC, Bennett CL, et al. Platelet transfusion for patients with cancer: clinical practice guidelines of the American Society of Clinical Oncology. J Clin Oncol 2001;19: 1519–38

64. Freireich EJ, Kliman A, Gaydos LA, et al. Response to repeated platelet transfusion from the same donor. Ann Intern Med 1963;50:277.

65. Daly PA, Schiffer CA, Aisner J, Wiernik PH. Platelet transfusion therapy: one-hour posttransfusion increments are valuable in predicting the need for HLA-matched preparations. JAMA 1980; 243:435.

66. Bishop JF, McGrath K, Wolf MM, et al. Clinical factors influencing the efficacy of pooled platelet transfusions. Blood 1988;71:383.

67. Murphy S. ABO blood groups and platelet transfusion. Transfusion 1988;28:401.

68. Duquesnoy RJ, Filip DJ, Rodey GE, et al. Successful transfusion of platelets 'mismatched' for HLA antigens to alloimmunized thrombocytopenic patients. Am J Hematol 1977;2:219.

69. Duquesnoy RJ, Vieira J, Aster RH. Donor availability for platelet transfusion support of alloimmunized thrombocytopenic patients. Transplant Proc 1977;9:519.

70. Yankee RA, Grumet FC, Rogentine GN. Platelet transfusion therapy: the selection of compatible platelet donors for refractory patients by lymphocyte HLA typing. N Engl J Med 1969;281:1208.

71. Moroff G, Garratty G, Heal JM, et al. Selection of platelets for refractory patients by HLA matching and prospective crossmatching. Transfusion 1992;32:633.

72. Heal JM, Blumberg N, Masel D. An evaluation of crossmatching, HLA, and ABO matching for platelet transfusions to refractory patients. Blood 1987;70:23.

73. Strauss RG. Neutrophil (granulocyte) transfusions in the new millennium. Transfusion 1998;38:710–2.

74. Bhatia S, McCullough JJ, Perry EH, et al. Granulocyte transfusions: efficacy in fungal infections in neutropenic patients following bone marrow transplantation. Transfusion 1994;34:226–32.

75. Walsh JH, Purcell RH, Morrow AG, et al. Post-transfusion hepatitis after open-heart operations: incidence after administration of blood from commercial and volunteer donor populations. JAMA 1970;211:261.

76. Evatt B, Gompaerts E, McDougal J, Ramsey R. Coincidental appearance of LAV/HTLV antibodies in hemophiliacs and the onset of the AIDS epidemic. N Engl J Med 1985;312:483.

77. Prince AM, Horowitz B, Brotman B. Sterilization of hepatitis and HTLV-III viruses by exposure to try (n-butyl) phosphate and sodium cholate. Lancet 1986;1:706.

78. Aronson, DL. The development of the technology and capacity for the production of factor VIII for the treatment of hemophilia A. Transfusion 1990;30:748.

79. Yaeger AS, Grumet FC, Hafleigh EB, et al. Prevention of transfusion-acquired cytomegalovirus infections in newborn infants. J Pediatr 1981;98:281.

80. Stagno S, Pass RF, Dworsky ME, et al. Congenital cytomegalovirus infection: the relative importance of primary and recurrent maternal infection. N Engl J Med 1982;306:945.

81. Miller WJ, McCullough J, Balfour HH, et al. Prevention of CMV infection following bone marrow transplantation: a randomized trial of blood product screening. Bone Marrow Transplant 1991;7(3):227.

82. Bowden RA, Sayers M, Flournoy N, et al. Cytomegalovirus immune globulin and seronegative blood products prevent primary cytomegalovirus infection after marrow transplantation. N Engl J Med 1986;314:1006.

83. Leitman SF, Holland PV. Irradiation of blood products: indications and guidelines. Transfusion 1985;25:293.

84. Button LN, DeWolf WC, Newburger PE, et al. The effects of irradiation on blood components. Transfusion 1981;21:419.

85. Thaler M, Shamiss A, Orgad S, et al. The role of blood from HLA-homozygous donors in fatal transfusion-associated graft-versus-host disease after open-heart surgery. N Engl J Med 1989;321:25.

86. Arsura EL, Bertelle A, Minkowitz S, et al. Transfusion-associated graft-versus-host disease in a presumed immunocompetent patient. Arch Intern Med 1988;148:1941.

87. Otsuka S, Kunieda K, Hirose M, et al. Fatal erythroderma (suspected graft-versus-host disease) after cholecystectomy. Transfusion 1989;29:544.

88. Tirindelli MC, Flammia G, Sergi F, et al. Fibrin glue for refractory hemorrhagic cystitis after unrelated marrow, cord blood, and haploidentical hematopoietic stem cell transplantation. Transfusion 2009;49:17–175.

89. Hess JR. Blood and coagulation support in trauma care. Hematology 2007; 187–91.

90. Shaz BH, Dente CJ, Harris RS, et al. Transfusion management of trauma patients. Anesth Analg 2009;108:1760–8.

91. Hartmann M, Sucker C, Boehm O, et al. Effects of cardiac surgery on hemostasis. Transf Med Rev 2006;20:230–41.

92. Bick RL. Hemostasis defects associated with cardiac surgery, prosthetic devices, and other extracorporeal circuits. Semin Thromb Hemost 1980;11:249.

93. Zimm AB, Hess JR. Current issues related to the transfusion of stored red blood cells. Vox Sang 2009;96:93–103.

94. Koch GC, Li L, Sessler DI, et al. Duration of red-cell storage and complications after cardiac surgery. N Engl J Med 2008;358:1229–31.

95. McCullough J. Principles of transfusion support before and after hematopoietic cell transplantation. In: Thomas ED, Blume KG, Forman SJ, editors. Hematopoietic Cell Transplantation. Oxford: Blackwell Science; 1999.

96. Sacher RA, Luban NLC, Strauss RG. Current practice and guidelines for the transfusion of cellular blood components in the newborn. Transfusion Med Rev 1989;3:39.

97. Petz LD, Garratty G, editors. Immune Hemolytic Anemias. 2nd ed. Philadelphia: Churchill Livingstone; 2004.

98. Aster RH, Jandl JH. Platelet sequestration in man. II. Immunological and clinical studies. J Clin Invest 1964;43:856.

99. McFarland JG, Frenzke M, Aster RH. Testing of maternal sera in pregnancies at risk for neonatal alloimmune thrombocytopenia. Transfusion 1989; 29:128.

100. Lalezari P. Alloimmune neonatal neutropenia. In: Engelfriet CP, von Loghem JJ, von dem Borne AEGKr, editors. Immunohematology. Amsterdam: Elsevier Science Publishers; 1984. p. 178.

101. Mercuriali F, Inghilleri G, Colotti MT, et al. Bedside transfusion errors: analysis of 2 years' use of a system to monitor and prevent transfusion errors. Vox Sang 1996;70:16–20.

102. FDA/CBER. Fatalities reported to FDA following blood collection and transfusion. Annual summary for fiscal year 2007. Online: http://www.fda.gov/BiologicsBloodVaccines/SafetyAvailability/ReportaProblem/TransfusionDonationFatalities/ucm118316.htm.

103. Osby MA, Saxen S, Nelson J, et al. Safe handling and administration of blood components. Arch Pathol Lab Med 2007;131:690–4.

104. Ryden SE, Oberman HA. Compatibility of common intravenous solutions with CPD blood. Transfusion 1975;15:250.

105. Davenport RD, Strieter RM, Kunkel SL. Red cell ABO incompatibility and production of tumour necrosis factor-alpha. Br J Haematol 1991;78:540–4.

106. Davenport RD, Burdick MD, Strieter RM, Kunkel SL. In vitro production of interleukin-1 receptor antagonist in IgG-mediated red cell incompatibility. Transfusion 1994;34:297–303.

107. Pineda AA, Brzica SM, Taswell HF. Hemolytic transfusion reaction: recent experience in a large blood bank. Mayo Clin Proc 1978;53:378.

108. Honing CL, Bove JR. Transfusion-associated fatalities: review of bureau of biologics reports, 1976–1978. Transfusion 1980;20:653.

109. Perkins HA, Payne R, Ferguson J, et al. Nonhemolytic febrile transfusion reactions: quantitative effects of blood components with emphasis on isoantigenic incompatibility of leukocytes. Vox Sang 1966;11:578.

110. Heddle NM, Klama L, Singer J, et al. The role of the plasma from platelet concentrates in transfusion reactions. N Engl J Med 1994;331:625–8.

111. Tobian AAR, King KE, Ness PM. Prevention of febrile nonhemolytic and allergic transfusion reactions with pretransfusion medication: is this evidence-based medicine? Transfusion 2008;48:2274–6.

112. Popovsky MA, Davenport RD. Transfusion-related acute lung injury: femme fatale? Transfusion 2001;41:312–5 (editorial).

113. Kleinman S, Caulfield T, Chan P, et al. Toward an understanding of transfusion-related acute lung injury: statement of a consensus panel. Transfusion 2004;44:1774–89.

114. Fung YL, Silliman CC. The role of neutrophils in the pathogenesis of transfusion-related acute lung injury. Transf Med Review 2009;23:266–83.

115. Palfi M, Berg S, Berling G. A randomized controlled trial of transfusion-related acute lung injury: is plasma from multiparous blood donors dangerous? Transfusion 2001;41:317–22.

116. Eder AF, Herron R, Strupp A, et al. Transfusion-related acute lung injury surveillance (2003–2005) and the

Transfusion medicine for pathologists

potential impact of the selective use of plasma from male donors in the American Red Cross. Transfusion 2007;47:599–607.

117. Chapman CE, Stainsby D, Jones H, et al. Ten years of hemovigilance reports to transfusion-related acute lung injury in the United Kingdom and the impact of preferential use of male donor plasma. Transfusion 2009;49:440–52.

118. Sandler SG. How I manage patients suspected of having had an IgA anaphylactic transfusion reaction. Transfusion 2006;46:10–3.

119. Eckrich RJ, Mallory DM, Sandler SG. Laboratory tests to exclude IgA deficiency in the investigation of suspected anti-IgA transfusion reactions. Transfusion 1993;33:488–91.

120. Alter HJ, Holland PV, Purcell RH, et al. Posttransfusion hepatitis after exclusion of commercial and hepatitis-B antigen-positive donors. Ann Intern Med 1972; 77:691.

121. Busch MP, Young MJ, Samson SJ, et al. Risk of human immunodeficiency virus (HIV) transmission by blood transfusions before the implementation of HIV-1 antibody screening. Transfusion 1991;31:4.

122. Vamvakas EC, Blajchman MA. Transfusion-related mortality: the ongoing risks of allogeneic blood transfusion and the available strategies for their prevention. Blood 2009;113: 3406–17.

123. Dodd RY. Germs, gels, and genomes: a personal recollection of 30 years in blood-safety testing. In: Stramer SL, editor. Blood safety in the new millennium. Bethesda, MD: American Association of Blood Banks; 2001. p. 99–121.

124. Dodd RY, Notari E 4th, Stramer SL. Current prevalence and incidence of infectious disease markers and estimated window-period risk in the American Red Cross blood donor population. Transfusion 2002;42:975–9.

125. Hollinger FB, Khan NC, Oefinger PA, et al. Posttransfusion hepatitis type A. JAMA 1983;250:2313.

126. Noble RC, Kane MA, Reeves SA, Roeckel I. Posttransfusion hepatitis A in a neonatal intensive care unit. JAMA 1984;252:2711.

127. Choo QL, Kuo G, Weiner AJ, et al. Isolation of a cDNA derived from a blood-borne non-A, non-B viral hepatitis genome. Science 1989;244:359.

128. Alter HJ, Purcell RH, Shih JW, et al. Detection of antibody to hepatitis C virus in prospectively followed transfusion recipients with acute and chronic non-A, non-B hepatitis. N Engl J Med 1989;321:1494.

129. Lackritz EM, Satten GA, Aberle-Grasse J, et al. Estimated risk of transmission of the human immunodeficiency virus by screened blood in the United States. N Engl J Med 1995;333:1721–25.

130. Schreiber GB, Busch MP, Kleinman SH. The risk of transfusion-transmitted viral infections. N Engl J Med 1996;334: 1685–90.

131. Cohen ND, Munoz A, Reitz BA, et al. Transmission of retroviruses by transfusion of screened blood in patients undergoing cardiac surgery. N Engl J Med 1989;320:1172.

132. Busch M, Garratty G. Applications of Molecular Biology to Blood Transfusion Medicine. Bethesda, MD: American Association of Blood Banks; 1997. p. 123–76.

133. Busch MP, Taylor PE, Lenes BA, et al. Screening of selected male blood donors for p24 antigen of human immunodeficiency type 1. Transfusion Safety Study Group. N Engl J Med 1990;323:1308–12.

134. Alter HJ, Epstein JS, Swenson SG, et al. Prevalence of human immunodeficiency virus type 1 p24 antigen in US blood donors – an assessment of the efficacy of testing in donor screening. HIV-antigen study group. N Engl J Med 1990;323: 1312–7.

135. Report of the Interorganizational Task Force on Nucleic Acid Amplification Testing of Blood Donors. Nucleic acid amplification testing of blood donors for transfusion-transmitted infectious diseases. Transfusion 2000;40: 143–59.

136. Busch MP, Kleinman SH, Stramer SL. Nucleic acid amplification testing of blood donations. In: Smit Sibinga CTh, Klein HG, editors. Moleuclar Biology in Blood Transfusion. Dordrecht: Kluwer Academic Publishers; 2000. p. 81–103.

137. Greenwalt TJ, Rios JA. To test or not to test for syphilis: a global problem. Transfusion 2001;41:1045–51.

138. Turner TB, Diseker TH. Duration of infectivity of Treponema pallidum in citrated blood stored under conditions obtaining in blood banks. Bull Johns Hopkins Hosp 1941;68:269.

139. Pealer LN, Martin AA, Petersen LR, et al. for the West Nile Virus Transmission Investigation Team. Transmission of West Nile virus through blood transfusion in the United States in 2002. N Engl J Med 2003;349:1236–45.

140. Peterson LR, Epstein JS. Problem solved? West Nile virus and transfusion safety. N Engl J Med 2005;353:516–7.

141. de Oliveira AM, Beecham MD, Montgomery SP, et al. West Nile virus blood transfusion-related infection despite nucleic acid testing. Transfusion 2004;44:1695–9.

142. Okochi K, Sato H. Adult T-cell leukemia virus, blood donors and transfusion: experience in Japan. Prog Clin Biol Res 1985;182:245.

143. Young C, Losikoff P, Chawla A, et al. Transfusion-acquired Trypanosoma cruzi infection. Transfusion 2007;47:540–4.

144. Galel S, Kirchhoff LV. Risk factors for Trypanosoma cruzi infection in California blood donors. Transfusion 1996;36: 227–31.

145. Tobler LH, Contestable P, Pitina L, et al. Evaluation of new enzyme-linked immunosorbent assay for detection of Chagas antibody in US blood donors. Transfusion 2007;47:90–6.

146. McQuiston JH, Childs JE, Chamberland ME, et al. Transmission of tick-borne agents of disease by blood transfusion: a review of known and potential risks in the United States. Transfusion 2000; 40:274–84.

147. Badon SJ, Fister RD, Cable RG. Survival of Borrelia burgdorferi in blood products. Transfusion 1989;29:581.

148. Mortimer PP, Luban NL, Kelleher JF, Cohen BJ. Transmission of serum parvovirus-like agent by clotting factor concentrates. Lancet 1983;2:482.

149. Koenigbauer UF, Eastlund T, Day JW. Clinical illness due to parvovirus B19 infection after infusion of solvent/detergent-treated pooled plasma. Transfusion 2000;40:1203–6.

150. Eschbach JW, Abdulhadi MH, Browne JK, et al. Recombinant human erythropoietin in anemic patients with end-stage renal disease: results of a phase III multicenter clinical trial. Ann Intern Med 1989;111:992–1000.

151. Evans R, Rader B, Manninen D. Cooperative multicenter EPO clinical trial group: the quality of life of hemodialysis recipients treated with recombinant human erythropoietin. JAMA 1990;263:825–30.

152. Spivak JL. Recombinant human erythropoietin and the anemia of cancer. Blood 1994;84:997–1004.

153. Bohlius J, Schmidlin K, Brillant C, et al. Recombinant human erythropoiesis-stimulating agents and mortality in patients with cancer: a meta analysis of randomized trials. Lancet 2009;373: 1532–42.

154. Fullerton DA, Campbell DN, Whitman GJ. Use of human recombinant erythropoietin to correct severe preoperative anemia. Ann Thorac Surg 1991;51:825–6.

155. Tremper KK, Friedman AE, Levine EM. The preoperative treatment of severely anemic patients with a perfluorochemical oxygen-transport fluid, fluosol-DA. N Engl J Med 1982;307:277.

156. Gould SA, Rosen AL, Sehgal R, et al. Fluosol-DA as a red-cell substitute in acute anemia. N Engl J Med 1986;314:1653.

157. Stowell CP, Levin J, Spiess BD, Windlow RM. Progress in the development of RBC substitutes. Transfusion 2001;41:287–99.

CHAPTER 39

Histocompatibility: HLA and other systems

PE Posch, CK Hurley

Introduction

The classical human leukocyte antigens (HLA-A, HLA-B, HLA-C, HLA-DR, HLA-DQ and HLA-DP) are an integral part of the maintenance of self integrity and of the specific immune response to microbial pathogens and malignancies. The HLA molecules display extensive variability (polymorphism) among their gene and protein sequences. HLA polymorphism is important to survival of the species, threatened with a large number of diverse pathogens with the potential to rapidly mutate to avoid the immune response. However, this diversity impedes the successful transplantation of tissues from one individual to another, especially transplantation of hematopoietic stem cells (HSC). Theoretically, HSC transplantation requires that the donor and recipient be identical (matched) for all classical HLA molecules in order to avoid immune recognition. Any disparity might cause graft rejection, where the donor's cells are destroyed by the recipient's immune system, or graft-versus-host disease (GVHD), where the donor's cells recognize the recipient's tissues as foreign and react to them. Yet, even in cases where the donor and recipient are HLA matched, graft-versus-host disease can occur. Thus, despite the progress made in our understanding of histocompatibility, it is evident that there are histocompatibility antigens that likely have a role in maintaining self integrity and in transplant outcome, in addition to the classical HLA molecules. We are now beginning to broaden our knowledge of what constitutes a histocompatibility antigen and of the immune system receptors that recognize these molecules.

The human major histocompatibility complex

History

What has become known as the major histocompatibility complex (MHC) was initially identified in the early 1900s, but it was not until the late 1930s that studies began to focus on graft acceptance (histocompatibility) and antigen response phenotypes (H-2) in different strains of mice.[1,2] In the 1950s, Dausset detected the first histocompatibility antigens in humans, the MHC class I antigens, with antibodies from multiply transfused patients.[3,4] These antibodies revealed in the human population differing patterns of binding to white blood cells (leukocytes) and each pattern of binding came to define a human leukocyte antigen (HLA) specificity.[5,6] These HLA specificities were later determined to be encoded by three distinct polymorphic loci, HLA-A, HLA-B and HLA-C. The human MHC class II antigens were initially described via their ability to stimulate the proliferation of T-cells from one individual when mixed with lymphocytes from a second individual.[7] Each pattern of T-cell reactivity (allorecognition) to a panel of homozygous typing cells (HTC) was assigned an HLA-D phenotype.[8] It is now known that the HLA-D phenotypes are due to T-cell allorecognition of the products of the MHC class II loci, primarily HLA-DR. HLA-DQ and HLA-DP make minor contributions to these phenotypes. The genes specifying both class I and class II antigens are tightly clustered in a single chromosomal region, the MHC.

Genomic organization

The human MHC is a genetic region located on the short arm of chromosome 6 (6p21.3) extending approximately 4 megabases (Mb) (Fig. 39.1). The MHC encodes over 250 genes and pseudogenes of which at least 150 are expressed as proteins.[9,10] This genetic complex is divided into three regions: (centromeric) class II, class III and class I (telomeric). Although the proteins encoded within the MHC participate in a variety of functions, approximately 40% are devoted to immune system functions.

The class II region (~1.2 Mb) contains at least 34 expressed genes and 16 pseudogenes and spans from SynGAP (Ras-GTPase-activating protein, centromeric) to TSBP (testis-specific basic protein, telomeric).[11] This region includes the

genes that encode for the classical class II molecules (HLA-DR, -DQ and -DP). In addition, gene products involved in MHC class I antigen processing (LMP2 and LMP7, the large multifunctional proteosome genes), peptide transport (TAP1 and TAP2, the transporter associated with antigen processing genes) and complex assembly (tapasin) and gene products involved in MHC class II complex assembly (HLA-DM and HLA-DO) are encoded in this region.

The class III region (~1 Mb) extends from NOTCH4 (transmembrane receptor involved in cell differentiation and development, centromeric) to MCCD1 (mitochondrial coiled-coil domain protein 1, telomeric).[12,13] On average, this region contains 1 gene every 10 kilobases (kb) and is the most gene dense region in the human genome with approximately 72% of it being transcribed. The class III region encodes at least 62 expressed genes including complement components (e.g., C2 and C4B), heat shock proteins (e.g., Hsp70-1 and Hsp70-2) and cytokines of the tumor necrosis factor family (e.g., TNF and LTA). Some individuals have duplications in the area encoding complement component C4B; thus, this area can vary in length.

The class I region (~1.85 Mb) from MICB (centromeric) to HLA-F (telomeric) encodes at least 118 genes; 57 expressed genes and 61 pseudogenes.[14] In some instances, an additional ~0.95 Mb to TRIM27 (tripartite motif 27, a transcription factor, telomeric) is included and called the extended class I region.[9] This region includes the classical class I genes (HLA-A, -B and -C) and the nonclassical class I genes (HLA-E, -F, and -G). This region also encodes the MHC class I chain-related (MIC) genes (MICA and MICB). The focus of this chapter is on the MHC encoded gene products involved in histocompatibility, primarily the classical human leukocyte antigens. Other MHC and nonMHC encoded genes that participate in histocompatibility are also covered.

The human leukocyte antigens

The classical human leukocyte antigens (HLA molecules) include the MHC class I molecules (HLA-A, -B and -C) and the MHC class II molecules (HLA-DR, -DQ and -DP). The primary function of these molecules is to bind small fragments of proteins (peptides) and present them on the surface of cells for immune system surveillance. The principal player in recognition of these HLA molecule + peptide complexes is the T-cell receptor (TCR) expressed by T-cells. Recognition by T-cells can lead to a plethora of immunologic outcomes including inflammation, antibody production and cellular cytotoxicity. At least two of the nonclassical class I molecules perform functions similar to the classical class I molecules, but are more specialized antigen presentation molecules. The following sections will discuss the genetics and structures of the classical HLA molecules, their function with respect to recognition by TCR and their identification, nomenclature and importance in HSC transplantation. Also included are sections on the nonclassical MHC class I molecules, additional MHC and nonMHC encoded histocompatibility antigens and on the receptors, other than the TCR, that recognize histocompatibility molecules as ligands.

Human Major Histocompatibility Complex
Chromosome 6

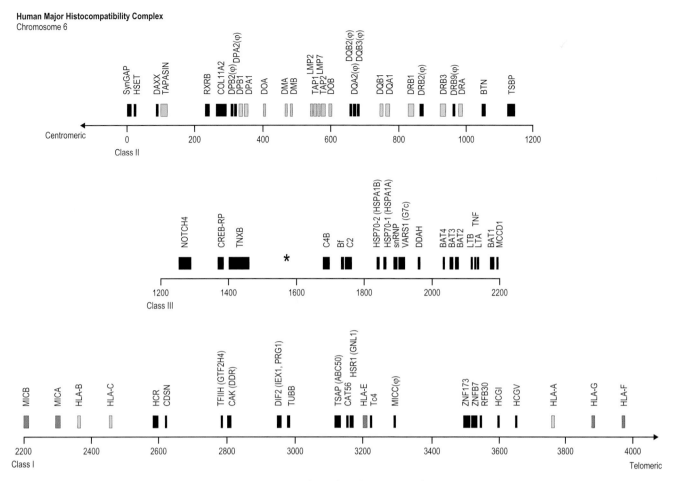

Fig. 39.1 Map of the human major histocompatibility complex (MHC) located on the short arm of chromosome 6. The map (drawn closely to scale) is divided into three regions (class II, class III and class I) and shows the relative positions of some of the MHC encoded genes and pseudogenes (ψ). The class II region encodes the expressed classical HLA class II molecules (yellow). The number of HLA-DR B (DRB) genes and pseudogenes differs for different haplotypes (DR52 haplotype shown; Fig. 39.2). Genes encoding protein products intimately involved in MHC class I and class II molecule assembly and in peptide processing and binding (green) also are shown. The class III region contains several immune system relevant genes and varies in length among individual chromosomes in the area encoding C4B (asterisk). The class I region encodes the classical HLA class I heavy chain proteins (yellow). This region also encodes the expressed nonclassical HLA class I genes (red) and MHC class I chain-related genes (blue). (*The figure was generated from data contained in references.[9,13]*)

Genomic organization

The heavy chains of the classical MHC class I (class Ia) molecules are encoded in the class I region of the MHC and associate with beta 2 microglobulin (encoded on chromosome 15) to form the mature class I molecule. The gene order within the MHC is shown in Fig. 39.1. Each of the classical MHC class I heavy chains is encoded by a single gene that is divided into 8 exons.[15] Exon 1 encodes the 5′ untranslated region (UTR) and the hydrophobic signal sequence. The signal sequence directs insertion of the protein into the membrane at the cell surface and is cleaved from the mature protein. The extracellular portion of the class I heavy chain is encoded by exons 2–4. Exon 5 encodes the transmembrane region and exons 6 and 7 encode the intracellular cytoplasmic tail. The 3′ UTR and the polyadenylation (poly(A)) site are encoded by exon 8. The mRNA, which is translated into protein, includes all eight exons after removal by splicing of the intervening sequences (introns).

The class II region of the MHC contains three subregions (centromeric) HLA-DP, -DQ and -DR (telomeric). Each encodes at least one cell surface class II molecule (Fig. 39.1). The class II molecules are noncovalently associated heterodimers that consist of an α chain and a β chain.[15,16] Each chain is encoded by a separate gene, an A gene for the α chain and a B gene for the β chain. The expressed HLA-DP heterodimer is encoded by the DPA1 and DPB1 genes. The HLA-DP subregion contains two DP pseudogenes, DPA2 and DPB2. The HLA-DQ subregion contains two A (DQA1 and DQA2) and three B (DQB1, DQB2 and DQB3) genes. The expressed HLA-DQ heterodimer is encoded by the DQA1 and DQB1 genes, while the remaining DQ genes are pseudogenes. Each individual has two copies of chromosome 6 and, thus, two copies of each of the expressed HLA-DP and HLA-DQ genes. These genes are polymorphic and, consequently, an individual can have two different expressed A genes and two different expressed B genes for HLA-DP and for HLA-DQ. While not all combinations form,[17] the products of some of these genes can associate in several αβ combinations, regardless of chromosomal origin. Therefore, an individual could express up to four different HLA-DP and up to four different HLA-DQ molecules.

MHC class II DR subregion

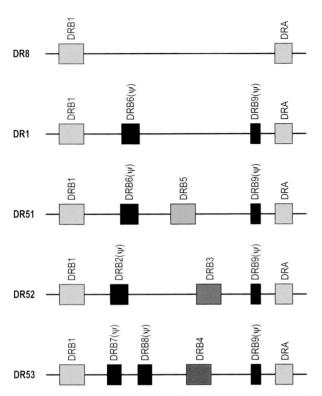

Fig. 39.2 Relative gene organization of the DR subregion of different DR haplotype groups. The protein products of the DRA and DRB1 genes (yellow) combine to form the primary expressed HLA-DR molecule. The protein products of the DRB5 (green), DRB3 (blue) and DRB4 (red) genes encoded by the DR51, DR52 and DR53 haplotype groups, respectively, also form expressed functional DR molecules in combination with the DRA polypeptide. The DRB pseudogenes (ψ) are shown in black. Table 39.4 lists the alleles associated with each haplotype.

The HLA-DR subregion is more complex.[18,19] A HLA-DR molecule composed of a conserved α chain encoded by the DRA gene and a polymorphic β chain encoded by the DRB1 gene is almost always present. This is the major class II molecule expressed on the cell surface. An additional eight DRB genes and pseudogenes have been identified in the HLA-DR subregion. The number of DRB genes present and the number of expressed DRB gene products is characteristic of each chromosome (haplotype) a person inherits (Fig. 39.2). For example, the DR1 haplotype carries two DRB genes, the expressed DRB1 gene and a DRB6 pseudogene. The DR8 haplotype carries only one DRB gene, the expressed DRB1 gene. Other DR subregion haplotypes can encode a second expressed HLA-DR molecule composed of the DRA gene product associated with a DRB3 gene product (DR52 molecule), a DRB4 gene product (DR53 molecule) or a DRB5 gene product (DR51 molecule) and can contain one to three DRB pseudogenes. The designations DR51, DR52 and DR53 are antibody (serologically) defined.

The A genes, which encode the α chains of class II molecules, contain five exons.[15,16] The 5′ UTR and hydrophobic signal sequence are encoded by exon 1, like the class I genes. Exons 2 and 3 encode the extracellular domains. Exon 4 encodes the connecting peptide, the transmembrane region,

the intracellular cytoplasmic tail and a portion of the 3′ UTR. The remainder of the 3′ UTR and the poly(A) signal are encoded by exon 5. Each class II β chain is encoded by a B gene divided into six exons. Exons 1–3 are similar to that of the A genes. Exon 4 encodes the connecting peptide and transmembrane region, while exon 5 encodes the cytoplasmic tail. The 3′ UTR and poly(A) signal are encoded by exon 6. All exons and introns are transcribed into RNA for the class II A and B genes. Again, introns are removed by splicing to form the mRNA that is translated into protein.

Diversity

The nucleotide sequences of many of the HLA genes differ among individuals. These sequence variants are termed alleles; genes with many alleles are termed polymorphic. Alleles of a locus may differ by a single nucleotide to many nucleotides potentially resulting in changes in the amino acid sequence of the protein specified by that gene. The classical HLA class I and class II loci are the most polymorphic loci in humans. The HLA-B and HLA-DRB1 loci have over 1100 and 650 known alleles, respectively (Tables 39.1, 39.2).[20,21] In contrast to non-HLA genes, the nucleotide differences found among HLA alleles are usually nonsynonymous (alter the amino acid sequence) and are focused in the exon(s) encoding the most functionally important region of the HLA molecule, the antigen binding site.[18] It is thought that this diversity has been maintained to provide the human population with the capacity to recognize a diverse repertoire of pathogenic peptides.[22–24] Unfortunately, the allelic differences in HLA molecules expressed on the cells of different individuals can be recognized as foreign when tissue is grafted from one individual to another.

Several mechanisms are hypothesized to have generated this HLA diversity over evolutionary time. The majority of the polymorphism is hypothesized to have arisen by the non-reciprocal exchange of short polymorphic regions or cassettes among alleles, a process referred to as gene conversion. As a result, the HLA alleles are patchworks of polymorphic cassettes, each cassette shared by some of the other alleles at the locus, embedded in a conserved framework (Fig. 39.3). Exchange of cassettes among alleles at different loci, reciprocal recombination involving the exchange of entire exons, and mutation also have contributed to HLA diversity.[18,25]

Each individual inherits two copies of the chromosome carrying the MHC, one from each parent, and thus has two copies of each gene in the MHC. Individuals who carry two identical alleles at a locus are homozygous; individuals with two different alleles at a locus are heterozygous. Because the HLA genes are located within a small genetic distance, they are usually inherited as a block unless separated by recombination. The block, a specific set of alleles at the multiple HLA loci inherited together from a parent, is termed a HLA haplotype. Fig. 39.4 illustrates the inheritance of HLA-A, -B, and -DRB1 alleles within a family. By convention, the paternal haplotypes are generally designated a and b and the maternal haplotypes, c and d. Thus, there are four possible MHC genotypes in the offspring: ac, ad, bc, and bd. Because the chances of inheriting a given genotype are random, the probability of occurrence of any one of the four genotypes is one in four in a mating. In a family with five children, at

Table 39.1 HLA class I alleles[a,b]

HLA-A	HLA-B		HLA-C
A*01010101–*0142	B*070201–*0783	B*510101–*5173	Cw*010201–*0128[c]
A*02010101–*0299 A*9201–*9286[d]	B*080101–*0842	B*520101–*5215	Cw*020201–*0228
A*03010101–*0359	B*130101–*1326	B*530101–*5318	Cw*030201–*0361
A*110101–*1147	B*1401–*1411	B*5401–B*5419	Cw*04010101–*0441
A*230101–*2321	B*15010101–*1599 B*9501–*9564[d]	B*550101–*5535	Cw*05010101–*0525
A*24020101–*2499	B*180101–*1837	B*5601–*5624	Cw*06020101–*0624
A*250101–*2509	B*2701–*2754	B*570101–*5722	Cw*070101–*0774
A*260101–*2640	B*350101–*3599	B*580101–*5822	Cw*080101–*0827
A*29010101–*2920	B*370101–*3715	B*5901–*5905	Cw*120201–*1222
A*300101–*3029	B*380101–*3819	B*670101–*6702	Cw*140201–*1412
A*310102–*3127	B*39010101–*3950	B*7301	Cw*150201–*1522
A*320101–*3220	B*400101–*4098	B*7801–*7806	Cw*160101–*1614
A*330101–*3326	B*4101–*4109	B*8101–*8104N	Cw*1701–*1705
A*340101–*3408	B*4201–*4212	B*8201–*8202	Cw*1801–*1803
A*3601–3604	B*44020101–*4474	B*8301	
A*4301	B*4501–*4509		
A*6601–*6610	B*460101–4621		
A*680101–*6848	B*47010101–*4705		
A*6901	B*480101–*4819		
A*7401–*7414N	B*490101–4905		
A*8001	B*5001–*5004		

[a]Listing of class I alleles assigned by July 2009.[20,21] The number of HLA class I alleles continues to increase as more individuals are studied. Alleles are defined by DNA sequencing. An expanded and updated table can be found at http://hla.alleles.org.

[b]Each column is independent. Each row lists the names of one to several alleles. For example, A*01010101–A*0142 includes alleles, A*01010101, A*01010102N, A*0102, A*0103, A*0104N for a total of 49 alleles whose names begin with A*01. The number of alleles included depends on the number and characteristics of the alleles described. The names of alleles are discarded if the nucleotide sequences are found to be in error. For example, alleles B*0701 and Cw*1301 have been deleted.

[c]'w' is added to avoid confusion with the complement genes. In 2010, the Nomenclature Committee removed the 'w' from the designation and added colons to separate fields so that Cw*010201 was renamed C*01:02:01 (Table 39.9).

[d]Since each field in the name of an allele can only be two digits in length, the over 100 alleles in the A*02 family have been designated A*02010101–A*0299 and A*9201–A*9286. In 2010, these alleles were renamed so that the series of alleles became A*02:01:01:01–A*02:186. B*15 alleles have also been designated in two series, B*15 and B*95. In 2010, these alleles were renamed B*15:01:01:01–B*15:164. Table 39.9 includes additional information on the changes in HLA nomenclature format that became effective in April 2010.

least two of the children will be MHC identical unless recombination has occurred.

The alleles in the MHC complex can be reshuffled by crossing over between homologous chromosomes during the generation of sperm or eggs. The frequency of recombination across the MHC from HLA-A to HLA-DPB1 can range from 0.7 to 4.3%.[26] Studies in humans suggest that there are several sites at which recombination preferentially occurs within the MHC, particularly between HLA-B and HLA-DRB1 and between HLA-DQB1 and HLA-DPB1.[26,27] Studies comparing MHC-identical sib pairs versus haplotype mismatched sib pairs and unrelated individuals show that recombination rates can vary up to sixfold between individu-als with different MHC haplotypes and suggest a genetic influence within the MHC on recombination rates.[26] On average, the frequency of recombination between HLA-A and HLA-B is 0.7%, between HLA-B and HLA-DRB1 is 1.0%, and between DQB1 and DPB1 is 0.8%. Recombinations between DQA1 and DRB1 loci and between B and C loci are very rare.

The HLA alleles and haplotypes found in individuals depend on their racial and ethnic backgrounds.[28,29] For example, the allele DRB1*0302 is found in African Americans, but is only rarely observed in individuals of northern European or Asian descent. Likewise, the frequency of a combination of alleles on a single copy of chromosome 6 can differ among population groups. Table 39.3 lists the ten

Table 39.2 HLA class II alleles[a,b]

DR	DQ	DP
DRA*0101–*010202[c]	DQA1*010101–0107[h]	DPA1*010301–*0110[j]
DRB1*010101–*0122[d]	DQA1*0201	DPA1*020101–*0204
DRB1*03010101–*0348	DQA1*030101–*0303	DPA1*0301–*0303
DRB1*040101–*0478	DQA1*040101–*0404	DPA1*0401
DRB1*07010101–*0717	DQA1*050101–*0509	DPB1*010101–*9901[k]
DRB1*080101–*0836	DQA1*060101–*0602	
DRB1*090102–*0908	DQB1*020101–*0205[i]	
DRB1*100101–*1003	DQB1*030101–*0325	
DRB1*110101–*1181	DQB1*0401–*0403	
DRB1*120101–*1219	DQB1*050101–*0505	
DRB1*130101–*1392	DQB1*060101–*0635	
DRB1*140101–*1490		
DRB1*15010101–*1533		
DRB1*160101–*1613N		
DRB3*01010201–*0113[e]		
DRB3*0201–*0224		
DRB3*030101–*0303		
DRB4*01010101–*0107[f]		
DRB4*0201N		
DRB4*0301N		
DRB5*010101–*0113[g]		
DRB5*0202–*0205		

[a]Listing of class II alleles assigned by July 2009.[20,21] The number of HLA class II alleles continues to increase as more individuals are studied. Alleles are defined by DNA sequencing. An expanded and updated table can be found at http://hla.alleles.org. A description of the nomenclature in this table can be found in Table 39.9.

[b]Each column is independent.

[c]Alleles of the DRA locus. The differences among these DR alpha chain alleles are not considered important for transplantation matching.

[d]Alleles of the DRB1 locus. Most haplotypes contain a DRB1 locus.

[e]Alleles of the DRB3 locus, the second expressed DR molecule in haplotypes carrying DRB1*03, *11, *12, *13, *14 alleles.

[f]Alleles of the DRB4 locus, the second expressed DR molecule in haplotypes carrying DRB1*04, *07, *09 alleles.

[g]Alleles of the DRB5 locus, the second expressed DR molecule in haplotypes carrying DRB1*15, *16 alleles.

[h]Alleles of the DQA1 locus. DQA1 allelic products pair with DQB1 allelic products to form the DQ molecule.

[i]Alleles of the DQB1 locus.

[j]Alleles of the DPA1 locus. DPA1 allelic products pair with DPB1 allelic products to form the DP molecule.

[k]Alleles of the DPB1 locus. The approach to naming DPB1 alleles was slightly different than that used for other loci because of the lack of serologic information.[20]

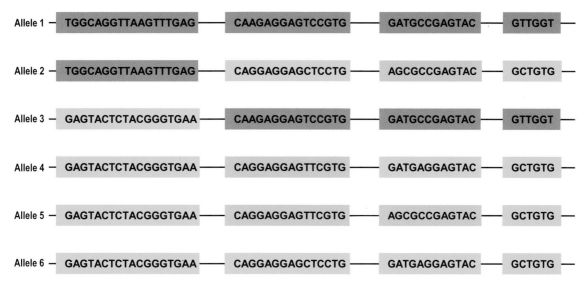

Fig. 39.3 Representation of a polymorphic exon of several HLA alleles. Each allele is a combination of conserved (solid line, nucleotides not shown) and polymorphic (colored blocks) nucleotide sequences. The polymorphic nucleotides form 'cassettes' which are shared among HLA alleles. The combination of cassettes within an HLA gene characterizes a specific allele. To identify the exact HLA alleles present in an individual, DNA-based typing must be able to identify these multiple cassettes and to link the cassettes to one another.

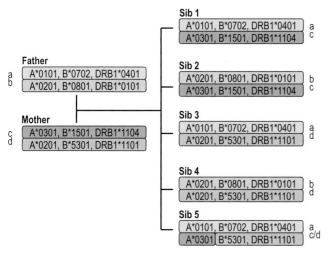

Fig. 39.4 The inheritance of HLA alleles and haplotypes within a family. Paternal haplotypes are labeled a,b; maternal haplotypes, c,d. Sibling 5 inherits a recombinant chromosome from the mother. Not all HLA genes are shown. The HLA nomenclature used in the figure is described in Table 39.9.

most common haplotypes identified in the African American population compared to the ranking of these haplotypes in several other US populations.[29] For example, the most common haplotype in African Americans is A*3001, Cw*1701, B*4201, DRB1*0302 found at a frequency of 1.5%. This haplotype was ranked 37th in Hispanic Americans but was not observed in this sampling of European Americans and Asian Americans.

There are, however, some alleles and haplotypes that are found in many populations. For example, the allele A*0201 is a common allele in many US populations, being found in 29.6% of European Americans, 12.5% of African Americans, 9.5% of Asian Americans and 19.4% of Hispanic Americans.[29] The most common haplotype in European Ameri-

cans, A*0101, Cw*0701, B*0801, DRB1*0301, is the second most frequent haplotype in African Americans and Hispanic Americans but is the 191st most frequent haplotype in Asian Americans.

When large databases of HLA typed individuals are analyzed, only a small percent of potential HLA phenotypes are found. Using serologic assignments from an unrelated donor registry, of the predicted 19 536 660 HLA-A,-B,-DR phenotypes, only 1.6% were observed.[30] This suggests that not all HLA allele combinations will be found. Indeed, some HLA haplotypes appear more frequently than expected. Linkage disequilibrium measures the degree of non-random association between alleles of separate loci. Apparently high disequilibrium across the DR-DQ subregion coupled with a lack of recombination have resulted in specific associations between DQA1 and DQB1 alleles and between DRB1 and DQ alleles although a single allele such as DQB1 may be associated with one of several partner alleles. For example, DQB1*0602 is found on the same chromosome as the DQA1 alleles DQA1*0102, or *0103 or *0104, but has not been observed with DQA1*0201, *0301, *0401, or *0501.[31,32] These associations may differ among individuals of different racial/ethnic backgrounds. For example, DRB1*0901 is associated with DQB1*0201 in African Americans but with DQB1*0303 in individuals of northern European descent. Within the DR subregion, specific allele combinations at the several DRB loci are associated with families of DR haplotypes (Fig. 39.2). For example, the DRB3 locus is found in haplotypes carrying specific DRB1 alleles including DRB1*0301, *1101, *1201, *1301, and *1401 alleles (Table 39.4). In the class I region, associations between HLA-B and -C alleles have also been noted.[29]

Extension of linkage disequilibrium across longer regions of the MHC has resulted in associations between specific class I and class II alleles. The associations of multiple alleles result in extended haplotypes.[33,34] The most well known extended haplotype is A*0101, Cw*0701, B*0801, DRB1*0301

Table 39.3 The ten most common African American haplotypes and their ranking in individuals of other ethnicities from a US registry[a,b]

	African Americans				Rank		
	A	C	B	DRB1	European American	Hispanic American	Asian American
1	3001	1701g	4201	0302	NA	37	NA
2	0101g	0701g	0801g	0301	1	2	191
3	6801g	0602	5802	1201g	NA	NA	NA
4	0301g	0702	0702g	1501	2	3	NA
5	3601	0401g	5301	1101	NA	1929	NA
6	3303	0401g	5301	0804	1046	210	NA
7	6802	0304	1510	0301	NA	98	NA
8	3402	0401g	4403	1503	2513	520	1799
9	2902	1601	4403	0701	5	1	NA
10	0201g	0501g	4402g	0401	3	28	406

[a]An expanded and searchable list of haplotypes from all four US populations is provided at http://bioinformatics.nmdp.org.[29]

[b]Haplotypes predicted at the allele level. The letter 'g' indicates a group of alleles that share the nucleotide sequence of exons encoding the antigen binding groove of the HLA molecule. For example Cw*1701g includes Cw*1701, Cw*1702, and Cw*1703. c NA, haplotype not observed in the population study.

Table 39.4 DR haplotypes[a]

DR molecules encoded	Expressed DR loci included in haplotype	DRB1 alleles associated with haplotype
DR, DR51	DRA, DRB1, DRB5	DRB1*15, *16
DR, DR52	DRA, DRB1, DRB3	DRB1*03, *11, *12, *13, *14
DR, DR53	DRA, DRB1, DRB4	DRB1*04, *07, *09
DR	DRA, DRB1	DRB1*01, *08, *10

[a]It should be noted that there are exceptions to these associations. For examples, DRB1*15 haplotypes have been observed that lack a DRB5 locus and some DRB5 positive haplotypes lack a DRB1 locus. In addition, some DRB1*01 haplotypes carry a DRB5 locus.

which is common in northern Europe, appearing at a frequency of approximately 5–15%.[28] It has been hypothesized that these associations may have been maintained in the population by selection, that is, associations between DR and DQ as well as associations within an extended haplotype might represent optimal combinations of immune response molecules. It is also likely that features of the genome structure limiting recombination or changes in the structure of the population, such as through admixture of different ethnic groups, have caused the linkage disequilibrium. Because alleles at various HLA loci are non-randomly associated, these associations enhance the frequency with which individuals share alleles across multiple HLA loci facilitating the selection of HLA identical individuals as tissue donors.

Expression

Classical MHC class I proteins are expressed by most nucleated cells, but the level of expression on the cell surface varies for different cell types. *Cis*-acting sequence blocks (enhancer A, interferon-stimulated response element (ISRE), W/S box, X box (previously known as site α) and Y box (previously known as enhancer B)) in the regulatory (promoter) region upstream of each class I gene control gene expression (Fig. 39.5A).[35] Each promoter sequence block binds numerous proteins (transcription factors) that regulate the level of transcription of the gene and ultimately the amount of protein at the cell surface. For example, enhancer A binds stimulating protein 1 (Sp1) and various members of the NF-κB/rel family of transcription factors. Collectively, the complex is termed NF-κB. Normal class I gene expression requires the coordinated action of each of these regulatory elements; however, disruption of any one sequence block reduces, but does not appear to ablate, MHC class I expression.

The amounts of HLA-A, -B and -C molecules expressed at the surface of a cell are not equal.[36] HLA-A and -B are abundant with HLA-A expressed at somewhat higher levels than HLA-B, in many instances. HLA-C is expressed at very low levels in comparison accounting for about 10% of cell surface class I molecules. This is due to sequence variations in the regulatory blocks of each class I locus (Fig. 39.5B) which alter the type and affinity of transcription factor binding. For example, only NF-κB/rel family members bind to enhancer A in the HLA-A promoter, while enhancer A in the HLA-B promoter binds SP1 in addition to NF-κB/rel family members. The inclusion of SP1 binding may lead to less efficient expression of the HLA-B gene. There are also allele specific differences in the nucleotide sequence of these regulatory elements such that, for example, different HLA-B alleles are expressed at different levels. Additionally, some HLA-B allele promoter regions encode an E box regulatory element that binds the transcription factors upstream stimulatory factor 1 (USF-1) and USF-2. The presence of the E box correlates with reduced basal expression levels of these HLA-B alleles.[35]

A MHC class I promoter

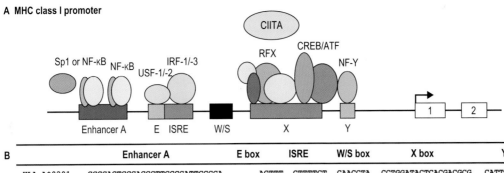

B

	Enhancer A	E box	ISRE	W/S box	X box	Y box
HLA-A*0201	GGGGAGTCCCAGCCTTGGGGATTCCCCA		AGTTT..CTTTTCT	CAACCTA	CCTGGATACTCACGACGCG	CATTGGGTGTC
HLA-B*3501	GGGGAGGCGCAGCGTTGGGGATTCCCCA	CACG AG	TTTCACTTCTTC	CAACCTA	CCAGGATACTCGTGACGCG	CATTGGGTGTC
HLA-B*3801	GGGGAGGCGCAGCATTGGGGATTCCCCA		AGTTTCACTTCTTC	CAACTTG	CCAGGATACTCGTGACGCA	CATTGGGTGTC
HLA-B*4201	GGGGAGGCGCAGCGTTGGGGATTCCCCA		AGTTTCACTTCTTC	CAACTTG	CCAGGATACTCGTGACGCG	CATTGGGTATT
HLA-C*0304	GGGGAGGCGCCGCGTTGAGGATTCTCCA		AGTTTCACTTCTTC	CAACCTG	CCTGAATACTCATGACGCG	CATTGGGTGTC
HLA-C*0401	GGGGAGGCGCCGCGTTGGGGATTCTCCA		AGTTTCACTTCTTC	CAACCTG	CCTGAATACTCATGACGCG	CATTGGGTGTC

C MHC class II promoter

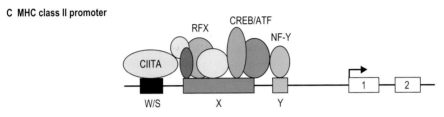

Fig. 39.5 (A–C) The promoter regions of the classical MHC class I and class II genes. (A) MHC class I gene expression is regulated by sequence blocks: enhancer A, E box, interferon-stimulated response element (ISRE) and the SXY module (W/S, X and Y boxes). Each block binds specific transcription factor complexes such as interferon response factor 1 and 3 (IRF-1/-3), regulatory factor X (RFX) and nuclear factor Y (NF-Y) that regulate expression. (B) Nucleotide sequences of each regulatory block of several MHC class I alleles compared to that of HLA-A*0201 with nucleotide variations underlined. Nucleotide sequence variations dictate the set of transcription factors that comprise each complex and the binding affinity of the complex to the regulatory block. These differences cause variations in the level of transcription of each class I gene and ultimately to differences in the level of specific MHC class I molecules expressed at the cell surface. (C) MHC class II gene expression is regulated by the SXY module. Again, each block of this module binds specific transcription factor complexes. Unlike class I gene expression, class II gene expression is entirely dependent on the class II transactivator (CIITA) (yellow). Similar to class I gene expression, differences in the nucleotide sequence of class II allele regulatory sequence blocks (examples not shown) ultimately affect the level of specific MHC class II molecules expressed at the cell surface. Transcription start site in (A) and (C) denoted with an arrow.

MHC class I gene expression can be up-regulated by various cytokines.[35,36] Interferon-γ (IFN-γ) performs a fundamental role in enhancing MHC class I expression by inducing increased gene transcription via transactivation of the ISRE. Again, locus and allele specific sequence differences in the ISRE result in different levels of transcriptional enhancement for each of the class I genes. Additionally, IFN-γ up-regulates expression of the class II transactivator (CIITA) further enhancing MHC class I gene expression. Other cytokines, such as tumor necrosis factor (TNF), can enhance the stimulatory effect of INF-γ on MHC class I gene expression via up-regulation of NF-κB that acts through enhancer A.

MHC class II protein expression is more limited than that of MHC class I. Cell surface HLA-DR, -DQ and -DP molecules are found primarily on professional antigen presenting cells (APC) and on other immune system cells such as T-lymphocytes.[36,37] Professional APC are bone marrow derived cells dedicated to the task of peptide presentation by MHC molecules and include B-lymphocytes, macrophages, dendritic cells, thymic epithelial cells and Kupffer cells. IFN-γ can induce class II expression in other cell types. Like the class I genes, the promoter regions of the class II genes contain the *cis*-acting sequence blocks W/S box, X box and Y box (termed the SXY module) that regulate gene expression (Fig. 39.5C). This is a conserved regulatory module present in the promoters of a wide range of genes involved in antigen presentation which functions as a single regulatory block. The X and Y boxes bind several ubiquitous transcription factors, such as regulatory factor X (RFX) and nuclear factor Y (NF-Y), respectively, in a complex termed the enhanceosome.[38,39]

Occupancy of the class II gene regulatory elements by the enhanceosome is absolutely required, but not adequate for expression and IFN-γ induction of the A and B genes of HLA-DR, -DQ and -DP. CIITA also is required for class II gene expression.[35,38] Cell type specific and IFN-γ induction of class II expression is the direct result of CIITA expression patterns. Constitutive expression of CIITA is confined to professional APC and other immune system cells and can be induced by IFN-γ in other cell types, paralleling expression of MHC class II. CIITA is recruited to the enhanceosome of the class II promoter by the S box. This is not the case for class I gene expression for which the S box apparently plays no role. All of the other transcription factors that regulate class II gene transcription are ubiquitously expressed and constitutively occupy the regulatory sequence blocks in the MHC class II gene promoters. Of interest, patients with bare lymphocyte syndrome (MHC class II deficiency) can have a defect in any one of a number of the transcription factors that bind to the SXY module or in CIITA. These patients still express MHC class I albeit at reduced levels.

HLA-DR, -DQ and -DP are not expressed at the same levels on cell surfaces, similar to expression of the different MHC class I molecules. HLA-DR is the most abundant MHC class II molecule expressed by cells. DRB1 is expressed at a higher level compared to DRB3 and DRB4.[40,41] HLA-DQ is expressed at reduced levels and HLA-DP is the least abundant cell surface class II molecule. Like the regulatory elements in the promoters of class I genes, there are both locus and allele specific sequence differences in the regulatory elements of the class II genes.[36] These sequence differences account for the dissimilar levels of class II molecule expression in two ways: 1) alter the binding affinity of the transcription factors and 2) allow binding of proteins that repress gene transcription of specific class II loci. For example, the X box in the HLA-DPA1 gene promoter region specifically binds the X box repressor protein which diminishes transcription of the HLA-DPA1 gene and reduces the overall level of HLA-DP on the cell surface.

Some pathogenic micoorganisms and many malignant cells down-regulate HLA gene expression to avoid recognition by the immune system.[42–44] For example, human cytomegalovirus (CMV) interferes with IFN-γ induction of MHC class I and class II gene expression.[45] To avoid detection by T-cells, many carcinomas and lymphomas lack cell surface HLA-A and HLA-B molecules due to defects in the expression or the binding of specific transcription factors to the promoter regulatory blocks of these genes. In many instances, expression of HLA-C in these malignant cells is unaffected, allowing the cell to avoid recognition by natural killer (NK) cells. In fact, alterations in MHC class I expression is very common (reported to be 70% or greater) in a variety of tumor types such as cervical, breast and colorectal cancers.[42]

Structure of class I and class II molecules

The classical class I molecules (HLA-A, -B and -C) are expressed on cell surfaces as a trimolecular complex. This complex is composed of the HLA class I polypeptide (heavy chain), beta 2 microglobulin (β2m) and a peptide. The MHC encoded class I heavy chains are glycosylated transmembrane proteins of approximately 340 amino acids (~44 kilodaltons (kD)) that belong to the immunoglobulin (Ig) superfamily of proteins.[15,46] The extracellular portion of the class I heavy chain is composed of the amino-terminal 275 amino acids. The following 40 amino acids make up the hydrophobic transmembrane region and the carboxy-terminal 25 amino acids comprise the intracellular cytoplasmic tail. As an aside, soluble isoforms of the classical HLA molecules are produced and may have immunoregulatory roles.[47]

The extracellular portion of the class I heavy chain is divided into three domains, termed α1, α2 and α3 (Fig. 39.6A). Each domain is encoded by a separate exon (exons 2–4, respectively) and is approximately 90 amino acids long.

The 3D structures of the extracellular portion of several class I molecules were resolved by X-ray crystallography.[48,49] The α1 and α2 domains fold together to form a groove (termed the antigen binding groove) distal to the cell membrane that consists of a floor of eight antiparallel beta strands topped by two alpha helices fashioned into the walls. The membrane proximal α3 domain folds into a structure which is similar to that of the constant region domains of immunoglobulins (antibodies). This domain is composed of two antiparallel beta sheets, one with four strands and one with three strands. The sheets are linked by a disulfide bond. β2m (~12 kD) is non-covalently associated with the α3 domain of the class I heavy chain and is required for cell surface expression. Its 3D structure is identical to that of the α3 domain of the heavy chain.

The peptide, the third component of the trimolecular complex, is generally 8–10 amino acids in length and non-covalently bound to the class I heavy chain.[48,49] It lies in the groove formed by the α1 and α2 domains (Fig. 39.6C). The peptide is anchored at its amino- and carboxy-terminal ends by non-covalent bonds to amino acid residues in the class I heavy chain. There are pockets along the groove which accommodate amino acid side chains at various positions along the peptide. The pockets are unique for each class I molecule because polymorphic residues from the α1 and α2 domains participate in their formation. Each pocket has specific physical and chemical characteristics that are determined by the conserved and polymorphic class I residues that form the pocket. These characteristics, in turn, dictate which amino acid side chains are accommodated at the corresponding peptide position. This defines the peptide binding motif of each class I molecule and defines the overall character of the set of peptides bound (Table 39.5).[50,51] For example, the protein encoded by A*1101 will accommodate a variety of 'small' amino acids at peptide postions 2, 3 and 6 and prefers basic amino acids at peptide position 9. However, each pocket does not make an equal contribution to peptide binding. Certain pockets, specific to each class I molecule, play a more predominant role and the corresponding peptide position is termed an anchor position. The preferred amino acids at an anchor position are termed anchor residues. Using the protein encoded by A*1101 again as an example, although peptide positions 2, 3 and 6 contribute to peptide binding, it is peptide position 9 that is the anchor position. Lysine and arginine are the anchor residues at this position with lysine preferred over arginine. It is of note that not all peptides that bind to an HLA molecule fully adhere to the defined peptide binding motif and that amino acids other than anchor residues can be found at anchor positions in these peptides. In the end, each class I molecule does bind a unique, large set of peptides and the peptide set shares particular sequence characteristics which are dictated by the amino acid residues that make up the groove of the HLA class I heavy chain.

There are benefits to determining the peptide binding motif for HLA molecules. For example, these motifs can be used to identify antigenic peptides from pathogen proteins as candidates for use in peptide based vaccines. As another example, expression of specific HLA allelic products is associated with an increased risk of developing many autoimmune diseases.[52,53] In most cases, this is thought to be the result

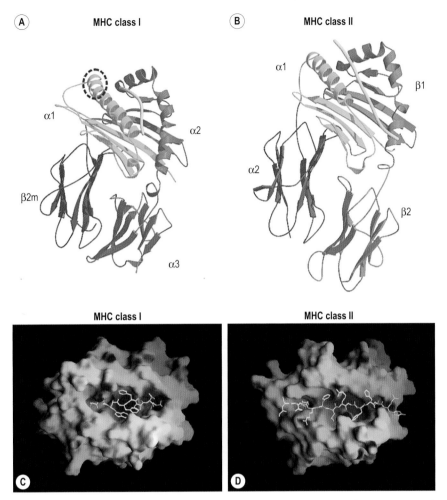

Fig. 39.6 (A–D) Classical MHC class I and class II structures. (A) Ribbon diagram of the extracellular portion of a representative classical MHC class I molecule encoded by HLA-A*0201. The antigen binding groove is formed by the α1 (green) and α2 (blue) domains of the class I heavy chain. An eight-stranded β pleated sheet (broad arrows) forms the floor of the groove which is overlaid on two sides by α helical walls (twists). The backbone of a peptide (yellow) is seen within the groove. The α3 domain (brown) of the class I heavy chain non-covalently associates with beta 2 microglobulin (β2m; red). The transmembrane region and cytoplasmic tail (not visualized) would extend toward the bottom of the figure. The relative position of the HLA-Bw4/Bw6 and NK KIR C1/C2 epitopes on the α1 helix is circled. (B) Ribbon diagram of the extracellular portion of a representative MHC class II molecule, HLA-DR1; DR(α,β1*0101). The antigen-binding groove is formed by first domains of the α chain (α1; green) and β chain (β1; blue), similar to that of MHC class I. The backbone of a peptide (yellow) is shown in the groove. The class II α chain α2 domain (red) and class II β chain β2 domain (brown) form structures similar to β2m and the class I heavy chain α3 domain, respectively. The transmembrane region and cytoplasmic tail (not visualized) would extend toward the bottom of the figure. Top view of the electrostatic surface of the antigen binding grooves of the (C) class I molecule and (D) class II molecule shown in A and B, respectively. Negatively and positively charged surfaces are denoted by red and blue, respectively. The respective peptides (yellow) are depicted as stick models showing the carbon backbone and side chains. Pockets binding amino acid side-chains of each peptide are clearly visible in each figure. Ribbon diagrams were generated with the program Molescript and electrostatic surface models were generated with the program Grasp on a Silicon Graphics workstation from Protein Data Bank accession codes 1b0g (MHC class I) and 1aqd (MHC class II).

of the differential binding capacity of HLA molecules for particular peptides. Thus, knowing the binding motif for a HLA molecule aids in the identification of the culprit peptide and allows for the design of synthetic peptides that mimic disease associated peptides for use in blocking autoimmune responses. Because the number of HLA allelic products is so large, algorithms have been developed for prediction of peptide binding to HLA molecules.[54–57]

The class II molecules are expressed on cell surfaces as a trimolecular complex, structurally analogous to the class I molecules, and consist of the class II α chain, the class II β chain and a peptide. Both the class II α (34 kD) and β (28 kD) chains are transmembrane glycoproteins and are Ig

superfamily members, comparable to the class I heavy chain.[15,16] The extracellular portion of the α and β chains are divided into two domains, the membrane distal α1 and β1 domains and the membrane proximal α2 and β2 domains. Similar to the class I heavy chains, each domain is encoded by a separate exon (exons 2 and 3, respectively) and is about 90 amino acids in length. Three additional regions complete each chain of the class II molecule; a connecting peptide of 12 amino acids which is highly hydrophilic and links the membrane proximal domain to the transmembrane region, a 23 amino acid hydrophobic transmembrane region and an intracellular cytoplasmic tail that consists of the carboxy terminal 8–15 amino acids.

Table 39.5 MHC class I and class II peptide binding motifs[a]

Allele	Relative amino acid position in peptide								
	1	2	3	4	5	6	7	8	9
A*0201		LMIVAT[b,c]		EPDG		LVI			VLIAM
A*0206		VQIL	ILPV	EPDG		LIVF			VLI
A*0101		TSM	DEAS						Y
A*1101		small[d]	small			small			KR
B*3701		DE			VI			FML	ILMF
Cw*0301		A	VIY	PE		FY			L
DRB1*0101	YFWILV			LMAIV		AG			LMAV
DRB1*1501	LVI			FYI			ILVMF		
DRB5*0101	FYLM			QVIM					RK
DQA1*0102[e] DQB1*0602						LIV			AGST
DPA1*0201[e] DPB1*0901	RK					AGL			LV

[a57]

[b]Amino acids denoted by single letter designation.

[c]Bold indicates amino acids that are optimal anchor residues. Normal face type indicates amino acids that are strong anchor residues. Strike through indicates that the amino acid is not allowed at that position.

[d]Small amino acids include: A, G, S, T, L, M, I, V, N.

[e]The alleles specifying both chains of the DQ and DP molecules contribute to the HLA antigen binding site and the characteristics of the bound peptides.

The 3D structures of the extracellular portion of several class II molecules have been determined by X-ray crystallography.[48,49,58] These structures are strikingly similar to that of class I molecules. The α1 and β1 domains fold together to form a peptide binding groove like the groove formed by the class I heavy chain α1 and α2 domains (Fig. 39.6B). The α2 and β2 domains of the class II chains fold to form Ig constant region domain like structures similar to that of the class I α3 domain and β2m.

The peptides that bind to class II molecules are anchored to the class II antigen binding groove by non-covalent bonds to the peptide backbone and by binding of peptide amino acid side chains into pockets along the groove (Fig. 39.6D), similar to the class I molecules.[49,58,59] Because of the polymorphic nature of the MHC class II proteins, each class II molecule, like each class I molecule, also binds a large set of peptides which share a peptide binding motif specific to that class II molecule (Table 39.5). The peptides that bind to class II molecules are heterogenous in length and generally 13–25 amino acids long. The low and open ends of the class II groove allow peptides of varying lengths to bind in an extended conformation with the ends of the peptide overhanging the ends of the groove. This is in contrast to the class I molecules which bind peptides of 8–10 amino acids. The ends of the class I groove are high and closed; thus, MHC class I molecules optimally accommodate shorter peptides whose ends are tucked into the groove (compare Fig. 39.6C and 39.6D).

Function

Peptide processing and binding

Mature cell surface class I molecules are formed in the endoplasmic reticulum (ER) with the aid of several resident ER proteins including tapasin, calnexin and calreticulin.[60,61] Initially, the class I heavy chain and β2m fold and associate facilitated by calnexin and calreticulin (Fig. 39.7). This complex then transiently associates with the transporter associated with antigen processing (TAP) where a peptide is loaded into the groove of the class I heavy chain. Finally, the trimolecular complex is dispatched to the cell surface.

Peptides, derived from both self (normal cellular) proteins (potential autoantigens) or foreign proteins (antigens), are generated in the cytosol by the proteosome.[60,61] The proteosome is a macromolecular structure that proteolytically cleaves proteins into peptides (a process termed antigen processing) and consists of members of the large multifunctional proteosome (LMP) family and other protein subunits. Two LMP family members (LMP2 and LMP7) are encoded in the class II region of the MHC. The proteosome is tightly associated with the TAP molecule which shuttles the peptides into the lumen of the ER.[60,61] TAP is formed by the association of the products of the TAP1 and TAP2 genes also encoded in the MHC class II region. Another MHC encoded gene product, tapasin, stabilizes the TAP heterodimers, links the class I heavy chain to TAP for peptide loading and facilitates loading of peptides onto the class I molecule. An

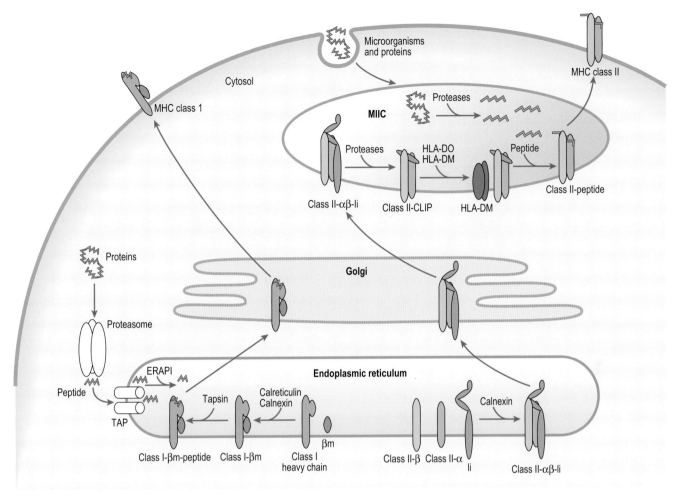

Fig. 39.7 MHC class I and class II peptide processing and binding. MHC class I peptide processing and binding is depicted in the left portion of the figure. Class I heavy chain (blue) and beta 2 microglobulin (β_2m) (lavender) fold and associate in the endoplasmic reticulum (ER) aided by resident ER proteins. Cytosolic derived proteins are converted into peptides (orange) by the proteosome, shuttled into the ER by the transporter associated with antigen processing (TAP) and trimmed by the ER aminopeptidase I (ERAPI) where they bind to the class I antigen binding groove. Stable class I + β_2m + peptide complexes are transported from the ER to the Golgi where the class I polypeptide is glycosylated. Mature MHC class I molecules then are shuttled to the cell surface. MHC class II peptide processing and binding is depicted in the right portion of the figure. Like MHC class I and aided by resident ER proteins, the class II α (green) and β (yellow) chains associate in the ER along with the invariant chain (Ii) (light gray). The class II $\alpha\beta$ + Ii complex is glycosylated as it is transported through the Golgi to the MHC class II compartment (MIIC). Here, proteases cleave Ii leaving only the Ii derived peptide CLIP bound to the class II binding groove (class II + CLIP). HLA-DM (dark gray) catalyzes the exchange of CLIP for peptides (orange) derived by proteolytic degradation from internalized microorganisms and proteins. Stable class II + peptide complexes then traffic to the cell surface and represent mature MHC class II molecules.

endoplasmic reticulum aminopeptidase plays a dual function in class I antigen presentation. It trims longer peptides that are more readily shuttled by TAP to the optimal length (8–9 amino acids) enhancing binding to class I molecules, but also destroys many peptides limiting the pool available for binding to class I.[62,63]

The class II α and β chains fold and associate in the ER with the assistance of resident ER chaperones such as calnexin (Fig. 39.7),[64] similar to class I molecules. Unlike class I, full maturation of the class II molecule does not take place in the ER. Instead, class II heterodimers are directed primarily to specialized endosomal compartments (MHC class II compartments, MIIC), or, in some instance, first traffic to the cell surface and then to the MIIC.[65] Once in the MIIC, peptides are loaded into the antigen binding groove and mature class II molecules are dispatched to the cell surface.

MHC class II molecules bind peptides derived from endocytosed microorganisms and from self and foreign proteins degraded by proteases in the endocytic pathway.[66] This is in contrast, yet complementary, to the peptides bound by MHC class I molecules. In general, class II molecules bind peptides from cell surface and extracellular sources, while class I molecules bind peptides from intracellular sources. Thus, proteins from the whole environment of a cell can be surveyed by the immune system. Invariant chain (Ii), a nonMHC encoded glycoprotein, plays a key role in facilitating this division of function.

Ii performs several functions in assuring proper antigen presentation by class II molecules. Ii chain serves as a chaperone in the folding and assembly of class II $\alpha\beta$ heterodimers and protects the class II peptide binding groove from binding peptide in the ER via a 25 residue internal peptide segment termed CLIP (class II associated invariant chain peptide).[65,66] Ii also provides the intracellular targeting signals that direct the complex to the MIIC. Under the acidic conditions of the MIIC, Ii is proteolytically cleaved and dissociates from the class II molecule, while CLIP remains bound to the class II antigen binding groove. CLIP is exchanged for antigenic peptides in a reaction catalyzed by HLA-DM, a resident MIIC protein that tightly associates with the class II heterodimer.[67–69] HLA-DM is a critical component in shaping the repertoire of peptides bound to class II molecules as it retains the class II molecules in the MIIC until a stable, high affinity complex between the class II molecule and a peptide is formed. In certain APC types, B-cells and thymic epithelial cells, another resident MIIC protein, HLA-DO, negatively regulates the actions of HLA-DM.[67,68]

Analogous to the MHC class II molecules, both HLA-DM and HLA-DO are class II related Ig superfamily members expressed as heterodimers that consist of an α chain and a β chain.[67–69] The HLA-DM and HLA-DO α and β chains are encoded by A and B genes, respectively, in the MHC class II region and regulation of these genes is similar to that of the MHC class II genes.[69] The 3D structure of HLA-DM resembles that of the MHC class II molecules except that its peptide binding groove is almost entirely obscured.[48]

Components of the peptide processing and binding pathways of MHC class I and class II molecules are a favorite target of disruption by many pathogens and malignant cells to avoid detection by the immune system.[42–44] For example, two proteins (US3 and US6) encoded by human CMV block cell surface expression of MHC class I molecules and thus, detection of the infected cell by cytotoxic T-cells. US3 binds to MHC class I molecules and retains them in the ER and US6 inhibits peptide transport into the ER by TAP. Lack of cell surface MHC class I, however, renders the CMV infected cell susceptible to lysis by NK cells. To circumvent NK cell recognition, CMV encodes a class I like decoy termed UL18 which is recognized by NK cells and inhibits their function.[45] Other pathogens and malignant cells employ a variety of unique strategies to block MHC expression.

T lymphocyte recognition of HLA molecules

The predominant function of classical MHC class I and class II molecules is to bind peptides from the cell's environment and present these peptides on the surface of the cell for inspection by the immune system. The archetypical receptor involved in the inspection process is the T-cell receptor (TCR) on T lymphocytes (Fig. 39.8). There are two types of TCR (αβ and γδ) both of which are multipolypeptide complexes that consist of a TCR α chain covalently paired with a TCR β chain or of a TCR γ chain covalently paired with a TCR δ chain tightly, but noncovalently, associated with several chains of the CD3 family (α, δ, ε, ζ, η).[70,71] The TCR chains are involved in the direct recognition of the HLA molecule and of the peptide bound to the HLA molecule.[71,72] CD3 is involved in the signaling process which activates the T-cell after recognition of the ligand by the TCR chains.[70]

T lymphocytes are classically divided into two groups based on expression of co-receptors (CD4 and CD8) which are intimately involved in recognition of the HLA molecule.[71,73] CD4 expressing (CD4+) T-cells are usually MHC class II restricted; that is, their TCR recognizes either an HLA-DR, -DQ or -DP molecule which all have a CD4 binding site (Fig. 39.8). CD8 expressing (CD8+) T-cells are generally MHC class I restricted recognizing either an HLA-A, -B or -C

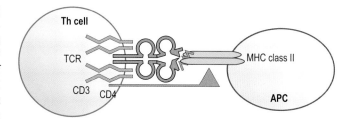

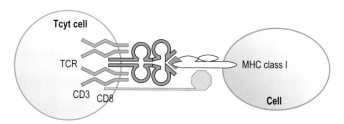

Fig. 39.8 CD4+ versus CD8+ T-cells. T-cells are classically divided into two groups based on their expression of either CD4 (top, dark gray) or CD8 (bottom, light gray). Both types of T-cell express the TCR (blue) and CD3 complex (CD3) (lavender). CD4+ T-cells are primarily of the helper phenotype (Th) and CD8+ T-cells are generally of the cytotoxic phenotype (Tcyt). The TCR expressed by CD4+ Th-cells is usually restricted to MHC class II molecules (green), while the TCR expressed by CD8+ Tcyt cells is generally restricted to MHC class I molecules (yellow). Peptide bound to each MHC molecule is depicted in orange.

molecule which all have a CD8 binding site. CD4 and CD8 enhance the interaction between the TCR and HLA molecule and provide signals, like the CD3 chains, to activate the T-cell.

The CD4/CD8 division in MHC restriction, for the most part, also extends to the general phenotypic function of the T-cell. CD4+ T-cells are mostly of the helper phenotype (helper T-lymphocyte; Th-cell). Th-cells are dedicated to the initiation and generation of immune responses to specific antigens, including antibody production by B-lymphocytes and cytotoxic cellular responses. CD8+ T-cells are usually of the cytotoxic phenotype (cytotoxic T-lymphocyte; Tcyt-cell) and are the principal component of the cytotoxic cellular response to specific antigens. Tcyt-cell recognition of a foreign peptide bound to a MHC class I molecule leads to killing of the abnormal or infected cell.

Like immunoglobulins, the TCR chains are encoded by novel genes formed by the combining of gene segments termed variable, diversity, joining and constant.[74,75] Multiple gene segment alternatives and variable joining lead to an enormous potential repertoire of TCR structures. The outcome of this diversity is the generation of a large pool of T-cells expressing a wide range of TCR that can recognize a wide variety of antigenic peptides. Simplistically, each T-cell, through its TCR, recognizes a specific MHC molecule (MHC restriction) in combination with a distinct peptide (antigen specific recognition) (Fig. 39.9). In actuality, a single TCR can recognize with different affinities many (estimated to be approximately 10^6) different MHC/peptide complexes that share common structural features.[72]

MHC class I and class II molecules are essential to the creation of the T-cell pool available for immune surveillance. T-cell maturation and selection occurs in the thymus in a

Antigen specific T cell recognition

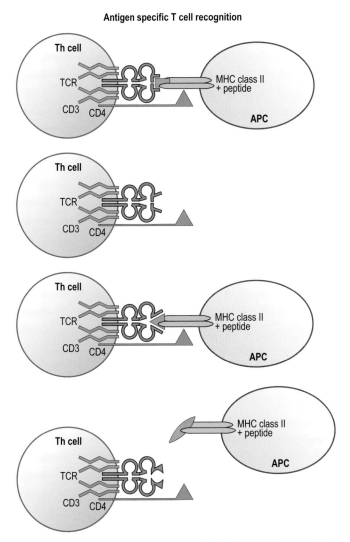

Fig. 39.9 T-cell recognition is antigen specific. The TCR (blue) expressed by different individual T-cells differ and, thus, each recognizes a specific peptide bound to a specific MHC molecule. In the example shown, the four CD4+ (dark gray) Th-cells have differing specificities for particular peptides (orange) due to variations in the sequence of their TCR. However, each recognizes their respective peptide bound to the same MHC class II molecule (green). The CD3 complex (CD3) is depicted in lavender.

process called thymic education.[76,77] In the thymus, T-cells are in contact with MHC class I and class II molecules that are complexed with a variety of self peptides. The TCR must be able to interact with a self MHC molecule complexed with a self peptide. Many T-cells have a TCR that is unable to bind to self MHC plus self peptides complexes and these die in the thymus. T-cells whose TCR has a low affinity interaction with and are partially activated by self MHC plus self peptide complexes (positive selection) are self tolerant and leave the thymus for peripheral tissues. These T-cells maintain some degree of partial autoreactivity and constitute the pool available for immune responses to foreign peptides. T-cells whose TCR has a high affinity for and are reactive to (autoreactive) these complexes are deleted (negative selection) from the T-cell pool via the generation of a variety of intracellular signals. It has become apparent in recent years that a subset of these autoreactive cells are not deleted from the thymus, but instead develop into regulatory T-cells

(Treg). Treg-cells are not themselves reactive to self antigens, but instead suppress the activity of other potentially autoreactive T-cells.[76,78]

The diversity of MHC molecule + self peptide complexes is central not only to the selection of a diverse repertoire of T-cells in the thymus, but also to the maintenance of the multiplicity of available T-cells in peripheral tissues.[79] Disruptions in this process can result in autoreactivity and autoimmune diseases. Other histocompatibility antigens (nonclassical MHC class I molecules, MHC class I related chains and CD1 molecules) are expressed in the thymus and by other tissues and likely help to select and maintain the available T-cell pool. In a human tissue transplant, amino acid sequence differences (mismatches) between any of the HLA molecules expressed by the cells of the donor and of the recipient, theoretically, can cause T-cell reactivity to the foreign HLA molecule. This reactivity can manifest itself as either graft rejection or GVHD and results because the T-cells were not educated for tolerance to the disparate HLA molecule.

The TCR is not the only receptor that binds MHC molecules as its ligand. Other receptors are discussed in the section on 'Other immune system receptors' and their interactions with MHC molecules regulate a variety of functions by immune system cells.

Allorecognition and transplantation

Allorecognition results when T-cells of one individual react to foreign (allogeneic) MHC molecules of another individual. There are three distinct pathways of allorecognition termed direct, indirect, and semi-direct[80,81] (Fig. 39.10). Direct allorecognition occurs when recipient T-cells recognize as foreign an intact allogeneic MHC molecule expressed by a donor cell.[81] Indirect allorecognition occurs when recipient T-cells recognize a self MHC molecule that has bound a peptide derived from the foreign MHC molecule which contains the amino acid difference(s). This type of allorecognition involves the uptake of grafted cellular material, from which the foreign MHC molecules are processed into peptides and bound to self MHC molecules via the normal MHC class I and class II peptide processing and binding pathways. The semi-direct pathway involves the uptake and surface expression of intact foreign MHC+peptide complexes by recipient APC. Since these APC can also process and present foreign MHC molecules as peptides, this enables both direct and indirect recognition of foreign MHC on the surface of the same APC by recipient T-cells. When immune cells are present in the graft, donor T-cells may recognize recipient MHC by these same pathways. These pathways may contribute differentially to the alloresponse over time.

Allorecognition is purely a transplantation phenomenon. Successful transplantation of tissues, especially HSC grafts, relies heavily on the HLA identity of the donor and the recipient.[82] Unfortunately, HLA mismatches between a donor and recipient are often unavoidable. Any HLA disparity has the potential to cause allorecognition which increases the risk of graft rejection or GVHD. However, not all HLA disparity leads to destructive alloreactive T-cell responses.

The frequency of T-cells of any individual that respond to allogeneic MHC is substantially greater than the frequency of T-cells that respond to a specific foreign antigen.[83] The

Direct allorecognition

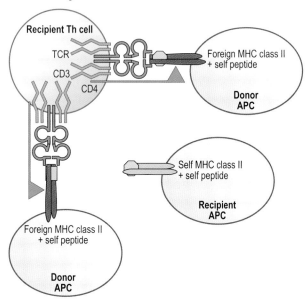

Indirect allorecognition

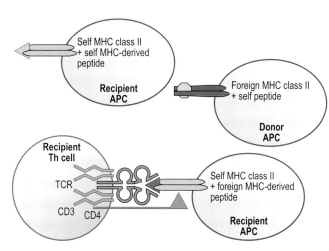

Fig. 39.10 Allorecognition is the recognition of and reaction to determinants of foreign MHC molecules by T-cells. Two of the types of allorecognition, direct (top) and indirect (bottom), are shown. In direct allorecognition (top), the TCR (blue) expressed by a CD4⁺ (dark gray) Th-cell is directly recognizing the differences of the foreign class II molecule (red) complexed with self peptides (yellow) which may or may not play a role in recognition of the complex. In indirect allorecognition (bottom), the TCR expressed by a CD4⁺ Th is recognizing a peptide (red) derived from the foreign class II molecule in complex with a self class II molecule (green). This peptide contains one or more amino acids that differ from the comparable peptide (green) derived from the self class II molecule.

high frequency of potentially alloreactive T-cells is most likely due to the fact that the available T-cell pool consists of T-cells that are inherently reactive to MHC molecules complexed with self peptides.[81,84] Furthermore, because the TCR itself is flexible, a single TCR is able to recognize multiple MHC+peptide complexes and to accommodate differences in structure.

Non-classical MHC class I molecules

The non-classical MHC class I (class Ib) molecules, HLA-E, HLA-F and HLA-G, are encoded in the class I region of the MHC (Fig. 39.1) and the proteins expressed by these genes are structurally similar to the classical class I molecules (class Ia). However, the class Ib molecules, in general, are noticeably less polymorphic and expressed at lower levels on cell surfaces than the class Ia molecules. These glycoproteins also display unique tissue distribution patterns and participate in specialized immune system functions. The impact of the class Ib molecules on immune responses directed toward foreign tissue is not yet known.

HLA-E

HLA-E shares many features with the classical class I molecules. Its gene is organized and regulated in a manner nearly identical to that of the class Ia genes and is highly transcribed in most nucleated cells.[85–87] HLA-E is expressed on cell surfaces as a trimolecular complex that includes the HLA-E heavy chain, β_2m and peptide and has a similar overall 3D conformation.[88–90] Assembly of the HLA-E molecule and binding of peptides requires all of the same ER components. Like the class Ia molecules, the peptides that bind to HLA-E are optimal at 9 amino acids in length.

In contrast to classical MHC class I genes, HLA-E is the least polymorphic of the MHC class I genes; nine alleles encoding three unique proteins.[21,87] Although high levels of HLA-E gene transcripts and intracellular protein are found in most cells, very little HLA-E protein is detected at cell surfaces. These observations are likely the consequence of the unique function of HLA-E, which has been well conserved across species. The peptide binding groove of HLA-E is highly hydrophobic and specializes in the binding of hydrophobic peptides primarily derived from the signal sequences of many of the classical class I molecules and HLA-G. These HLA-E + signal sequence complexes serve as the ligand recognized by some members of the CD94/NKG2 family of NK cell receptors. Recognition of HLA-E by CD94/NKG2 family members regulates NK cell mediated lysis of a potential target cell. The coordinate expression of HLA-E with classical MHC class I molecules and the binding of peptides derived from their signal sequences provides a means for NK cells to monitor the efficacy of expression and translation of the classical class I genes which is often disrupted in malignant and virally infected cells.

Recently, it has been documented that HLA-E also plays a role in antigen presentation to T-cells expressing $\alpha\beta$ TCR. HLA-E restricted CD8⁺ cytotoxic T-cells have been isolated that recognize peptides from pathogens such as CMV, *Salmonella* and *Mycobacterium*.[91] Further, the crystal structure of the interaction of a TCR with HLA-E/CMV peptide complex was recently solved.[89] Thus, HLA-E is important not only in NK cell (innate), but also in T-cell (adaptive) immune responses. Whether HLA-E affects transplantation outcome is yet to be determined.

HLA-F

HLA-F remains the most mysterious of the class Ib molecules. Like HLA-E, HLA-F also shares properties associated with the classical MHC class I molecules.[85] Its gene is highly transcribed in a variety of cell types such as B-cells, tonsil, spleen and thymus, but not as ubiquitously as expression of the classical MHC class I genes.[92] The HLA-F heavy chain associates with β_2m and possibly to several of the ER components involved in class Ia molecule assembly, but these data are conflicting.[92,93]

Contrary to the class Ia genes, polymorphisms reported in the HLA-F gene are limited; 21 alleles have been described.[21] The HLA-F protein has only been detected intracellularly in normal tissues in which its gene is transcribed, but it has been detected on the surface of transformed B-cell and monocyte cell lines[93] and may have a unique pathway for its transport to the cell surface.[94] It has not been determined whether HLA-F binds peptides, although 3D models suggest that the HLA-F antigen binding groove could accommodate peptides. One report has shown an interaction of HLA-F with leukocyte immunoglobulin-like receptors on the surface of B-cells and monocytes suggesting that HLA-F may have a role in the regulation of these cell types.[92] However, more work needs to be done before the function of HLA-F is fully discerned.

HLA-G

HLA-G is less analogous to the classical class I molecules than HLA-E and HLA-F. Regulation of the HLA-G gene is unique.[85] First, the sequence of the SXY module is divergent from the other class Ia and class Ib genes, is not responsive to CIITA and may not bind components of the enhansosome. Second, part of the ISRE is deleted and is replaced with a SP1 binding site. Thus, HLA-G is not IFN-γ inducible. Although less polymorphic than the classical class I genes, HLA-G is the most polymorphic of the class Ib genes with 44 alleles that encode 14 unique proteins.[21,91] Assembly and expression of the HLA-G trimolecular complex (HLA-G heavy chain, β_2m and peptide) is identical to classical MHC class I molecules.[95] The 3D structure of HLA-G is analogous to that of the class Ia molecules and HLA-E, but the number of contacts between HLA-G and the bound peptide is greater than class Ia molecules and is more deeply buried.[96] The peptides bound to HLA-G appear to be less diverse than class Ia molecules and their presentation to T-cells is not known as HLA-G restricted T-cells have not been identified.[97]

HLA-G has other unique features. Six different HLA-G proteins (isoforms) are expressed as a result of alternative splicing of its mRNA. HLA-G1 is the full length isoform that is membrane bound and associated with β_2m. There are three other membrane bound isoforms of HLA-G (HLA-G2, -G3 and -G4) that lack various extracellular domains. Alternative mRNA that includes intron 4 produces the two soluble isoforms of HLA-G, HLA-G1sol and HLA-G2sol. All isoforms appear to bind peptides and, thus, may be functional, but the G1 isoform is the most predominant *in vivo*.[97]

HLA-G is the primary histocompatibility molecule expressed during pregnancy and its expression appears to be restricted to trophoblasts of the fetal placenta.[97] HLA-E and HLA-F are also expressed, but classical class I molecules are not expressed in the trophoblasts.[85] HLA-G has a dual role in maternal tolerance of the fetus.[97] First, HLA-G provides a signal sequence peptide for expression of HLA-E which, in turn, regulates maternal NK cell recognition of fetal tissue.

Second, HLA-G, particularly the homodimeric form, regulates the functional interaction of a variety of immune system cells with fetal tissue by serving directly as the ligand for members of the leukocyte immunoglobulin-like receptor family, LILRB1 and LILRB2, which are expressed by professional APC of the myeloid lineage and by some lymphocytes.[98,99] HLA-G also may serve as the ligand for the NK cell receptor KIR2DL4.[100]

Other potential histocompatibility molecules

MHC class I chain-related molecules (MIC)

The genes encoding the MHC class I chain-related molecules (MIC) are located in the class I region of the MHC centromeric to HLA-B (Fig. 39.1).[101] MICA and MICB are relatively polymorphic.[21,102] To date, 67 alleles of MICA that encode 56 unique proteins and 30 alleles of MICB that encode 19 unique proteins have been described.

Several features are unique to MICA and MICB. Expression of MICA and MICB is up-regulated in response to stress because of a heat shock response element in the promoter region of their genes.[101] In fact, the promoter regions of the MICA and MICB genes do not contain any of the classical MHC class I regulatory elements (Fig. 39.5). Instead, their promoters share homologies with the heat shock protein 70 promoter. MICA and MICB protein expression is limited to endothelial cells, fibroblasts and epithelial cells primarily in the gastrointestinal tract and thymus and does not require association with β_2m, peptide or TAP.[103] The 3D structure of the extracellular domains of MICA revealed that the folding resembles that of the class Ia molecules, but that the overall orientation of these domains is dissimilar.[104] The MICA α1 and α2 domains are tilted to expose a portion of the underside of the groove, as well as the groove itself to interactions with receptors. The peptide binding groove is mostly obscured and unlikely to bind peptide antigens.

MICA and MICB serve as ligands for NKG2D, an activating NK cell receptor.[101,103] The interaction of NKG2D with the MIC molecules leads to NK cell mediated lysis of the epithelial cell. In fact, MIC expression is up-regulated in a wide variety of epithelial tumors such as melanoma, colon and kidney and it has been shown that the response to these cells is mediated through the interaction of NKG2D with MICA and MICB.[105] MICA and MICB also may play a role in solid organ transplantation. Both molecules have been found to be expressed on epithelial and endothelial cells of transplanted kidney, heart and pancreas that show evidence of rejection and/or cellular injury.[106] Further, the presence of MIC-specific antibodies in solid organ transplant recipients shows an association with graft failure.[107] Thus, MIC molecules appear to be transplantation antigens that can mediate an alloresponse by NK cells and B-cells that leads to graft rejection.

CD1 molecules

CD1 is a family of proteins whose nonpolymorphic genes are encoded on an MHC paralogous region on chromosome 1.[108] CD1 molecules are structurally close to MHC class I molecules at the gene and protein levels, while they are functionally close to MHC class II molecules as CD1 molecules associate with invariant chain and utilize the class II antigen presentation pathway.[65,109] Like both MHC class I and class II molecules, CD1 molecules present antigens to T-lymphocytes for immune recognition.

Five CD1 molecules have been described which are classified into two groups based on sequence homology and tissue distribution.[108] Members of group I (CD1a, -b, -c, -e) are expressed primarily on professional APC, such as dendritic cells and B-cells, and on cortical thymocytes; while members of group II (CD1d) are expressed on most cells of hematopoietic origin and on hepatocytes, keratinocytes and intestinal epithelium. The crystal structures of CD1a, CD1b and CD1d reveal a general conformation similar to MHC class Ia molecules except that the antigen-binding grooves are narrower, deeper and very hydrophobic.[108,110] There are two deep pockets at either end of the groove that accommodate the lipid tails of lipid antigens. The depth of these pockets varies (CD1d has the deepest and CD1a has the shallowest), conferring different lipid antigen binding characteristics on each of the CD1 molecules. Several lipid antigens have been identified from bacterial, synthetic and self sources. For example, CD1b binds mycolates derived from mycolic acid of *Mycobacterium* species, while CD1a binds lipopeptides also from mycobacteria. Lipid antigens also have been identified from *Borrelia burgdorferi* (Lyme disease) and *Sphingomonas*.

Group I CD1 molecules present lipid antigens to T-cells that express either γδ TCR or αβ TCR.[108,110] CD1d (group II) is the ligand primarily for invariant NK T-cells (iNKT). iNKT cells are usually double negative (CD4⁻/CD8⁻) or CD4⁺ T-cells that express a specific αβ TCR (Vα24-Jα18 with Vβ11) together with receptors found on NK cells, CD161 (NK-RP1A) in particular. iNKT cells develop in the thymus from double positive (CD4⁺/CD8⁺) T-cells like other T-cells, but require interaction with CD1d in the thymus for their differentiation and maturation. iNKT cells play a large role in enhancing the immune response to certain microbial pathogens by stimulating APCs, T-cells and B-cells. These cells can also be directly cytotoxic. Because the CD1 molecules are not polymorphic, they are unlikely to have an impact on donor selection for tissue transplantation.

Minor histocompatibility antigens

Clinically significant GVHD is observed in HLA identical sibling transplants of HSC implicating histocompatibility antigens specified by genes other than the classical HLA genes in the allorecognition of foreign tissue.[111] These so-called minor histocompatibility antigens (mHag) were identified coincident with the major histocompatibility antigens. mHag are peptides derived from self proteins, other than HLA, whose sequence differs among individuals in the population. Theoretically, any polymorphic protein that differs between the tissue donor and recipient has the potential to provide a peptide which functions as a mHag. Many mHag loci have been described in humans utilizing mHag specific T-cell clones in cytotoxicity assays. However, only a handful of peptides derived from these loci have been identified (Table 39.6).[112,113] The frequency of the mHags alleles varies in different population groups and some can be quite common.[114] The peptides containing the variant amino acid(s) are processed through the normal MHC class I and class II antigen presentation pathways, are bound to an HLA molecule and are recognized as foreign by T-cells.[111,115]

Table 39.6 Examples of human minor histocompatibility antigens[a]

Minor antigen	Sequence[b]	Source protein	Tissue distribution	HLA restriction[c]	Characterization of antigenicity
HA-1	VL**H**DDLLEA VL**R**DDLLEA	Gene locus KIAA0223	Hematopoietic cells Solid tumors	HLA-A*0201 HLA-B*4001	HA-1 R variant does not bind HLA molecules
HA-2	YIGSVLISV	Myosin 1G	Hematopoietic cells	HLA-A*0201	Not determined
H-Y	SP**S**VDKA**R**AEL SP**A**VDKA**Q**AEL	SMCY SMCX	Ubiquitous	HLA-B*0702	Females do not carry a Y chromosome and react to variant male peptide
ACC-1	DYLQ**Y**VLQI DYLQ**C**VLQI	BCL2A1	Hematopoietic cells Solid tumors	HLA-A*24	ACC-1 C variant does not elicit a T-cell response
HA-3	VTEPG**T**AQY VTEPG**M**AQY	AKAP13	Ubiquitous	HLA-A*03	HA-3 M variant is not immunogenic
HB-1	EEKRGSL**H**VW EEKRGSL**Y**VW	HB-1 gene	Cancerous B cells[d]	HLA-B*4402 HLA-B*4403	Both peptides are immunogenic

a113-115

[b]Bold denotes variant amino acid residues in peptides.

[c]HLA molecules other than those listed may bind each mHag, but studies have not been performed.

[d]High levels of expression in B-cell acute lymphoblastic leukemia and in small percentage of B-cell lymphomas and undifferentiated B-cell leukemias. Also high expression levels in EBV-transformed B-cells. Very low levels of expression detected in normal B-cells and in testis.

The HLA alleles expressed by a donor and recipient determine whether a mHag might contribute to allorecognition in transplantation. Furthermore, the contribution of a mHag on transplant outcome might be contingent on the sex of the donor and recipient and on the type of tissue transplanted (Table 39.6). HLA alleles are important because each HLA allelic product binds peptides that fit a specific binding motif and, thus, each mHag is only bound by certain HLA molecules. Therefore, the mHag(s) of significance differ widely depending on which HLA alleles are carried by the tissue donor and recipient (transplant pair). For example, mHag HA-1 could have an impact if the donor or recipient expresses HLA-A*0201 and there is HA-1 disparity between the transplant pair.[113,115] Recognition of the H allelic form of the HA-1 peptide bound to the A*0201 encoded molecule stimulates allorecognition. HA-1 would be of no consequence to the graft when, for instance, both donor and recipient are homozygous for HLA-A*0101, as HA-1 is not able to bind to this HLA-A molecule and consequently is never presented to T-cells. The HA-1 R peptide does not elicit an immune response. HA-1 also can be used to demonstrate the importance of the type of tissue involved in the transplant. HA-1 is expressed only on cells of hematopoietic origin. Therefore, HA-1 most likely would not be pertinent in the case of a kidney transplant, even if the transplant pair expresses HLA-A*0201, since HA-1 would not be expressed by the transplanted kidney.

It is now apparent that mHags not only have an impact on the development of GVHD, but also can be beneficial in generating a graft versus tumor (GVT) response[111–113,115] as cancer cells of both hematopoietic and epithelial origin have been found to aberrantly express mHag. Once characterized, mHags can be included in matching protocols when they are pertinent to transplantation of tissue or to the elimination of residual malignant disease.[112]

Other immune system receptors that recognize histocompatibility molecules as their ligands

In addition to the TCR, several families of receptors interact with histocompatibility molecules. The quest to find a receptor(s) involved in NK cell discrimination of normal cells from malignant and infected cells led to the identification and characterization of the first two receptor families (killer cell immunoglobulin-like receptors and CD94/NKG2). Members of these two families were found to recognize specific groups of MHC class I molecules and regulate NK cell function. Since these initial findings, another family of receptors (leukocyte immunoglobulin-like receptors) has been identified and characterized. These receptors are expressed by many immune system cell types and appear to regulate a variety of immune cell functions.

Killer cell immunoglobulin-like receptors

The killer cell immunoglobulin-like receptors (KIR) are, at least, a 14 member family of proteins expressed by NK cells and a subset of T-cells.[116] Like the HLA molecules and TCR, KIR belong to the immunoglobulin (Ig) protein superfamily

and possess either 2 (KIR2D) or 3 (KIR3D) glycosylated extracellular Ig like domains (Fig. 39.11). The type of signal (activating or inhibiting) generated by a KIR is dictated by its cytoplasmic tail. Members that generate inhibitory signals, preventing cytotoxicity and cytokine release, have a long cytoplasmic tail (e.g., KIR3DL1 and KIR2DL2) which contains immunoreceptor tyrosine based inhibitory motifs (ITIM). Binding of the inhibitory KIR to its ligand leads to phosphorylation of the tyrosine residue in each ITIM and ultimately to inhibition of NK and T-cell functions. Activating KIR family members have a short cytoplasmic tail without ITIM (e.g., KIR2DS1 and KIR3DS1). Instead, these members associate via a conserved positively charged residue in their transmembrane regions with an adaptor protein, often DAP12, that contains immunoreceptor tyrosine-based activation motifs (ITAM) in its cytoplasmic tail. Interaction of an activating KIR with its ligand causes phosphorylation of the ITAM in the adaptor which may lead to activation of NK and T-cell functions. Since NK and T-cells express multiple activating and inhibiting receptors including KIR, cellular function is finely regulated and represents an integration of signals.[117]

Classical MHC class I molecules serve as the ligand for several of the KIR family members (Fig. 39.11).[116,118] Some KIR with two extracellular Ig like domains interact with groups of HLA-C molecules.[116,119] Almost all HLA-C molecules can be divided into one of two groups (C1 and C2) based on the presence of a shared (public) epitope determined by amino acid residue 80 in the α1 domain of the HLA-C molecule.[120] The C1 group (e.g. Cw1 encoded by Cw*010201) has an asparagine at residue 80 and the C2 group (e.g. Cw2 encoded by Cw*020201) has a lysine at residue 80. C1 group molecules are ligands for KIR2DL2 and KIR2DL3, while C2 group molecules are ligands for KIR2DL1. A KIR with three extracellular Ig like domains, KIR3DL1, interacts with a group of HLA-B molecules carrying the Bw4 public epitope. HLA-G is recognized by KIR2DL4.[100] Ligands for some KIR have not been identified.

The genes encoding KIR are located in the leukocyte receptor complex on chromosome 19.[121] Haplotypes vary in the number of KIR genes they encode.[122] One common haplotype includes only seven of the 14 KIR genes: KIR3DL3, KIR2DL3, KIR2DL1, KIR2DL4, KIR3DL1, KIR2DS4, and KIR3DL2. Other haplotypes include more of the stimulatory KIR genes. In addition to gene content variability, the KIR genes are polymorphic.[123] For example, there are over 50 KIR3DL1 alleles. KIR3DL1 allelic variation alters its level on the cell surface and impacts the affinity of interaction with its HLA ligand.[124]

At the level of the individual NK cell, only a subset of the KIR genes carried by an individual are expressed.[125] During development, individual NK cells acquire specific KIR, apparently at random so that an individual who carries KIR2DL1 and KIR2DL3, for example, will have NK cells that express only KIR2DL1, only KIR2DL3, and KIR2DL1+KIR2DL3. This variegated expression increases the sensitivity of the NK cells to the loss of individual HLA molecules during tumorgenesis or viral infection. Because KIR and HLA genes are found on different chromosomes, individuals may carry a KIR gene yet lack its cognate HLA ligand. For example, an individual may express KIR3DL1 but not express an HLA-B molecule carrying a Bw4 epitope. To avoid autoreactivity by absence of a

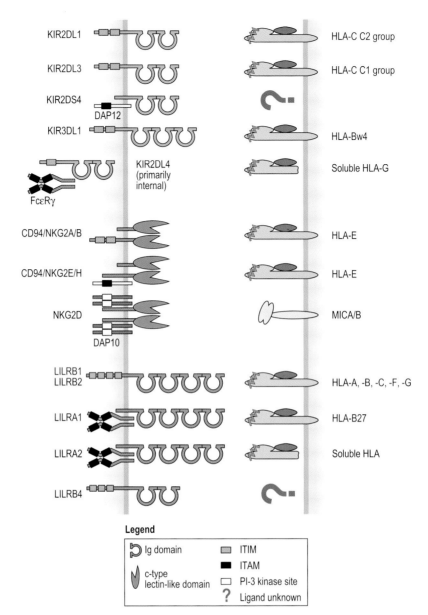

Fig. 39.11 Examples of the three receptor families that recognize HLA molecules as their ligands. The killer cell immunoglobulin-like receptors (KIR, green, top) have either two or three extracellular Ig like domains. Inhibitory KIR have long cytoplasmic tails and signal via immunoreceptor tyrosine based inhibitory motifs (ITIM, gray box). Activating KIR with short cytoplasmic tails associate with a signaling protein called DAP12 (yellow) that has an immunoreceptor tyrosine based activation motif (ITAM) (black box) in its cytoplasmic tail. KIR2DL4 has an ITIM but is activating by associating with Fc epsilon receptor gamma chains (FcεRγ, magenta) that contain ITAM in their cytoplasmic tails. The ligands for many of the KIR are groups of class I HLA molecules (heavy chain, light green; β$_2$m, blue; peptide, orange). For example, KIR2DL1 recognizes group 2 HLA-C class I molecules; KIR2DL3 recognizes group 1 HLA-C class I molecules; KIR3DL3 recognizes HLA-B class I molecules with a HLA-Bw4 public epitope (Fig. 39.6, Table 39.8); and KIR2DL4 recognizes soluble HLA-G. The ligands for some KIR are unknown (denoted by question mark). NKG2A, -B, -C, -E and -H (orange, center) are expressed as heterodimers with CD94. NKG2D is expressed as a homodimer. Like the KIR, inhibitory members contain ITIM in their cytoplasmic tails, while activating members associate with DAP12. The exception is NKG2D, an activating receptor, which associates with another signaling protein called DAP10 (lavender) that possesses a phosphatidylinositol-3 (PI-3) kinase binding site (white box) instead of an ITAM. The ligand for all CD94/NKG2 heterodimers is the non-classical MHC class I molecule, HLA-E. NKG2D recognizes the MHC class I chain-related A and B (MICA/B) molecules (light blue). The leukocyte immunoglobulin-like receptors (LILR) have either two or four extracellular Ig like domains (cyan, bottom). Again, inhibitory members possess ITIM in their cytoplasmic tails. Activating members associate with FcεRγ (magenta) like KIR2DL4. LILRB1 and LILRB2 recognize a variety of HLA molecules. HLA-B27 allelic products are the ligand for LILRA1 and LILRA2 recognizes soluble HLA molecules. The ligand(s) for other family members is not known.

ligand, it is thought that individual NK cells are educated by interaction with MHC class I molecules and that this process controls the functional responsiveness of the NK cells.[126] In KIR3DL1 positive, HLA-Bw4 negative individuals, NK cells expressing KIR3DL1 as their only inhibitory receptor will be hyporesponsive, unable to react to the absence of the HLA-Bw4 ligand.[127]

Specific KIR genes have been associated with susceptibility or resistance to a variety of infectious and autoimmune diseases.[118] The impact of NK cells, and inhibitory KIR in specific, in eradicating residual malignant disease was first noted in T-cell depleted haploidentical HSC transplants.[128] Subsequent studies have underscored the difficulty in predicting NK alloreactivity in the context of differing transplantation protocols and recent studies have continued to investigate the utility of considering KIR when selecting a HSC donor.[129] In general, algorithms to predict NK alloreactivity have focused on KIR and HLA genotypes of the donor and the recipient.[130] The goal is to select a donor expressing an inhibitory KIR ligand for a patient who does not express the ligand for that receptor, for example, to select a KIR2DL1 positive donor for a patient who is negative for the HLA-C2 group. It is then expected that donor NK cells, released from their inhibition, will attack residual malignant cells expressing NK cell activating ligands. Observations of NK reactivity in HSC transplantation have lead to clinical trials using adoptive immunotherapy with NK cells for patients with myeloid leukemia and with solid tumors.[131]

CD94 and NKG2

CD94 and the NKG2 family (NKG2A-NKG2F and NKG2H) are primarily transmembrane glycoproteins and their genes are encoded in the NK complex on chromosome 12.[132] NKG2A, NKG2C, NKG2E and NKG2F share greater than 94% protein sequence homology in their extracellular domains. NKG2A, 2C and 2E are expressed as covalently linked heterodimers with CD94. NKG2B and NKG2H are alternative mRNA splice products of the NKG2A and NKG2E genes, respectively, and also are expressed as heterodimers with CD94. NKG2F does not form heterodimers with CD94 and is expressed in intracellular compartments. NKG2D is discussed separately below.

Like the KIR, CD94/NKG2 heterodimers and NKG2F are expressed by NK cells and subsets of CD8+ T-cells and can either inhibit or activate cellular functions.[132] The action of the CD94/NKG2 heterodimeric receptors is determined by the NKG2 family member. CD94/NKG2A and CD94/NKG2B are inhibitory with two ITIM in their cytoplasmic tails. NKG2C, NKG2E and NKG2H lack ITIM in their cytoplasmic tails and, like activating KIR, are associated noncovalently with DAP12 and are activating receptors. NKG2F, although intracellular, also associates with DAP12 and is an activating receptor.

All of the CD94/NKG2 heterodimers recognize the non-classical class I molecule HLA-E as their ligand; NKG2A/B and NKG2E/H with equal affinity and NKG2C with tenfold less affinity.[132] Polymorphism has not been demonstrated in these receptors, nor is it likely since their ligand, HLA-E, is highly conserved in the population. On the other hand, it has been demonstrated that the sequence of the bound peptide can affect CD94/NKG2 recognition of HLA-E.[132,133] This could have consequences on the regulation of NK and T-cell recognition of tissues in transplantation, particularly stimulating a GVT response, especially since there is polymorphism in the HLA class I signal sequences bound by HLA-E.[132]

NKG2D shares only ~20% protein identity with other NKG2 family members and is expressed as a homodimer on the cell surface of NK, γδ T-cells and subsets of CD4+ and CD8+ T-cells.[134,135] NKG2D is an activating receptor and signaling is achieved by association with two dimers of DAP10 carrying phosphatidylinositol-3 kinase binding sites in their cytoplasmic tails. The ligands for NKG2D are MICA and MICB. There is now evidence that the interaction of NKG2D with its ligands may play a role in the transplantation of tissues, particularly with respect to graft rejection of solid organ transplants.[134]

Leukocyte immunoglobulin-like receptors

The leukocyte immunoglobulin-like receptors (LILR) or immunoglobulin-like transcripts (ILT) are a multigene family located on the long arm of chromosome 19 closely linked to the KIR genes.[136] Eleven expressed LILR members have been identified, ten of which are glycosylated transmembrane proteins and one being a glycosylated soluble molecule.[136,137] The LILR, like the KIR, belong to the Ig superfamily and have either two or four Ig-like extracellular domains (see Fig. 39.11). There are inhibitory (LILRB1-5) and activating (LILRA1-6) receptors, similar to the KIR and CD94/NKG2 receptor families. Inhibitory LILR have long cytoplasmic tails that contain two to four ITIM and activating LILR have short cytoplasmic tails devoid of known signaling motifs. Activating LILR associate with the Fc epsilon receptor γ chain which contains an ITAM in its cytoplasmic tail.

LILR expression varies widely on immune system cells, but they are found primarily on APC of the myeloid lineage such as macrophages and dendritic cells[136-138] as well as on B-cells and on subsets of NK and T-cells. Two of the inhibitory LILR, LILRB1 and LILRB2, interact with HLA-A, -B, -C, -F, and -G molecules, but their specificities for HLA allelic products and affinities differ. Two of the activating LILR also bind class I molecules. LILRA1 binds some allelic products of HLA-B*27 and LILRA2 binds soluble class I molecules. There is a fair degree of polymorphism in the LILR genes which clusters in several discrete areas of the extracellular domains[136] which could be the reason for the differences in allelic specificity and affinity for class I molecules.

Evidence is beginning to mount for a possible role of LILRs in transplantation. The inhibitory LILR mediate potent tolerogenic effects on immune responses.[137,138] Thus, engagement of these receptors on APCs presenting alloantigens can result in down-regulation of the alloresponse. For instance, LILR recognition of HLA-G in kidney transplant patients was shown to be associated with a reduction in T-cell alloproliferation and induction of a regulatory/suppressive T-cell population. The full extent of LILR involvement in transplantation requires further study.

Techniques for the identification of HLA polymorphism

Selection of individuals expressing the same HLA molecules (an HLA identical or matched donor) has been used to decrease the detrimental immune response during transplantation of human tissues. HLA alleles and consequent differences in the HLA proteins can be identified through a variety of testing methods including serology, cellular assays, and DNA based detection methods. This process is termed tissue or HLA typing. The methods and quality control for typing have been described.[139] HLA typing and other histocompatibility testing is categorized as high complexity testing in the US. Clinical laboratory improvement amendments (CLIA) and histocompatibility testing laboratories are accredited through the American Society for Histocompatibility and Immunogenetics (ASHI), the European Federation for Immunogenetics (EFI) and other organizations.

Serologic detection of class I and class II allelic products

Lymphocyte microcytotoxicity testing has been used for HLA typing since the 1960s; however, typing for HSC transplantation is performed mainly by DNA-based testing. The HLA serologic phenotype is determined by testing unseparated lymphocyte preparations or T-lymphocytes (for HLA-A, -B, -C) or enriched B-lymphocytes (for HLA-DR, -DQ) for the presence of specific HLA molecules as detected by a panel of well-characterized HLA antibody preparations (alloantisera or monoclonal antibodies).[139] Lymphocytes are incubated with a panel of antibody reagents. If the lymphocytes carry a cell surface HLA molecule recognized by a complement-fixing antibody, the antibody binds to the cells and the cells are subsequently lysed by the addition of complement in excess. Following termination of the reaction and staining to distinguish live from dead cells, the percent lysis of the cells is determined for each antibody reagent using a microscope and a numerical grade is assigned (e.g., 1 = 0–10% lysis, 6 = 51–80%, 8 = 81–100%). Scores of 6–8 indicate that the specific HLA molecule detected by the antibody reagent is present.

The antibodies used to detect specific HLA molecules (or 'specificities') are derived primarily from the sera of alloimmunized individuals including multiparous women, transplant recipients, and multi-transfused patients. Because of the complex reactivity patterns of alloantisera, several alloantisera are used to define each specificity. To address this complexity, monoclonal antibodies detecting HLA specificities have been generated; however, the availability of these reagents is limited.

Cellular detection of HLA disparity

Cellular assays were historically used to detect HLA differences between individuals, but are not commonly used today. The response of one cell (responder) in tissue culture to the foreign histocompatibility molecules on the surface of a second cell (stimulator) is called the mixed leukocyte culture (MLC) or mixed lymphocyte reaction (MLR).[140] The response is made unidirectional by preventing cells from one of the two individuals from replicating by treating those cells with radiation or an alkylating agent prior to addition to the culture. The MLC represents a summation response of a responder cell to differences in the HLA class II molecules (HLA-DR, -DQ, and -DP) encoded by the irradiated stimulator cell haplotypes. The response to DR molecules predominates. The use of cellular assays to determine the similarity between two individuals has declined significantly because DNA based testing procedures can now be used to identify class II disparity between individuals and because the MLC can be influenced by a variety of factors including the health of the individuals contributing the cells, the patient's disease, and the history of prior transfusion.[141]

Other cellular assays measure the frequency of cytotoxic or helper T-lymphocytes in the potential HSC donor. Limiting dilution is used to isolate and measure the frequency of T-lymphocyte precursors which respond to recipient cells. The differences stimulating these responses are thought to be HLA class I differences or minor histocompatibility antigens for cytotoxic precursors and HLA class II differences for helper precursors. The correlation between the precursor frequency and transplantation outcome is controversial;[142,143] thus, DNA-based testing is more commonly used to identify HLA disparity between potential donor and recipient.

DNA-based identification of class I and class II alleles

DNA-based methods target differences in the nucleotide sequences of alleles for HLA typing. Commercial kits employing all of the methodologies described below are available although some laboratories continue to design their own reagents. Any cell with a nucleus can be used as a source of DNA; however, DNA is usually prepared from a small quantity (0.2–1 ml) of whole blood. Alternative sample types such as epithelial cells from a buccal swab might provide a more reliable source of genomic DNA in patients with hematologic malignancies,[144] in patients treated with immune suppressive agents or in patients who have been transfused.[145] The sensitivity of detection of HLA alleles is enhanced greatly by the amplification of DNA encoding HLA genes using the polymerase chain reaction (PCR) (Fig. 39.12). Many typing reactions utilize PCR primer sequences that are broadly specific and are shared by all alleles at an HLA locus. Other typing procedures utilize primer sets that are narrowly specific and are shared by only a subset of alleles at a locus. In this way, the laboratory can isolate large quantities of specific HLA alleles for identification as described below.

Sequence specific priming (SSP)

One method of typing uses a large panel of pairs of amplification primers.[146,147] Each pair of primers anneals to a limited number of potential alleles. In the subsequent PCR, only certain primer pairs will amplify the DNA from a given individual. Amplification is detected by electrophoresis in an agarose gel or, if the DNA is labeled with a dye during amplification, by fluorescence. The HLA alleles carried by an individual are then determined by the pattern of positive and negative amplifications with the primer panel using a knowledge of which alleles amplify with which primer pairs.

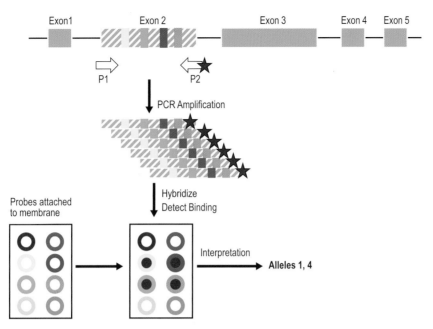

Fig. 39.12 One procedure used for DNA-based typing is sequence specific oligonucleotide probe hybridization. An HLA gene is amplified by the polymerase chain reaction using primers (P1, P2) that flank the polymorphic exon (in this example, exon 2 of DRB1). The DNA is labeled (indicated by a star) during amplification. The labeled DNA is hybridized to a series of oligonucleotide probes that are fixed to a solid support (membrane, microspheres or plate). Each probe detects a polymorphic region of exon 2 (indicated by colored blocks). The denatured DNA binds to those probes that contain sequences complementary to HLA allele sequences contained within the amplified DNA. Binding of the labeled DNA is detected by a variety of methods. The positive and negative probe hybridization results are interpreted by comparison of the nucleotide sequences of the probes with the sequences of known HLA alleles to determine those present in the sample.

Sequence-specific oligonucleotide probe hybridization (SSOPH)

It is possible to use the binding of synthetic single stranded DNA molecules (i.e., probes) to identify HLA alleles.[148,149] A panel of probes, each capable of identifying a short polymorphic region found in a group of HLA alleles, is hybridized to denatured PCR amplified DNA. Specific alleles are identified through the use of several probes and/or the use of SSP followed by hybridization with several probes. Fig. 39.12 illustrates the technique using a format where the oligonucleotide probes are bound to a solid support. The pattern of hybridization, including which probes bound and which did not, can be read to determine the nucleotide polymorphisms present or absent. Comparison of this result with the known sequences of alleles at the locus will predict the HLA alleles present or absent.

Sequence-based typing (SBT) of genomic DNA

A final method of identification of HLA alleles involves the direct determination of the DNA sequences of the HLA alleles carried by an individual.[150,151] Alleles are identified by sequencing following PCR amplication. The choice of PCR primers determines whether the alleles will be isolated separately based on sequence polymorphisms (using SSP) or whether the two alleles of a locus will be characterized as a mixture. The choice of primers also determines which segments of the gene are sequenced; most testing focuses on the exons encoding the antigen binding site of the HLA molecules (exons 2 and 3 for class I genes and exon 2 for class II genes). The presence of two alleles in the sequencing reaction is indicated by the presence of two half-height peaks at each polymorphic nucleotide position. Sequencing is the most powerful approach to determine if two individuals share the same HLA alleles.

Measurement of sensitization to histocompatibility differences

Individuals may become sensitized to foreign histocompatibility molecules through transfusion, pregnancy or prior transplantation. Sensitization may result in the presence of HLA specific antibodies and/or significant numbers of cytotoxic T-cells which may cause lysis of cells expressing the sensitizing foreign HLA molecules. If a pre-sensitized patient, such as a patient with severe aplastic anemia who has received prior blood transfusions, undergoes transplantation with tissue expressing the foreign HLA molecules targeted by the immune system, the pre-existing antibodies or T-cells may cause destruction of the graft. Antibodies are detected prospectively by incubation of serum from the putatively sensitized individual with a panel of HLA antigens.[152] There are several approaches used to measure alloreactive antibodies which vary in sensitivity and in the level of information provided on the specificity of the antibodies. Assays today are likely to utilize isolated HLA molecules bound to a solid support, often a multi-wall plate or microspheres, in ELISA, flow cytometry, or Luminex[153] formats. The screening assay identifies the presence of IgG antibodies specific for particular HLA antigens and the extent of sensitization to foreign

HLA molecules in general (i.e., a measurement of panel (or percent) reactive antibody (PRA)).

Once a potential tissue donor has been selected, patient antibodies specific for cells of the donor are detected in a donor-specific cross-match in a microcytotoxicity or flow cytometry-based assay.[152] In some centers, a patient with an HLA mismatched donor with a positive donor directed cross-match (i.e., patient sensitized to donor) would be considered at increased risk for graft failure after HSC transplantation.[154,155] As an aside, while sensitization to paternal HLA antigens inherited by the child can occur in the mother during pregnancy, exposure of the child to the non-inherited maternal antigens (NIMA) may lead to tolerance.[156]

HLA assignments

HLA terminology is assigned by a World Health Organization (WHO) Committee for HLA Nomenclature. Several different naming systems are in use, each the result of the technology used to identify HLA diversity: serologic, cellular, or DNA based. The nomenclature is described on the website http://hla.alleles.org.[21] Since not all tissue typing techniques identify specific HLA alleles, the assignments are called HLA 'types'. Individuals who differ at the level of resolution of each test are assigned different HLA 'types'. For example, an individual tested by serology might express HLA types HLA-A1 and -A2 (heterozygous) while another individual might express HLA-A2 and -A74. Within the limits of resolution of the serologic technique, the two individuals in this example share one HLA-A type (A2) but differ for the second (A1 vs. A74). Within the limits of DNA-based testing, however, these individuals may differ in the A2 allele carried by each individual, for example A*0204 and A*0207. Likewise, two individuals typed by DNA-based methods as DRB1*04, *11 may differ for the alleles they carry.

Serologic specificities

Historically, serological and cellular reagents were used to define HLA types. These reagents defined specificities (or determinants) localized to one or several HLA molecules; these specificities were used as surrogates of alleles. The specificities identified through these methods were defined and standardized during international workshops in which typing reagents and cells were exchanged among participating laboratories and a consensus reached on the definition of each specificity[6] (Table 39.7). These specificities were named by the HLA molecule and by a numerical designation based on the order of discovery. As additional reagents were identified, serologically defined specificities were often subdivided (i.e., 'split'). For example, the serologic specificity HLA-B5 defined in the 1967 international workshop was subdivided into HLA-B51 and -B52 as a result of the reagents tested in the 1975 workshop. Table 39.7 lists the broader, shared (supertypic) specificities for the current 'split' (subtypic) specificities.

The numbering system used to define HLA 'types' is based on the date of assignment so that the relationships among various types is not immediately clear. Thus, for example, subdivisions of B5 were assigned as B51 and B52 since they were the 51st and 52nd serologic specificities to be assigned.

Their relationship to B5 is not immediately clear unless their more complete nomenclature, B51(5) and B52(5), is provided. The assignments associated with the HLA-A and HLA-B serologic specificities are further complicated because it was not initially appreciated that these were specified by two different loci. Thus, the naming system is based on a single numerical series[5,6] such that numerical designations of HLA-A include HLA-A1, -A2, -A3, -A9, -A10, -A11, etc. while the HLA-B designations include the remaining numbers in the series, HLA-Bw4, -B5, -Bw6, -B7, -B8, -B12, etc.

The HLA-Bw4 and -Bw6 serologic specificities are broad, supertypic determinants which reside on the same molecule as the B locus subtypic specificities. HLA-B locus molecules (and some HLA-A locus molecules) characteristically carry either Bw4 or Bw6 specificities. In the case of Bw4 and Bw6, the use of the 'w' in the designation indicates the shared nature of the determinant. The region of the HLA-B molecule carrying the Bw4/Bw6 specificities has been identified to lie in the α1 alpha helix between amino acid residues 77 and 83 (Fig. 39.6A).[157,158] (A similarly located epitope identified by NK cell reactivity divides the HLA-C molecules in to group 1 and group 2[116,119,120].)

Antibody reactivity patterns have been used to group HLA-A and HLA-B molecules into cross-reactive epitope groups (CREG).[159–161] Examples of CREGs are listed in Table 39.8. An antigenic determinant (epitope) shared among members of a CREG is called a public specificity. Class I molecules within a CREG share one or more determinants that are not shared by molecules in another CREG. These groupings have been used as the basis for matching schemes for selection of solid organ donors[162,163] and to predict the reactivity of HLA-specific antibodies in sensitized patients.[160] In contrast, in HSC transplantation, mismatching schemes based on CREGs or other shared epitopes have been shown not to impact survival or the occurrence of GVHD.[164,165]

Limitations in serologic testing reagents have resulted in inconsistent assignments of some HLA types.[166] This can complicate the selection of HLA matched donors from HSC donor registries and umbilical cord blood banks. With the increased use of DNA based HLA typing and its increased resolution and consistency, these difficulties are expected to disappear as the number of DNA typed donors and cord blood units increases.

DNA-based allele designations

Nucleotide sequencing has been used to identify the many alleles encoding the HLA molecules. Each HLA allele is designated by the name of the gene followed by an asterisk and a multiple digit number indicating the allele.[20] Additional and optional letters added to the end of the numerical designation relate to the expression of the allele at the protein level. The present nomenclature system is summarized in Tables 39.1, 39.2, and 39.9 and is described below.

Currently, allele names may contain four two-digit fields. The first two-digit field was originally based on the serologic type of the resultant molecule. Thus, the first HLA-A allele characterized from a cell bearing the HLA-A1 serologic specificity was assigned as A*0101 and the first HLA-B allele characterized from a cell bearing the HLA-B8 serologic specificity was assigned as B*0801. Identification of new alleles

Table 39.7 HLA class I and class II specificities defined by serology[a,b]

A	B	C	DR	DQ
A1	B5	Cw1[e]	DR1	DQ1
A2	B7	Cw2	DR103[d]	DQ2
A203[d]	B703	Cw3	DR2	DQ3
A210[d]	B8	Cw4	DR3	DQ4
A3	B12	Cw5	DR4	DQ5(1)
A9	B13	Cw6	DR5	DQ6(1)
A10	B14	Cw7	DR6	DQ7(3)
A11	B15	Cw8	DR7	DQ8(3)
A19	B16	Cw9(w3)	DR8	DQ9(3)
A23(9)[c]	B17	Cw10(w3)	DR9	
A24(9)	B18		DR10	
A2403[d]	B21		DR11(5)	
A25(10)	B22		DR12(5)	
A26(10)	B27		DR13(6)	
A28	B2708[d]		DR14(6)	
A29(19)	B35		DR1403[d]	
A30(19)	B37		DR1404[d]	
A31(19)	B38(16)		DR15(2)	
A32(19)	b39(16)		DR16(2)	
A33(19)	B3901[d]		DR17(3)	
A34(10)	B3902[d]		DR18(3)	
A36	B40		DR51[f]	
A43	B4005[d]		DR52[f]	
A66(10)	B41		DR53[f]	
A68(28)	B42			
A69(28)	B44(12)			
A74(19)	B45(12)			
A80	B46			
	B47			
	B48			
	B49(21)			
	B50(21)			
	B51(5)			
	B5102[d]			
	B5103[d]			
	B52(5)			
	B53			
	B54(22)			
	B55(22)			
	B56(22)			
	B57(17)			

Table 39.7 Continued

A	B	C	DR	DQ
	B58(17)			
	B59			
	B60(40)			
	B61(40)			
	B62(15)			
	B63(15)			
	B64(14)			
	B65(14)			
	B67			
	B70			
	B71(70)			
	B72(70)			
	B73			
	B75(15)			
	B76(15)			
	B77(15)			
	B78			
	B81			
	B82			
	Bw4[g]			
	Bw6[g]			

[a20] DP is difficult to define by serology.

[b]Each column of the table is independent and unrelated to the other columns.

[c]() indicates the broad serologic specificity so that A9 is the broad serologic specificity of A23 and A24. The serologic type may be listed without the broad specificity. For example, both A23(9) and A23 are correct designations.

[d]The associated antigens can be considered variants of the broad serologic specificity. These serologic specificities were once thought to detect the product of a specific HLA allele. For example, the A203 serologic specificity was thought to be located on a molecule encoded by an allele in the A2 family, A*0203. It is now thought that it is unlikely that a serologic reagent will detect the product of only a single allele.

[e]'w' is added to avoid confusion with the complement genes.

[f]DR51, DR52, and DR53 are serologic specificities associated with a number of DR serologic types as described in Table 39.4.

[g]Bw4 and Bw6 are serologic specificities found on multiple HLA-B and some HLA-A molecules (Table 39.8).

from other A1 or B8 positive cells led to the assignment of alleles A*0102 and B*0802. The second two-digit field of the allele name indicates the order of discovery. Alleles that share digits in the first field of their name share extensive sequence homology. This sequence similarity is also a criterion for nomenclature assignment and may take precedence over the serologic association in assigning an allele name.

Since most allelic differences lie within the antigen-binding groove of the HLA molecule, it is theoretically possible that these differences will stimulate allorecognition. There are two exceptions in which different allele names may not indicate different HLA molecules: 1) alleles which differ in their DNA sequence but do not differ in their encoded polypeptides are designated by sharing the digits in the first two fields of their allele names and are distinguished by the two digits in the third field of their name (e.g., B*070201, B*070202, B*070203). The differences among alleles in these clusters are not important to consider in transplantation matching since these alleles encode the same HLA proteins. 2) Alleles which have identical nucleotide sequences in their coding regions but differ in the nucleotide sequences outside of the coding region (i.e., in 5′ regulatory regions or introns) are designated by a sharing of the digits in the first three fields of their allele names and are distinguished by the two digits in the fourth field of their name (e.g., A*01010101 and A*01010102N).

The differences among alleles in these clusters may or may not be important to consider in transplantation matching depending on the effect of the sequence difference. Allelic differences that result in loss of protein expression are important considerations in the selection of a donor while

Table 39.8 HLA class I cross-reactive epitope groups[a]

CREG	Antigen specificities included
1C	A1, 3, 11, 23, 24, 29, 30, 31, 36, 80
2C	A2, 23, 24, 68, 69, B57, 58
5C	B51, 52, 18, 35, 46,49, 50, 53,57, 58, 62, 63, 75, 76, 77, 71, 72, 73, 78
7C	B7, 8, 13, 27, 54, 55, 56, 60, 61, 41, 42, 47, 48, 59, 67, 81, 82
8C	B8, 18, 38, 39, 64, 65, 59, 67
10C	A25, 26, 34, 66, 11, 68, 69, 32, 33, 43, 74
12C	B44, 45, 13, 49, 50, 37, 60, 61, 41, 47
Bw4[b]	B13, 27, 37, 38, 44, 47, 49, 51, 52, 53, 57, 58, 59, 63, 77, A23, A24, 25, 32
Bw6[b]	B7, 8, 18, 35, 39, 41, 42, 45, 46, 48, 50, 54, 55, 56, 60, 61, 62, 64, 65, 67, 71, 72, 73, 75, 76, 78, 81, 82

[a][159,160] The inclusion of HLA specificities within a CREG is not standard (i.e., CREG nomenclature has not been assigned by consensus of the HLA community) although there is considerable overlap between the various groupings reported in the literature.

[b]A listing of antigens carrying Bw4 and Bw6 specificities can be found at http://hla.alleles.org. Not all alleles encoding a specific antigen may carry the usual Bw4 or Bw6 epitope. For example, B*0736, an allele whose product appears to carry the B7 serologic specificity,[168] carries a Bw4 epitope rather than the Bw6 epitope carried by most of the B*07 allelic products. See also B*2715 in Table 39.11.

a difference which has no impact on the expression of the allele is not an important consideration.

Alleles that are not expressed as proteins at the cell surface may have a single letter, N, appended to their names (e.g., A*01010102N) to indicate 'null'. Null alleles are important to consider in transplantation since individuals who carry a null allele are functional homozygotes. For example, an individual who carries A*01010102N, A*0207 alleles would be serologically typed as A2 only compared to an individual who carries A*01010101, A*0207 who would be serologically typed as A1,A2. Other designations (e.g., L, S, Q) signify alterations in HLA expression and are described on the HLA nomenclature website (http://hla.alleles.org).[21]

While this chapter was being written, the HLA nomenclature underwent a revision to allow an extension of the number of digits designating each field in an allele name and to use colons to separate the fields making up the designation. Examples of the new nomenclature are shown in Table 39.9.

National Marrow Donor Program® (NMDP) DNA nomenclature

The ability to distinguish among alleles (the level of resolution) by DNA-based typing methods is controlled by the choice and number of reagents used and the typing technique. Large scale volunteer donor typing for a HSC registry or umbilical cord blood bank is usually carried out at low to intermediate resolution in which the alleles at each HLA locus are narrowed down to a few possibilities. For example, the HLA-DRB1 test results of a volunteer might narrow the possible alleles at this locus to DRB1*1301 or 1320 and to DRB1*0403 or *0406 or *0407 or *0411 or *0417. In order to include these possibilities within their database, the

Table 39.9 An explanation of HLA nomenclature[a]

Locus	*	Serologic type/allele family (Field 1)	Order discovered (Field 2)	Variation in DNA but not protein sequence (Field 3)	Variation in DNA sequence outside of coding regions (Field 4)	Expression character	Nomenclature prior to April 2010	Revised nomenclature effective April 2010
A	*	01	01	01	01		A*01010101	A*01:01:01:01
A	*	01	01	01	02	N	A*01010102N	A*01:01:01:02N
A	*	01	01	02			A*010102	A*01:01:02
A	*	01	02				A*0102	A*01:02
A	*	01	04			N	A*0104N	A*01:04N
A	*	02	01	01	01		A*02010101	A*02:01:01:01
A	*	02	101				A*9201[b]	A*02:101
A	*	02	102				A*9202[b]	A*02:102

[a]HLA nomenclature is assigned by the World Health Organization (WHO) Nomenclature for Factors of the HLA System Committee. At the time this chapter was written, each field in the allele name was limited to two digits. Because of the rapid increase in new alleles, the Committee will revised the nomenclature in April 2010 to allow each field to include an unlimited number of digits with the fields separated by colons. For example, A*01010101 was renamed A*01:01:01:01.

[b]When the next A*02 related allele after A*0299 was discovered, it was assigned the allele designation A*9201 to keep the number of digits in each field to two digits. When the new nomenclature became effective, these alleles were renamed to reflect their A*02 origin. A*9201 became A*02:101 and A*9202 was renamed A*02:102.

Table 39.10 Patient and potential donor HLA assignments and level of match

	HLA assignment	Method of testing	Level of match with patient
Patient	A*0101,*6801	DNA	Alleles encode A1 and A68(28) antigens[a]
Donor 1	A1,68	Serology	*Potentially* identical at the allele level since it is not known which of the many A*01 and A*68 alleles this donor carries
Donor 2	A*01XX[b], *68XX[b]	DNA	*Potentially* identical at the allele level since it is not known which of the many A*01 and A*68 alleles this donor carries
Donor 3	A*0101, *6801	DNA	Identical at the allele level (high resolution match)
Donor 4	A*0102, *6801	DNA	Allele *mis*match with a different protein encoded by A*0101 vs. A*0102
Donor 5	A*0201, *6801	DNA	Antigen-level *mis*match; the difference in alleles A*0101 vs. A*0201 leads to the expression of different serologic antigens
Donor 6	A*01AB[b],*6801	DNA	*Potentially* identical at the allele level since it is not known which of the two alleles designated by AB (A*0101 or A*0102) the donor carries

[a]169

[b]A listing of the letter codes can be found on the NMDP web site http://bioinformatics.nmdp.org. In the NMDP registry, a typing such as A*01 will be listed A*01XX where XX indicates that any allele which begins with A*01 (such as A*0101, A*0102, A*0103, or A*0104N) is potentially present. Likewise, AB is an NMDP code that indicates multiple allele possibilities.[167]

NMDP has developed a letter coding system for these multiple allele combinations. Thus, the combination DRB1*1301 or 1320 is designated DRB1*13VS where VS means 01 or 20 and DRB1*0403 or *0406 or *0407 or *0411 or *0417 is designated DRB1*04DZ (DZ means 03 or 06 or 07 or 11 or 17). The letter codes are purely descriptive, with codes being created only for allele combinations which have been observed during HLA testing. A listing of codes can be found on the NMDP website (http://bioinformatics.nmdp.org); the NMDP codes are used internationally in the exchange of HLA information among registries and cord blood banks.[167]

Limitations in the assignment of HLA alleles

Since identification of HLA alleles may often be based on partial nucleotide sequence information obtained through the use of a small set of primers and probes, it is possible that the interpretation of the assay results will miss alleles which were unknown at the time of the typing.[168] For example, the identification of the DNA sequence GGTAAG-TATAAG encompassing codons 11–14 in the DRB1 gene was once interpreted to mean that the individual carried the allele DRB1*0701 since only DRB1*0701 was known to carry that polymorphic sequence cassette. In 1998, two new alleles were described which also carry this sequence, DRB1*0703 and DRB1*0704. Thus, individuals tested prior to 1998 and characterized as carrying DRB1*0701 might alternatively carry DRB1*0703 or DRB1*0704. The continued discovery of new HLA alleles has significant implications for the HLA assignments since HLA types of individuals are stored and used for many years in HSC registries or cord blood banks. Since a patient may be HLA typed during the initial evaluation of treatment options but donor selection and transplant may not be the first line of therapy, the clinical laboratory should update the HLA assignments for that patient when the decision to seek an unrelated donor is made. Patients

with newly described or rare alleles may require additional search strategy assistance.

Because of the similarity among HLA alleles, a DNA-based assay may assign several alternative genotypes; for example, a patient may carry the genotype A*01010101 + A*02010101 or the genotype A*0114 + A*9204 or the genotype A*0236 + A*3604. While clinical laboratories are required to report all alternative genotypes, the laboratory may indicate that one of the genotypes is more likely based on the expected frequencies of HLA alleles in the population group to which the patient belongs. The decision to perform additional HLA testing to determine which genotype is indeed carried by an individual is a decision made by the transplant center and its clinical laboratory and should be based on a sound knowledge of the HLA profile of the relevant human population.

Correlation between serologic specificities and DNA-based allele assignments

Today, patients requiring HSC transplants are often typed by DNA-based technologies while registries and banks of potential donors include many serologically typed volunteers or cord blood units. Thus, a HSC registry's matching algorithm must be designed to compare a variety of HLA assignments and to determine the potential for an allele match. Table 39.10 provides some examples of the association between HLA types. In many cases, digits in the first field of the allele name are based on the serologic assignment of the HLA molecule so, for example, alleles such as A*0101 and A*6801 correspond to A1 and A68, respectively. In addition, several alleles may encode the same serologic type, such as B*2701, *2702 and *2703, which all encode a HLA-B molecule carrying a B27 serologic specificity (Table 39.11).

It is important to note, however, the many examples where the associations between an allele and the serologic type of the HLA molecule encoded by that allele are not known or

Table 39.11 Association between some of the HLA-B*27 alleles and serologic specificities[a]

Allele	Serologic specificity[b]
B*2701	B27
B*2702	B27
B*2703	B27
B*2708	B2708 [Sera detecting B7 are positive; most B27 sera are negative; neural network predicts B27.]
B*2711	B27 [B27 sera are positive; some B40 sera are positive; neural network predicts an undefined[c] antigen.]
B*2712	Undefined [Most B27 sera are negative, sera detecting both B7 and B27 are positive; some B40 sera are positive; neural network predicts an undefined antigen.]
B*2715	Undefined [B27 sera are negative, Bw4 instead of usual Bw6; neural network predicts B27.]

[a]169

[b]Based on serologic typing of specific B*27 allelic products. Data in [ ] describes unusual serologic patterns or the prediction of serologic typing based on an artificial neural network.

[c]Undefined indicates that the allelic product does not have a known serologic specificity.

are apparently different. For example, even though B*2708 encoded a molecule which bore a B7 serologic determinant, it was found to have a closer structural relationship to alleles in the B*27 group which took precedence in the assignment of the allele name. In this case, the name of the allele cannot be used to predict the serologic type of its allelic product. Information on the serologic assignments associated with each HLA allele is routinely updated and reported.[169] This 'dictionary' can be found in a searchable format at http://www.ebi.ac.uk/imgt/hla/dictionary.html.

Identification of HLA in clinical situations

Autoimmunity

Autoimmune diseases are characterized by an abnormal immune response to self antigens. Many of these diseases are associated with the presence of specific HLA types.[52,53] The association of HLA-DQ2 and DQ8 with celiac disease is one example. This disease is a chronic inflammatory disease developing in response to ingested wheat gluten or related proteins.[170] The majority of patients carry DQ2 and a minority DQ8. Yet, since only a fraction of individuals with DQ2 or DQ8 develop celiac disease, HLA-DQ is most likely just one out of several genetic and/or environment factors that combine to cause susceptibility to the disease.

A variety of mechanisms involving the HLA molecule have been evoked to explain the observed HLA-disease associations. One hypothesis suggests that a peptide from a pathogen which mimics a self peptide binds to the HLA molecule associated with the disease to initially stimulate autoreactive T-cells. A second hypothesis suggests that disease occurs as the result of altered thymic selection in which self reactive

T-cells escape selection in the thymus as a result of poor self peptide binding properties of the disease-associated HLA molecules. Still another hypothesis suggests that it is not the HLA molecule itself, but the product of another as yet unknown gene within the MHC which affects susceptibility. It is likely that the immune mechanisms resulting in a loss of tolerance to self antigens will vary among autoimmune diseases; thus, elucidation of the role that HLA plays will await the unraveling of each complex disease.

Drug hypersensitivity

Hypersensitivity to several drugs has been associated with specific HLA alleles: 1) the HIV reverse transcriptase inhibitor abacavir and B*5701; 2) the gout prophylactic allopurinol and B*5801; and 3) the antiepileptic carbamazepine and B*1502. Hypersensitivity to abacavir has been linked to HLA antigen presentation to T-lymphocytes although it is not yet known how abacavir or its by-products create the novel antigen triggering the response.[171]

Cell, tissue and organ transplantation

Allogeneic grafts of HSCs, organs and other tissues have been everyday life-saving procedures since the mid 20th century.[4] The necessity for HLA matching of donor and recipient differs for each type of graft. For HSC transplantation, close matching for HLA is required for successful outcome. For kidney transplantation, close matching increases the likelihood of long-term organ survival,[172] but survival of grafts in mismatched donor–recipient pairs is also good. For logistical reasons, HLA matching plays a smaller role in transplantation of organs other than HSC and kidneys and outcome relies on management of graft rejection using immune suppression. Grafts of non-viable tissues rarely take HLA matching into consideration, as these non-viable tissues are generally used either temporarily (skin) or as 'scaffolding' for replacement with autologous tissue.

Solid organ transplantation

According to the US Department of Health's Organ Procurement and Transplantation Network (OPTN) data, as of 22 May 2009 (http://optn.transplant.hrsa.gov), there were 27 961 transplants of organs in 2008 in the United States. Of these, 16 517 were kidney transplants. Included in this number are 6217 transplants from living donors. All of the other reported transplants were from cadaveric donors.

The OPTN is a nationwide system for organ sharing authorized by the US Congress through the National Organ Transplant Act of 1984. One of the primary purposes for nationwide organ sharing is to provide an opportunity for avoiding HLA mismatches that might result in graft loss in a sensitized patient.[173,174] Organs are allocated based on the best opportunity for successful outcome both for patients local to the organization that obtained the cadaveric organ and for patients located nationwide.

Platelets

Platelet transfusions are required for clinical conditions where bleeding occurs or is threatened and there is a low platelet count. The clinical decision to transfuse platelets is made more difficult because patients can become refractory to platelet transfusion due to allosensitization to HLA antigens and platelet-specific antigens.[175] Platelets express significant amounts of HLA class I antigens (but not class II antigens) and can be readily destroyed by platelet-directed antibodies. Immune sensitization can be reduced by removing leukocytes from the transfused product; however, the patients may be allosensitized prior to platelet transfusions because of pregnancies or prior transfusion of blood products.

For patients who do become sensitized, transfusions from HLA-compatible donors can be life saving. Practically, this is accomplished by finding donors who share the HLA-A, -B types of the patient or who have fewer of the shared types (i.e. are homozygous for one or more of the class I loci). Selection of donors expressing HLA antigens that are not detected by the patient's alloantibodies is a second alternative. Before transfusion, lymphocytes or platelets from the prospective donor can be tested with serum from the patient to detect sensitization. Donors can also be screened for platelet alloantigens.

HSC transplantation

Successful HSC grafts could not be achieved until donors adequately matched for HLA could be identified. The first successful grafts in the United States were performed in 1968 using HLA-matched sibling donors to treat patients with immune deficiency diseases.[4,176] By the mid 1970s, it was established that marrow transplants from sibling donors could save the lives of people with a number of diseases. Unfortunately, only 30% of patients needing a transplant had HLA-matched siblings. Transplant physicians and families began to seek ways to identify alternate donors. The first successful transplant from an unrelated donor was in 1975, for a patient with severe combined immunodeficiency.[177]

Unrelated donor registries and umbilical cord blood banks

Today, over 60 registries of HLA typed potential adult HSC donors in 44 countries and 42 umbilical cord blood banks in 26 countries include over 13 million volunteer donors and cord blood units (http://www.bmdw.org). In the United States, the C. W. Bill Young Cell Transplantation Program, authorized by Congress through the Stem Cell Therapeutic and Research Act of 2005, is a nationwide system supporting those patients seeking an unrelated donor. The 'Be The Match' national registry, operated by the NMDP, lists 7 million donors in its database and has facilitated over 30 000 transplants (http://www.marrow.org). In any given month, there is an average of 3000 patients searching the 'Be The Match' registry. While a donor search usually begins within the country of origin of the patient, searches failing to identify a donor can extend to foreign registries and banks. Many registries have established cooperative relationships with one another to facilitate searches of these international resources. In 2007, almost 40% of transplants facilitated through the NMDP were performed with bone marrow or peripheral blood stem cells (PBSC) from a donor in another

country. US donors of marrow or PBSC facilitated 623 transplants in other countries; this was 30% of the donations through the NMDP. An international voluntary organization of registries and banks worldwide, the World Marrow Donor Association (WMDA), has published policies and procedures for these international exchanges[178,179] (http://www.worldmarrow.org).

Testing of unrelated donors is conducted in stages. Initially a blood sample or buccal swab from an adult volunteer is obtained at HSC donor drives following informed consent. Samples collected for the NMDP are sent to a repository for aliquoting and distribution. One of the aliquots is sent to an HLA testing laboratory for identification of the key HLA types, HLA-A, -B, -DRB1 and sometimes HLA-C, using intermediate resolution DNA-based testing. The majority of the sample is retained in the repository for future additional testing. A similar process is used for umbilical cord blood, although the initial resolution of HLA typing may be higher due to limitations in the quantity of the cord blood which may preclude further testing.

Search strategies for donor identification

Ideally, HLA testing and a donor search are initiated for a patient with the diagnosis of one of over 20 diseases routinely treatable through HSC transplantation.[180] Testing of the patient, siblings and parents should be used to identify a HLA matched sibling donor since the observed probability of a sibling match is 30%. The family typing will also confirm the patient's HLA types and define the linkage of alleles at multiple loci, that is, define haplotypes. If the patient does not have a matched sibling, testing of the extended family, such as cousins, may identify an HLA matched related donor.[181] Selection of an HLA haploidentical relative may also be an alternative.[182]

Typing of HLA-A, -B and -DR (-DRB1) is routinely performed. Within a family, only minimal resolution typing using serology or DNA-based testing is required to establish the segregation of the inherited HLA complex and to identify HLA recombinants. The exceptions are families in which similar alleles are segregating within the family or parents are not available or when HLA mismatched relatives are being evaluated for donation. In these cases, higher resolution testing using DNA-based methods as well as testing of other MHC loci is recommended.

In the US, an initial search of the 'Be The Match' registry for an unrelated donor or a cord blood unit can be undertaken by any physician by contacting the NMDP headquarters; however, formal searches in which the patient has a reasonable likelihood of proceeding to transplantation and during which specific donors are contacted for additional evaluation may only be undertaken by an NMDP accredited transplant center. Referrals to such centers can be obtained through the NMDP. Submission of patient HLA typing information for HLA-A, -B, -C and -DR (DRB1) is preferred; the greater the resolution of the initial testing, the more likely it is that an accurate picture of the availability of HLA allele-matched donors will be obtained. In families, HLA alleles are inherited so that siblings who have inherited identical chromosomes have identical HLA alleles. In comparison, unrelated individuals carry a diverse collection of alleles found embedded within a large number of haplotypes. Thus, the identification of unrelated individuals who carry identical HLA alleles requires higher resolution typing approaches of both patient and selected donors.

The search report from the 'Be The Match' registry includes information on the likelihood that each potential donor or cord blood unit will carry the same HLA alleles as the searching patient. This information is useful especially when confronted with a large number of potential matches and can assist the transplant center in selecting a few potential donors for extended HLA typing.

An additional tool in the search process is a database listing HLA phenotypes available on most registries worldwide provided through Bone Marrow Donors Worldwide (BMDW)[183] (http://www.bmdw.org). This listing is frequently useful for rapidly estimating the likelihood of finding an HLA matched donor for a specific patient. BMDW should be used to provide supplementary information since not all registry updates are incorporated into the BMDW database and not all donors listed in BMDW will be suitable or available. The BMDW search report, coupled with a knowledge of allele and haplotype frequencies in world populations, can assist the physician in determining the usefulness of and strategy for a search of worldwide registries.

A list of HLA types from potentially matched volunteers is provided by a registry or bank to the patient's physician. From this list of potential matches, the physician selects donors for additional HLA testing. Guidelines for unrelated adult donor selection have been published by the NMDP.[184] Guidelines for HLA matching for the transplantation of umbilical cord blood are not yet clear; a literature review and summary of the current status has been published by the NMDP.[185] Adult volunteer donors are contacted to determine whether they are interested in continuing participation. More than one potential donor should be evaluated since some may be unavailable for any of a number of reasons such as inability to locate the donor or donor's poor health. Extended HLA typing may include a higher level of resolution for the four primary HLA loci or the testing of additional loci such as HLA-DQB1 and/or -DPB1. These additional tests are used to identify the best matched donor if several HLA-A, -B, -C, -DRB1 matched donors are available. To ensure that the selected donor or umbilical cord blood unit carries the HLA type shown on the search report (i.e., to confirm identity), a low resolution HLA typing of two or more loci should be performed on a fresh blood sample from the adult donor or on an attached segment from the umbilical cord blood unit. Searches for the best HLA match for a patient must be balanced with the timing of the transplant in relationship to disease stage since survival is reduced as the disease advances.

Histocompatible matches for HSC transplantation

At a minimum, HSC transplant centers attempt to match HLA-A, -B, -C and -DRB1 assignments of patient and potential donor since these loci have been shown to be clinically important in outcome.[82,184] This level of match is sometimes referred to as an 8/8 allele match – two assignments at HLA-A, two at HLA-B, two at HLA-C, and two at HLA-DRB1. (A mismatch for a single allele is termed a 7 of 8 match, and so on.) The impact of mismatching likely differs depending on a variety of recipient factors including disease, treatment and age, as well as the source of the HSC; however, comprehensive guidelines are lacking at present.[184] One source of stem cells which may offer a reduced risk of severe GVHD is umbilical cord blood. The relative immaturity of these cells may permit more HLA mismatching.[185] In addition, an umbilical cord blood unit is more readily available than an adult donor for a patient with an urgent need for transplantation. Selection factors that HSC transplant centers use to identify the best donor for a particular patient are based on criteria that improve the likelihood of successful transplant outcome. In addition to HLA, these may include donor age, cytomegalovirus infection status, large donor size for large patients, and matching for ABO red blood cell type, although the relative importance of these criteria is still unclear.[184]

Today, most patients can find closely matched volunteer donors, although the likelihood of finding a matched donor varies depending on the frequency that various HLA haplotypes are found. Some individuals have thousands of identical volunteers listed on donor registries, while other individuals have no matches. Lack of a well-matched donor is not a contraindication to transplantation, however. Although HLA matching for alleles of HLA-A,-B,-C, and -DRB1 is preferred, an unrelated donor with a limited number of mismatches or a suitable cord blood unit may be acceptable alternatives compared to alternative therapies.[184,185]

Summary

The classical human leukocyte antigens bind antigenic peptides, stimulating specific immune responses to microbial pathogens and malignant cells. These molecules also play a primary role in determining the outcome of the transplantation of tissues from one individual to another. Now it is known that the classical HLA molecules have additional roles in the immune system and are the ligand for many different receptors and that other molecules also participate in a variety of these functions. Transplantation outcome will only improve from the benefits of continued research efforts in these areas of study.

References

1. Snell GD. Studies in histocompatibility. Science 1981;213:172–8.

2. Benacerraf B. Role of MHC gene products in immune regulation. Science 1981; 212:1229–38.

3. Dausset J. The Nobel Lectures in Immunology. Lecture for the Nobel Prize for Physiology or Medicine, 1980. The major histocompatibility complex in man. Past, present, and future concepts. Science 1981;213:1469–74.

4. Groth CG, Brent LB, Calne RY, et al. Historic landmarks in clinical transplantation: Conclusions from the consensus conference at the University of California, Los Angeles. World J Surg 2000;24:834–43.

5. Payne R, Tripp M, Weigle J, et al. A new leukocyte isoantigen system in man. Cold Spring Harbor Symp Quant Biol 1964;29:285–95.

6. van Rood JJ. HLA and I. Annu Rev Immunol 1993;11:1–28.

7. Bach FH, Hirschhorn K. Lymphocyte interaction: a potential histocompatibility test in vitro. Science 1964;143:813–4.

8. Thorsby E, Piazza A. Joint report from the sixth international histocompatibility workshop conference. II. Typing for HLA-D (LD-1 or MLC) determinants. In: Kissmeyer-Nielsen F, editor. Histocompatibility Testing. Copenhagen: Munksgaard; 1975. p. 414–58.

9. Horton R, Gibson R, Coggill P, et al. Variation analysis and gene annotation of eight MHC haplotypes: the MHC Haplotype Project. Immunogenetics 2008;60(1):1–18.

10. MHC Sequencing Consortium. Complete sequence and gene map of a human major histocompatibility complex. Nature 1999;401:921–3.

11. Beck S, Trowsdale J. Sequence organization of the class II region of the human MHC. Immunol Rev 1999;167: 201–10.

12. Xie T, Rowen L, Aguado B, et al. Analysis of the gene-dense major histocompatibility complex class III region and its comparison to mouse. Genome Res 2003;13(12):2621–36.

13. Milner CM, Campbell RD. Genetic organization of the human MHC class III region. Front Biosci 2001;6: D914–D926.

14. Shiina T, Tamiya G, Oka A, et al. Genome sequence analysis of the 1.8Mb entire human MHC class I region. Immunol Rev 1999;167:193–9.

15. Auffray C, Strominger JL. Molecular genetics of the human major histocompatibility complex. Adv Hum Genet 1986;15:197–247.

16. Kappes D, Strominger JL. Human class II major histocompatibility complex genes

and proteins. Annu Rev Biochem 1988;57:991–1028.

17. Kwok WW, Kovats S, Thurtle P, Nepom GT. HLA-DQ allelic polymorphisms constrain patterns of class II heterodimer formation. J Immunol 1993;150:2263–72.

18. Little A-M, Parham P. Polymorphism and evolution of HLA class I and class II genes and molecules. Rev Immunogenetics 1999;1:105–23.

19. Bontrop RE. Comparative genetics of MHC polymorphisms in different primate species: duplications and deletions. Hum Immunol 2006; 67(6):388–97.

20. Marsh SG, Albert ED, Bodmer WF, et al. Nomenclature for factors of the HLA system, 2004. Tissue Antigens 2005; 65(4):301–69.

21. Robinson J, Waller MJ, Parham P, et al. IMGT/HLA and IMGT/MHC: sequence databases for the study of the major histocompatibility complex. Nucleic Acids Res 2003;31(1):311–4.

22. Martin MP, Carrington M. Immunogenetics of viral infections. Curr Opin Immunol 2005;17(5):510–6.

23. Meyer D, Single RM, Mack SJ, et al. Signatures of demographic history and natural selection in the human major histocompatibility complex loci. Genetics 2006;173(4):2121–42.

24. Prugnolle F, Manica A, Charpentier M, et al. Pathogen-driven selection and worldwide HLA class I diversity. Curr Biol 2005;15(11):1022–7.

25. Yeager M, Hughes AL. Evolution of the mammalian MHC: natural selection, recombination, and convergent evolution. Immunol Rev 1999;167: 45–58.

26. Cullen M, Perfetto SP, Klitz W, et al. High-resolution patterns of meiotic recombination across the human major histocompatibility complex. Am J Hum Genet 2002;71(4):759–76.

27. Jeffreys AJ, Holloway JK, Kauppi L, et al. Meiotic recombination hot spots and human DNA diversity. Philos Trans R Soc Lond B Biol Sci 2004;359(1441): 141–52.

28. Solberg OD, Mack SJ, Lancaster AK, et al. Balancing selection and heterogeneity across the classical human leukocyte antigen loci: a meta-analytic review of 497 population studies. Hum Immunol 2008;69(7):443–64.

29. Maiers M, Gragert L, Klitz W. High-resolution HLA alleles and haplotypes in the United States population. Hum Immunol 2007;68(9):779–88.

30. Mori M, Beatty PG, Graves M, et al. HLA gene and haplotype frequencies in the North American population – the National Marrow Donor Program Donor

Registry. Transplantation 1997; 64(7):1017–27.

31. Begovich AB, Klitz W, Steiner LL, et al. HLA-DQ haplotypes in 15 different populations. In: Kasahara M, editor. The major histocompatibility complex: evolution, structure and function. Tokyo: Springer-Verlag; 2000. p. 412–26.

32. Klitz W, Maiers M, Spellman S, et al. New HLA haplotype frequency reference standards: high-resolution and large sample typing of HLA DR-DQ haplotypes in a sample of European Americans. Tissue Antigens 2003;62(4): 296–307.

33. Yunis EJ, Larsen CE, Fernandez-Vina M, et al. Inheritable variable sizes of DNA stretches in the human MHC: conserved extended haplotypes and their fragments or blocks. Tissue Antigens 2003;62(1): 1–20.

34. Traherne JA, Horton R, Roberts AN, et al. Genetic analysis of completely sequenced disease-associated MHC haplotypes identifies shuffling of segments in recent human history. PLoS Genet 2006; 2(1):e9.

35. Van den Elsen PJ, Holling TM, Kuipers HF, van der Stoep N. Transcriptional regulation of antigen presentation. Curr Opin Immunol 2004;16(1):67–75.

36. Van den Elsen PJ, Gobin SJP, Van Eggermond MC, Peijnenburg A. Regulation of MHC class I and II gene transcription: differences and similarities. Immunogenetics 1998;48(3): 208–21.

37. Mach B, Steimle V, Martinez-Soria E, Reith W. Regulation of MHC class II genes: lessons from a disease. Annu Rev Immunol 1996;14:301–31.

38. Muhlethaler-Mottet A, Krawczyk M, Masternak K, et al. The S box of major histocompatibility complex class II promoters is a key determinant for recruitment of the transcriptional co-activator CIITA. J Biol Chem 2004; 279(39):40529–35.

39. Gobin SJ, van Zutphen M, Westerheide SD, et al. The MHC-specific enhanceosome and its role in MHC class I and beta(2)-microglobulin gene transactivation. J Immunol 2001;167(9): 5175–84.

40. Emery P, Mach B, Reith W. The different level of expression of HLA-DRB1 and -DRB3 genes is controlled by conserved isotypic differences in promoter sequence. Hum Immunol 1993;38: 137–47.

41. Leën MPJM, Gorski J. DRB4 promoter polymorphism in DR7 individuals: correlation with DRB4 pre-mRNA and mRNA levels. Immunogenetics 1997; 45(6):371–8.

42. Garcia-Lora A, Algarra I, Garrido F. MHC class I antigens, immune surveillance,

and tumor immune escape. J Cell Physiol 2003;195(3):346–55.

43. Lilley BN, Ploegh HL. Viral modulation of antigen presentation: manipulation of cellular targets in the ER and beyond. Immunol Rev 2005;207:126–44.

44. Kaufmann SH, Schaible UE. Antigen presentation and recognition in bacterial infections. Curr Opin Immunol 2005; 17(1):79–87.

45. Lin A, Xu H, Yan W. Modulation of HLA expression in human cytomegalovirus immune evasion. Cell Mol Immunol 2007;4(2):91–8.

46. Kimball ES, Coligan JE. Structure of class I major histocompatibility antigens. Contemp Top Mol Immunol 1983;9: 1–63.

47. Adamashvili I, Kelley RE, Pressly T, McDonald JC. Soluble HLA: patterns of expression in normal subjects, autoimmune diseases, and transplant recipients. Rheumatol Int 2005;25(7): 491–500.

48. Maenaka K, Jones EY. MHC superfamily structure and the immune system. Curr Opin Struct Biol 1999;9:745–53.

49. Madden DR. The three-dimensional structure of peptide-MHC complexes. Annu Rev Immunol 1995;13:587–622.

50. Stevanovic S. Structural basis of immunogenicity. Transpl Immunol 2002;10(2–3):133–6.

51. Hickman HD, Luis AD, Buchli R, et al. Toward a definition of self: proteomic evaluation of the class I peptide repertoire. J Immunol 2004;172(5): 2944–52.

52. Jones EY, Fugger L, Strominger JL, Siebold C. MHC class II proteins and disease: a structural perspective. Nat Rev Immunol 2006;6(4):271–82.

53. Thorsby E, Lie BA. HLA associated genetic predisposition to autoimmune diseases: genes involved and possible mechanisms. Transpl Immunol 2005; 14(3–4):175–82.

54. Hattotuwagama CK, Doytchinova IA, Flower DR. Toward the prediction of class I and II mouse major histocompatibility complex-peptide-binding affinity: in silico bioinformatic step-by-step guide using quantitative structure-activity relationships. Methods Mol Biol 2007;409:227–45.

55. Sturniolo T, Bono E, Ding J, et al. Generation of tissue-specific and promiscuous HLA ligand databases using DNA microarrays and virtual HLA class II matrices. Nat Biotechnol 1999;17(6): 555–61.

56. Nielsen M, Lundegaard C, Blicher T, et al. Quantitative predictions of peptide binding to any HLA-DR molecule of known sequence: NetMHCIIpan. PLoS Comput Biol 2008;4(7):e1000107.

57. Stevanovic S, Lemmel C, Hantschel M, Eberle U. Generating data for databases – the peptide repertoire of HLA molecules. Novartis Found Symp 2003; 254:143–55.

58. Lee KH, Wucherpfennig KW, Wiley DC. Structure of a human insulin peptide-HLA-DQ8 complex and susceptibility to type 1 diabetes. Nat Immunol 2001;2(6): 501–7.

59. Zavala-Ruiz Z, Strug I, Anderson MW, et al. A polymorphic pocket at the P10 position contributes to peptide binding specificity in class II MHC proteins. Chem Biol 2004;11(10): 1395–402.

60. Garbi N, Tanaka S, van den BM, et al. Accessory molecules in the assembly of major histocompatibility complex class I/peptide complexes: how essential are they for CD8(+) T-cell immune responses? Immunol Rev 2005;207: 77–88.

61. Van Kaer L. Major histocompatibility complex class I-restricted antigen processing and presentation. Tissue Antigens 2002;60(1):1–9.

62. York IA, Chang SC, Saric T, et al. The ER aminopeptidase ERAP1 enhances or limits antigen presentation by trimming epitopes to 8–9 residues. Nat Immunol 2002;3(12):1177–84.

63. Serwold T, Gonzalez F, Kim J, et al. ERAAP customizes peptides for MHC class I molecules in the endoplasmic reticulum. Nature 2002;419(6906): 480–3.

64. Pieters J. MHC class II restricted antigen presentation. Curr Opin Immunol 1997;9:89–96.

65. Gelin C, Sloma I, Charron D, Mooney N. Regulation of MHC II and CD1 antigen presentation: from ubiquity to security. J Leukoc Biol 2009;85(2):215–24.

66. Watts C. The exogenous pathway for antigen presentation on major histocompatibility complex class II and CD1 molecules. Nat Immunol 2004;5(7):685–92.

67. Brocke P, Garbi N, Momburg F, Hammerling GJ. HLA-DM, HLA-DO and tapasin: functional similarities and differences. Curr Opin Immunol 2002; 14(1):22–9.

68. Karlsson L. DM and DO shape the repertoire of peptide-MHC-class-II complexes. Curr Opin Immunol 2005; 17(1):65–70.

69. Alfonso C, Karlsson L. Nonclassical MHC class II molecules. Annu Rev Immunol 2000;18:113–42.

70. Kuhns MS, Davis MM, Garcia KC. Deconstructing the form and function of the TCR/CD3 complex. Immunity 2006;24(2):133–9.

71. Rudolph MG, Stanfield RL, Wilson IA. How TCRs bind MHCs, peptides, and coreceptors. Annu Rev Immunol 2006;24:419–66.

72. Armstrong KM, Piepenbrink KH, Baker BM. Conformational changes and flexibility in T-cell receptor recognition of peptide-MHC complexes. Biochem J 2008;415(2):183–96.

73. Gao GF, Rao Z, Bell JI. Molecular coordination of alphabeta T-cell receptors and coreceptors CD8 and CD4 in their recognition of peptide-MHC ligands. Trends Immunol 2002;23(8): 408–13.

74. Rowen L, Koop BF, Hood L. The complete 685-kilobase DNA sequence of the human β T cell receptor locus. Science 1996;272:1755–62.

75. Xiong N, Raulet DH. Development and selection of gammadelta T cells. Immunol Rev 2007;215:15–31.

76. Von Boehmer H. Selection of the T-cell repertoire: receptor-controlled checkpoints in T-cell development. Adv Immunol 2004;84:201–38.

77. Starr TK, Jameson SC, Hogquist KA. Positive and negative selection of T cells. Annu Rev Immunol 2003;21:139–76.

78. Maggi E, Cosmi L, Liotta F, et al. Thymic regulatory T cells. Autoimmun Rev 2005;4(8):579–86.

79. Goldrath AW, Bevan MJ. Selecting and maintaining a diverse T-cell repertoire. Nature 1999;402:255–62.

80. Afzali B, Lombardi G, Lechler RI. Pathways of major histocompatibility complex allorecognition. Curr Opin Organ Transplant 2008;13(4): 438–44.

81. Felix NJ, Allen PM. Specificity of T-cell alloreactivity. Nat Rev Immunol 2007; 7(12):942–53.

82. Lee SJ, Klein J, Haagenson M, Baxter-Lowe LA, et al. High-resolution donor-recipient HLA matching contributes to the success of unrelated donor marrow transplantation. Blood 2007;110(13):4576–83.

83. Lindahl KF, Wilson DB. Histocompatibility antigen-activated cytotoxic T lymphocytes. II. Estimates of the frequency and specificity of precursors. J Exp Med 1977;145(3): 508–22.

84. Archbold JK, Macdonald WA, Burrows SR, et al. T-cell allorecognition: a case of mistaken identity or deja vu? Trends Immunol 2008;29(5):220–6.

85. Gobin SJ, Van den Elsen PJ. Transcriptional regulation of the MHC class Ib genes HLA-E, HLA-F, and HLA-G. Hum Immunol 2000;61(11):1102–7.

86. Posch PE, Borrego F, Brooks AG, Coligan JE. HLA-E is the ligand for the natural killer cell CD94/NKG2 receptors. J Biomed Sci 1998;5:321–31.

87. Sullivan LC, Clements CS, Rossjohn J, Brooks AG. The major histocompatibility complex class Ib molecule HLA-E at the interface between innate and adaptive immunity. Tissue Antigens 2008;72(5): 415–24.

88. Petrie EJ, Clements CS, Lin J, et al. CD94-NKG2A recognition of human leukocyte antigen (HLA)-E bound to an

HLA class I leader sequence. J Exp Med 2008;205(3):725–35.

89. Hoare HL, Sullivan LC, Pietra G, et al. Structural basis for a major histocompatibility complex class Ib-restricted T cell response. Nat Immunol 2006;7(3):256–64.

90. O'Callaghan CA, Bell JI. Structure and function of the human class Ib molecules HLA-E, HLA-F and HLA-G. Immunol Rev 1998;163:129–38.

91. Sullivan LC, Hoare HL, McCluskey J, et al. A structural perspective on MHC class Ib molecules in adaptive immunity. Trends Immunol 2006;27(9):413–20.

92. Lepin EJ, Bastin JM, Allan DS, et al. Functional characterization of HLA-F and binding of HLA-F tetramers to ILT2 and ILT4 receptors. Eur J Immunol 2000; 30(12):3552–61.

93. Lee N, Geraghty DE. HLA-F surface expression on B cell and monocyte cell lines is partially independent from tapasin and completely independent from TAP. J Immunol 2003;171(10):5264–71.

94. Boyle LH, Gillingham AK, Munro S, Trowsdale J. Selective export of HLA-F by its cytoplasmic tail. J Immunol 2006; 176(11):6464–72.

95. Munz C, Nickolaus P, Lammert E, et al. The role of peptide presentation in the physiological function of HLA-G. Cancer Biol 1999;9:47–54.

96. Clements CS, Kjer-Nielsen L, Kostenko L, et al. Crystal structure of HLA-G: a nonclassical MHC class I molecule expressed at the fetal-maternal interface. Proc Natl Acad Sci USA 2005;102(9): 3360–5.

97. Apps R, Gardner L, Moffett A. A critical look at HLA-G. Trends Immunol 2008; 29(7):313–21.

98. Shiroishi M, Kuroki K, Rasubala L, et al. Structural basis for recognition of the nonclassical MHC molecule HLA-G by the leukocyte Ig-like receptor B2 (LILRB2/LIR2/ILT4/CD85d). Proc Natl Acad Sci U S A 2006;103(44):16412–7.

99. Apps R, Gardner L, Sharkey AM, et al. A homodimeric complex of HLA-G on normal trophoblast cells modulates antigen-presenting cells via LILRB1. Eur J Immunol 2007;37(7):1924–37.

100. Rajagopalan S, Bryceson YT, Kuppusamy SP, et al. Activation of NK cells by an endocytosed receptor for soluble HLA-G. PLoS Biol 2006;4(1):e9.

101. Bahram S. MIC genes: from genetics to biology. Adv Immunol 2000;76:1–60.

102. Bahram S, Inoko H, Shiina T, Radosavljevic M. MIC and other NKG2D ligands: from none to too many. Curr Opin Immunol 2005;17(5):505–9.

103. Collins RW. Human MHC class I chain related (MIC) genes: their biological function and relevance to disease and transplantation. Eur J Immunogenet 2004;31(3):105–14.

104. Li P, Willie ST, Bauer S, et al. Crystal structure of the MHC class I homolog MIC-A, a gamma/delta T cell ligand. Immunity 1999;10:577–84.

105. Seliger B, Abken H, Ferrone S. HLA-G and MIC expression in tumors and their role in anti-tumor immunity. Trends Immunol 2003;24(2):82–7.

106. Suarez-Alvarez B, Lopez-Vazquez A, Baltar JM, et al. Potential role of NKG2D and its ligands in organ transplantation: new target for immunointervention. Am J Transplant 2009;9(2):251–7.

107. Zou Y, Stastny P. The role of major histocompatibility complex class I chain-related gene A antibodies in organ transplantation. Curr Opin Organ Transplant 2009;14(4):414–8.

108. Silk JD, Salio M, Brown J, et al. Structural and functional aspects of lipid binding by CD1 molecules. Annu Rev Cell Dev Biol 2008;24:369–95.

109. Lawton AP, Kronenberg M. The third way: progress on pathways of antigen processing and presentation by CD1. Immunol Cell Biol 2004;82(3):295–306.

110. Cohen NR, Garg S, Brenner MB. Antigen presentation by CD1 lipids, T cells, and NKT cells in microbial immunity. Adv Immunol 2009;102:1–94.

111. Simpson E, Scott D, James E, et al. Minor H antigens: genes and peptides. Transpl Immunol 2002;10(2–3):115–23.

112. Hambach L, Spierings E, Goulmy E. Risk assessment in haematopoietic stem cell transplantation: minor histocompatibility antigens. Best Pract Res Clin Haematol 2007;20(2):171–87.

113. Goulmy E. Minor histocompatibility antigens: from transplantation problems to therapy of cancer. Hum Immunol 2006;67(6):433–8.

114. Spierings E, Hendriks M, Absi L, et al. Phenotype frequencies of autosomal minor histocompatibility antigens display significant differences among populations. PLoS Genetics 2007; 3(6):e103.

115. Falkenburg JH, van de Corput L, Marijt EW, Willemze R. Minor histocompatibility antigens in human stem cell transplantation. Exp Hematol 2003;31(9):743–51.

116. Lanier LL. NK cell recognition. Annu Rev Immunol 2005;23:225–74.

117. Bryceson YT, March ME, Ljunggren HG, Long EO. Activation, coactivation, and costimulation of resting human natural killer cells. Immunol Rev 2006;214: 73–91.

118. Bashirova AA, Martin MP, McVicar DW, Carrington M. The killer immunoglobulin-like receptor gene cluster: tuning the genome for defense. Annu Rev Genomics Hum Genet 2006;7:277–300.

119. Colonna M, Spies T, Strominger JL, et al. Alloantigen recognition by two human natural killer cell clones is associated

with *HLA-C* or a closely linked gene. Proc Natl Acad Sci USA 1992;89:7983–5.

120. Mandelboim O, Reyburn HT, Vales-Gomez M, et al. Protection from lysis by natural killer cells of group 1 and 2 specificity is mediated by residue 80 in human histocompatibility leukocyte antigen C alleles and also occurs with empty major histocompatibility complex molecules. J Exp Med 1996;184(3): 913–22.

121. Trowsdale J. Genetic and functional relationships between MHC and NK receptor genes. Immunity 2001;15(3): 363–74.

122. Hsu KC, Chida S, Dupont B, Geraghty DE. The killer cell immunoglobulin-like receptor (KIR) genomic region: gene-order, haplotypes and allelic polymorphism. Immunological Reviews 2002;190(1):40–52.

123. Robinson J, Waller MJ, Stoehr P, Marsh SG. IPD – the Immuno Polymorphism Database. Nucleic Acids Res 2005;33(Database Issue):D523–D526.

124. Yawata M, Yawata N, Draghi M, et al. Roles for HLA and KIR polymorphisms in natural killer cell repertoire selection and modulation of effector function. J Exp Med 2006;203(3):633–45.

125. Andersson S, Fauriat C, Malmberg JA, et al. KIR acquisition probabilities are independent of self-HLA class I ligands and increase with cellular KIR expression. Blood 2009;114(1):95–104.

126. Jonsson AH, Yokoyama WM. Natural killer cell tolerance licensing and other mechanisms. Adv Immunol 2009;101: 27–79.

127. Brodin P, Karre K, Hoglund P. NK cell education: not an on-off switch but a tunable rheostat. Trends Immunol 2009;30(4):143–9.

128. Ruggeri L, Capanni M, Urgani E, et al. Effectiveness of donor natural killer cell alloreactivity in mismatched hematopoietic transplants. Science 2002;295:2097–100.

129. Witt CS. The influence of NK alloreactivity on matched unrelated donor and HLA identical sibling haematopoietic stem cell transplantation. Curr Opin Immunol 2009;21(5):531–7.

130. Grzywacz B, Miller JS, Verneris MR. Use of natural killer cells as immunotherapy for leukaemia. Best Pract Res Clin Haematol 2008;21(3):467–83.

131. Passweg JR, Huard B, Tiercy JM, Roosnek E. HLA and KIR polymorphisms affect NK-cell anti-tumor activity. Trends Immunol 2007;28(10):437–41.

132. Borrego F, Masilamani M, Marusina AI, et al. The CD94/NKG2 family of receptors: from molecules and cells to clinical relevance. Immunol Res 2006;35(3):263–78.

133. Sullivan LC, Clements CS, Beddoe T, et al. The heterodimeric assembly of the CD94-NKG2 receptor family and

implications for human leukocyte antigen-E recognition. Immunity 2007;27(6):900–11.

134. Burgess SJ, Maasho K, Masilamani M, et al. The NKG2D receptor: immunobiology and clinical implications. Immunol Res 2008;40(1):18–34.

135. Lopez-Larrea C, Suarez-Alvarez B, Lopez-Soto A, et al. The NKG2D receptor: sensing stressed cells. Trends Mol Med 2008;14(4):179–89.

136. Brown D, Trowsdale J, Allen R. The LILR family: modulators of innate and adaptive immune pathways in health and disease. Tissue Antigens 2004; 64(3):215–25.

137. Anderson KJ, Allen RL. Regulation of T-cell immunity by leucocyte immunoglobulin-like receptors: innate immune receptors for self on antigen-presenting cells. Immunology 2009; 127(1):8–17.

138. Katz HR. Inhibition of inflammatory responses by leukocyte Ig-like receptors. Adv Immunol 2006;91:251–72.

139. American Society of Histocompatibility and Immunogenetics Laboratory Manual. 4.2 ed. 2008.

140. Reinsmoen NL, Zeevi A. Evaluation of the cellular immune response in transplantation. In: Detrick B, Hamilton RG, Folds JD, editors. Manual of Molecular and Clinical Laboratory Immunology. Washington DC: ASM Press; 2006. p. 1228–43.

141. Mickelson EM, Longton G, Anasetti C, et al. Evaluation of the mixed lymphocyte culture (MLC) assay as a method for selecting unrelated donors for marrow transplantation. Tissue Antigens 1996;47:27–36.

142. Spencer A, Szydlo RM, Brookes PA, et al. Bone marrow transplantation for chronic myeloid leukemia with volunteer unrelated donors using ex vivo or in vivo T-cell depletion: major prognostic impact of HLA class I identity between donor and recipient. Blood 1995;86: 3590–7.

143. Wang XN, Taylor PR, Skinner R, et al. T-cell frequency analysis does not predict the incidence of graft-versus-host disease in HLA-matched sibling bone marrow transplantation. Transplantation 2000; 70(3):488–93.

144. Sayer DC, Smith LK, Krueger R, Chrisitansen FT. DNA sequencing-based HLA typing detects a B-cell ALL blast-specific mutation in HLA-A(*)2402 resulting in loss of HLA allele expression. Leukemia 2004;18(1):174–6.

145. Jacobbi LM, Blackwell P. Guidelines for specimen collection, storage and transportation. In: Hahn AB, Land GA, Strothman RM, editors. ASHI Laboratory Manual. American Society for Histocompatibility and Immunogenetics; 2000.

146. Schaffer M, Olerup O. HLA-AB typing by polymerase-chain reaction with sequence-specific primers: more accurate, less errors, and increased resolution compared to serological typing. Tissue Antigens 2001;58(5):299–307.

147. Welsh K, Bunce M. Molecular typing for the MHC with PCR-SSP. Rev Immunogenetics 1999;1:157–76.

148. Kimura A, Dong RP, Harada H, Sasazuki T. DNA typing of HLA class II genes in B-lymphoblastoid cell lines homozygous for HLA. Tissue Antigens 1992;40: 5–12.

149. Cao K, Chopek M, Fernandez-Vina MA. High and intermediate resolution DNA typing systems for class I HLA-A, -B, -C genes by hybridization with sequence specific oligonucleotide probes (SSOP). Rev Immunogenetics 1999;1:177–208.

150. Scheltinga SA, Johnston-Dow LA, White CB, et al. A generic sequencing based typing approach for the identification of HLA-A diversity. Hum Immunol 1997; 57(2):120–8.

151. McGinnis MD, Conrad MP, Bouwens AGM, et al. Automated, solid-phase sequencing of DRB region genes using T7 sequencing chemistry and dye-labeled primers. Tissue Antigens 1995;46:173–9.

152. Zachary AA, Houp JA, Vega R, et al. Evaluation of the humoral response in transplantation. In: Detrick B, Hamilton RG, Folds JD, editors. Manual of Molecular and Clinical Laboratory Immunology. Washington, DC: ASM Press; 2006. p. 1215–27.

153. Fulton RJ, McDade RL, Smith PL, et al. Advanced multiplexed analysis with the FlowMetrix system. Clinical Chemistry 1997;43:1749–56.

154. Mickelson EM, Petersdorf E, Anasetti C, et al. HLA matching in hematopoietic cell transplantation. Hum Immunol 2000;61:92–100.

155. Ottinger HD, Rebmann V, Pfeiffer KA, et al. Positive serum crossmatch as predictor for graft failure in HLA-mismatched allogeneic blood stem cell transplantation. Transplantation 2002; 73:1280–5.

156. van den Boogaardt DE, van Rood JJ, Roelen DL, Claas FH. The influence of inherited and noninherited parental antigens on outcome after transplantation. Transpl Int 2006; 19(5):360–71.

157. Wan AM, Ennis PD, Parham P, Holmes N. The primary structure of HLA-A32 suggests a region involved in formation of the Bw4/Bw6 epitopes. J Immunol 1986;137:3671–4.

158. Toubert A, Raffoux C, Boretto J, et al. Epitope mapping of HLA-B27 and HLA-B7 antigens by using intradomain recombinants. J Immunol 1988;141(7): 2503–7.

159. Rodey GE, Fuller TC. Public epitopes and the antigenic structure of the HLA

molecules. Crit Rev Immunol 1987;7:229–67.

160. Rodey GE, Neylan JF, Whelchel JD, et al. Epitope specificity of HLA class I alloantibodies. I. Frequency analysis of antibodies to private versus public specificities in potential transplant recipients. Hum Immunol 1994;39: 272–80.

161. Rodey GE. HLA Beyond Tears. 2nd ed. Durango CO: De Novo; 2000.

162. Thompson JS, Thacker LR. CREG matching for first cadaveric kidney transplants (TNX) performed by SEOPF centers between October 1987 and September 1995. Southeastern Organ Procurement Foundation. Clin Transplant 1996;10:586–93.

163. Takemoto SK, Cecka JM, Terasaki PI. Benefits of HLA-CREG matching for sensitized recipients as illustrated in kidney regrafts. Transplant Proc 1997;29(1–2 PT 5):1417.

164. Wade JA, Hurley CK, Takemoto SK, et al. HLA mismatching within or outside of cross-reactive groups (CREGs) is associated with similar outcomes after unrelated hematopoietic stem cell transplantation. Blood 2007;109(9): 4064–70.

165. Duquesnoy R, Spellman S, Haagenson M, et al. HLAMatchmaker-defined triplet matching is not associated with better survival rates of patients with class I HLA allele mismatched hematopoietic cell transplants from unrelated donors. Biol Blood Marrow Transplant 2008;14(9): 1064–71.

166. Noreen HJ, Yu N, Setterholm M, et al. Validation of DNA-based HLA-A and HLA-B testing of volunteers for a bone marrow registry through parallel testing with serology. Tissue Antigens 2001; 57(3):221–9.

167. Bochtler W, Maiers M, Oudshoorn M, et al. World Marrow Donor Association guidelines for use of HLA nomenclature and its validation in the data exchange among hematopoietic stem cell donor registries and cord blood banks. Bone Marrow Transplant 2007;39(12):737–41.

168. Hurley CK. Acquisition and use of DNA-based HLA typing data in bone marrow registries. Tissue Antigens 1997;49:323–8.

169. Holdsworth R, Hurley CK, Marsh SG, et al. The HLA dictionary 2008: a summary of HLA-A, -B, -C, -DRB1/3/4/5, and -DQB1 alleles and their association with serologically defined HLA-A, -B, -C, -DR, and -DQ antigens. Tissue Antigens 2009;73(2):95–170.

170. Sollid LM. Coeliac disease: dissecting a complex inflammatory disorder. Nat Rev Immunol 2002;2(9):647–55.

171. Chessman D, Kostenko L, Lethborg T, et al. Human leukocyte antigen class I-restricted activation of CD8+ T cells provides the immunogenetic basis of a

systemic drug hypersensitivity. Immunity 2008;28(6):822–32.

172. Opelz G, Dohler B. Effect of human leukocyte antigen compatibility on kidney graft survival: comparative analysis of two decades. Transplantation 2007;84(2):137–43.

173. Takemoto SK, Zeevi A, Feng S, et al. National conference to assess antibody-mediated rejection in solid organ transplantation. Am J Transplant 2004; 4(7):1033–41.

174. Zachary AA, Montgomery RA, Leffell MS. Defining unacceptable HLA antigens. Curr Opin Organ Transplant 2008; 13(4):405–10.

175. Hod E, Schwartz J. Platelet transfusion refractoriness. Br J Haematol 2008; 142(3):348–60.

176. Thomas ED. A history of haematopoietic cell transplantation. Br J Haematol 1999; 105(2):330–9.

177. O'Reilly RJ, Dupont B, Pahwa S, et al. Reconstitution in severe combined immundeficiency by transplantation of marrow from an unrelated donor. N Engl J Med 1977;297:1311–8.

178. Hurley CK, Raffoux C. World Marrow Donor Association: international standards for unrelated hematopoietic stem cell donor registries. Bone Marrow Transplant 2004;34(2):103–10.

179. Gahrton G, van Rood JJ, Oudshoorn M. The World Marrow Donor Association (WMDA): its goals and activities. Bone Marrow Transplant 2003;32(2):121–4.

180. Ljungman P, Urbano-Ispizua A, Cavazzana-Calvo M, et al. Allogeneic and autologous transplantation for haematological diseases, solid tumours and immune disorders: definitions and current practice in Europe. Bone Marrow Transplant 2006;37(5):439–49.

181. Schipper RF, D'Amaro J, Oudshoorn M. The probability of finding a suitable related donor for bone marrow transplantation in extended families (see comment by Kollman). Blood 1996;87:800–4.

182. Koh LP, Chao N. Haploidentical hematopoietic cell transplantation. Bone Marrow Transplant 2008;42(Suppl 1): S60–3.

183. Oudshoorn M, van Leeuwen A, v.d.Zanden HG, van Rood JJ. Bone Marrow Donors Worldwide: a successful exercise in international cooperation. Bone Marrow Transplant 1994;14:3–8.

184. Bray RA, Hurley CK, Kamani NR, et al. National marrow donor program HLA matching guidelines for unrelated adult donor hematopoietic cell transplants. Biol Blood Marrow Transplant 2008;14 (9 Suppl):45–53.

185. Kamani N, Spellman S, Hurley CK, et al. State of the art review: HLA matching and outcome of unrelated donor umbilical cord blood transplants. Biol Blood Marrow Transplant 2008;14(1): 1–6.

Subject Index

Page numbers followed by "f" indicate figures, "t" indicate tables, and "b" indicate boxes.

Notes
  vs. indicates a comparison or differential
    diagnosis
  To save space in the index, the following
    abbreviations have been used:
    ALL – acute lymphoblastic leukemia/
      lymphoma
    AML – acute myeloid leukemia
    CLL – chronic lymphoid leukemia
    CML – chronic myeloid leukemia
    CMML – chronic myelomonocytic
      leukemia
    MDS – myelodysplastic syndromes

A

A9 gene, 317
ABCB7 gene, 227t, 228
ABH antigens, 601–603
  metastases, 602
  platelets, 525
  tumors, 602–603
ABL1 gene, 322
Abnormal localization of immature
    precursors (ALIP), 311–312, 312f
Abnormal oxygen binding, hemoglobin
    disorders, 151–152
ABO blood group, 601–603
  antigens, 601–602, 601f
    A_1, 601
    A_2, 601
    soluble, 601–602
  crossmatching, 625–626
  hemolytic disease of the newborn, 602
  incompatibility, transfusion reactions,
    632
  leukemia, 602
  von Willebrand disease type 1, 557
Absolute reticulocyte count, 6–7
Acanthocytes ('spur' cells), anemias, 107–109,
    108f, 109t
Accelerated phase (AP)
  chronic myelogenous leukemia, 364f–365f,
    366
  polycythemia vera, 341, 342f–343f
Aceruloplasminemia, 189–190
Acidemia
  methylmalonic, neutropenia, 250
  propionic, neutropenia, 250
Acidified serum lysis test (Ham test),
    congenital dyserythropoietic anemia
    type 2, 238–239
Acidurias
  methylmalonic, vitamin B_{12} deficiency,
    205–206
  orotic, macrocytic anemias, 208

aCML *see* Atypical chronic myeloid leukemia
    (*BCR–ABL1* negative)(aCML); Atypical
    chronic myeloid leukemia(*BCR–ABL1*
    negative)(aCML)
Acquired amegakaryocytic thrombocytopenia,
    527–528
Acquired aplastic anemia, 213–219
  classification, 217, 217t
  clinical course, 217
  clinical presentation, 216–217
  clonal evolution, 217
  definition, 213
  differential diagnosis, 213, 214t
    hairy cell leukemia *vs.*, 213
    hypoplastic myelodysplastic syndrome
      vs., 213
  etiology, 214–215
    drugs, 214, 214t
    industrial/domestic chemicals, 214,
      214t
    viral infections, 214–215
  hematology, 215–216
  incidence, 213
  medical history, 216–217
  pathophysiology, 215
    autoimmune causes, 215
    microenvironment, 215
    stem cells, 215
  prevalence, 213
  treatment, 217–219
    anabolic steroids, 218
    cyclophosphamide, 218
    growth factors, 218
    immunosuppression, 218
    stem cell transplantation, 218–219
Acquired coagulation inhibitors, 573
Acquired erythrocytosis, 336–337
  independent of hypoxia, 336–337
    erythropoietin, 336
    post-transplant renal erythropoiesis,
      336
    tumors, 336–337
  secondary to hypoxia, 335f, 336
Acquired hemolytic anemia, 157–172
  clinical features, 157–158
  hemolysis mechanisms, 158–160
    complement-mediated, 158–160, 159f
    Fc receptor-mediated, 158–159
    mechanical damage, 158
  historical aspects, 157
  laboratory features, 157–158, 158t
  symptoms, 157
  see also Immune hemolytic anemia;
    Non-immune hemolytic anemia
Acquired hyperfibrinolysis, 576
Acquired lymphopenia, 258–259

Acquired metabolism abnormalities
  folate deficiency, 207
  vitamin B_{12} deficiency, 205
Acquired myeloperoxidase deficiency, 255
Acquired neutropenia, 250
Acquired pure red cell aplasia, 219
Acquired α thalassemias, 145
Acquired thrombophilia, 591–592
Acquired von Willebrand disease, 577
Activated partial prothrombin time (APTT),
    479, 481–482
  correction tests, 480
    logical uses, 483–484, 484b
    misleading results, 482, 482b
    mixing tests, 480–481
    thrombolytic agents, 568
    von Willebrand disease, 554
Activated protein C resistance, 590
Activation complex, protein C, 587
Activation, platelets, 526
Active bleeding, hemostasis disorders, 478
Acute basophilic leukemia, 284
Acute chest syndrome, sickle cell disease, 148
Acute erythroid leukemia, 283, 283f
Acute hemorrhage, neutrophilia, 253
Acute infections
  eosinopenia, 256
  neutrophilia, 252–253
Acute leukemias
  bleeding disorders, 576
  chronic myelogenous leukemia *vs.*, 369
  see also specific types
Acute lymphoblastic leukemia/lymphoma
    (ALL), 289–297
  B-cell, 292–293, 294t, 295f
    molecular genetics, 296
  classification, 289–290
  clinical presentation, 289–290
  cytochemistry, 290–291, 291f
  cytogenetics, 293, 295t
  cytology, 290–291, 290f
  diagnosis, 289
  histopathology, 290–291, 291f
  immunophenotypic diagnosis, 291–292,
    292f
  mixed phenotype, 297–300
    classification, 297
    clinical presentation, 297
    cytogenetics, 300
    cytology, 298, 299f
    histopathology, 298
    immunophenotype, 300
    molecular genetics, 300
  molecular genetics, 293–296, 296t
    minimal residual disease monitoring,
      296–297, 297f–298f